MW01069427

Encyclopedia of Sex and Sexuality

Encyclopedia of Sex and Sexuality

Understanding Biology, Psychology, and Culture

VOLUME I: A–M

Heather L. Armstrong, Editor

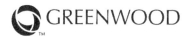

An Imprint of ABC-CLIO, LLC
Santa Barbara, California • Denver, Colorado

Library of Congress Cataloging-in-Publication Data

Names: Armstrong, Heather L., editor.
Title: Encyclopedia of sex and sexuality : understanding biology, psychology, and culture / Heather L. Armstrong, editor.
Description: Santa Barbara, California : Greenwood, [2021] | Includes bibliographical references and index. |
Identifiers: LCCN 2020024424 (print) | LCCN 2020024425 (ebook) | ISBN 9781440847684 (v. 1 ; hardcover ; alk. paper) | ISBN 9781440847691 (v. 2 ; hardcover ; alk. paper) | ISBN 9781610698740 (set ; hardcover ; alk. paper) | ISBN 9781610698757 (ebook)
Subjects: LCSH: Sex—Encyclopedias. | Sex (Biology)—Encyclopedias. | Sex (Psychology)—Encyclopedias.
Classification: LCC HQ21 .E647 2021 (print) | LCC HQ21 (ebook) | DDC 306.703—dc23
LC record available at https://lccn.loc.gov/2020024424
LC ebook record available at https://lccn.loc.gov/2020024425

ISBN: 978-1-61069-874-0 (set)
978-1-4408-4768-4 (vol. 1)
978-1-4408-4769-1 (vol. 2)
978-1-61069-875-7 (ebook)

25 24 23 22 21 1 2 3 4 5

This book is also available as an eBook.

Greenwood
An Imprint of ABC-CLIO, LLC

ABC-CLIO, LLC
147 Castilian Drive
Santa Barbara, California 93117
www.abc-clio.com

This book is printed on acid-free paper ∞

Manufactured in the United States of America

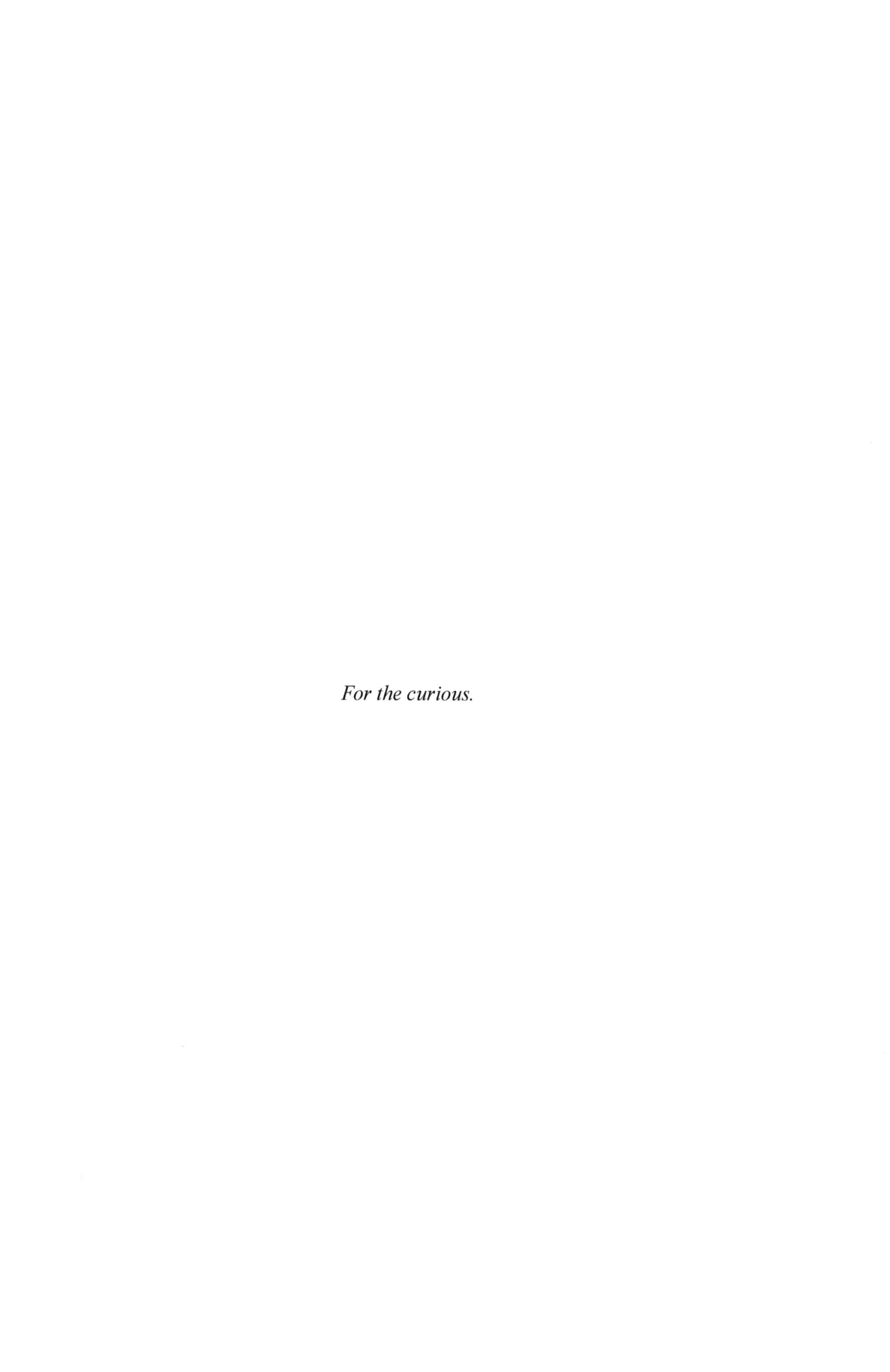

For the curious.

Contents

Introduction

Sex is a funny thing. In some ways, it's everywhere. We see it in the media, in advertisements, in movies and TV shows, and in the headlines of many newspapers and magazines. Comedians joke about it, as do most of us with our friends and partners. With the explosion of the internet, sexual imagery is just a click away, and an available sexual partner can be found within seconds with just a swipe on an app. Sex is seemingly all around us, but how much do we really know about it?

When I began studying sex as an undergraduate student, I was fascinated by the juxtaposition of how something could simultaneously be all around us, and (supposedly) something that nearly everyone desires, yet still be something that felt taboo and sometimes shameful. Everyone has some kind of relationship with sex, even those of us who have never had sex or who don't desire sex. Because of this, I believe that it is every individual's right to be accurately informed about sex, sexual health, and sexuality. It is by having this scientific and accurate information that people can make the best choices for their own sexual health and well-being.

Unfortunately, sex education is often woefully lacking, if it even occurs at all. Because of this, rumors circulate about how sex is "supposed" to be, and many of us rely on things we hear from peers and the media and from what we see on TV, in the movies, and online. As I'm sure you well know, these are rarely accurate sources of information. As a result, sexual myths and sexual double standards begin to be believed as fact, and this, coupled with a lack of accurate, science-based sexual education, often means that people are unsure and misinformed, which can lead to sexual shame, guilt, and dysfunction. The good news is that often, just by learning more about sex, sexuality, and sexual health, these problems and difficulties can be improved if not fixed completely.

So, this encyclopedia is for every person of every sex, gender, orientation, preference, and everything in between. In over 460 entries, written by nearly 150 sexuality experts, these volumes aim to provide a brief introduction and summary to a wide variety of topics related to sexuality. The authors present an overview of the latest research representing the current evidence-based understanding of the area. In addition, at the end of each entry, you will find a section with suggestions for further readings. Some of these are academic articles, others are books or websites, so it is hoped that these resources will be accessible to a variety of readers.

That said, our understanding of sexuality has changed drastically in the past few decades, and new research and theories are continuously developed. As such, new information that was not available at the time this book was written will continue to be produced, so anyone with a particular interest should continue to explore the state of the science beyond these pages.

As with all encyclopedias, these volumes were not written to be read cover to cover but rather to provide a general overview on a wide variety of topics related to sexuality. Some topics are biological, others are psychological, some are behavioral, and others are social and cultural. Sex can be good, but it can also be bad, and sometimes it can be both at the same time. To reflect this, entries include both positive and negative aspects of sex and sexuality.

The scope of human sexuality is infinite, so inevitably some things will be missing from these volumes, but I hope that we have covered a sufficiently broad range of topics so that everyone who is studying—or just as importantly, everyone who is even slightly curious about—sex will find something of interest and maybe even learn something new about this sometimes taboo, but deeply integral, part of who we are as human beings.

Heather L. Armstrong, PhD

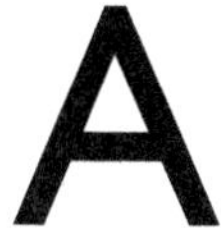

Abortion, Elective

Voluntary termination of a pregnancy without a medical necessity is considered an elective abortion. The National Abortion Federation (NAF) states that half of all pregnancies in the United States are unintended, and about half of these (1.3 million) are terminated through an elective abortion. The Guttmacher Institute estimates that 35 percent of all women of reproductive age in the United States will have an abortion by the time they reach the age of forty-five. About 19 percent of these are elected by women between the ages of fifteen and nineteen, while 33 percent of elective abortions are performed on women between twenty and twenty-four years old. Women thirty years and older account for 25 percent of all abortions.

Most women who seek elective abortion are unmarried. The NAF reports that the majority of women who choose to abort a pregnancy do so for economic reasons—either because of a lack of adequate income to start a family or the inability to support more children. Women also seek abortion when pregnancy causes significant medical complications or when they discover that their child will have severe birth defects that will compromise its life. Roughly 13,000 women each year choose abortion because they have become pregnant as a result of rape or incest.

Abortions are performed around the world, with varying degrees of regulation and standards for safety. In the United States, abortion laws went into effect by state beginning in 1821, when Connecticut passed the first law banning the practice. The Roman Catholic Church declared its prohibition of any kind of abortion in 1869, driving further bans on the practice around the world. By 1900, every state in the United States had some form of antiabortion law.

Originally, these laws had some basis in practicality. Like all surgeries performed before antiseptic procedures became widespread, abortions could be dangerous for the patient, frequently leading to infections, sepsis, and death. Surgeries became far safer in the early to mid-1900s, but by this time abortion had become a moral issue rather than a medical one. Women had to seek the procedures in secret, often from people who were not medical professionals. Deaths from back-alley abortions were common well into the second half of the twentieth century.

Legislators had other motivations for banning abortion that went beyond medical protection and morality. Prejudices against the massive influx of arriving immigrants led state governments to decide that native-born U.S. citizens should have as many children as possible, to maintain white Anglo-Saxon dominance in the face of swelling Irish, Italian, Eastern European, and Asian populations.

In 1973, the U.S. Supreme Court's landmark *Roe v. Wade* decision determined that the right to privacy granted by the Fourteenth Amendment extended to a woman's decision to have an abortion and that a woman has a right to an abortion until "viability," the point in the pregnancy at which the fetus can live outside the womb. This decision disallowed some of the state and federal restrictions on abortion, essentially legalizing abortion across the country. Abortions could now be performed in doctors' offices, gynecological clinics, and hospitals, with the medical supervision required to handle complications and keep patients safe.

Roe v. Wade did not end the controversy over abortion rights, however. The question of viability became the lynchpin for debate on either side of the abortion issue, creating two political camps based on "pro-choice" and "pro-life" points of view. The pro-choice movement focuses on a woman's right to choose whether or not to have a child, while the pro-life movement advocates the right of the fetus to be born. As the terms "pro-choice" and "pro-life" have taken on moral connotations that further polarize the debate, the media have relabeled the two sides as "abortion rights" and "antiabortion."

The abortion rights side of the debate centers on the issue of viability and the medical fact that fetuses that are aborted during the first trimester of pregnancy cannot exist independently outside of the womb. It asserts that a woman must have control over her own body, making the right to have an abortion a civil rights issue. Abortion rights activists see the government's intervention in women's reproductive choices as the first step on a slippery slope, one that could lead to forcing women to use contraception or mandating the number of children women must or must not have.

The antiabortion side sees abortion as the act of taking a human life, making an abortion the murder of a fetus. This side offers adoption as a viable alternative to abortion, pointing to the statistic that 1.5 million American families are looking to adopt a child at any given time. Some on the antiabortion side promote abstinence as the only viable method of birth control, objecting to medical contraception because it prevents the formation of an embryo by killing the egg or sperm before conception can take place. Others on the antiabortion side believe contraceptives are an acceptable means of preventing unwanted pregnancy.

Supreme Court decisions and some state laws continue to work toward restricting abortions, even as *Roe v. Wade* continues to stand. A law passed by Congress in 2003 and upheld by the Supreme Court in 2007 banned late-term abortions (called "partial-birth abortions" by their political opponents). In 2011, Texas—the leading state on the antiabortion side of the debate—passed a law requiring all women seeking an abortion to make at least two visits to an abortion facility, one of which must include an ultrasound within twenty-four hours before the abortion. In 2013, a new Texas law closed all but eight abortion clinics throughout the state because they did not provide hospital-level treatment or facilities, shutting down thirteen clinics in rural areas. In October 2014, the U.S. Supreme Court blocked some of the provisions of this law.

In 2011, 2012, and 2013, thirty states enacted a total of 205 new antiabortion statutes, banning private insurance coverage of abortion procedures and setting limits on abortions using medications. More than half of the laws passed targeted regulation of abortion providers (known as TRAP laws). These require women seeking abortions to travel to hospitals or hospital-like clinics at which doctors have admitting privileges at area hospitals.

Randi Minetor

See also: Abortion, Medical; Abortion, Risks of; Abortion, Surgical; Abortion, Therapeutic (Medically Necessary); Abortion, Unsafe; Abortion Legislation; Emergency Contraception; Hyde Amendment; *Roe v. Wade*; Sexual Rights.

Further Reading

Boonstra, H. D., & Nash, E. (2014). A surge of state abortion restrictions puts providers—And the women they serve—In the crosshairs. *Guttmacher Policy Review, 17*(1). Retrieved from https://www.guttmacher.org/gpr/2014/03/surge-state-abortion-restrictions-puts-providers-and-women-they-serve-crosshairs

Cole, G. F., & Frankowski, S. (Eds.) (1987). *Abortion and protection of the human fetus: Legal problems in a cross-cultural perspective* (Vol. 1). Boston, MA: Martinus Nijhoff.

Haney, J. (2009). *The abortion debate: Understanding the issues.* Berkeley Heights, NJ: Enslow.

McBride, D. E., & Keys, J. L. (2018). *Abortion in the United States: A reference handbook.* Santa Barbara, CA: ABC-CLIO.

Abortion, Late-Term

A late-term abortion is a medical procedure that terminates pregnancy after the twentieth week of gestation. The exact stage at which an abortion becomes late term has not been clearly defined by the medical community. A very small percentage (about 1 percent) of abortions occur after the twentieth week and typically are required because the pregnant patient's health or life is at risk or because serious fetal abnormalities have been detected. While all forms of abortion have been the subject of controversy in the United States, late-term abortion is the most controversial. This is due to the fact that a fetus aborted in a late-term abortion is usually more fully developed and sometimes viable. Late-term abortions can take different forms, with the most common procedures being dilation and extraction (D&E), labor-induced abortion, and intact dilation and extraction (IDX).

IDX was a common late-term abortion procedure before it was made illegal after the passage of the Partial-Birth Abortion Act of 2003. It takes place in four stages. First, the cervix is dilated over a few days to accommodate the size of the fetus. Once the cervix is sufficiently dilated, the fetus is placed in position for a footing breech either manually or through the use of forceps. The fetus is then removed by the doctor through a series of stages. This procedure may be referred to as "partial-birth abortion," although the American Medical Association does not consider that to be a medical term.

While D&E is similar to IDX, they are distinct procedures. Prior to a D&E procedure, the doctor will insert a cervical dilator into the cervix to help dilate the cervix for twenty-four hours. Once the cervix is dilated, the remainder of the procedure typically takes thirty minutes. The doctor uses an instrument to keep the uterus in place and passes a cannula—a hollow tube—into the uterus. The cannula, which is attached to a bottle and pump, is then used to remove tissue from the uterus. If there are larger pieces of tissue in the uterus that the cannula cannot handle, forceps are used to remove them. A curved instrument called a curette and suction may also be used during the procedure to remove tissue from the lining of the uterus. Once all the tissue is removed from the uterus, it is examined by the doctor to make sure the procedure is complete. D&E is difficult to perform after twenty weeks of gestation and is more commonly used at earlier stages of pregnancy.

A labor-induced abortion is a procedure in which a substance is administered to the fetus to cause a medically induced stillbirth. Before beginning the procedure, the doctor will sometimes dilate the cervix using a cervical dilator to reduce the risk of complications. Once the cervix is dilated, the doctor will inject a substance—a salt solution, drug, or chemical compound—into the amniotic fluid surrounding the fetus or directly into the fetus. This induces a stillbirth, and the fetus is typically delivered within twenty-four hours of the injection. Once the fetus has been delivered, the doctor may scrape the uterus with a curette to ensure that all the tissue has been removed. Labor-induced abortions become more difficult to perform the later the stage of pregnancy.

Abortion is a generally safe medical procedure, although the risk of complications increases the further along the patient is in her pregnancy. Some complications that can occur during a late-term abortion include heavy bleeding, blood clots in the uterus, infection, pain and discomfort, and injury to the cervix or other organs. Following an abortion, the patient may experience a variety of emotions, such as relief, sadness, guilt, and anger. However, it is important to note that in general, late-term abortion is not associated with any negative physical health outcomes, and the consequences of the pregnancy proceeding typically pose more serious health risks than termination.

A woman may decide to undergo a late-term abortion procedure for a number of reasons, including health complications, fetal birth defects, or not realizing she was pregnant until late in the pregnancy. Late-term abortions are the rarest of all abortion procedures, making up an average of just 1.2 percent of all abortions that take place in the United States.

Late-term abortions have been the subject of intense controversy in the United States since abortions were made legal through the U.S. Supreme Court's ruling in *Roe v. Wade* in 1973. However, the Supreme Court's ruling did allow states to impose greater restrictions on late-term abortion procedures taking place after fetal viability than on abortions occurring at earlier stages of gestation. As of 2014, twenty-one states have passed laws prohibiting abortions performed at the point of fetal viability, and three states have laws prohibiting abortion during the third trimester. Nine states prohibit abortion after twenty weeks' gestation based on the argument that the fetus can feel pain by that point, although the scientific validity of this argument has been challenged by the medical community. If a state places a ban on late-term abortion, the law must contain an exception for abortions "necessary to preserve the life or health" of the pregnant person in order to be constitutional in accordance with the Supreme Court's ruling in *Roe v. Wade*.

In 2003, Congress passed, and President George W. Bush signed into law, the Partial-Birth Abortion Act of 2003. This law prohibits IDX late-term abortion procedures, referred to in the text of the legislation as "partial-birth abortion." Under this legislation, if a doctor performs an abortion using IDX, they would receive a fine or be imprisoned for up to two years. The constitutionality of the Partial-Birth Abortion Act was challenged in 2007 in the Supreme Court case *Gonzales v. Carhart*. Prior to reaching the Supreme Court, three federal district and circuit courts had ruled the act to be unconstitutional. However, in a 5–4 decision, the Supreme Court ruled that the act was constitutional since it clearly outlines which abortion procedure is banned and thus does not place an undue burden on women who are seeking a late-term abortion.

Abortion providers have often been the targets of terrorism and violence carried out by antiabortion activists. In 2009, Dr. George Tiller, one of the nation's leading abortion providers, was shot and killed while attending church in Wichita, Kansas. Tiller was murdered by Scott Roeder, an antiabortion activist, who was sentenced to life in prison. Previously, Tiller's clinic had been bombed in June 1986, and in 1993 he was shot in both arms outside a clinic in Wichita by antiabortion activist Shelley Shannon, who was sentenced to eleven years in prison for attempted murder.

Renee Dubie

See also: Abortion, Elective; Abortion, Medical; Abortion, Risks of; Abortion, Surgical; Abortion, Therapeutic (Medically Necessary); Abortion, Unsafe; Abortion Legislation; *Roe v. Wade*; Sexual Rights.

Further Reading

Herring, M. Y. (2003). *The pro-life/choice debate.* Santa Barbara, CA: Greenwood.

McBride, D. E., & Keys, J. L. (2018). *Abortion in the United States: A reference handbook.* Santa Barbara, CA: ABC-CLIO.

Abortion, Medical

Medical abortion is the use of medication to end an early-stage pregnancy. It is highly effective and is usually safe up to twelve weeks from the first day of the last menstruation, although some places may restrict its use to earlier in the pregnancy. Medical abortion may be therapeutic (medically necessary to protect the life and health of the pregnant patient) or elective. Early medical abortion is considered very safe, with low risk of serious side effects or complications. It enables pregnancy termination to occur in one's home without surgical intervention or the risk of public exposure and violence that may accompany a clinic visit.

Medications used to induce abortion include steroid hormone drugs such as mifepristone, prostaglandin hormone drugs such as misoprostol, and chemotherapy drugs such as methotrexate. The exact combination depends on the prescribing physician's preference, the specific prescription medication, presence of pregnancy complications or fetal abnormalities, and the patient's medical history and condition. Treatment may consist entirely of oral tablets or may combine oral tablets with vaginal suppositories. Muscle relaxants, clotting agents, and analgesics (painkillers) may also be prescribed.

Medical abortion typically requires an office visit to determine the exact stage of pregnancy and the patient's overall health. A blood or urine test, pelvic exam, and ultrasound are generally performed to confirm gestational age and screen for serious medical complications. All U.S. board-certified family practice physicians must offer counseling regarding abortion, adoption, and parenting options to prospective abortion patients. In addition, some states require that patients receive antiabortion counseling and information regarding fetal development. The attending physician usually gives the medication to the patient directly, along with instructions for use, rather than writing a prescription.

A medical abortion may take one to three days to complete and includes strong cramping, vaginal bleeding, and other physical effects similar to a natural miscarriage. A follow-up appointment is required to ensure expulsion of all uterine contents. Patients are cautioned to avoid driving, operating heavy machinery, and all intense physical activity during the course of the abortion, and to avoid sexual intercourse for a minimum of two weeks following treatment. Fertility may resume before the next menstrual period, so patients must institute an effective birth control method immediately. Normal menstruation should resume within six weeks.

Potential side effects and complications include nausea, vomiting, diarrhea, fever, chills, fatigue, severe abdominal pain, severe bleeding, shock, retained tissue, and infection, as well as negative reactions to specific medications (such as unforeseen allergic reaction). Serious side effects or complications may require additional medical treatment, such as emergency care, antibiotics, or follow-up surgery in the case of retained tissue.

Though considered very safe and effective, medical abortion has been a source of significant controversy in the United States because it allows discrete, safe pregnancy termination in the privacy of one's home. Abortifacient pharmaceuticals have been widely available since the 1970s but were not legally available in the United States for most elective abortions until 2000. As localities limit access to abortion, black-market "abortion pills," primarily imported from Latin America, are becoming popular, but these carry significantly more risk.

Angela Libal

See also: Abortion, Elective; Abortion, Risks of; Abortion, Surgical; Abortion, Therapeutic (Medically Necessary); Abortion, Unsafe; Abortion Legislation; Emergency Contraception; *Roe v. Wade*; Sexual Rights.

Further Reading

Guttmacher Institute. (2019). *State laws and policies: Medication abortion.* New York: Guttmacher Institute. Retrieved from https://www.guttmacher.org/state-policy/explore/medication-abortion

Jacobson, J. D., & Zieve, D. (Eds.). (2018). Abortion—Medical. Retrieved from http://www.nlm.nih.gov/medlineplus/ency/article/007382.htm

University of California, San Francisco. (2019). Medical abortion. Retrieved from https://www.ucsfhealth.org/treatments/medical-abortion

WHO Reproductive Health Library. (2016). *Medical methods for first trimester abortion: RHL summary.* Geneva: World Health Organization.

Abortion, Risks of

Induced abortion is therapeutic (necessary for the health of the pregnant person) or elective termination of pregnancy through surgical procedure or medication. Legal first-trimester abortion is considered one of the safest medical procedures, with a complication rate of less than 1 percent for surgical abortion and around 2 percent for abortion by medication. Abortions performed after the first trimester use different procedures and carry different and greater risks. They are not typically performed on an elective basis. Illegal abortion carries different and far greater risks.

"Surgical abortion" is a misleading term because these abortions do not involve cutting. A more appropriate term is "procedural abortion." Procedural abortions may be performed in a physician's office, hospital, or clinic. They do not require sterile, operating-room conditions. Potential complications of procedural abortion include uterine infection, retained tissue from incomplete abortion, and cervical damage during dilation. Uterine infection is treated with antibiotics. Retained tissue requires further extraction to prevent infection and severe bleeding. Cervical damage is rarely treated and may not be apparent at the time of the procedure. Aspiration abortion (removal of fetal tissue through suction) carries a uterine perforation risk of less than 0.01 percent.

Potential risks of medical abortion include side effects such as extreme pain and gastrointestinal distress, and complications such as severe bleeding, shock, retained tissue, and adverse reactions to the medication used. Side effects may be treated with analgesics (painkillers). Severe complications require emergency care, and retained tissue requires procedural abortion. Very rarely, medical abortion may fail to terminate pregnancy. Research findings vary regarding whether abortifacient medications cause significant fetal damage and birth defects if such pregnancies are continued.

Retained tissue is the greatest risk of procedural and medical abortion. It can cause continued, heavy bleeding and sepsis (potentially fatal blood infection). However, the combined risk of all incomplete abortion complications is less than 0.24 percent.

Due to controversy surrounding abortion, many inaccurate claims regarding its effects on patients' physical health and future fertility have been perpetuated. However, most of these claims have been disproven by research involving hundreds of thousands of women. Many claims were based on older surgical techniques, such as dilation and curettage, which are rarely used in a modern medical setting; on illegal abortions; or on abortions performed after the first trimester. Late-term abortions are almost always performed to preserve the life or health of the pregnant patient or chosen due to severe, often fatal fetal abnormalities. Their risks are very different from those associated with first-trimester, elective abortion.

According to a 2009 article in the *Journal of the American Board of Family Medicine*, "when abortion is safe and legal, [the patient's] chances of getting pregnant and staying pregnant in the future are not affected by the abortion. There is no increase in rates of ectopic pregnancy, spontaneous abortion, preterm birth, or low birth weight, and no association with an increase in breast cancer risk" (Lyus, Gianutsos, & Gold, 2009). At least one study conducted in China has shown an association between first-trimester aspiration abortion and an increased risk of less than 2 percent for first-trimester miscarriage in future pregnancies. However, this risk was greatest in pregnancies occurring within three months of an abortion.

Some women experience depression following abortion. This may be attributed to and complicated by multiple factors, including feelings of rejection by family members or faith communities, lack of support from a significant other for continuing pregnancy or pressure to terminate, adverse life circumstances associated with the choice to terminate, and a sense of loss of the pregnancy itself. A 2008 study in Denmark suggests that women past their teen years who lack social support and counseling are at greatest risk for abortion-related depression. Lack of social support strongly affects women in communities that condemn abortion. These women may become victims of social judgment, condemnation, abuse, and violent attacks.

Angela Libal

See also: Abortion, Elective; Abortion, Medical; Abortion, Surgical; Abortion, Therapeutic (Medically Necessary); Abortion, Unsafe; Abortion Legislation; Emergency Contraception; *Roe v. Wade*; Sexual Rights.

Further Reading

Alaska Department of Health and Social Services. (2019). Possible medical risks or complications of abortion. Retrieved from http://dhss.alaska.gov/dph/wcfh/Pages/informedconsent/abortion/risks

Louisiana Department of Health. (n.d.). Abortion & pregnancy risks. Retrieved from http://dhh.louisiana.gov/index.cfm/page/915/n/275

Lyus, R. J., Gianutsos, P., & Gold, M. (2009). First trimester procedural abortion in family medicine. *Journal of the American Board of Family Medicine, 22*(2), 169–174.

Pedersen, W. (2008). Abortion and depression: A population-based longitudinal study of young women. *Scandinavian Journal of Public Health, 36*(4), 424–428.

Sun, Y., Che, Y., Gao, E., Olsen, J., & Zhou, W. (2003). Induced abortion and risk of subsequent miscarriage. *International Journal of Epidemiology, 32*(3), 449–454.

Abortion, Surgical

Surgical abortion is a method of ending a pregnancy by manually removing the fetus and placenta from the womb. Also known as suction-aspiration or vacuum-aspiration abortion, a surgical abortion can be performed on a pregnancy of up to sixteen weeks. If the fetus is between sixteen and twenty-four weeks old, a less common and more complicated surgical procedure, known as dilation and evacuation, or D&E, is necessary.

A pregnant individual may choose to have a surgical abortion for the same reasons one might choose to have a medical abortion (one induced by medication): for personal reasons, because the pregnancy is harmful to their health, because the fetus has a genetic problem or birth defect, or because the pregnancy resulted from rape or incest.

Although a suction-aspiration abortion procedure typically lasts only five to ten minutes (a D&E usually lasts ten to twenty minutes), additional time is needed for talking with the health care provider, undergoing a physical exam, reading and signing forms, allowing time for anesthetics to take effect, and recovering afterward. As a result, most surgical abortions require three to six hours at a clinic, depending on the clinic and the age of the fetus.

Once a person has decided to have a suction-aspiration abortion, they are given pain medication—typically some combination of ibuprofen, valium, and Vicodin. If they are more than eleven weeks pregnant, they may also receive misoprostol, a drug that softens the cervix. Oral medications for those who are fewer than twelve weeks pregnant require forty-five minutes to an hour to take effect; misoprostol takes two to three hours to take effect and is therefore administered before oral medications.

Many abortion providers also inject a numbing agent into or near the cervix. Less commonly, a general sedative or anesthetic may be given. The opening of the cervix is then stretched (dilated) using a series of rods of increasing diameter. Some clinics may instead use an absorbent dilating rod that slowly stretches the cervical opening over the course of several hours, but this must be given to the patient the day before the abortion procedure. Some may also prescribe medications that chemically dilate the cervix. In addition, those undergoing surgical abortion are usually prescribed an antibiotic to prevent infection.

After an examination of the patient's uterus and cervix to ensure that all medications have taken effect and the cervix is properly dilated, a tube is inserted into the uterus via the cervix. A machine or handheld device then suctions blood and fetal tissue from the uterus. A medical instrument known as a curette is sometimes used to ensure that the uterus is empty or to remove any remaining tissue. The use of this device can result in the abortion being termed a D&C, for dilation and curettage.

After one to three hours of recovery time, the patient can return home and typically may resume work or school the following day, though recovery after a later-term surgical abortion may take a few days. Doctors recommend refraining from sexual intercourse, or placing any object in the vagina, for at least one week.

Most people who have surgical abortions experience cramps similar to menstrual cramps for one to two days, though some may experience longer or more pronounced periods of discomfort. Vaginal bleeding or spotting may continue for up to ten days, and menstrual pads, rather than tampons, must be used to absorb the blood.

Surgical abortions are considered very safe. The risk of death from childbirth is eleven times higher than the risk of death from an abortion carried out in the first twenty weeks of pregnancy. The risk of death from childbirth and abortion are roughly equal when an abortion occurs after more than twenty weeks of pregnancy. In general, the more advanced the pregnancy, the greater the risk of complications.

Surgical abortion risks may include blood clots, very heavy bleeding, allergic reactions to medications, infections, injury to the cervix or uterus, scarring of the inside of the uterus, incomplete abortion (in which some tissue remains inside the uterus), and failure to terminate the pregnancy. In rare cases, the patient may have complications from an undetected ectopic pregnancy.

Many people also experience strong emotions after an abortion. These may include relief, sadness, anger, regret, or guilt. Although any negative feelings typically fade, it is important to seek professional counseling if they continue for a longer period of time. However, it is important to note that in general, abortion is not associated with any negative or physical health outcomes.

Terri Nichols

See also: Abortion, Elective; Abortion, Medical; Abortion, Risks of; Abortion, Therapeutic (Medically Necessary); Abortion, Unsafe; Abortion Legislation; Emergency Contraception; *Roe v. Wade*; Sexual Rights.

Further Reading

Jacobson, J. D., & Zieve, D. (Eds.). (2018). Abortion—Surgical. Retrieved from https://www.nlm.nih.gov/medlineplus/ency/article/002912.htm

Paul, M., Lichtenberg, E. S., Borgatta, L., Grimes, D. A., & Stubblefield, P. G. (1999). *A clinician's guide to medical and surgical abortion.* London: Churchill Livingstone.

Planned Parenthood. (2019). In-clinic abortion. Retrieved from https://www.plannedparenthood.org/learn/abortion/in-clinic-abortion-procedures

Abortion, Therapeutic (Medically Necessary)

In the United States, "therapeutic abortion" refers to medically necessary termination of pregnancy. It includes all abortions performed to preserve the life and physical health of the pregnant patient and may include abortions performed due to severe, incurable, irreversible, and usually fatal conditions of the fetus. However, some countries, such as the United Kingdom and Canada, use the term "therapeutic abortion" to refer to all elective abortions.

Therapeutic abortion may become necessary due to pregnancy complications, fetal defects, or maternal health conditions. It is usually performed at any stage prior to fetal viability (the ability of the fetus to survive outside the uterus); however, in the case of severe conditions of the fetus, therapeutic abortion may also be performed after the age of technical viability. When physical defects are not present and the fetus is potentially viable, pregnancy interruption may be performed by early labor induction or cesarean surgery, with effort to preserve the life of the infant.

Viability is considered to begin at twenty-four weeks. Survival at this stage is around 50 percent and depends entirely on major medical intervention. The risk of permanent disability or impairment increases significantly the further the fetus is from being full term (considered a minimum of thirty-seven weeks' gestation).

The technique used to induce therapeutic abortion depends on the type of problem and stage of gestation. First-trimester therapeutic abortions are usually accomplished with abortifacient medication or vacuum extraction. Second- and third-trimester therapeutic abortions are accomplished by early induction of labor or surgical dilation of the cervix and extraction of the fetus, placenta, and associated tissue. Feticidal drugs may be injected directly into the amniotic sac or fetus. A few life-threatening conditions such as ectopic and molar pregnancy may require additional surgery and medication, such as chemotherapy drugs.

Pregnancy complications that require therapeutic abortion include ectopic pregnancy, when the amniotic sac lodges inside a fallopian tube rather than the uterus; fetal death without expulsion, or retained miscarriage; and gestational trophoblastic disease (GTD), also called hydatidiform or hydatid mole, or molar pregnancy. Molar pregnancy may exist with or without a fetus. It is an abnormal, cancer-like growth of placental cells throughout the uterus, which may penetrate the uterine wall or invade other parts of the body. Roughly 20 percent of GTD cases develop into an actual cancer called choriocarcinoma. Fetuses in all these cases are not viable.

Complications of pregnancy that may require therapeutic abortion if they occur prior to fetal viability include placenta previa with hemorrhage, placenta abruption, preeclampsia, hemolysis with elevated liver enzymes and low platelet count (HELLP) syndrome, and eclampsia. Placenta previa occurs when the placenta grows into the muscular wall of the uterus. It usually requires surgical birth and may require hysterectomy to prevent fatal hemorrhage. When it causes hemorrhage before fetal viability, therapeutic abortion and emergency hysterectomy may be necessary. Placenta abruption occurs when the placenta detaches from the uterine wall. It can cause fatal blood loss to the pregnant individual and kill the fetus by cutting off oxygen and nutrition. Preeclampsia, HELLP syndrome, and eclampsia are potentially fatal hypertensive disorders that affect multiple systems in the pregnant patient's body and necessitate ending a pregnancy.

Rare maternal complications that may require therapeutic abortion include advanced cervical cancer; uterine rupture or sepsis caused by severe, degenerating fibroid tumors; life-threatening hyperemesis gravidarum (uncontrollable, continuous vomiting resulting in clinical dehydration); advanced cardiovascular disease; advanced renal failure; and serious autoimmune disease caused by fetal antigens.

Abortion is considered therapeutic when the fetus carries fatal disorders or defects such as Tay-Sachs disease or anencephaly or when it has a disorder likely to result in fatal or severe, irreversible effects, such as trisomy 18, trisomy 13, or congenital rubella syndrome.

Abortions are considered elective rather than therapeutic when they are performed due to fetal abnormalities with unpredictable prognosis for the infant. Selective termination of fetuses with Down syndrome has been particularly criticized due to favorable outcomes for children living with Down syndrome who receive early medical, behavioral, and developmental intervention. Critics note that much of the information provided to prospective parents of fetuses affected by Down syndrome is based on outdated material. This material dates to an era before modern surgical and intervention techniques. It may overestimate negative outcomes for physical defects such as heart and gastrointestinal malformations, which can typically be corrected with surgical intervention, and it may overstate levels of intellectual disability, which can be strongly moderated by early behavioral, developmental, and educational intervention.

Angela Libal

See also: Abortion, Elective; Abortion, Medical; Abortion, Risks of; Abortion, Surgical; Abortion, Unsafe; Abortion Legislation; Emergency Contraception; *Roe v. Wade*; Sexual Rights.

Further Reading

Breborowicz, G. H. (2001). Limits of fetal viability and its enhancement. *Early Pregnancy, 5*(1), 49–50.

Jacobson, J. D., & Zieve, D. (Eds.). (2018). Hydatidiform mole. Retrieved from http://www.nlm.nih.gov/medlinepls/ency/article/000909.htm

Jauniaux, E., Gillerot, Y., & Hustin, J. (2001). Placental and fetal cancers. In E. R. Barnea, E. Jauniaux, & P. E. Schwartz (Eds.), *Cancer and pregnancy* (6–20). London: Springer London.

Mayo Clinic. (2019). Placental abruption. Retrieved from https://www.mayoclinic.org/diseases-conditions/placental-abruption/symptoms-causes/syc-20376458

Mayo Clinic. (2019). Preeclampsia. Retrieved from https://www.mayoclinic.org/diseases-conditions/preeclampsia/symptoms-causes/syc-20355745

Abortion, Unsafe

Unsafe abortion is intentional termination of pregnancy in the absence of a trained, competent clinician; adequate, sanitary medical facilities; or both. It may be illegal or legal and may be performed by the pregnant individual, a nonmedical practitioner, an inadequately trained or incompetent clinician, or a trained clinician working in unsafe conditions. Unsafe abortions are a leading cause of death for pregnant women worldwide, where they account for 13 percent of global pregnancy-related deaths and take the lives of 68,000 women and girls per year worldwide. Approximately 18.4 million unsafe abortions with 67,500 deaths occur annually in developing countries. Developed countries account for 500,000 unsafe abortions and 500 or fewer deaths annually.

Approximately one-fifth of all pregnancies end in abortion. This statistic is stable throughout the world regardless of the overall birth rate and regardless of whether abortion is legal in a region or not. Half of these abortions are unsafe. Currently, about one-quarter of the world's population lives in areas where abortion is prohibited, and many more live in areas without access to skilled practitioners or sanitary conditions that meet minimum medical standards.

Unsafe abortions may be induced by drug overdose; oral ingestion or vaginal insertion of herbs or other traditional remedies; insertion of objects through the cervix and into the uterus; oral consumption or vaginal insertion of caustic chemicals; physical or extreme sexual abuse; or prolonged, vigorous physical activity.

They may also be induced by unsafe or unapproved use of pharmaceuticals or with inappropriate or unsanitary surgical or procedural equipment.

The most common cause of death from unsafe abortion is sepsis (blood infection) from retained tissue. Other causes of death include fatal infection by genital flora, sexually transmitted infection pathogens, or wound-infecting bacteria such as *Clostridium*; heavy bleeding or hemorrhage from drugs, chemicals, suppositories, retained tissue, or uterine damage; uterine perforation with bowel injury, damage to other organs, or shock; and poisoning or drug overdose. Unsafe abortion can also cause chronic infection or inflammation, permanent disability, pelvic inflammatory disease, infertility, extreme genital trauma, and reproductive tract abscesses.

Unsafe abortion has an extremely high social and economic cost beyond the direct loss of lives. In some regions, these abortions account for half or more of hospital admissions and annual expenditures. In addition, they take an incalculable social, economic, and emotional toll on communities and families—especially children left motherless.

Legalization of abortion has no impact on rates of pregnancy and birth—access to effective contraception and women's ability to insist on contraceptive use does. However, legalization of abortion and easy access to safe, early abortion dramatically reduces annual numbers of unsafe abortions. Modern medicine's ability to perform safe, first-trimester abortion is now so advanced that where trained clinicians, appropriate equipment, and sanitary facilities are available, deaths are virtually nonexistent—however, many blockades to access exist even in regions where abortion is technically legal. Blocks to access include distance; cost; excessive bureaucratic regulations imposed on patients (such as waiting periods, requirements for multiple written medical referrals, or parental consent); excessive bureaucratic regulations imposed on clinics (such as requiring that facilities have complete operating rooms and the ability to perform general anesthesia—neither of which is necessary for early-term abortions); lack of equipment and pharmaceuticals; lack of dependable, safe water supplies, fuel, and power; lack of clinicians, facilities, and emergency care; hostility toward, ostracism, and condemnation of women who seek abortion; and harassment and violence targeted at abortion providers and patients.

Lack of access to prompt and appropriate emergency medical care contributes to unsafe abortion deaths. In the *British Medical Bulletin* in 2003, Dr. David A. Grimes wrote, "Perhaps the greatest danger of all is indifference—or overt disdain. The lack of commitment on the part of medical and nursing staff to provide prompt, attentive and emotionally supportive care indirectly dooms women whose lives could easily be saved. Many women who reach medical facilities are met with suspicion and hostility, and their treatment deferred while other more 'suitable' candidates receive medical attention." In addition, women who face legal repercussions may not seek emergency care until it is too late.

Abortion is the most common surgical procedure for U.S. women, and approximately one-third have an abortion at some point in their lives. The annual death rate from legal abortion in the United States is less than one in one hundred thousand. Yet, according to the *New York Times*, in 2010, "In 87% of the counties in the U.S., where a third of women live, there is no known abortion provider."

Angela Libal

See also: Abortion, Elective; Abortion, Medical; Abortion, Risks of; Abortion, Surgical; Abortion, Therapeutic (Medically Necessary); Abortion Legislation; Emergency Contraception; *Roe v. Wade*; Sexual Rights.

Further Reading

Barot, S. (2001). Unsafe abortion: The missing link in global efforts to improve maternal health. *Guttmacher Policy Review, 14*(2), 24–28.

Bazelon, E. (2010, July 14). The new abortion providers. *New York Times*, p. MM30.

Grimes, D. A. (2003). Unsafe abortion: The silent scourge. *British Medical Bulletin, 67*(1), 99–113.

Haddad, L. B., & Nour, N. M. (2009). Unsafe abortion: Unnecessary maternal mortality. *Review of Obstetric Gynecology, 2*(2), 122–126.

World Health Organization. (2019). Preventing unsafe abortion. Retrieved from https://www.who.int/en/news-room/fact-sheets/detail/preventing-unsafe-abortion

Abortion Legislation

Abortion has been practiced throughout history as a means of controlling unwanted or unsafe reproduction. In the United States, abortion legislation began on the state level in 1821 and has continued to the present day. Legislation began as a means of protecting women from life-threatening, amateur abortion practices, but as the general public became polarized on the issue in the later 1800s, states began passing laws to criminalize all forms of abortion.

The first abortion legislation in the United States was passed in Connecticut in 1821 and was a law to prevent women from taking poison to terminate a pregnancy after the fourth month. Over the next thirty-five years, most states allowed abortion or classified it as a misdemeanor. This position met its first major challenge in 1856, when gynecologist and antiabortion advocate Horatio Robinson Storer started the "physicians' crusade against abortion," persuading the American Medical Association (AMA) to create the Committee on Criminal Abortion. The committee presented a report in 1859 that led the AMA to petition state and territory legislatures to ban elective abortions. Their campaign met with considerable success: by 1880, nearly every state and territory had passed legislation making most forms of abortion a criminal act. Adding fuel to the fire, the Roman Catholic Church declared its prohibition of any kind of abortion in 1869, driving further bans on the practice around the world.

The AMA's campaign made an impact on the national level as well. On March 3, 1873, Congress passed the Comstock Law, an act for the "suppression of trade in, and circulation of, obscene literature and articles of immoral use." The act made it illegal to send materials including contraceptives, abortion-inducing drugs, and information about abortions and other "obscene" topics through the U.S. Postal Service. The Comstock Law made it virtually impossible for women to obtain information about options for abortion. By the 1880s, most abortions were illegal across the United States, unless they were necessary "to save the life of the woman."

In the late nineteenth century, as the women's suffrage movement began to gain momentum, antiabortion legislation became a way for all-male legislatures to control women and negate their rights to make choices involving their own bodies. At the same time, male obstetricians began to see midwives—often the practitioners of abortions—as threats to their livelihood. The eugenics movement added more pressure to the debate against abortion, demanding that white women continue to reproduce to keep other races from gaining ground in the United States.

Even with all these forces in play, doctors estimated that in the 1890s, more than two million abortions were performed in the United States each year. While women with discretionary income could travel to another country or find a reputable doctor who would perform the procedure, poor women resorted to dangerous methods. Back-alley abortionists often demanded large sums of money and rejected precautions like anesthesia and sterilization so they could finish the job faster. Women often were abused or raped in the course of seeking an abortion. The poorest women could not afford even these unsanitary and dangerous practices, so they attempted their own procedures. The coat hanger became the symbol of secret do-it-yourself abortions, often resulting in severe internal damage to the women who used these methods.

This situation continued into the 1960s, when the feminist movement brought illegal abortions into the public eye. The movement made incremental gains as some states passed laws allowing women to obtain abortions if they were victims of rape or incest or if they were younger than fifteen. In general, however, abortion had become a felony in forty-nine states by 1969. The first meaningful change in legislation came in 1970, when Hawaii and then New York allowed abortion on demand through the twentieth week (Hawaii) or twenty-fourth week (New York) of pregnancy if a doctor performed the procedure in a medical facility. Soon several other states passed similar laws, but women in the majority of states still had to make their own way in finding someone to perform an abortion illegally.

All this changed on January 22, 1973, when the U.S. Supreme Court passed the landmark *Roe v. Wade* decision. The decision determined that the right to privacy granted by the Fourteenth Amendment extended to a woman's decision to have an abortion and that a woman has a right to an abortion until "viability," the point in the pregnancy at which the fetus can live outside the womb. This decision disallowed some of the state and federal restrictions on abortion, essentially legalizing abortion across the country. Abortions now could be performed in doctors' offices, gynecological clinics, and hospitals, with the medical supervision required to handle complications and keep patients safe.

This decision did not end the dispute, however—in fact, it provided the point of coalescence that created the "pro-life" and "pro-choice" factions that keep the debate active today. The two sides argue over the question of viability and whether life begins well into the pregnancy or at the point of conception. This controversy led to the passage of the Hyde Amendment in 1976, just three years after *Roe v. Wade* legalized abortion. The Hyde Amendment banned Medicaid funding for abortion unless the pregnancy endangered a woman's life. Before Hyde, 294,000 women annually received Medicaid funding for their abortions—roughly one-third of all women seeking to terminate a pregnancy.

In 1980, the Supreme Court upheld the Hyde Amendment, opening the door to new legislation on abortion rights. A series of cases that came before the court throughout the 1980s and 1990s found state laws limiting abortion rights to be unconstitutional, allowing minors to petition the court for permission to have an abortion, eliminating waiting periods before abortions, and disallowing the declaration that "life begins at conception." In 1996, a law to ban so-called partial-birth abortions, or abortions performed using the dilation and evacuation method, passed Congress but was vetoed by President Bill Clinton.

Since the 2010 midterm election, states have adopted 231 new abortion restrictions. The year 2014 became pivotal in the passage of new state laws restricting access to abortion—as well as laws expanding that access. The 2010 passage of the Affordable Care Act brought new focus to the abortion debate, as the law included the potential for government and private insurance funding of abortion procedures. According to the Guttmacher Institute, major abortion restrictions fell into four basic categories: targeted regulation of abortion providers (known as TRAP), limits on providing medications that cause abortion, bans on private insurance coverage of abortion, and bans on abortions after twenty weeks from fertilization.

Randi Minetor

See also: Abortion, Elective; Abortion, Medical; Abortion, Risks of; Abortion, Surgical; Abortion, Therapeutic (Medically Necessary); Abortion, Unsafe; Emergency Contraception; Hyde Amendment; *Roe v. Wade*; Sexual Rights.

Further Reading

Boonstra, H. D., & Nash, E. (2014). A surge of state abortion restrictions puts providers—And the women they serve—In the crosshairs. *Guttmacher Policy Review, 17*(1). Retrieved from https://www.guttmacher.org/gpr/2014/03/surge-state-abortion-restrictions-puts-providers-and-women-they-serve-crosshairs

Cole, G. F., & Frankowski, S. (Eds.). (1987). *Abortion and protection of the human fetus: Legal problems in a cross-cultural perspective* (Vol. 1). Boston: Martinus Nijhoff.

Haney, J. (2009). *The abortion debate: Understanding the issues*. Berkeley Heights, NJ: Enslow.

McBride, D. E., & Keys, J. L. (2018). *Abortion in the United States: A reference handbook*. Santa Barbara, CA: ABC-CLIO.

Abstinence

When discussing sex, abstinence generally means abstaining from sex or not having sexual intercourse. This means people who are abstinent (or practice abstinence) may avoid any sexual contact at all or may only engage in certain sexual or genital activities. Some people abstain from engaging in penile-vaginal intercourse but engage in oral sex or penile-anal sex. People may also completely abstain from any type of sexual contact. Because of the wide variety of what constitutes "sex," the practice of abstaining from some sexual behaviors to prevent pregnancy is called selective abstinence.

People have the choice to abstain from sexual activity (or specific types of sexual activities). Abstinence can be a beneficial way of engaging with one's sexuality should a person choose to do so. For some people, practicing abstinence can help express one's sexuality more fully, prevent the spread of sexually transmitted infections, and prevent unwanted pregnancy.

Sexuality education in the United States has often focused on abstinence. Abstinence-only or abstinence-only-until-marriage education teaches about abstaining from sex (or sexual activity) until marriage. These programs may also teach that abstinence is the only moral choice and often do not include information on contraceptive methods or safe ways to explore sexual touch or expression. Abstinence-based or abstinence-plus education has a strong abstinence message but also includes information on condoms and other forms of contraception. Comprehensive sexuality education generally includes abstinence as one of many ways of expressing one's sexuality. These programs often recognize abstinence as a way for people to express their values about sexuality within their own sexual practices.

The debate about how abstinence should be incorporated into sexuality education often involves shame. When people are given a strong message about abstaining from sexual intercourse, they may experience shame around sexual activity (Crawford & Popp, 2003). Whether the shame comes from double standards or being told that sexual activity makes a person "dirty," shame around sexuality has the potential to result in sexual difficulty later in life. These messages may intentionally or unintentionally perpetuate shame and guilt and can affect people whether the sexual activity was wanted or unwanted.

Ultimately, whether or how someone practices abstinence is a choice that each person makes for themselves.

Mark A. Levand

See also: Celibacy; Contraception; Double Standards, Sexual; Religion, Diversity of Human Sexuality and; Sex Education; Virginity.

Further Reading

Crawford, M., & Popp, D. (2003). Sexual double standards: A review and methodological critique of two decades of research. *Journal of Sex Research, 40*(1), 13.

Cushman, N., Kantor, L. M., Schroeder, E., Eicher, L., & Gambone, G. (2014). Sexuality education: Findings and recommendations from an analysis of 10 United States programmes. *Sex Education, 14*(5), 481–496.

Hastings, A. S. (1998). *Treating sexual shame: A new map for overcoming dysfunction, abuse, and addiction.* Northvale, NJ: Jason Aronson.

Hock, R. R. (2016). *Human sexuality* (4th ed.). New York: Pearson.

Acquired Immunodeficiency Syndrome (AIDS)

Acquired immunodeficiency syndrome (AIDS) is a chronic, and potentially deadly, health condition caused by the human immunodeficiency virus (HIV). HIV is a virus that is spread through certain bodily fluids. Once in the system, if left untreated, HIV attacks the body's immune system and may weaken it so that the body can no longer fight off other infections and diseases. Although there is presently no cure for HIV, not everyone who contracts HIV ultimately develops AIDS. AIDS is recognized by the World Health Organization (WHO) as the most severe stage of HIV infection; it may develop if medications, also known as antiretroviral therapy (ART), are not taken (WHO, 2017). An AIDS diagnosis describes the point at which the immune system is so weak that it is susceptible to opportunistic infections that would normally be controlled by a healthy immune system. It is estimated that about thirty-seven million people worldwide are living with HIV, and roughly 1 million people died of AIDS-related illnesses in 2016 (UNAIDS, 2017). Further, in 2016, 1.8 million new infections were diagnosed (UNAIDS, 2017). While HIV or AIDS exists in all countries around the world, it is especially prevalent in sub-Saharan Africa.

Even with the increasing accessibility to comprehensive sexual education, there are many misconceptions about how HIV is transmitted. Due to the fact that HIV is transmitted through bodily fluids, many people incorrectly think that HIV can be transmitted by any and all bodily fluids, which is not the case. HIV cannot be transmitted by the sharing of toilets, food, or drink; by insects or pets; or by sweat, tears, or saliva; and it is not airborne or waterborne (i.e., transmitted by air or water) (CDC, 2018a). HIV can be transmitted through contact with HIV-positive blood (e.g., blood transfusions, organ or tissue transplants, sharing intravenous needles) and through contact with the sexual bodily fluids of someone living with HIV (e.g., vaginal and seminal fluids, including preejaculate fluid) (CDC, 2018a). This means that HIV can be transmitted through both penetrative sex (e.g., vaginal or anal sex) and nonpenetrative sex (e.g., oral sex). It is also possible that a mother who is living with HIV may pass the virus to a child during pregnancy, childbirth, or breastfeeding, if proper precautions are not taken. HIV is transmitted by contact with mucous membranes, damaged tissue, or direct contact with the bloodstream (CDC, 2018a). However, the spread of HIV can be prevented. People who are living with HIV and who take their medication as prescribed are unable to pass on the virus (CDC, 2017). Further, if someone is at risk of being in contact with the virus—for example, if their sexual partner(s) has HIV—they can take preexposure prophylaxis (PrEP) medication, which reduces the chances of contracting the virus by more than 90 percent (CDC, 2018b). Also, safer sex methods, such as the use of condoms and dental dams, can reduce the potential for transmission of HIV and other sexually transmitted infections (STIs). It is also important to be regularly tested for STIs, as many, including HIV, may not have any noticeable symptoms of infection.

Although the disease was observed in the United States by the Centers for Disease Control (CDC) in 1981, the term "AIDS" was not introduced until 1982. Prior to the term being coined, it was initially referred to by the afflicting opportunistic infections and soon after by the use of marginalizing misnomers based on the most notably affected populations. Outdated and inappropriate classification phrases such as "4H Disease" (i.e., disease affecting homosexuals, heroin users, hemophiliacs, and Haitians) and "GRID" (i.e., "gay-related immune deficiency") were briefly used; however, these are misleading and discriminatory, since AIDS is not isolated to any specific group of people. It does, however, show that preexisting social prejudices surrounding marginalized communities catalyzed a wide spread of misinformation regarding HIV and AIDS. Socially constructed notions of "immoral" behavior (e.g., homosexuality, drug use) and "uncleanliness" perpetuated victim blaming, and those who were living with HIV faced stigma, prejudice, and hostility. The prevalence of such discrimination may also be a contributing factor to the initial lack of public support for AIDS research. As more and more people outside of these marginalized groups became infected, it became clear that HIV and AIDS do not discriminate, and anyone can be affected. Thanks to international medical intervention and increasing AIDS awareness advocacy efforts, like World AIDS Day, which has been held every year on December 1 since 1988, rates of infection have steadily declined (WHO, 2017). Unfortunately, many people still hold negative attitudes and prejudice toward people living with HIV, and this HIV stigma contributes to discrimination, isolation, fear, and abuse toward people living with AIDS. Further, people may be afraid to be tested for fear of the stigma and discrimination they may face if diagnosed with HIV.

With greater public support over recent decades, significant scientific developments continue to improve treatment of HIV and associated symptoms as well as to reduce and prevent transmission. While cure efforts continue to be actively explored, advances in pharmaceutical interventions for people who are living with HIV have led to many available options for ART. Preventative medications, known as preexposure prophylaxis, are also more widely available. PrEP is a daily prescription medication for people who are HIV-negative and who are at "ongoing substantial risk for HIV infection" (e.g., in an ongoing sexual relationship with an HIV-positive partner who is not virally suppressed with ART, using or sharing illicit drug injection equipment) (CDC, 2018b). Combination prevention that includes multiple prevention strategies, such as using PrEP in addition to condoms, may further decrease risk of transmission.

As the world continues to strive toward a safe and reliable cure, proper medical education continues to spearhead advocacy work and public dialogue against the discrimination of people living with HIV or AIDS. These efforts, in addition to scientific advances, have helped AIDS move from a "terminal" illness to a "chronic" yet manageable disease.

Ilyssa Boseski

See also: Human Immunodeficiency Virus (HIV); Sexually Transmitted Infections (STIs).

Further Reading

Centers for Disease Control and Prevention. (2017). *HIV treatment as prevention.* Retrieved from https://www.cdc.gov/hiv/risk/art/index.html

Centers for Disease Control and Prevention. (2018a). *About HIV/AIDS.* Retrieved from https://www.cdc.gov/hiv/basics/whatishiv.html

Centers for Disease Control and Prevention. (2018b). *PrEP.* Retrieved from https://www.cdc.gov/actagainstaids/basics/prep.html

UNAIDS. (2017). *UNAIDS data 2017.* Retrieved from http://www.unaids.org/sites/default/files/media_asset/20170720_Data_book_2017_en.pdf

U.S. Department of Health and Human Services, National HIV/AIDS Strategy. (2016). *HIV/AIDS Basics*. Retrieved from https://www.aids.gov/

World Health Organization. (2017). *WHO HIV/AIDS fact sheet*. Retrieved from http://www.who.int/mediacentre/factsheets/fs360/en/

Adolescent Sexuality

The World Health Organization describes adolescence as the transitional period between childhood and adulthood that can range from ages ten to nineteen years. The adolescence time period is also known as the time after puberty has started. There has been much debate around the actual years of adolescence as it is ever-changing, so these time periods are estimates of the transitional period. During this period, individuals will go through many different physical, mental, sexual, and psychological changes. Adolescents go through their own self-development; many will feel a strong urge for independence from their parents or caregivers, and most have to start making tough decisions for themselves as they begin to prepare for adulthood. This is a highly critical time of life that is filled with internal and external transitions.

During adolescence, many different physical changes take place, and some can be different for boys and girls. For both sexes during this time, usually referred to as puberty, the endocrine glands start to produce hormones that aid in the development of secondary sex characteristics. For girls, the ovaries start to increase production of estrogen and progesterone. Girls also grow taller, their hips get wider, they start having vaginal secretions, and they grow hair on their body. Breasts also develop, and typically girls will have their first menstrual period, also known as menarche. For boys, the testicles start to increase their production of testosterone, and during the beginning of adolescence, both testes enlarge. This is followed by growth in height, hair on the body, increased shoulder width, growth of the penis, night ejaculations, and deepening of the voice. As these changes occur, teenagers can feel uncomfortable with their bodies, may feel as though they are developing either too fast or too slow compared to their peers, and can experience lots of fluctuations in their mood and temperament. During the adolescent years, it is very typical for individuals to go through mood swings. These mood swings, or rushes of emotions and feelings, are in part due to the influx of sex hormones that flood the body during this transitional time.

As Erik Erikson's development stages would suggest, in the beginning of adolescence, individuals are starting to process the idea of identity versus identity diffusion. This means that they are building upon the stages they have already completed (trust versus mistrust, autonomy versus shame and doubt, initiative versus guilt, and industry versus inferiority), and after conquering these stages, they are starting to build their own identity. When teenagers enter the development stage of adolescence, they are still seeing the world as black and white with no gray areas. This can make it difficult for them to understand the relationship between their behavior and its consequences. Adolescents tend to have a difficult time imagining life in the future and are much more grounded in their present life, which is why they have difficulty thinking about the future consequences of their actions. However, toward the later stages of adolescence, individuals are able to start understanding the concept of their future. They can also start to solve complex problems and start to understand what other people are thinking on a social basis. This does not mean that they are no longer impulsive; however, this characteristic will lessen as they develop.

Adolescence can lead individuals to question relationships in their life, and they will often try to break away from their parents' authority. During this time, adolescents are still dependent on their parents in a lot of different ways, but most are fighting this to try to find their own independence. They are also trying to figure out where they belong in their social worlds, and their peer groups will become the most important influence on their lives. This can have positive or negative effects, depending on their peers. Adolescents will also want to start forming stronger bonds with same- and other-sex friends, and eventually most will start to develop strong feelings toward sexual and romantic partners.

As mentioned, adolescence is when most people start to feel sexual attraction toward others. This can be an emotional time when people may be overwhelmed with their newfound affection, and, consequently, individuals may find it difficult not to give in to peer pressure, and they may engage in high-risk behavior. Sexual arousal also starts to take place during this time, which may lead to very uncomfortable moments for adolescents and potentially their caregivers. Most individuals will start to masturbate and explore their sexuality. It is important for caregivers not to overreact to this behavior but instead to approach it in a calm and understanding manner. Making sure adolescents and caregivers have access to comprehensive and appropriate sex education is an important aspect of this transitional phase.

Adolescence happens at different stages for different people. While the physical aspects of the transition tend to happen earlier for most, the intellectual, social, and emotional aspects often occur much later in this transitional time. Even though adolescence can be trying for everyone, with time, the adolescent will start to understand their own body and emotions. Parents and caregivers should take the time to remember that their children and loved ones are going through drastic physical and mental changes, and they need love and support even when they do not act like it.

Amanda Baker

See also: Childhood Sexuality; Gender Identity Development; Puberty; Sex Hormones; Sexuality across the Life Span; Sexuality among Older Adults; Sexuality among Younger Adults.

Further Reading

Allen, B., & Waterman, H. (2019). *Stages of adolescence.* Retrieved from https://www.healthychildren.org/English/ages-stages/teen/Pages/Stages-of-Adolescence.aspx

Basso, M. J. (2003). *The underground guide to teenage sexuality* (2nd ed.). Minneapolis: Fairview Press.

Harris, R. H., & Emberley, M. (2009). *It's perfectly normal: Changing bodies, growing up, sex, and sexual health.* Somerville, MA: Candlewick Press.

World Health Organization. (2015). *Adolescent development.* Retrieved from http://www.who.int/maternal_child_adolescent/topics/adolescence/dev/en/

Adrenarche

Adrenarche means "awakening of the adrenal glands." It is a prepuberty shift in the body's production of adrenal hormones. Adrenarche only occurs in certain species of primate, including humans, and is related to the maturation of a specific area, the zona reticularis in the adrenal cortex (the outer portion of the adrenal glands).

Androgenic hormones (so-called masculinizing hormones) control adrenarche and its characteristic body changes. These body changes include the initial growth of pubic and other body hair, called axillary hair; development of adult body odor due to changes in the composition of sweat; changes in the skin's sebaceous glands with increased production of skin oils, which can cause hormonal (microcomedonal) acne; heightened emotionality and mood swings; bone maturation; and growth in height. In boys, it is also associated with an increase in circulating testosterone and a decrease in sex-hormone binding globulin, a blood protein that prevents the body from using sex hormones.

Although characterized by physical events typically associated with puberty, adrenarche is a separate developmental stage. Puberty is sexual and reproductive maturation. Adrenarche is a shift in adrenal hormones that occurs independent of puberty. It typically begins by age nine, though its resultant physical changes may take longer to appear. Puberty usually begins within several years following the onset of adrenarche.

The characteristic hormonal features of adrenarche include a steady level of circulating cortisol, a constant rate of cortisol production, an increase in adrenal androgens in the urine, and an increase in circulating adrenal androgens. Adrenarche does not directly lead to puberty nor to sexual and reproductive maturity. Neither its causes nor its purpose is completely understood. It does not appear to be triggered by any known sex-related hormones, including the gonadotropins, prolactin, or estrogen, or by adrenocorticotropic ("adrenal cortex–growing") hormone. While adrenal androgens increase during adrenarche, levels of other hormones remain constant.

The relationship of adrenarche to puberty is unknown. While abnormal levels of adrenal androgens have been associated with precocious (early-onset) puberty in some boys, some children with adrenal insufficiency (lower-than-normal adrenal hormone production) still begin puberty at a normal age, while others fail to undergo normal puberty even when treated with supplementary hormones. Though it causes changes associated with puberty and may play a role in its onset, adrenarche does not appear to be required for puberty to begin.

Premature adrenarche is considered a medical condition that should be addressed by an endocrinologist. However, there is little agreement on what qualifies as "premature": some say before age eight in girls and nine in boys; others say before age six or even five. Unlike precocious puberty, children who experience premature adrenarche do not exhibit reproductive capability, and they can otherwise develop normally. Yet, premature adrenarche is of concern because it may signal a more serious health problem, such as an adrenal tumor. Early adrenarche is common in obese children and in children who experienced intrauterine growth restriction, which shows a possible relationship between adrenarche and fetal, infantile, or early childhood body fat levels and body mass.

Angela Libal

See also: Androgen Insensitivity Syndrome; Androgens; Andropause; Puberty; Sex Hormones; Testosterone.

Further Reading

Boston Children's Hospital. (2019). Premature adrenarche. Retrieved from http://www.childrenshospital.org/conditions-and-treatments/conditions/p/premature-adrenarche

Forest, M. G., David, M., & Sempe, M. (1982). Does adrenarche really play a determining role in pubertal development? A study of the dissociations between adrenarche and gonadarche. The failure of dehydroepiandrosterone sulfate treatment in delayed adrenarche. *Annals of Endocrinology, 43*(6), 465–495.

Parker, L. N. (1991). Adrenarche. *Endocrinology and Metabolism Clinics of North America, 20*(1), 71–83.

Adultery

Often seen as synonymous with "marital infidelity" or "cheating," "adultery" refers to sex with a person or people other than one's spouse, primarily in a monogamous marriage. Originating from a religious background, adultery has been seen as engaging in extramarital sexual relations. Those who engage in adultery, often called adulterers, have historically been punished in many different ways, including socially, financially, and legally. Because of the common use of "adultery" in the Christian Bible, much religious connotation is placed on the word, often followed by moral judgment. In this context, the morality of adultery is closely tied to what Christians believe to be the purpose of marriage—that is, primarily, sexual exclusivity and procreation.

In a strict sense, adultery entails a sense of sexual transgression. It is assumed that the other spouse would most certainly not approve of the sexual activity outside of the marriage. Components such as spousal permission or involvement begin calling into question the assumed moral wrongness of such a sexual relationship, perhaps more in line with consensual nonmonogamy, while others may still refer to the activity as adultery.

In a broader sense, the primary focus is on the breach of the marital contract. Because monogamous marriages are often assumed to be sexually exclusive, any sexual contact outside of one's spouse is seen as infidelity or cheating. When couples practice communication about sexual desires and needs, what is considered cheating can be more clearly defined and less assumed by both parties. What constitutes cheating or infidelity for a particular couple may not be universally considered a breach of contract. For example, one couple may feel that holding hands with other people or giving a massage can be a form of cheating, while other couples may agree that intense kissing or manual sexual stimulation does not constitute infidelity but vaginal-penile intercourse does. It is important to note that sexual activity is intrinsically tied to adultery. While someone can engage in physical or emotional infidelity, the strict meaning of adultery is of a sexual nature.

There have been many thoughts on why people seek connection outside of their marriage. In his book *The Marriage Clinic*, John Gottman (1999) discusses the reasons people cheat on their spouses. After summarizing many different studies, he points to feeling unloved as a common theme in what causes infidelity. This reasoning is often what guides therapeutic practices that help couples work through instances of extramarital affairs. Fife, Weeks, and Stellberg-Filbert (2013) suggest that couples can use therapy to focus on forgiveness in situations of infidelity. They suggest four key components to be used with couples: empathy, humility, commitment, and apology.

Empathy and nondefensive listening allow for the partners to better understand each other's positions. They can better understand their partner's experience and begin to see them as fallible rather than as a genuinely bad person. Humility allows the partners to recognize their own role in the situation and decreases blaming. Acknowledging the damage that was done is an important aspect of being humble. Commitment to the relationship can be helpful for a couple to remember, as well as thinking of past memories, closeness, connection, and shared life goals. Finally, apology is the honest acknowledgment of a wrongdoing. Pledging to stay committed and faithful and asking for forgiveness are often crucial parts of apology.

The work of therapist Esther Perel (2014) suggests a more nuanced and complicated view of why affairs happen. She adds to the discussion with her new book, *The State of Affairs*, on the topic of affairs and why people engage in adultery. Perel identifies much of the literature and current dialogue around sex and sexuality involved in an affair and pleads for the movement away from demonizing and stigmatizing such behavior, claiming that this only causes more confusion and misconception around the subject. She points to numerous causes of infidelity, such as tainted love, revenge, unfulfilled longings, or simply lust. One of her main talking points about infidelity is that the quest for a new lover is less than the want for a new self—that people cheat because they are tired of the self they have become. Her further research may be helpful for uncovering useful future therapeutic practices. Whether adultery is strictly interpreted with religious connotations or broadly recognized, the reality remains that it can affect partnered relationships.

Mark A. Levand

See also: Cheating and Infidelity; Marriage; Monogamy; Open Marriage.

Further Reading

Fife, S. T., Weeks, G. R., & Stellberg-Filbert, J. (2013). Facilitating forgiveness in the treatment of infidelity: An interpersonal model. *Journal of Family Therapy, 35*(4), 343–367.

Gottman, J. M. (1999). *The marriage clinic: A scientifically-based marital therapy.* New York: W. W. Norton & Company.

Perel, E. (2014). Changing the view on infidelity. Retrieved from http://www.estherperel.com/2014/03/changing-the-view-on-infidelity/

Perel, E. (2017). *The state of affairs: Rethinking infidelity.* New York: Harper.

Advertising, Sex in

Most people have heard the phrase "sex sells," which expresses the fact that advertisers use sexual images and messages to draw attention to the products they try to sell. In 2017, advertising expenditures in the United States amounted to over $206 billion. Advertising attempts to inform, position, convince, reinforce, differentiate, and ultimately sell products and services, and sexualized ads often contribute to these goals.

Researchers at the University of Georgia reviewed ads in six popular magazines and categorized them based on the models' clothing, or the amount of skin shown, and the amount of physical contact between models. Between 1983 and 2003, the amount of advertisements containing sexual imagery almost doubled, from 15 percent to 27 percent of advertisements. The products most likely to use sexual imagery were alcohol, entertainment, and beauty products.

Using sex to sell goes back to the beginning of modern advertising in the late 1800s. An early example is collectible advertising cards, similar to baseball cards, which many nineteenth-century tobacco companies put in packages of cigarettes. These images showed women in revealing costumes at a time when street clothes completely covered women from neck to toe. Early in the twentieth century, Woodbury's Facial Soap was the product most frequently cited as the first important campaign that used sex to sell. The text, along with a picture of a romantic couple and the tag line, "A Skin You Love to Touch," was so provocative that some women's magazine readers canceled their subscription when the ad appeared.

Today, sexualized images and messages are in television shows, movies, books and magazines, music, and, of course, on the internet. With pervasive and increasingly frank sexual depictions everywhere in popular culture, advertisers sometimes push the limits with ads that border on explicit erotica. Various strategies are used to stimulate consumers sexually. Nudity is an obvious tool that has been used since the beginning of corporate marketing. Models are shown baring their bodies to various degrees, wearing lingerie, swimwear, underwear, or nothing at all.

The vast majority of advertisements use models who are physically attractive. The suggestion is that if you use whatever product they are promoting, you will be as attractive as the models. Advertisers may provoke consumers' anxiety about their own appearance in order to prompt the purchase of the product or service.

Sexual behavior is often suggested in advertising, especially in sex-related products, like erectile dysfunction drugs or condoms. More subtle suggestions of sexual behavior are in eye contact, flirting, or movement often used in ads for beauty products or alcohol. Another strategy using sex to sell is to refer to sexual objects or events through innuendo or double entendres. An example is the 1960s shaving cream commercial that used a woman's voice saying, "Take it off. Take it all off." A further subtle tactic is to embed subliminal sexual content in advertisements. An ad may have nonsexual objects arranged in such a way that they represent sexual body parts, or words like "sex" may be embedded in the image in an unobtrusive way.

A benefit that consumers derive from sexualized ads is often a form of wish fulfillment. When someone buys the product, they may feel more attractive, they may feel more likely to engage in sexual behavior or enjoy the encounter more, or they may feel sexy or sensual, with increased self-esteem. If the consumer buys and uses the product as directed, they may hope to find themselves in the sexual situation depicted in the ad. Beyond associating sex with a product, advertisers also use sex to position brands as sexual and to imply that sex-related benefits can come to consumers who purchase the brand's goods.

Critics of sexualized advertising have pointed out the objectification of the body, which is viewed as dehumanizing. This is especially apparent in advertising where the models are posed in passive positions or when only body parts are shown. Another criticism is about how these ads define who is sexual. Almost never are the "sexy" models older, imperfect, overweight, or disabled. The models chosen for sexualized ads are usually young, attractive, and fit, with ideal features and bodies. This can lead the consumer to develop a poor body image because their body varies so much from the presented ideal.

With increasing sexual images and messages in advertising, there is the suggestion that it is normal to be sexually aroused, alluring, and active at all times. The effect on consumers is that they suspect they are somehow dysfunctional or lacking if they are not as sexually responsive and interested as the people in the advertisements. Despite the criticisms of sex in advertising, it has been proven effective over the decades, and advertisers are sure to continue using it.

Michael J. McGee

See also: Media and Sexuality; Physical Attractiveness; Sexualization.

Further Reading

Reichert, T., & Lambiase, J. (Eds.). (2014). *Sex in advertising: Perspectives on the erotic appeal.* New York: Routledge.

Statista. (2018, April). *Media advertising spending in the United States from 2015 to 2021 (in billion U.S. dollars).* Retrieved from http://www.statista.com/statistics/272314/advertising-spending-in-the-us/

Advocate, The

The Advocate is an American lesbian, gay, bisexual, and transgender interest bimonthly magazine and website. The magazine was founded in 1967 and is the oldest and largest LGBTQ+ publication in the United States, founded before the Stonewall riots. Both magazine and website focus on news, politics, opinion, and arts and entertainment of interest to LGBTQ+ people.

The Advocate was first published in Los Angeles as a local newsletter by the activist group Personal Rights in Defense and Education (PRIDE). The newsletter was inspired by police raids and brutality, specifically one such instance on a Los Angeles gay bar, the Black Cat Tavern, on January 1, 1967. By early 1968, PRIDE was struggling financially, so Richard Mitch and Bill Rau paid the group one dollar for ownership of the paper. In 1969, the newspaper was renamed *The Advocate*, and 40,000 copies were being printed for each issue by 1974.

The Advocate was bought by David Goodstein, an investment banker from San Francisco, in 1974. Under his direction, *The Advocate* began to be published twice a month and focused on providing information and covering events important to the LGBTQ+ community; it also began to have advertisements from more mainstream sponsors. In 1985, Goodstein died from complications after surgery for bowel cancer. Soon after his death, and beginning with the October 1, 1985, issue, the magazine was transformed from a newspaper format to a standard magazine format.

Editor in chief Richard Rouilard was the first to feature straight celebrities on the cover in the 1980s and early 1990s. After Rouilard's death from AIDS, Jeff Yarbrough became editor in chief and continued this trend. Under the leadership of Judy Wieder, its first female editor in chief (1996–2002; editorial director, 2002–2006), *The Advocate* won numerous awards and set multiple sales records. Under her direction, *The Advocate* also published many coming-out interviews with LGBTQ+ celebrities like Ellen DeGeneres, George Michael, and Chastity Bono, which increased the popularity and exposure of the magazine.

By 2008, the print edition of *The Advocate* could no longer compete with local weekly LGBTQ+ newspapers and the internet, so it switched the magazine from a biweekly to a monthly publication. *The Advocate* print version continues to be published and is available but is now published bimonthly with six issues per year.

Lauren Ewaniuk

See also: Gay Rights Movement; LGBTQ+; Stonewall Riots.

Further Reading

The Advocate. (2019). Retrieved from https://www.advocate.com

Afterplay

Afterplay is the set of interactions that occur after a sexual experience. Afterplay, also referred to as postcoital play, spans a wide variety of possible activities, including cuddling, holding hands, kissing, talking, stroking, massaging, or reengaging in sexual acts like oral sex, mutual masturbation, outercourse, or intercourse. Interactions can be sensual, affectionate, or sexual, and each person can decide in which behaviors they are interested. What they all have in common is that afterplay behaviors are meant to increase the sense of connection and safety between partners.

There are many researched benefits to afterplay. Afterplay is often used as a bonding tool between partners to increase intimacy. The period after sex can be a vulnerable time and is a critical time for promoting relationship satisfaction among partners. When sex is enjoyable, the release of the neurotransmitters oxytocin and dopamine creates feelings of closeness and pleasure and lowers the stress hormone cortisol, which helps create intimacy within a relationship. Partners often naturally use the time following sex to reinforce their commitment to one another, provide feedback on their experience, and demonstrate their feelings toward the other. Research on afterplay within long-term partnerships suggests that it can aid in feelings of sexual satisfaction, especially when following an orgasm. Research also suggests that for women, the experience of afterplay can improve their experience of the sexual encounter, whereas men may experience more indirect benefits, such as increasing the likelihood of future sexual activity. It has also been reported that the more time people spend engaging in postsex affectionate behaviors like afterplay, the higher their sexual and relationship satisfaction. Further, spending more time being caring and affectionate gave people more satisfaction overall than being sexual. This could be explained by humans' interactive nature, the different emotional benefits associated with sex, or the relative lack of intimacy in many social relationships. Regardless of the reasons, research consistently demonstrates that afterplay can promote relationship development and healing from traumas like infidelity, and can increase individual well-being.

In addition, kink communities consider afterplay a necessary part of power-exchange scenes. They may refer to afterplay as aftercare, a more nuanced experience of postcoital activity that has less to do with increasing arousal and more to do with creating safety, maintaining trust, and lowering anxiety. In these communities, afterplay is negotiated before any sexual activity has taken place to ensure that the needs for afterplay are clear and an agreement about fulfillment of those needs can be reached.

Not everyone feels equally inclined to participate in afterplay as their partners. While many people enjoy ongoing engagement after sex, some people feel overstimulated by extended contact after a sexual encounter. Some may find afterplay too intimate and are therefore unwilling to participate if their sexual partner is not someone with whom they want a romantic bond. Others may not enjoy nonsexual touch, may feel restless during afterplay, or may want to receive rather than give care. All these positions can prevent afterplay from occurring, which may provide a challenge when one sexual partner is seeking it and the other or others are uninterested.

Even for those who do enjoy afterplay, barriers can exist. The most common reasons for not engaging in as much afterplay as wanted are fatigue and a lack of communication between partners about their desires.

Research shows that the most positive reports of afterplay come from people who are future oriented and prone to pursuing long-term committed relationships. Therefore, people who do not meet these criteria may not reap the same benefits from afterplay as their counterparts or may not experience the same desire to engage in postcoital activity.

Shadeen Francis

See also: Foreplay; Intimacy, Sexual and Relational; Kink; Touching, Sexual Arousal and.

Further Reading

Denes, A. (2012). Pillow talk: Exploring disclosures after sexual activity. *Western Journal of Communication, 76*(2), 91–108.

Denny, N. W., Field, J. K., & Quadagno, D. (1984). Sex differences in needs and desires. *Archives of Sexual Behaviors, 13*(3), 233–245.

Hughes, S. M., & Kruger, D. J. (2011). Sex differences in post-coital behaviours in long and short term mating: An evolutionary perspective. *Journal of Sex Research, 48*(5), 496–505.

Muise, A., Giang, E., & Impett, E. A. (2014). Post sex affectionate exchanges promote sexual and relationship satisfaction. *Archives of Sexual Behavior, 43*(7), 1391–1402.

Age of Consent

"Age of consent (AoC)" is a legal term that defines when minors (persons younger than eighteen years old) can engage in sexual intercourse without fear that their sex partner might potentially be arrested, prosecuted, and jailed. In the United States, AoC is the age state law determines a young person is intellectually and emotionally responsible enough to fully appreciate the consequences of sexual intercourse (or other activities) such that they can make a truly informed decision, free of the undue influence or social pressure of older adults.

The concept of AoC dates back hundreds of years to British law. In 1275, the Westminster 1 Statute established the AoC at twelve years. This was born out of the public's concern that young girls were largely ignorant of the potential consequences of intercourse, such as sexually transmitted infections, pregnancy, and a lowered social standing (bad reputation). Furthermore, young girls were believed to be susceptible to deception. As such, the law had to protect them from those who might entice them into sexual activity. Protection came in the form of arrest, legal prosecution, and lengthy jail sentences upon conviction. In the past, this idea of protection was so important that advocacy groups such as the Women's Christian Temperance Union preferred the term "age of protection" rather than "age of consent." "Statutory rape" is the modern term to describe sex between an older person and an individual under the AoC. Historical terms included "ravish," "abuse," "ruin," and "seduce," among others. This is where the term "jail bait" comes from: a girl identified as under the AoC and who—at least in the eyes of others—appears interested in sex.

In the United States, the AoC depends on where you live; each state determines its own. In the past, some AoCs were as low as seven. Presently, the AoC ranges between sixteen and eighteen nationwide. A somewhat similar term is "age of majority," the age at which you can legally sign a contract—to purchase a car or join the military, for example. The age of majority is eighteen in all states, except Alabama and Nebraska, where it is nineteen.

Historical criticism of a legally enforceable AoC included (1) the belief that AoC was unique to each girl, based on when she developed her secondary sex characteristics (pubic hair, breasts, menstruation), (2) fears that young working girls would blackmail their male bosses with the threat of false rape accusations, and (3) that male chivalry was sufficient protection.

The historical focus on girls has led to a gender disparity. In some states, the AoC for boys is younger than for girls, in part due to the belief that the consequences are less severe for boys. Although many laws with such gender disparities have been deemed unconstitutional, the Supreme Court has allowed those related to AoC to stand.

Today, whether AoC violations are prosecuted, as well as potential punishments if convicted, vary state to state and depend on the age difference between partners. Some states allow for a wide age gap. Utah, where the AoC is eighteen, allows up to a ten-year age difference between partners before prosecution. In other words, a seventeen-year-old could have sex with a twenty-seven-year-old and prosecution would be unlikely. Other states, in contrast, allow no age gap and have stiffer penalties when violators are much older. For example, in New York the AoC is seventeen. An eighteen-year-old male who has sex with a sixteen-year-old female could be charged with a misdemeanor and face up to one year in jail, even if both parties wanted to participate in the sexual activity. If the man were twenty-five, he could be prosecuted for a felony and face up to ten years' incarceration.

In the 1970s, the federal government essentially extended the concept of AoC from sex to all reproductive health care services with the passage of the Title X Family Planning Program. This law initially allowed poor girls age twelve or older to consent to federally funded contraception, sexually transmitted infection treatment, prenatal visits, adoption counseling, infant care, and abortions. Since then, states have established limits on such services, either raising the AoC or else mandating parental notification or consent.

David J. Reynolds

See also: Adolescent Sexuality; Childhood Sexuality; Intercourse; Puberty; Sexual Consent; Statutory Rape.

Further Reading

Clarke, P. (2018). *Age of consent by state.* Retrieved from http://www.legalmatch.com/law-library/article/age-of-consent-by-state.html

Gardener, H. H. (1895, November). A battle for sound morality: Final paper. *The Arena*, p. 410.

Guttmacher Institute. (2018). *An overview of minors' consent law.* Retrieved from https://www.guttmacher.org/state-policy/explore/overview-minors-consent-law

Michael M. v. Sonoma County Superior Court. 450 U.S. 464 (1981).

Old Bailey Proceedings Online. (2011, April 17). Trial of Stephen Arrowsmith, sexual offenses: Rape, December 11th, 1678. (t16781211). Retrieved from www.oldbaileyonline.org, version 6.0, accessed April 22, 2017.

Ploscowe, Morris. (1951). *Sex and the law.* New York: Prentice-Hall.

Robertson, S. (2015). *Age of consent laws. Children and youth in history.* Sydney, Australia: University of Sydney. Retrieved from http://chnm.gmu.edu/cyh/case-studies/230

Women's Christian Temperance Union. (1887, January 13). Petition. *Union Signal.*

Agender

Agender is a nonbinary gender identity. The prefix "a-" means "without" and generally refers to the lack of some characteristic. In relation to gender, "agender" refers to someone who identifies as not having a gender or gender identity. Other terms that are related to agender include, but are not limited to, "genderless," "gender neutral," "gendervoid," "nongendered," "genderblank," and "genderfree." These terms are not well represented in the literature as "agender" is a newer identity term, but within the community, particularly online in social media spaces, "agender" and related terms are currently being refined, defined, and used by individuals. Similar to the flags of other identities within the LGBTQ+ spectrum, there is an agender flag that is comprised of black, gray, white, and green stripes.

As mentioned above, little published research on agender individuals exists. To date, there have been no large published studies, so it is unknown how many people identify as agender; however, in an unpublished, informal 2016 online study of 3,055 nonbinary-identified individuals across the globe, just over 30 percent of the sample identified their gender as agender.

Agender individuals are not a monolithic group and report different interpretations of this identity in relation to their own gender(s) or lack thereof. The potential range of interpretations of agender include, but are not limited to, persons who have no gender; are gender neutral, indicating potentially having a gender that is neither male nor female or both male and female; having a gender that is not aligned with any common socially defined gender category; a reflection that society does not have any words to describe a person's own gender; identifying more as a person or human than as a gendered being; not feeling strongly attached to gender as a defining characteristic in one's own life; and refusing to label one's own gender. These various interpretations of the term also mean that agender individuals may present socially (in terms of clothing, body styling, etc.) in various ways, including more traditionally masculine or feminine presentations. Similarly, pronoun usage varies within the agender community, with some individuals using nongendered language to refer to themselves.

While some agender individuals may also identify as transgender, many do not. Likewise, some agender individuals may engage in steps, medical or otherwise, so that their body more accurately represents their identity. Some agender individuals have also fought for legal recognition of their genderless status, and, in some cases, this has been legally recognized by the government.

Jay A. Irwin

See also: Asexuality; Bigender; Gender; Binary Gender System; Gender Diversity; Gender Identity; Genderqueer; LGBTQ+; Nonbinary Gender Identities; Pronoun Usage.

Further Reading

cassolotl. (2016). NB/GQ survey 2016: The worldwide results. Retrieved from http://cassolotl.tumblr.com/post/137953257500

Nonbinary wiki. (n.d.). Retrieved from nonbinary.org

O'Hara, M. E. (2017, April 28). Judge grants Oregon resident the right to be genderless. *NBC News*. Retrieved from http://www.nbcnews.com/feature/nbc-out/judge-grants-oregon-resident-right-be-genderless-n736971

Papisova, V. (2016, January 20). What it means to identify as agender. *Teen Vogue*. Retrieved from http://www.teenvogue.com/story/what-is-agender

Shumer, D. E., & Araya, A. (2019). Endocrine care of transgender children and adolescents. In L. Poretsky & W. C. Hembree (Eds.), *Transgender medicine* (165–181). New York: Humana Press.

American Association of Sexuality Educators, Counselors and Therapists (AASECT)

The American Association of Sexuality Educators, Counselors and Therapists (AASECT) is a nonprofit association of professionals who work in sexual health. It was founded by Patricia Schiller, a lawyer and psychologist, in 1967. AASECT's mission is to advance the highest standards of professional practice for sexuality educators, counselors, and therapists. Its offices are in Washington, D.C.

As Patricia Schiller, the founder of AASECT, wrote, "Education appears to be the best means by which to remedy or prevent harm that comes from misinformation, and negative attitudes about sexuality" (Schiller, 1981). At the time that AASECT was founded, the sexual revolution was in full swing. The Food and Drug Administration had approved the birth control pill in 1960, which allowed women to have sexual intercourse without fear of pregnancy. The women's rights movement was making progress toward greater equality with men, and the civil rights movement was contributing to equality among the races. More people were having sex outside of marriage, and gay and lesbian people were increasing their advocacy for acceptance. By the early 1970s, homosexuality was removed from the American Psychiatric Association's manual of mental disorders, and abortion was legalized throughout the United States.

All these movements created opportunities for sexual fulfillment and freedom but also challenges for people who wanted clear boundaries for personal behavior. Many people were seeking information about sexuality, and some were concerned about their relationships in these changing times. Previous generations had been quieter about sex, and individuals often found it difficult to talk about sex with one another. In the new era of openness about sexuality, many people looked for professional help, and AASECT was where they could find it.

AASECT provides professional development through their annual conferences, institutes, and publications, and they certify professional members in the fields of sexuality education, counseling, and therapy. In order to become AASECT-certified, a professional must receive extensive education and supervision, and all members must abide by the organization's code of ethics.

AASECT members include doctors, nurses, social workers, psychologists, clergy members, lawyers, sociologists, marriage and family counselors, family planning counselors, and students. These individuals share an interest in promoting understanding of human sexuality and healthy sexual behavior.

Sexuality educators work in schools, colleges, social service agencies, and a variety of other spaces. Sex counselors often work in health care settings. Sex therapists may work in their private offices, in group practices, or in other clinical locations. There are approximately 1,800 members of the association at any given time.

In their "Vision of Sexual Health," AASECT affirms the fundamental value of sexuality as an inherent, essential, and beneficial dimension of being human. It opposes all psychological, social, cultural, legislative, and governmental forces that would restrict, curtail, or interfere with the fundamental values of sexual health and sexual freedom that they espouse. AASECT also opposes all abuses of sexuality, including, but not limited to, harassment, intimidation, coercion, prejudice, and the infringement of any individual's sexual and civil rights.

Michael J. McGee

See also: Gay Rights Movement; Psychosexual Therapy; Sex Education; Sexual Health; Sexual Rights.

Further Reading

American Association of Sexuality Educators Counselors and Therapists. (2014). Code of ethics and conduct for AASECT-certified members. Retrieved from http://www.aasect.org/code-ethics

American Association of Sexuality Educators, Counselors and Therapists. (n.d.). Retrieved from http://www.aasect.org

Schiller, P. (1981). *The sex profession: What sex therapy can do.* Washington, DC: Chilmark House.

Anal Intercourse

Anal intercourse, or anal sex, generally refers to the insertion of an erect penis into a person's anus and rectum for sexual pleasure. It incorporates thrusting of the penis inside the anus in the same way as vaginal intercourse. However, it is not limited to the insertion of the penis into the anus but can also incorporate fingers, various sex toys (some with the specific purpose, such as butt plugs and anal beads), and oral sex performed on the anus (also termed "anilingus" or colloquially known as "rimming").

There are numerous nerve endings within the region of the anus, and inside the rectum, which can make anal sex pleasurable for both men and women. For a woman to perform anal sex on a partner, which has been termed "pegging," she might use a sex toy or wear a strap-on dildo to insert into her partner's anus with the woman then performing the thrusting action with the toy or dildo.

As with any other form of sexual act, anal intercourse also carries risks of contracting sexually transmitted infections (STIs). Sexual acts involving the anus and rectum may carry higher risks than other forms of sexual behavior because the tissue in this area of the body is delicate and easily damaged as it is not naturally self-lubricating. Any tear of this tissue could lead to increased risk of acquiring an STI. As such, commercial lubricants can be used and may reduce the risk of tearing and increase pleasure for both parties.

Anal sex is commonly associated with gay men; indeed, early depictions of anal sex through art have commonly associated the act with male homosexuality. However, the assumption that anal sex is primarily engaged in by men with other men is somewhat of a stereotype, as research has shown that not all gay men engage in anal sex. Anal intercourse is common among all people of all sexual orientations.

Because of the many pleasurable nerve endings in the anus, orgasm can be achieved through anal sex. For men, orgasm through anal sex may also be associated with stimulation of the prostate. However, some people may find anal intercourse to be uncomfortable or even painful. For some, commercial lubricants may increase comfort and pleasure, but for others, discomfort and pain may still occur. It is also possible that this pain may be attributed to psychological factors, such as socially learned myths about all forms of anal intercourse being painful or even the pure anticipation and expectation that it will be painful. If an individual expects anal intercourse to be painful, they may become tense, which can increase any pain and discomfort they feel.

Anal sex has often been considered a taboo subject, and various views are expressed among individuals as well as in cultures and religions. Some religions teach that the only "true" purpose of sexual interaction is procreation and as such consider nonprocreative sex acts like oral sex, masturbation, and anal sex to be "wrong." Some countries also have laws against anal sex among men; in these countries, anal sex may be punishable by corporal or even capital punishment. Consequently, anal sex may be seen as illegal or immoral and may be considered by some as an unnatural act.

Yet there are other views that anal sex is just as natural as any other form of sexual activity. Some mammals in the animal kingdom participate in anal intercourse, which suggests that it is a very natural act. People who engage in anal sex do so for many reasons: they enjoy it, it feels pleasurable, and it enhances their sex lives.

Callum E. Cooper and Lesley-Ann Smith

See also: Homosexuality; Intercourse; Sex Toys; Sexually Transmitted Infections (STIs); Sodomy Laws.

Further Reading

Gillibrand, R., & Turner, K. (2013). "Let's talk about sex": A post-structuralist discourse analysis into the meanings and experiences of anal sex for gay men. *Psychology of Sexualities Review, 4*, 54–67.

Herbenick, D., Reece, M., Schick, V., Sanders, S. A., Dodge, B., & Fortenberry, J. D. (2010). Sexual behaviour in United States: Results from a national probability sample of men and women ages 14–94. *Journal of Sexual Medicine, 7*, 255–265.

McBride, K. R., & Fortenberry, J. D. (2010). Heterosexual anal sexuality and anal sex behaviours: A review. *The Journal of Sex Research, 47*(2–3), 123–136.

Androgen Insensitivity Syndrome

"Androgen insensitivity syndrome" is an umbrella term for several congenital conditions where the body does not respond, or does not respond fully, to androgens. Androgens are the group of sex hormones that are responsible for masculinizing the body (the Greek root for "male" is "andro-"). Testosterone is the most well-known, but dihydrotestosterone, androstenedione, and dehydroepiandrosterone (DHEA) are also androgens. When someone has androgen insensitivity, they are less responsive to these hormones, which produce the signals that cause the body to masculinize.

Androgen insensitivity syndromes are part of a group of conditions that are collectively referred to as disorders of sexual development or differences of sexual development (DSDs). DSDs are all conditions where sexual development differs from the standard developmental pathways expected of XX females and XY males. Although it is commonly taught that sexual development is determined by whether people have two X chromosomes or an X and a Y chromosome, this is too simplistic. Sexual development depends on several factors, one of the most important of which is the body's ability to produce and respond to androgens.

All androgen insensitivity syndromes are caused by androgen receptor gene mutations. As such, these conditions are inherited and tend to run in families. Because the androgen receptor gene is on the X chromosome, androgen insensitivity is considered to be an X-linked trait. That means that familial androgen insensitivity follows the maternal line. More than 1,000 mutations associated with androgen insensitivity have been identified to date.

There are three types of androgen insensitivity syndrome—complete, partial, and mild. Individuals with complete androgen insensitivity syndrome (CAIS) have no ability to respond to androgens at all. People born with CAIS have the XY chromosomes associated with male infants but appear to be typical female infants at the time of birth. During childhood, they develop normally, and their condition may not be discovered until they reach puberty and do not menstruate or grow pubic or underarm hair.

Young women with CAIS have internal testes instead of ovaries and do not have a uterus, which means they are unable to have children; however, they are otherwise typical women. Because young women with CAIS have testes instead of ovaries, the condition was historically known as testicular feminization syndrome. However, we now know that androgen insensitivity is caused by mutations in the gene that codes for the androgen receptor and is not caused by problems with the testes.

Individuals with partial or mild androgen insensitivity syndrome have some ability to respond to androgens. As such, the symptoms of these conditions are more variable. At the time of birth, individuals with partial androgen insensitivity syndrome (PAIS) may have bodies that appear anywhere from completely female to almost typically male. As such, infants with PAIS may be categorized as either male or female at the time of birth, depending on the extent of their androgen insensitivity.

Individuals with androgen insensitivity syndrome are generally quite healthy, and there is not generally any need for medical treatment prior to puberty. Historically, many infants with ambiguous genitalia were subject to genital surgeries, usually designed to make the genitals appear more feminine. However, there has been a move against these surgeries, except in cases where the procedures are medically necessary. This is, in part, because the surgeries can cause permanent problems in sexual functioning solely for aesthetic outcomes.

After puberty, most individuals with PAIS or CAIS have their testes removed, in part due to an elevated risk of testicular cancer. For young women with CAIS, leaving the testes in place can also cause enlargement of the clitoris and fusion of the labia. Some women with CAIS may also need to use vaginal dilation to increase their vaginal depth if they are interested in vaginal intercourse. Later in life, hormone replacement therapy may also be needed to maintain overall health.

Androgen insensitivity syndrome is a rare condition, affecting only around thirteen in every hundred thousand people. However, androgen insensitivity has taught scientists a great deal about the role of hormones in gender identity formation. Specifically, individuals with this condition have provided evidence that gender identity formation may be, at least in part, responsive to prenatal hormone exposure in the brain.

Gender assignment for individuals with PAIS is largely based on whether or not the infant clearly has a penis at the time of birth. The presence or absence of a penis is directly related to how well the body was able to respond to testosterone levels in the prenatal environment. Research has consistently shown that individuals with PAIS who are assigned as female at the time of birth generally have a female gender identity, and those who are assigned as male generally have a male gender identity. Studies on other conditions suggest that this is not simply because of how the individuals are raised. Instead, it appears to be, at least in part, because the extent of masculinization of an infant's genitals also reflects the extent of masculinization of that infant's brain.

Elizabeth R. Boskey

See also: Androgens; Chromosomal Sex; Congenital Adrenal Hyperplasia; DHEA; 5-Alpha-Reductase Deficiency; Hypogonadism; Intersexuality; Sex Hormones; Testosterone.

Further Reading

Chen, M. J., Vu, B. M., Axelrad, M., Dietrich, J. E., Gargollo, P., Gunn, S., … Karaviti, L. P. (2015). Androgen insensitivity syndrome: Management considerations from infancy to adulthood. *Pediatric Endocrinology Reviews, 12*(4), 373–387.

Gottlieb, B., Beitel, L. K., Nadarajah, A., Paliouras, M., & Trifiro, M. (2012). The androgen receptor gene mutations database: 2012 update. *Human Mutation, 33*(5), 887–894.

Kolesinska, Z., Ahmed, S. F., Niedziela, M., Bryce, J., Molinska-Glura, M., Rodie, M., … Weintrob, N. (2014). Changes over time in sex assignment for disorders of sex development. *Pediatrics, 134*(3), e710–e715.

Kon, A. A. (2015). Ethical issues in decision-making for infants with disorders of sex development. *Hormone and Metabolic Research, 47*(5), 340–343.

Mendoza, N., & Motos, M. A. (2013). Androgen insensitivity syndrome. *Gynecological Endocrinology, 29*(1), 1–5.

Wisniewski, A., & Aston, C. E. (2015). A cross-section study of the ontogeny of gender roles in women with DSD. *Current Pediatric Review, 11*(1), 27–35.

Androgens

Androgens are hormones commonly referred to as the "male sex hormones," though they also occur, in small amounts, in females. The two most important androgens, in terms of their physiological effects, are testosterone and androsterone. Chemically, androgens are classified as steroids, as are the "female sex hormones," estrogen and progesterone. Steroids are fat molecules, formed from cholesterol, that have a core structure made of three rings of six carbon atoms and one ring of five carbon atoms.

During fetal development, androgens prompt the development of the testes (or testicles), penis, prostate, and other male physical traits. They are the chemical compounds that cause a fetus to become male rather than female. In the growing boy, only small amounts of androgens are secreted prior to puberty.

When a male reaches puberty, the testes begin to secrete large amounts of androgens. The adrenal glands of both males and females, and the ovaries (sex organs of females), also begin to secrete more androgens at puberty, though still in much smaller amounts than the testes. The puberty-related ramp-up in androgen production is medically referred to as the "adrenarche," though that term is not commonly used. Female bodies typically produce about one-twelfth as much androgen as do male bodies.

As puberty progresses, androgens cause the testes and penis to grow in size and to mature sexually. These hormones also prompt male sexual behaviors, such as interest in sexual intercourse and masturbation (both characteristic of the "sex drive"). Androgens further cause the development of other secondary sexual characteristics in males, such as a deepened voice (caused by the lengthening and thickening of vocal cords), beard growth, body hair growth, and increased muscle and bone mass.

In females, androgens have more subtle influences on sexual characteristics and behavior, such as the growth of pubic and underarm hair and an elevated sex drive. However, some androgens are converted through metabolic processes into estrogens, which are the main hormones that cause female secondary sexual characteristics.

As some men age, androgens influence the regression of hair on the scalp, leading to baldness. Still other physiological factors influenced by androgens, in both men and women, include kidney size, red blood cell production, skin pigments, sweat gland activity, and sebaceous (oil) gland activity.

Androgen molecules produce their physiological changes by binding to receptors on the surfaces of cells or to receptors inside cells that then move into the cell nuclei (DNA-containing central part). These cellular processes lead to a series of chemical reactions that initiate hormone secretion, tissue maturity, or other biochemical changes.

Testosterone is the most active male sex hormone. Most testosterone is produced by the connective tissue cells surrounding the sperm-producing tubules in the testes. Those connective tissue cells are known as the cells of Leydig. The secretion of testosterone by the Leydig cells is primarily regulated by the secretion of luteinizing hormone by the pituitary gland in the brain.

Androsterone plays a supportive role for the functions of testosterone as well as for other physiological processes in the body. Androsterone and certain other androgens—including androstenedione, dehydroepiandrosterone (DHEA), and dehydroepiandrosterone sulfate (DHEA sulfate)—are produced mainly in the adrenal cortex, the outer portion of the adrenal glands, on the kidneys. The testes and ovaries also produce some of these hormones. DHEA and DHEA sulfate can be converted into testosterone or androstenedione in other body tissues, including the skin, fat, muscle, and brain.

In men, it is normal for androgen production to gradually decrease with age, typically beginning in the thirties. However, androgen deficiency refers to abnormal conditions that occur when too few androgen compounds are produced in the male body, leading to various health problems. Symptoms of androgen deficiency may include a low sex drive, fatigue, depression, weak erections, reduced ejaculate, gynecomastia (breast development), an increase in abdominal fat, a reduction in body hair, and decreased muscle and bone mass.

Low androgen levels are often the effect of physical problems. For example, some males are born with malfunctioning or nonfunctioning testes. This may be the result of failure of the testes to descend into the scrotum, a blocked blood supply, or a chromosomal abnormality called Klinefelter syndrome. Some males sustain damage to the testes as a result of trauma, or they require orchiectomies (testicle removal) for health problems, such as testicular cancer. Tumors and other disorders of the pituitary gland or hypothalamus (parts of the brain that regulate testicular function) may also cause low androgen levels in men.

In any of these or other cases in which males do not produce sufficient androgen, testosterone or androgen replacement therapy is necessary for the individuals to develop and maintain functioning reproductive organs and normal sperm cells. The hormones can be administered as injections, pills, creams, gels, patches, or implants. Androgen replacement may also be used as treatment for men who have low sex drives. Surgical procedures, such as tumor removal, may be required to cure some cases of androgen deficiency.

Low androgen levels are sometimes caused by exposure to chemical compounds in the environment known as androgen disrupters or androgen blockers, which can interfere with the effects of androgens by blocking hormone secretion, receptor binding, or genital development and function. These problems may begin as early as fetal development, or they may occur during childhood or adulthood. Research suggests that some of these disruptive compounds are phthalates, which are found in a variety of consumer products, including skin lotions, perfumes, adhesives, pesticides, plastics, and electronic components.

In women, medical problems develop when too many androgen compounds are produced in the body. Excess androgen levels in women can lead to the irregular occurrence or premature end of menstrual periods, acne, and physical changes resembling male secondary sexual characteristics, such as growth of facial and body hair, balding, a deepened voice, increased muscle mass, decreased breast size, and enlargement of the clitoris.

Excess androgen levels in women can be caused by glandular or ovarian disorders, including Cushing syndrome (a pituitary gland disorder), congenital adrenal hyperplasia, polycystic ovary syndrome, and benign or malignant tumors in the adrenal glands or ovaries. Treatment for women with any of these disorders depends on the patient's particular condition, but various medications or surgical procedures are often necessary.

In addition to their use as hormone therapy for males who produce insufficient amounts, androgens are used as treatments for a number of other disorders. Prescription androgen-based medications are a common treatment for women with breast cancer. Physicians may also prescribe androgen medications for people with anemia, certain skin problems, and abnormally delayed growth.

Yet another use of androgens is as hormone therapy for transgender people who are transitioning from female bodies to male bodies. For transgender people who are transitioning from male bodies to female bodies, androgen-blocking medications are used as part of their hormone therapy.

Androgen drugs referred to as "anabolic steroids" have been used by some athletes to build muscle strength. However, such use can result in serious physical and psychological side effects—including cardiovascular problems, liver damage, testicular shrinkage, and increased aggression ("roid rage")—especially when unsupervised by a physician.

A. J. Smuskiewicz

See also: Adrenarche; Androgen Insensitivity Syndrome; Andropause; Estrogen; Hormone Replacement Therapy; Progesterone; Puberty; Sex Hormones; Testosterone; Testosterone Replacement Therapy.

Further Reading

The hormones: Androgens. (n.d.). Retrieved from http://e.hormone.tulane.edu/learning/androgens.html

Lee, G. (2018). Phthalates: What you need to know. Retrieved from https://www.babycenter.com/0_phthalates-what-you-need-to-know_3647067.bc

Mayo Clinic. (2019). Androgen (oral route, parenteral route, subcutaneous route, topical application route, transdermal route). Retrieved from http://www.mayoclinic.org/drugs-supplements/androgen-oral-route-parenteral-route-subcutaneous-route-topical-application-route-transdermal-route/description/drg-20069341

Androgyny

Androgyny is defined as the expression of both "masculine" and "feminine" characteristics by an individual. The nature of androgyny is controversial, with competing perspectives, namely, biological, psychological, and sociological. In many ways, "androgyny" is an outdated term. The term "gender nonconformity" is better fitting as it accurately reflects the physical, social, and psychological components that make up an individual's gender identity as well as the social treatment of a nonnormative gender expression.

"Androgyny" is a term that has been used to describe a wide variety of behaviors, characteristics, and appearances that are gender-ambiguous or gender-nonconforming. That is, "androgyny" is often used today to describe a person whose gender is difficult to determine based on their appearance. An alternative term to "androgyny" is "gender-role transcendence," which captures the individual's right to maintain the freedom to express their gender as they wish rather than on the basis of popularly held definitions of "masculinity," "femininity," and "androgyny."

From a biological standpoint, the term "androgyny" was incorrectly used to refer to the co-occurrence of both male and female physical traits in one individual, which is correctly referred to as "intersex." For example, an individual who has a vagina and a penis is considered intersex as they possess typically ascribed male and female sex organs. Intersex individuals were once referred to as hermaphrodites; however, this term has drastically declined in popularity because it is considered by many to be stigmatizing. Although it remains unknown the exact percentage of people who are intersex, it has been estimated that 2 percent of newborns may be intersex.

Contrary to the aforementioned biological viewpoint of androgyny, a sociological framework emphasizes the behavioral aspects of androgyny, such as the individual's way of dress and mannerisms, which embodies traditional attributes of more than one gender. For example, a female individual who dresses in suits that are traditionally associated with masculinity may be considered androgynous. Relatedly, from a psychological perspective, androgyny refers to an individual's gender identity, which may include both "masculine" and "feminine" characteristics. Sandra Bem, the developer of the Bem Sex-Role Inventory (BSRI), was one of the earliest proponents of psychological androgyny as it relates to gender identity and psychological well-being. The BSRI has four classifications of gender identity: masculine, feminine, androgynous, and undifferentiated. Further, as early as 1977, Bem asserted that she is of the opinion that androgynous men and women are more flexible and psychologically healthy than rigidly "masculine" or "feminine" individuals. Today, the BSRI is widely used to measure gender in psychological research.

Androgyny has not always been a widely recognized concept in mainstream culture. The term appeared for the first time in the context we use it today in Plato's seminal book *Symposium*. Androgynous gender expression has received much attention in popular media over the past century. Earlier popular examples include Elvis Presley performing wearing makeup in the 1950s and male artists David Bowie and Prince incorporating feminine dress into their performance wardrobe in the 1970s and 1980s. Today, many people in the fashion industry celebrate androgyny in their design and marketing efforts. In addition, many people nowadays dress androgynously as a statement of individuality and style.

Androgynous and gender-nonconforming individuals often face stigma and discrimination because they are perceived as violating "normative" gender norms and roles. These experiences of stigma and discrimination can take a toll on health and well-being. Indeed, studies show that experiencing discrimination leads to high levels of psychological distress among androgynous individuals. Although one's androgynous identity is often conflated with being gay or lesbian, it is important to distinguish between one's gender identity and sexual orientation. This distinction also has implications for the health of androgynous individuals, as it was found that androgyny has negative implications for one's well-being, even more so than a nonheterosexual orientation. A better understanding of attitudes toward androgyny and further investigation of factors contributing to the endorsement of such negative attitudes is needed in order to better advocate for the rights and equal treatment of marginalized androgynous and gender-nonconforming populations.

Ariel A. Friedman and Nadav Antebi-Gruszka

See also: Agender; Bigender; Cisgender; Femininity; Fluidity, Gender; Gender Roles, Socialization and; Genderqueer; Intersexuality; Masculinity; Stereotypes, Gender.

Further Reading

Bem, S. L. (1981). Gender schema theory: A cognitive account of sex typing. *Psychological Review, 88*(4), 354–364.

Bem, S. L., & Lewis, S. A. (1975). Sex role adaptability: One consequence of psychological androgyny. *Journal of Personality and Social Psychology, 31*(4), 634–643.

Blackless, M., Charuvastra, A., Derryck, A., Fausto-Sterling, A., Lauzanne, K., & Lee, E. (2000). How sexually dimorphic are we? Review and synthesis. *American Journal of Human Biology, 12*(2), 151–166.

Lippa, R. A. (2001). On deconstructing and reconstructing masculinity–femininity. *Journal of Research in Personality, 35*(2), 168–207.

Pleck, J. H. (1995). The gender-role strain paradigm: An update. In R. F. Levant & W. S. Pollack (Eds.), *A new psychology of men* (11–32). New York: Basic Books.

Rieger, G., & Savin-Williams, R. C. (2012). Gender nonconformity, sexual orientation, and psychological well-being. *Archives of Sexual Behavior, 41*(3), 611–621.

Skidmore, W. C., Linsenmeier, J. A., & Bailey, J. M. (2006). Gender nonconformity and psychological distress in lesbians and gay men. *Archives of Sexual Behavior, 35*(6), 685–697.

Toomey, R. B., Ryan, C., Diaz, R. M., Card, N. A., & Russell, S. T. (2010). Gender-nonconforming lesbian, gay, bisexual, and transgender youth: School victimization and young adult psychosocial adjustment. *Developmental Psychology, 46*(6), 1580–1589.

Andropause

Andropause, also known as late-onset hypogonadism, is a condition in men with low levels of testosterone that results in a decrease in erections, lower sexual desire, and possible erectile dysfunction. Andropause is often compared to female menopause because it occurs at similar times and ages as menopause, commonly between forty and sixty years old. Andropause is the process of a decrease in testosterone hormone levels in a male. It is a gradual decrease over time and leads to a decline in fertility in men; however, it does not lead to a complete loss of fertility, which differs from females after menopause. Therefore, males can still produce sperm and father children during and after andropause. Andropause contributes to a decline in sexual function, meaning a lower desire to engage in sexual activities, which leads to a lower frequency of sexual intercourse for males as they age. There is also a decrease in sperm count in a male's semen and reduced amounts of semen, which results in smaller amounts of ejaculate during orgasm. The male hormone testosterone contributes to many of the defining male features that are developed during puberty, such as more hair production, a deeper voice, and an increase in muscle development. Therefore, when a man goes through andropause and his testosterone levels decrease, it is natural that some of the features that are developed during puberty will also be influenced by andropause.

Andropause affects male sexual function and contributes to some physical changes. As the body ages and testosterone levels begin to decline, men typically see a change in their muscle mass, bone density, and strength. Male bodies become less capable of meeting strenuous physical demands that could have been met years prior. It is common to start to see increased body fat, specifically in the stomach and waist areas of the body, in men experiencing andropause as men experience decreased physicality and energy levels. Men may also experience hot flashes, although these are more often associated with women going through menopause. Due to the decreased testosterone levels in the blood, the body is not able to regulate temperature as efficiently as it could during younger years. Men who experience hot flashes may go from feeling a normal body temperature to feeling as if they are burning up in a short period of time. Additional physical changes include changes in hair structure and growth and changes in one's skin.

There are mental symptoms of andropause that are similar to the mental symptoms of women going through menopause. Men experiencing andropause may experience depressive symptoms, lack of energy, and possible mood swings. During andropause, there are many hormonal changes happening inside of the body. Every year, testosterone levels are falling, which may have a negative impact on the person's perceptions of his own manhood. Sexual desire may decrease, the body may not be as physically fit as it had been years prior, and men may not have the energy they once had, which could lead to the depressive symptoms experienced by some men during andropause.

Similar to menopause in women, andropause is a natural part of life and does not necessarily need to be treated medically. Many times, outside treatments do not have a significant effect on the symptoms of andropause, possibly because the symptoms are a part of getting older, which is not reversible. In addition, if a man seeks medical attention to treat his symptoms, a misdiagnosis could occur because there are many other conditions associated with low testosterone levels.

Andropause in males and menopause in females serves a similar purpose: to make changes to a person's body to transition them out of the reproduction phase of life and into a later adulthood phase. This may mean the body reverting to some of the ways that it was before a person went through puberty. Some ways andropause is similar to puberty are the changing hormone levels, the physical and sexual changes, and emotional changes. Mood swings are common in both puberty and in andropause and can be one of the symptoms that can lead a man to seek medical guidance. Males go through many physical changes during puberty as well as during andropause. During puberty, boys may be growing more hair in different places, developing a deeper voice, and experiencing an increase in libido. However, during andropause, physical changes may include a decrease in hair production, a production of more gray hairs, and a decrease in libido. Some men may choose to use hormone replacement treatments to try and slow this process of aging appearances. However, hormone replacement treatments can be risky and are only a temporary fix for symptoms of aging. Andropause is a natural process that occurs in males with varying levels of impact, as it is a part of getting older in men.

Casey T. Tobin

See also: Androgens; Erection; Fertility; Hormone Replacement Therapy; Hot Flashes; Hypogonadism; Menopause; Sexuality among Older Adults; Testosterone; Testosterone Replacement Therapy.

Further Reading

Araujo, A. B., Mohr, B. A., & McKinlay, J. B. (2004). Changes in sexual function in middle-aged and older men: Longitudinal data from the Massachusetts male aging study. *Journal of American Geriatric Society, 52*, 1502–1509.

LeVay, S., Baldwin, J., & Baldwin, J. (2018). *Discovering human sexuality* (4th ed.). Sunderland, MA: Sinauer Associates.

Mayo Clinic. (2017). Male menopause: Myth or reality? Retrieved from https://www.mayoclinic.org/healthy-lifestyle/mens-health/in-depth/male-menopause/art-20048056

Preston, R. (2014). *How to cope with male menopause: The andropause mystery revealed.* Charleston, SC: CreateSpace.

Anorgasmia

"Anorgasmia" is a medical term that describes the persistent delay in, or absence of, orgasm after a prolonged sexual arousal. It can affect people of any gender or sex, and for biological males, it is usually experienced as delayed ejaculation rather than an inability to ejaculate.

Anorgasmia can be classified four ways: lifelong, acquired, situational, and generalized. Someone with lifelong anorgasmia has never experienced orgasm, while acquired anorgasmia refers to someone who may have experienced one or more orgasms in the past but currently does not. Situational anorgasmia occurs when someone can only experience orgasm under specific circumstances (e.g., with a specific sexual activity or partner). Generalized anorgasmia occurs when someone cannot experience orgasm in any situation. While lifelong and generalized anorgasmia seem similar, the person with the former might be able to experience orgasm with more education or different attitudes and behaviors. For this reason, some people prefer to use the term "preorgasmic," since it acknowledges the potential for orgasm to occur.

The *Diagnostic and Statistical Manual of Mental Disorders* includes both female and male orgasmic disorder, defining the condition as involving difficulty in achieving orgasm, substantially decreased intensity of orgasm, or both.

Anorgasmia can be frustrating because the myth persists that orgasm comes naturally and easily to everyone who is sexually active. Orgasm may be difficult to experience if people

- are unfamiliar with their sexual anatomy
- do not understand what an orgasm is
- do not feel free to express themselves sexually (e.g., they may feel embarrassed by their sexual interest and responses)
- have underlying emotional issues or cultural messages that impede sexual pleasure
- fear getting pregnant or getting a sexually transmitted infection
- focus only on a partner's needs
- spend too little time on arousal and stimulation
- are in an unhealthy or unsafe sexual relationship
- have a history of sexual abuse and/or intimate partner violence
- take medication that reduces desire, such as some blood pressure medications, antihistamines, and some antidepressants

- have a medical condition that affects the sexual response cycle, such as diabetes or a neurological disease
- have had medical treatment affecting the sexual organs or nerves involved in orgasm
- have poor circulation throughout the body, particularly to the genitals
- experience hormonal changes that decrease sexual desire, increase time necessary for arousal, or decrease the intensity of sexual response
- overindulge in alcohol and some nonprescription drugs

Orgasm involves a balance of physical, emotional, and psychological factors. For many people, difficulties in one or more of those areas can only be overcome with education and practice; other people may find it helpful to consult a physician or sex psychotherapist.

Barring medical or serious psychological factors, overcoming anorgasmia is often a matter of learning more about one's body and sexual responses. One of the best forms of self-education is masturbation, during which people can learn what kind of sexual touch they find enjoyable. If they have partners, they can then describe or demonstrate to their partners what they enjoy.

Some people may experience orgasm yet discount their experience because it differs from the "fireworks" portrayed in mass media and explicit films. It can be helpful to understand that everyone experiences orgasm differently, and the expressions of orgasm portrayed in media and adult film are often overdramatic and unrealistic.

Learning how to experience orgasm may require private, interruption-free time as well as a basic understanding of sexual anatomy. For example, most females do not experience orgasm through vaginal penetration; rather, they require direct clitoral stimulation. Males may find their orgasm enhanced with stimulation of the scrotum as well as the penis. In general, older adults require longer and more direct stimulation of the genitals in order to experience arousal and orgasm.

Melanie Davis

See also: Arousal; *Diagnostic and Statistical Manual of Mental Disorders* (*DSM*); Ejaculation; Orgasm; Sexual Disorders, Female; Sexual Disorders, Male.

Further Reading

Jenkins, L. C., & Mulhall, J. P. (2015). Delayed orgasm and anorgasmia. *Fertility and Sterility, 104*(5), 1082–1088.

Laan, E., & Rellini, A. H. (2011). Can we treat anorgasmia in women? The challenge to experiencing pleasure. *Sexual and Relationship Therapy, 26*(4), 329–324.

Antigay Prejudice

Antigay prejudice involves negative beliefs and behaviors directed at individuals who identify as, or are perceived to be, gay, lesbian, bisexual, queer, or otherwise varying from the heterosexual norm. Antigay prejudice may also be directed toward transgender youth and adults and those who engage in same-sex sexual behaviors, whether or not the individual identifies as a sexual minority. Further, antigay prejudice may be directed toward individuals who do not conform to gender expectations in dress or behavior, or to the family members of sexual-minority individuals. For example, the child, parent, sibling, or friend of a person who is, or is perceived as, other than heterosexual may also be the recipient of antigay prejudice, without regard to the recipient's sexual orientation or gender identity.

Antigay prejudice ranges from subtle exclusion to physical violence and systemic discrimination. It may be expressed through derogatory speech and other behaviors, such as discrimination in employment, housing, inheritance, and other civil rights such as marriage or the adoption of children by same-gender couples. Antigay prejudice is widespread and observed across many cultural contexts. Several studies of hate speech and physical violence in the United States in the 1980s and 1990s indicated that a majority of gay and lesbian respondents had been targeted by others with antigay remarks, and a significant portion of adults reported one or more incidents of physical violence related to perceptions of their sexual orientation. Some studies indicate that the incidence of violence against sexual minorities may be declining in the United States; however, it is still common. In many U.S. states and several other countries, individuals may be legally prosecuted for engaging in same-sex sexual activities, and in some countries, individuals may receive the death penalty for participation in same-sex sexual behaviors.

Antigay prejudice may develop through exposure to implicit and explicit negative messages about sexual minorities from family members, peers, and cultural and religious communities. Early studies of antigay prejudice focused on what is now considered traditional homophobia or homonegativity. These forms of homonegativity may be expressed in derogatory statements about gay men and lesbian women, such as "lesbians are sick" or "gay men shouldn't be allowed to teach school." In contrast, modern homonegativity is often characterized by statements indicating that sexual minorities should not receive special treatment or that sexual minorities ask for too much accommodation from other members of the society.

Overall, research in this field indicates that receiving antigay prejudice from others contributes to negative mental health outcomes among sexual-minority individuals, including depression, anxiety, substance abuse, and intimate partner violence. Researchers have also explored the impact of internalized homophobia/homonegativity, defined as negative attitudes and prejudices that sexual-minority individuals may express toward themselves as the result of repeated exposure to these negative messages. Consequently, studies of antigay prejudice have noted more negative attitudes toward sexual-minority people than heterosexual people, among both heterosexually identified and sexual-minority participants. That is, sexual-minority individuals often report more negativity toward other sexual-minority individuals than toward heterosexuals. Research on internalized prejudice, particularly internalized homonegativity, has noted correlations between this internalized antigay prejudice and higher rates of substance abuse and sexual compulsivity. Thus, antigay prejudice, whether from outside or inside the self, appears to be deleterious to mental health for many sexual-minority people.

Research in this area has also revealed gender and cultural differences in antigay prejudice. Overall, studies indicate that men report more antigay attitudes than women, and men are more likely to report stronger antigay attitudes toward gay men than toward lesbian women. Some studies have noted differences between African American and European American adults' attitudes, with African American adults reporting more antigay attitudes than those of white peers. However, studies indicate that African American and European American adults are equally likely to engage in discriminatory behavior toward sexual minorities. Thus, while attitudes may differ among cultural groups, the intent to discriminate against sexual minorities appears to be roughly the same between these two groups. Also, there may be generational differences in attitudes and behaviors, with younger adults and adolescents reporting lower levels of antigay prejudice than older adults. Antigay attitudes and behaviors appear to be shifting in many cultural and religious groups, with a growing acceptance of same-sex marriage, parenting, and other civil rights within the United States and many other countries.

Elizabeth A. Maynard

See also: Biphobia; Don't Ask, Don't Tell; Heterosexism; Homophobia; Homophobia, Internalized; Homosexuality; Religion, Diversity of Human Sexuality and; Sexual Assault; Transphobia.

Further Reading

Herek, G. (Ed.). (1998). *Stigma and sexual orientation: Understanding prejudice against lesbians, gay men, and bisexuals.* Thousand Oaks, CA: SAGE.

Herek, G. (2000). The psychology of sexual prejudice. *Current Directions in Psychological Science, 9*, 19–22. doi: 10.1111/1467-8721.00051

Morrison, M. A., & Morrison, T. G. (2003). Development and validation of a scale measuring modern prejudice toward gay men and lesbian women. *Journal of Homosexuality, 43*(2), 15–37. doi: 10.1300/J082V43n02_02

Aphrodisiac

An aphrodisiac is a substance that is said to increase one's sexual desire and arousal. Aphrodisiacs are often used to improve many aspects of personal sexual experiences and romantic health and can be utilized to increase sexual desire. An aphrodisiac may be a way to increase sexual performance or pleasure during a sexual experience. Or, it can be used to draw in others for love and affection. While it is nice to think about substances or objects that can magically boost one's libido or make someone fall in love, there are not many substances that are proven to have this effect. While science may not be able to prove a sexual connection, personal experiences fuel the existence and effectiveness of these substances. People's belief in the success of using an aphrodisiac is what fuels more people to try them. Aphrodisiacs can be a variety of items, such as objects, foods, plants, or even illicit drugs.

The story of the creation of aphrodisiacs is not certain. But, it is known that people have been devising many different substances as aphrodisiacs for a long time. The name "aphrodisiac" comes from the Greek goddess Aphrodite, the goddess of love, beauty, pleasure, and procreation. It is fitting that the sexually enhancing nature of these items were named after her. There have been many different plants and animals that have been proposed as aphrodisiacs, from potatoes to skinks (a type of lizard), from Spanish flies to mandrake roots, and from chocolate to cucumbers. It seems like humans were and still are fascinated with the idea of improving sexual desire and performance. Using aphrodisiacs is one way that people seek to improve sexual pleasure.

There is limited research on the effectiveness of utilizing aphrodisiacs to increase sexual desire and arousal. Suggested aphrodisiacs such as rhino horns and oysters are likely only thought to have sex-boosting characteristics because they look like a penis or a vulva (the idea being that if the item resembles the texture or structure of sexual organs, it is also associated with increased sexual desire and stimulation). Some people may experience an increase in their sexual desire when they eat oysters, but it is most likely their belief or desire to have it work that is responsible, rather than an actual effect on their hormones. This placebo effect is so powerful that people are convinced that eating oysters will "put them in the mood."

A well-known aphrodisiac is dark chocolate. It is thought to increase sexual desire through three different mechanisms. The first mechanism is an amino acid called L-arginine, which increases nitric oxide to promote better blood flow. It is thought that better blood flow, specifically to the genitals, could increase desire. The second mechanism is through phenylethylamine, a chemical in your brain that is involved in the feelings of pleasure and happiness. This aspect could be one that helps draw one into falling in "love," a claim of aphrodisiacs. The third aspect refers to dark chocolate acting as an energy booster, and if one has more energy, one will also have more desire. Most aphrodisiacs are backed by little to no scientific evidence; however, many aphrodisiacs are shaped and supported by individual experiences.

While most aphrodisiacs are harmless, some can be very dangerous. Some people use illicit drugs to enhance their sexual desire and performance. Cocaine, for example, can increase sexual stimulation. However, routine use of cocaine can hinder the ability to have an orgasm, which is the opposite of its intended aphrodisiac use. A common recreational psychoactive drug 3,4-methylenedioxy-methamphetamine (MDMA/Ecstasy/Molly) has an impact on serotonin, a hormone that affects mood. Initial use of Ecstasy may increase feelings of sexual arousal, but repeated use could damage serotonin receptors and have a negative effect on mood. By constantly flooding the brain with serotonin, one's body can no longer produce its own serotonin and will become dependent on the drug to sustain the hormone, leading to possible addiction. While some illicit drugs may be initially aphrodisiac-like in nature, they can have serious consequences.

While most aphrodisiacs have no scientific backing, one substance does have some scientific backing. Ginseng has been used to treat sexual dysfunction, primarily in men, but there has been an increase in the number of women who use it. Red ginseng has been used in Asian countries for over 2000 years, with many claiming health benefits, one benefit being of aphrodisiac nature. It has been used to treat erectile dysfunction in men and more recently has been used to help boost sexual drive in postmenopausal women. While there are a limited number of studies exploring the mechanisms of red ginseng and erectile dysfunction, it is suggested that higher levels of nitric oxide may increase sex drive. For men, nitric oxide relaxes the corpus cavernosum and helps promote blood flow to the genital region. When the corpus cavernosum fills with blood, an erection occurs. Therefore, red ginseng could provide an aphrodisiac-like effect for men with erectile dysfunction. Red ginseng helps postmenopausal women in a very similar way, releasing nitric oxide to promote blood flow not only overall but specifically to the vaginal region to increase stimulation.

Casey T. Tobin

See also: Arousal; Desire; Pheromones.

Further Reading

LeVay, S., Baldwin, J., & Baldwin, J. (2018). *Discovering human sexuality* (4th ed.). Sunderland, MA: Sinauer Associates.

Maier, T. (2009). *Masters of sex*. New York: Basic Books.

Rätsch, C., & Müller-Ebeling, C. (2013). *The encyclopedia of aphrodisiacs: Psychoactive substances for use in sexual practices*. Rochester, VT: Inner Traditions/Bear.

Arousal

Sexual arousal is a construct without a widely accepted definition. When used in a nonsexual context, "arousal" refers to the creation of excitement, awakening, or a strong response. Sexual arousal, then, is the experience of sexual excitement, awakening, or response. It is a series of physical, psychological, and affective changes that prime an organism for sexual activity.

Sexual arousal has historically referred to a central physiological state. Among males, penile erection in the presence of erotic stimuli has been used as a way to operationalize sexual arousal. Among females, researchers and sexologists have had greater difficulty measuring arousal. Some visible signs of female arousal are lubrication of the vagina and swelling of the clitoris, labia, and nipples.

Researchers have also looked to hormones to determine arousal. Testosterone levels in both sexes are implicated in the physiology of sexual arousal. People with naturally low testosterone levels, or levels that decrease due to normal aging, report fewer experiences of sexual arousal. In females, other hormones that contribute to sexual arousal are estradiol and estrogen.

Like hormones, chemical substances can significantly affect the expression and function of arousal. Common inhibitors of arousal are smoking, the excessive use of alcohol, heart medications, psychotropic medications, and narcotics. Overall wellness is important to arousal; therefore, maintaining good physical health supports sexual function. Blood flow problems, heart or lung disease, low energy, suppressed immune function, and diabetes are all associated with issues in arousal.

While the foundational research on sexual arousal focused primarily on the genitals, more recent studies have considered the role that psychological function plays in arousal. Arousal is said to occur first in the mind, spurring from thoughts of psychological arousal, and then is felt in the body. Arousal changes the neurotransmission of chemicals in the forebrain and brainstem to promote changes in the genitalia, particularly the increased sensitivity and thus increased pleasure. As arousal builds, the relationship between mind and body becomes a feedback loop: psychological arousal produces physiological changes in receptivity that, in turn, support and maintain the initial psychological arousal. The brain registers conscious and subconscious sexual stimuli such as attractiveness, fantasy, sexual context, a sexual advance, or innuendo. This is a subjective experience; it doesn't matter how much stimuli there is if the context is wrong. The brain processes the sexual stimuli and creates the motivation for an aroused state, which is what is experienced as sexual desire. Sexual desire inspires individuals to act on their psychological arousal, often leading to some form of sexual experience.

Psychological factors can preclude a person from experiencing arousal by blocking the neurological signals that allow genital and somatic arousal responses. Some common psychological barriers to arousal are nonsexual distractions, feelings of sexual ineptitude, anxiety, lack of physical awareness, and psychological traumas such as social exclusion or sexual abuse.

The feedback cycle between the brain and the somatic system is also mediated by emotions; when the emotional experience of arousal is pleasurable, the somatic changes will reflect that. Sexologist Rosemary Basson (2003) concluded that when an emotionally satisfying sexual stimulus is added to an otherwise neutral psychological state, it promotes sexual desire, physical satisfaction, and emotional intimacy. If the emotional experience is not enjoyable, a negative feedback cycle turns off the parts of the brain receptive to sexual stimuli. The change in receptivity is experienced as physical discomfort and emotional unease, such as embarrassment, anger, sadness, fear, and shame.

Some scientists believe that positive affect is necessary to promote sexual arousal. The more positive factors present in any potentially sexual experience, the more likely arousal is to occur. The fewer positive factors, the more likely there are to be barriers to arousal. One such example is depression, which inhibits sexual arousal by reducing the available levels of prosexual neurochemicals serotonin and dopamine and promoting the cue-blocking hormone norepinephrine. This limits the possibility of arousal by limiting the psychological capacity to register sexual stimuli as well as limiting the motivation to act on any sexual stimuli registered in the brain. Researchers Wincze and Carey (2015) found that factors like good emotional health, attraction toward partner, a positive sexual attitude, a focus on pleasure, good self-esteem, and a sense of ease and comfort all allow for arousal to occur.

Shadeen Francis

See also: Desire; Erection; Sex Hormones; Sexual Disorders, Female; Sexual Disorders, Male; Touching, Sexual Arousal and; Vaginal Lubrication.

Further Reading

Basson, R. (2003). Biopsychosocial models of women's sexual response: Applications to management of "desire disorders." *Sexual and Relationship Therapy, 18*(1), 107–115.

Benson, E. (2003, April). The science of sexual arousal: Psychologists are gaining new insights into sexual arousal with the help of innovative research methods. *The Monitor, 34*(4). Retrieved from http://www.apa.org/monitor/apr03/arousal.aspx

Madsen, P. (2012, December 13). Put your attention on sexual arousal, not orgasm. Retrieved from https://www.psychologytoday.com/blog/shameless-woman/201212/put-your-attention-sexual-arousal-not-orgasm

Sachs, B. D. (2007). A contextual definition of male sexual arousal. *Hormones and Behavior, 51*(5), 569–578.

Wincze, J. P., & Carey, M. P. (2015). *Sexual dysfunction: A guide for assessment and treatment* (3rd ed.). New York: Guilford Press.

Artificial Insemination

Artificial insemination (AI) is a technique in which artificial methods are used to insert sperm directly into a woman's cervix, uterus, or fallopian tubes. It is used as a treatment for infertility of either the man or the woman in a mixed-sex couple. It can also be used in other circumstances. For example, the technique allows a woman in a same-sex relationship to become pregnant through the use of donor sperm.

Physicians typically recommend AI as the first attempt to treat infertility. If this relatively simple procedure does not result in pregnancy, more advanced, complex techniques for treating infertility are attempted.

Among the most common forms of infertility that AI is used to treat are cases in which men have abnormally low sperm levels or other sperm abnormalities. For example, some men have sperm cells that are too weak to "swim" through the cervix and reach a fallopian tube, where fertilization typically occurs.

Other forms of infertility that AI may be able to overcome are cases in which women have certain abnormalities of their reproductive organs, such as endometriosis, in which the lining of the uterine wall grows outside the uterus. Artificial insemination is also an option for women with a condition called unreceptive cervical mucus, in which mucus in the cervix is unusually thick, blocking the sperm from passing into the uterus and fallopian tubes. Yet another condition for which AI is useful is semen allergy, in which ejaculation into the vagina causes severe irritation, burning, and swelling in the woman's body.

For women who cannot produce viable eggs, AI can still be performed using the male partner's sperm. But instead of injecting the sperm into that woman, they are injected into another woman, called the surrogate mother. If the surrogate mother's egg is fertilized by the male's sperm, she bears the child for the couple, relinquishing the infant upon birth.

For AI to be successful, the woman must be ovulating at the time the procedure is performed. Ovulation urine tests, blood tests, or ultrasonography can be used to determine when this is happening. The woman may be prescribed fertility drugs to make her ovaries release multiple eggs, increasing the chances that at least one egg will be fertilized by the sperm. The use of fertility drugs also raises the chances of multiple births. In some cases, the physician may induce ovulation with an injection of human chorionic gonadotropin, a type of hormone.

The man provides a semen sample by masturbating into a cup—ideally after he has refrained from ejaculation for several days (so that his sperm count is high).

The semen sample is "washed" in a laboratory process to enhance the chances of fertilization. This process involves removing certain chemical compounds that may cause discomfort for the woman; adding a chemical that separates out the most active, healthy sperm cells; and collecting and concentrating those sperm cells through centrifugation.

Some women undergoing AI use donor sperm instead of sperm from a male partner. Donor sperm are obtained from certified laboratories, commonly called sperm banks, where the samples are kept frozen and preserved until needed. Such samples are thawed prior to their use in AI. Donor sperm may be used when there is no male partner, when the male partner has abnormal sperm, or when the male partner is known to carry genes than could pass diseases or birth defects to the offspring.

The sperm sample is placed into the woman's body with a catheter, which is inserted up through the vagina while the woman lies on an examination table with her legs spread. Her legs are secured in stirrups, and her vagina is kept open with a speculum, the same kind of tool used to perform a Pap smear.

Depending on the woman's particular condition, different variations of AI may be performed. The most frequently used form of AI is intrauterine insemination (IUI), in which the sperm are released into the uterus as close to the fallopian tubes as possible. This uterine insemination makes it easier for the sperm to swim into a fallopian tube to fertilize an egg released by an ovary. In some cases, the sperm may actually be placed into a fallopian tube.

The IUI technique is more likely to be successful than an older AI technique called intracervical insemination (ICI), in which the sperm are released into the cervix. The ICI technique requires the sperm to swim farther to reach the fallopian tubes, reducing the chance of fertilization.

After the AI procedure, the woman is usually instructed to remain on her back for fifteen to forty-five minutes to allow the sperm to more easily reach their target. The entire process typically requires less than an hour in a physician's office or clinic, with the actual AI technique taking only a couple minutes. Temporary minor side effects of the procedure may include light bleeding from the vagina and cramping. If the woman is taking fertility drugs, she is usually advised to keep taking the drugs for about another week. A pregnancy test is taken about two weeks after the AI procedure.

Artificial insemination fails more often than it succeeds. On average, the chances of becoming pregnant with one AI procedure ranges from about 5–20 percent, with the use of fertility drugs raising the chances closer to 20 percent or slightly higher. The technique is less likely to result in pregnancy if the woman is older than age forty, if the woman has severe endometriosis, if the fallopian tubes are blocked or damaged (such as from infection), or if either the egg or sperm have multiple problems (such as abnormal shape and size and, for sperm, weak movement).

Some couples try the AI procedure several times before turning to more advanced—and more expensive—infertility treatment techniques, such as in vitro fertilization (IVF). In IVF, an egg is combined with a sperm in the laboratory, and the resulting embryo is transferred into the woman's uterus. As an historical note, modern methods of AI began in the 1970s as a result of the "sperm washing" techniques developed for IVF.

A. J. Smuskiewicz

See also: Assisted Reproductive Technology; Conception; Infertility; Intracytoplasmic Sperm Injection; Ova Donation; Surrogate Mothers.

Further Reading

Ding, K. (2017). Fertility treatment: Intrauterine insemination (IUI). Retrieved from http://www.babycenter.com/0_fertility-treatment-artificial-insemination-iui_4092.bc

Mayo Clinic. (2019). Intrauterine insemination (IUI). Retrieved from http://www.mayoclinic.org/tests-procedures/intrauterine-insemination/basics/definition/prc-20018920

Asexuality

Asexuality is a sexual orientation, as are heterosexuality, bisexuality, pansexuality, and other sexual identities, such as being gay, lesbian, or queer. The term "ace" is sometimes used as an abbreviation of the term "asexual." People who identify as asexual do not experience sexual attraction to other people, although they often experience emotional or romantic attraction to others. This is different from celibacy, which is when people choose not to be sexually active with other people for a variety of reasons, like religion or focusing on other life activities, but still experience sexual attraction. Rather, asexuality is an internal sense of not being attracted to others in a sexual manner. Asexuality is considered an identity; as with other identities, there is no test to confirm someone is asexual. People may use this identity by itself or with other asexual identities (such as demisexual or graysexual) to be more specific about their identity, or in combination with other identities (such as being an asexual lesbian or a demisexual heterosexual) to explain who they are romantically or emotionally attracted to. Asexual people may be single, dating, partnered, or married, either to other asexual individuals or to those who do experience sexual attraction.

Research has shown that although there is sometimes confusion, with lack of sexual behavior being an indicator of asexuality, the most accurate predictor of asexuality is when an individual states that they do not feel sexually attracted to others. This corroborates that people may be sexually active even though they do not experience sexual attraction for a variety of reasons, including social pressure, nonconsensual sexual experiences, experimenting, and to please a partner who does experience sexual attraction. Despite the fact that it is not listed as a psychological disorder in the *Diagnostic and Statistical Manual*, some people feel that asexuality is problematic. While there are some medical and psychological issues that have symptoms that may be similar to asexuality (such as low testosterone in women or hypoactive sexual desire disorder), asexuality itself is not problematic from either a psychological or physical perspective.

Although there is no urge to act on attraction to others in a sexual way, some asexual individuals may still masturbate, without a specific sexual attraction to someone, to seek individual sexual release, while others do not experience sexual arousal at all. Like other sexual orientations, many asexual people report knowing of their sexual orientation since they were young and not having experienced the sexual attraction to others that their peers were experiencing. Still others come into this identity at a later point in their life.

Within the realm of asexuality, there are additional terms that more specifically describe individuals' experiences and identities. While "asexuality" is used both as an umbrella term for those who do not experience much or any sexual attraction toward others and as a specific identity for people who have absolutely no sexual attraction, "demisexual" and "graysexual/gray-ace" are also used to identify those who do not often experience sexual attraction but who may feel sexual attraction to specific people or in specific circumstances. Additional terms may be created and used by individuals or groups who feel the need to create language more authentic to their own experiences.

Shanna K. Kattari

See also: Bisexuality; Heterosexuality; Homosexuality; Pansexuality; Queer; Questioning; Romantic Attraction and Orientation; Sexual Orientation.

Further Reading

Asexual Awareness Week. (n.d.). Retrieved from http://asexualawarenessweek.com

Asexual Visibility and Education Network. (n.d.). Retrieved from http://www.asexuality.org/home

Bogaert, A. F. (2015). Asexuality: What it is and why it matters. *Journal of Sex Research, 52*(4), 362–379.

Decker, J. (2014). *The invisible orientation: An introduction to asexuality.* New York: Skyhorse.

Van Houdenhove, E., Gijs, L., T'Sjoen, G., & Enzlin, P. (2015). Asexuality: A multidimensional approach. *The Journal of Sex Research, 52*(6), 669–678.

Assisted Reproductive Technology

Assisted reproductive technology (ART) is the use of laboratory or clinical procedures to manipulate gametes (i.e., eggs and sperm) or embryos for reproductive purposes. It most commonly refers to the handling of both male and female gametes outside the human body (Mneimneh et al., 2013). When a couple's or individual's infertility cannot be treated with medication, surgery, or other techniques, they may choose ART. A variety of methods are available depending on the needs of the individual(s) and can include retrieval (removing egg or sperm from the body), cryopreservation (i.e., freezing) of gametes, manipulating and monitoring fertilization, genomic testing, donor gametes, assisted hatching, gamete/embryo cryopreservation, gestational surrogacy, and tracking the early stages of pregnancy.

Spermatozoa, the male gametes, more commonly known as sperm, are produced in the testicles and are expelled from the penis through ejaculation. Sperm retrieval is the process of collecting sperm by means of masturbation, epididymal aspiration, or testicular biopsy. Generally, surgical removal of sperm may be required for those who have had a vasectomy, have a blockage or structural abnormality, have reduced or absent testicular function, or who experience retrograde ejaculation. If the testicles are not producing sperm or living sperm cells cannot be obtained, donor sperm may be used to create an embryo. For most ART procedures, sperm is examined for its concentration, motility, morphology, and presence of antisperm antibodies. Fertility specialists analyze the quality and concentration of the sperm and level of antibodies in order to recommend the optimal process for fertilization.

Methods of extracting motile sperm from semen were developed in the 1960s and were designed to remove dead sperm, debris, proteins, and prostaglandins from the sample. Currently, this purification system is used when preparing sperm for any ART procedure, including cryopreservation. While not technically ART (only male gametes are manipulated ex vivo), intrauterine insemination (IUI) is a frequently used fertility treatment. IUI is the process of placing sperm inside a woman's uterus in an effort to have more sperm reach the fallopian tubes, which can improve the chance of fertilization. This long-used method is generally less expensive, invasive, and involved than ART procedures. The first account of successful IUI is from 1785, and 1909 marks the first pregnancy using IUI and donor sperm.

In vitro fertilization (IVF) is the process of preparing and pairing male and female gametes in a sterile lab environment for the purposes of making an embryo. The IVF cycle begins with administration of follicle-stimulating hormone and luteinizing hormone to the female, which stimulates the ovary to mature multiple follicles. Follicles are monitored via ultrasound and, when ready, patients are injected with human chorionic gonadotropin, which matures oocytes. Before ovulation occurs, oocytes are aspirated from the ovary using a thin needle and suction device. Once removed from the body, oocytes are graded for their maturity and prepared for insemination.

Insemination involves putting both gametes together in the same environment, which is usually a drop of media inside a bath of oil. The whole environment, contained inside a small petri dish, is then placed in a tri-gas incubator that is regulated to mimic the uterine environment. In instances where there are few or low-quality sperm, or if there have been failed attempts to fertilize, intracytoplasmic sperm injection (ICSI) is used for insemination. ICSI is the process of directly injecting a single healthy sperm cell into the mature oocyte. Since fertilization does not guarantee successful pregnancy, often multiple eggs are fertilized.

Combined gametes are monitored over the next several days for fertilization, blastocyst development, and the release of the embryo (hatching) from the residual oocyte membrane. Assisted hatching occurs when a hole is put in the membrane to allow the embryo to become free. All embryos are graded based on their appearance, and those deemed highest in quality are transferred into the uterus. Additional medications, such as progesterone, may be recommended at the time of egg retrieval or embryo transfer to support uterine lining and receptiveness to embryo implantation. Approximately two weeks after embryo transfer, female patients take a pregnancy test, and positive results are monitored for several weeks.

In some situations, oocytes, sperm, and embryos may need to be cooled and stored in liquid nitrogen for future use. This multistep process is called cryopreservation and can store cells long term without decreasing their quality.

Gestational surrogacy is the act of becoming pregnant with a child that is genetically unrelated to the carrying mother. The originating embryo can be from one, both, or neither of the intended parents and has been created with one or more ART procedures. Surrogacy, like using donor gametes, involves in-depth screening, selection, and legal processes that can be expensive.

Genomic testing usually occurs in patients who have unexplained infertility. Carriers of structural chromosomal abnormalities can experience infertility, recurrent miscarriages, or chromosomally unbalanced offspring. Genomic testing can help clarify the source of infertility and inform treatment options.

Darci Shinn

See also: Artificial Insemination; Conception; Fertility; Fertility Drugs; Follicle-Stimulating Hormone; Infertility; Intracytoplasmic Sperm Injection; Luteinizing Hormone; Ova Donation; Surrogate Mothers.

Further Reading

Centers for Disease Control and Prevention. (2019). *Infertility FAQs.* Retrieved from http://www.cdc.gov/reproductivehealth/infertility/index.htm

Fertility Coalition. (2019). *Getting the timing right.* Retrieved from http://yourfertility.org.au/for-women/timing-and-conception

Jones, R. E., & Lopez, K. (2006). *Human reproductive biology* (3rd ed.). New York: Academic Press.

Mneimneh, A. S., Boulet, S. L., Sunderam, S., Zhang, Y., Jamieson, D. J., ... Kissin, D. M. (2013). States monitoring assisted reproductive technology (SMART) collaborative: Data collection, linkage, dissemination, and use. *Journal of Women's Health, 22*(7), 571–577.

Association of Black Sexologists and Clinicians

Conceptualized and created in 2014 by Dr. James C. Wadley of Lincoln University, the Association of Black Sexologists and Clinicians (ABSC) emerged from the input of twenty-seven black scholars, clinicians, and educators dedicated to formal and informal sexual health dialogue and research about persons of African descent. The organization seeks to bring together professionals who are interested in addressing intersectionality, sensitive issues, and social justice. A welcoming and affirming organization, the ABSC facilitates informed sexuality discourse through its scholarly, interdisciplinary refereed inquiry, the *Journal of Black Sexuality and Relationships.* The mission of the organization is as follows: "The Association of Black Sexologists and Clinicians promotes the sexual health of individuals, couples, families, and communities by advocating for culturally sensitive research, informed clinical practice, and culturally sensitive educational curricula. The organization seeks to foster ongoing dialogue in an effort to reduce and or prevent adverse sexual health outcomes. As a welcoming and affirming organization, we advocate for sexual, racial, and gender equality" (ABSC, 2020).

The vision of the organization is to change or enhance the way intersectionality is thought about. In addition, the ABSC strives to offer research, clinical, and educational opportunities that focus on and include race and sexuality. As an organization, it seeks to empower communities by "engaging, informing, dialoguing, learning and collaborating about sexual health issues" (ABSC, 2020). Finally, the ABSC aims to build and sustain community involvement of black professionals in the field of human sexuality and mental health; to engage in ongoing dialogue, both formally and informally, about social and sexual health issues that affect black communities; to develop and support programs and policies that reduce sexual health disparities among black communities through prevention, education, and clinical response; to create local, national, and international networks for members; and to be a research, educational, and clinical resource for initiatives relating to mental and sexual health.

The ABSC hosted its first formal event, Black Families, Black Relationships, Black Sexuality Conference, in Philadelphia in October 2015. There were over one hundred proposals accepted, and approximately 150 people from as far west as Alaska to as far east as Kenya attended. Participants who attended the event shared their work that was specifically devoted to the affective, cognitive, and behavioral experiences of persons of African descent. The keynote speakers for this inaugural event included Drs. Loretta Sweet Jemmott, Juan Battle, and Robert Weiss. The conference also included a "Black Family Reunion," held at Lincoln University, where participants had a chance to network.

In April 2016, the ABSC hosted its first Spring Roundtable Series in the U.S. Virgin Islands. In collaboration with the University of the Virgin Islands and several Caribbean organizations and media outlets, Black Americana attracted scholars and clinicians from various institutions and mental health agencies within the United States who shared their research and clinical best practices.

In August 2017, the ABSC and Cape Peninsula University of Technology hosted its first International Lecture Series in Cape Town, South Africa. Scholars devoted to research, education, policy, or clinical interventions targeted at persons of African descent were invited to share their work at this epic event. The organization continues to hold events around the world.

The official publication of the ABSC is the *Journal of Black Sexuality and Relationships*. The journal is a scholarly, peer-reviewed publication for researchers, clinicians, educators, and policy makers that explores and discusses issues related to black sexuality, including how it has evolved and how it affects and interacts with interpersonal relationships. *Journal of Black Sexuality and Relationships* is an interdisciplinary journal, and contributors and readers come from a range of fields. The concept and study of sexuality is broad and combines elements of psychology, sociology, cultural anthropology, law, and biology among others. For those of African ancestry, other factors, such as slavery, the black feminist movement, black womanist movement, and the evolution and role of homophobia or heterosexism must also be considered as these affect not only individuals but also larger social and cultural environments. The quarterly journal discusses the sexual health interests of persons of African descent, which traditionally has been an overlooked and underrepresented group within sexual health research and literature.

James Wadley

See also: Black Sexuality; Sexology.

Further Reading

Association of Black Sexologists and Clinicians. (2020). About us. Retrieved from http://www.theabsc.com/about-us/

Wadley, J. (2014). Editor's note: The *Journal of Black Sexuality and Relationships* is finally here. *Journal of Black Sexuality and Relationships, 1*(1), vii–xv.

Wadley, J. (2014). Editor's note: "We have a lot of work to do . . .": The emergence of the Association of Black Sexologists and Clinicians. *Journal of Black Sexuality and Relationships, 1*(2), vii–xvi.

Wadley, J. (2015). Editor's note: It's time . . . *Journal of Black Sexuality and Relationships, 1*(3), vii–xi.

Attachment Theory of Love

The attachment theory of love posits that a person's attachment relationship to their primary caregiver as a child influences how the person will bond with others in adult romantic and intimate relationships. Attachment theory was shaped by British psychologist, psychiatrist, and psychoanalyst John Bowlby (1969) and further developed by American Canadian developmental psychologist Mary Ainsworth in 1965 with her famous experiment known The Strange Situation. Bowlby defined attachment as "the bond that ties" the child and their primary caretaker, and through behavioral interactions of the caretaker and child, attachment schemas and behaviors are exchanged to strengthen (or weaken) the bond. Attachment behaviors between the infant and caretakers include eye contact, touch, crying, grasping, smiling, vocalizing, and reaching.

These behaviors also help create attachment schemas, collective implicit memories organized in networks within the brain to help infants determine if the environment around them is safe and if the caretakers they are bonding with are going to protect them from danger through a goal-corrected control system. Within this system, infants use attachment behaviors to determine how close the caretaker is to the infant in terms of proximity. For example, if an infant cries or makes certain physical movements and the caretaker responds and is aware of what the child needs (to be fed, to have a diaper changed, to respond to facial cues), the infant will feel more secure internally and externally within their environment. If the caretaker does not meet these needs, the infant will see the environment as insecure, thus creating fear within the infant.

Ainsworth's experiment The Strange Situation consisted of her taking various pairings of infants and their mothers, separating the two by having the infants explore unfamiliar settings without the mother, then having the mothers return to reunite with their infants. Depending on the infant's reaction upon their mother's return, they were given a label of their attachment style: secure, avoidant, anxious-ambivalent, or disorganized. In general, it was found that children who were more securely attached to their mothers were able to be soothed when the mother returned to the room. Children who were avoidantly attached ignored their mothers upon return. Those who were anxious-ambivalent seemed to be more stressed when their mothers returned due to lack of internalized safety, and the infants who had a disorganized attachment style demonstrated chaotic and self-injurious behaviors due to internalizing their mother's unresolved trauma and grief issues.

These attachment styles can be used to theorize as to how these infants will develop intimate relationships with other adults when they are older. Based on the experiences they internalized as children from their parents, they can be securely attached, anxiously attached, or avoidantly attached within their relationships. Securely attached relationships, where the person has internalized their caretaker's ability to comfort them, occur when people allow their partners to get close to them without fear of abandonment. Those who are anxiously attached are concerned that their partners will not want to get as close as they would like, and they experience jealousy and fear that their partner will not return feelings of love. Finally, those who are avoidantly attached see love and relationships as temporary, are not comfortable with intimacy, and do not wish to be dependent on another person, thus having a low expectation that the relationship will last. Overall, it is expected that relationships with people who are securely attached will last longer, and those who are anxiously or avoidantly attached are more likely to experience shorter and less emotionally fulfilling relationships.

Shane'a Thomas

See also: Intimacy, Sexual and Relational; Lee's Theory of Love Styles; Love; Sternberg's Triangular Theory of Love.

Further Reading

Cozolino, L. (2010). *The neuroscience of psychotherapy: Healing the social brain.* New York: W. W. Norton & Company.

Harwood, R. L., Miller, J. G., & Irizarry, N. L. (1995). *Culture and attachment: Perceptions of the child in context.* New York: Guilford Press.

Lehmiller, J. J. (2014). *The psychology of human sexuality.* Hoboken, NJ: Wiley-Blackwell.

B

Bacterial Vaginosis

Bacterial vaginosis (BV) is an imbalance of the vaginal ecosystem caused by changes in the vaginal pH and a resultant overgrowth of many types of anaerobic bacteria. BV is not a vaginitis—meaning there is no inflammation of the actual cells lining the vagina. BV is also sometimes referred to as "Gardnerella vaginalis," as this particular type of bacteria is often found in high numbers in those women with BV.

BV is characterized by an unusual vaginal discharge that can be a grayish-white color and usually thinly adheres to the vaginal wall. There can be a small or large amount of discharge, and it can sometimes be frothy in appearance. It can also have a fishy smell, which can cause embarrassment for some women and affect their sexual relationships. Some women may also experience burning, itching, or pain. However, up to half of women with BV do not experience any symptoms. Presence of BV can increase susceptibility to sexually transmitted infections (STIs), and it is possible to have both BV and other STIs.

BV is the most common cause of vaginal infection in women of childbearing age worldwide. BV is not seen in postmenopausal women unless they commence hormone replacement therapy, when some women find that BV recurs. The bacteria use estrogen as part of their survival and reproduction inside the vagina, so without estrogen, there is no BV.

Debate continues on whether the condition is sexually transmitted or not because male partners do not report symptoms or test positive for the various bacteria that are present with BV. BV can also occur in women who are sexually inexperienced. However, what is clear is that in sexually active women, BV is related to sexual activity, even if it is not (yet) considered to be a sexually transmitted infection. Women who have BV may pass BV to female sex partners.

The normal pH (level of acidity or alkalinity) of the vagina is ≤ 4.5. This acidic environment is hostile to microbes and sperm alike—a protective factor at one of the potentially vulnerable entry points into the body. The acid (H_2O_2) is hydrogen peroxide and is produced by *Lactobacilli*, which are also known as "normal flora" or healthy bacteria that live in the vagina. Anything that reduces the numbers of these friendly bacteria also changes the amount of acid produced and therefore alters the vaginal pH. Many things can cause this imbalance in the vaginal ecology to occur, including antibiotic use, vaginal douching, semen, menstruation, and use of perfumed soaps, shower gel, or bubble bath.

Semen has an alkaline pH, perhaps as an evolutionary response to assist some sperm to survive the hostile acidity of the vagina. But as a consequence, when semen is present in the vagina, the pH increases, resulting in a more bacteria-friendly environment where small amounts of bacteria can multiply and cause BV.

Menstruation similarly increases the pH of the vagina, and some women find that menstrual blood can also wash out some of the bacteria that make the acid. This depends on the amount of blood and *Lactobacilli* present and how quickly the *Lactobacilli* are able to recover. This may also depend on the particular species of *Lactobacilli* that are present, with some women being more susceptible to recurrent BV compared to others.

Antibiotic medication used to treat other bacterial infections can also unintentionally wipe out or reduce the population of *Lactobacilli* in the vagina, so some women experience a BV episode while taking antibiotics.

Management of BV includes treating the types of bacteria that cause the unwanted bacterial overgrowth and encouraging growth of the healthy bacteria. Normalizing the pH of the vagina by using an acid-based intravaginal medication, such as a gel-based product, may also be helpful. The vagina may also be repopulated with *Lactobacilli.*

Recurrences of BV are common, and this can be very distressing for women and their partners. Reducing the amount of semen ejaculated into the vagina through the use of condoms or withdrawal can help to reduce reoccurrence in some women. Women should also avoid using perfumed soaps or bubble bath, and they should not use vaginal deodorants, washes, or douches.

Kelwyn Browne

See also: Douching; Sexually Transmitted Infections (STIs); Vagina; Vaginal Secretions; Vaginitis.

Further Reading

Centers for Disease Control. (2017). Bacterial vaginosis—CDC fact sheet. Retrieved from https://www.cdc.gov/std/bv/stdfact-bacterial-vaginosis.htm

National Health Service. (2019). Bacterial vaginosis. Retrieved from https://www.nhs.uk/conditions/bacterial-vaginosis/

Spiegel, C. A. (1991). Bacterial vaginosis. *Clinical Microbiology Reviews, 4*(4), 485–502.

Barrier Contraceptive Methods

Barrier contraceptive methods reduce the risk of conceiving an unintended pregnancy by inserting a barrier between sperm and the female reproductive tract during sexual intercourse. Many, but not all, confer the added benefit of reducing the risk of contracting or spreading sexually transmitted infections (STIs) by preventing each partner's bodily fluids from contacting the other's mucous membranes. While the role of barrier devices in contraception specifically applies to mixed-sex couples, their role in reducing STI risk applies to all sexual partners regardless of gender or orientation.

The main benefit of barrier methods is that they are not ingested, and therefore they have a very low risk of triggering adverse physical effects. They do not alter fertility in the long term, have no rebound period between intentional discontinuation and ability to achieve pregnancy, do not affect hormone levels within the body, are 100 percent reversible, and do not interfere with the menstrual cycle.

Specific methods vary in effectiveness, convenience, and availability. Some require a prescription or a medical office visit to size and fit the device. Others require concurrent use of pharmaceutical spermicide. Not all of them cover an adequate area of skin to prevent the spread of some STIs. Persons with latex allergies can have a severe reaction to some barrier contraceptives, and certain methods have triggered toxic shock syndrome in some women.

In addition, there are social and personal drawbacks to barrier contraceptive use for some individuals and couples. Some methods are associated with an actual or perceived loss of sensation during intercourse. Some individuals feel that the need to carry a barrier device on one's person, request its use, or pause to apply it interferes with spontaneity. Further, all barrier methods, with the exception of the insertive (male) condom, require the receptive partner to pause sexual relations and properly insert and position the device.

Social issues, issues of personal agency, and interpersonal power dynamics within relationships may complicate the use of barrier methods for some populations. Partners in abusive relationships may be unable to request or enforce the use of a barrier device. Since it is obvious to a partner when these devices are in use, a person in such a relationship does not have the option to control contraception (or STI risk) over a partner's objection. Some persons, such as adolescents, may encounter logistical problems, such as access and expense, when attempting to purchase barrier devices. By nature, barrier methods are typically nonbiodegradable, and most involve packaging, so they may be objectionable to some consumers on environmental or ethical grounds. Finally, barrier method use in the United States is complicated by lack of comprehensive sex education and accurate medical information. Sex education curricula that focus on abstinence tend to dramatically overstate failure rates for barrier methods, and young people may be strongly discouraged from learning proper usage techniques and subjected to social stigma when they seek further information.

Barrier contraceptive devices include the insertive (male) condom, receptive (female) condom, diaphragm, cervical cap, and contraceptive sponge. Failure rates listed here are annual rates for couples correctly using a method for each and every episode of sexual intercourse. Higher failure rates are based on inconsistent or incorrect usage.

Insertive condoms are tight-fitting latex or polyurethane sheaths that cover the erect penis. With perfect use, they have a failure rate of one in fifty (2%) or fewer, making them one of the most effective contraceptive methods. Receptive condoms are loose tubes inserted into the vagina with a ringed entrance that partially covers the vulva. With perfect use, their failure rate is one in twenty (5%). Diaphragms and cervical caps are latex or silicone cups that are inserted into the vagina to cover the mouth of the uterus. They require a prescription and custom fitting, must be used with pharmaceutical spermicides, and carry some risk of toxic shock syndrome. Their failure rate with perfect use is one in eighteen (5.6%); although failure rates are higher among those who have previously been pregnant.

Contraceptive sponges contain spermicide and are inserted into the vagina. Their failure rate with perfect use is greater than one in ten (10%) and also increases after previous pregnancy.

Angela Libal

See also: Cervical Cap; Condoms, Female (Receptive); Condoms, Male (Insertive); Contraception; Diaphragm; Pregnancy; Sexually Transmitted Infections (STIs); Spermicides; Sponge, Contraceptive.

Further Reading

Centers for Disease Control and Prevention. (2019). Contraception: Birth control methods. Retrieved from https://www.cdc.gov/reproductivehealth/contraception/index.htm

U.S. National Institutes of Health. (2017). What are the different types of contraception? Retrieved from https://www.nichd.nih.gov/health/topics/contraception/conditioninfo/types

Basson, Rosemary

Dr. Rosemary Basson is a clinical professor in the department of psychiatry at the University of British Columbia (UBC). She is also the director of the sexual medicine program at UBC. Basson is most notably recognized for creating a circular model of sexual response, as she felt that traditional linear models did not often apply to women.

Basson started her career in the medical field in 1973, helping young men with spinal cord injuries. This experience made her want to learn more about sexual functioning. She continued to work as a generalist in family medicine until 1986, when she began a fellowship at UBC in the sexual medicine unit. Here she met her mentor and cofounder of the sexual medicine unit, George Szasz.

Basson's most notable achievement has been the creation of a circular model of sexual response, which she first published in 2000. Her model acknowledges how emotional intimacy, sexual stimuli, and relationship satisfaction affect female sexual response. In the model, arousal is mediated by feelings of being desired, the partner's behavior toward the female, and the woman's body image and mood. This model also reflects overlapping desire and arousal phases and focuses on females becoming more aroused during a sexual experience rather than assuming that desire must always be present before the beginning of a sexual act. Because of this, the model also recognizes that desire is not mandatory to initiate sex, as sometimes sex is initiated for other reasons, such as to feel more connected to the partner.

In 2010, Basson's research was able to show that there were no androgen differences between women with and without hypoactive sexual desire disorder. Instead she was able to investigate and discover that females with low sexual desire had low serum levels of a hormone (dehydroepiandrosterone or DHEA) that is produced in the adrenal gland and helps in the production of other hormones, including testosterone and estrogen. Her further research discovered that women with low or absent sexual desire and arousal had markers of hypothalamic pituitary adrenal dysregulation, which are strong indicators of chronic stress in the early life stages, thus displaying that this chronic stress is linked to low or absent sexual desire.

Basson has devoted her career to helping normalize female sexuality and does so through research in many different areas. Her other research projects include studying how different therapy techniques can be used to help individuals suffering from vestibulodynia and sexual interest or arousal disorders.

Basson has over ninety peer-reviewed publications, many around the human sexual response detailed above. She has dedicated her career to helping to reframe, rename, and decrease stigma associated with sexual dysfunctions. She has also been a strong opponent of the use of Viagra-like drugs to help "cure" female sexual arousal difficulties. Due to her work, Basson has written many articles, book chapters, and manuals for students to better understand sexual function and dysfunction. She is very involved in teaching undergraduate, graduate, and postgraduate courses.

Amanda Baker

See also: Arousal; Desire; Desire Disorders; Female Sexuality; Masters and Johnson Four-Stage Model of Sexual Response; Sexual Dysfunction, Treatment of.

Further Reading

Basson, R. (2000). The female sexual response: A different model. *Journal of Sex and Marital Therapy, 26*(1), 51–65.

Basson, R. (2001). Using a different model for female sexual response to address women's problematic low sexual desire. *Journal of Sex and Marital Therapy, 27*(5), 395–403.

Basson, R. (2002). A model of women's sexual arousal. *Journal of Sex and Marital Therapy, 28*(1), 1–10.

Basson, R. (2007). Sexual desire/arousal disorders in women. In S. R. Leiblum (Ed.), *Principles and practice of sex therapy* (25–53). New York: Guilford Press.

Basson, R., McInnes, R., Smith, M. D., Hodgson, G., & Nandan, K. (2002). Efficacy and safety of sildenafil citrate in women with sexual dysfunction associated with female sexual arousal disorder. *Journal of Women's Health and Gender-Based Medicine, 11*(4), 367–377.

BDSM

Some people derive sexual pleasure from displays of power or inflicting (sadism) or receiving (masochism) pain (physical or psychological) in a sexual context. A host of terms has been used to describe these interests, the most popular of which are "bondage and discipline (B&D)," "dominance and submission (D&S or D/S)," and variations of "sadism," "masochism," or "sadomasochism," often abbreviated as S&M, S/M, or simply SM. In the late 1990s, people who shared these interests increasingly adopted the term "BDSM," a term that combines all of these (B&D, D&S, S&M) to describe their activities.

Surveys in the last few decades indicate that as much as 10 percent of the American population may have sexual fantasies that involve some degree of masochism or sadism. How many people act on these fantasies is unknown, but the number of people actively involved in the BDSM community—that is, people who belong to local BDSM organizations, subscribe to BDSM magazines, participate in online chat areas devoted to BDSM, or attend any of several dozen BDSM conventions—grew steadily in the twentieth century. Nonetheless, the organized BDSM community in the United States remains relatively small, perhaps numbering in the low tens of thousands.

Renaissance writer Giovanni Pico della Mirandola (1463–1494) was among the first to comment on sexual sadism and masochism when he described a friend who needed prostitutes to flog him so that he could perform sexually. By the Victorian era, brothels that specialized in flagellation operated in most of Europe's major cities, and scenes of flagellation or other forms of sexual sadism and masochism commonly appeared in erotic literature. John Cleland's *Memoirs of a Woman of Pleasure* (1749), for example, contains scenes in which protagonist Fanny Hill whips customers and is in turn whipped by them, and flagellation developed as a niche market for nineteenth-century erotic literature.

Several early sexologists interviewed people who derived sexual pleasure from inflicting or receiving pain or cruelty. Richard von Krafft-Ebing (1840–1902) coined the terms "sadism" and "masochism" in the fifth edition of his book *Psychopathia Sexualis* in 1890, deriving "sadism" from Donatien Alphonse François, Marquis de Sade (1740–1814), a French writer famous for literary works that mixed violent sexuality with religious and political polemics. Krafft-Ebbing named its opposite "masochism," after Austrian writer Leopold von Sacher-Masoch (1836–1895), several of whose novels, particularly *Venus in Furs* (1870), featured sexually submissive men and dominant women. Krafft-Ebing labeled both sadism and masochism pathologies and presented several case studies of people whose masochistic or sadistic interests significantly disrupted their lives. Iwan Bloch (1872–1922) was somewhat less pejorative in his work, and Havelock Ellis (1859–1939) described several happily married couples whose sex lives included masochistic and sadistic activities in *Love and Pain* (1903).

Discussions of masochistic and sadistic sexual activities appeared periodically in several general interest magazines, including *The Englishwoman's Domestic Magazine* during the Victorian era and *London Life* in the 1920s and 1930s. It was not until after World War II (1939–1945), though, that dedicated fetish and BDSM magazines appeared. The first of them, *Bizarre*, was launched by John Willie, a pseudonym for John Alexander Coutts (1902–1962), in 1946 and spawned a host of imitators in the 1950s. By the 1960s, many BDSM and fetish magazines published personal ads that allowed readers with similar sexual interests to find one another. These correspondence networks laid the foundation for the increasingly visible BDSM community that emerged in the 1970s in the United States and Western Europe.

Sexual sadism received only brief mention in the first edition of the American Psychiatric Association's *Diagnostic and Statistical Manual of Mental Disorders* (*DSM*, 1952), which lumped it with other sexual "pathologies," including fetishism, homosexuality, pedophilia, and transvestism. The next edition, *DSM-II* (1968), continued this practice, listing sexual sadism with other "sexual deviations" in which a person's sexual interest was directed toward particular objects or "sexual acts not usually associated with coitus, or toward coitus performed under bizarre circumstances as in necrophilia, pedophilia, sexual sadism, and fetishism" (*DSM-II*, 1968). Revisions championed by psychologist John Money (1921–2006) substituted the less pejorative term "paraphilia" for "perversion" in the 1980 edition (*DSM-III*), but *DSM-III* and *DSM-IIIR* (1987) continued to reflect negative judgments of sexual sadism, sexual masochism, and fetishism along with a host of other maligned sexual behaviors. They also failed to clearly differentiate between consensual and nonconsensual sexual sadism, seeing either as acceptable criteria for a diagnosis of mental illness. As BDSM community leaders pointed out, the *DSM* evinced no engagement with actual BDSM practitioners or the organized BDSM community. It provided no discussion of the safety practices of its members or even descriptions of BDSM activities.

Public awareness of BDSM activities increased steadily in the 1970s as bars that catered to gay sadomasochists opened; the first BDSM organizations formed in New York, Chicago, and San Francisco; and BDSM imagery, what the press labeled "SM chic," appeared in fashion shows, magazines, and other venues. By the mid-1980s, more than a hundred BDSM organizations had formed in American cities. A national organization, the National Leather Association (NLA), formed in 1986. Among its goals was to eliminate the pejorative characterization of BDSM activities by both the general public and mental health professionals—characterizations reflected in the 1980 film *Cruising* about a police officer (played by Al Pacino) pursuing a serial killer targeting the BDSM community.

Members of the NLA and other BDSM organizations explained that their sexual activities were "safe, sane, and consensual," the latter being particularly important in differentiating BDSM from criminal violence. Large BDSM events employed "dungeon monitors" to keep participants safe, and those in a submissive role could call out a "safe word" to halt activity in the event of problems. Educating BDSM practitioners in safe practice became one of the primary goals of BDSM organizations, as well as several BDSM publications, most notably *DungeonMaster*, which launched in 1979.

In the early 1990s, leading BDSM organizations campaigned for revisions to the *DSM* that would reflect actual BDSM practice, an effort made urgent by several legal cases involving BDSM activity, particularly the 1987 Operation Spanner case, in which British police arrested sixteen men for their consensual BDSM activities. Charged with assault and other crimes, twelve of the men were convicted after the judge refused to accept consent as a defense. Appeals, supported by funds raised by the NLA and other North American and British BDSM groups, continued for a decade but repeatedly failed.

Efforts to revise the *DSM* proved more successful. Both *DSM-IV* (1994) and *DSM IV-TR* (2000) included revisions that reduced the negative characterizations of sexual masochism and sexual sadism and defined them as problematic only if they caused "clinically significant distress or impairment in social, occupational, or other important areas of functioning" (*DSM IV-TR*, 2000). Nonetheless, the *DSM* continued to conflate consensual and nonconsensual activities until its fifth edition. *DSM-V* (2013) substantially changed its approach, differentiating between paraphilias, which were "unusual sexual interests," and people with paraphilic disorders, who harmed themselves or others. Exhibiting a paraphilia, such as fetishism, masochism, or sadism, does not justify or require clinical intervention. *DSM-V* reserved the term "sexual sadism disorder" specifically for nonconsensual actions—that is, people who violated the norms of BDSM behavior and were likely guilty of criminal violence. These changes in the *DSM* resulted from both a successful campaign by the National Coalition for Sexual Freedom, which revived the BDSM community's *DSM* revision campaign, and changing popular perceptions of BDSM. The best-selling novel *Fifty Shades of Grey* (2011) introduced millions of Americans to BDSM sexuality, while references to BDSM sexuality became increasingly common in the media. Comedian Stephen Colbert, for example, regularly made jokes that relied on BDSM terminology, such as safe words.

The BDSM community itself changed dramatically in the first decades of the twenty-first century. A climate of growing acceptance combined with the ease of disseminating practical BDSM information and finding likeminded people on the internet meant that many BDSM publications and organizations lost subscribers and members. Many shut down entirely, among them *DungeonMaster*. In their place, websites such as FetLife became centers for much BDSM discussion. Nonetheless, numerous local BDSM organizations continue to thrive, and many American cities boast an annual BDSM convention.

Stephen K. Stein

See also: Diagnostic and Statistical Manual of Mental Disorders (*DSM*); Kink; Krafft-Ebing, Richard von; Paraphilias.

Further Reading

American Psychiatric Association. (2013). *Diagnostic and statistical manual of mental disorders* (5th ed.). Arlington, VA: American Psychiatric Publishing.

Moser, C., & Kleinplatz, P. J. (2005). DSM-IV-TR and the paraphilias: An argument for removal. *Journal of Psychology and Human Sexuality, 17*(3–4), 91–109.

Stein, S. (2012). *Twenty-five years of living in leather: The National Leather Association, 1986–2011.* Daytona Beach, FL: Adynaton.

Stoller, R. J. (1991). *Pain and passion: A psychoanalyst explores the world of S&M.* New York: Plenum Press.

Thompson, B. (1994). *Sadomasochism: Painful perversion or pleasurable play.* New York: Cassell.

Weinberg, T. S. (Ed.). (1995). *S&M: Studies in dominance and submission.* New York: Prometheus.

Benign Prostatic Hyperplasia

Benign prostatic hyperplasia (BPH) is the enlargement of the prostate gland. BPH is found in 50 percent of people with prostates over the age of fifty. The incidence of BPH increases with every year over fifty, making BPH a common condition. The prostate gland is a part of the reproductive system; it secretes prostate fluid, which is found in semen. The muscles of the prostate gland also help to project seminal fluid into the urethra during ejaculation. The prostate is located directly below the bladder and the urethra, the tube-like structure that carries urine from the bladder during urination, passes through the center of the prostate gland. Therefore, enlargement of the prostate creates a smaller hole for the urethra to fit into and can cause the urethra to pinch or become obstructed.

There are several possible explanations for why the prostate enlarges. One hypothesis involves hormone-driven growth, specifically testosterone (T) and dihydrotestosterone (DHT). In some cases of BPH, high levels of T and DHT are present; however, this is not true for every case of BPH. Another hypothesis involves chronic inflammation from infection or trauma to the prostate.

The obstruction caused by BPH can produce several different clinical urinary symptoms, including a weak or intermittent urine stream, nocturia (i.e., urinating at night), dribbling of urine at the end of urination, and the inability to empty the bladder. When the bladder does not empty urine properly, it becomes more susceptible to bladder infections, bladder stones, and even kidney damage.

BPH symptoms present in ways that can be disruptive to the sufferer's everyday life. Painful, unpredictable, and frequent urination can interrupt sleep, work hours, and intimacy between partners. Therefore, BPH can have a far reach, affecting not only someone's physical health but also their psychological well-being. For others, these lower urinary tract symptoms (LUTS) are not bothersome and are barely noticeable. The size of the prostate does not always indicate the severity of the LUTS that someone may experience; the symptoms can be a very personal and subjective experience.

The American Urological Association (AUA) has developed a symptom score to objectively measure the severity of LUTS typically caused by BPH. The AUA separates the LUTS briefly described above into seven distinct symptoms: urinary frequency, intermittent stream, urinary urgency, weak stream, straining to urinate, incomplete emptying, and nocturia. Each of these seven symptoms are rated on a scale of 0–5, and the total score indicates clinically mild (0–6), moderate (7–19), and severe (20–35) symptoms.

There are several ways to diagnose BPH, including the digital rectal examination (DRE). The DRE consists of inserting a finger into the patient's anus, where the lobes of the prostate can be felt through the wall of the lower rectum. The DRE can also check for indications of prostate cancer and is also used as a cancer screening tool. The other diagnostic tool used for BPH is to measure the prostate specific antigen (PSA) levels in one's blood. PSA is an antigen that is only made by prostate gland tissue. High PSA serum blood levels indicate that there is an abundance of prostatic tissue present, which would occur with BPH. However, high PSA can also indicate prostate cancer. BPH is so common among people with prostates over the age of fifty that it is not uncommon for PSA levels to rise with age. In a young person, a higher PSA level may indicate prostate cancer as they are less likely to have BPH, whereas the same PSA level in someone in their seventies may more likely be due to BPH.

Another diagnostic tool for BPH is to measure someone's postvoid residual—that is, to measure the bladder's volume before and immediately following thorough urination. If the bladder has a high postvoid residual, this could mean that the bladder is not emptying correctly due to a BPH-produced obstruction of the urethra. Cystourethroscopy is a procedure where a flexible microscope is fed through the urethra and into the bladder and is also used to identify BPH. Individually, these diagnostic tools may also indicate other disorders; however, used together, they paint a reliable portrait of BPH.

Once diagnosed, there are several possible interventions to treat BPH. The typical first line of treatment is medication therapy paired with a healthy diet and lifestyle changes. Dual therapy is the combination of two classes of medications that work together to keep the urethra open and to reduce the size or muscle capacity of the prostate. These medications have relatively mild side effects, including dry mouth, dizziness, and retrograde ejaculation. If dual therapy does not work to modify LUTS, then surgical intervention may be considered to shrink, shave, or remove the prostate entirely via prostatectomy.

Another treatment for BPH is watchful waiting, which is recommended by the AUA for those with mildly rated symptoms. Watchful waiting involves close symptom monitoring paired with regular DREs and other screening tools to observe any changes in symptoms that may necessitate further intervention; watchful waiting is not recommended for those with severely rated LUTS or known possible complications. BPH can become a complex urological condition with a nuanced symptom presentation, and treatment plans may differ from person to person depending on their condition.

Cassia Araujo-Lane

See also: Prostate; Prostate Cancer; Prostatectomy; Prostatitis.

Further Reading

Foster, H. K., Barry, M. J., Gandhi, M. C., Kaplan, S. A., Kohler, T. S., Lerner, L. B., … McVary, K. T. (2019). *Benign prostatic hyperplasia: Surgical management of benign prostatic hyperplasia/lower urinary tract symptoms* (2018, amended 2019). Linthicum, MD: American Urological Association.

Kim, E. H., Larson, J. A., & Anriole, G. L. (2016). Management of benign prostatic hyperplasia. *Annual Review of Medicine, 67*(1), 137–151.

Mayo Clinic. (2019). Benign prostatic hyperplasia (BPH). Retrieved from https://www.mayoclinic.org/diseases-conditions/benign-prostatic-hyperplasia/symptoms-causes/syc-20370087

Shvartzman, P., Borkan, J. M., Stoliar, L., Peleg, A., Nakar, S., Nor, G., & Tabenkin, H. (2001). Second-hand prostatism: Effects of prostatic symptoms on spouses' quality of life, daily routines and family relationships. *Family Practice, 18*(6), 610–613.

Te, A. E., & Chughtai, B. (2014). Benign prostatic hyperplasia. In S. A. Kaplan & K. T. McVary (Eds.), *Male lower urinary tract symptoms and benign prostatic hyperplasia* (191–200). New York: John Wiley & Sons.

Benjamin, Harry

Dr. Henry (Harry) Benjamin (1885–1986) was born in Berlin, Germany, on January 12, 1885. Benjamin became the founding father of the study and treatment of transsexualism. He started his career working on slowing the aging process and then moved into working in the world of transgender care. During his career, he helped outline treatment protocols for sex reassignment surgery and hormone therapy that are still closely followed years after his passing. Benjamin was a champion for providing appropriate transgender care instead of labeling individuals with psychiatric disorders.

Benjamin attended the University of Rostock and the University of Berlin and graduated with his medical degree from the University of Tubingen in Germany in 1912. Shortly after, in 1913, he moved to the United States to work with a new treatment for tuberculosis. Benjamin opened a general medical practice in New York City and focused on treating the aging population via hormones and surgery. During his time at this practice, he focused on some of his interests in the fields of endocrinology, gerontology, and sexology. In 1935, Benjamin became licensed to practice medicine in California and, for a time, had a summer practice in Los Angeles and San Francisco.

While treating his aging patients in New York City, one of his male clients asked for hormones and disclosed to Benjamin that he was a cross-dresser. Benjamin noticed after giving him the hormone medication that he was a lot calmer and happier. Benjamin took this discovery and moved forward with a whole career to help transsexuals receive care for hormones and surgery. Benjamin was also one of the charter members of the Society for the Scientific Study of Sexuality.

Benjamin published *The Transsexual Phenomenon* in 1966, which was the first book on gender identity for a medical audience. In the book, he outlined an affirmative treatment path that he pioneered. Benjamin would give talks at hospitals and schools to help spread his research and first coined the term "transsexual." In 1979, the Harry Benjamin International Gender Association was formed and created the first standard of care for transsexual individuals, with Benjamin leading the way. Later the title of the organization was changed to the World Professional Association of Transgender Health, and it is still active to this day.

In 1974, Benjamin officially retired from his medical practices. In August 1986, he passed away in New York City at 101 years old. Benjamin was married to his bride, Gretchen, for sixty years, and they had no children. During his career, Benjamin worked with many notable scholars, such as Dr. Alfred Kinsey and Dr. Magnus Hirschfeld.

Amanda Baker

See also: Gender Identity; Gender Transition; Sex Reassignment Surgery; Society for the Scientific Study of Sexuality (SSSS); Transgender; Transsexual; World Professional Association for Transgender Health (WPATH).

Further Reading

Archives Online at Indiana University. (2019). *The Harry Benjamin collection.* Retrieved from http://webapp1.dlib.indiana.edu/findingaids/view?doc.view=entire_text&docId=VAC1594

Benjamin, H. (1966). *The transsexual phenomenon.* New York: Julian Press.

Ihlenfeld, C. L. (2004). Harry Benjamin and psychiatrists. *Journal of Gay and Lesbian Psychotherapy, 8*(1–2), 147–152.

Meyer, W., III, Bockting, W. O., Cohen-Kettenis, P., Coleman, E., DiCeglie, D., Devor, H., … Wheeler, C. C. (2001). The Harry Benjamin International Gender Dysphoria Association's standards of care for gender identity disorders, sixth version. *Journal of Psychology and Human Sexuality, 13*(1), 1–30.

Bigender

"Bigender" refers to a gender identity in which the individual is neither exclusively male nor female but rather a fluid mix of male and female identities, frequently shifting from one to the other, or a simultaneous combination of male and female identities. Each bigender individual tends to feel and express bigenderism in a unique way.

"Bigender" is one of many terms that have sprung from the LGBTQ+ community in its attempts to describe diverse people whose gender identities fall somewhere between the "male" and "female" of the traditional binary gender system. Many psychologists consider bigenderism as one of the facets of the multifaceted concept of transgenderism. Such complex ideas are recognition of the reality that not all people fit psychologically or physically into the strict categories of being a "man" or a "woman." The causes and prevalence of bigenderism—like those of other varieties of transgenderism—are unknown.

Some bigender people also identify with the descriptive expressions "gender fluid" or "gender flexible." Other descriptive terms that may be applied to some bigender people—with various degrees of overlap—include "pangender" (literally meaning "all genders"), "polygender" ("many genders"), "trigender" (referring to male, female, and any of various "third genders"), and "genderqueer" (meant to be a comprehensive term for all genders other than male and female).

The overlapping meanings of these terms can seem very confusing to people who identify with the binary gender system. However, for many individuals who do not fit neatly into that traditional system, the meanings of these terms are understandable, and they seem more appropriate and applicable to their own lives than "male" or "female."

Bigender people may sometimes feel like one gender and at other times like another gender, depending on their mood and the situation of the moment. They may express the gender that they are feeling at any given time by the way they dress and behave. An individual might dress like a man one day and a woman the next. Or an individual might prefer to wear gender-neutral clothing on a daily basis—or to even express a simultaneous combination of distinctly male and distinctly female genders, such as having a beard and wearing a dress.

Many bigender people reject the gender-related pronouns of "he," "she," "his," and "her." Some prefer the gender-neutral "they" and "their." Others have proposed new, alternative pronouns, including "zie" and "hir."

Bigender people typically do not desire hormonal or surgical treatment to physically transition from one distinct gender to another.

A. J. Smuskiewicz

See also: Agender; Binary Gender System; Childhood Gender Nonconformity; Fluidity, Gender; Gender; Gender Diversity; Gender Identity; Genderqueer; Nonbinary Gender Identities; Two-Spirit.

Further Reading

Nestle, J., Howell, C., & Wilchins, R. (Eds.). (2002). *GenderQueer: Voices from beyond the sexual binary*. New York: Alyson Books.

Sycamore, M. B. (2006). *Nobody passes: Rejecting the rules of gender and conformity*. Berkeley, CA: Seal Press.

Wickham, K. N. (2011). *The other genders: Androgyne, genderqueer, non-binary gender variant*. Charleston, SC: CreateSpace.

Binary Gender System

The binary, or bipolar, gender system is the system for classifying gender and sex into the two distinct categories of male and female. It is the dominant, traditional gender system in most world cultures—but not the only gender system. Several cultures have long recognized alternative gender systems. In the United States and many other countries, the traditional binary gender system is beginning to make room for systems recognizing multiple gender identities.

The binary gender system may seem obvious. Most people are born distinctly male or distinctly female, and men and women traditionally wear distinct types of clothing and traditionally have distinct roles in society. Furthermore, the traditional teachings of most major religions, including Judaism, Christianity, and Islam, reinforce the concept of only two genders. However, not all people fit neatly into one gender or the other.

Intersex people are born with sexual characteristics that are not distinctly male or female. Some intersex people have unusual chromosomes that do not match the typical XX of females or the XY of males. Transgender people are people whose psychological gender identity does not match their physical gender, leading some to get hormonal and surgical treatments to change their bodies. Bigender people may sometimes self-identify as male and other times as female, alternately dressing and behaving as one gender or the other, or they may simultaneously feel like both genders. Pangender, polygender, trigender, and other transgender people may consider themselves to be various mixes of genders.

People with alternative gender conditions vary psychologically and, in some cases, physically, from simply "male" or simply "female." Although many causes of physical intersex conditions are known to be related to unusual genetic variations, the causes of most alternative gender identities are unknown. They may be related to biochemical factors that are present at birth or that develop later in life, they may be associated with certain experiences in life, or they may be partly biochemical and partly experience based. Only limited scientific research has been published on this topic.

Among the world cultures that have long recognized nonbinary gender systems are some Native American tribes and some peoples in South Asia. The English term "two-spirit" is broadly applied to individuals who are accepted in various Native American cultures as having a gender that is neither male nor female. Each of these cultures has its own native expression to refer to these individuals, such as the Lakota *winyanktehca* or *winkte*. In some cultures, two-spirit people dress and behave as the gender opposite to their physical gender. In other cultures, they fulfill "third-gender" or "fourth-gender" roles, which may be associated with special spiritual powers.

In India, "hijra" is the term applied to individuals who were born with male or intersex physical traits but live as females. They are socially recognized as a third gender and are allowed to marry men. There are believed to be more than five million hijra in India. Similar groups of "third-sex" individuals are recognized in Pakistan, Bangladesh, and certain other Asian countries.

The growing prominence of transgender people in popular culture and LGBTQ+ communities of the United States and other Western nations is a direct challenge to continued adherence to the binary gender system. The increasing rejection of traditional male and female social roles has also challenged the binary gender system. For example, today, as compared to previous decades, more women are the main income earners in families, and more men stay at home raising children. Further evidence of this nonbinary shift in popular culture came in 2014 when the Facebook online social network unveiled fifty-six gender identities for users to choose from.

Professional psychological perspectives on gender in the West have also shifted. In 2013, the American Psychiatric Association (APA) discarded the diagnostic term "gender identity disorder" in favor of "gender dysphoria" in the fifth edition of its *Diagnostic and Statistical Manual of Mental Disorders* (*DSM-V*). The APA made the change partly to remove the stigma associated with "disorder," noting that "gender nonconformity is not in itself a mental disorder."

A. J. Smuskiewicz

See also: Agender; Bigender; Childhood Gender Nonconformity; Gender; Gender Diversity; Gender Identity; Gender Roles, Socialization and; Nonbinary Gender Identities; Two-Spirit.

Further Reading

Jacobs, S.-E., Thomas, W., & Lang, S. (Eds.). (1997). *Two-spirit people: Native American gender identity, sexuality, and spirituality*. Champaign: University of Illinois Press.

Nanda, S. (1998). *Neither man nor woman: The hijras of India*. Boston: Cengage Learning.

Nestle, J., Howell, C., & Wilchins, R. (Eds.). (2002). *GenderQueer: Voices from beyond the sexual binary*. New York: Alyson Books.

Wickham, K. N. (2011). *The other genders: Androgyne, genderqueer, non-binary gender variant*. Charleston, SC: CreateSpace.

Biological Sex

The term "biological sex" is commonly used to discuss a person's primary sex characteristics (also referred to as "sex traits") and other components of their anatomy and body. This includes primary sex characteristics such as a uterus, penis, vagina, or testes, but is also understood to include one's chromosomes, the appearance of one's chest, and more. While all these comprise what makes up one's "biological sex," biological sex is often reduced to be a euphemism for genitals—often when discussing transgender people or how one's legal sex is determined before and at the time of birth. Because of this, more and more individuals are shifting from using the term "biological sex" to discussing specific components of anatomy or using the phrase "sex assigned at birth" or "current sex traits." In addition, many components of one's biology and anatomy are able to be altered via surgery or hormone replacement therapy (HRT). Indeed, Sari M. Van Anders states, "Genitals are not a definitive marker of gender or sex precisely because they can be altered" (2014). Therefore, one's biological sex is not a fixed component nor a great indicator of their gender, reproductive capacity or desire, or transition/transgender status.

While many are familiar with the view that gender is a social construct (that is, ideas and norms around gender can vary from culture to culture, and these understandings of gender—what it means to be a man, a woman, or another gender—can have differing impacts depending on the context one lives in), fewer understand "biological sex" to be a social construct. However, when one considers the number of individuals with intersex conditions—individuals born with biology and anatomy that does not align with Western society's current understanding of being a biological man or woman—the argument can certainly be made. It is currently estimated by the Intersex Society of North America (2019) that about one person in one hundred is born with sex characteristics that naturally vary from what is commonly thought to align with female or male.

Often, when a baby is born with genitals and hormone levels that do not align with Western society's binary understanding of anatomy, they are subjected to surgeries (or HRT) at birth, during adolescence, or during or after the onset of puberty. Altering sex traits at birth due to natural variances that occur did not become a practice until after biology emerged as an organized discipline in European and U.S. culture, around the turn of the nineteenth century. At this time, scientists who were beginning to grow their knowledge of this natural variation also grew the authority to declare certain bodies "abnormal and in need of correction." Because these practices and norms emerged from white conceptions of science, bodies, and health, the sexing of bodies and altering of sex traits has racial underpinnings.

People of any gender or sex assigned at birth might currently have sex traits or anatomy that do not align with societal expectations for their gender. For example, a transgender man might have a uterus, ovaries, and cervix, and therefore need to be regularly screened for cervical cancer. Transgender women, whether or not they are undergoing HRT, could develop breast cancer. Transgender, cisgender, and gender-expansive individuals might use language other than "biological sex" or "(fe)male reproductive system" to describe their anatomy. To better reflect and respect individuals' autonomy over their bodies, more inclusive phrases such as "people with prostates" or "individuals with higher levels of estrogen" can be used when referring to individuals of all genders with these characteristics.

Vern Harner

See also: Biological Theories of Sexual Orientation; Chromosomal Sex; Gender; Gender Transition; Hormone Replacement Therapy; Hypogonadism; Intersexuality; Sex Chromosomes; Sex Hormones; Sex Reassignment Surgery; Sexual Dimorphism; Transgender.

Further Reading

Fausto-Sterling, A. (2000). *Sexing the body: Gender politics and the construction of sexuality.* New York: Basic Books.

Intersex Society of North America. (2019). Retrieved from http://www.isna.org

Van Anders, S. (2014). Bio/logics. *TSQ: Transgender Studies Quarterly, 1*(1–2), 33–35.

Biological Theories of Sexual Orientation

Various theories attempt to explain how sexual orientation is determined, often with a particular focus on understanding homosexuality, or same-gender orientation (SGO). An estimated 2.4 percent of the population maintains a homosexual orientation, making this a significant sexual minority. Research into the origins of SGO engages the nature-nurture debate that is often seen in discussions of human development. Biological theories present a "nature" perspective, viewing SGO as the expression of inborn biological characteristics. In contrast, the "nurture" perspective is reflected in theories that view SGO as developing from psychological or social environmental factors or as a matter of individual choice. A combined approach to development of sexual orientation may also be assumed, with biological factors creating a predisposition toward this trait and environmental elements facilitating its development.

There is considerable research evidence of a biological influence on sexual orientation, though no "gay gene" or other singular identifying physical attribute has been, or is likely to be, found. Some of the most convincing research for a genetic basis for SGO focuses on family patterns of this trait. Other research suggests that existence of SGO is influenced by prenatal exposure to certain hormones or other conditions, as are other physical attributes that differ between persons with SGO and the overall population.

One notable family study found that 9 percent of men who have gay brothers also maintain a SGO. This is roughly four times the occurrence rate in the general population, lending support for the notion of a genetic connection with SGO. Male twin studies provide further evidence for this notion. Where one *identical* twin had a homosexual orientation, the second twin also reported a SGO 52 percent of the time. In the case of *fraternal* twins, the rate was 22 percent, and for adopted brothers the rate was 11 percent. Similar findings were noted in female twin studies of SGO. These results support the role of genetics in determining SGO, as higher levels of shared genetics resulted in stronger agreement in sexual orientation. At the same time, they illustrate that genetics are not the sole determinant of SGO, as even identical twins were concordant only 52 percent of the time.

Family studies also reveal that gay men are more likely to have a later birth order and specifically more likely to have older brothers. The number of younger siblings or older sisters was not found relevant, but the number of older brothers influenced the likelihood of SGO such that each additional older brother raised the odds by 33 percent. Further study of this phenomenon led to the development of the "fraternal birth order" hypothesis, which proposes that maternal immune systems may react to a male child by generating antibodies and that this effect becomes more likely with each successive male fetus. The theory proposes that prenatal exposure to these antibodies influences the development of sexual orientation. Other research suggests that prenatal exposure to hormones under certain conditions, particularly testosterone, may influence brain development in a manner that creates a predisposition toward SGO.

Where the above theories suggest that prenatal exposure to antibodies or hormones creates a predisposition to SGO, the specific mechanism for this has not been uncovered. Despite this, some research has noted physical and cognitive differences between heterosexual and homosexual men that may also be explained by these theories. The "fraternal birth order" hypothesis is supported by findings that gay men are not only more likely to have older brothers; they are also more likely to be shorter in height. Further, the height difference is likely to be greater when two or more older brothers exist. Other research notes physical differences in finger size as well as in brain structure between homosexual and heterosexual men. Cognitive differences in performance of language and special processing tasks have also been noted.

Future research to explore these theories may be influenced by changing assumptions regarding the nature of sexual orientation. Options beyond the traditional homosexual/heterosexual dichotomy may be incorporated, and assumptions that orientation will remain fixed across the life span may also be challenged.

Mary McClure

See also: Homosexuality; Romantic Attraction and Orientation; Sex Differentiation of the Brain and Sexual Orientation; Sexual Identity; Sexual Orientation.

Further Reading

Maucieri, L., & Stone, M. (2008). Adler's interpretation of same-gender orientation from a neurobehavioral perspective. *Journal of Individual Psychology, 64*(2), 214–223.

Mustanski, B. S. (2002). A critical review of recent biological research on human sexual orientation. *Annual Review of Sex Research, 13*(1), 89.

Rahman, Q., & Wilson, G. D. (2003). Born gay? The psychobiology of human sexual orientation. *Personality and Individual Differences, 34*(8), 1337–1382.

Biphobia

Bisexuality is a sexual orientation whereby a person experiences emotional, sexual, romantic, or physical attractions to more than one gender or sex. Although bisexual people make up the largest proportion of the LGBTQ+ community, they experience significant stigmatization, exclusion, and invalidation by lesbian, gay, and straight communities. In many cultures, such as in the United States, individuals are often socialized to think with binary or mutually exclusive categories for social identities (e.g., gay, lesbian, or straight). Some people experience significant discomfort when interacting with someone who does not fit neatly into binary categories. This discomfort can at times be the foundation for insensitivity and discrimination. Bisexual individuals, for example, may experience a unique form of prejudice called biphobia.

"Biphobia" is a term coined by Kathleen Bennett (1992) to describe "prejudice against bisexuality" and "the denigration of bisexuality." Biphobia has at least two dimensions: instability and intolerance. The instability dimension of biphobia is the perception that bisexuality is a denial of a lesbian, gay, or straight identity and thus is not a stable or legitimate sexual orientation. The intolerance dimension of biphobia represents the extent to which others are hostile toward those who identify as bisexual, perceiving them, for example, as a threat to society. Furthermore, "biphobia" is considered related to "homophobia," "transphobia," and other terms that describe the intolerance and discrimination faced by those who are sexual and gender minorities. Importantly, biphobia is meant to capture a unique phenomenon that involves the oppression and stereotypes experienced specifically by bisexual people.

Biphobia may pervade the everyday experiences of bisexual people. Bisexual individuals are often misunderstood and misrepresented in society and the media. They might be erroneously depicted as promiscuous, as traitors to the LGBTQ+ community, as too afraid to fully "come out" as their "true" sexual orientation, as "going through a phase," or simply as confused about their identity. Family and friends are not immune to perpetuating biphobia, as they might also ask hurtful questions based on assumptions and stereotypes. The consequences of biphobia often result in bisexual individuals experiencing significant isolation from both straight and LGBTQ+ communities. Research also suggests that biphobia is associated with increased rates of negative health outcomes, including anxiety, depression, suicide ideation and attempts, and substance use for bisexual people compared to their straight, lesbian, and gay peers.

Research has historically focused on the high rates of mental illness that bisexual individuals experience without much attention to protective factors that may buffer against negative health outcomes. Identifying factors that protect against the harmful effects of biphobia is needed to inform bisexual-specific prevention and intervention efforts. Although it is important to acknowledge the risk factors and health disparities affecting bisexual individuals, equally important is recognizing that many bisexual individuals are doing well and flourishing in their lives.

G. Nic Rider and Korey L. Watkins

See also: Antigay Prejudice; Bisexuality; Homophobia; Homophobia, Internalized; LGBTQ+; Sexual Orientation; Transphobia.

Further Reading

Bennett, K. (1992). A both/and option for an either/or world. In E. R. Weise (Ed.), *Closer to home: Bisexuality and feminism* (205–232). Seattle: Seal Press.

Bisexual Resource Center. *Mental health in the bisexual community: Biphobia, bi erasure, and getting help.* (n.d.). Retrieved from http://biresource.org/wp-content/uploads/2016/11/Mental_Health_Biphobia_Brochure.pdf

Brewster, M. E., & Moradi, B. (2010). Perceived experiences of anti-bisexual prejudice: Instrument development and evaluation. *Journal of Counseling Psychology, 57*(4), 451–468.

Dodge, B., Herbenick, D., Friedman, M. R., Schick, V., Fu, T.-C., Bostwick, W., … Sandfort, T. G. (2016). Attitudes toward bisexual men and women among a nationally representative probability sample of adults in the United States. *PLoS ONE, 11*(10), e0164430.

Eliason, M. J. (1997). The prevalence and nature of biphobia in heterosexual undergraduate students. *Archives of Sexual Behavior, 26*(3), 317–326.

Obradors-Campos, M. (2011). Deconstructing biphobia. *Journal of Bisexuality, 11*, 207–226.

Ochs, R. (1996). Biphobia: It goes more than two ways. In B. Firestein (Ed.), *Bisexuality: The psychology and politics of an invisible minority* (217–239). New York: SAGE.

Birth Control Pills, Estrogen-Progestin

Estrogen-progestin birth control pills are oral contraceptives containing forms of two female hormones—estrogen and progesterone (progestin is a synthetic version of progesterone). The estrogen in these pills is usually in the form of estradiol, which is the main kind of natural estrogen in the female body.

Estrogen-progestin pills are commonly called "the combination pill" to distinguish them from oral contraceptives containing only progestin, commonly called "the minipill." The combination pill contains a higher dose of progestin than the minipill. Most people who use oral contraceptives take some type of combination pill, which was initially approved by the U.S. Food and Drug Administration in 1960.

There are many types of combination pill available. Most pills are sold in packages that contain enough pills to take one every day for either one month or three months. They are available under several proprietary (brand) names. Many combination pills are designed to vary the relative doses of estrogen and progestin throughout the month. Some brands require taking a pill every day. Other brands may require skipping doses or taking placebo pills for one week out of every month in order for menstruation to occur. Many brands include some pills with iron supplements or other inactive ingredients.

Physicians recommend that different versions of combination pills be chosen depending on various personal factors, such as age, any existing medical conditions, and how frequently menstruation is desired to occur (also called withdrawal bleeding, this is a shedding of uterine lining that happens when inactive pills are taken).

The combination of estrogen and progestin in oral contraceptives works to block ovulation; to thin the endometrial lining of the uterus, preventing any fertilized eggs from implanting; and to thicken the mucus of the cervix, blocking sperm from entering the uterus. Together, these three effects are a very effective way to prevent pregnancy. The combination pill is generally more effective at preventing pregnancy than the minipill, with a failure rate of less than 1 percent when used correctly. The minipill does not block ovulation as well as the combination pill, and it must be taken at almost the exact same time every day to be optimally effective. The combination pill, by contrast, has more flexibility in the time it can be taken—with a several-hour window on any given day. There are other potential advantages to using the combination pill, such as reduced emotional distress before any menstrual periods that may occur, less painful menstrual periods, reduced acne, and, in older people, improved bone density.

Despite the greater effectiveness of the combination pill, some people prefer to take the minipill because it is less likely to carry certain health risks associated with the estrogen or higher doses of progestin as in the combination pill. Potential combination-pill risks include increased risk of uterine cancer, blood clots, heart attack, stroke, diabetes, and migraine headaches, as well as reduced milk supply in those who are breastfeeding. Because of the enhanced cardiovascular risk, many physicians recommend that those who smoke and are over thirty-five avoid using combination pills. Obese people and those with a family history of heart disease or stroke may also want to avoid these pills. Yet another disadvantage of the combination pill is that it may continue to interfere with fertility for two or three months after use is stopped. A return to normal fertility happens more quickly when the minipill is stopped. Estrogen-progestin pills, like all forms of hormonal birth control, do not protect against sexually transmitted infections, including HIV.

Minor side effects associated with combination pills include light vaginal bleeding (or "spotting"), nausea, vomiting, diarrhea, breast tenderness, and weight gain. More serious adverse effects that may occur are dizziness or faintness, numbness in an arm or leg, coughing up blood, vision problems, and depression.

Besides their use in birth control, estrogen-progestin pills are also commonly used in hormone replacement therapy to manage the unpleasant symptoms associated with menopause.

A. J. Smuskiewicz

See also: Birth Control Pills, Progestin-Only; Contraception; Estrogen; Hormone Replacement Therapy; Ovulation; Progesterone; Synthetic Hormones.

Further Reading

Eig, J. (2014). *The birth of the pill: How four crusaders reinvented sex and launched a revolution.* New York: W.W. Norton & Company.

May, E. T. (2011). *America and the pill: A history of promise, peril, and liberation.* New York: Basic Books.

Birth Control Pills, Progestin-Only

Progestin-only birth control pills are oral contraceptives containing only the hormone progestin, a synthetic version of the natural female hormone progesterone. They are commonly called the minipill to distinguish them from oral contraceptives containing both progestin and estrogen (the combination pill). The minipill contains a lower dose of progestin than the combination pill. Progestin-only pills have the generic name norethindrone and are sold in packages containing twenty-eight daily tablets.

The effects of progestin-only pills include thinning of the endometrial lining of the uterus and thickening of the cervical mucus. The thickened mucus serves to block sperm from entering the uterus and fertilizing any eggs that were released by the ovaries during ovulation. Furthermore, the pills suppress ovulation in at least half the menstrual cycles of the user.

Progestin-only pills offer an oral contraception alternative for people who may experience problems with the higher doses of progestin or the estrogen in combination pills. Unlike the combination pill, the minipill does not interfere with the milk supply of people who are breastfeeding. In addition, the minipill is less likely than the combination pill to increase the risks of cardiovascular disease, such as heart attack and stroke, and diabetes. Thus, it is safer to use for those with a history of blood clots, high blood pressure, diabetes, and smoking. Still other advantages of the minipill over the combination pill are that it does not carry the estrogen-related risks of uterine cancer or migraine headaches and that fertility quickly returns to normal after use of the minipill is stopped. Minipills are also considered safer for older women.

A disadvantage of the minipill is that it is not as effective as the combination pill at preventing pregnancy. Statistics indicate that one to thirteen of every hundred minipill users become pregnant in the first year of use. Its efficacy is enhanced by sticking to a strict schedule of taking the pill at the exact same time every day. A delay of as little as three hours from the normal daily pill-taking time increases the chance of pregnancy during the following two days. The minipill, like all forms of hormonal contraception, does not protect against sexually transmitted infections.

Although adverse health effects are less common with the minipill than with the combination pill, some people do experience minor side effects. Such minor effects, which typically dissipate after the first few months of use, include irregular menstrual cycles, sore breasts, headache, nausea, dizziness, acne, and weight gain. Depression and discoloring of facial skin are less common adverse effects. Some physicians discourage use of the minipill for people with a history of breast cancer, liver disease, or unexplained vaginal bleeding, or for people taking anticonvulsant drugs (such as for epilepsy) or antituberculosis drugs.

Some people may take progestin pills as part of hormone replacement therapy (HRT) to manage the symptoms of menopause. However, HRT typically includes estrogen as well as progestin.

A. J. Smuskiewicz

See also: Birth Control Pills, Estrogen-Progestin; Contraception; Hormone Replacement Therapy; Ovulation; Progesterone.

Further Reading

Bennet, J., & Pope, A. (2009). *The pill: Are you sure it's for you?* Sydney, Australia: Allen & Unwin.

Pelton, R. (2013). *The pill problem: How to protect your health from the side effects of oral contraceptives.* Portland, OR: BookBaby.

Bisexuality

Bisexuality is a sexual orientation in which people report sexual or romantic attraction to people of both male and female genders or sexes. Some bisexual people report that they are attracted to people regardless of gender, and as such, there may be some similarity between bisexuality and pansexuality. Some bisexual individuals report being sexually attracted to both men and women but only romantically attracted to one sex or gender or the other. Alternatively, some may be romantically attracted to both sexes or genders but may only experience sexual desire for either the same or other sex or gender. Finally, some bisexual people report experiencing attraction to both sexes or genders throughout their lives, whereas others experience attraction to either sex or gender at different times, and, as such, bisexuality for some people may be associated with sexual fluidity.

There are different ways to measure sexual orientation in general and bisexuality specifically. Depending on how the question is asked, more or fewer people may report elements of bisexuality. For example, if asked, more people will report ever having experienced sexual attraction to both men and women than will report having had sex with both male and female partners. Fewer people still will report having a bisexual sexual identity.

There are many myths and misconceptions about bisexuality, and many people hold negative attitudes toward bisexuality and bisexual people. This is referred to as binegativity or biphobia. For example, some people wrongly believe that bisexuality does not exist and that people who say they are bisexual are confused, in denial, or still in the closet about really being gay. Men who identify as bisexual are especially likely to experience stigma and discrimination from people who think that their bisexual identity label is a phase on the way to acknowledging a gay identity, while women who identify as bisexual are often assumed to be "really straight" and just experimenting or behaving bisexually for attention-seeking purposes. Personal accounts from bisexual individuals, as well as support from sexual orientation research, has clearly indicated that bisexuality is a sexual orientation, like being straight, gay, or lesbian.

There are other myths about the sexual behavior and preferences of bisexual people. For example, many people believe that in order to be bisexual, people have to have sexual partners of both genders or sexes. Consequently, many people believe that bisexual people are hypersexual and cannot, and do not want to, be in a monogamous relationship. Because of this mistaken belief that all bisexual people are hypersexual, many people also believe that bisexual people are responsible for spreading HIV and other sexually transmitted infections.

These and other negative beliefs about bisexual people may be held by members of both the LGBTQ+ communities as well as by heterosexual communities. Because of this "double discrimination," bisexual people tend to experience worse mental and physical health outcomes compared to other people. Some research has shown that personally knowing a bisexual person, or knowing more about bisexuality in general, may help to disconfirm these negative stereotypes and may lead to more positive attitudes toward bisexual people.

Heather L. Armstrong

See also: Biphobia; Fluidity, Sexual; Pansexuality; Romantic Attraction and Orientation; Sexual Identity; Sexual Orientation.

Further Reading

Armstrong, H. L., & Reissing, E. D. (2014). Attitudes toward casual sex, dating, and committed relationships with bisexual partners. *Journal of Bisexuality, 14*(2), 236–264.

de Bruin, K., & Arndt, M. (2010). Attitudes toward bisexual men and women in a university context: Relations with race, gender, knowing a bisexual man or woman and sexual orientation. *Journal of Bisexuality, 10*, 233–252.

Eliason, M. (2001). Bi-negativity: The stigma facing bisexual men. *Journal of Bisexuality, 1*, 137–154.

Eliason, M. J. (1997). The prevalence and nature of biphobia in heterosexual undergraduate students. *Archives of Sexual Behavior, 26*, 317–326.

Eliason, M. J., & Raheim, S. (1996). Categorical measurement of attitudes about lesbian, gay, and bisexual people. *Journal of Gay and Lesbian Social Services, 4*, 51–65.

Fahs, B. (2009). Compulsory bisexuality? The challenges of modern sexual fluidity. *Journal of Bisexuality, 9*, 431–449.

Gustavson, M. (2009). Bisexuals in relationships: Uncoupling intimacy from gender ontology. *Journal of Bisexuality, 9*, 407–429.

Herek, G. M. (2002). Heterosexuals' attitudes toward bisexual men and women in the United States. *Journal of Sex Research, 39*, 264–274.

Hinrichs, D. W., & Rosenberg, P. J. (2002). Attitudes toward gay, lesbian, and bisexual persons among heterosexual liberal arts college students. *Journal of Homosexuality, 43*, 61–84.

Israel, T., & Mohr, J. J. (2004). Attitudes toward bisexual women and men: Current research, future directions. *Journal of Bisexuality, 4*, 117–134.

Kleese, C. (2005). Bisexual women, non-monogamy and differentialist anti-promiscuity discourses. *Sexualities, 8*, 445–464.

Lannutti, P. J., & Denes, A. (2012). A kiss is just a kiss? Comparing perceptions related to female-female and female-male kissing in a college social situation. *Journal of Bisexuality, 12*, 49–62.

McLean, K. (2004). Negotiating (non)monogamy: Bisexuality and intimate relationships. *Journal of Bisexuality, 4*, 83–97

Mint, P. (2004). The power dynamics of cheating: Effects on polyamory and bisexuality. *Journal of Bisexuality, 4*, 55–76.

Mohr, J. J., & Rochlen, A. B. (1999). Measuring attitudes regarding bisexuality in lesbian, gay and heterosexual populations. *Journal of Counseling Psychology, 46*, 353–369.

Mulick, P. S., & Wright, L. W., Jr. (2002). Examining the existence of biphobia in the heterosexual and homosexual populations. *Journal of Bisexuality, 2*, 45–64.

Spalding, L. R., & Peplau, L. A. (1997). The unfaithful lover: Heterosexuals' perceptions of bisexuals and their relationships. *Psychology of Women Quarterly, 21*, 611–625.

Steffans, M. C., & Wagner, C. (2004). Attitudes toward lesbians, gay men, bisexual women, and bisexual men in Germany. *Journal of Sex Research, 41*, 137–149.

Black Sexuality

A number of scholars, clinicians, and educators have emerged over the years to conceptualize the physiological, psychological, sociological, spiritual, aesthetic, identity, cultural, reproductive, recreational, and human developmental processes that occur for persons of African descent. These professionals have considered some of the transhistorical factors that have evolved into present-day functioning of those who fall within the African diaspora and how they build, maintain, and sever relationships. Moreover, there are many narratives and manuscripts that focus on the affective, cognitive, and behavioral experiences of those people who identify or consider themselves to have black heritage. Some professionals agree that a set of behaviors, ideas, assumptions, and feelings is inextricably woven into the history of Africa and the traumatic experiences of ancestors who survived the Middle Passage. From these works, it may be inferred that the sexual expression of persons of African descent is socially constructed, represents a continuum of social functioning, and contains several conceptual strands, including (but not limited to) race, socioeconomic status, religion, media, education, and identity. Since sexuality is the intersection of cognition, affect, behavior, and desire, black sexuality uses race to further describe the experiences of persons who identify with African heritage or describe themselves as being a part of the African diaspora.

Black sexuality is about *being and action*, and those intentional or unintentional movements are reflective of the history of Africa and migration (voluntary and coerced) of Africans around the world. The evolution of these sexual phenomena has enabled an unmistakable resilience of people who have a history of being marginalized. At the same time, black sexuality is fluid and gracefully enriched by music, art, dance, food, and various cultural traditions. It is important to remember that there is no single black sexuality in that it should never be considered a monolith or essentialist by design. Rather, there are relativistic sexualities that change as a result of individual and collective governance and are influenced by a myriad of contextual factors, including time, context, and circumstance.

From a Western perspective, some of those who identify with African ancestry have had to demonstrate creative fortitude in relation to managing oneself as well as the relationships that one is a part of. Because of racism, systemic oppression, white supremacy, segregation, war, and underemployment, the perceived and experienced sexual expression of those of African descent is sometimes distorted and based on debilitating stereotypes, myths, and unfounded assumptions. These belief systems have created and maintained cultural expectations that affect individual functioning within and outside of relationships.

The literature also describes various sociopolitical constructs (e.g., issues of socioeconomic status, systemic oppression) that are particular to this community. In the United States, more than 25 percent of black Americans live below the poverty line. Underemployment, lack of education, and insufficient access to resources restricts decision making around sexuality and relationships and reduces life satisfaction. Reduced employment and underemployment pose challenges for some and significantly affect well-being as well as one's familial, acquaintance, and romantic relationships. In addition, if there is a lack of education, some individuals may be unaware about various forms of contraception or resources that could potentially empower or shift relationship formation and maintenance. Systemic oppression as a result of overt and covert forms of racism creates structural barriers that restrict or reduce access to opportunities for black individuals, couples, and families. These structural inequalities create additional stress on individuals. Low self-esteem, self-efficacy, and self-worth can affect how positively one feels about the sexual and relational decisions that one makes.

Perceptions, attitudes, and opportunities have shifted over the past three centuries. Partially crafted from colonialism, coerced transatlantic migration, slavery, war, separated families, public distortions and myths, restrictive laws, social inequities, and systemic oppression from white supremacy, black sexuality manifests the cultural ethos of resilience, strength, and agility that shapes individual, couple, and community sexual expression. It is the product of black history, art, music, informed scholarship, public policy, and informal discourse that has affected the cognition, affect, and intimate behaviors of persons of African descent and those who serve this unique population.

One major influence that has shaped black sexual expression is the unique history of slavery and the relationships of black families with whites, which is captured in the literature. Over the years, perceptions and attitudes have changed about blacks (e.g., extrarelational sex, same-sex relationships, autoeroticism), while others have remained unchanged (e.g., beliefs about incest). Moreover, stereotypes and unfounded assumptions of the sexual expression of those of African descent that existed before and after the antebellum period are still maintained by other ethnic groups as well as by some black individuals. These stereotypes have created disproportionate expectations and do not allow for the collective experience to be reconceptualized into more individualized experiences and interactions.

Another significant factor that has a tremendous impact on the sexual expression and relationships of persons of African descent is the history of racism, segregation, lack of education, and escalating unemployment. These pervasive and debilitating phenomena have negatively affected how some people of African heritage form and maintain romantic and familial relationships.

A possible third contributor in the formation and maintenance of black relationships has been the tragic outbreak of HIV infection. Since the mid-1980s, HIV transmission has taken on pandemic proportion among men who have sex with men, heterosexual black women, and adolescents. Because of this, partner availability and selection, intimacy between individuals, and family systems have all been negatively influenced. Prevention research and education continue to advocate for individuals to practice safer sex and get tested regularly.

Another important factor that has influenced the sexual expression of blacks is the increased television viewing, internet consumption, and use of social media in the acquisition and exchange of information. The expanded capacity to share information, engage in courtship and relational maintenance, and be presented with idealized depictions of aesthetics has enabled colorism, ageism, feelings of entitlement, and diminished communication skill sets. The increased number of roles for black actors in television and movies that depict a greater range of black relationships have contributed to the expanded understanding of experiences.

It is also noteworthy that black sexuality has been influenced over the past decade by the election of the United States' first black president. Not only was his election historically significant, but President Barack Obama has endorsed same-sex relationships. Given the history of homophobia and heterosexism in the black community, the endorsement by the president enabled a significant shift in public acknowledgment and acceptance of same-gender-loving relationships.

The black church also continues to evolve. As a medium for congregating, worshiping, and networking, the black church has always maintained a powerful position in communities that have faced marginalization and social challenges. For some individuals, the black church has been a place for refuge when circumstances seemed difficult to manage. Regarding sexuality, the black church has been considered conservative in promoting abstinence from sex until after marriage and refraining from masturbation and prohibiting same-sex relationships. The use of spirituality to humiliate or even condemn individuals or communities based on assumptions or breaches of cultural expectations has had a profound influence on many individuals for over four centuries. The rebuke by black church officials and congregants has discriminated against, oppressed, and rejected many individuals who have struggled to reconcile their sexual expression with their religious affiliation.

Over the last twenty years or so, black church leaders have begun to have conversations about the continuum of sexuality and how it does or does not intersect with religious dogma and traditions. While there are any number of systemic barriers and sanctions that still exist for LGBTQ+ people within black churches, leaders are beginning to acknowledge that black relationships come in a variety of constellations and that ostracizing one member or group is destructive and counterproductive to keeping families intact and functional. The movement toward acceptance of safer sex (e.g., consensual and protected) before marriage and acknowledgment of same-gender-loving individuals and people engaging in autoeroticism continues to change black churches as they become more welcoming and affirming institutions.

Finally, there are a number of scholars and books devoted to black sexuality, and there are organizations (e.g., Association of Black Sexologists, Women of Color Sexual Health Network) that have emerged to address the range of these phenomena through research, clinical practice, education, and policy.

James Wadley

See also: Association of Black Sexologists and Clinicians; Down Low; LGBTQ+; Religion, Diversity of Human Sexuality and; Tuskegee Syphilis Study.

Further Reading

Battle, D. J., & Barnes, D. S. L. (Eds.). (2009). *Black sexualities.* New Brunswick, NJ: Rutgers University Press.

Fausto-Sterling, A. (2000). *Sexing the body.* New York: Perseus Books.

Irvine, J. (1994). *Sexuality across cultures.* San Francisco: Josey-Bass.

Wadley, J. (2014). Editor's note: The Journal of Black Sexuality and Relationships is finally here. *Journal of Black Sexuality and Relationships, 1*(1), vii–xv.

Wadley, J. (2014). Editor's note: "We have a lot of work to do . . .": The emergence of the Association of Black Sexologists and Clinicians. *Journal of Black Sexuality and Relationships, 1*(2), vii–xvi.

Wilson, P. (1986). African American culture and sexuality. *Journal of Social Work and Human Sexuality, 4,* 29–46.

Born This Way Foundation

The Born This Way Foundation is a United States–based nonprofit organization established in 2012. The foundation was designed to promote youth empowerment and foster self-expression. In addition to other targeted groups, Born This Way aims to help troubled LGBTQ+ teens. Musical recording artist Stefani Germanotta—more commonly known by her stage name, Lady Gaga—and her mother, Cynthia Germanotta, are its founders; the organization was named after Lady Gaga's second studio album, *Born This Way,* which became an anthem of sorts for the LGBTQ+ communities.

Born This Way was officially founded in 2012. It is a partnership between Lady Gaga and three main organizations: the Berkman Center for Internet and Society at Harvard University; the California Endowment, a private foundation aimed at providing access to quality, affordable health care for all; and one of the largest private foundations in the United States, the John T. and Catherine T. MacArthur Foundation, which works to support creative endeavors and movements aimed at fostering a more peaceful world. Run by Lady Gaga and Germanotta as joint directors, the foundation was founded on three tenets: safety, which means creating a safe environment to celebrate individuality; skills, which means promoting useful skills for civic engagement and expression; and opportunity, which means providing ways for people to work toward empowerment and inclusion in their local communities. The goal of the three is to create a more accepting society and a "kinder, braver world."

The organization's kick-off event was held at Harvard University on February 29, 2012, and was attended by a host of student leaders and panel experts as well as such distinguished guests as Oprah Winfrey, world-renowned physician and author Deepak Chopra, and U.S. Department of Health and Human Services secretary Kathleen Sebelius. The event was streamed live via the internet. In speaking out about the foundation and its roots, Lady Gaga said that the impact of the title single from her album had inspired her to delve deeper into the ideas of youth empowerment and prejudicial attitudes toward sexuality, among other issues. At the launch, Gaga revealed that the organization was already embarking on its first activity, sponsorship of the Born Brave Bus, which would travel the country to provide an interactive experience for young people to connect with likeminded peers and local community resources and to access information about topics such as antibullying and suicide prevention. In its first year, the tour bus hit twenty-three events in eighteen cities and was seen by more than twenty thousand people. To continue the momentum created by the Born Brave Bus, the foundation also began Born Brave Groups, a grassroots collective of local groups led by teens or young adults wanting to make a difference in their communities. The Born This Way website was also created to promote the foundation's message and provide a forum for information sharing among peers. It currently boasts approximately half a million users.

Despite its initial positive reception, Born This Way came under attack in 2014 for allegedly keeping and spending more money than it donates as a charity. According to tax information, more than half of the $2.6 million in revenues gained in 2012 went to operation expenses, and only a few thousand dollars were given out in grant money. Lady Gaga and Germanotta immediately defended the organization, stating that it was never intended to fund other charities; rather it was built to "conduct charitable activities directly" and that Lady Gaga herself gave personal funds to launch the organization she believes in so passionately. The official website also clarified that none of the directors and officers were compensated for their work with the foundation.

Tamar Burris

See also: Adolescent Sexuality; LGBTQ+.

Further Reading

Born This Way Foundation. Retrieved from https://bornthisway.foundation

Iddon, M., & Marshall, M. L. (2014). *Lady Gaga and popular music: Performing gender, fashion, and culture.* New York: Routledge.

Monster, M. (2013). *Lady Gaga: The message of Born This Way.* South Paris, ME: G.O.A.T. Publishing.

Bornstein, Kate

Kate Bornstein (Katherine Vandam Bornstein) is a transgender author, educator, playwright, gender theorist, and performance artist, born in New Jersey in 1948, who uses the pronouns "ze" and "hir." These are gender-neutral pronouns used in lieu of "he," "him," "she," "her," "they," "them," and so on (e.g., ze was born in 1948 and lives with hir partner).

Best known for hir work around gender, particularly moving away from the gender binary, Bornstein has several books published, including hir famous *Gender Outlaw: On Men, Women, and the Rest of Us* (1994), *My Gender Workbook: How to Become a Real Man, a Real Woman, the Real You, or Something Else Entirely* (1998), *Gender Outlaws: The Next Generation* (with S. Bear Bergman, 2010), and, most recently, Bornstein's own autobiography, *A Queer and Pleasant Danger: The True Story of a Nice Jewish Boy Who Joins the Church of Scientology, and Leaves Twelve Years Later to Become the Lovely Lady She Is Today* (2012). Ze travels around the world sharing hir story of hir transition of first becoming a woman and then hir realization that ze identified as gender nonconforming, as well as being open about hir history with anorexia, borderline personality disorder, and posttraumatic stress disorder.

Bornstein is often cited in conversations about radical gender, and hir books are frequently found on college feminist and gender studies reading lists. *Gender Outlaw* helped to reframe the conversation around gender to move beyond the idea of men versus women and to be more inclusive of the diversity of gender that exists in the world. *My Gender Workbook*, while actually including worksheets, is also a more advanced glimpse into the nuances of gender identity, gender expression, and gender presentation, supporting individuals in exploring their own gender but also helping those newer to the gender conversation to better understand the spectrum of gender.

Bornstein is also well known for hir engagement around issues of self-harm and suicide within many communities and the particularly elevated levels within the transgender and gender-nonconforming community. Hir book *Hello Cruel World: 101 Alternatives to Suicide for Teens, Freaks, and Other Outlaws* provides people, particularly young people, with support systems that can be options for them when in depressive and suicidal places. Bornstein also includes conversation around suicide prevention when performing and presenting at colleges, high schools, and youth conferences.

While mostly recognized for hir work on gender, sex, sexuality, and suicide prevention, Bornstein is also fairly vocal about hir past as a now ex-communicated member of the Church of Scientology. Ze details in hir writing about how the genderless construct of an immortal soul really appealed to hir during hir grappling with hir own gender and felt supportive in a way that Judaism (how Bornstein was raised) never had. Given Bornstein's choice to speak out about the church, as well as being publicly out around hir gender, ze is now considered a "suppressive person" by the church.

Shanna K. Kattari

See also: Binary Gender System; Gender; Gender Dysphoria; Pronoun Usage; Transgender.

Further Reading

Bornstein, K. (1994). *Gender outlaw: On men, women, and the rest of us.* New York: Psychology Press.

Bornstein, K. (1998). *My gender workbook: How to become a real man, a real woman, the real you, or something else entirely.* New York: Psychology Press.

Bornstein, K. (2012). *A queer and pleasant danger: The true story of a nice Jewish boy who joins the Church of Scientology, and leaves twelve years later to become the lovely lady she is today.* Boston: Beacon Press.

Bornstein, K., & Bergman, S. B. (2010). *Gender outlaws: The next generation.* Berkeley, CA: Seal Press.

Pasulka, Nicole. (2012, May 5). "A queer and pleasant danger": Kate Bornstein, trans Scientology survivor. *Mother Jones.* Retrieved from http://www.motherjones.com/media/2012/04/kate-bornstein-gender-outlaw-queer-and-pleasant-danger-interview

Breast, Female

The female breasts are two roundish masses of tissue that overlay the pectoral muscles of a woman's chest. Breasts appear during puberty and vary widely in size and shape from one individual to another. Although their function is to secrete milk to feed newborns, breasts have become a highly sexualized part of the female body in today's culture.

The female breasts contain much fatty tissue, connective tissue, ligaments, ducts, lymph nodes, and other structures. Small oval structures called lobules, each containing numerous tiny sacs called alveoli, spread throughout each breast in a branching network from the nipple. The lobules are connected to one another with ducts (thin tubes), which transport milk secreted by glands in the alveoli to the nipples during breastfeeding.

Fatty and connective tissues surround the lobules and ducts. The size of the breasts is mostly determined by the amount of fat in them. The fatty tissue tends to increase and become denser with age as a result of hormonal changes. At the same time, the glandular and ductal tissues decrease and become less dense with age. Because of these hormonal factors and other biochemical and physical factors related to aging, the size and shape of breasts change throughout life. Breasts generally tend to sag as a woman enters middle age.

The nipple of a breast is filled with nerves that make it very sensitive to touch and other stimuli, and it tends to become more erect during sexual arousal, breastfeeding, and exposure to cold. The dark area surrounding the nipple is called the areola. It contains sweat glands that secrete moisture to act as a lubricant for breastfeeding.

When a girl begins to reach puberty—usually sometime between the ages of ten and twelve—her body starts producing more of the female hormones estrogen and progesterone. These hormones stimulate the growth of the breasts and the breasts' ability to secrete milk.

The eventual size of the breasts is largely determined by genetic factors that influence fatty tissue development, and it bears no relation to ability to breastfeed. Small breasts can generally produce as much milk as large breasts.

In a rare condition called amastia, one or both breasts may fail to develop. This condition is usually associated with birth defects involving the absence of pectoral muscles or other anatomical abnormalities. Treatment involves the surgical construction of breasts using implants and the patient's available tissue.

Breast cancer is the most common form of cancer in women, developing in about one in eight women. Breast cancer is characterized by abnormal lumps that develop in breast tissue. If diagnosed and treated early, breast cancer can often be cured with a combination of surgery, chemotherapy, and radiation therapy. Depending on the extent of the malignancy, surgery might be either a lumpectomy (removal of the tumor and surrounding tissue) or a mastectomy (removal of the entire breast and sometimes nearby lymph nodes).

Not all breast tumors are cancerous. Some breast tumors, such as cysts and fibroadenomas, are benign (noncancerous). These tumors can usually be successfully removed with surgery. Hyperplasia is a condition in which cells multiply abnormally in the breast ducts or lobules. This condition is usually noncancerous, though it raises the risk for the later development of breast cancer. Surgical interventions, as well as biopsies to check for cancer signs, are usually performed in patients with hyperplasia.

Other abnormal tissue developments in breasts include fat necrosis (lumps of scar tissue that develop in response to injuries in the fatty parts of breasts), intraductal papillomas (wart-like masses that grow inside ducts, sometimes leading to bloody leakage from the nipple), and calcifications (calcium deposits). Surgery and biopsies are usually performed in these cases.

Breasts are subject to a variety of infections, especially as a result of breastfeeding. In such cases—known as mastitis—abscesses (pus-filled wounds) or cellulitis (spreading redness) may develop. Antibiotics are prescribed for breast infections.

Cancer and other diseases of the breasts can be most successfully treated if they are detected and diagnosed in an early stage. That is why women should regularly (about once a month) perform careful self-inspections of their breasts. Such inspections include looking and feeling for lumps, swellings, skin changes, or any other abnormalities on or in the breasts and adjoining underarm tissue. Any unexplained changes should be referred to a physician.

Depending on the expert consulted, women over age forty or fifty should get mammograms (X-ray examinations of breast tissue) once a year or once every other year to look for early signs of cancer or other problems. Findings that are suspicious may require follow-up tests to pinpoint the diagnosis. Such tests may include ultrasound examinations, magnetic resonance imaging, and biopsies.

The most popular form of cosmetic surgery in the United States is breast augmentation, in which the breasts are enlarged through the use of implants. In 2014, more than 280,000 such surgeries were performed in the United States. Breast reconstruction is a similar surgery, but it is performed on women who have had their natural breasts removed in mastectomies, usually because of cancer. About 93,000 breast lifts (mastopexies)—to elevate sagging or drooping breasts—were performed in 2014 in the United States. That same year, more than 110,000 breast reduction surgeries were performed on women, most of whom had breasts so large that they caused neck or back pain.

A. J. Smuskiewicz

See also: Breast Cancer; Breastfeeding; Estrogen; Galactorrhea; Progesterone; Puberty.

Further Reading

Canadian Cancer Society. (2019). The breasts. Retrieved from http://www.cancer.ca/en/cancer-information/cancer-type/breast/breast-cancer/the-breasts/

Stöppler, M. C. (2019). Breast (anatomy and function). Retrieved from https://www.emedicinehealth.com/breast/article_em.htm#facts_on_the_breast

Breast Cancer

Breast cancer is the abnormal, uncontrolled multiplication of cells within the breast. It is the most common type of cancer among women in the United States, and it also occurs among some men.

Breast cancer usually originates in the milk ducts or glands of the breast. The cancerous cells then spread through channels within the breast. The two main types of breast cancer are classified as noninvasive and invasive. Noninvasive, or in situ, breast cancer remains within the breast tissue. Invasive breast cancer spreads out of the breast to other parts of the body through the blood or lymph system.

Roughly one in eight women in the United States will have breast cancer during their lives. The prevalence in men is much less than this. Only about 1 percent of all breast cancer cases occur in men.

In 2014, there were approximately 230,000 newly diagnosed cases of breast cancer in the United States, representing about 14 percent of all new cancer cases. Some 40,000 people died from breast cancer in 2014.

With treatment for their breast cancer, about eight of every ten women will survive more than five years after diagnosis, and about five of ten women will survive more than ten years.

The risk of breast cancer becomes greater with age, especially after age fifty. This disease is most frequently diagnosed between the ages of fifty-five and sixty-four.

A woman's risk for breast cancer is increased by the inheritance of mutations in either of two genes known as BRCA1 and BRCA2. Approximately 1 in 200 women has at least one of these mutated genes. These same mutations also increase the risk for ovarian cancer. Genetic screening tests—in the form of blood tests—can detect the presence of these genes. A woman with either of the genes may choose to have her breasts or ovaries surgically removed preemptively to prevent the possible development of cancer.

The actress Angelina Jolie drew attention to this issue when she underwent breast and ovary removal to avoid the development of cancer, which her mother, grandmother, and aunt all died from. However, it should be kept in mind that having the BRCA1 or BRCA2 gene does not guarantee a woman will develop breast or ovarian cancer; the genes merely raise the risk for these cancers. For a woman whose mother, sister, or daughter had breast cancer, her own risk of having the disease is increased two to three times.

Only about 10 percent of breast cancer cases are inherited. The majority of cases result from other, unknown causes. Some of these possible causes include exposure to high levels of radiation, obesity, a high-fat diet, and heavy alcohol use.

Research indicates that the longer a woman is exposed to high levels of the female sex hormone estrogen, the greater the chance that she will get breast cancer. Estrogen levels are affected by the menstrual cycle, by childbirth, by breastfeeding, and by other factors. The risk of breast cancer is elevated for females who start menstruating before age twelve, who have their first child after age thirty-five, who have never had children, who have never breastfed, and who stop menstruating after age fifty-five.

Overall, non-Hispanic white women are at the highest risk of breast cancer development. Among women aged forty to fifty, however, African American woman are at greater risk than white women.

Some studies suggest that breast cancer risk is increased by the use of birth control pills and by hormone replacement therapy. However, other studies have found no such associations.

The main symptom of breast cancer is an abnormal but painless lump in one of the breasts. Doctors advise women to regularly inspect their breasts for unusual lumps. If anything out of the ordinary is detected in breast shape, appearance, or texture, the women should consult a physician. Many doctors also recommend that women older than age forty get an annual mammogram, a type of X-ray procedure that can detect breast cancer before lumps become noticeable.

If a lump or other unusual feature is detected, further tests are needed to distinguish malignant, cancerous tissue from benign, noncancerous tissue. Images from mammography or ultrasonography can sometimes indicate this difference, but a biopsy is usually needed to verify the malignant or benign nature of the tissue.

Breast cancer, if detected early, is one of the most treatable forms of cancer. The specific treatment depends on the extent to which the cancer has spread in the patient. If the cancer is confined to a small area, the cancerous tissue and surrounding tissue can be removed in a surgical procedure called a lumpectomy. This procedure allows the surgeon to preserve the breast. Follow-up radiation therapy and chemotherapy can then kill any possible remaining cancer cells.

If the cancerous area has spread too widely, the entire breast will be removed in a procedure called a mastectomy. In both a lumpectomy and a mastectomy, the surgeon also typically removes lymph nodes from the adjoining armpit. Examination of the lymph nodes will indicate if the cancer is likely to recur in other parts of the body. Even with a mastectomy, radiation therapy or chemotherapy may be necessary. Some drugs work by killing cancer cells directly, others work by preventing estrogen and other hormones from promoting cancer cell growth, and still others work by prompting the body's immune system to attack cancer cells.

In approximately one of five cases, cancer reappears in other parts of the body in women who were treated for breast cancer. Such metastatic breast cancer can sometimes be controlled with chemotherapy.

A. J. Smuskiewicz

See also: Breast, Female; Cervical Cancer; Estrogen; Ovarian Cancer; Uterine Cancer.

Further Reading

Canadian Cancer Society. (2019). What is breast cancer? Retrieved from http://www.cancer.ca/en/cancer-information/cancer-type/breast/breast-cancer

Lesh, M. (2013). *Let me get this off my chest: A breast cancer survivor over-shares.* StoryRhyme.com Publishing.

National Cancer Institute. (n.d.). Cancer stat facts: Female breast cancer. Retrieved from http://seer.cancer.gov/statfacts/html/breast.html

Breastfeeding

Breastfeeding is feeding infants or young children human milk. Its physiological process includes milk production, letdown, and ejection. Each component is influenced by hormonal and physical cues. Human milk provides complete nutrition for human infants and immune protective factors specific to their immediate environments. Breastfeeding was subject to considerable medical and social condemnation in the twentieth century and continues to be a subject of social contention.

Breast tissue develops during puberty and matures during pregnancy, usually by the twenty-eighth week of gestation. At labor onset, the pituitary gland begins releasing prolactin and oxytocin, which stimulate glandular milk production, letdown into the milk ducts, and ejection from the nipples. An infant's nursing mechanically stimulates milk ejection and hormonally stimulates increased production. Appropriate latch is necessary for adequate milk withdrawal, productive stimulation, and infant nutrition. Inappropriate latch is the most common cause of maternal pain and inadequate infant feeding.

Milk composition changes over time. For around seventy-two hours following birth, clear, sticky colostrum is produced, which is primarily immune factors, protein, minerals, and fat-soluble vitamins. No additional nutrition is required until two to four days postpartum, when regular milk appears. "Mature milk" appears seven to fourteen days postpartum and continues until the nursing child is approximately two years of age, when composition shifts to "toddler milk." Milk produced by mothers of premature infants is more nutrient-dense than that of mothers of full-term infants, and it remains "immature" longer.

Lactation may be induced without pregnancy by various programs involving breast preparation, nutrition, frequent nipple stimulation, and sometimes pharmaceutical aids. Induced lactation is usually more successful for those who have given birth and breastfed in the past and may provide between 25 percent and 50 percent of an infant's nutritional needs. Induced lactation has been promoted as a way to ensure survival of orphaned and abandoned infants in underdeveloped countries. However, child welfare workers typically condemn it for foster and adoptive infants in the United States.

World Health Organization (WHO) guidelines state that exclusive breastfeeding beginning within one hour of birth and continuing until six months of age, with continued breastfeeding until at least age two, is ideal for all infants and essential for reducing infant morbidity and mortality worldwide. According to WHO, universal breastfeeding would prevent more than eight hundred thousand infant deaths every year, primarily because of breastfeeding's cleanliness, antibiotic properties, nutrition, and availability.

Breast milk cannot be contaminated during nursing because it travels straight into the infant's body. The areolas secrete antimicrobial compounds through the Montgomery glands that protect infants from being exposed to pathogens on the nipples. In contrast, infant formula contains microorganisms and must be mixed with clean water, which a large percentage of the world's population lacks. Use of unsafe water to mix infant formula is among the leading causes of infant mortality worldwide.

Breast milk contains maternal white blood cells that kill invading microorganisms in the infant's digestive tract, immunoglobulin that prevents pathogens from entering the infant's body through the intestines, enzymes and proteins that kill pathogens, sugars that coat the infant's intestine and prevent bacterial penetration, growth factors that speed intestinal lining maturation, bile enzymes that break down fat, and colonies of normal human digestive flora.

Human milk completely and specifically meets all infant nutritional needs except for vitamin D, which the skin produces when exposed to sunlight. While infant formulas produced under food safety regulations in developed countries contain nutrient proportions similar to human milk, they are made from vegetable products and animal milks and subjected to substantial processing to produce expensive products that are harder to digest and lack immune factors. Pure animal milks and vegetable-based milk substitutes are inappropriate for human infants under one year of age and will cause health problems, including severe anemia and intestinal bleeding.

Most mothers who nurse on demand, express milk when separated, and do not offer supplemental formula feedings can completely meet infant nutritional needs. When formula feedings are introduced, lactation may be reduced, which can endanger infant survival if formula access is lost, such as during natural disasters. Watering down of infant formula to stretch supplies is a significant factor in infant malnutrition and disease in the developing world and among impoverished families in developed countries.

While these considerations are most critical to persons in developing countries or impoverished conditions, the safety, ideal nutrient composition, and free availability of breast milk, combined with the bonding and neurological and emotional stimulation of the breastfeeding relationship, are optimal for infant health regardless of region or economic circumstance.

Breastfeeding benefits maternal health by reducing risk of postpartum hemorrhage and postpartum depression, enabling swift loss of pregnancy-related weight (because extra calories are needed to produce breast milk), and reducing lifelong cancer and metabolic disease risks.

Despite WHO's clear guidelines and a preponderance of evidence for breastfeeding's benefits, U.S. rates of breastfeeding hover around 80 percent at birth. Rates drop below 20 percent for exclusive breastfeeding by six months of age.

From the 1930s through the 1970s, U.S. obstetric and pediatric medicine actively tried to eradicate breastfeeding due to widespread opinion that it was unscientific, unsanitary, and nutritionally inadequate, supported by social norms that discouraged any exposure or discussion of the female breast. During this time, women birthing in hospitals were routinely given hormone injections to prevent lactation, often without their knowledge or consent.

Between the 1930s and 1950s, physicians instructed mothers to feed newborns powdered, evaporated, or condensed cow milk combined with corn syrup. Aggressive global marketing of powdered commercial infant formulas began in the 1950s, and by 1970 only about one in five U.S. mothers had ever breastfed.

In the 1970s, feminist-initiated movements to improve childbirth health care and maternal support raised breastfeeding rates. Rates continued to rise through the end of the twentieth century. However, they appear to be declining once again.

Economic pressures; cultural, religious, and social stigmas; and certain health conditions can challenge breastfeeding. Working apart from one's infant necessitates milk expression, or "pumping," which can be painful and is impossible if privacy and storage facilities are lacking. While most U.S. states protect breastfeeding, some individuals continue to face stigmas that discourage breast exposure or sexualize breasts to the point where they feel psychologically unable to breastfeed. Mothers in the adoption process may be banned from nursing under rules meant to prevent sexual abuse. Nursing is sometimes economically stigmatized as a sign that a mother "can't afford" formula.

Health conditions that interfere with milk production include insufficient glandular tissue, which can occur naturally or arise from injury, breast reduction, or anticancer surgery; maternal malnutrition, stress, and physical overexertion; and thyroid diseases, especially Hashimoto disease. Maternal chemotherapy, active tuberculosis, and HIV infection can potentially make breast milk unsafe.

Angela Libal

See also: Breast, Female; Oxytocin.

Further Reading

Breastfeeding USA. (2019). Breastfeeding articles. Retrieved from https://breastfeedingusa.org/content/article/breastfeeding-information-articles

La Leche League International. (2019). Retrieved from https://www.llli.org

National Institutes of Health. (2019). Breastfeeding. Retrieved from https://medlineplus.gov/breastfeeding.html

World Health Organization. (2009). The physiological basis of breastfeeding. In World Health Organization, *Infant and young child feeding: Model chapter for textbooks for medical students and allied health professionals.* Geneva: World Health Organization. Retrieved from http://www.ncbi.nlm.nih.gov/books/NBK148970/

World Health Organization. (2017). 10 facts on breastfeeding. Retrieved from http://www.who.int/features/factfiles/breastfeeding/en/

Wright, A. L., & Schanler, R. J. (2001). The resurgence of breastfeeding at the end of the second millennium. *The Journal of Nutrition, 131*(2), 4215–4255.

Bulbourethral Glands

The bulbourethral glands are two small exocrine glands found in the male reproductive systems of most mammals. In humans, the glands are about the size of peas and are found below the prostate gland and on either side of the urethra at the base of the penis. The bulbourethral glands are also known as Cowper's glands, because they were first discovered by English anatomist William Cowper in the 1600s. Their main function is to produce a clear mucus-like secretion known as the preejaculate fluid. The preejaculate helps prepare the urethra for the safe passage of sperm during an ejaculation.

The bulbourethral glands consist of several lobules composed of acini and ducts that conduct secretions out of the lobules. A thin fibrous membrane surrounds the lobules and holds the gland together. A duct about one inch long carries the secretions to the urethra. As an individual ages, the bulbourethral glands decrease in size.

When sexually stimulated, the bulbourethral glands begin to produce the preejaculate, a clear liquid with a consistency like mucus. The preejaculate is an alkaline solution that neutralizes any acidic urine left in the urethra, which would be harmful to sperm. The preejaculate also helps to moisturize and lubricate the urethra and its external orifice to allow the sperm to be ejaculated without mechanical damage. During penile-vaginal sex, it also helps prepare the environment in the vagina to be more hospitable for sperm.

The preejaculate secreted by the bulbourethral glands averages about 5 percent of the total ejaculate, although some individuals produce much more. A controversy exists about whether sperm can be present in the preejaculate. Many mixed-sex couples practice withdrawal before ejaculation as a form of birth control. If the preejaculate includes sperm cells, pregnancy might result.

The bulbourethral glands also produce prostate-specific antigen (PSA), which is used as an indicator for prostate cancer. High levels of PSA produced by these glands can produce false-positive prostate cancer diagnoses.

Analogous structures to the bulbourethral glands among females are known as Bartholin's glands.

Tim J. Watts

See also: Ejaculation; Penis; Preejaculate Fluid; Prostate; Prostate Cancer.

Further Reading

Barclay, T. (2017). Cowper's gland. Retrieved from http://www.innerbody.com/image_repmov/repo16-new2.html

Chughtai, B., Sawas, A., O'Malley, R. L., Naik, R. R., Ali Khan, S., & Pentyala, S. (2005). A neglected gland: A review of Cowper's gland. *International Journal of Andrology, 28*(2), 74–77.

Healthline. (2015). Bulbourethral gland (Cowper's gland). Retrieved from http://www.healthline.com/human-body-maps/bulbourethral-cowpers-gland

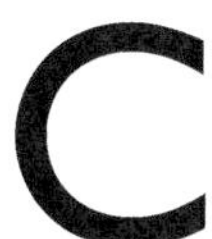

Castration

Castration involves the destruction or excision of testicles. The practice originated in primitive cultures from a desire to control animal populations. Castrated males cannot reproduce, and they exhibit reduced aggression. Human castration began as a way to control slaves. Owners believed the practice led to an elevated level of compliance. Subsequently, the practice became associated with dynamics of sexual pleasure. "Eunuch" is the word often associated with a castrated human.

Eunuchs existed in ancient Rome. The term "eunuch" typically refers to a male slave castrated at a young age. In many cases, castration involved the removal of the testicles and the penis. Eunuchs would engage in sex with masters and arrange events such as orgies. When having sex with a master, eunuchs would often dress in female attire and simulate the sounds of a woman losing her virginity. Literature implies that women also used eunuchs as tools for sexual gratification. Castration became less common as Christianity spread through the Western world, but castration for purposes of celibacy continued for men interested in certain vocations within the church. Sources indicate that the use of eunuchs in Middle Eastern countries persisted through the early twentieth century. There have been modern-day reports of eunuchs working as prostitutes in south Indian cities. In addition, there are currently online cyber communities supporting male castration and eunuch-based sexual fantasies.

Early forms of castration were crude. They involved crushing the testicles with a mallet or removing them with a sharp blade. Medical processes involving surgery and the use of chemicals currently characterize castration. Chemical castration involves giving males antiandrogen therapy, which decreases the functional activity of the testicles and penis and is a common treatment for advanced prostate cancer; approximately five hundred thousand men in North America have been surgically or chemically castrated as a result of prostate cancer.

Some research also indicates that castration may decrease illicit desires exhibited by sex offenders. In the United States, various states attempted to legalize castration as a therapeutic and punitive measure for sex offenders through the 1970s and 1980s. One of the first was Maine. In 1979, a castration bill failed, but the legislature approved funding for the study of the effectiveness of chemical castration. Failures to pass castration legislation occurred in other states. However, in 1997, a California bill went into effect requiring repeat child sex offenders to undergo chemical castration before prison release. Offenders can forego chemical castration if they voluntarily endure surgical castration. Other states with similar laws now include Iowa, Georgia, Montana, Oregon, Wisconsin, Texas, and most recently Louisiana. Proponents argue for its effectiveness, and chemical castration for sex offenders exists in other countries around the world. Organizations such as Amnesty International have designated the practice of castrating sex offenders a violation of basic human rights.

Jason S. Ulsperger

See also: Male Sexuality; Medical Treatment of Sex Offenders; Prostate Cancer; Sexual Slavery; Sterilization; Testicles.

Further Reading

Deshotels, T., & Forsyth, C. J. (2007). Postmodern masculinities and the eunuch. *Deviant Behavior, 28*(3), 201–218.

Handy, A., Wassersug, R. J., Ketter, J. T., & Johnson, T. W. (2015). The sexual side of castration narratives. *The Canadian Journal of Human Sexuality, 24*(2), 151–159.

Sreenivasan, S., & Weinberger, L. E. (2016). Surgical castration and sexual recidivism risk. In A. Phenix & H. M. Hoberman (Eds.), *Sexual offending* (769–777). New York: Springer.

Taylor, G. (2000). *Castration: An abbreviated history of Western manhood.* New York: Routledge.

Casual Sex

"Casual sex" refers to sexual activity that takes place outside the context of a long-term romantic relationship. Casual sex can take numerous forms, from one-night stands to friends with benefits. Interest in this activity varies across persons, but it can be predicted by a number of factors, including gender and personality. Although casual sex is widely believed to be on the rise and is thought to be linked primarily to negative outcomes, research paints a different and far more complicated picture.

There are several distinct types of casual sex, which vary in terms of the nature and frequency of sexual contact between partners, the extent of their communication, as well as whether the partners consider themselves to be friends. For instance, some researchers distinguish between one-night stands, "booty calls," and friends with benefits.

One-night stands are exactly what they sound like—a singular sexual encounter, usually between people who do not know each other very well. By contrast, booty calls are like one-night stands, except that they occur on a repeat basis. Finally, friends with benefits involve two people who have a simultaneous friendship and sexual relationship but are not romantically involved.

On the surface, one-night stands might appear to be the prototypical type of casual sex; however, they are actually the least common in practice. Research suggests that most casual sex occurs between people who have at least some history between them as opposed to people who just met.

Several studies have found that men are more interested in casual sex than are women. For instance, when college students are approached by an attractive stranger who propositions them for sex, men are far more likely to say yes than women. However, this does not mean that women are uninterested in casual sex. In fact, other research has found that, under certain circumstances, women are almost as likely to say yes to casual sex as men, such as when propositioned by someone who appears to be highly sexually competent or skilled.

Women are far less likely than men to reach orgasm during casual sex, a phenomenon that has been dubbed the "orgasm gap." In light of this, it is perhaps not surprising that women are more likely than men to take anticipated pleasure into account when making decisions about casual sex.

Beyond gender, attitudes toward casual sex are also related to personality. For instance, persons with an unrestricted sociosexual orientation, or people who have an easier time separating sex from emotion, tend to have more casual sex, but they also enjoy their experiences more.

Casual sex is thought to have increased dramatically in recent years. Indeed, millennials are often referred to as "the hookup generation." However, a closer look at the research suggests that this view is inaccurate. In fact, millennials are actually having less sex with fewer partners compared to generations past.

Casual sex is also widely thought to be a risky behavior, both physically and psychologically. For instance, casual sex is believed to significantly increase the risk of contracting sexually transmitted infections (STIs). However, the degree to which casual sex affects people's risk for STIs depends on numerous factors, including the specific sexual activities they engage in, their sexual communication skills, and their consistency of condom use. Categorizing the inherent riskiness of casual sex is thus more complicated than it first appears because not all casual sex is created equal.

With respect to the psychological effects of casual sex, it appears that casual sex is linked to negative outcomes for some but not others. These effects appear to be contingent, at least in part, on one's reasons for having casual sex in the first place. For instance, casual sex is linked to negative outcomes for people who say they did it in order to feel better about themselves but not for people who did it because they wanted to experience pleasure.

The psychological effects of casual sex also depend on one's gender, such that men are more likely than women to look back on these experiences positively. The "orgasm gap" is likely part of the reason behind this gender difference; however, it may also have to do with men and women having different motivations and reasons for casual sex. Alternatively, it could be the product of a sexual double standard that penalizes women more than men for having casual sex.

Justin J. Lehmiller

See also: Double Standards, Sexual; Friends with Benefits; Hookup Culture; Serial Monogamy; Sexually Transmitted Infections (STIs).

Further Reading

Clark, R. D., & Hatfield, E. (1989). Gender differences in receptivity to sexual offers. *Journal of Psychology & Human Sexuality, 2*, 39–55.

Conley, T. D. (2011). Perceived proposer personality characteristics and gender differences in acceptance of casual sex offers. *Journal of Personality and Social Psychology, 100*, 309–329.

Garcia, J. R., Reiber, C., Massey, S. G., & Merriwether, A. M. (2012). Sexual hookup culture: A review. *Review of General Psychology, 16*, 161–176.

Regan, P. C., & Dreyer, C. S. (1999). Lust? Love? Status? Young adults' motives for engaging in casual sex. *Journal of Psychology and Human Sexuality, 11*, 1–24.

Vrangalova, Z. (2015). Does casual sex harm college students' well-being? A longitudinal investigation of the role of motivation. *Archives of Sexual Behavior, 44*, 945–959.

Wentland, J. J., & Reissing, E. D. (2011). Taking casual sex not too casually: Exploring definitions of casual sexual relationships. *Canadian Journal of Human Sexuality, 20*, 75–89.

Celibacy

The term "celibacy" has been used differently by various people. Some use "celibacy" to mean a lifestyle of refraining from sexual intercourse. Others refer to celibacy as abstinence from all sexual contact. When referring to priests in today's society, often in Catholicism, celibacy is seen as the renunciation of marriage or living a nonmarried life. Depending on the context, celibacy can simply mean not getting married, refer to abstaining from sexual contact, or both. The sexual contact can include any sexual experiences or penile-vaginal sexual intercourse specifically. This is often determined by the contextual use of the word.

Most religious traditions have a philosophy on celibacy that often stems from asceticism—self-discipline concerning various pleasures (eating, drinking, satiating a sexual appetite, etc.). These practices are often embarked on to gain spiritual enlightenment or direction. Some religions may require religious leaders or communities to be celibate (e.g., Catholicism and Jainism), while others hold celibacy to be a more temporary tool (e.g., Brahmacarya [brahmacharya] in Hinduism—abstaining from sex for a period of time while studying the Vedas, the religion's holy texts). An indicator of how an individual or group may define celibacy will be their philosophical view on sexuality.

There is a more recent social movement centered around people who are celibate but not by choice. Seemingly gaining its name from the misplaced American cultural value regarding when people are "supposed" to have sex, involuntary celibates identify themselves as people who have never been in a situation where sex with another person has presented itself, or if they have previously had sex, as people who do not currently have opportunities to have sex. A study by Donnelly, Burgess, Anderson, Davis, and Dillard (2001) first studied this phenomenon through an online survey. The researchers further labeled people virginal celibates (having never had sexual experiences or partners), single celibates (having had sexual experiences but no current partner), and partnered celibates (being currently partnered and having had past sexual experiences). While little research has been done on the group, there seems to be an online involuntary celibate community, often abbreviated to the "incel" community.

The definition of celibacy can fluctuate depending on the perspective of the individual or group using it. Some groups may use the word to imply certain sexual behaviors because of how they view the function of sex and sexuality (e.g., in

Catholicism celibacy is defined as no marriage, which is equated to no sex). With "celibacy" meaning abstaining from marriage, sex, or both, the term can be used to describe a wide array of sexual or marital situations in which people may find themselves.

Mark A. Levand

See also: Abstinence; Marriage; Religion, Diversity of Human Sexuality and; Virginity.

Further Reading

Delhaye, P. (1967). Celibacy, history of. In *New Catholic encyclopedia* (Vol. 3, 369–374). New York: McGraw-Hill.

Donnelly, D., Burgess, E., Anderson, S., Davis, R., & Dillard, J. (2001). Involuntary celibacy: A life course analysis. *Journal of Sex Research, 38*(2), 159–169.

Fox, T. C. (1995). *Sexuality and Catholicism.* New York: George Braziller.

Westheimer, R. K. (2000). *Encyclopedia of sex.* New York: Continuum.

Cervical Cancer

Cervical cancer is cancer of the cervix, the lower part of the uterus. This cancer can affect either of the two main types of cells in the cervix—the squamous cells in the exocervix (near the vagina) or the glandular cells in the endocervix (near the main body of the uterus). These two cell types meet in an area called the transformation zone.

Approximately 90 percent of cervical cancers affect squamous cells. Such cancer is known as squamous cell carcinoma, and it usually begins to develop in the transformation zone. Most other types of cervical cancer, known as adenocarcinoma, affect the glandular cells. This cancer usually develops in the mucus-producing cells of the cervix. Some types of cervical cancer affect both squamous and glandular cells.

According to the American Cancer Society, about 12,900 new cases of cervical cancer are diagnosed, and about 4,100 women die from cervical cancer each year in the United States.

The risk for cervical cancer increases between the ages of twenty and fifty, when most cases are diagnosed. Risk is also related to ethnicity, with Hispanic women at the greatest risk followed by—in descending order—African Americans, Asians and Pacific Islanders, whites, and Native Americans. Research suggests that some cases are associated with an inherited condition that makes the immune system less able to resist infection from human papilloma virus (HPV). Infection with certain strains of this sexually transmitted infection, which can also cause genital warts, can cause cervical cancer if left untreated. Two HPV types (16 and 18) cause 70 percent of cervical cancers, but there are at least fourteen types of HPV that can cause cancer.

Certain lifestyle factors are associated with increased risk for cervical cancer, including smoking, a diet low in fruits and vegetables, being overweight, and long-term use of birth control pills. In addition, women are at elevated risk if they have had three or more pregnancies, if they were younger than seventeen during their first pregnancy, and if their mothers were given the drug diethylstilbestrol (DES) when they were pregnant. DES was used between 1940 and 1971 to prevent miscarriage.

In its early stages, cervical cancer usually does not produce noticeable symptoms. But after the cancer establishes itself in a relatively large area of the cervix, symptoms commonly develop. These symptoms may include abnormal vaginal bleeding and other unusual vaginal discharges and pain during intercourse. Because identical symptoms could be caused by other conditions, a medical diagnosis is necessary to determine the cause.

Doctors advise people who have a cervix to get regular Pap tests, or Pap smears, so that cellular changes in cervical tissue can be found and addressed in either precancerous or early cancerous stages. Although not all precancerous conditions develop into cancer, doctors usually recommend treatment at the precancerous stage to minimize the risk. Pap tests can also detect HPV infection.

If a Pap test reveals suspicious results in the form of abnormal cervical cells, additional tests are needed to arrive at a definitive diagnosis. In a colposcopy pelvic examination, the interior of the cervix is inspected with a magnifying instrument called a colposcope, and a small piece of tissue is removed for a biopsy. Biopsies of cervical tissue can reveal clear evidence of squamous cell carcinoma, adenocarcinoma, or other cervical cancer under microscopic examination.

If cancer is confirmed, various imaging tests can be performed to determine the stage of cancer development and, thus, the most appropriate treatment strategy. Such tests could include computed tomography, magnetic resonance imaging, and positron emission tomography.

Because HPV infection can cause cervical cancer, preventing HPV infection is crucial to preventing cervical cancer. Thus, condoms and other safer sex practices should be used during sexual activity. Vaccinations against HPV are recommended for all children, usually around age nine to twelve, before they are exposed to the virus. If not vaccinated at that age, people can be vaccinated as adults.

Treatment for cervical cancer is most successful when begun in its early stages. As previously indicated, the early stages of this cancer can be detected by getting regular Pap tests. The use of the Pap test as a screening tool is credited with reducing the death rate from cervical cancer by more than 50 percent from 1985 to 2015. Cervical cancer development is classified into nine stages, with five-year survival rates for these stages ranging from 93 percent to 15 percent.

Once cancer is diagnosed and its stage of development is determined, a treatment strategy can be initiated. The four main treatment options are surgery, radiation therapy, chemotherapy, and targeted therapy. Some combination of these therapies is usually used.

Many kinds of surgical procedures are available, ranging from destruction of abnormal tissue with a focused laser beam to removal of the uterus and adjoining tissues in a radical hysterectomy. In advanced cases, in which the cancer has spread widely, even more radical surgery—involving removal of the vagina, bladder, rectum, and part of the colon—may be necessary.

Radiation therapy might be administered in the form of external beams or as an internal radiation source placed near the cancerous tissue. Medications commonly used in general cervical cancer treatment include cisplatin, carboplatin, and paclitaxel. In targeted therapy, medications are selected for their effectiveness in targeting specific biological changes that occur in cervical cancer. For example, drugs known as angiogenesis inhibitors block the development of new blood vessels that cancer tumors need to grow.

A. J. Smuskiewicz

See also: Breast Cancer; Cervix; Human Papillomavirus (HPV); Hysterectomy; Ovarian Cancer; Pap Smear; Uterine Cancer.

Further Reading

Canadian Cancer Society. (2019). Cervical cancer. Retrieved from http://www.cancer.org/cancer/cervical-cancer.html

National Cancer Institute. (2019). Cervical cancer—Patient version. Retrieved from http://www.cancer.gov/types/cervical

Cervical Cap

The cervical cap is a barrier method birth control device, shaped like a cup and made of silicone, that is inserted into the vagina to cover the cervix.

The cervical cap is available in three sizes: small (for those who have never been pregnant), medium (for those who have had an abortion or a cesarean delivery), and large (for those who have delivered vaginally). These devices can be purchased with a doctor's prescription at a drugstore or clinic for roughly $75 USD —with an additional cost of about $17 USD for the recommended spermicide to be used with the cap.

To be most effective, the cervical cap should be used with a spermicide cream or jelly, which is applied onto the device. The spermicide stops the movement of sperm, while the cervical cap blocks the sperm from entering the uterus and fertilizing the egg.

Before inserting the cervical cap in the vagina, some spermicide is placed in the dome and along the rim of the cap. The cap is then inserted into the vagina while standing, sitting, or lying in a comfortable position. The cap is inserted with the dome side facing downward. The device must be inserted all the way in to completely cover the cervix.

Before each instance of sexual intercourse, it is important to make sure the cap is still properly positioned. If additional spermicide is thought to be necessary, it can be inserted deep into the vagina without removing the device. After intercourse, the cap should be left in place for at least six hours. It should not be left in place for more than forty-eight hours at a time.

The cervical cap should be thoroughly washed with mild soap and warm water after removal. It can be reused and will remain effective for as long as two years. The cap should be regularly inspected for small holes or weak spots, which may be signs that a replacement cap is needed.

The effectiveness of the cervical cap at preventing pregnancy is greatest for those who have never been pregnant or who have never given birth vaginally. However, even if these conditions are met, the one-year failure rate is quite high:

approximately 14 percent will become pregnant. Among those who have given birth vaginally, 29 percent become pregnant each year. The cap's effectiveness can be further enhanced if a condom is also used.

The cervical cap offers some advantages compared with various other methods of birth control. It does not interfere with an individual's natural hormone balance, and it can be safely used during breastfeeding. It can be conveniently carried in a purse or pocket until it is needed; then it is immediately effective on insertion. Its effects are immediately reversible on removal, as it does not affect fertility. In most cases, neither the user nor their partner can feel the device.

There are several disadvantages with using the cervical cap. It cannot be used during menstruation. Some also experience difficulty in inserting the device, and some may find that the device gets pushed out of place during sexual intercourse. Failure rates for cervical caps are relatively high compared to other birth control methods because the cap's effectiveness is heavily dependent on proper positioning. Because the cervical cap requires a prescription, it is less readily available than other forms of birth control. Finally, the cervical cap offers no protection against sexually transmitted infections.

A. J. Smuskiewicz

See also: Barrier Contraceptive Methods; Cervix; Spermicides.

Further Reading

Mayo Clinic. (2019). Cervical cap. Retrieved from https://www.mayoclinic.org/tests-procedures/cervical-cap/about/pac-20393416

Planned Parenthood. (2019). Cervical cap. Retrieved from https://www.plannedparenthood.org/learn/birth-control/cervical-cap

Cervical Mucus Method

The cervical mucus method is a way of gauging fertility by carefully monitoring the secretions that collect on the cervix and vagina throughout the menstrual cycle, then using this information to determine when pregnancy is most likely to occur. Some couples use this method to avoid pregnancy; others use it to help them conceive. Like most other forms of birth control, the cervical mucus method is not failsafe. Every female fertility cycle is different, so using any of these methods requires careful observations over several menstrual cycles.

Also known as the ovulation method or the Billings method, the cervical mucus method requires that the appearance and consistency of cervical secretions be checked several times a day. Ideally this is done by inserting clean fingers into the vagina to check the color and texture of the mucus on them, although those who are more experienced with this method may check their mucus by wiping the vaginal opening with tissue prior to urination or by observing secretions on their underwear. All observations should be marked on a calendar each day until the patterns of cervical discharge are very familiar.

In general, days when the cervical mucus is either absent or scanty, cloudy, and sticky are days on which pregnancy is less likely to occur. Days when cervical discharge is abundant and similar to raw egg white (stretchy, clear, and slippery)

are days when pregnancy is more likely because this type of mucus indicates the time around ovulation. Mucus patterns may also change around or during certain events, including

- breastfeeding
- cervical surgery
- douching or use of other "feminine hygiene" products
- perimenopause
- use of hormonal contraceptives, including emergency contraception
- use of spermicides
- sexually transmitted infection
- vaginitis or a yeast infection

Because menstrual cycles can vary widely, and because this method is an imprecise way of determining fertility, nearly a quarter of women—twenty-three out of one hundred—will become pregnant unintentionally in the first year with typical use of this method as a form of birth control. Unintended pregnancy rates drop to three out of one hundred annually for those who know their body's cycle well and who use the cervical mucus method perfectly.

When using the cervical mucus method or other fertility awareness–based methods (FAMs) to avoid pregnancy, couples must still practice abstinence or use another form of contraception during the ten to seventeen days in each cycle when a woman is most likely to become pregnant. Many women also use the cervical mucus method in conjunction with other FAMs, such as the basal temperature method and the calendar method, to increase its effectiveness. When the cervical mucus and basal temperature methods are used together, they are sometimes known as the symptothermal or muco-thermal method.

Terri Nichols

See also: Cervix; Fertility; Fertility Awareness Methods of Contraception; Ovulation; Vaginal Secretions.

Further Reading

Mayo Clinic. (2019). Cervical mucus method for natural family planning. Retrieved from https://www.mayoclinic.org/tests-procedures/cervical-mucus-method/about/pac-20393452

Weschler, T. (2015). *Taking charge of your fertility: The definitive guide to natural birth control, pregnancy achievement, and reproductive health.* New York: HarperCollins.

Cervix

The cervix is the lower portion of the uterus just above the vagina. It has the same layers as the uterus, perimetrium, myometrium, and endometrium. The composition and physiology is different within the cervix. For example, the myometrium in the cervix is thinner since the need for strength is not as great as in the uterus.

Another example is that the cervical endometrium is not separated into a functional and basal layer. Within the uterus, the functional layer grows through the menstrual cycle and then is shed when there is no implantation of a fertilized egg. The basal layer is the base that is always present. Since implantation should not occur within the cervical endometrium, it does not grow and therefore does not need to be shed.

The cervix itself can be divided into several sections, though the entirety is only about an inch in length. The top of the cervix is called the internal cervical os, which is the opening between the cervix and the uterus. The middle portion in called the cervical canal, which connects the vaginal cavity to the uterine cavity. The last portion, the external cervical os, is where the cervical canal opens to the vagina. Also like the uterus, the cervix can vary in sizes between people. It can also vary in size in the same person depending on whether or not that person is pregnant. Typically during pregnancy the cervix will increase in size. This is the area that must flatten and open in order for the fetus to pass from the uterus to the vagina.

While the cervix does not host a growing fetus, it does have implications in the process of menstruation, pregnancy, and childbirth. There are glands within the endometrium that secrete mucus. Depending on where a person is in their menstrual cycle, the cervical mucus will be of different consistencies. These correspond to fertility throughout the cycle. A person is most fertile when they observe mucus that is similar in color and consistency to egg whites. This type of mucus allows sperm to swim more easily. Another type of mucus is watery and slippery; while this also helps sperm swim, it is not preferable to the egg-white consistency. Mucus types that indicate a drop in fertility include a creamy yellow or white mucus that resembles moisturizing lotion. Another type is a thick, chunky mucus with the consistency of glue. Both of these also cause a drop in fertility because they make it difficult for the sperm to travel through the cervix. Because of mucus's implications in fertility, one method of birth control is to monitor the secretions to see when fertility is less likely.

Rebecca Polly

See also: Cervical Cancer; Cervical Cap; Cervical Mucus Method; Fertility; Fertility Awareness Methods of Contraception; Pregnancy; Uterus.

Further Reading

Jordan, J. (2006). *The cervix.* Boston: Wiley-Blackwell.

Lowry, I. (2011). *A woman's disease: The history of cervical cancer.* New York: Oxford University Press.

Chancroid

Chancroid is the name given to one type of genital ulcer seen in both men and women; however, it is more commonly seen in men. Chancroid is caused by the bacteria *Haemophilus ducreyi,* which is transmitted primarily through sexual activity, although nonsexual transmission is also possible. Worldwide, the number of chancroid cases is decreasing, with rare exceptions in North India and Malawi.

Because of its rare occurrence, it may be misdiagnosed as genital herpes, and testing is needed to determine the presence of the bacteria. Antibiotics are usually effective in curing chancroid.

Due to the sexually transmitted nature of the bacteria, most people who acquire the infection are sexually active adults. However, there are cases of nonsexual transmission of *Haemophilus ducreyi* in some countries where the lesion appears in nongenital parts of the body, such as on the lower legs of children. In addition, an infected person can infect another part of their own body if they touch their genital lesion and then touch another part of their body without first washing their hands. Transmission is not possible through healthy intact skin, so the bacteria must find a way through the skin barrier, such as an abrasion that happens when kids play. Sex frequently involves friction and vigorous movement, and even with natural and added lubricant sufficient for comfort and pleasure, abrasions can occur. These small tears in the vaginal, vulval, anal, or penile skin are the entry points for *Haemophilus ducreyi.*

While some cases of *Haemophilus ducreyi* may be asymptomatic, most people develop a visible lesion (chancroid) within three to seven days after exposure. Unlike the syphilis ulcer, chancroid is often painful in those who get it, and it has a ragged edge with a soft base, whereas syphilis often has a relatively hard base to the ulcer. This led early doctors to refer to soft and hard chancres (lesions) to differentiate chancroid (soft lesion) from syphilis (hard lesion). Now clinics use blood tests plus a swab test of the ulcer to determine which bacteria is the cause. Mixed infections are also possible, in which syphilis and chancroid (or other ulcer-causing microbials, such as herpes) are present in the same ulcer. Multiple ulcers are also possible with chancroid, as is a painful lump in the groin (inguinal lymphadenopathy), which may burst and spill pus if not treated early.

Chancroid, like other ulcerative sexually transmitted infections (STIs), such as herpes and syphilis, increases the risk of acquisition and transmission of HIV. The chancroid ulcer can increase susceptibility to HIV for HIV-negative individuals. Among people living with HIV, chancroid has been associated with treatment failure, and, as such, lesions may take longer to heal.

Prevention of chancroid infection is the same as for the other STIs—namely, using condoms during sexual contact and intercourse and avoiding sex if a genital ulcer is present. Fortunately, chancroid is treatable with antibiotics, and symptoms usually disappear after one to two weeks of treatment. There are both injectable and oral forms of antibiotic. If the infection has caused a swelling in the groin (inguinal lymphadenopathy), then additional treatment to drain the swelling may be needed.

Kelwyn Browne

See also: Herpes; Human Immunodeficiency Virus (HIV); Sexually Transmitted Infections (STIs); Syphilis.

Further Reading

Bong, C. T., Hareziak, J., Katz, B. P., & Spinola, S. M. (2002). Men are more susceptible than women to pustule formation in the experimental model of Haemophilus ducreyi infection. *Sexually Transmitted Diseases, 29*(2), 114–118.

Centers for Disease Control. (2015). Chancroid. *2015 sexually transmitted diseases treatment guidelines*. Atlanta: Centers for Disease Control.

Lautenschlager, S., Kemp, M., Christensen, J. J., Mayans, M. V., & Moi, H. (2017). 2017 European guideline for the management of chancroid. *International Journal of STD and AIDS, 28*(4), 324–329.

Cheating and Infidelity

Infidelity occurs when one or both parties in an agreed-upon relationship engage in behaviors that cross the decided boundaries of said relationship with an outside individual. According to various studies, cheating is quite common; more than 30 percent of men and 20 percent of women in the United States have reported cheating in their lifetime. Other literature suggests that cheating is especially common in younger people, and prevalence of cheating may be rising among college-aged adults.

It is valuable to note that infidelity is not defined in one specific way. For some, infidelity can be classified as engaging in genital intercourse with an outside partner. Others define infidelity as nongenital sexual exchanges with an outside partner (which include, but are not limited to, oral sex, kissing, hugging, holding hands, fondling, etc.). Even so, others may classify nonsexual behaviors, such as withholding information, lying in a relationship, flirting, and emotionally bonding with an outside partner, as forms of infidelity.

Various personality traits (i.e., extroversion, neuroticism, openness, conscientiousness, and agreeableness) can contribute to individuals engaging in infidelity. Researchers have found that a desire for sex, anger toward a partner, feeling neglect in the relationship, and dissatisfaction in the relationship served as predictors for cheating in a relationship. While conscientiousness and openness were not found to significantly affect infidelity, neuroticism was associated with a partner's likelihood to neglect their primary partner and engage in outside relationships. Low agreeableness and neuroticism were linked to the heightened potential for anger in relationships. This means that if one partner is more prone to please their mate and is insecure about the status of their relationship, this may influence said partner to resent and abandon the relationship. Finally, dissatisfaction in a relationship was found to correlate with higher levels of individual extraversion, which suggests that those who prefer interaction with others may become bored with a dyadic (two-person partnered) pairing and may seek stimulation from outside partners.

Infidelity can have a variety of effects on individuals in dyadic relationships. While some may assume that infidelity only affects the partner being cheating on, research highlights that cheating may have negative effects on both the cheating partner and the partner being cheated on. For some, cheating may lead to personal shame and guilt related to potentially damaging the relationship, contributing to the suffering of one's partner, or potentially enjoying the extradyadic (outside) relationship. These feelings of guilt and shame could potentially lead the cheating partner to experience anxious and depressive symptoms. On the other hand, the individual being cheated on could experience depressive symptoms that relate to feelings of jealousy, distress, and betrayal.

When it comes to the infidelity experienced by gender, research highlights that men and women are more prone to cheat in different ways. Studies highlight that men and women also experience infidelity-related distress differently. While men are more likely to engage in sexual, or physical, infidelity, women have been found to be more likely to engage in emotional infidelity that involves an emotional connection with an outside partner (Martins et al., 2016). Similarly, in heterosexual relationships, men have reported feeling more distressed when their female partners have engaged in sexual infidelity. Conversely, women in heterosexual relationships have reported higher levels of distress when their male partners have engaged in emotional relationships with outside partners.

Little research exists around gay, lesbian, and bisexual (GLB) individuals and infidelity experiences. Nevertheless, the research that does exist suggests that some GLB persons may be less concerned with their partners engaging in physical, or sexual, extradyadic relationships. The rationale behind this is that because GLB individuals have, for so long, been sexually oppressed, they have now found comfort in having relationships that are more welcoming of outside sexual partners. That said, research highlights that GLB individuals may experience greater distress when their partners engage in emotional infidelity. This finding may speak to the fact that GLB individuals have recently been given the social space to freely engage in relationships that go beyond the physical; therefore, emotional cheating may lead to an increased experience of betrayal, sadness, and depressive symptoms.

While infidelity among adolescents is highly underinvestigated, there exists a breadth of research that highlights the way in which adults perceive, participate in, and are affected by infidelity. Some studies communicate that adolescents mainly conceptualize infidelity, and the distress associated with cheating, through their own experiences and through the experiences of their peers. Due to this, the adolescent experience should be given greater attention. Observing adult, emerging adult, and adolescent relationships may highlight unique patterns and dynamics and may provide a glimpse into the ways in which these relationship structures develop over the life span.

Shadeen Francis and Patrick R. Grant

See also: Adultery; Marriage; Monogamy; Open Marriage; Polyamory.

Further Reading

Barta, W. D., & Kiene, S. M. (2005). Motivations for infidelity in heterosexual dating couples: The roles of gender, personality differences, and sociosexual orientation. *Journal of Social and Personal Relationships, 22*(3), 339–360.

Frederick, D. A., & Fales, M. R. (2016). Upset over sexual versus emotional infidelity among gay, lesbian, bisexual, and heterosexual adults. *Archives of Sexual Behavior, 45*(1), 175–191.

Furr, R. E. (2006). *Infidelity in adolescent romantic relationships* (Unpublished master's thesis). University of Tennessee, Tennessee. Retrieved from http://trace.tennessee.edu/utk_gradthes/1556

Leeker, O., & Carlozzi, A. (2014). Effects of sex, sexual orientation, infidelity expectations, and love on distress related to emotional and sexual infidelity. *Journal of Marital and Family Therapy, 40*(1), 68–91.

Martins, A., Pereira, M., Andrade, R., Dattilio, F. M., Narciso, I., & Canavarro, M. C. (2016). Infidelity in dating relationships: Gender-specific correlates of face-to-face and online extradyadic involvement. *Archives of Sexual Behavior, 45*(1), 193–205.

Norona, J. C., Khaddouma, A., Welsh, D. P., & Samawi, H. (2015). Adolescents' understandings of infidelity. *Personal Relationships, 22*(3), 431–448.

Schützwohl, A. (2004). Which infidelity type makes you more jealous? Decision strategies in a forced-choice between sexual and emotional infidelity. *Evolutionary Psychology, 2*(1), 121–128.147470490400200.

Child Sexual Abuse

Child sexual abuse (CSA) is a form of sexual abuse in which children are the victims. Recently, this form of assault has gained a lot of media and research attention. In 2005, nearly 10 percent of all child abuse cases involved some sort of sexual abuse, which equals more than 83,000 CAS victims in 2005 alone. Importantly, many instances of CSA are not reported, so these were just the incidents that the authorities are aware of. Adult survivors of CSA are starting to speak up more for themselves and are helping to shed light on this issue. Statistics show that one in seven girls and one in twenty-five boys are sexually abused before they turn eighteen.

CSA can be any form of sexual activity with a minor, and the definition is very broad and varies by country and by state. A child cannot give consent of any kind to perform sexual acts. Further, CSA can occur in many forms and does not have to involve physical contact. Types of CSA can include, but are not limited to, digital interactions (e.g., sexting, chatting, or phone calls that are sexual in nature); fondling or touching the child; exposing oneself to the child; masturbating in front of or forcing the child to masturbate; intercourse of any kind (oral, vaginal, or anal); having, seeing, or sharing any type of images or videos of children with sexual content; sex trafficking; or any other sexual misconduct that can be harmful to a child. Any of these actions can lead an individual to suffer legal consequences, and each U.S. state has its own legal definition of CSA.

Knowing warning signs of CSA can be helpful, but each individual is different, and sometimes the warning signs are not easily detected. Signs can be physical, behavioral, and/or emotional. Most common physical signs are difficulty walking or sitting; bloody, torn, or stained underclothes; bleeding, bruises, or swelling of the genital region; pain, itching, or burning in the genital region; frequent urinary tract or yeast infections; eating issues; vomiting; bowel problems; sexual behavior problems; substance abuse; anger or aggression; and suicidal behaviors. Some of the common behavioral and emotional signs are moving away from or seeming threatened by physical contact; depression or posttraumatic stress disorder; suicidal thoughts, especially in teenagers; self-harm; phobias; behavior problems in school; changes in hygiene (not bathing enough or bathing too much); running away; overly protective of siblings; nightmares or bedwetting; and inappropriate sexual knowledge or behaviors for their age range. These are just some of the warning signs as each individual will react differently to being victimized.

The effects of CSA can extend into the individual's life far beyond their childhood years. Sexual abuse can leave children with a lack of trust, feelings of shame and guilt, and oftentimes can lead to self-harming behaviors. Many victims continue to suffer from depression, low self-worth, and many more psychological and emotional problems. CSA can also cause problems with romantic relationships later on in life and can make survivors more likely to experience domestic violence as adults.

According to RAINN, 93 percent of victims of CSA know their abuser. This means that the majority of abusers are people the child knows, such as a parent, sibling, other relative, teacher, coach, babysitter, and so on. This is not a "stranger danger" epidemic as many may think it is. Abusers manipulate the child to keep secrets, which oftentimes leads them to feel guilty about what is taking place. Abusers may also threaten the child with punishment or with harm to a loved one. It is important to support the child when they do open up about the abuse and make sure they know they are believed.

The first line of protection is for a child to have an open and supportive dialogue with their parents or caretakers so that they know they have someone to talk to about even the toughest subjects. Children should also be taught that they can say no, and they need to understand their own body parts and who can see them. Children also need to be reassured that they are not in trouble and are not blamed for what has happened to them. There are many helpful websites, such as RAINN.org, that give talking points and education around having conversations with children. If you suspect a child is being abused, report this to local law enforcement or child protective services.

If you suspect something, there are two different hotlines that are available to provide support in this matter: the National Child Abuse Hotline at 1-800-4-A-CHILD (422-4453) and the National Sexual Assault Hotline at 1-800-656-HOPE (4673). You can also chat online at online.rainn.org. Support is available 24-7 for those in need (RAINN, 2019).

Amanda Baker

See also: Childhood Sexuality; Incest; Pedophilia; Rape, Abuse and Incest National Network (RAINN); Roman Catholic Church Sexual Abuse Scandal; Sexual Abuse.

Further Reading

Darkness to Light. (2017). *Child sexual abuse statistics: The issue of child sexual abuse.* Retrieved from http://www.d2l.org/wp-content/uploads/2017/01/all_statistics_20150619.pdf

Davis, L. (1988). *The courage to heal: A guide for women survivors of child sexual abuse.* New York: Perennial Library.

Herman, J. L. (1997). *Trauma and recovery.* New York: Basic Books.

RAINN. (2019). *Child sexual abuse.* Retrieved from https://www.rainn.org/get-information/types-of-sexual-assault/child-sexual-abuse

Townsend, C., & Rheingold, A. A. (2013). *Estimating a child sexual abuse prevalence rate for practitioners: A review of child sexual abuse prevalence studies.*

Charleston, SC: Darkness to Light. Retrieved from https://www.d2l.org/wp-content/uploads/2017/02/PREVALENCE-RATE-WHITE-PAPER-D2L.pdf

U.S. Department of Health and Human Services, Administration on Children, Youth, and Families. (2007). *Child maltreatment 2005.* Washington, DC: U.S. Government Printing Office.

Childhood Gender Nonconformity

Gender nonconformity occurs when one's outward expression of interests, clothing, or behavior differs from cultural expectations based on the person's birth-assigned sex. Gender nonconformity differs from gender dysphoria (i.e., distress in reaction to the incongruence between internal experience of gender and birth-assigned sex) in that gender nonconformity relates to behavior, while gender dysphoria relates to internal distress. Some people who are gender nonconforming do not experience dysphoria regarding their birth-assigned sex, while others do.

For many, gender identity development progresses as a predictable developmental process that includes gender stability (i.e., gender identity is the same across time) occurring around age three, and gender consistency (i.e., self-recognition of gender identity remaining consistent across situations) occurring between ages four and seven. Prior to developing gender consistency, a child's understanding of gender identity is often based on observable displays of expression (e.g., clothing, hairstyle, and interests), which are influenced by cultural social-role norms. However, research examining experiences of gender-nonconforming and gender-dysphoric children suggests that gender identity development can be a dynamic process that may not follow a predictable progression. While childhood gender nonconformity has been associated with developing a lesbian, gay, bisexual, or other sexual minority sexual identity, as well as transgender gender identity development, not all gender-nonconforming children will identify with these communities.

Gender nonconformity exists on a spectrum or continuum, with some children exhibiting strong nonconformity and others exhibiting less. Once children reach preschool age, culturally based gender stereotypes begin to solidify and form rigid gender rules that are reinforced over the life span. Such stereotypical gender rules have negative social implications for gender-nonconforming children, including rejection and ridicule by others and family disapproval and abuse. These experiences often place gender-nonconforming children at higher risk for emotional and behavioral issues than their gender-conforming peers.

Research examining mental health protective factors for gender-nonconforming people suggests that parental acceptance of gender identity and expression in childhood and adolescence increases positive and decreases negative health outcomes in adulthood. Other research suggests that social acceptance of gender nonconformity can be mediated by early education and ongoing exposure to the diversity of gender expression and identity. What this boils down to is gender diversity is a cultural issue influenced by social constructs that are taught and continually reinforced by societal gender rules. In order for gender-nonconforming children to develop to their full potential, they need to feel valued and seen as a legitimate part of the cultures in which they live. Such a shift in culture begins with normalizing and educating everyone about the complexities of gender and sexual development beyond the historical binary view.

Rachel Becker-Warner, Leonardo Candelario-Pérez, G. Nic Rider, and Dianne Berg

See also: Binary Gender System; Childhood Sexuality; Gender; Gender Dysphoria; Gender Expression; Gender Identity; Gender Identity Development; Gender Roles, Socialization and; Nonbinary Gender Identities; Stereotypes, Gender; Stereotypes, Sexual; Transgender.

Further Reading

Becerra-Culqui, T. A., Liu, Y., Nash, R., Cromwell, L., Flanders, W. D., Getahun, D., … Goodman, M. (2018). Mental health of transgender and gender nonconforming youth compared with their peers. *Pediatrics, 141*(5), e20173845.

Brill, S., & Pepper, R. (2008). *The transgender child: A handbook for families and professionals*. San Francisco: Cleis Press.

Bussey, K., & Bandura, A. (1999). Social cognitive theory of gender development and differentiation. *Psychological Review, 106*(4), 676–713.

Ehrensaft, D. (2016). *The gender creative child: Pathways for nurturing and supporting children who live outside gender boxes*. New York: The Experiment.

Huston, A. C. (1983). Sex typing. In E. M. Hetherington (Ed.), *Handbook of child psychology: Socialization, personality, and social development* (387–467). New York: Wiley.

Kohlberg, L. (1966). A cognitive-developmental analysis of children's sex-role concepts and attitudes. In E. E. Maccoby (Ed.), *The development of sex differences* (82–173). Stanford, CA: Stanford University Press.

Kowalski, K. (2007). The development of social identity and intergroup attitudes in young children. In O. N. Saracho & B. Spodek (Eds.), *Contemporary perspectives on social learning in early childhood education* (51–84). Charlotte, NC: Information Age.

Lev, A. I. (2005). Disordering gender identity: Gender identity disorder in the DSM-IV-TR. *Journal of Psychology and Human Sexuality, 17*, 35–69.

Martin, C. L., & Ruble, D. N. (2004). Children's search for gender cues: Cognitive perspectives on gender development. *Current Directions in Psychological Science, 13*, 67–70.

National Center for Gender Spectrum Health. (2019). Retrieved from https://www.sexualhealth.umn.edu/national-center-gender-spectrum-health

Roberts, A. L., Rosario, M., Corliss, H. L., Koenen, K. C., & Austin, S. B. (2012). Childhood gender nonconformity: A risk indicator for childhood abuse and posttraumatic stress in youth. *Pediatrics, 129*(3), 410–417.

Ruble, D. N., Taylor, L. J., Cyphers, L., Greulich, F. K., Lurye, L. E., & Shrout, P. E. (2007). The role of gender constancy in early gender development. *Child Development, 78*, 1121–1136.

Ryan, C., Russell, S. T., Huebner, D., Diaz, R., & Sanchez, J. (2010). Family acceptance in adolescence and the health of LGBT young adults. *Journal of Child and Adolescent Psychiatric Nursing, 23*, 205–213.

Siegal, M., & Robinson, J. (1987). Order effects in children's gender-constancy responses. *Developmental Psychology, 23*(2), 283–286.

Silverberg, C. (2015). *Sex is a funny word: A book about bodies, feelings and YOU.* New York: Seven Stories Press.

Thorne, B. (1993). *Gender play: Girls and boys in school.* New Brunswick, NJ: Rutgers University.

Wallien, M. S. C., & Cohen-Kettenis, P. T. (2008). Psychosexual outcome of gender-dysphoric children. *Journal of the American Academy of Child & Adolescent Psychiatry, 47*(12), 1413–1423.

Zucker, K. J., & Bradley, S. J. (1995). *Gender identity disorder and psychosexual problems in children and adolescents.* New York: Guilford.

Zucker, K. J., Bradley, S. J., Kuksis, M., Pecore, K., Birkenfeld-Adams, A., Doering, R. W., … Wild, J. (1999). Gender constancy judgments in children with gender identity disorder: Evidence for a developmental lag. *Archives of Sexual Behavior, 28*, 475–502.

Zucker, K. J., Wood, H., Singh, D., & Bradley, S. J. (2012). A developmental, biopsychosocial model for the treatment of children with gender identity disorder. *Journal of Homosexuality, 59*, 369–397.

Childhood Sexuality

Humans are born with an innate sense of sexual pleasure, and sexual development starts even before birth. From birth, boys are able to experience erections, and girls' vaginas are able to lubricate. This can be very uncomfortable information for most adults to comprehend. Childhood sexuality has been studied for centuries by the likes of Sigmund Freud and Alfred Kinsey, but recently (in the 2000s) more attention has been paid to childhood sexuality due in part to the surge of research on childhood sexual abuse. Here we will go over healthy sexual development in children (birth to twelve years old) and warning signs of unhealthy sexual development and offer information for parents, caregivers, and counselors.

It is important to understand what healthy sexual development looks like in childhood. Children of all ages are curious by nature and want to learn more about themselves and the world around them. This is true for many things, including their bodies and sexuality. At a young age, children start to explore their own bodies and may be curious about other bodies, especially those that are different from their own. This behavior is not sexually motivated, as children at this age do not have the concept of sexuality that develops in later life. Instead, they are motivated by curiosity, and it is important to remember that this curiosity is perfectly normal, and overreacting can lead to shame and guilt in the child, which can have effects lasting into adulthood. Below, some healthy behaviors and their associated ages are described.

From birth to age four, babies and young children use their senses to explore and quickly learn that certain areas of their bodies are more pleasurable to touch than others. During this time, parents may see children exploring and touching their genitals, rubbing their genitals with their hands or objects, showing off their genitals, trying to touch breasts, having a desire to be naked, trying to watch others when they are undressing, asking questions about bodies, and talking to their peers about bodily functions. Children still wearing diapers will oftentimes touch their genitals while their diapers are being changed. Around age two or three, children will start to understand their own gender and some of the differences between genders as they begin to develop their own gender identity.

Between the ages of four and six years, children may touch themselves on purpose (sometimes in front of others), attempt to see others naked, imitate dating behavior such as kissing or holding hands, talk about genitals and use "naughty" words, and explore their bodies with their peers.

Between the ages of seven and twelve years old, children will masturbate and explore their genitals mainly in private, play games with children that involve sexual behaviors (e.g., kissing games like Spin the Bottle), attempt to see others naked, look at sexualized pictures, watch or listen to sexual content, want more privacy, and begin to develop sexual attraction to others. As children reach this age, their curiosity is still high, but they tend to become more private about their exploration. They also become more curious about adult behavior and may start to copy what they see adults doing.

Sometimes children's behavior falls outside the realm of typical sexual exploration. Signs of potentially unhealthy behavior include behaviors that are beyond the child's developmental stage; involve threats, force, coercion, or aggression; involve children of wide age ranges; and provoke negative emotional reactions in the child. If behavior is taking place with any of these signs, it could be a warning of sexual trauma or problematic sexual behavior.

It is common for parents and caregivers to become worried about their children's behavior, especially if they have not been taught what to expect and what is considered developmentally healthy. It is important to remember that it is common for children who play together often to become curious about each other. If the children are around the same age and the sex play is unplanned, infrequent, voluntary, and easily stopped, then it can generally be considered typical childhood sexual play and exploration. How an adult reacts to seeing children involved in sexual play can make a big difference. It is important for adults to stay calm, composed, and nonjudgmental. A parent or caregiver can use this time as a teaching moment for the child or children. Open-ended questions asked in a calm voice are encouraged when discussing what took place. When children are engaged in honest, open, and educational discussion, they will learn the importance of healthy sexual expression and behavior. As parents, it is important to have ongoing healthy sexuality conversations with children as they grow and mature.

Amanda Baker

See also: Adolescent Sexuality; Child Sexual Abuse; Childhood Gender Nonconformity; Gender Identity Development; Sexual Health; Sexuality across the Life Span.

Further Reading

American Academy of Pediatrics. (2016). *Sexual behaviors in young children: What's normal, what's not?* Retrieved from https://www.healthychildren.org/English/ages-stages/preschool/Pages/Sexual-Behaviors-Young-Children.aspx

Cavanagh Johnson, T. (1999). *Understanding your child's sexual behavior: What's natural and healthy.* Oakland, CA: New Harbinger.

Dowshen, S. (2014). *Understanding early sexual development.* Retrieved from http://kidshealth.org/parent/growth/sexual_health/development.html

National Child Traumatic Stress Network. (2009). *Sexual development and behavior in children.* Retrieved from http://nctsn.org/nctsn_assets/pdfs/caring/sexualdevelopmentandbehavior.pdf

SexInfo Online. (2018). *Childhood sexuality.* Retrieved from http://www.soc.ucsb.edu/sexinfo/article/childhood-sexuality

Thanasiu, P. L. (2004). Childhood sexuality: Discerning healthy from abnormal sexual behaviors. *Journal of Mental Health Counseling, 26*(4), 309–319.

Chlamydia

Chlamydia is a sexually transmitted infection (STI) caused by the gram-negative bacterium *Chlamydia trachomatis*. It can infect the penis, vagina, cervix, anus, urethra, eye, or throat. According to the Centers for Disease Control and Prevention (CDC), it is the most commonly reported STI in the United States.

Chlamydia can be spread from the anus, penis, mouth, or vagina of an infected individual. It is typically transmitted through sexual contact by an infected partner. On rare occasions, touching the eye after touching an infected body part can cause transmission.

Transmission occurs when the *Chlamydia trachomatis* bacterium infect mucus membranes. Ejaculation does not have to occur for the disease to be transmitted. It is also possible for chlamydia to be passed from a pregnant person to their fetus during delivery. This can result in pneumonia or conjunctivitis in a newborn.

Chlamydia is also known as the "silent" infection because most infected individuals are asymptomatic. For people who experience symptoms, they can begin as early as five days after exposure, or they may not appear for several weeks. Rectal infection can potentially cause proctitis symptoms, while chlamydia eye infections may cause conjunctivitis, and throat infections can cause soreness.

For infected females, symptoms may include yellowish vaginal discharge, abdominal pain, bleeding between menstrual periods, painful intercourse, and irritation. Symptoms of cervicitis and urethritis are common. Males infected with chlamydia also commonly experience urethritis, often accompanied with pus or a milky or watery urethral discharge. Less frequently, males may experience epididymis. Males and females may experience frequent or painful urination.

Chlamydia can be diagnosed by a health care professional in several ways. If an individual is exhibiting symptoms, it might be possible to make a visual diagnosis. They may also use a swab to get cell samples from the penis, cervix, urethra, or anus. Urine can also be tested to detect the infection.

It is important to treat chlamydia, as it can result in severe complications. In females, if left untreated, it can spread from the cervix to the uterus and fallopian tubes, causing pelvic inflammatory disease, damage to the oviducts, chronic pelvic pain, and infertility.

Chlamydia infection can be cured through antibiotic treatments such as azithromycin or doxycycline. Any person taking antibiotics should abstain from sexual activity for at least seven days to prevent spreading the infection. According to the

CDC, people who were treated for chlamydia should be retested three months after treating the initial infection.

Several measures can be taken to prevent contracting or transmitting chlamydia. Abstaining from sexual intercourse will prevent transmission. For sexually active individuals, using condoms and other barriers can greatly reduce the risk of transmission. Getting regularly tested for STIs can also help prevent the spread of the infection.

If someone has chlamydia, treatment and partner notification can help prevent complications from the infection as well as transmission to others. According to the CDC, persons diagnosed or being treated with chlamydia should tell all sexual partners within sixty days of the diagnosis or onset of symptoms.

Sarah Gannon

See also: Infertility; Pelvic Inflammatory Disease (PID); Safer Sex; Sexually Transmitted Infections (STIs); Testing, STI.

Further Reading

Centers for Disease Control and Prevention. (2016). *Chlamydia: CDC fact sheet (detailed).* Retrieved from http://www.cdc.gov/std/chlamydia/stdfact-chlamydia-detailed.htm

Centers for Disease Control and Prevention. (2017). *Chlamydia.* Retrieved from https://www.cdc.gov/std/chlamydia/default.htm

Jones, R. E., & Lopez, K. H. (2014). *Human reproductive biology* (4th ed.). San Diego, CA: Academic Press.

Mayo Clinic. (2019). *Chlamydia trachomatis.* Retrieved from https://www.mayoclinic.org/diseases-conditions/chlamydia/symptoms-causes/syc-20355349

Planned Parenthood (2019). *Chlamydia.* Retrieved from https://www.plannedparenthood.org/learn/stds-hiv-safer-sex/chlamydia

Chromosomal Sex

"Chromosomal sex" refers to the physical sexual characteristics that an individual has as a result of the chromosomes in their cells. Sexual characteristics may be male, female, or intersex (a mix of male and female). Chromosomes are threadlike structures that carry genes, sequences of molecules made of deoxyribonucleic acid (DNA). Combinations of different types of genes, each made of specific combinations of DNA, determine physical and behavioral characteristics that offspring inherit from parents.

Sex is not the same as gender. "Gender" refers to the sense an individual has of being male, female, or any other gender identity. Some people may have the physical sexual characteristics of a male but the psychological gender identity of a female or vice versa.

An individual's physical sex is set at conception, the moment after sexual intercourse, when the egg cell is fertilized by the sperm cell. The egg and the sperm each contain twenty-three chromosomes, including one chromosome that determines the offspring's sex. The sex chromosome carried by the egg cell is called an X chromosome because of its X-like shape. The sperm cell may have either an X sex chromosome or a Y sex chromosome (also named based on its shape). If a sperm with an X chromosome fertilizes the egg, the offspring will have female

(XX) chromosomes. If a sperm with a Y chromosome fertilizes the egg, the offspring will have male (XY) sex chromosomes.

Chromosome-caused sexual differences become obvious during puberty, which starts at approximately age ten to twelve in females and age twelve to fourteen in males. The physical changes of either male or female sexual development are triggered by the increased production of chemical substances called hormones, which are coded for by genes on the X or Y chromosome. Male sexual development, including facial hair and a deeper voice, is triggered by the hormone testosterone. Female sexual development, including breast growth and wider hips, is triggered by the hormone estrogen.

Not all people are born with either XX or XY chromosomes. In some cases, a parent's sperm or egg cells are generated in an abnormal process of cell division called nondisjunction. If such parental sex cells become fertilized, the offspring's cells will have less than, or more than, the usual number of chromosomes. The general name for such abnormal chromosome conditions is aneuploidy. The most common type of aneuploidy in human beings is an intersex condition called Klinefelter syndrome, in which individuals are born with an extra X chromosome (resulting in an XXY chromosome combination). These individuals usually have male genitalia along with enlarged breasts, sparse facial and body hair, and other typically female physical traits. Klinefelter syndrome occurs in from 1 in 500 to 1 in 1000 newborn males.

In contrast to the chromosomal basis of sex determination, gender identity is determined by a combination of biochemical factors present at birth, ways in which individuals are raised during childhood, and cultural influences. Evidence suggests that gender identity is set by about age four or five in most individuals, though some individuals continue to explore their gender identity into adulthood. Some influences on a child's gender identity include their preferred types of toys, clothes, and chores, as well as pop culture influences like television shows, music, and fashion trends. Individuals whose psychological gender differs from their physical sex may identify as transgender. Some transgender people undergo hormone and surgical treatments so that their physical sex matches their gender identity.

A. J. Smuskiewicz

See also: Biological Sex; Intersexuality; Sex Chromosomes; Sex Hormones; X Chromosome; Y Chromosome.

Further Reading

Beasley, C. (2005). *Gender and sexuality: Critical theories, critical thinkers.* Thousand Oaks, CA: SAGE.

Fausto-Sterling, A. (2012). *Sex/gender: Biology in a social world.* London: Routledge.

Richardson, S. S. (2013). *Sex itself: The search for male and female in the human genome.* Chicago: University of Chicago Press.

Circumcision

Circumcision is a surgical procedure done to remove the foreskin that covers the tip of the penis. This is usually done within ten days after birth, with painkilling medicine applied to the penis beforehand. It is fairly common in the Muslim world and in Israel, South Korea, the United States, and parts of Southeast Asia and Africa. Almost all boys in the Middle East and Central Asia are circumcised. It is fairly rare in Europe, Latin America, parts of Southern Africa and Oceania, and other parts of Asia. After the newborn period, circumcision is a more complex procedure, more costly, and more likely to incur complications like infection.

Circumcision is usually an elective surgery performed for religious or cultural reasons. Circumcision is part of religious law in Judaism and is a traditional practice in Islam, Coptic Christianity, and the Ethiopian Orthodox Church. About 37–39 percent of males worldwide are circumcised, about half for religious or cultural reasons. At the turn of the twentieth century, a circumcised penis became a mark of distinction in the United States. It was considered a sign of good breeding, sound hygiene, and middle-class medicine. This was primarily a social convention and not supported by medical necessity, although circumcision was considered by some as a remedy for many conditions, including epilepsy, paralysis, malnutrition, disruption of the digestive organs, chorea, convulsions, hysteria, and other nervous disorders, in addition to a curb to masturbation.

There are some individuals and advocacy groups who are opposed to circumcision, saying that it should not be done without the child's consent, that it has the potential to reduce sexual pleasure, and that it risks causing injury to the penis. In the United States, the rate of complications with newborn circumcision is low, ranging between 0 percent and 3 percent. There are places (e.g., Iceland, South Africa, Germany, Denmark, San Francisco) where legislators have introduced bills to outlaw the procedure, but these laws have not been passed. According to the Centers for Disease Control and Prevention, the rates of circumcision in the United States declined from the 1970s to the early 1990s but have been increasing since the late 1990s, and currently about 60 percent of newborn boys are circumcised.

The American Academy of Pediatrics (AAP) says the benefits of circumcision outweigh the risks. The AAP leaves the circumcision decision up to parents and supports the use of anesthetics for infants who have the procedure. They have identified research on some of the health benefits of circumcision, including

- a slightly lower risk of urinary tract infections
- some protection from penile cancer
- reduced likelihood of developing sexually transmitted infections, including HIV
- a reduced risk for cervical cancer in female partners of circumcised men

The World Health Organization says circumcision reduces the risk of heterosexual men contracting HIV by around 60 percent. In Tanzania, which has a high rate of HIV infection, it has been suggested that any uncircumcised member of Parliament should be circumcised as a way to raise awareness of the health benefits of circumcision. In Kenya, some top politicians volunteered for the procedure in 2008 as a way of inspiring men from their districts to do the same. There are a few other medical reasons for circumcision, including phimosis, a condition where the foreskin is so tight that it prohibits retraction of the foreskin over the head (glans) of the penis. This can make it difficult to clean under the foreskin, leading to the glans becoming infected or inflamed (balanitis), and it may also cause a lack of sensation during sexual intercourse.

Michael J. McGee

See also: Female Genital Cutting; Foreskin; Penis; Phimosis; Religion, Diversity of Human Sexuality and; Sexually Transmitted Infections (STIs).

Further Reading

American Academy of Pediatrics Task Force on Circumcision. (2012). Circumcision policy statement. *Pediatrics, 130*(3), 585.

Bailey, R. C., Egesah, O., & Rosenberg, S. (2008). Male circumcision for HIV prevention: A prospective study of complications in clinical and traditional settings in Bungoma, Kenya. *Bulletin of the World Health Organization, 86*, 669–677.

Centers for Disease Control and Prevention (CDC). (2011). Trends in in-hospital newborn male circumcision—United States, 1999–2010. *Morbidity and Mortality Weekly Report, 60*(34), 1167.

Gollaher, D. L. (2000). *A history of the world's most controversial surgery.* New York: Basic Books.

Morris, B. J., Wamai, R. G., Henebeng, E. B., Tobian, A. A., Klausner, J. D., Banerjee, J., & Hankins, C. A. (2016). Estimation of country-specific and global prevalence of male circumcision. *Population Health Metrics, 14*(1), 4.

Cisgender

"Cisgender" is a term popularized in the mid-2010s to refer to individuals whose gender identity matches their physical sex. Individuals who were born physically male and gender identify as male, and individuals who were born physically female and gender identify as female, are considered to be cisgender. This term began being used by many LGBT activists, as well as by academics, to distinguish the sexual identification of the majority of the population from that of the minority of people who identify themselves as nonbinary, gender diverse, or transgender. A transgender female is an individual who was born physically male but whose gender identity is female, and a transgender male is an individual who was born physically female but whose gender identity is male.

Most estimates suggest that more than 99 percent of the people in the United States have a gender identity that coincides with their physical sex—that is, they are cisgender—and that roughly 0.5 percent of Americans consider themselves transgender.

Prior to the sociopolitical and cultural popularization of transgender awareness in the United States and other Western nations, the term "cisgender" was not widely known. The expression was adopted by some activists and scholars based on the Latin meaning of "cis," which is "on this side of"—in contrast to "trans," which means "on the other side of." The editors of the Oxford dictionaries added "cisgender" to their publications in 2013. However, biologist Dana Leland Defosse of the University of Minnesota is on record as using the term as early as 1994.

Many linguistic authorities express doubts about the widespread and long-term use of "cisgender" as a description for the gender identification of the majority of the population. They note that whereas "trans" has long been used as a generally understood prefix for many words—such as transport, translate, and transparent—the preface "cis" has never been generally understood or widely used in the English language. As lexicographer Kerry Maxwell has noted, if a newly minted word is not "user-friendly"—easy and comfortable to use, familiar, and understandable—it is unlikely to have longevity within the culture.

A. J. Smuskiewicz

See also: Gender; Gender Diversity; Gender Identity; Transgender.

Further Reading

Blank, P. (2014, September). Will "cisgender" survive? *The Atlantic.* Retrieved from http://www.theatlantic.com/entertainment/archive/2014/09/cisgenders-linguistic-uphill-battle/380342/

Brydum, S. (2015, July). The true meaning of the word "cisgender." *The Advocate.* Retrieved from http://www.advocate.com/transgender/2015/07/31/true-meaning-word-cisgender

Chalabi, M. (2014). Why we don't know the size of the transgender population. Retrieved from http://fivethirtyeight.com/features/why-we-dont-know-the-size-of-the-transgender-population/

Steinmetz, K. (2014, December). This is what "cisgender" means. *Time.* Retrieved from http://time.com/3636430/cisgender-definition/

Civil Union

On June 26, 2015, in a historic 5–4 ruling, the U.S. Supreme Court ruled that states cannot ban same-sex marriage, thus allowing same-sex couples to marry. Prior to this momentous ruling, same-sex couples struggled to gain the same rights as mixed-sex couples to form long-term unions. One way that gay rights advocates and politicians tried to circumvent hostility toward what was termed "gay marriage" was to create another type of union. Civil unions, or domestic partnerships in some states, became the alternative. A civil union is a legal status that provides some of the same protections as civil marriage, but these protections are only provided at the state level. Federal provisions, such as Social Security benefits and tax breaks for married couples, are unavailable to couples of civil unions. Vermont created the first civil union law in 2000, and several other states followed suit in the following years. Other states that passed civil union laws include Colorado, Hawaii, Illinois, New Jersey, Connecticut, Delaware, New Hampshire, and Rhode Island. When same-sex marriage was legalized in Vermont, Connecticut, Delaware, New Hampshire, and Rhode Island, civil unions were converted to marriages.

Proponents of civil unions said that these unions would help to solve certain problems faced by same-sex couples, such as hospital visitation rights and the transfer of property. It was a way to give same-sex couples equality while avoiding the controversial issue of religion and marriage. However, there were many differences between civil unions and civil marriages. Civil marriage is defined as a legal status conferred by and recognized by governments all over the world with certain rights, obligations, and protections. But it is also a cultural institution; it is recognized as the ultimate expression of love and commitment between two people.

Civil marriages are recognized in all fifty states. And although civil unions have legal status, these unions were recognized only within the states that had legalized civil unions. Married couples can obtain a divorce in any state in which they reside; however, couples in a civil union could only end the relationship in states that recognize these civil unions. The federal government gives over 1,100 legal protections, including the right to take a leave from work to care for a family member, the right to sponsor a spouse to immigrate to the United States, income tax deductions and credits, Medicaid benefits, and Social Security benefits, which can often mean the difference between poverty and financial security in a couple's retirement years. Civil unions did not have these legal protections. Because the federal government did not recognize civil unions, many state and federal governmental functions were not clearly defined, including such issues as taxation, pension protections, insurance for families, and Medicare and Medicaid benefits. Finally, couples in civil unions lived a second-class status. The word "marriage" mattered to many proponents of gay marriage. Even if there were no differences between civil unions and civil marriages, gay marriage proponents believed that the separate status for gay people conveyed inequality.

Amy Reynolds

See also: Gay Rights Movement; Marriage; Same-Sex Marriage.

Further Reading

Eskbridge, W. N., Jr. (2002). *Equality practice: Civil unions and the future of gay rights.* New York: Routledge.

Krieger, D. (2014). Denmark's civil unions: One giant leap for mankind. *Wilson Quarterly.* Retrieved from https://www.wilsonquarterly.com/quarterly/summer-2014-1989-and-the-making-of-our-modern-world/denmarks-civil-unions-one-giant-leap-for-mankind/

Soloman, M. (2014). *Winning marriage: The inside story of how same-sex couples took on the politicians and pundits—And won.* Lebanon, NH: University Press of New England.

Clitoris

The clitoris is an organ found in biological females whose sole purpose is to provide sexual pleasure—the only organ in either males or females with this sole function. The clitoris is analogous to the male penis. Both organs develop from the same fetal structure, and both are composed of a glans, a shaft (containing two cavernous bodies), and crura anchoring them into the pubic bone. The external portion of the clitoris, the glans, is located at the top of the vulva, underneath the clitoral hood as a fibro-vascular cap. The glans, which is often considered incorrectly to be the entire clitoris and is often referred to as button-like, is external, whereas the shaft and crura are internal. The glans is usually the size and shape of a pea, although there is much variation, and some are much larger or smaller. The internal portion of the clitoris is actually much larger than people might expect and expands through the body on either side of the vaginal opening. As a whole, the clitoris is comprised of the glans, the hood, the clitoral body, two clitoral crura, and the vestibular bulbs.

As a fetus grows and develops during pregnancy, the sexual organs develop from a part known as the "genital tubercle." If the fetus is male, the tubercle develops into the penis. If the fetus is female, it first develops into two separate corposa carnova. They then combine into the clitoris as the fetus develops further.

When compared to the penis, the clitoris has a similar anatomical structure. The penis has been seen anatomically as an extended clitoris that contains a urethral opening (while the urethra in female anatomy lies between the clitoris and the vagina). The head or glans of the penis and the clitoris are both highly sensitive to stimulation and are major sources of sexual pleasure. Due to the external location of the glans of the clitoris, it is easily sexually stimulated. The clitoris is estimated to contain more than 8,000 nerve endings and is often argued to have as many as twice the number as the penis (although the debates and opinions vary).

In some cultures, the clitoris is removed for a variety of social and religious reasons; this may be known as female genital cutting, female genital mutilation, or female circumcision. The World Health Organization has recognized Africa as having the greatest prevalence of this practice, with millions of women having undergone the procedure. Such practices are outlawed in many places around the world, including Britain, the United States, Canada, France, Norway, Sweden, and Switzerland.

For many years, the clitoris was not well understood and was considered by some to be a rudimentary nonfunctioning part of the body. During the 1960s and 1970s, understanding of the clitoris began to change, due in part to the influence of feminist activists, and this contributed to a new vision of female sexuality and the female orgasm. Previously, there had been long-standing myths that women's orgasms came purely through vaginal stimulation. Sigmund Freud argued that clitoral stimulation (through masturbation) represented an immature stage of development, and for a woman to achieve maturity, her sexual interests must shift to the vagina. However, we now know that contrary to many beliefs (especially in previous decades) the more common cause of orgasm in females is through clitoral stimulation and not vaginal penetration. Interestingly, because the bulbs of the clitoris lie on either side of the vagina, stimulation can often occur through vaginal penetration, which may have led to the assumption of vaginal penetration being the cause of orgasm. Many sex toys for women focus on clitoral stimulation through vibration or combine vibration with vaginal penetration.

Callum E. Cooper

See also: Erogenous Zones; Female Genital Cutting; Female Sexuality; Orgasm; Sex Toys.

Further Reading

Davis, D. K., McCafferty, C., & Momoh, C. (2005). *Female genital mutilation.* London: Radcliffe.

Dutta, D. C. (2014). *Textbook of gynecology.* London: JP Medical.

Freud, S. (1991). *Introductory lectures on psychoanalysis.* London: Penguin.

O'Connell, H. E., Sanjeevan, K. V., & Hutson, J. M. (2005). Anatomy of the clitoris. *The Journal of Neurology, 174*, 1189–1195.

Pomeroy, W. B. (1986). *Girls and sex.* Middlesex, UK: Penguin.

Colposcopy

Colposcopy is a gynecological procedure used to more closely examine the cervix for signs of abnormality and disease after a Pap smear (a screening test for cervical cancer) has come back with abnormal results. The colposcopy procedure is both well regarded in the medical industry and fairly common practice—each year, approximately 2–3 million colposcopies are performed in the United States alone.

A special low-powered microscope called a colposcope is used to perform a colposcopy. During the procedure, a patient will lie face up on the exam table with legs spread, much like during a regular pelvic exam. An instrument called a speculum is inserted into the vagina to keep the vaginal walls open and make the cervix more visible. Then, the colposcope is placed a few inches away from the vaginal opening and is used to conduct a magnified examination of the vagina, vulva, and cervix. If a practitioner sees any abnormal or suspicious-looking cell growth, a small sample of tissue (biopsy) is collected and sent for laboratory testing. It is not unusual for several samples to be collected from different areas of the vagina and cervix during a colposcopy. It usually takes one to two weeks to confirm the results of the biopsy.

There are several reasons to perform a colposcopy following an abnormal Pap smear. The procedure may be recommended if irregular vaginal bleeding is occurring or if an abnormal growth has appeared on the cervix or vagina. A colposcopy may also be recommended if a woman has genital warts or human papillomavirus, a common sexually transmitted infection that can cause cervical cancer. Any inflammation or irritation in the cervix may also be cause for a colposcopy. The test can reveal abnormal patterns in the blood vessels, swollen or atrophied areas of the vagina and cervix, precancerous changes in the tissues, and the presence of both vaginal and vulvar cancer. Although procedural risks are minimal, a colposcopy can result in such complications as infection, severe pelvic pain, and heavy vaginal bleeding.

The colposcopy was first introduced in Germany in 1924. Gynecologist and researcher Dr. Hans Hinselmann spent several years experimenting with different colposcopy techniques as he looked to find ways to detect cervical cancer in its earliest stages. Although early colposcopy tools proved unwieldy and difficult to use, by the 1950s a more advanced colposcope had been invented, and by the 1960s the procedure was being performed in the United States and elsewhere. Although Hinselmann is hailed for pioneering the colposcopy, he is also reviled by many, as it has been brought to light that much of his experimentation (aided by Nazi SS doctor Eduard Wirths) occurred in concentration camps during World War II and ended in often painful death for the subjects. In addition to his controversial colposcopy work, at the end of World War II, Hinselmann was also found guilty of forced sterilization of Roma (Gypsy) women in Germany.

Although the origins of the colposcopy are clouded with atrocious acts, the procedure has in modern times become the "gold standard" for cervical cancer detection and is nearly universally accepted as the most effective follow-up screening for cervical cancer after a Pap smear. In many developing nations where colposcopies are not as readily available, cervical cancer remains a leading cause of death from cancer, accounting for about 190,000 deaths per year.

Tamar Burris

See also: Cervical Cancer; Cervix; Human Papillomavirus (HPV); Pap Smear.

Further Reading

Hollen, K. H. (2004). *The reproductive system.* Westport, CT: Greenwood.

Paludi, M. A. (2014). *The Praeger handbook on women's cancers: Personal and psychological insights.* Westport, CT: Praeger.

Coming Out

The concept of "coming out" was derived from the idea that one needed to "come out of the closet," or become unhidden around their sexual orientation, particularly if they identified as other than heterosexual (gay, lesbian, bisexual, queer, and others). While originally applied only to sexual orientation, "coming out" can now refer to expressing any sexual- or gender-minority identity. Coming out is first a personal, then public, affirmation of one's sexual orientation or other identity, which involves many steps of personal growth and development but can also involve other alternative lifestyles.

Though the phrase "coming out" was not used, the idea that one should be publicly open about their sexual orientation has been credited to Karl Heinrich Ulrichs. Born in 1825 in Germany, through his study and discovery of his own homosexuality, Ulrichs felt strongly about being public about his identity, though it was illegal. Though his family urged him to change his ways because they were against God, he "defended his homosexuality as natural and said that because God had given him his same-sex drive, he had the 'right to satisfy it'" (Bullough, 1994, p. 35).

The coming-out process, when speaking about personally and publicly revealing one's sexual orientation or other identity, is different for everyone and may vary according to socioeconomic status, immigrant status, race, class, and other societal oppressing factors. In *Homosexual Identity Formation: Testing a Theoretical Model* (1984), theorist Vivienne Cass, through research, identified six stages of the coming-out process for people identifying as homosexual: identity confusion, identity comparison, identity tolerance, identity acceptance, identity pride, and identity synthesis. These steps proceed from the individual questioning their own sexual orientation, comparing their experience to that of other gay or queer individuals, and eventually moving to find pride and support in who they are as a gay or queer person.

For people who identify as transgender or gender nonconforming, there may be a more complicated and longer process for people to feel congruency in their sexual and gender identities. Dr. Aaron Devor (2004) created *Witnessing and Mirroring: A Fourteen Stage Model of Transsexual Identity Formation*, which gave a look into the proposed development of a person identifying as transgender: abiding anxiety, identity confusion about originally assigned gender and sex, identity comparisons about assigned gender and sex, discovery of transsexualism, identity confusion about transsexualism, identity comparisons about transsexualism, tolerance of transsexual identity, delay before acceptance of transsexual identity, acceptance of transsexualism identity, delay before transition, transition, acceptance of posttransition gender and sex identities, integration, and pride. Again, these steps may be seemingly complete but do vary with time and ability for each person as with the gay or queer coming-out process.

Coming out as polyamorous, or participating in an alternative lifestyle such as kink or BDSM (bondage and discipline/dominance, submission/sadism and masochism) may also involve a process where people who engage in these relationships want to be public; some may also just want to be out and open with family and friends. Revealing this information may have some of the same consequences as coming out as gay, queer, or transgender, such as losing support of family and friends. Individuals going through the coming-out process may also require some support, either professionally or from friends and family.

Some people decide to come out publicly immediately after personally realizing their sexual or gender identity. For others, the process takes more time. People come out within these various identities depending on several factors—most importantly, safety. For example, coming out or being public about a nonmonogamous or polyamorous relationship can have negative implications if the people involved have kids. For instance, if someone outside of their relationship sees their relationship structure as a danger to the traditional family structure, they may report the parents to social services. Transgender people who are out may experience violence and discrimination; some may even be denied housing or employment. Coming out as a gay teenager within a household that believes in a religion that speaks against homosexuality may cause the loss of stable housing for that child as well as loss of family or friend support for that individual.

Though coming out can be a difficult experience for many, there are some ways to find support in the process so that feelings and situations around coming out can be more manageable. First, finding a support group with other people who are experiencing the same process is helpful in alleviating overwhelming feelings of isolation, sadness, or depression. Individual therapy can be helpful, as can family or couples therapy with a therapeutic service provider who is able to address the particular needs at hand. The internet has provided increased visibility of various sexual- and gender-minority orientations, identities, and lifestyles, and examples of people coming out can be found on platforms such as YouTube, helping put names, faces, and voices to a variety of experiences in the privacy of one's own space.

Shane'a Thomas

See also: Gender Diversity; Gender Identity; Homosexuality; Polyamory; Queer; Questioning; Sexual Identity; Sexual Orientation; Transgender; Ulrichs, Karl.

Further Reading

Bullough, V. (1994). *Science in the bedroom: A history of sex research.* New York: Basic Books.

Cass, V. (1984). Homosexual identity formation: Testing a theoretical model. *The Journal of Sex Research, 20*, 143–167.

Devor, A. (2004). Witnessing and mirroring: A fourteen stage model of transsexual identity formation. *Journal of Gay & Lesbian Psychotherapy, 8*, 41–67.

Yarber, W. L., Sayad, B. W., & Strong, B. (2010). *Human sexuality: Diversity in contemporary America* (7th ed.). New York: McGraw-Hill.

Commission on Obscenity and Pornography

The Commission on Obscenity and Pornography—officially called the President's Commission on Obscenity and Pornography—was a group established by Congress in 1967, with its eighteen members appointed by U.S. President Lyndon B. Johnson in 1968, to examine the possible relationships between obscene and pornographic materials and antisocial behavior. The commission was also charged with determining whether more effective methods were needed to limit the availability of such materials. The group released its final report in 1970 to Congress and President Richard M. Nixon.

Members of the commission were considered to be experts in law, medicine, religion, or culture. The commission's chair was William B. Lockhart, an ordained minister of the Disciples of Christ Church and Dean of the School of Law at the University of Minnesota.

The commission tasked Danish criminologist Berl Kutchinsky with performing a scientific study on the criminal effects of pornography. Kutchinsky published his results in 1970 as *Studies on Pornography and Sex Crimes in Denmark*. His findings indicated that the legalization of pornography in Denmark did not lead to an increase in sex-related crimes.

Reflecting the results of Kutchinsky's study, the commission's *Report of the Commission on Obscenity and Pornography*, released in late 1970, found no evidence that obscene or pornographic materials harmed individuals or led to social problems or criminal actions among youth or adults. It concluded that no legal restrictions on adult access to such materials were needed and that any existing restrictions on such access be repealed. The commission further recommended that sex education be provided in schools, that children's access to pornography remain restricted, and that more studies on pornography be funded.

A minority block of the commission, led by Charles Keating, an attorney named to the commission by President Nixon to replace a Johnson-appointed member who had resigned, drafted its own report opposing the majority's conclusions, calling them "moral anarchy." Moreover, both the U.S. Senate, which was dominated by Democrats, and President Nixon, a Republican, rejected the commission's findings and recommendations.

The congressional and White House reactions to the commission's report can best be understood when placed in the context of the generally socially conservative nature of the times. President Nixon had been elected in 1969 on a platform of restoring "law and order" to a nation reeling in youthful rebellion against the Vietnam War and the traditional social conventions of the older generation, which was still in charge of most institutions.

Over the succeeding years, society's attitudes have changed. In the internet age, pornography is far easier and cheaper to access today than it was in the 1970s. The commission's findings are now seemingly accepted by most people in the much more sexually permissive modern-day United States. And the commission's findings continue to influence government policy and laws regarding obscenity and pornography.

A. J. Smuskiewicz

See also: Pornography; Sex Education.

Further Reading

Brenner, R. (2011, May). Sins of commission: The 40th anniversary of the illustrated presidential report of the Commission on Obscenity and Pornography. *Huffington Post.* Retrieved from https://www.huffpost.com/entry/sins-of-commission-the-fo_b_779849?guccounter=1

Kemp, E. (Ed.). (1970). *The illustrated presidential report of the Commission on Obscenity and Pornography.* San Diego, CA: Greenleaf Classics.

Communication, Sexual

Sex is everywhere—from movies and TV to advertisements and magazines. On a daily basis, messages about sex are communicated to people by the media and society at large. But, despite messages about sex being so common, people find it difficult to talk about sex. Sexual communication is, at its most basic level, any information related to sex and sexuality that we send out or receive. This information can come from the media, as mentioned, but it also comes from partners, friends, and other important people, such as parents and family. Some people will also receive messages about sex in more formal settings like schools or religious associations. All this information shapes a person's understanding and beliefs about sexuality, which in turn shapes how sex is communicated in general.

Many people find talking about sex to be uncomfortable and difficult; they may even feel embarrassed or ashamed. While there are many possible reasons for this, there are some general ones too. Talking about sex is seen as taboo by many people in Western culture, and the attitudes and norms of society often influence what individuals think and how they behave. Past experiences can also influence how people feel when they talk about sex. Children who are taught at a young age that sex is something negative that should be avoided often grow up believing these messages and may find it more difficult to discuss the topic with others (like their partners and even their doctors) when older. However, even people who have relatively positive views about sex often experience discomfort when talking about their sexuality with others. Talking about sex, especially with a partner whose opinion is valued, can be a very vulnerable experience and can leave one open to the possibility of rejection.

Because many people feel uncomfortable talking about sex, most sexual communication in intimate relationships occurs nonverbally. Rather than using words to express sexual interest, behaviors like sexual touching or removing clothing are often used to initiate sex. While this strategy often works, it can also be problematic. Talking about sex with one's sexual partners is important for many reasons. To begin with, talking about sex is important for health and the health of one's partners. Ideally, before engaging in sexual activities, partners should discuss things like condom use, birth control, and other safer sex practices to prevent the transmission of sexually transmitted infections and unintended pregnancies. Numerous studies have shown that couples who talk about using condoms are more likely to actually use them. Talking about sex can also help to increase sexual enjoyment and satisfaction. Researchers have found that when one partner is able to explain their sexual preferences to their partner, the partner's understanding increases, leading to greater sexual satisfaction. By discussing what one likes, wants, and even things they would like to try, sex becomes more fun and pleasurable. Talking about sex among partners has also been shown to increase satisfaction within the relationship and to build intimacy among partners. Talking about sex in a positive and productive way with one's partner may even have a greater impact on relationship satisfaction than other types of communication between partners. It should also be noted that sexual communication is important for all couples, and there are no differences in communication between same-sex and mixed-sex couples.

Given that sexual communication can have a significant effect on personal lives and on the success of one's relationships, it is important to consider what makes sexual communication effective. First, it is important to recognize that the beliefs and experiences of both partners will affect what they think and say about sex. So, if one partner wishes to discuss sex in an open and frank manner, while the other partner tends to be more reserved, the couple may face communication difficulties right from the start. Therefore, people need to be aware of their own sexual communication style as well as the style of the person with whom they are speaking. Second, expectations about sexual communication matter. If people begin a difficult discussion expecting it to go poorly, research suggests that it might; on the contrary, positive expectations may be more likely to result in a positive conversation. Finally, how partners relate to each other during sexual conversations also affects the success of the discussion. Good listening skills, being able to take the other's perspective into consideration, and being aware of how messages and tone of voice affect sensitive sexual conversations are a few things that can improve sexual communication. Fortunately for those who dread talking about sex with their partners, communication skills can be learned and developed throughout the course of one's life, making it easier to have these discussions and potentially leading to a more satisfying sex life and better relationships.

Heather L. Armstrong

See also: Advertising, Sex in; Contraception; Media and Sexuality; Sex Education; Sexual Health; Sexual Satisfaction; Sexually Transmitted Infections (STIs).

Further Reading

Downey, G., Freitas, A. L., Michaelis, B., & Khouri, H. D. (1998). The self-fulfilling prophecy in close relationships: Rejection sensitivity and rejection by romantic partners. *Journal of Personality and Social Psychology, 75*, 545–560.

Holmberg, D., & Blair, K. L. (2009). Sexual desire, communication, satisfaction, and preferences of men and women in same-sex versus mixed-sex relationships. *Journal of Sex Research, 46*, 57–66.

MacNeil, S., & Byers, E. S. (2009). Role of sexual self-disclosure in the sexual satisfaction of long-term heterosexual couples. *Journal of Sex Research, 46*, 3–14.

Montesi, J. L., Fauber, R. L., Gordon, E. A., & Heimberg, R. G. (2010). The specific importance of communicating about sex to couples' sexual and overall relationship satisfaction. *Journal of Social and Personal Relationships, 28*, 591–609.

Noar, S. M., Carlyle, K., & Cole, C. (2006). Why communication is crucial: Meta-analysis of the relationship between safer sexual communication and condom use. *Journal of Health Communication: International Perspectives, 11*, 365–390.

Rehman, U. S., & Fallis, E. E. (2014). Sexual communication. In C. F. Pukall (Ed.), *Human sexuality: A contemporary introduction.* Don Mills, ON: Oxford University Press.

Rehman, U. S., Janssen, E., Newhouse, S., Heiman, J., Holtzworth-Munroe, A., Fallis, E., & Rafaeli, E. (2011). Martial satisfaction and communication behaviors during sexual and nonsexual conflict discussions in newlywed couples: A pilot study. *Journal of Sex & Marital Therapy, 37*, 93–103.

Vannier, S. A., & O'Sullivan, L. F. (2011). Communicating interest in sex: Verbal and nonverbal initiation of sexual activity in young adults' romantic dating relationships. *Archives of Sexual Behavior, 40*, 961–969.

Companionate Love

Companionate love is a construct created by psychologist Robert Sternberg as part of his triangular theory of love. According to Sternberg's model, there are three components to love: intimacy, passion, and commitment. Intimacy represents the emotional component of love that describes the closeness and affection people have for each other. Passion is the motivational aspect of love. Commitment is the decision to love and to maintain that love. Sternberg combined these three components into a triangle, and the components combine to produce different types of love. Companionate love is the combination of intimacy and commitment but not passion.

Companionate love is defined as an intimacy and affection felt when caring deeply for a person, without the experience of passion or arousal in the person's presence. This passion may have faded over time or possibly was not present in the early stages of the relationship. Despite its absence, the relationship continues. An example of this type of relationship would be a married couple who do not have sex but share interests and enjoy each other's company. Their marriage to one another signifies their commitment to one another, and the depth of their emotional bond represents their shared intimacy despite the lack of a sexual relationship. In reflection of this construct, Professor Beverley Fehr notes that the foundational components of companionate love may underlie all types of love. For example, the love between parent and child, the love of a caretaker for their pet, or the love between longtime friends might match the general concept of companionate love, even though not holding the title. Sternberg emphasizes that the addition of long-term allegiance is the key differentiation between this relationship and a deep friendship. Partners in this type of relationship are matched counterparts that complement and support one another.

Relationship psychologist Judith Wallerstein was interested in discovering how couples determined relationship satisfaction in a marriage. To investigate this, she conducted a qualitative study on couples whose marriages survived conflict and were considered happy and successful. Wallerstein identified four types of "good marriages," each having a unique set of characteristics and challenges. In Wallerstein's conceptualization, companionate marriage is the most common type of relationship among younger couples as well as the most difficult to maintain. Companionate loves are described as newer loves, at whose core is a friendship and trust in an equal partnership. Wallerstein found that these relationships require high levels of self-confidence, self-awareness, and the patience to postpone gratification. Partners in a companionate love marriage value friendship and equality and strive toward a balance between their home life and work life. While deep affection and commitment are the foundations, the primary long-term risk is for the relationship to degenerate into a relationship resembling a brother-sister bond. Sternberg, however, believed that companionate love was not youthful or undeveloped but thought instead that at its healthiest, it represented a deep, mature, affectionate attachment between people who love, like, and respect each other.

Shadeen Francis

See also: Attachment Theory of Love; Consummate Love; Intimacy, Sexual and Relational; Lee's Theory of Love Styles; Love; Marriage; Sternberg's Triangular Theory of Love.

Further Reading

Aronson, E., Wilson, T. D., & Akert, R. M. (2010). *Social psychology* (7th ed.). Upper Saddle River, NJ: Prentice Hall.

Ashford, J., & LeCroy, C. (2009). *Human behavior in the social environment: A multidimensional perspective.* Toronto: Nelson Education.

Fehr, B. (1995). Love. In D. Levinson (Ed.), *Encyclopedia of marriage and the family.* New York: Macmillan.

Sternberg, R. J. (1986). A triangular theory of love. *Psychological Review, 93,* 119–135.

Compulsivity, Sexual

Compulsive sexual behavior is defined by the Society for the Advancement of Sexual Health as a "persistent and escalating pattern of sexual behavior acted out despite increasing negative consequences to self and others." This behavior is often one that the individual feels is outside of voluntary control and may involve risky behavior, the desire to limit one's sexual behaviors or the consequences of those behaviors, and the use of sexual fantasies or obsessions as primary coping strategies for life stresses. Individuals often report spending excessive amounts of time being sexual, obtaining sex, hiding sexual behavior, or recovering from sexual experiences. Important social, occupational, financial, or social responsibilities may be neglected due to the sexual behavior.

Sexual compulsivity can lead to relational, occupational, legal, financial, emotional, spiritual, and physical distress. For example, isolation, impairment in the relationship with the primary sexual partner, impaired job performance, job loss, criminal convictions for illegal sexual behaviors, financial strain if sex and sexual materials are paid for, depression, anxiety, guilt, spiritual strain, and sexually transmitted infections are common outcomes.

Sexually compulsive behaviors may include anonymous, voyeuristic, exhibitionistic, intrusive, or exploitive sex. Some seductive role sex, pain exchange sex, and fantasy sex behaviors may also be used in compulsive ways. Compulsive sex may be both free and paid sex and may include sex trades and bartering.

Research suggests that there is no single cause for sexually compulsive behavior. It is often helpful to consider several biological, psychological, social, and spiritual contributors to compulsive behavior. From a biological perspective, both testosterone and serotonin may play important roles in compulsive sexual behaviors. Classical and operant conditioning may powerfully reinforce specific sexual behaviors to the point that they are engaged in habitually. Many individuals report that sexual behaviors may create dissociative psychological experiences or represent reenactment of past conflicts and traumas (both sexual traumas and other traumas, such as combat-related posttraumatic stress disorder). Some individuals find that sexually compulsive behavior arises in response to cultural or religious sexual prohibitions. Sexual compulsivity has been found to be comorbid (co-occurring) with other conditions, such as other sexual disorders (dysfunctions and paraphilias), mood and anxiety disorders, chemical dependency, and eating disorders.

Diagnosis of sexually compulsive behavior can be difficult, as individuals are often reluctant to disclose sexual behaviors to others. Clinicians often begin by assessing the amount of time that the individual spends each day and week engaged in sexual behaviors and the extent to which they have noticed negative relational, occupational, legal, financial, emotional, and spiritual consequences as a result of sexual behaviors. Screening tests and assessment questionnaires may also be used, such as the Sexual Addiction Screening Test and the Sexual Compulsivity Scale. The *Diagnostic and Statistical Manual of Mental Disorders, Fifth Edition* (*DSM-5*) does not include a diagnosis for sexual compulsivity among its descriptions of substance-related and addictive disorders, though some individuals with sexual compulsivity may display symptoms consistent with the paraphilic disorders. In its newest edition, the World Health Organization's *International Classification of Diseases, Eleventh Revision* included compulsive sexual behavior disorder as an impulse control disorder.

A consultation with a mental health professional that specializes in sexual concerns is recommended before determining if an individual is engaging in sexually compulsive behavior. Successful treatment usually assumes that all behaviors, including compulsive sexual behaviors, are engaged in by the individual for good reasons; identifying and addressing the client's needs and motivators is important. Emphasis may be placed on addressing common motivators for compulsive sexual behaviors, such as excitement, comfort (reduce stress, reward, relax), and escape (dissociation, trance, avoidance, mood regulation), as well as psychological motivators such as affirmation, helplessness, power, and revenge. Interventions target decreasing the frequency of compulsive behaviors, preventing use, methods to change behavior "in the moment," and strategies to alter behavior after a relapse. Specific interventions vary according to the client's needs and may include mindfulness practices, ending destructive relationships, prescriptive masturbation, journaling, cognitive restructuring, and identification of coping strategies for use when the client is upset (bored, angry, anxious, lonely, or tired). Treatment may be offered in inpatient hospital settings, partial hospitalization programs, outpatient counseling, twelve-step groups, and online programs. Treatment may be focused on the individual, couple, family, or group.

Elizabeth A. Maynard

See also: Hypersexuality; *International Classification of Diseases, Eleventh Revision (ICD-11)*; Out-of-Control Sexual Behavior; Pornography Addiction.

Further Reading

Carnes, P., Green, B., & Carnes, S. (2010). The same yet different: Refocusing the Sexual Addiction Screening Test (SAST) to reflect orientation and gender. *Sexual Addiction & Compulsivity: The Journal of Treatment & Prevention, 17*(1), 7–30.

Dodge, B., Reece, M., Cole, S. L., & Theo, G. M. (2004). Sexual compulsivity among heterosexual college students. *Journal of Sex Research, 41*(4), 343–350.

Kalichman, S. C., & Cain, D. (2004). The relationship between indicators of sexual compulsivity and high risk sexual practices among men and women receiving services from a sexually transmitted infection clinic. *The Journal of Sex Research, 41*, 235–241.

Kalichman, S. C., & Rompa, D. (1995). Sexual sensation seeking and sexual compulsivity scales: Reliability, validity, and predicting HIV risk behaviors. *Journal of Personality Assessment, 65*, 586–602.

Society for the Advancement of Sexual Health. (2019). Retrieved from www.sash.net

Conception

Conception, strictly speaking, is initiated with the fertilization by a male's sperm (spermatozoon) with a female's egg (ovum), which eventually results in pregnancy. "Conception," however, is a term that is somewhat variable with respect to definition and connotation. To refer to a moment of conception is somewhat a misnomer as it is actually a process that usually occurs over a forty-eight-hour span.

The sperm and egg are, respectively, the male and female gametes produced by meiosis. They are haploid cells, each containing twenty-three chromosomes, or half the total needed to form a new individual.

An array of complex circumstances in both male and female bodies is necessary for conception to occur. In female bodies, a viable egg must be stimulated to mature in an ovarian follicle by follicle-stimulating hormone, which is secreted by the pituitary gland. Estrogen levels must increase to trigger the thickening of the lining of the uterus; as the levels of estrogen increase, the pituitary will begin secreting luteinizing hormone, which causes the follicle to rupture and release the mature egg, a process referred to as ovulation. Ovulation generally occurs around twelve to fourteen days before the beginning of the next menstrual cycle. The ruptured follicle then begins to release progesterone, at which point it becomes known as the corpus luteum. Estrogen and progesterone cause the endometrium to thicken. The released egg, hopefully, is drawn into the fallopian tube, also known as the oviduct.

In male bodies, sperm are produced in the seminiferous tubules of the testes, stimulated by testosterone. Mature sperm are stored in the epididymis. From there, they travel through the vas deferens, where they are mixed with fluids secreted from the seminal vesicles; this fluid contains a simple sugar, fructose, to help nourish the sperm. More substances are added to the fluid mixture from the prostate gland; these mainly serve to help neutralize the harsh acidity of the female's vagina. The bulbourethral glands, also known as the Cowper's glands, release substances that help to neutralize the environment within the male's urethra. During penile-vaginal sex, ejaculation, a complex process in itself, sends millions of sperm into a vagina. Approximately 40 million sperm are released in each healthy ejaculate, with at least 30 percent having normal morphology and at least 50 percent moving forward for an optimal probability of conception to occur.

For conception to occur, one viable sperm must have access to a mature egg, which is usually flowing down the fallopian tube toward the uterus. The survival time of sperm in the female reproductive tract is highly variable but can last for several days, which means that the fertile period lasts for several days on either side of ovulation. The head of the sperm produces enzymes that permit it to bore through the jelly coating that surrounds the egg. The sperm head that successfully penetrates into the plasma membrane of the egg detaches its tail (flagellum) as it enters the egg's yolk (ooplasm). A chemical reaction is then initiated to form the perivitelline membrane around the egg to prevent any additional sperm from penetrating. For conception to occur, the sperm head must successfully penetrate the cumulus oophorous and corona radiate cells and bind to the zona pellucida inside the egg. The nucleus of the sperm decondenses after penetration in synchrony with the nucleus of the egg, creating two pronuclei. The fusion of genetic material from the sperm and egg, known as syngamy, occurs after the membranes of the two pronuclei are broken down.

The fusion of the sperm and the egg, begun by fertilization, produces a zygote. The zygote begins as a single diploid cell, which contains a total of forty-six chromosomes. It makes its way through the fallopian tube for three to four days until it reaches the uterus. The zygote must then implant itself into the uterine wall, which typically happens about seven to ten days after ovulation. About five days after the zygote is formed, it transforms into a blastocyst; about fourteen days later, it normally becomes an embryo. By the ninth week, it has usually grown into a fetus.

Victor B. Stolberg

See also: Contraception; Ejaculation; Fertility; Fertility Awareness Methods of Contraception; Infertility; Ova; Pregnancy; Safer Sex; Sperm.

Further Reading

Aslam, I., & Fishel, S. (1996). The use of spermatids for human conception. In V. Hansson, F. O. Levy, & K. Taskén (Eds.), *Signal transduction in testicular cells* (272–286). Berlin: Springer-Verlag.

Bongso, A., Ho, J., Fong, C.-Y., Ng, S.-C., & Ratnam, S. (1993). Human sperm function after coculture with human fallopian tubal epithelial cell monolayers: In vitro model for studying cell interactions in early human conception. *Archives of Human Andrology, 31*(3), 183–190.

Ford, N. M. (1991). *When did I begin? Conception of the human individual in history, philosophy and science.* Cambridge: Cambridge University Press.

Condoms, Female (Receptive)

The receptive condom, sometimes also called the "female condom" or internal condom, is a barrier contraceptive method that can be used to prevent unintended pregnancy and the transmission of sexually transmitted infections (STIs). The name "female condom" is a misnomer as receptive condoms can be used vaginally or anally by people of any sex or gender.

A receptive condom is a tube-shaped device that goes into the vagina or anus and creates a physical barrier between sexual partners to block sperm and STI transmission. It is usually made of polyurethane, a nonlatex synthetic material. The receptive condom has two rings, one at each end. When used vaginally, the interior ring and shaft of the condom is inserted into the vagina, and the outer ring is held outside the body. The interior ring can be placed behind the pubic bone to help keep the condom in place. The outer ring is placed outside the vagina. If used anally, the interior ring should be removed before the condom is inserted and the outer ring held outside the body. Once inserted, the ring is placed over the anus.

It is important to use a commercial lubricant when using receptive condoms as this will help to prevent the condom from tearing or being dislodged, and it will increase pleasure and sensation if a partner's penis is being used for sexual stimulation. A spermicide may be added to the condom if additional contraceptive protection is needed or desired. It is important not to also use an insertive condom while using a receptive condom, as using both can lead to tearing and decreased effectiveness of both devices.

When used perfectly, the receptive condom is 95 percent effective at preventing pregnancy; however, with typical use, it is only about 79 percent effective. That means that over the course of one year, if one hundred fertile females use the receptive condom as their only method of birth control, twenty-one of them will become pregnant.

The receptive condom offers many benefits. As mentioned, it can help prevent unintended pregnancy and transmission of STIs. Also, because the receptive condom is larger than the insertive condom, some material of the condom is placed around the opening of the vagina or anus and covers the skin in this area. This means that the receptive condom can help prevent some STIs that can be transmitted via skin-to-skin contact, such as HPV or herpes. The receptive condom can also be inserted up to eight hours ahead of sexual activity, and since it is typically made of polyurethane, it can be used by people with latex allergies or sensitivities. While they are not as common as insertive condoms, they can be purchased online or in stores without a prescription.

While their use is largely beneficial, there are some potential drawbacks of the receptive condom to consider. The biggest drawback is that they are more expensive than the insertive condom, although they are cheaper than hormonal forms of birth control. In addition, some people may not like their appearance. Receptive condoms may also make a crinkly noise during intercourse, although this may be reduced by using commercial lubrication. Internal condoms are not reusable, so a new one is needed for every sexual encounter.

Heather L. Armstrong

See also: Barrier Contraceptive Methods; Condoms, Male (Insertive); Lubricants; Pregnancy; Sexually Transmitted Infections (STIs); Spermicides.

Further Reading

Planned Parenthood. (2019). Internal condom. Retrieved from https://www.plannedparenthood.org/learn/birth-control/internal-condom

Society of Obstetricians and Gynaecologists of Canada. (2019). Female condom. Retrieved from https://www.sexandu.ca/contraception/non-hormonal-contraception/#tc2

Sutton, K. S., & Chalmers, B. (2017). Contraception and pregnancy options. In C. F. Pukall (Ed.), *Human sexuality: A contemporary introduction* (2nd ed.). Don Mills, ON: Oxford University Press.

Condoms, Male (Insertive)

An insertive condom provides protection against sexually transmitted infections (STIs) and pregnancy during sexual activities. Barrier methods of birth control create a separation between an egg and sperm so that pregnancy is prevented. An insertive condom, also sometimes called a "male condom," fits over an erect penis, securing to the base of the penis. As such, partners' bodily fluids cannot be mixed, which greatly reduces the risk of HIV and other STI transmission as well as pregnancy. Insertive condoms can also be used with shared sex toys to reduce the risk of STIs.

An insertive condom is made from thin materials. It is soft, flexible, and rolls out to become a sheath. It may be made from several different types of materials, including latex (which is most common), polyurethane, or processed animal tissue. It may be used for oral sex, anal sex, or vaginal sex. Condoms come in a variety of different textures, colors, sizes, and shapes. Some come lubricated and others do not. There are many options depending on preference and the desired use for the condom. For example, condoms may be flavored or colored. These should not be used for anal or vaginal sex but may be a great option for oral sex or nonpenetrative sex play. Polyurethane or animal tissue condoms may be an option for people who have a latex allergy. However, animal tissue condoms do not protect against STIs, as the material of the condom is porous and so viruses and bacteria are able to pass through; as such, they may only be used for pregnancy prevention. Polyurethane condoms protect against both STIs and pregnancy. When used correctly, insertive condoms are very effective, and their use has greatly increased since the 1980s. With perfect use, condoms are 98 percent effective at preventing pregnancy. With typical use, they are 85 percent effective at preventing pregnancy.

There are many benefits of using insertive condoms. They are quite easy to obtain, as they are available at grocery stores, pharmacies, and online; they are also commonly provided for free at various health clinics and schools. Condoms are also relatively inexpensive and do not cause harmful side effects, so long as you or your partner are not allergic to the material you choose for the condom. Insertive condoms may be a great addition to safer sex practices that include another form of birth control, such as a hormonal method, in order to protect against STIs and further decrease risk of pregnancy.

Despite all the benefits of using condoms, some people may complain that a condom dulls sensation. If this is a problem, users are encouraged to try a different size, shape, or brand as different condoms fit and feel differently, so usually this problem can be solved by finding the right condom for the user. In addition, some people may find it to be disruptive to put a condom on while in the heat of the moment. Sexual communication and incorporating applying the condom as part of foreplay can make using a condom a positive part of the sexual experience. Users should also be aware that an insertive condom might break or slip during sex, and this risk is elevated during anal sex. Using proper lubrication decreases this risk.

Condom use is very common among adolescents and young adults. The 2009 National Survey of Sexual Health and Behavior shows that condom use decreases with age, and this is true for all relationship statuses.

As mentioned previously, some people think that condoms diminish sensation. However, a study conducted by Debby Herbenick, a researcher at the Center for Sexual Health Promotion at Indiana University, found that Americans aged fourteen to ninety-four from all across the country mostly disagree with that assertion. Instead, most participants noted that sex with a condom is just as pleasurable and exciting as sex without a condom. Many younger people even responded that having sex with a condom is more pleasurable than having sex without one.

Only about 10 percent of men need an extra-large condom. If an extra-large condom is used when it is not necessary, the condom is more likely to slip and fall off during intercourse. If a standard size condom does not roll down to the base of the penis, an extra-large condom is needed.

Condoms have expiration dates on the packaging, and these must be checked prior to use. In addition, condoms are very thin; therefore, the package must be opened carefully. It's important to avoid using teeth or nails to open the package, as this may result in tearing or puncturing the condom, which makes it useless. While holding the tip of the condom, the condom may be rolled down to the base of the penis. It is important that the base of the penis is dry so that the condom can grip to the base and not slip. Holding the tip of the condom allows room for the semen and prevents the condom from breaking from the force of thrusting. Once the condom is on, any air bubbles in the condom should be pushed out to reduce the likelihood of breakage. If the condom was put on the wrong way and was not able to be rolled down, the condom should be thrown away and another should be used. A new condom should also be used for every sexual encounter and when changing from anal sex to vaginal sex or from anal sex to oral sex. When the sexual encounter is over, the base of the condom should be held while the penis is removed from the vagina or anus in order to prevent any semen from dripping out. The condom can then be thrown away in the garbage. Condoms should be stored in a cool, dry place in order to maintain their effectiveness.

Amanda Manuel

See also: Barrier Contraceptive Methods; Condoms, Female (Receptive); Lubricants; Pregnancy; Safer Sex; Sexually Transmitted Infections (STIs); Spermicides.

Further Reading

Herbenick, D., & Stoddard, G. (2012). *Great in bed.* New York: DK.

Joannides, P. (2012). Birth control: Sperm v. egg. In P. Joannides (Ed.), *Guide to getting it on* (6th ed., 713–773). Waldport, OR: Goofy Foot Press.

Yarber, W., Sayad, B., & Strong, B. (2010). *Human sexuality: Diversity in contemporary America* (7th ed.). New York: McGraw-Hill.

Congenital Adrenal Hyperplasia

Congenital adrenal hyperplasia describes a group of seven autosomal recessive conditions that affect the function of the adrenal glands. More than 95 percent of these cases are caused by a mutation in the gene for 21 hydroxylase. The classic understanding of congenital adrenal hyperplasia is a condition where XX infants are exposed to elevated levels of testosterone during development and are born with external genitalia that may appear to be male. Specifically, they may have a greatly enlarged clitoris that resembles a penis. This presentation is known as the virilizing form of congenital adrenal hyperplasia. XY infants with the virilizing form of congenital adrenal hyperplasia also show signs of excess androgen production. These include rapid skeletal growth, early growth of pubic hair, and being sexually precocious.

There is also what is known as the salt-wasting form of congenital adrenal hyperplasia. Unlike the virilizing form, which does not have a major impact on infant health, the salt-wasting form can be life-threatening. If not detected early, through neonatal screening, infants with the salt-wasting form of congenital adrenal hyperplasia are at high risk of dying within the first two weeks of life. The functional difference between the two types of congenital adrenal hyperplasia is that individuals with the salt-wasting form have no enzyme activity from 21 hydroxylase, and individuals with the virilizing form have enough enzyme activity (1–2 percent) to maintain levels of aldosterone that are sufficient for health. There are also what are known as "cryptic" forms of congenital adrenal hyperplasia that have no, or minimal, symptoms but are diagnosed through genetic testing. The mutations that cause cryptic congenital adrenal hyperplasia reduce enzyme activity only by approximately half.

Other genes where mutations cause congenital adrenal hyperplasia lead to what are referred to as nonclassic forms of the condition, which resemble the 21 hydroxylase varieties to varying degrees. One exception is cases of congenital adrenal hyperplasia caused by mutations in the 17-alpha-hydroxylase gene, where children appear to be female at the time of birth but never develop secondary sexual characteristics during adolescence. Treatment for all forms of congenital adrenal hyperplasia is based on the principal of regulating abnormal hormone production—suppressing excess and supplementing where production is insufficient. This reduces both the abnormally fast growth and the sexual precocity associated with the condition.

Congenital adrenal hyperplasia is considered to be a disorder of sexual development (also known as a difference of sexual development) because of the effects it has on infant genitalia. Historically, many surgeons have recommended genital surgery for XX infants with congenital adrenal hyperplasia to make their genitals appear more feminine. More recently, there has been growing concern that performing such surgeries during infancy has the potential to both deny patients their autonomy and risk permanently impairing their sexual function. Nonetheless, early surgery remains recommended for cases of extreme virilization by the Endocrine Society guidelines that were released in 2010. Those guidelines note that the presumed values of early surgery are "reducing parental anxiety and easing acceptance of the child's congenital anomaly, avoiding stigmatization of a girl with masculinized genitals, and avoiding the psychological trauma of genital surgery during adolescence" (Speiser et al., 2010).

One of the concerns sometimes brought up in discussions of the appropriateness of genital surgery for XX individuals with congenital adrenal hyperplasia is the likely gender identity development of these children as they grow to adulthood. Research has generally suggested that XX individuals with congenital adrenal hyperplasia identify as girls, although as girls with more male-type behaviors than XX individuals without congenital adrenal hyperplasia. Newer research suggests that these children are significantly more likely to have gender identity scores in the male domain than their peers but that it is still rare for these children to take on a male gender identity and role.

There is limited research suggesting that many young women with congenital adrenal hyperplasia have a preference for early surgery. However, much of the literature supporting early genital surgery focuses on managing parental distress rather than on how the surgery affects patient outcomes. In part, this is because there has not yet been sufficient research to determine whether sexual and psychological outcomes are better for individuals with congenital hyperplasia who undergo genital surgery early, late, or not at all.

Most arguments against early genital surgery focus on patient autonomy, sexual health, and gender identity formation. These are concerns that may not seem salient to parents who are faced with raising an infant whose differences make them hesitant or uncomfortable. They are also hard to address or assess before the infant reaches adolescence or adulthood. Finally, these arguments require acknowledging that pleasure is an important component of sexual health. This is something that can be both difficult and uncomfortable for parents and providers to discuss in the context of infant and child health. Sexual pleasure may have been codified into the World Health Organization's definition of sexual health since 2002, but it is still a long way from being considered universally relevant to clinical practice.

Elizabeth R. Boskey

See also: Androgen Insensitivity Syndrome; Androgens; Biological Sex; Chromosomal Sex; 5-Alpha-Reductase Deficiency; Intersexuality; Sex Reassignment Surgery.

Further Reading

Berenbaum, S. A., Beltz, A. M., Bryk, K., & McHale, S. (2018). Gendered peer involvement in girls with congenital adrenal hyperplasia: Effects of prenatal androgens, gendered activities, and gender cognitions. *Archives of Sexual Behavior, 47*(4), 915–929.

El-Maouche, D., Arlt, W., & Merke, D. P. (2017). Congenital adrenal hyperplasia. *Lancet, 390*(10108), 2194–2210.

Jesus, L. E. (2018). Feminizing genitoplasties: Where are we now? *Journal of Pediatric Urology, 14*(5), 407–415.

Pasterski, V., Zucker, K. J., Hindmarsh, P. C., Hughes, I. A., Acerini, C., Spencer, D., ... Hines, M. (2015). Increased cross-gender identification independent of gender role behavior in girls with congenital adrenal hyperplasia: Results from a standardized assessment of 4- to 11-year-old children. *Archives of Sexual Behavior, 44*(5), 1363–1375.

Speiser, P. W., Azziz, R., Baskin, L. S., Ghizzoni, L., Hensle, T. W., Merke, D. P., ... White, P. C. (2010). Congenital adrenal hyperplasia due to steroid 21-hydroxylase deficiency: An Endocrine Society clinical practice guideline. *Journal of Clinical Endocrinology and Metabolism, 95*(9), 4133–4160.

World Health Organization. (2002). *Defining sexual health: Report of a technical consultation on sexual health, 28–31 Jan 2002.* Geneva: WHO.

Consummate Love

The triangular theory of love is a model created by psychologist Robert Sternberg in 1984. Sternberg's theory of love holds that love can be understood in terms of a triad of complementary components that together form the vertices of a triangle. The three components of the theory are intimacy, passion, and commitment. Each component represents a unique and important aspect of love. Intimacy refers to the closeness, connection, and emotional bond in relationships. Passion is described as the drive that leads to sexual activity as well as physical attraction and arousal. The third component is commitment, which is the decision to sustain a relationship. The three components of love interact with each other to create eight different relationship types by having one, two, three, or none of the components. Consummate love is the relationship resulting from having all three components present at one time: a relationship containing intimacy, passion, and commitment. This type of love sits at the very center of the triangle, because it is said to be the ideal type of love.

Consummate love is considered the complete form of love between partners. Satisfaction, mutual understanding, support, and concern for the other are major components of this relationship type. These relationships are a healthy example of balance of self and other, with each person contributing positively to the growth of the other and to the future of the relationship. Each component is necessary to the experience of this balance. Passion develops quickly and creates the motivational energy needed to kindle the relationship and to keep it feeling fun and progressive. Intimacy bonds people closer together and creates the feeling of love that inspires people to stay together. Intimacy develops slowly over time and, therefore, requires commitment to increase and intensify. Commitment begins at zero when people first meet and grows until it levels off in a long-term relationship, if supported by passion and intimacy.

Not all loves will reach the level of consummate love. Sternberg cautions that while few may ascend to this peak on the relationship hierarchy, maintaining a consummate love may be more difficult than achieving it. For example, if intimacy is lost over time, the relationship may shift into a less stable pattern, and the other components may be jeopardized without the grounding influence of an intimate emotional connection. However, building greater intimacy may lead to greater passion or commitment, just as greater commitment may lead to greater intimacy and so forth. Whenever the relationship begins to falter, strengthening any point may help elevate and restabilize the triangle. In knowing about these components of love, Sternberg believes that couples may be better able to avoid impending pitfalls in their relationship, work on the areas in need of improvement, or recognize when it is time for a relationship to end.

Shadeen Francis

See also: Attachment Theory of Love; Companionate Love; Intimacy, Sexual and Relational; Lee's Theory of Love Styles; Love; Sternberg's Triangular Theory of Love.

Further Reading

Sternberg, R. J. (1986). A triangular theory of love. *Psychological Review, 93*, 119–135.

Sternberg, R. J. (1988). Triangulating love. In R. J. Sternberg & M. Barnes (Eds.), *The psychology of love* (119–138). New Haven, CT: Yale University Press.

Sternberg, R. J., & Grajek, S. (1984). The nature of love. *Journal of Personality and Social Psychology, 47*, 312–329.

Contraception

"Contraception" refers to all strategies and methods meant to prevent ovulation, prevent sperm from fertilizing the egg, or if fertilization occurs, prevent the fertilized egg from implanting into the uterus. The overall goal is to prevent pregnancy while improving sexual health and well-being. Because 95 percent of sexual activity is practiced for reasons other than procreation, contraception is of prime importance for many people. At the same time, because contraception separates the notions of sexuality and procreation, it continues to raise social, political, ethical, and economic issues in many countries and states. Moreover, although women are the main users of contraceptive methods and have the main responsibility for carrying out contraceptive strategies, the fact remains that conception requires the coming together of two gametes, one male and one female. Despite this fact, the social norms that guide contraception decisions persist in reflecting gender inequalities such that women usually carry the burden of conception decision making on their own. A more inclusive approach would be to acknowledge that both those who possess a vagina and ovaries and those who possess a penis and testicles should be concerned about contraception when they engage in sexual relations.

For women, the fertile period begins at puberty, with the beginning of menstruation. Puberty starts around age twelve years, and menopause, the point at which menstruation ends, occurs around age fifty years. Consequently, a woman is typically fertile about thirty to forty years during her lifetime. The fertile period for men is less well defined because unlike egg production in women, sperm production does not end at a certain age. Men can be fertile into their very advanced years, although their reproductive capacity (in terms of sperm count and spermatozoa motility and morphology) diminishes with age, along with their fertility. Therefore, people who engage in heterosexual relations but do not want to have children generally end up practicing some form of contraception for lengthy periods of time.

The ideal contraceptive is 100 percent effective, convenient, safe, free of adverse side effects, completely reversible, maintenance-free, and affordable (and ideally, free). Furthermore, it should not inhibit sexual activity, and it should be culturally acceptable and protect against sexually transmitted infections (STIs). Unfortunately, this contraceptive method has not yet been invented, which is why the choice of contraceptive strategy or method usually involves a compromise. In practice, a contraceptive strategy or method is selected in light of several factors, such as accessibility, cost, social acceptability, safety, and health risks. A large variety of contraceptive methods is available. Hormonal methods prevent ovulation, thicken the cervical and endometrial mucus to block sperm from entering the uterus, and thin the lining of the uterus to prevent a fertilized egg from implanting. Intrauterine devices are small devices that are inserted into the uterus, where they remain for several years. They act by interrupting the sperm's ability to reach the egg. Barrier methods are physical methods that prevent contact between sperm and ovum, such as a condom or diaphragm. Natural methods do not involve medications, devices, or surgery. Instead, fertility signals are identified and interpreted so that the partners can abstain from penile-vaginal intercourse during the fertile window. Surgical methods, such as a tubal ligation or vasectomy, are generally irreversible and block the passage between sperm and egg. In addition, people often combine methods, for example, using a hormonal method with a condom to prevent STIs.

Contraceptive methods have been around for a long time. Historians and archaeologists have found evidence of contraceptive use by ancient civilizations. Down through the ages, methods have ranged from coitus interruptus (i.e., withdrawal), condoms, vaginal douches, the calendar method, and other barrier methods such as the diaphragm and the cervical cap. The contraceptive pill was first developed in 1960, in the face of impassioned social resistance. At the time, access to the pill required the husband's permission and approval as well as the doctor's. It took repeated battles for women to win the right to make their own choices about contraception and family planning. Since then, several new methods have been developed, refined, and marketed, providing a wider range of choices. When selecting a contraceptive method, the most important criteria for North American women have been reported to be effective prevention of pregnancy (79%), effective prevention of HIV and STIs (67%), and convenience (49%). Fewer than one-quarter of women (22–24%) prioritized a method that was both hormone-free and inexpensive.

In the United States, Canada, and elsewhere around the world, social changes have pushed women to delay having a first child up to an average age of thirty years. This suggests that women who have sexual relations with male partners are exposed to the risk of unintended pregnancy for at least half their life span. Health care clinicians and professionals can play a key role in contraceptive decision making by providing comprehensive and practical information to help women and their partners select and use the method that best fits their needs, priorities, and values. The discussion should also include personal behaviors and circumstances, and in a broader sense, medical, financial, and regulatory problems. All these issues can discourage individuals from obtaining, using, and continuing their preferred conceptive method.

Sylvie Lévesque

See also: Barrier Contraceptive Methods; Birth Control Pills, Estrogen-Progestin; Birth Control Pills, Progestin-Only; Cervical Cap; Cervical Mucus Method; Conception; Condoms, Female (Receptive); Condoms, Male (Insertive); Contraceptive Implants; Contraceptive Injectables; Contraceptive Patch; Diaphragm; Emergency Contraception; Essure Coil; Fertility; Fertility Awareness Methods of Contraception; Intrauterine Device (IUD); Pregnancy; Safer Sex; Sexually Transmitted Infections (STIs); Spermicides; Sponge, Contraceptive; Sterilization; Teen Pregnancy; Tubal Ligation; Vaginal Ring; Vasectomy; Withdrawal Method.

Further Reading

Black, A., Guilbert, E., Costescu, D., Dunn, S., Fisher, W., Kives, S., ... Todd, N. (2015). Consensus canadien sur la contraception (1ere partie de 4). *Journal of Obstetrics and Gynaecology Canada, 37*(10), 939–942.

Briggs, P., Kovacs, G., & Guillebaud, J. (Eds.). (2013). *Contraception: A casebook from menarche to menopause.* Cambridge: Cambridge University Press.

Glasier, A., & Gebbie, A. E. (2008). *Handbook of family planning and reproductive healthcare* (5th ed.). London: Churchill Linvingstone.

Liu, K., Case, A., Cheung, A. P., Sierra, S., AlAsiri, S., Carranza-Mamane, B., ... Hemmings, R. (2011). Âge génésique avancé et fertilité. *Journal of Obstetrics and Gynaecology Canada, 33*(11), 1176–1177.

Marshall, C., Guendelman, S., Mauldon, J., & Nuru□Jeter, A. (2016). Young women's contraceptive decision making: Do preferences for contraceptive attributes align with method choice? *Perspectives on Sexual and Reproductive Health, 48*(3), 119–127.

McVeigh, E., Guillebaud, J., & Homburg, R. (2013). *Oxford handbook of reproductive medicine and family planning.* Oxford: Oxford University Press.

Society of Obstetricians and Gynaecologists of Canada. (2019). Sex & U. Retrieved from www.sexandu.ca

Taylor, H. S., McVeigh, E., Aldad, T. S., Homburg, R., & Guillebaud, J. (2012). *Oxford American handbook of reproductive medicine.* New York: Oxford University Press.

van Lusen, R. H. W. (2013). Myths and misconceptions about sex and con(tra)ception. In P. Briggs, G. Kovacs, & J. Guillebaud (Eds.), *Contraception: A casebook from menarche to menopause.* Cambridge: Cambridge University Press.

Contraceptive Implant

In 1991, the first subdermal long-term reversible contraceptive methods were used in the United States to prevent pregnancy. These contraceptive implants consisted of six matchstick-sized tubes that released hormones into the body for five years. They were taken off the market in 2002, reportedly due to injuries resulting from the difficulty of removing the implant.

A new contraceptive implant was approved by the Federal Drug Administration in 2006. This new implant is much smaller than the previous version, containing just one flexible plastic matchstick-sized tube. A second version of the new implant came out shortly after the first, the only difference being an easier insertion and the ability to track the implant in the body.

The contraceptive implant works by releasing the synthetic hormone progestin etonogestrel directly into a person's bloodstream for three years. These hormones work to prevent pregnancy primarily by preventing ovulation. They also thicken the cervical mucus, preventing sperm from entering the uterus.

In order to get the contraceptive implant, a person needs to go to a health care provider to discuss the method. The health care provider will collect the person's medical information and conduct a physical exam; they can then perform the procedure. During the procedure, the inside of the upper arm is numbed with a painkiller, and the contraceptive implant is surgically inserted under the skin. This procedure typically takes a few minutes.

After three years, a person needs to go back to their health care provider, who will numb the area again, make a tiny cut under the skin, and remove the implant. If the person wanted to continue using the contraceptive implant, the provider can insert another one at that appointment. If someone wanted to get the implant removed prior to the full three years, they would just need to make an appointment with their health care provider.

The contraceptive implant is known to have positive and negative side effects. One common side effect is irregular uterine bleeding within the first six months to one year of use. After this, most people report having fewer and lighter periods. Less common side effects include headaches, nausea, slight weight gain, mood swings, sore breasts, or a change in sexual desire.

The contraceptive implant is one of the most effective methods of birth control. Testing indicates it only has a 0.05 percent failure rate. Since it is a long-acting method, there is little chance for human error. Any person with the implant needs to make sure they get it removed after three years, as after this time the amount of hormones in the implant subside.

The contraceptive implant is a relatively safe method of birth control, though hormones affect different bodies in different ways. It can be used by people who cannot use synthetic forms of estrogen. Sometimes the implant may become dislodged from the section under the arm where it was inserted; this is rare and usually due to an error by the doctor. If this happens, the implant will still work to prevent pregnancy; it just might be more difficult to locate and remove. Because of this, the newest version of the implant has been built with a tracker so that the implant can be more easily found if it becomes dislodged.

Sarah Gannon

See also: Contraception; Contraceptive Injectables; Intrauterine Device (IUD); Pregnancy; Sex Hormones; Synthetic Hormones.

Further Reading

Bedsider. (2018). Implant. Retrieved from https://www.bedsider.org/methods/implant #details

Jones, R. E., & Lopez, K. H. (2014). *Human reproductive biology* (4th ed.). San Diego, CA: Academic Press.

Palomba, S., Falbo, A., Di Cello, A., Materazzo, C., & Zullo, F. (2012). Nexplanon: The new implant for long-term contraception. A comprehensive descriptive review. *Gynecological Endocrinology, 28*(9), 710–721.

Planned Parenthood. (2019). Birth control implant. Retrieved from https://www.plannedparenthood.org/learn/birth-control/birth-control-implant-implanon

Contraceptive Injectables

Contraceptive injectables function in similar ways as oral contraceptives. Most contain only the hormone progestin; over time, this hormone is released into the bloodstream in order to prevent pregnancy. A few newer types of injectables include both progestin and estrogen. Contraceptive injectables are highly effective, easy to use, and can be used by most healthy female individuals. There are currently no contraceptive injectables approved for use in male individuals, but clinical trials to develop this are ongoing.

Contraceptive injectables work by preventing ovulation. They also thicken the cervical mucus, which helps prevent sperm from entering into the female reproductive system, preventing fertilization. Combination injectables also change the uterine environment by thinning the lining of the uterus, which makes it more difficult for implantation to occur if fertilization does take place.

Contraceptive injectables are highly effective. Progestin-only injectables are between 97– 99.7 percent effective. This means that one to three out of every hundred women who use contraceptive injectables as their only means of contraception will become pregnant within one year of use. Combination injectables are slightly less effective, between 94–99 percent effective.

In order to be effective and prevent pregnancy, a person using the progestin-only type of contraceptive injectable needs to get the shot every eight to thirteen weeks, depending on the type used. A person using the combination injectable needs to get the shot every twenty-eight to thirty days (once a month). If a contraceptive injectable is given for the first time during the first five days of a person's menstrual cycle, it is effective immediately after it is injected. If the first dose is given at any other point during the menstrual cycle, another form of contraception, such as condoms, should be used for seven days in order to prevent pregnancy.

There are several benefits of contraceptive injectables. Because they are injected in a doctor's office or sexual health clinic, the individual does not need to remember to take a pill every day. Further, there is no preparation needed prior to sex, such as making sure to have condoms or putting another type of barrier method in place, and there are no interruptions during sexual activity. This also makes them very discreet so the individual can be in complete control of their reproductive health. Some forms of contraceptive injectable have also been approved for helping with the symptoms of endometriosis.

As with all medications, there can be some side effects. A common side effect is irregular bleeding or "spotting," although this tends to get better over time, and some individuals may stop menstruating entirely. Some individuals also report weight gain, mood swings, abdominal pain, dizziness, headache, and fatigue. For individuals who wish to become pregnant after using contraceptive injectables, it may several months, and in some cases up to a year, for fertility to return to normal, depending on the type of injectable used. Combination injectables tend to have fewer side effects than progestin-only injectables. Finally, progestin-only contraceptive injectables have been found to be associated with a loss of bone mineral density, so it is recommended that they not be used for an extended period of time.

Contraceptive injectables do not protect against sexually transmitted infections (STIs) and so a barrier method of STI protection, such as condoms, should also be used.

Heather L. Armstrong

See also: Birth Control Pills, Estrogen-Progestin; Birth Control Pills, Progestin-Only; Contraception; Estrogen; Ovulation; Pregnancy; Progesterone; Sex Hormones; Synthetic Hormones.

Further Reading

Centers for Disease Control and Prevention. (2020). Contraception. Retrieved from https://www.cdc.gov/reproductivehealth/contraception/index.htm

Mayo Clinic. (2020). Depo-Provera (contraceptive injection). Retrieved from https://www.mayoclinic.org/tests-procedures/depo-provera/about/pac-20392204

National Health Service. (2018). The contraceptive injection. Retrieved from https://www.nhs.uk/conditions/contraception/contraceptive-injection/

Contraceptive Patch

In 2001, the Food and Drug Administration approved the use of the transdermal patch, or the birth control patch. The birth control patch is thin, beige, and made of plastic. It sticks to the skin, providing a continuous flow of hormones into the bloodstream, and is used to prevent pregnancy.

A person places a new birth control patch on their skin once a week for three consecutive weeks, followed by one week with no patch. The patch releases synthetic estrogen (ethinyl estradiol) and progesterone (norelgestromin). These hormones work to prevent pregnancy primarily by preventing eggs from leaving the ovaries. The hormones also prevent sperm from meeting an egg by thickening the cervical mucus.

In order to get the contraceptive patch, a person needs to consult with a health care provider and receive a prescription. Once the patches are obtained from a drugstore or pharmacy, a person can place the sticky part of the patch on the skin of the torso (avoiding the breasts), stomach, upper outer arm, back, or buttocks. It is recommended to use the palm to press the patch onto the skin for ten seconds.

At the end of each week, the patch is removed and a new one is placed on a different area of skin. Once a patch has been used for the full week, it should be sealed and thrown in the trash. After changing patches for three weeks, a person then goes patchless for the fourth week when, typically, menstruation is experienced.

The birth control patch is known to have both positive and negative side effects. A common side effect of the patch that users report experiencing is lighter and shorter periods. The patch may also prevent acne and improve menstrual cramping. Some negative side effects include bleeding between periods, nausea, vomiting, and swollen or tender breasts. Typically, these side effects will cease after the first few months of use. Sometimes, long-term side effects might include a negative skin reaction on the area where the patch is placed, vaginal irritation, increased vaginal discharge, or a change in sexual desire.

The patch is very effective in preventing pregnancy and is more than 99 percent effective with perfect use, meaning that a new patch is placed on the correct area of skin on the correct day each week. This ensures the appropriate levels of hormones are circulating in a person's body. With inconsistent use, the patch is 91 percent effective in preventing pregnancy. When someone chooses to stop using the patch, the ability to become pregnant returns quickly.

The patch is a relatively safe method of birth control. However, in some cases and in certain bodies, it may come with more severe risks. These risks are rare but include high blood pressure, gallstones, liver tumors, and jaundice.

Sarah Gannon

See also: Contraception; Contraceptive Implant; Contraceptive Injectables; Pregnancy; Sex Hormones.

Further Reading

Bedsider. (2019). The patch. Retrieved from http://bedsider.org/methods/the_patch#details_tab

Courtney, K. (2006). The contraceptive patch. *AWHONN Lifelines, 10*(3), 250–254.

Jones, R. E., & Lopez, K. H. (2014). *Human reproductive biology* (4th ed.). San Diego, CA: Academic Press.

Planned Parenthood. (2019). Birth control patch. Retrieved from https://www.plannedparenthood.org/learn/birth-control/birth-control-patch

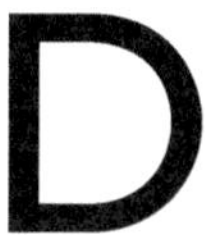

Date Rape

The term "date rape" originally distinguished rapes that occur in an intimate setting with a known person—such as on a date—from rapes perpetrated by strangers. A more appropriate term is "acquaintance rape." While these terms are meant to distinguish between rapes committed by known versus unknown assailants, they are also used to differentiate between "forcible" rape and rapes in which severe physical injuries are not otherwise sustained.

The distinction between forcible rape and date rape is foggy and often at the discretion of reporting officers. Most rapes where the victim knows the assailant are classified as date rapes, regardless of whether additional physical violence was used, as over 50 percent of acquaintance rape victims report using force to try to stop the rape. Since the FBI only collects statistics regarding forcible rape, there may be pressure for various institutions to minimize sexual attacks by classifying them as "date rapes."

The majority of acquaintance rapes occur in nonsexual settings between persons who do not have a sexual relationship. They typically occur when a victim and perpetrator are alone, and they are most common at parties, during visits or study sessions, in cars, or in isolated workplace areas. Only around 13 percent of acquaintance rapes occur during dates. Gang rape—the rape of one person by multiple perpetrators at the same time or in close succession—is presumed to be least common, though all forms are underreported, and neither acquaintance nor gang rape are specifically counted under federal reporting guidelines.

Acquaintance rape may include alcohol or drug intoxication. This may be environmental (such as during a party), or the perpetrator may intentionally give alcohol or drugs to the victim to lower their resistance, select a victim based on their level of intoxication, or drug the victim without their knowledge.

At least one in six women, and possibly as many as one in three, are raped at some point in their lives. The perpetrator and victim know one another in over 90 percent of cases. Fewer than 5 percent of victims report rape to the police. Native American women, who account for slightly over 1 percent of the population, suffer a 35 percent rate of rape; black women, at 13 percent of the population, suffer an 18 percent rate; and white women, at 77 percent of the population, suffer a 17 percent rate. Most acquaintance rape victims are females between the ages of sixteen and twenty-four, and most perpetrators are classmates or friends. Current and past boyfriends are the second-most-common class of perpetrator, and friends of the family and friends' family members are third.

Until 2012, the FBI only recognized attacks against women by men as rape. Estimates of male rape victims are based on self-reports and indicate that as many as one in thirty-three men experience rape at some point in their lives and that up to one-tenth of acquaintance rape victims may be male.

Forcible rape of men is most frequently committed by men who self-identify as heterosexual against men who are perceived to be gay or feminine. Accurate statistics regarding the demographics of victims and perpetrators in male-victim acquaintance rapes are not yet available.

While evidence presented in 2000 by authors Jerrold Greenberg, Clint Bruess, and Debra Haffner indicate that up to 6 percent of rape perpetrators may be female, this percentage appears to include women who participate with male partners in the rape of other women or men as well as women who perpetrate intimate-partner violence within same-gender relationships. Statistics regarding rape of men by women are lacking.

While over one-third of lesbian-identified women and over one-tenth of gay-identified men report being victims of coerced sex, this statistic neither specifically addresses acquaintance rape nor indicates the gender of perpetrators.

Acquaintance rape—along with a host of other sexual crimes, such as harassment, stalking, sexual battery, and unwelcome exposure—occurs much more frequently in association with college campuses than in the general population, with an estimated one in four female college students suffering rape during their time at school. This may be due to a sense of liberty and privacy on the part of perpetrators and a perception of female college students as being alone and vulnerable.

Like all forms of rape, campus rape is underreported, and most statistics come from surveys and self-reports. Acquaintance rape occurs most frequently at the beginning of the school year and primarily targets first- and second-year female students. About 10 percent of campus rapes occur in fraternity housing. Of the remainder, slightly over half occur off-campus, and just under half occur in dorm rooms. According to students' self-reports, campus rape accounts for at least one rape per week on college campuses, though only around 2,500 are reported annually for all campuses nationwide.

Self-reports of perpetrators indicate that a minority of men account for the majority of campus rapes. Virtually all men who acquaintance rape do so more than once, and most who successfully evade report become serial rapists (defined as committing four or more rapes). A study conducted by David Lisak and Paul Miller indicates that serial rapists commit around 90 percent of all campus acquaintance rapes, averaging six each. The assumption is that, as perpetrators get away with rape, they gain confidence and go to greater lengths to strategize and plan their attacks and to groom and isolate potential victims. Athletic teams and fraternities have a strong association with campus rape and account for at least 55 percent of reported gang rapes.

Established intervention strategies tend to focus on the behavior of potential victims, and when given on college campuses, they typically occur at a point in the school year when most acquaintance rapes have already occurred. Colleges may also avoid or downplay rape awareness and prevention to avoid the impression that their campuses are risky. Campus rape statistics, however, make it clear that more effective interventions are necessary.

One strategy based on studying the psychology of rape perpetrators is to train nonrapist men to recognize rapist behavior and intervene on behalf of victims. Like successful antibullying strategies, this creates advocates by eliminating the phenomenon of silent bystanders. Another strategy is to train women and vulnerable others to recognize warning signs in potential perpetrators. For example, most acquaintance rapists engage in victim grooming where they "court" intend victims in a way that is subtly intrusive and aggressive, persistently violating personal space until the uneasiness this engenders "wears off" and they can isolate their victims.

Angela Libal

See also: Rape; Rape, Abuse and Incest National Network (RAINN); Rape Shield Laws; Rape Trauma Syndrome; Sexual Abuse; Sexual Assault; Sexual Harassment; Statutory Rape.

Further Reading

Girls Health. (2015). What is rape and date rape? Retrieved from http://girlshealth.gov/safety/saferelationships/daterape.html

Greenberg, J. S., Bruess, C. E., & Haffner, D. W. (2000). *Exploring the dimensions of human sexuality.* Sudbury, MA: Jones and Bartlett.

Lisak, D., & Miller, P. (2002). Repeat rape and multiple offending among undetected rapists. *Violence and Victims, 17*(1), 73–84.

Sampson, R. (2002). *Acquaintance rape of college students.* Washington, DC: U.S. Department of Justice, Office of Community Oriented Policing Services.

Solnit, R. (2013, January 24). A rape a minute, a thousand corpses a year. *The Nation.* Retrieved from http://www.thenation.com/article/172408/rape-minute-thousand-corpses-year

U.S. Centers for Disease Control and Prevention. (2019). The National Intimate Partner and Sexual Violence Survey (NISVS). Retrieved from http://www.cdc.gov/violenceprevention/nisvs/

Dating

"Dating" is a term that emerged in the early twentieth century as a new iteration of courtship. In order to appreciate the magnitude of the shift from dating to courtship, and all the factors affecting this change and resulting from it, one must first understand courtship. Courtship describes the process leading up to marriage and procreation, which includes mate selection, relationship formation, and partnership. At various times and geographical locations, different things are valued in the selection of a mate, and the process by which one is selected varies as well. In cultures where arranged or assisted marriage is practiced, spouses may be chosen in infancy or childhood, so courtship could occur in childhood or at the time of marriage. In these locales, "dating" may not exist at all.

Prior to industrialization, family served a very specific economic function, and children were needed to help perform agricultural labor. At this time, the average life span was shorter, and fertility rates were higher. Adults married at a young age and could expect to raise many children before they died. Because marriage was valuable economically to both families, the family of origin was important in guiding young people into relationships and evaluating the suitability of a mate. The emphasis was on family worth (or name) and economic stability. Since women were expected to be financially dependent on their husbands, a good suitor was a male who would be able to be a good provider (Bailey, 1989).

After industrialization, work moved from the family to the factory, resulting in a gendered division of labor within the family and a more defined class system. It was during this time that women were encouraged to actualize their "natural" instincts of childbearing. Despite the lack of necessity to have more hands on the farm, this ideology kept fertility rates high. Also during this time, the family of origin was the judge of appropriate mates for both men and women. Dating, or courtship, during these times took place with the family present. Young adults would meet at family, school, or church functions, and they rarely spent time together without a chaperone. Courting at this time was regulated by the family; it was a social norm for young men to "call" on young women and socialize with the young woman and her mother. Control of this process belonged to the women, as they established days and times to receive callers, and it was they who invited callers to visit. Calling was enmeshed within the middle class, as middle-class homes had parlors where young women could receive callers. Dating first emerged among the working class, who often lived in dwellings that did not facilitate calling, so working-class youth were forced to socialize outside of the home.

The advent of the automobile at the turn of the twentieth century gave opportunity for affluent youth to spend time together socially without supervision. However, the affordability of the Model T Ford expanded this access to the middle class, which enabled young men to take young women out on "dates." This brought courtship out of the home and into public and marked the beginning of the shift away from the family as the regulators of young adults' choices of mates, since this period also marked the emergence of media giving advice on dating and relationships. This advice, often in the form of magazine articles or etiquette manuals, served as a referent against which people judged behavior and made decisions.

In addition to the shift out of the home, dating had other significant aspects relating to the control of the date. Dates required money and places to go, such as theaters and dance halls. In fact, something was often considered a date when money was spent, and it was the man's money spent on the woman. This is important, as control of the date shifted to the man by virtue of his paying for it as well as it taking place in the public, male, sphere. Etiquette at this time instructed women not to pay or offer to pay for dates and instructed that there were certain places where "respectable" women should not go.

In the nineteenth century, dating was framed in language relating to home and family, while in the next century, these metaphors shifted to those relating to capitalism. As American society was experiencing abundance, the emphasis in dating was also abundance: youth were instructed to date as many people as possible, and those without dates faced stigma. Not only was having a date important, but one gained status from having the "right" date. The right man was one with financial resources and the ability to pay for many dates. The right girl was one who was popular and highly sought after by others. Youth would "rate" their peers to determine popularity and suitability. "Rating and dating" echoed the themes of competition inherent in capitalism, and the public nature of dating allowed for this competition to be enacted in view of others, reinforcing the significance of the peer group as an appraiser of status and popularity. Being seen out with a highly popular young woman afforded the young man status, while "getting stuck" with one partner on the dance floor, by not having another man cut in, was a catastrophic marker of unpopularity for young women.

Rating and dating, and the spirit of competition within dating, remained common until World War II. During the war years, most young men went to war, so the ratio of women to men changed. Competition flourished when there were more available men, but during and after the war, women outnumbered "marriageable" men. Economically, too, the trend shifted from competition to scarcity, and this was reflected in dating changes. After the war, the concept of "going steady," or only dating one person with the intention of hopefully marrying, emerged. The average age at marriage began to decline after a rise during the Depression, as the fear of being alone encouraged youth to marry young, which encouraged dating at younger ages than before. By 1950, children as young as twelve experienced "going steady," and among older youth, having a steady partner was the marker of status and popularity.

Steady relationships, and the public consumption they encouraged, remained popular until the 1960s, when there was widespread social change. Feminism took root, and many of the conventional restrictions on young adult behavior, specifically young women's behavior, relaxed. Young people began to spend time in mixed-sex groups, and mechanisms for relationship formation changed as well. The availability of oral contraception affected patterns of relationships and intimacy, since it allowed people the availability of sexual intercourse without concern of pregnancy. In spite of these changes, conceptions of dating remained fairly consistent through the 1990s.

Media has been used to assist dating and mate selection since the 1960s, but the advent of the internet has expanded this with the introduction of online dating, which allows users to expand their network of potential partners as well as to manage self-presentation in the hopes of attracting a mate. The use of internet technology is continuing to expand, allowing for users of all social classes, and as it does, so does social acceptance of internet dating and the decrease of stigma associated with it. The proliferation of online dating sites, and the specificity of such sites, allows people to seek out partners with very specific characteristics, as there are sites designed to find a partner with a specific religion, income, height, and even health status, such as having HIV or HSV, which may help to offset some of the perceived risks that are associated with online dating.

Internet technology also fosters a sense of instant gratification, and this has also affected dating trends, encouraging the shift to hooking up among emergent adults. Hookups allow people to engage in sexual activity without the time or monetary expenditure involved in dating, and social media technology facilitates communication to arrange for such encounters as well as providing a platform for peers to comment on one's relationship. For these reasons, hookup culture has become quite prominent as a mechanism for relationship formation, in some circumstances replacing traditional dating.

Many studies of dating and courtship focus on youth and emergent adults. Recent work has begun to examine the process of dating in midlife. Adults reentering the dating scene after the end of a long-term relationship are often challenged by a cultural emphasis on partnering and a focus on physical appearance. Older individuals may be influenced by courtship norms from their youth and, thus, may be unprepared to negotiate contraception use. This makes older adults specifically vulnerable to sexually transmitted infections. Adults in midlife often approach dating with an emphasis on gains and losses and may partner up for the purposes of companionship, financial assistance, a need for a caretaker, or sexual gratification. Midlife women who are financially stable may fear a partner will take advantage of or manipulate them. For midlife adults, the internet is also perceived as risky, leading women to engage in different kinds of dates to increase safety, such as the interview date, a public meeting to evaluate safety in hopes of a subsequent romantic date, or the companion date, a platonic friend to socialize with, devoid of physical intimacy.

Rachel Kalish

See also: Adolescent Sexuality; Casual Sex; Dating, Cross-Cultural Comparison of; Friends with Benefits; Hookup Culture; Marriage; Online Dating; Serial Monogamy; Sexual Revolution.

Further Reading

Bailey, B. L. (1989). *From front porch to back seat: Courtship in twentieth century America.* Baltimore: Johns Hopkins University Press.

Bergdal, A. R., Kraft, J. M., Andes, K., Carter, M., Hatfield-Timajchy, L., & Hock-Long, L. (2012). Love and hooking up in the new millennium: Communication technology and relationships among urban African American and Puerto Rican young adults. *Journal of Sex Research, 49,* 570–582.

Bogle, K. A. (2008). *Hooking up: Sex, dating and relationships on campus.* New York: New York University Press.

Couch, D., & Liamputtong, P. (2008). Online dating and mating: The use of the internet to meet sexual partners. *Qualitative Health Research, 18,* 268–279.

England, P., & Thomas, R. J. (2007). The decline of the date and the rise of the college hook up. In A. S. Skolnick & J. H. Skolnick (Eds.), *Family in transition* (14th ed., 151–162). Boston: Allyn & Bacon.

Laner, M. R., & Ventrone, N. A. (2000). Dating scripts revisited. *Journal of Family Issues, 21,* 488–500.

Lichtenstein, B. (2012). Starting over: Dating risks and sexual health among midlife women after relationship dissolution. In L. M. Carpenter & J. DeLamater (Eds.), *Sex for life: From virginity to Viagra, how sexuality changes throughout our lives* (180–197). New York: New York University Press.

Waller, W. (1937). The rating and dating complex. *American Sociological Review, 2,* 727–734.

Dating, Cross-Cultural Comparison of

Dating is a system whereby persons who are not currently in a civil or religious marriage develop a mutual romantic attachment to one another through a series of personal encounters. When dating is defined by strict cultural norms with the specific intention of facilitating a marriage, it is referred to as courtship. The intention, trajectory, length, and expectations of dating tend to change significantly over time and to vary across cultures.

Broadly defined, "dating" may include a constellation of relationships ranging from friendly group recreational outings to one-on-one intimate partnerships that include cohabitation and childrearing. Traditionally, "dating" refers to a mate selection process, the ultimate intention of which is civil or religious marriage. The types of behaviors that constitute dating, and the extent to which these behaviors are encouraged, tolerated, or forbidden, vary powerfully between different ethnic, social, and religious cultures even within a single time and place.

In the traditional dating-as-prelude-to-marriage system, it is predominantly young, never-married persons who date. As social expectations shift, the dating demographic expands. As age of first marriage rises and fewer people ever marry, it is now common throughout the United States for persons in all age groups from puberty onward to engage in dating relationships. This includes single, divorced, and widowed persons, regardless of their intentions to marry or remarry. It may also include polyamorous people—persons who simultaneously engage in multiple committed relationships—regardless of their current marital status.

Since the Christianization of the Roman Empire and the European Conquest, dating and courtship have been confined to heterosexual, or mixed-sex, pairings throughout most of the world. However, in most industrialized nations, it is now possible for people to date and court within their own gender openly and with relative freedom.

Since the 1950s, it has been common for persons in most ethnic groups within the United States to begin dating in their early teens but not marry until much later: typically in their early twenties for Latin Americans, late twenties for whites, and late twenties to early thirties for blacks. In traditional Asian homes where education is highly valued, young people often do not begin dating until their undergraduate studies are well underway or completed and they are considered ready to marry, typically in their early twenties. In general, same-sex dating tends to commence at a later age, often after the individuals have begun living independently.

In cultures that practice arranged marriages, an acquaintanceship period similar to courtship or dating may or may not be present. In some Orthodox Jewish communities, parents and professional matchmakers bring couples together. Traditionally, the relationship begins with betrothal, approximately one year before the wedding. At betrothal, the marriage contract is signed, and the man (or couple) is expected to spend the upcoming year purchasing a home and otherwise preparing economically to set up a household. In traditional communities, actual cohabitation and sexual relations do not begin until the wedding. If a couple finds themselves incompatible during betrothal, they can leave the relationship but must do so through a formal religious divorce proceeding. In non-Orthodox communities, the formal betrothal ceremony may be retained but is usually performed on the same day as the wedding ceremony.

Certain fundamentalist Christian movements within and outside the United States also practice arranged marriages, which are usually negotiated by the couple's fathers. In many traditional Asian cultures, families negotiate with one another to bring couples together. In some cases, the active players are the parents; in others, all older immediate and extended relatives expect to participate in the matchmaking. In many cultures, including Korean, Chinese, and Laotian, the couple is introduced and may begin to date once the match is approved, and each partner has veto power; but in a few cultures, such as many from India, the couple does not traditionally meet until the wedding.

Where dates occur also varies between cultures. In dominant American culture, dating activities and locations primarily vary with the age of participants. For young adolescents, dating partners may primarily spend time with one another at school or during other group social activities without any formal "dates" occurring at all. Older teens with access to transportation may go on formal or informal dates by themselves or with larger groups of friends. College-age teens and adults might spend time together in residences, go on formal dates, or engage in public social activities together. Independent adults may extend the dating relationship indefinitely, going on formal and informal dates, splitting time between each other's residences, and eventually cohabitating.

In some cultures, parents expect their children's dates to be chaperoned. Young Mormon couples, for example, are expected to primarily see each other at church and during church-oriented group activities. Korean girls traditionally bring a female friend to chaperone public dates, while it is considered indecent for unmarried Japanese and Chinese couples to be seen alone in public at all. In these cases, dates either take place in groups or within the family home. Among these cultures, all physical displays of affection are strongly discouraged, and unaccompanied public dates typically signal a couple's intention to marry.

Norms for establishing a dating relationship, and the expected outcome of such relationships, change dramatically throughout time. For example, in the nineteenth century, middle- and upper-class white people established dating relationships at the woman's invitation, with her parents' permission. Her suitors would visit her in her parents' home under their eye; "keeping steady company" and being seen together in public were tantamount to announcing engagement. With the rise of the automobile and public entertainment in the 1920s, dating became a public, unchaperoned activity, but being seen with different dating partners remained the norm until a couple was engaged. Which gender could initiate dating varied based on local culture, socioeconomic class, and ethnic group. It was not until after World War II that "going steady" became the norm and women were expected to wait for men to initiate dating.

In contemporary American culture, a person may ask another on a date regardless of gender, though expectations vary somewhat with region and cultural identification. The expectation that men will take the initiative to establish a heterosexual dating relationship is more common among black and Latin Americans than among whites, and among teenagers and older adults than young and middle-aged adults.

In some communities, such as among certain very traditional South American cultures, custom requires a male to gain permission from a female's parents before commencing a dating relationship; in others, such as African American, non-Orthodox Jewish, and some Korean and Chinese American communities, being introduced to a dating partner's parents and family signals the seriousness of the relationship and possibly the intent to marry. This is in contrast to many traditional Asian, Orthodox Jewish, and certain fundamentalist Christian communities, where heterosexual couples are introduced to one another by the parents.

For LGBTQ+ persons, establishing a dating relationship can have additional complications, since it often involves sensitive information such as determining the sexual orientation, and sometimes the gender, of the person of interest and possibly coming out oneself, which in some communities may still carry the actual risk of violent attack or extreme social censure.

Traditionally, the purpose of dating was to assess potential heterosexual marriage partners. However, as the stigma attached to sexual relationships between unmarried people declines, the purposes of dating and types of dating relationships have multiplied. For mixed-sex couples, dating may now lead to cohabitation and childrearing outside of marriage or may be entered into for temporary companionship or casual sex. For same-sex couples, dating may now be conducted openly with the express purpose of eventually marrying and establishing a family—dramatic shifts that have slowly developed since the sexual revolution of the 1960s and 1970s.

When sex is considered acceptable, and between whom, is the most emotionally charged issue associated with dating. According to the Pew Research Center, as of 2014, sex between unmarried persons is considered morally unacceptable by 30 percent of the U.S. population and 46 percent of persons globally, while homosexuality is considered morally unacceptable by 37 percent of persons in the United States and 59 percent of persons globally (Poushter, 2014). These opinions, combined with those on associated issues such as contraception (7 percent unacceptable in the United States and 14 percent worldwide) and divorce (22 percent unacceptable in the United States and 24 percent worldwide) affect when sex is considered appropriate, types of sex considered acceptable, and expectations regarding how sex fits into a couple's plans to marry.

The fact that only 46 percent of U.S. children now live in households with two married, heterosexual parents who have only been married to each other testifies that statements regarding the acceptability of various sexual, partnership, and reproductive choices only represent broad generalizations. Typically, however, stigma against sex outside of marriage is much stronger the younger a couple is and relaxes the further they move into adulthood and financial independence. Stigma against nonmarital sex also tends to relax for persons who are divorced, widowed, or LGBTQ+; for persons of dominant racial and ethnic groups and higher socioeconomic classes; and in urban, multiethnic populations.

In some populations, such as certain LGBTQ+ and heterosexual subcultures, it is relatively common for a sexual encounter to occur outside of a dating relationship or to signal the beginning of a dating relationship. In others, sex is popularly considered acceptable after a certain level of commitment has been established, either by completing a certain number of formal dates, dating for a certain period of time, exchanging specific tokens of affection, or announcing an engagement. A growing number of people, especially those in urban areas, place more importance on cohabitating or coparenting as indicators of relationship commitment and stability than on traditional expressions such as engagement or marriage.

Sex outside of marriage is considered least acceptable in traditional Asian and Asian American communities; fundamentalist Christian and Islamic communities; and Orthodox Jewish, Mormon, and Hindu communities, where even sexual expression within marriage is strictly governed by rules regarding modesty, chastity, and family relationships.

Considering the extent to which moral expectations around sexual expression vary based on age, ethnicity, culture, religion, sexual orientation, level of education, and subculture, expectations regarding the timing and acceptability of sex within dating relationships are likely to continue to rapidly evolve and fluctuate with overall shifts in global and U.S. society.

Angela Libal

See also: Dating; Hookup Culture; Marriage, Cross-Cultural Comparison of; Online Dating; Polyamory; Public Displays of Affection.

Further Reading

Jackson, P. B., Kleiner, S., Geist, C., & Cebulko, K. (2011). Conventions of courtship: Gender and race differences in the significance of dating rituals. *Journal of Family Issues, 32*(5), 629–652.

Poushter, J. (2014). What's morally acceptable? It depends on where in the world you live. Retrieved from http://www.pewresearch.org/fact-tank/2014/04/15/whats-morally-acceptable-it-depends-on-where-in-the-world-you-live/

Sex Info Online. (2018). The history of dating in America. Retrieved from https://sexinfo.soc.ucsb.edu/article/history-dating-america

Wang, W., & Parker, K. (2014). Record share of Americans have never married as values, economics and gender patterns change. Retrieved from http://www.pewsocialtrends.org/2014/09/24/record-share-of-americans-have-never-married/

Demisexuality

Demisexuality describes a sexual orientation in which sexual attraction and expression are based on a strong emotional and personal connection rather than on physical appearance or sexual desire. Demisexuality is often placed under the umbrella of asexuality and has been considered a way to further describe those who may not readily experience sexual attraction and desire.

Those who identify as asexual make up about 1 percent of the world's population, and it is thought that those who identify as demisexual represent a steadily increasing portion of this group. The term "demisexual" comes from the idea that the orientation is "halfway" between sexual and asexual; yet this is not to suggest that demisexuals have half, or somehow incomplete, sexualities. As with all sexual orientations, demisexuality will be different for different people. Some demisexuals may only experience attraction to a handful of people (or less) during their lives. And while some demisexuals may report at times experiencing strong sexual desire, their expression of sexual attraction and desire is based on an established emotional connection. Hookups, excessive sexual experimentation, one-night stands, and even flirting may not be desirable to those with a demisexual orientation.

Demisexuality has been gaining visibility around the world, thanks largely to internet communities like the Asexual Visibility and Education Network (AVEN) and Asexuality India. These platforms have increased the opportunity for individuals to learn, discuss, and meet other individuals with similar lived experiences and identities. Members of the demisexual community advocate to increase visibility and representation of demisexuals in media, politics, education, and advocacy to bring greater awareness of demisexuality and representation of demisexual-identified folk in society.

Despite growing awareness, little research exists about demisexuality or the experiences of those who identify as demisexual. As such, much of the information available comes from personal accounts in brief op-eds as well as other print and online articles. Further study of demisexuality may help individuals navigate their own experiences with demisexuality and may help promote increased understanding and acceptance of this sexual orientation.

Shadeen Francis and Patrick R. Grant

See also: Asexuality; Sexual Orientation.

Further Reading

D'Silva, M. D. (2017, December 4). Are you a demisexual? *DNA*. Retrieved from https://www.dnaindia.com

Hosie, R. (2017, August 28). What is demisexuality? *The Independent*. Retrieved from https://www.independent.co.uk

Kumar, S. (2017, March 18). Meet India's newest sexual minority: The asexuals. *The Hindustan Times*. Retrieved from https://www.hindustantimes.com

Williams, M. (2016, November 2016). I'm demisexual: It takes me a while to feel physical attraction. *The Washington Post*. Retrieved from https://www.washingtonpost.com

Dental Dam

Dental dams are square pieces of latex or silicon-based material that can be used during oral sex on the penis, vulva, vagina, and anus to prevent the spread of sexually transmitted infections (STIs). Many people are unaware that STIs can be spread through oral-genital contact; however, transmission is possible for many STIs, including herpes, gonorrhea, and chlamydia. Dental dams are available in a variety of colors, and some may be flavored.

By design, dental dams are used by dentists to isolate teeth or parts of the mouth for certain procedures. The dams help keep the area dry to improve the performance of adhesives and composite materials. They also prevent instruments or parts of drilled teeth from falling into the oral cavity of the patient. Dental dams are also important protection for the patient and the dental team from body fluids that could carry infectious bacteria or viruses. Because of their ability to prevent transfer of fluids, dental dams have also become popular among some for use in oral-genital and oral-anal sex to help prevent the transmission of diseases, including HIV.

Dental dams allow a person to stimulate the genitals or anus of their partner without the risk of contact with bodily fluids, which can carry STIs. In order to use a dental dam, the sheet is spread over the vulva or anus and can be held in place by either partner's hands. Because the material of the dam is very thin, sexual stimulation with the tongue and mouth can be performed without the risk of STI transmission. Experts recommend that dams be disposed of after one use to prevent possible infection. It is also important never to flip the dam over, so only one side must be used.

Despite the benefits of using dental dams, they can be hard to find to purchase. If a dental dam is not available, a condom can be used by cutting off both ends of the condom and then cutting up the length of the condom and rolling it out into a square. This square can then be placed over the genitals or anus before oral sex.

Latex dams may cause irritation for those with latex allergies, so silicon and polyurethane dams are also available.

Tim J. Watts

See also: Condoms, Female (Receptive); Condoms, Male (Insertive); Oral Sex; Sexually Transmitted Infections (STIs).

Further Reading

Centers for Disease Control and Prevention. (2016). Dental dam use. Retrieved from https://www.cdc.gov/condomeffectiveness/Dental-dam-use.html

Galan, N. (2018). Dental dams: Everything you need to know. Retrieved from https://www.medicalnewstoday.com/articles/323768.php

Desire

Sexual desire (also known as libido or sex drive) is considered to be an individual's psychological state where there is a want, need, desire, or appetite for sexual activity of some kind. It is a term that might seem straightforward but actually encompasses physiological drives and processes, cognitions, behaviors, emotions, motivations, subjective experiences, and many other unknown factors. The exact physiological, cognitive, emotional, and behavioral mechanisms that create and interact with sexual desire are not yet fully understood. However, it has been said that desire (an appetite for sexual activity) to some extent can be compared with hunger (an appetite for food). An individual may feel hunger due to internal cues (a memory of food or growling stomach) or external cues (walking past a bakery or a friend asking if they want lunch), but whether or not they take action to seek out food to sate this appetite depends on many factors. These include the level of hunger they are feeling, their ability to tolerate this hunger, the individual's proximity to food, their emotions relating to food in that moment, their thoughts about food, past experiences with food, the motivation to physically source food, and ultimately a decision about whether to eat or not. While sexual desire is thought of as the desire for sex, it is ultimately one of many factors that determine whether an individual will engage in sexual activity or not.

Sexual desire has typically been considered to be spontaneous and the first phase of the human sexual response; however, it is now known that it can also be experienced as responsive. Responsive desire is desire that occurs at any point in the sexual response cycle, with individuals (particularly females) being able to feel aroused without desire and to experience desire as a response to arousal. This means that desire does not always need to be present prior to the commencement of sexual activity as many individuals choose to engage in sexual behavior without, or prior to, any sense of sexual desire. However, as sexual activity continues, desire often begins or increases in response to the sexual situation.

The current understanding of the mechanisms of sexual desire is extremely limited, but there is some knowledge about some of the cognitive, behavioral, and physiological aspects of this state. Historically, the cognitive element of desire has been considered to be sexual fantasy, although this has been expanded to include many other internal sexual cues that may lead to sexual desire, including thoughts and memories. Sexual fantasies or daydreams can occur during or outside of sexual activity, can be spontaneous or intentional, and can include any mental imagery that is arousing to the individual.

Behind these cognitive elements of desire are complex mixes of physiological mechanisms, including hormones and neurotransmitters, that serve to make sexual desire possible. At the start of the sexual response cycle is a release of steroid hormones such as norepinephrine and oxytocin, which cause the individual to pay more attention to sexual cues. Dopamine and melanocortin assist with the stimulation of attention and desire and downregulate the inhibitory systems, meaning that the individual is more likely to act on their desire. Following sexual reward (often orgasm but may be other rewards, such as a sense of bonding or emotional warmth), endocannabinoids and serotonin begin the refractory period and give the individual a sense of satiation or satisfaction.

Despite these mechanisms, it is not actually necessary for desire to be present prior to engaging in sexual activity, as research indicates that 82 percent of all females and 60 percent of men will regularly participate in sexual activity without desire. This is an important distinction, as desire is commonly equated to the amount of sexual activity in which a person engages. Regardless, researchers have historically measured levels of desire through frequency of sexual activity, with the assumption that if desire is present it will lead to sexual behavior. In reality, desire is more closely related to the hunger analogy provided above with many factors influencing whether the experience of sexual desire turns into actual sexual activity. It is also important to note that sexual desire includes desire for sexual activity of any type, including fantasy alone, masturbation, and sexual acts with other individuals.

One question that is often raised is "How much desire is normal?" Research has found that levels of sexual desire vary widely from one person to the next and also vary dramatically for some individuals from day to day as well as at different times in their lives. Many things influence an individual's sexual desire, including their age, health, psychological well-being, beliefs, stress and fatigue, relationship status, and relationship satisfaction. A "normal" level of sexual desire can only be determined by considering each individual's own particular set of circumstances.

Rebecca Frost

See also: Arousal; Desire, Models of; Desire Discrepancy; Desire Disorders; Fantasy, Sexual and Erotic.

Further Reading

Bancroft, J. (2010). Sexual desire and the brain. *Sexual and Relationship Therapy, 25*(2), 172–188.

Basson, R. (2002). Rethinking low sexual desire in women. *BJOG: An International Journal of Obstetrics & Gynaecology, 109*(4), 357–363.

Beck, J. G., Bozman, A. W., & Qualtrough, T. (1991). The experience of sexual desire: Psychological correlates in a college sample. *The Journal of Sex Research, 28*(3), 443–456.

Kaplan, H. S. (1979). *Disorders of sexual desire.* New York: Simon and Schuster.

Leitenberg, H., & Henning, K. (1995). Sexual fantasy. *Psychological Bulletin, 117*(3), 469–496.

Pfaus, J. G. (2009). Pathways of sexual desire. *The Journal of Sexual Medicine, 6*(6), 1506–1533.

Desire, Models of

There is not currently one all-encompassing sexual desire model but instead several different models of sexual desire, including the triphasic model introduced by Helen Singer Kaplan (1979) and Rosemary Basson's circular model of female sexual response (2000). The triphasic model can be considered as a timeline of the human sexual response with desire as one of the "phases," while the circular model was developed as a model of female sexual response and includes both spontaneous and responsive sexual desire.

Helen Singer Kaplan's model of sexual response was based on the four-phase model proposed previously by Masters and Johnson. Importantly, Masters and Johnson's model did not include sexual desire. The four phases of this model are excitement, plateau, orgasm, and resolution. Kaplan revised this model to include the three stages of desire, excitement, and orgasm.

Within the linear models, desire was traditionally considered as the original appetite for sexual activity and the first phase of the sexual response. Arousal was then considered to be the second phase and the physiological aspect of the beginning of sexual response. Although desire and arousal were described as two separate phases, there is now some confusion as to whether these are two distinct or overlapping experiences, and some researchers are now considering these to be so highly linked that they need to be considered together.

Despite their widespread acceptance, the linear models of sexual response as proposed by Kaplan and Masters and Johnson have been found lacking, especially when applied to the female experience. After many years of conducting clinical work with women with low desire, Rosemary Basson (2000) arrived at a new model of sexual response, which may be more representative of sexual response, especially for females. In keeping with more contemporary theory and research showing the overlap between desire and arousal, as well as research on women's motivations for sex, this model is based more on intimacy and emotion than the pure behavioral and physiological model proposed by Masters and Johnson. The circular model highlights that people, especially females, are often sexually neutral at the beginning of a sexual experience and that they may choose to engage in sexual activity for one of many reasons (sexual or otherwise). In response to the beginning of sexual activity, they then experience subjective or physiological arousal, which then leads to experiencing desire to continue with the sexual experience. The most important change in Basson's model is the introduction of the idea that people may be more likely to experience "responsive" (desire that occurs after arousal or the start of sexual activity) rather than "spontaneous" desire (where desire is present and drives the sexual activity). It is believed that sexual satisfaction or nonsexual rewards such as emotional intimacy that occur as a result of being responsive and experiencing sexual activity is reinforcing and will facilitate the recurrence of responsiveness in future sexual experiences.

Rebecca Frost

See also: Arousal; Basson, Rosemary; Desire; Desire Discrepancy; Desire Disorders; Johnson, Virginia; Kaplan, Helen Singer; Kaplan's Triphasic Model; Masters, William H.; Masters and Johnson Four-Stage Model of Sexual Response.

Further Reading

Basson, R. (2000). The female sexual response: A different model. *Journal of Sex & Marital Therapy, 26*(1), 51–65.

Basson, R. (2002). Rethinking low sexual desire in women. *BJOG: An International Journal of Obstetrics & Gynaecology, 109*(4), 357–363.

Kaplan, H. S. (1979). *Disorders of sexual desire.* New York: Simon and Schuster.

Masters, W. H., & Johnson, V. E. (1966). *Human sexual response.* Toronto: Bantam Books.

Meana, M. (2010). Elucidating women's (hetero)sexual desire: Definitional challenges and content expansion. *Journal of Sex Research, 47*(2–3), 104–122.

Desire Discrepancy

Sexual desire discrepancy is most often defined as differing levels of sexual desire between two partners. Therefore, in a relationship where one partner reports a greater desire for sexual activity than their partner, a desire discrepancy is said to exist. While sexual desire discrepancy is not always distressing in relationships, it has been found to be the most distressing sexual issue that couples face. This is largely due to the negative impact that desire discrepancy has on sexual and relationship well-being and satisfaction. Often, this discrepancy in desired frequency of sexual activity is associated with more obvious negative impacts in relationships of longer duration.

Similar to other sexual health problems, sexual desire discrepancy can occur for many reasons. Because of the many contributing factors, it is best to use an approach that includes an assessment of biological, psychological, and sociocultural factors (known as a biopsychosocial approach) to understand these layers of influence. For instance, when a couple experiences conflict and distress because of a discrepancy around sexual desire or sexual activity, one might first look at biological factors at play: hormones, medical issues, current medications, weight, physical ability, and so on. Next, one might explore psychological wellness: each individual's mental health, symptoms of anxiety, depression, body image, or self-esteem. In addition, one would want to explore social and cultural factors that might affect sexual desire: current stage of life (e.g., pregnancy, early parenthood), external stressors (e.g., job stress, financial strain), cultural or religious factors (e.g., restrictive attitudes about sex, history of sexual shaming), gender roles, and relational dynamics (e.g., power differences, conflict, fighting). Together any or all of these factors can interact and affect sexual desire.

It is important to note that, historically, issues of sexual desire have been seen as an individual issue. In dealing with sexual desire discrepancy, however, the primary objective is to focus on the distress caused by the discrepancy, therefore making it a relational problem. Depending on the factors that have contributed to and exacerbated the sexual desire discrepancy, sex therapy treatment focuses on assisting both partners in addressing underlying concerns; improving communication, connection, and intimacy; and addressing any other co-occurring sexual or mental health issues. For instance, often when a male partner experiences low desire, it is coupled with an ejaculatory or erectile issue. Therefore, it is also necessary to address the extenuating sexual health concerns during the treatment process.

Abby Girard

See also: Desire; Desire, Models of; Desire Disorders; Psychosexual Therapy.

Further Reading

Bridges, S. K., & Horne, S. G. (2007). Sexual satisfaction and desire discrepancy in same-sex women's relationships. *Journal of Sex & Marital Therapy, 33*(1), 41–53.

Mark, K. P., & Murray, S. H. (2012). Gender differences in desire discrepancy as a predictor of sexual and relationship satisfaction in a college sample of heterosexual romantic relationships. *Journal of Sex & Marital Therapy, 38*(2), 198–215.

Desire Disorders

There is no commonly agreed on definition of what constitutes "normal" sexual desire; however, the American Psychiatric Association's *Diagnostic and Statistical Manual, Fifth Edition* (*DSM-5*) includes two desire disorders: female sexual interest/arousal disorder and male hypoactive sexual desire disorder. While the diagnostic criteria differ for males and females, both are disorders that can be diagnosed when an individual experiences abnormally low sexual desire as well as distress as a result of their level of desire.

There is a lack of research into disorders of sexual desire, despite their high prevalence, and there is a false prevailing belief in the clinical community that sexual disorders are well understood. Desire dysfunction (the presence of symptoms without distress) and disorders are the most prevalent of female sexual dysfunctions and disorders, having been found to occur in 26 percent to 55 percent of the population depending on measurement; they are less prevalent (approximately half as common) but potentially more distressing in men. One of the most obvious differences in sexual behavior between males and females is their disparate levels of desire, with 51.4 percent of men experiencing sexual desire at least daily compared to 7 percent of women. A less pronounced result occurs when measuring desire for sexual activity, with 23 percent of men desiring to have sex daily or more often compared to only 8.3 percent of women. Of course, any diagnosis of a desire disorder needs to be placed within the context of the large but normal range of an individual's desire across age, stage of life, and relationship factors. It requires the clinician to judge whether the deficiency or absence of desire is sufficient to diagnose the disorder within the context of that individual's life circumstances, even though little is known about the distinctions between normal, healthy levels of desire and levels that constitute a dysfunction. Therefore, many clinicians now consider desire disorders to frequently be an issue of desire discrepancy within a couple rather than a disorder of the individual.

Low sexual desire is considered notoriously difficult to treat by clinicians from many backgrounds, including psychology, psychiatry, and gynecology. To date, there has been limited controlled research into the treatment of desire disorders, and no medications are currently proven to be effective for treating desire disorders. Trials for psychological therapy have shown only moderate effects. Currently, popular treatments for desire disorders include cognitive behavioral therapy, sensate focus, mindfulness-based treatments, and emotion-focused therapy for couples.

Rebecca Frost

See also: Desire; Desire, Models of; Desire Discrepancy; *Diagnostic and Statistical Manual of Mental Disorders (DSM)*; Sensate Focus; Sexual Disorders, Female; Sexual Disorders, Male.

Further Reading

American Psychiatric Association. (2013). *Diagnostic and statistical manual of mental disorders* (5th ed.). Arlington, VA: America Psychiatric Association.

Basson, R. (2002). Rethinking low sexual desire in women. *BJOG: An International Journal of Obstetrics & Gynaecology, 109*(4), 357–363.

Beck, J. G., Bozman, A. W., & Qualtrough, T. (1991). The experience of sexual desire: Psychological correlates in a college sample. *The Journal of Sex Research, 28*(3), 443–456.

Brotto, L. A. (2010). The DSM diagnostic criteria for hypoactive sexual desire disorder in women. *Archives of Sexual Behavior, 39*(2), 221–239.

Brotto, L. A. (2010). The DSM diagnostic criteria for hypoactive sexual desire disorder in men. *The Journal of Sexual Medicine, 7*(6), 2015–2030.

Heiman, J. R. (2002). Psychologic treatments for female sexual dysfunction: Are they effective and do we need them? *Archives of Sexual Behavior, 31*(5), 445–450.

Rissel, C. E., Richters, J., Grulich, A. E., Visser, R. O., & Smith, A. M. A. (2003). Sex in Australia: Selected characteristics of regular sexual relationships. *Austraian and New Zealand Journal of Public Health, 27*(2), 124–130.

Shifren, J. L., Monz, B. U., Russo, P. A., Segreti, A., & Johannes, C. B. (2008). Sexual problems and distress in United States women. *Obstetrics & Gynecology, 112*(5), 970–978.

DHEA

Dehydroepiandrosterone (DHEA) is a hormone produced in the adrenal glands and brain of the human body. Once adults reach the age of thirty, levels of natural DHEA usually begin to decline. In addition, DHEA levels can also be affected by certain medications. Research suggests that low DHEA levels may be connected to depression, fatigue, and other conditions. DHEA can be produced by extracting certain chemicals from wild yams and soy and is touted as a dietary supplement to aid with weight loss, antiaging, and muscle building, among other functions. It can be taken in tablet or capsule form and is sometimes used in a topical cream or lotion.

DHEA is considered a "parent hormone"; it leads to the production of sex hormones (androgens and estrogens). These hormones decline with age, and DHEA supplements can be used to rebuild their levels. Because of this, there have been a number of claims made about the health benefits of DHEA and the potential that DHEA supplements have for addressing issues associated with aging and hormone imbalances. Athletes and others may take DHEA as a dietary supplement to help build muscle mass and increase energy, although the National Collegiate Athletic Association, the National Football League, and Major League Baseball have all banned the use of this supplement by their athletes. Some people take DHEA to help prevent heart disease, diabetes, and other diseases. Older women who are no longer menstruating may take DHEA to help build bone density and improve menopausal symptoms. DHEA has also been recommended by some to help decrease "age spots" on the skin and as a way to improve memory and brain functions in older adults. Others tout DHEA as a cure for depression and a way to fight chronic fatigue. The Food and Drug Administration (FDA) is currently investigating DHEA as a potential treatment for such conditions as osteoporosis, which is a condition that leads to fragile, weakened bones.

When taken in small doses for short periods of time, DHEA is considered to be a relatively safe supplement. For example, a dose of between 5 and 450 milligrams for a six-week period has been suggested as a possible treatment for depression, and a dose of 50 milligrams a day for three months has been recommended as a possible treatment for fibromyalgia. To use DHEA to treat infertility, between 25 and 80 milligrams daily for four weeks to six months is the suggested dosage. Side effects of such short-term usage may include hair loss, acne, sleep problems, nausea, and blood pressure changes. Women sometimes experience irregular menstruation, increased facial hair, and changes to breast size when taking DHEA. Men may sometimes experience breast tenderness, increased aggression, and changes in the size of their testes. At higher doses or with longer periods of use, the risk of such side effects increases, as does the risk of prostate, breast, and ovarian cancer, along with the possibility of liver and cholesterol problems.

Scientists first discovered DHEA in 1934. The FDA banned it in 1985 due to unproven safety and effectiveness issues; however, the ban was removed in 1994, and DHEA supplements became available in the United States shortly thereafter. There is still a great deal to learn about DHEA as a supplement, and research is not yet conclusive regarding its use for most functions. Because the potential long-term effects of DHEA supplements are still unknown and the hormone may interact with other medications being taken, it is always advised to seek the counsel of a medical professional before taking DHEA.

Tamar Burris

See also: Androgens; Andropause; Estrogen; Menopause; Sex Hormones; Testosterone.

Further Reading

Cavanaugh, J. C., & Cavanaugh, C. K. (2009). *Aging in America*. Westport, CT: Praeger.

Nyborg, H. (1994). *Hormones, sex, and society: The science of physicology*. Westport, CT: Praeger.

Diagnostic and Statistical Manual of Mental Disorders (DSM)

The *Diagnostic and Statistical Manual of Mental Disorders* (*DSM*) is a comprehensive listing of mental disorders and the necessary criteria that must be met in order to diagnose each psychiatric illness. The first edition of the *DSM* was published in 1952 and aligned with the then current *International Classification of Diseases* (*ICD-6*) published in 1948. The goal of the *DSM* was clinical in nature, with the hopes that researchers and clinicians would use the classification system to promote validity and reliability among diagnoses of mental disorders. The *DSM* has had multiple revisions since the first edition was published (*DSM, DSM-II, DSM-III, DSM-III-R, DSM-IV, DSM-IV-TR, DSM-5*), the most current of which is *DSM-5* published in 2013. The inclusion and criteria of sexual disorders in the *DSM* has evolved over time.

In the original *DSM*, sexual disorders were conceptualized through the lens of Sigmund Freud and viewed as manifestations of subconscious desires. In later editions of the *DSM*, revisions to the classification and diagnostic criteria for sexual disorders were influenced by biology and biochemistry. These revisions integrated empirical evidence into the conceptualization of sexual disorders in a more objective manner. Although the goal was to utilize empirical evidence for the classification of psychiatric disorders, social biases have historically influenced the inclusion of sexual and gender minorities as mental illnesses. For example, homosexuality was listed as a paraphilic sexual disorder in a number of editions. This was corrected in 1973, when the American Psychiatric Association deleted homosexuality from the list of paraphilias. This iteration was not without its flaws, however. Ego-dystonic homosexuality, a disorder described as the stress an individual experiences due to their sexual orientation, was listed in the *DSM* after the removal of homosexuality as a paraphilia. Ego-dystonic homosexuality was later removed from the *DSM* in 1986. Paraphilic sexual disorders have also evolved over time in the *DSM*, from originally being termed as "perversion" to an understanding in today's cultural climate that a paraphilia by itself does not equate to a mental health disorder. For a paraphilia to be considered a disorder, it must now cause personal distress or involve an unconsenting party.

DSM-5 was published in 2013 after several years of research and revisions by thirteen work groups with expertise in various areas. *DSM-5* is highly regarded not only in the United States but across the world and has been translated into eighteen different languages. Within the *DSM-5*, mental health diagnoses related to sex are primarily encompassed within the sexual dysfunctions or paraphilic disorders categories. Other conditions that may be a focus of clinical attention, a section in the *DSM-5*, include topics related to sex, including relationship distress with partner, child sexual abuse, sexual abuse from a partner, sexual abuse by nonpartner, and problems related to unwanted pregnancy.

Sexual dysfunctions include delayed ejaculation, erectile disorder, female orgasmic disorder, female sexual interest/arousal disorder, genito-pelvic pain/penetration disorder, male hypoactive sexual desire disorder, premature (early) ejaculation, substance/medication-induced sexual dysfunction, other specified sexual dysfunction, and unspecified sexual dysfunction. Sexual dysfunctions arise when an individual has difficulty engaging in sexual behaviors or experiencing sexual satisfaction. Multiple factors may influence the conceptualization and diagnosis of sexual disorders, including characteristics of the individual, partner, relationship, culture, religion, or ongoing medical issues. Sexual dysfunction may also be the result of a different primary mental health diagnosis (e.g., depression) and is then better conceptualized as a symptom of that mental health disorder as opposed to a separate sexual disorder diagnosis.

Paraphilic disorders include voyeuristic disorder, exhibitionistic disorder, frotteuristic disorder, sexual masochism disorder, sexual sadism disorder, pedophilic disorder, fetishistic disorder, transvestic disorder, other specified paraphilic disorder, and unspecified paraphilic disorder. Paraphilias are classified as their own subset of disorders within the paraphilic disorders category in the *DSM-5*. Dozens of paraphilias have been identified and linked to paraphilic disorders; however, the *DSM-5* only classifies the most commonly occurring or destructive in terms of legal ramifications. However, "other specified paraphilic disorder" and "unspecified paraphilic disorder" are available for clinician use if one of the eight identified paraphilias is not appropriate.

Lauren G. Masuda and Stephen K. Trapp

See also: BDSM; Child Sexual Abuse; Freud, Sigmund; Gender Dysphoria; *International Classification of Diseases, Eleventh Revision (ICD-11)*; Paraphilias; Premenstrual Dysphoric Disorder (PMDD); Sexual Abuse; Sexual Disorders, Female; Sexual Disorders, Male.

Further Reading

American Psychiatric Association. (2013). *Diagnostic and statistical manual of mental disorders: DSM-5*. Washington, DC: American Psychiatric Association.

American Psychiatric Association. (2019). *DSM history*. Retrieved from https://www.psychiatry.org/psychiatrists/practice/dsm/history-of-the-dsm

American Psychiatric Association. (2019). *Sexual dysfunctions*. Retrieved from http://dsm.psychiatryonline.org/doi/full/10.1176/appi.books.9780890425596.dsm13

Pappas, S. (2013). The history of sex in the DSM. *Live Science*. Retrieved from http://www.livescience.com/28380-history-of-sex-dsm.html

Diamond, Milton

Milton Diamond is a sexologist who specialized in the study of intersexuality and the role of neurology in determining the sexual and gender identities of individuals. He taught anatomy and reproductive biology at the University of Hawaii medical school before his retirement at the end of 2009. Diamond is most famous for his investigation of the John/Joan case of a boy raised as a girl because of his physical condition. The results of Diamond's research showed that nurture and social context cannot change the sexual and gender identities with which a person is born.

Diamond was born on March 6, 1934, in the Bronx, New York City. His parents were European Jews who had emigrated from Ukraine after World War I. Diamond's father ran grocery stores for a living. He purchased failing stores, built them up, and then sold them for a profit. When Diamond was in junior high, the family moved to Manhattan. Diamond had always enjoyed school and was admitted to the Bronx High School of Science. The experience awakened a love of science, which he was anxious to pursue. He entered college in January 1951 and joined the Reserve Officers Training Corps to help pay his way. Diamond majored in physics at City College of New York but chose a minor in biology. He became one of the first undergraduate students there to receive a bachelor of science degree in biophysics, in 1955. After three years in the U.S. Army, Diamond entered graduate school at the University of Kansas. He graduated with a PhD in anatomy and psychology. His first job was teaching at the University of Louisville School of Medicine, where he completed two years of study toward an MD degree. In 1967, Diamond was hired by the John A. Burns School of Medicine at the University of Hawaii as professor of anatomy and reproductive biology.

Diamond's primary area of research was gender identity and how it was determined. He became interested in the so-called John/Joan case. John Money, a psychologist and sex researcher, had become famous for his writings about the case and his involvement in it. Identical twin boys were born in 1966 in Winnipeg. One boy lost most of his penis in a circumcision accident. Money convinced the parents that the child could be raised as a girl, after surgery to remove his male reproductive organs. Hormone treatments would complete the transformation. The child was not to be told the truth. Money believed that gender could be determined by a child's upbringing. He wrote extensively about the success of the process, leading to many other children undergoing the same procedures.

Diamond searched for years to find out more about the John/Joan case. He believed that a person's gender was determined in the brain before birth. Eventually, Diamond made contact with a psychiatrist who had treated the child. He found that Money's description of success was misleading. The child raised as a girl displayed many male traits and was very troubled. Eventually, the parents admitted the truth. The young person resumed his male identity and eventually had surgery to restore most of his male characteristics. After interviewing the man, Diamond published his findings in 1997, refuting Money's theories. John Colapinto, a journalist, collaborated with the man to tell his tragic story in *As Nature Made Him: The Boy Who Was Raised as a Girl*, in 2000. Unfortunately, the experience drove the subject of the study to commit suicide in 2004, two years after his twin committed suicide.

Diamond's theories were validated by the case. He continued to research and publish extensively on gender and sexual identity issues and the social effects associated with them. He became well known as a supporter of gay, transgender, and intersex rights, since he taught that their identities were not selected or influenced by their surroundings but were the result of biology. Diamond became the director of the Pacific Center for Sex and Society. He received many awards for his work and served as president of the International Academy of Sex Research. Diamond retired from teaching in 2009.

Tim J. Watts

See also: Intersexuality; Money, John; Reimer, David; Sexology.

Further Reading

Colapinto, J. (2000). *As nature made him: The boy who was raised as a girl.* New York: HarperCollins.

Diamond, M., & Sigmundson, H. K. (1997). Management of intersexuality: Guidelines for dealing with persons with ambiguous genitalia. *Archives of Pediatrics & Adolescent Medicine, 151*(10), 1046–1050.

Diamond, M., & Sigmundson, H. K. (1997). Sex reassignment at birth: Long-term review and clinical implications. *Archives of Pediatrics & Adolescent Medicine, 151*(3), 298–304.

Diaphragm

A diaphragm is a method of birth control that does not offer any protection against sexually transmitted infections (STIs). The diaphragm blocks the entrance to the uterus, thus preventing sperm from reaching and fertilizing an egg. Diaphragms are used in conjunction with spermicides, which help in the prevention of pregnancy.

Lemons, tissue paper, wool, beeswax, silver, seaweed, and rock salt have all been used in the past to cover the cervix in an attempt to prevent pregnancy. The idea was to block the cervix so that sperm that have entered the vagina during vaginal intercourse cannot swim through the cervix to get to an egg that might be waiting. Similarly, the diaphragm is a kind of birth control called a barrier contraceptive method (which also include condoms). The first versions of the modern diaphragm were introduced in the early 1800s, and the diaphragm was further modernized when Charles Goodyear developed a process called vulcanization, which involves a chemical reaction that makes rubber more durable. Safer than barriers made of natural material, rubber became the most common type of diaphragm.

The U.S. government passed a law in 1873 called the Comstock Act, which made it illegal to send "obscene, lewd, or lascivious" material through the mail. This meant that it was illegal to mail anything having to do with birth control, including information about diaphragms. As a result, contraceptives became more difficult to obtain, and their use was limited to wealthy people who could get around the restrictive laws. This lasted until Margaret Sanger, a birth control and women's rights activist, entered the picture. Sanger spent time in Europe in the early 1900s and tried to import diaphragms into the United States. When this was blocked by the Comstock Act, she fought back by smuggling them into the country in 1923.

Modern diaphragms are made of silicone and have a thin, flexible rim that fits over the cervix. Users fill them with spermicide and then place them over the cervix as early as two hours before intercourse. They should be left in place six to eight hours after intercourse. With precise use, six in one hundred women will still get pregnant while using a diaphragm as their only method of birth control in the first year of use. Realistically, it is more probable that sixteen in one hundred women will get pregnant while using a diaphragm over the course of a year.

In order to get a diaphragm, one needs to be fitted by a medical care provider because diaphragms come in different sizes depending on body size and anatomy. In order to determine the appropriate size, the medical care provider will insert a gloved middle and index finger into the patient's vagina. This helps measure the vagina to determine the correct diaphragm diameter. A fitting ring will then be inserted into the vagina to confirm that the measurements are correct. A properly fitted diaphragm is held in place by the pubic bone and the rear wall of the vagina. A diaphragm that fits correctly will not move around at all and should not be noticed by the person wearing it. If a diaphragm is too big, it may be uncomfortable. If a diaphragm is too small, it can fall out. Either way, an incorrectly sized diaphragm will not protect against pregnancy as well as one that fits properly. If a diaphragm user experiences weight gain or loss of fifteen pounds or more, gets pregnant, or is breastfeeding, they will need to be refitted for a new diaphragm to confirm proper fit.

The diaphragm is small, portable, reusable, and relatively inexpensive. A diaphragm is nonpermanent, and it will not affect the menstrual period. It can also be inserted up to two hours before intercourse, which may be less disruptive to intimacy with a sexual partner. Also, a partner will not necessarily feel the diaphragm and may not even know that one is being used.

The downsides to using a diaphragm are (as noted earlier) that it provides no protection against STIs (such as HIV, herpes, gonorrhea, or chlamydia), it has to be fitted and prescribed by a health care provider, and proper insertion can be difficult or uncomfortable. Because proper placement and use of spermicide are so important, the risk of incorrect use of this form of birth control is relatively high, thus increasing the chance of pregnancy. Also, diaphragms can increase the risk of urinary tract infections. People who have a history of toxic shock syndrome (a very serious but rare bacterial infection) should not use diaphragms.

Kristen Kelly and Dawn S. Tasillo

See also: Barrier Contraceptive Methods; Cervix; Contraception; Sexually Transmitted Infections (STIs); Spermicides.

Further Reading

Allen, R. E. (2004). Diaphragm fitting. *American Family Physician, 69,* 97–100.

Grimes, J. A., Smith, L. A., & Fagerberg, K. (2013). *Sexually transmitted disease: An encyclopedia of diseases, prevention, treatment, and issues.* Santa Barbara, CA: Greenwood.

Tone, A. (2001). *Devices and desires: A history of contraceptives in America.* New York: Hill and Wang.

Disabilities, Sexual Function and

The definition of "disability" depends on the framework used to define it. For example, in medical terms, a disability is a physical, sensory, emotional, and/or cognitive impairment that affects an individual's ability to perform daily tasks that are conceived to be within the norm of human capacity. This definition of disability is often described as a medical model of disability. In the past thirty years or so, in social science, another model of disability has been developed to contrast the medical model. The social model of disability, as it is commonly known in social sciences, defines disability as the social and systemic barriers encountered by people whose bodies do not fall under what is considered the norm of human capacity. The social model of disability sees disability not as an individual impairment, linked to someone's physical, sensory, emotional, and/or cognitive capacity, but rather as a social problem that stems from our conception of what is normal. Understanding that there are contrasting models of disabilities is essential before discussing disabilities and sexual functioning given that the definition also influences the understanding of the sex and sexualities of people with disabilities.

Regardless of the model adopted, medical or social, the range of issues with sex and sexuality faced by people with disabilities can be vast given that it involves a population with a wide range of different physical, sensory, emotional, and/or cognitive conditions and barriers. In addition, people with disabilities also have other dimensions of their identities linked, for example, to their gender, class, race and ethnicity, religion and spirituality, sexuality, and geographic location. Further, people with disabilities might have been born with a disability or acquired one through an accident or aging. Sometimes those are referred to as lifelong versus acquired disabilities. The combination of these identities and experiences means that people with disabilities cannot be conflated under one umbrella and that they face a range of sexual functioning issues. However, there are some common threads among those identities and experiences, which have increasingly been researched and described by a range of scholars both in disability studies and in sex research.

For example, children and young people with disabilities are usually seen as vulnerable and often do not receive adequate sexual health education, if they receive any sex education at all. The lack of education often leaves children and young people with disabilities more vulnerable to abusive behaviors. While evidence shows that children and young people with disabilities generally experience higher levels of physical and sexual abuse, it also shows that often they are uninformed and unequipped to deal with those experiences given their lack of sexual health knowledge. Historically, many children and young people with disabilities also experienced being sent to residential, specialist schools where the possibilities for abuse were generally higher given the lack of close parental supervision and the dependence on the adults who were both providing care and perpetrating abusive behaviors. Considering children and young people with disabilities as inherently vulnerable, and as such incapable of making decisions around their sexuality, especially if they have learning disabilities, has frequently led to parents and medical providers making decisions over their reproductive issues, from implanting birth control without the young person's consent or knowledge, or sterilization, which particularly affects those young people who are assigned female at birth. Controlling the ability to reproduce for people with disabilities has historically also led to legislative bans that prohibited people with certain disabilities to marry.

The conceptualization of people with disabilities as vulnerable, and therefore as needing to be both protected and controlled, also affects adults with disabilities. The literature in disability studies clearly indicates that people with disabilities are often infantilized—that is, reduced to childlike beings without sex or sexuality. This means that often doctors do not discuss sex and sexuality with people with disabilities, often overlooking testing and counseling for sexual health conditions. The infantilization of people with disabilities also means that they usually do not have access to essential sexual health services and education, such as HIV prevention, testing, and treatment, or sexual abuse survivors' groups. Given that people with disabilities, like other groups marginalized by society, experience higher rates of substance use, which also affects sexual behaviors and experiences, the lack of access to essential services affects their well-being and ability to develop and maintain healthy sexualities. Lack of access and infantilization also lead to invalidating the identities of people with disabilities who are also transgender, gender nonconforming, lesbian, gay, bisexual, pansexual, or asexual. Those identities are usually seen as being outside of mainstream culture and identities, and often people with disabilities are questioned on whether they identify in those ways because they cannot conform to societal expectations around gender and sexuality. Further, people with disabilities who identify as LGBTQIA usually have difficulties accessing services and resources for those populations due to physical, emotional, linguistic, and cognitive barriers.

Sexual functioning is also often defined in a way that is not inclusive of a wide range of bodies, including sensory, emotional, and cognitive differences. This means that there is very little information for people with disabilities to access around sex and sexuality. For example, people who might need to make physical adaptions in order to have sex with another person might not have information about props available, different positions, or even the possibility of timing pain medication or muscle relaxants in a way that facilitates their ability to have a sexual encounter. People who might need to access different communication tools to express their boundaries and needs might not know that there are handouts, exercises, and models of communicating their sexual boundaries and desires that might be better suited to their needs. Sexual health information and sex education in braille for blind and visually impaired people, or in sign language for deaf people, are rare and often nonexistent. Disability advocates have been raising awareness about those issues globally, and, currently, issues affecting the sexual functioning of people with disabilities are being considered both in legislative arenas as well as in social sciences and medical education. Movies like *The Sessions* (2012) have also brought some of those issues to the attention of the general public, showing that having a disability does not neutralize a person's sexuality.

Alex Iantaffi

See also: Asexuality; Gender Diversity; Sex Education; Sexual Health; Sexual Identity; Sexuality among Older Adults; Surrogate, Sexual.

Further Reading

Barker, M. J., & Iantaffi, A. (2015). Social models of disability and sexual distress. In H. Spandler, J. Anderson, & B. Sapey (Eds.), *Madness, distress and the politics of disablement* (139–152). Bristol: Policy Press.

Barnes, C. (2000). A working social model? Disability, work and disability politics in the 21st century. *Critical Social Policy, 20*(4), 441–457.

Bonnie, S. (2004). Disabled people, disability and sexuality. In J. Swain (Ed.), *Disabling barriers, enabling environments* (124–132). Los Angeles: SAGE.

Greenwood, N. W., & Wilkinson, J. (2013). Sexual and reproductive health care for women with intellectual disabilities: A primary care perspective. *International Journal of Family Medicine, 2013*, 1–8.

Iantaffi, A. (2013). Sexuality and disability. In *The sexualization report.* Retrieved from https://thesexualizationreport.wordpress.com/section-1-sexuality/sexuality-and-disability/

Iantaffi, A., & Mize, S. (2015). Disability. In *The Palgrave handbook of the psychology of sexuality and gender* (408–426). London: Palgrave Macmillan UK.

Kaufman, M., Silverberg, C., & Odette, F. (2007). *The ultimate guide to sex and disability: For all of us who live with disabilities, chronic pain, and illness.* San Francisco: Cleis Press.

McRuer, R., & Mollow, A. (Eds.). (2012). *Sex and disability.* Durham, NC: Duke University Press.

Rainey, S. S. (2011). *Love, sex, and disability: The pleasures of care.* Boulder, CO: Lynne Rienner Publishers.

Dodson, Betty

The title of Betty Dodson's first book, *Liberating Masturbation: A Meditation on Selflove* (1974), is an excellent framework to understand her importance in the field. Her bold approach to sex education has freed many women to experience their own sexuality in a way they might not have done without learning from Dodson. She was the author of multiple books and videos that teach people about sexuality with a no-nonsense approach. Her style was genuine, open, and fearless. Many women have claimed that after reading one of her books, watching one of her videos, or attending one of her talks, they developed a completely new appreciation for their vulvas and that the shame they previously felt melted away. Dodson offered Bodysex Workshops for women to address genital shame and learn masturbatory techniques. Through her work, she earned the title "Godmother of Masturbation."

Dodson did not begin her career as a sex educator but instead as a trained artist. Born in 1929, she went to New York City in 1950 to receive a formal education in fine arts. Because of her artistic talent, she was hired to draw women's lingerie and undergarments for department store advertisements. It was not until 1965, when she met Grant Taylor (who became her patron), that she began pursuing her own sexual self-discovery. Her erotic artwork landed her a show at the Wickersham Gallery in New York City in 1968. Amid the women's movement of the 1960s and 1970s, Dodson realized that although women were gaining new power in the United States, most did not understand their sexual selves, instead subscribing to the idea that a man will know what to do with her body in order for her to receive sexual pleasure. With a slideshow of multiple color pictures of female genitals and a bag of masturbatory devices, she began traveling the country, teaching women about their vulvas. In 1973, at the NOW Sexuality Conference, more than a thousand women gathered to learn from Dodson. She taught women that there is huge variation in vulvas and that the differences are beautiful.

Dodson authored several books, articles, and videos and also created a masturbatory and Kegel exercise device, "the barbell." In 1992, she received a doctorate degree from the Institute for the Advanced Study of Human Sexuality. She received the Public Service Award from the Society for the Scientific Study of Sexuality in 2011 and also received the Masters and Johnson Award from the Society for Sex Therapy and Research. Not only did she appear on multiple television shows, such as *The View*, but she was also the subject of many articles. Dodson conducted Bodysex Workshops for more than thirty years and continued these workshops until her death in October 2020 as sex coaching in her private practice. She and her business partner, Carlin Ross, continue to educate others about sexuality through their website: www.dodsonandross.com. Dodson was widely known and respected for her amazing contributions to the field of sexuality.

Karen S. Beale

See also: Female Sexuality; Kegel Exercises; Masturbation; Sex Education; Vulva.

Further Reading

Dodson, B. (1996). *Sex for one: The joy of selfloving.* New York: Three Rivers Press.

Dodson, B. (2016). *Sex by design: The Betty Dodson story.* CreateSpace.

Dodson, B. (Producer) & Schoen, M. (Director). (2007). *Betty Dodson: Her life of sex and art.* Dodson Schoen Films.

Don't Ask, Don't Tell

In 1993, President Bill Clinton suspended a former military policy that completely banned lesbian, gay, and bisexual (LGB) personnel from service and enacted a new policy that was hoped to breed more tolerance of sexual minorities in the military. Entitled the "Don't Ask, Don't Tell" policy, it was similar to the previous policy in that it did not allow known LGB personnel to join the military but was dissimilar in that the military was no longer permitted to ask potential enlistees if they were LGB, hence the name Don't Ask, Don't Tell. However, under this new policy, if an enlistee kept their sexuality to themselves during enlistment and then decided to come out as LGB at a later date while serving, they could still be dismissed from the military.

Those that supported the ban on LGB personnel in the military believed that these personnel would receive special treatment, which would undermine unit cohesion, morale, performance, and readiness capability. While many military officials held negative believes that LGB personnel were in some way unfit to serve, no supporting evidence that LGB personnel undermine military performance at any level has been found, though many studies have taken place within the military. In fact, militaries across the world that include LGB personnel have shown that military performance is not hindered, even in situations where troops still hold negative prejudices and homophobic attitudes.

Rather than increasing tolerance, Don't Ask, Don't Tell led to greater experiences of discomfort, fear, and embarrassment in regard to the disclosure of sexual orientation in the military, even under anonymous conditions. There was serious underreporting of victimization, such as sexual assault and harassment, and a belief that there were fewer options for assistance available for LGB military members. From the implementation of Don't Ask, Don't Tell in 1993 to its repeal in 2011, over 14,000 service members, were discharged from the military under this policy. During this time, an assumption of inappropriate homosexual contact was all that was needed for an investigation of personnel to begin. However, since the policy did not define what behaviors would justify an inquiry or what grounds would lead to discharge, there was little uniformity in its implementation.

In 2010, President Barack Obama announced his intention to repeal the law that denied LGB Americans the right to serve in the military. A long process began as government officials started taking apart the language of Don't Ask, Don't Tell. Not only was there a lack of supporting evidence to show that LGB troops led to poor morale and unit cohesion; there was a tremendous amount of evidence indicating that the number of troops that were removed from service due to Don't Ask, Don't Tell dropped after 2001. This showed the willingness to retain LGB troops during wartime. The cost for training troops was also considered, as many well-trained individuals were removed from service due to Don't Ask, Don't Tell, which resulted in a loss of federal money and time. The policy also affected military recruitment as supporters of the LGB community and their loved ones refused to consider military service, which caused recruitment of less-qualified enlistees. Lastly, troops who were suspected of violating Don't Ask, Don't Tell were routinely held until after completion of overseas deployments, thus serving the interests of the government.

Eventually, through court proceedings, it was determined that Don't Ask, Don't Tell violated both the First and Fifth Amendments of the United States Constitution and, as of September 20, 2011, the repeal of the policy within all military services was announced by the undersecretary of defense. This order called "for all military service members to treat each other with dignity and respect regardless of sexual orientation and that all services should strive to promote an environment that is free from personal, social, or any type of institutional barriers that might arise due to sexual orientation" (Burrelli, 2012). Repeal of Don't Ask, Don't Tell means that personnel who were discharged under this policy will be given the opportunity to reenlist and complete their military service in the way initially intended.

Linda D. Hinkle

See also: Antigay Prejudice; Biphobia; Homophobia; Homosexuality; LGBTQ+; Sexual Orientation.

Further Reading

Belkin, A. (2003). Don't ask, don't tell: Is the gay ban based on military necessity? *Parameters, 33*(2), 108–119.

Burks, D. (2011). Lesbian, gay, and bisexual victimization in the military. *American Psychologist, 66*(7), 604–613.

Burrelli, D. (2010). *"Don't ask, don't tell": The law and military policy on same-sex behavior* (CRS Report No. R40782). Washington, DC: Congressional Research Service.

Burrelli, D. (2012). *The repeal of "don't ask, don't tell": Issues for Congress* (CRS Report No. R42003). Washington, DC: Congressional Research Service.

Feder, J. (2013). *"Don't ask, don't tell": A legal analysis* (CRS Report No. R40795). Washington, DC: Congressional Research Service.

Double Standards, Sexual

A double standard occurs when two groups are judged differently for engaging in the same behavior. A sexual double standard involves different standards of sexual permissiveness for men and women and is often used to differentiate appropriate behaviors for both. Sexual double standards are often used as a tool to stratify different groups and are often deployed as a mechanism through which some behaviors, when demonstrated by certain people, are denigrated or stigmatized. Beliefs about appropriate expressions of sexuality and gender factor into sexual decision making and can even supersede an actor's own desires, for example encouraging a young woman to curtail her own desires to maintain a good reputation, or leading young men to make judgments about female peers that may foster negative treatment or slut shaming. For this reason, sexual double standards are a powerful form of social control.

Mary Crawford and Danielle Popp (2003) conducted a review of two decades of research on the sexual double standard, illuminating the methodological challenges of measuring the concept but also demonstrating how common the double standard is, as seen through many studies of adolescents and young adults. This review shows that while the traditional, or orthodox, heterosexual double standard, prohibiting women from having sex outside of marriage, is waning, in its place have emerged different iterations of sexual double standards, which "are local and subcultural constructions rather than a universal mandate" (Crawford & Popp, 2003). This is supported by more current research that demonstrates the existence of the double standard in subcultures such as the collegiate hookup culture.

Sexual double standards often focus on appropriate sexuality for women, while men experience more permissiveness regarding their sexual behaviors. The sexual double standard is often found in regard to three issues: appropriateness of sexuality in different forms of relationships, number of previous sex partners, and suitability for someone as a mate instead of a date.

These intertwined issues all have implications for women's sexual identity and agency and affect contraception negotiation and sexual assault. Previous sexual experience, including casual sex, is often used to scrutinize a woman's assertion of sexual assault, even with the existence of rape shield laws. This affects many survivors' choice to come forward with a rape case.

Men are allowed freedom to have sex anytime, but women are judged for having sex outside of a relationship. In fact, a man may see a woman as ineligible to be his girlfriend because of her choice to engage in casual sex, even if the casual sex was with him. Women with higher numbers of partners, regardless of whether they were boyfriends or not, are also judged more harshly. Determination of the suitability of a woman as a potential relationship partner often hinges on how restrictive she is sexually. Young men may desire a more sexually experienced woman as a temporary sex partner but would not even consider a serious relationship with her because of her permissiveness.

The sexual double standard makes women much more circumspect about when to engage in sex and with whom. Concerns about reputation may make women less apt to initiate conversations about sex or contraception, limiting their sexual agency and autonomy as well as their safety. As such, sexual double standards may lead women to relinquish their sexual autonomy in order to maintain social desirability.

Rachel Kalish

See also: Binary Gender System; Casual Sex; Female Sexuality; Hookup Culture; Madonna/Whore Dichotomy; Male Sexuality; Sexual Expression; Slut Shaming; Stereotypes, Gender; Stereotypes, Sexual.

Further Reading

Crawford, M., & Popp, D. (2003). Sexual double standards: A review and methodological critique of two decades of research. *Journal of Sex Research, 40*, 13–27.

Hamilton, L., & Armstrong, E. A. (2009). Gendered sexuality in young adulthood: Double binds and flawed options. *Gender and Society, 23*(5), 589–616.

Reid, J. A., Elliot, S., & Webber, G. R. (2011). Casual hookups to formal dates: Refining the sexual double standard. *Gender and Society, 25*(5), 545–568.

Reiss, I. L. (1967). *The social context of premarital sexual permissiveness.* New York: Holt, Rinehart and Winston.

Douching

Some women mistakenly believe that vaginal douching is an important part of feminine hygiene and consider douching a method to prevent or even treat sexually transmitted infections (STIs). Some people, mostly men who have sex with men, also practice rectal douching as a method to clean the anus and rectum prior to engaging in receptive anal sex. Medical professionals, however, recommend against douching, especially vaginal douching, because it can be harmful and lead to irritation and infection. Douching is the practice of flushing a stream of water or water-based fluid into the vaginal or anal cavity via an inserted tube. An attached bulb or bag is used to hold the fluid, and squeezing that bulb forces the contents into the vagina or rectum under varying amounts of pressure. The terminology "douche" comes from the French verb for showering (*doucher*). The fluid content is usually either plain water, a home mixture of water and vinegar, or a commercially available product that can be purchased over the counter (without a prescription) at common drugstore chains.

The origins of douching are unclear but date back to ancient times. Douching is a practice that has been prevalent across various national and cultural backgrounds and throughout many parts of the world. In fact, in the nineteenth century, it was a commonly recognized means of postcoital birth control in a time when little else was available. The theory was that irrigating the vagina after sexual intercourse would flush away the sperm, thus preventing pregnancy. However, this was not (and still is not) an effective means of contraception. In the twentieth century, douching was popularized as a cleansing method during a new wave of body and odor awareness that dawned during the late Victorian era. This theme continued via advertising practices through the 1980s with television commercials for douching products.

However, with new medical knowledge and greater understanding of vaginal health in the last twenty to thirty years, it is now understood that vaginal douching does more harm than good. Public health pressure has helped to remove the false and misleading advertising from the general viewing audience, and more communities are becoming aware of its dangers. While medical knowledge and sexual health education were limited in the past, it is now known that the vagina is a self-contained environment that is fully capable of, and was designed to, clean itself. Cervical and vaginal mucus clear out blood, sperm, and other debris by themselves without any help, and if disturbed and interrupted from doing this work, many problems can arise.

Vaginal douching has been found to have several unintended consequences, as it has been directly linked to various infections as well as pregnancy- and birth-related problems. Complications occur both because of the force or pressure involved with injecting the fluid and because douching strips the vagina of healthy and normal bacteria and protective mucus.

Pelvic inflammatory disease (PID) and STIs are seen more frequently in those who douche than in those who do not. The risk of PID grows higher the more frequently douching occurs. Bacterial vaginosis (BV) is 2.5 times more likely to occur in women who douche. BV is a condition of discharge and odor directly caused by the overgrowth of abnormal and unhealthy bacteria in the vagina, which can occur when the normal bacteria are removed during the act of douching. Women who douche frequently also have higher risks for pregnancy-related complications such as premature labor and low-birth weight babies as well as higher risk of ectopic pregnancies. Rectal douching is safer than vaginal douching as the rectum does not have the same delicate flora balance; however, damage to tissue from incorrect technique can occur.

Overall, approximately one out of every three women in the United States douche on a regular basis, and in some studies, up to 75 percent have done so at least once; there is some variation in frequency of douching by age, race, ethnicity, and education. The prevalence of rectal douching is less known; however, in one study, half of the gay men surveyed reported douching at least once. Generally, the reasons why women report douching include hygiene, after a period, after sex, or because they believe it will treat or prevent infection or discharge. While some teens surveyed in one study were aware that having some discharge is normal, outdated and misinformed cultural and family beliefs surrounding vaginal douching practices still persist.

Lara E. Stewart

See also: Anal Intercourse; Bacterial Vaginosis; Vagina; Vaginal Secretions.

Further Reading

Grimes, J. A., Smith, L. A., & Fagerberg, K. (2013). *Sexually transmitted disease: An encyclopedia of diseases, prevention, treatment, and issues.* Santa Barbara, CA: Greenwood.

Newton, D. E. (2009). *Sexual health: A reference handbook.* Santa Barbara, CA: ABC-CLIO.

Noor, S. W., & Rosser, B. R. (2014). Enema use among men who have sex with men: A behavioral epidemiological study with implications for HIV/STI prevention. *Archives of Sexual Behavior, 43*(4), 755–759.

Tepper, M. S., & Owens, A. F. (Eds.). (2006). *Sexual health.* Santa Barbara, CA: Praeger.

Down Low

The down low (DL) typically refers to a man who is, or claims to be, involved in a heterosexual relationship with a woman and who develops romantic feelings or becomes sexually intimate with another man without his female companion's knowledge. Publicly, the man has a companionate or romantic relationship with a woman and is typically able to acknowledge this arrangement to family, peers, and colleagues, while his feelings or sexual behavior with another man remains a secret. Being on the DL can refer to men being in a relationship with a woman but secretly having fantasies about being sexual with another man, having clandestine romantic feelings or attachment to another man, or, as previously mentioned, privately engaging in intimate behaviors (e.g., kissing, hugging, petting, oral sex, anal sex). The heterosexist assumption follows that the man with whom the man has sex knows about the relationship with the woman. Paradoxically, the woman with whom the man has sex does not know about the other man or any feelings associated with that relationship.

For centuries, men have been having romantic feelings for or having sex with men without their female partners knowing. However, it was only in the mid-1990s that this phenomenon became more public when associated with black men. Some African American communities rejected this because of negative sentiments about same-sex relationships, homophobia within and outside of the black church, and pervasive heterosexist discourse. However, more people started talking about the DL during this time in an attempt to explain and pathologize black relationships, as the prevalence of HIV was increasing among black women. It was assumed that black men on the DL were having intimate relationships with women and secretly with men, which resulted in greater exposure to sexually transmitted infections including HIV. Depictions by media and other social institutions suggested that black men would callously prey on unsuspecting women and then not be forthcoming with potential male partners about their sexual history and HIV status. This stereotype created much tension and apprehension between some black men and women who had an interest in developing intimate relationships with another. Some literature suggests that men are afraid to adopt sexual identity labels other than heterosexual out of fear of public backlash or scrutiny.

The general discourse around black men on the DL has continued to contribute to homophobic and heterosexist attitudes in many communities. Secrecy of fantasies, feelings, and behaviors is necessary in order to maintain concurrent heterosexual and same-gender-loving relationships. The effects and implications of racism and systemic oppression have created tension in the black community between some men and women. Debilitating belief systems and stereotypes of black men being hypersexual, animalistic, and unable to control their sexual impulses continues to be maintained both within and external to black communities. It is believed that men on the DL are sexually insatiable and unable to have enough sex with females or males, and they are seen as selfish, self-centered, and greedy. Because of this faulty assumption, some black women are fearful of forming or maintaining relationships with black men because of the notion of secret encounters with other men. Some black men are equally concerned about being given the social latitude to examine having romantic or sexual feelings for other men and the diminished possibility of receiving support.

Some scholars have pointed out that women can also be on the down low such that they publicly maintain a heterosexual relationship with a man but engage in intimate encounters or have romantic feelings for women. According to Phillips (2005), society's conservative attitudes toward sexuality "contribute to black women's silence around their own sexual desires and relationships, obscuring the amount and type of sex that black women actually have. Due to its enforcement of silence, this 'culture of respectability' contributes to the oppression of black women's sexuality, sexual agency, and access to sexual health care."

Critically, sexism and patriarchy make women's sexuality less of a priority than men's sexual expression. There is a tendency to negate, minimize, or ridicule the feelings and behaviors of women. There is a greater risk of male-to-female sexually transmitted infection than there is from female to female. More research needs to be done that examines women who are in heterosexual relationships and are sexually intimate with women without their male partners knowing. Finally, research on DL women and men needs to take into account that the phenomenon may be a deflection from the acknowledgment of HIV transmission.

James Wadley

See also: Black Sexuality; Heterosexism; Homophobia; Human Immunodeficiency Virus (HIV); Intimacy, Sexual and Relational; Same-Sex Attraction and Behavior; Sexual Identity.

Further Reading

Ford, C. L., Whetten, K. D., Hall, S. A., Kaufman, J. S., & Thrasher, A. D. (2007). Black sexuality, social construction, and research targeting "The Down Low" ("the DL"). *Annals of Epidemiology, 17*(3), 209–216.

Hammonds, E. (1994). Black (w)holes and the geometry of black female sexuality. *Differences, 6*(2–3), 126–145.

Malebranche, D. J. (2008). Bisexually active black men in the United States and HIV: Acknowledging more than the "down low." *Archives of Sexual Behavior, 37*(5), 810–816.

Phillips, L. (2005). Deconstructing "down low" discourse: The politics of sexuality, gender, race, AIDS, and anxiety. *Journal of African American Studies, 9*(2), 3–15.

Drag

Drag involves a person performing a gender identity that does not correspond to cultural standards of biological sex. It has a long history. Historically, men presented themselves as women in the theater. However, this was often a necessity since women were typically not permitted on stage. It is important to note that throughout history, because of cultural restrictions on same-sex relationships, men and women were pushed into appearing in drag so that they could safely go to public places with their partners. Contemporary drag has a different focus. People now dress as the other sex in their personal lives to gain gender self-realization. In addition, drag queens and kings participate in public shows to challenge socially constructed gender norms. It is also possible for a person to wear the typical clothing of the opposite sex as a matter of preference related to comfort or sexual desire, though not all scholars would consider these instances to be drag.

Because understanding of gender is growing, classifying drag can be complicated. Cross-dressing and drag have similarities in that they both involve gender bending by wearing clothing typical of the other sex. However, depending on the source referenced, there is a strong directive to keep the two separate. In the cross-dressing community, where participants are largely straight, "drag" can serve as an acronym for "Dressed As a Girl" or "Dress Resembling A Girl." Alternatively, the term "drab" represents "Dressed As a Boy." Cross-dressers, historically known as transvestites, want to achieve feelings of normality while passing as the other sex in public settings, and many feel comfortable moving between gender presentations depending on the situation. In the context of nonheterosexual communities, drag explicitly concerns queens and kings who are predominantly gay and lesbian. While one goal of engaging in this performance art is to entertain others, there are also intentional exaggerations of long-standing gender stereotypes to downplay traditional binary ideals while highlighting gender fluidity.

Drag has a long history. Greek mythology notes that Hercules may have dressed as a woman. Aphroditus was a masculine god who donned female attire. In celebrations of the deity, followers would theatrically dress in other-sex attire as a form of worship. In ancient Greece, soldiers would dress as women to gain access to strategic locations and to avoid capture. Other historical military-based examples also exist. Consider Hua Mulan dressing as a man to take her father's place in the army and Joan of Arc wearing male soldier attire in the Hundred Years' War. In addition, British reporter Dorothy Lawrence took the name Denis Smith and participated in World War I. Some European folktales focus on drag, and many cultures have rituals reflecting the practice. For instance, some North American Mennonite groups have young men dress as mischievous characters, some in feminine clothing, around New Year's Eve. The men raid community houses, play music and tricks, and demand money, food, or drink. Cross-cultural dynamics of dress can provide interesting insight on gender and power. Consider the Scottish tradition of men wearing kilts, which leads some men to feel objectified when women make suggestive comments or raise their skirt-type garments without consent. Debates about identity, sexual preference, and motives exist with all these examples. Regardless, they seem to fall under the classification of drag from the cross-dressing community perspective.

Drag as related specifically to the LGBTQ+ community has roots in the late 1800s. During this time, people in American and British dance halls, early forms of nightclubs, began to perform as drag queens and kings to entertain patrons. Some scholars argue that when a man would first wear a woman's dress, people would say it would "drag" the floor until he became comfortable with it. Nearly a century later, organized groups of flamboyant attendees at gay-friendly establishments, such as the Club Kids, would make wearing clothing that challenges gender dynamics customary. Scholars imply that prominent entertainers in the late 1900s helped to promote the acceptance of drag themes in wider culture. This includes, but is not limited to, David Bowie, Boy George, Grace Jones, and Annie Lenox. The foundation they laid opened the door for drag personalities such as RuPaul to achieve success not only in the music industry but also with product sponsorships, movies, and television.

Today, drag shows predominantly occur in LGBTQ+-associated nightclubs. Costumes for drag queens involve corsets, jumpsuits, and dresses with boots or heeled shoes. Wigs, intricately applied makeup, and sometimes body paint accentuate the presentation. For drag kings, male attire is essential. However, engaging in rituals associated with the application of faux facial hair and binding of the breasts is key as well. Drag shows can involve monologues, skits, lip-synching of popular music, and dancing. Audience participation is encouraged, and comedy at the expense of viewers is commonplace. Though queens give the impression of confidence on stage, research shows that some experience considerable performance anxiety. Their onstage personas can help to shield them from fears. Performers will adopt a stage name for shows and character traits to match. The name typically plays on popular culture themes for a sexualized, comedic effect. For example, names of former contestants on *RuPaul's Drag Race* include Rebecca Glasscock, Madame LaQueer, Jiggly Caliente, and Kandy Ho. Some shows have a pageant format that allows for winners in smaller communities to move up to larger venues to compete for prestigious titles such as Miss Continental USA, which occurs over Labor Day weekend in Chicago. People are generally more familiar with drag queens as compared to kings. Drag kings are more likely to perform in groups and keep performances located around one specific geographic location. In both cases, performers frequently give the money generated from shows to community groups supporting LGBTQ causes.

Scholars argue that drag shows provide a form of political protest against homophobia and heteronormativity. However, critics contend that they also support existing power structures when they emphasize and reward physical characteristics that create oppression in the first place. In other words, drag queen shows can focus too much on narrow understandings of femininity and fail to foster acceptance and respect for multiple femininities. This could be one reason some people in the gay community discriminate against drag queens. On the other hand, king shows provide the acceptance of a wider understanding of gender with participants not only being lesbians but also straight women, queer women, trans men, and masculine-gendered women.

Jason S. Ulsperger

See also: Gender Expression; Gender Identity; LGBTQ+; Transvestite.

Further Reading

Berkowitz, D., Belgrave, L., & Halberstein, R. (2008). The interaction of drag queens and gay men in public and private spaces. *Journal of Homosexuality, 52*, 11–32.

Brennan, N., & Gudelunas, D. (2017). *RuPaul's drag race and the shifting visibility of drag culture: The boundaries of reality TV.* New York: Palgrave Macmillan.

Garber, M. (2012). *Vested interests: Cross-dressing and cultural anxiety.* New York: Routledge.

Greaf, C. (2016). Drag queens and gender identity. *Journal of Gender Studies, 25*, 655–665.

Greenhill, P., & Tye, D. (2014). *Unsettling assumptions: Tradition, gender, and drag.* Boulder, CO: University Press of Colorado.

Knutson, D., Koch, J., Sneed, J., & Lee, A. (2018). The emotional and psychological experiences of drag performers: A qualitative study. *Journal of LGBT Issues in Counseling, 12*, 32–50.

Kramer, G., & Bernstein, R. (2017). *Drags.* New York: KMW Studio.

Senelick, L. (2000). *The changing room: Sex, drag, and theatre.* New York: Routledge.

Dysmenorrhea

Dysmenorrhea is painful cramping during menstruation. It is a common problem, affecting around 50 percent of postpubescent women. The condition is most regularly seen in people between the ages of twenty and twenty-four, and symptoms often decrease with age. In the United States, about 10–20 percent of those affected by dysmenorrhea have severe pain that leaves them unable to participate in everyday functions like work and school for several days each month. Those who smoke or who entered puberty at a young age (under eleven) are at greater risk for dysmenorrhea, as are those who have irregular menstrual cycles or heavy bleeding during their period.

There are two types of dysmenorrhea: primary dysmenorrhea and secondary dysmenorrhea. The first occurs in otherwise healthy individuals and is usually seen in younger adults. The menstrual pain felt as a result of primary dysmenorrhea is not related to uterine or other issues. While the cause is not entirely known, the increased level of hormone-like substances (prostaglandins) during menstruation is thought to play a role in the condition. Prostaglandins are the natural substances that trigger the uterus to contract and expel menstrual blood. So far, research has shown that the higher the level of prostaglandins, the greater the chance of dysmenorrhea.

Secondary dysmenorrhea is a condition that typically develops in people older than twenty-five as a result of problems associated with the uterus or pelvic organs. These individuals have usually had normal, relatively pain-free menstruation until the onset of their uterine or pelvic disorders. Issues that may trigger secondary dysmenorrhea include uterine fibroids, which are noncancerous growths in the uterus; pelvic inflammatory disease, a bacterial infection in the pelvic organs; and endometriosis, a condition in which uterine lining tissues mistakenly implant and grow on the fallopian tubes, ovaries, or elsewhere outside of the uterus. Stress and anxiety are also factors that may trigger secondary dysmenorrhea.

The symptoms of dysmenorrhea include an intense throbbing or aching in the lower abdomen, sharp pains that come and go, and a persistent ache that radiates through the lower back and legs. Some people also experience diarrhea, nausea, headaches, or dizziness during menstruation as a result of dysmenorrhea. Although dysmenorrhea itself does not lead to other medical conditions, the underlying issues that cause secondary dysmenorrhea may if left untreated. For example, endometriosis can lead to fertility issues, and pelvic inflammatory disease may increase the risk of ectopic pregnancy, a sometimes life-threatening problem that occurs when a fertilized egg implants outside of the uterus.

A pelvic exam should be able to show whether an individual has primary dysmenorrhea or secondary dysmenorrhea. If the exam reveals no irregularities or abnormalities, the problem is most likely primary dysmenorrhea. Primary dysmenorrhea is often treatable with home remedies like a low-sugar, low-sodium, and no-caffeine diet, or increased stress-reducing activity such as yoga and meditation. Warm showers and baths and over-the-counter anti-inflammatory medication are also often recommended. If the pain is severe, a medical practitioner may recommend prescription anti-inflammatory medication and pain relievers or birth control pills. If secondary dysmenorrhea is suspected, a doctor may recommend additional tests such as an ultrasound, a CT scan, or other imaging tests. In addition, a complete blood count test can be used to pinpoint infections and other such problems. Laparoscopic outpatient surgery can also be used to explore the pelvic region and reproductive organs for signs of fibroids, endometriosis, cysts, and other issues that may be creating the painful menstrual cramps. This is usually only recommended for a small percentage of women who have not responded to other tests and treatments.

Evidence shows that dysmenorrhea was a known problem in ancient civilizations such as Egypt and Greece. Early practitioners applied aromatic oils and ointments to treat inflammation and pain associated with the problem. Roman physicians wrote extensively about their use of asparagus root to relieve menstrual pain. By the nineteenth century, dysmenorrhea was seen as a common but serious problem, though the suspected causes were wide and varied. In 1938, a connection between ovulation and dysmenorrhea was made, followed by the discovery of increased prostaglandins creating menstrual pain in 1965. Over time, different courses of treatment were prescribed and studied. Newer research has shown that calcium channel-blocking agents are helpful in decreasing pain associated with dysmenorrhea. Experimentation has also revealed that transcutaneous electrical nerve stimulation, a noninvasive procedure in which electrical impulses are used to block pain in the pelvis, may also be effective for some people.

Tamar Burris

See also: Menstruation; Premenstrual Dysphoric Disorder (PMDD); Premenstrual Syndrome (PMS).

Further Reading

Gannon, L. R. (1985). *Menstrual disorders and menopause.* Westport, CT: Praeger.

Hollen, K. H. (2004). *The reproductive system.* Westport, CT: Greenwood.

Dyspareunia

"Dyspareunia" is a medical term referring to the symptom of pain with sexual intercourse. It is commonly used in reference to painful intercourse in both men and women and can include pain as a result of physical, psychological, and combined causes.

Apart from use as a medical term, dyspareunia also has a history of being classified as a type of mental disorder. In a previous edition of the *Diagnostic and Statistical Manual of Mental Disorders* (*DSM*), dyspareunia was included as a sexual disorder, and one that applied to both men and women. The *DSM* criteria for this diagnosis included (1) pain that occurs before, during, or just after intercourse; (2) the presence of distress or interpersonal difficulty as a result of the condition; and (3) the condition is not caused by vaginismus (involuntary spasm of the muscles of the vagina), insufficient lubrication, use of a drug or medication, or another psychological or medical condition.

However, the fifth edition of the *DSM* does not include dyspareunia. Instead, both it and vaginismus have been removed and replaced with the term genito-pelvic pain/penetration disorder (GPPPD). GPPPD is classified as a sexual dysfunction, but in the *DSM-5* it only applies to women. In addition to pain with intercourse, this diagnosis also includes women who experience difficulty with vaginal penetration or fear or anxiety about pain with penetration even if they do not experience pain.

In the more common usage of the term, "dyspareunia" describes the symptom of pain with intercourse and requires further assessment to determine the cause. Assessment includes a thorough medical history, visual examination, and tests for physical causes.

In both men and women, causes of dyspareunia include sexually transmitted infections, skin disorders, allergy to latex condoms or spermicide, bladder disorders, and pelvic floor dysfunction (a condition where the muscles supporting the reproductive organs are either too tight or too loose, both of which may cause pain). In women, some additional causes of dyspareunia include endometriosis, vaginismus, vulvodynia, vaginal atrophy, lack of lubrication, adhesions, hormonal changes from perimenopause or menopause, and traumatic childbirth.

Some additional causes of dyspareunia in men include prostatitis (infection of the prostate gland), Peyronie's disease (a condition where the penis has an abnormal shape when erect), and phimosis (where the foreskin is too tight).

The prevalence of dyspareunia is unknown due to the fact that there are multiple conditions that include dyspareunia as a symptom, and many cases go unreported. Dyspareunia is more common in women, and there is little research about the condition in men.

Treatment for dyspareunia varies depending on the cause and may include medication for sexually transmitted infections, surgery for endometriosis, and pelvic floor physical therapy (e.g., for conditions including pelvic floor dysfunction, prostatitis, and vaginismus). Regardless of the cause, a multidisciplinary approach is recommended, including sex therapy for psychological factors and to address the impact of painful intercourse on the individual and his or her relationships.

Adrienne M. Bairstow

See also: Diagnostic and Statistical Manual of Mental Disorders (*DSM*); Endometriosis; Menopause; Pelvic Floor Muscles; Phimosis; Prostatitis; Psychosexual Therapy; Sexual Dysfunction, Treatment of; Sexually Transmitted Infections (STIs); Vaginal Lubrication; Vaginismus; Vulvodynia.

Further Reading

American Psychiatric Association. (2000). *Diagnostic and statistical manual of mental disorders* (4th ed., text rev.). Washington, DC: Author.

American Psychiatric Association. (2013). *Diagnostic and statistical manual of mental disorders* (5th ed.). Washington, DC: Author.

Goldstein, A., & Burrows, L. J. (2009). Sexual pain disorders in women. Retrieved from http://www.issm.info/news/review-reports/sexual-pain-disorders-in-women/

Mayo Clinic. (2019). Painful intercourse (dyspareunia). Retrieved from http://www.mayoclinic.org/diseases-conditions/painful-intercourse/basics/definition/CON-20033293?p=1

E

Ejaculation

Ejaculation can occur in both penises and vulvas. (Female ejaculation is discussed in a separate entry.) Ejaculation in both cases involves the expulsion of fluids from the genitals, usually produced in response to sexual excitement. It may or may not accompany an orgasm. Even though orgasm and ejaculation are widely believed to be the same, they are in fact separate events, and one is not guaranteed by the presence of the other.

For penises, ejaculation is usually the result of excitement and is the mechanism that allows sperm (semen) to leave the body. The testes are the home of sperm production, and ejaculate for penises is comprised of a tiny amount of sperm produced in the testes. The fluids that house the sperm travel from the testes via the vas deferens, a tube connecting the testes to the prostate, where it mixes with prostatic fluid and fluid from the seminal vesicles before heading out the urethra for an ejaculation. The process of ejaculation is helped by clear, extra-slippery fluid from the bulbourethral glands. This substance is known as preejaculate fluid (commonly known as precum).

Because the majority of the ejaculate is comprised of seminal fluid and prostatic fluid, it is still possible to have ejaculations after a vasectomy because the majority of the fluid comes from the prostate gland. The vasectomy only prevents sperm from mixing with the other ejaculation fluids. Penis ejaculation happens when the bulbospongiosus and ischiocavernosus muscles contract to help propel the ejaculate from the urethra. Penis ejaculate usually travels two to three inches outside the body after having traveled two feet within the body to make its way outside. Ejaculate may carry sexually transmitted infections such as HIV.

Sometimes males wake in the morning with sticky underwear or sheets after ejaculating in their sleep. This is called a wet dream, or nocturnal emission, and it is totally normal, especially during puberty. Sometimes while sleeping, the penis becomes erect and ejaculates. It may or may not be accompanied by erotic dreams or rubbing on the bed while sleeping. Wet dreams are common and tend to become less frequent with age. Ejaculation can occur even without erections present.

Premature ejaculation (when someone ejaculates sooner than they would like) is a common physical sexual problem experienced by around 30 percent of people with penises worldwide. Delayed ejaculation (when someone does not ejaculate despite sufficient sexual stimulation) is also a common problem. Frequent ejaculation may be linked to a decreased risk of prostate cancer.

Cyndi Darnell

See also: Female Ejaculation; Nocturnal Emissions; Orgasm; Penis; Preejaculate Fluid; Premature Ejaculation; Retrograde Ejaculation; Semen.

Further Reading

Carson, C., & Gunn, K. (2006). Premature ejaculation: Definition and prevalence. *International Journal of Impotence Research, 18*(S1), 5–13.

Gottlieb, S. (2004). Frequent ejaculation may be linked to decreased risk of prostate cancer. *BMJ, 328*, 857.

Montorsi, F. (2005). Prevalence of premature ejaculation: A global and regional perspective. *The Journal of Sexual Medicine, 2*, 96–102.

Pryor, J. P. (2002). Orgasmic and ejaculatory dysfunction. *Sexual and Relationship Therapy, 17*(1), 87–95.

Waldinger, M. D. (2017). Physiology of ejaculation. In S. Minhas & J. Mulhall (Eds.), *Male sexual dysfunction: A clinical guide* (8–13). West Sussex: John Wiley & Sons.

Ellis, Albert

Albert Ellis (1913–2007), while best known as one of the main pioneers of the cognitive revolution in psychotherapy with his approach of rational emotive behavior therapy (REBT), was a key force in the sexual revolution of the 1950s and 1960s. He was one of the founders, and first president, of the Society for the Scientific Study of Sexuality and the first major cognitive behavioral sex therapist. One of his main goals was to make the field of sexology a respectable and vital area of science.

Ellis was born in Pittsburgh, Pennsylvania, and moved to New York with his family when he was an infant. New York remained his home base for the rest of his life. Throughout his teens and young adult years, he researched any and all studies and books about sex and sexuality that he could find. A main source for his readings was the New York Public Library. His expertise on sex, sexuality, "nonconforming" sexual behavior, and more drew people seeking help with issues that included, or were related to, their sex activities with others, masturbation, relationships, and marriage. As a result of his success in helping his clients suffer less anxiety and concern about sex and relationship issues, and their consequential greater harmony and contentment, he founded the Love and Marriage Problems Institute in 1939 for research and therapy.

Because there were no academic programs offering courses about sexuality and relationships at this time, Ellis completed the master's and PhD programs at Columbia University's Teachers College clinical psychology program. He completed writing *The Case for Promiscuity* in 1938, which was considered by publishers to be too liberal for that time; consequently, it was first published in 1965.

From the late 1930s onward, Ellis fought vigorously in talks, books, and articles against censorship, the ignoring of sexual liberty, and other social restrictions. He presented in favor of free love, premarital sex, easy divorce, same-sex relationships, birth control, equal rights for women, equal rights for gay people, interracial relationships and marriage, liberation of sex laws, and other aspects in favor of sexual freedom. Few others dared to talk about such topics in those years, and he was considered a renegade, maverick, and worse by many people with conservative views. He wrote many articles on sex and love, which were published in journals and popular magazines, and gave many talks and workshops on sex and psychotherapy. His first book, *The Folklore of Sex*, was published in 1951, followed by many more volumes and articles about sex and love topics.

Ellis became a renowned sexologist, clinician, and writer and often corresponded with Alfred Kinsey (1894–1956) and other notables in the field. Kinsey consulted with Ellis and interviewed him for some of his reports and studies. Others in the field, including John Money and Harry Benjamin, were influenced by Ellis, respected his work, and often cited him. By 1954, Ellis had published at least forty-six articles, two books, and two anthologies and was the American editor of the pioneering journal the *International Journal of Sexology*. In 1957, Ellis founded and was the first president of the Society for the Scientific Study of Sexuality, and he produced more best-selling books on sex and love, making him one of the most influential writers and speakers of the American, European, British, and Australian sex revolution of the 1960s. His public fame flourished in the 1960s following publications that included his best-selling books: *Sex without Guilt* (1958), *The Art and Science of Love* (1960), *The Intelligent Woman's Guide to Dating and Mating* (1963), and *Sex and the Single Man* (1963).

Despite being frequently invited to write for magazines and to appear on radio and television talk shows, his views were at times censored. Some magazine editors rejected his articles, saying they were too bold or controversial. Some radio programs on which he spoke were not rebroadcast because management deemed his views, such as saying that masturbation and sex were desirable, too radical and controversial. On a couple of occasions when he appeared on television programs and espoused premarital sex relations, the Federal Communications Commission took those programs temporarily off the air.

As the 1960s progressed, and in the decades that followed, Ellis became known more for his revolutionary work in psychotherapy, but his reputation as a sexologist continued, and he was often criticized for his controversial views. He disagreed with Freud that sex problems are major causes of general emotional problems and asserted that general human disturbance is much more likely to lead to sex problems than vice versa. His REBT approach teaches techniques and methods of minimizing emotional disturbance and maximizing joy in life and significantly contributes to assisting those with sexual problems and dysfunctions.

Ellis considered some of his main contributions to the fields of sex, love, and marriage to be his vigorous assertions that masturbation was not harmful and shameful but beneficial for most people; that mutual consenting premarital sex for adults, and the use of contraception, was not immoral; and that unconventional sexual behavior was not perverse or deviant and that "sexual abnormality" is usually a myth. Additional contributions that he considered significant included his being a pioneering feminist, one of few mid-twentieth-century psychologists to strongly advocate gay liberation, and his, along with Kinsey's, disputing of the sacredness of the so-called vaginal orgasm.

Ellis was married three times: his first two marriages ended in divorce, yet good friendships with his ex-wives endured. He was in a long-term open relationship following those marriages and finally enjoyed marriage with the woman he called the greatest love of his life, Australian psychologist Debbie Joffe Ellis, until his passing in 2007.

Debbie Joffe Ellis

See also: Benjamin, Harry; Kinsey, Alfred; Money, John; Sexology; Sexual Revolution; Society for the Scientific Study of Sexuality (SSSS).

Further Reading

Ellis, A. (2010). *All out: An autobiography!* Amherst, NY: Prometheus Books.

Ellis, A., & Ellis, D. J. (2011). *Rational emotive behavior therapy.* Washington, DC: American Psychological Association.

Reiss, I. L., & Ellis, A. (2002). *At the dawn of the sexual revolution.* Walnut Creek, CA: Altamira Press.

Ellis, Henry Havelock

Henry Havelock Ellis (1859–1939) was a physician, writer, and sexologist. To some, he is considered the founding father of the psychology of sex. In his early career as a newly qualified medical doctor in the 1880s (having graduated from St. Thomas' Hospital Medical School, which is now King's College London), Ellis found himself working as the acting midwifery clerk in the London slums on the south side of Westminster Bridge. The job further emphasized his interests in research and knowledge on sex and sexual behavior. Even though Ellis wrote on a variety of topics, he is most noted for his work on sex, particularly his seven-volume work entitled *Studies in the Psychology of Sex* (published from 1897 to 1928). These volumes caused an outpouring of books on similar topics in the rest of psychology and social science (even self-help books), as the topic was clearly of popular interest.

In his professional capacity, Ellis served as president of the Galton Institute, joined the Fellowship of the New Life in 1983, and is credited with introducing the concepts of narcissism and autoeroticism, which were later taken on by psychoanalysis and further developed by Sigmund Freud. Naturally, Ellis and Freud shared correspondence on their work on sex and psychoanalysis—even though differences of opinion occurred.

Ellis was known for his own sexual problems throughout his life. During his time at boarding school, around the age of fourteen, he was bullied and forced by one particular boy to act like a horse. Pushed over and forced onto all fours, he was mounted by the fellow pupil who rode on Ellis's back around the dorm and dug his heels into Ellis with homemade spurs. Apparently, Ellis put up no resistance, and this resulted in Ellis experiencing associated wet dreams (seminal emissions during sleep) far into life as a result of these "mental wounds," as they were described.

Later in life, once he became a doctor and an established author, Ellis was often ridiculed by friends for being a leading authority on sex but not having had sex for the first time until the age of thirty-two. In 1891, at the age of thirty-two, he married English writer and female rights activist Edith Lees. Together they shared what many would consider a peculiar relationship, as Edith was openly lesbian (or arguably bisexual) and had frequent affairs with women, of which Ellis was seemingly aware. Ellis idolized Edith, and she became the central focus of his own autobiography, entitled *My Life*, which many reviewers have said focused more on Edith than Ellis and appears to end at the point of Edith's death in 1916. For a long time after his marriage to Edith, Ellis suffered from erectile dysfunction. It was not until he was in his sixties that he discovered that he was still able to become aroused when observing women urinating. This was apparently associated with his early experiences as the acting midwifery clerk, where on one occasion of attending a delivery, the pregnant woman concerned had apparently urinated on Ellis during the birth. Ellis reported in his personal notes and private life that he gained some pleasure from this act.

Having published some fifty books in his lifetime, Ellis has been credited with being the coauthor (with J. A. Simonds) of the first medical textbook on homosexuality, entitled *Sexual Inversion* (1897). Ellis did not consider homosexuality a disease, unnatural, nor a crime. However, in reading this book today, there are significant age gaps between some of the case studies of male-on-male relationships, which today would be considered child abuse. Ellis even published on, and provided some of the initial framework for, transgender psychology.

He became somewhat of a household name in his time due to his writings, being widely known in public as the infamous sex psychologist. With sex being somewhat of a taboo subject in England in the late nineteenth to early twentieth century, a lot of negative reviews were received for his books. Some boasted of having burned Ellis's books, while others expressed feeling dirty and wrong for having read the material. In their day, Ellis's books would have been seen as highly controversial. Read in the current context, Ellis's writings on sex present nothing more than academic observations of sexual processes and behavior. Yet, at the time, he was seen as a purveyor of pornography.

Ellis conducted most of his research and writings in his study in his Brixton flat, where he also saw "patients" (or clients), who came to him to discuss various sexual problems they had, typically within marriage. Some who visited him for such counsel reported him to be a tall, shy, and reserved man in a home office surrounded by books and furniture. Much like Sigmund Freud, Ellis also corresponded with his patients by post, which at one point led to a considerable number of letters being received.

Following the death of Ellis's wife, Edith, in 1916, he spent the last twenty years of his life in a close relationship with Françoise Delisle. Moving from France to England to become a schoolteacher of French, Delisle reignited some of Ellis's early interests in metaphysics and materialism. She notes in her autobiographies—of which she published three—that sex dwindled in their relationship, but conversations on the topic and many others were constant. Delisle noted discussions and experiences of psychic phenomena between Ellis and herself, instances that some would describe as telepathic, involving hallucinations of Ellis or "bilocation." Following Ellis's death in his home in Suffolk in 1939, Delisle discussed in great detail three specific instances of encountering apparitions of Ellis and sittings with mediums, the latter after having consulted with Sir Oliver Lodge. All this is noted in her third autobiography, *The Return of Havelock Ellis*, published in 1968.

Today, Ellis remains an important historical figure in sexology, especially due to the amount of publications he produced and his establishment of some of the solid foundations that have served as the basis for the field of sexology. However, much like Sigmund Freud, his work on sex has not stood the test of time, with modern thought and a vast array of research findings changing the way we view and understand who we are and the world we live in. Several Ellis biographies have been published with varying reviews. Certainly, one of the better pieces to offer a full and detailed coverage of Ellis's life was published in 1979, entitled *Havelock Ellis: Philosopher of Sex* by Vincent Brome.

Callum E. Cooper

See also: Freud, Sigmund; Sexology.

Further Reading

Brome, V. (1979). *Havelock Ellis: Philosopher of sex*. London: Routledge & Kegan Paul.

Cooper, C. E. (2015). Havelock Ellis' involvement in psychical research. Paper presented at the joint 58th Annual Parapsychological Association Convention and 39th International Conference of the Society for Psychical Research (pp. 50–51, book of abstracts), University of Greenwich, UK.

Delisle, F. (1946). *Friendship's odyssey*. London: Heinemann.

Delisle, F. (1968). *The return of Havelock Ellis*. London: Regency Press.

Ellis, H. (1940). *My life*. London: Heinemann.

Eysench, H. J., & Wilson, G. (1979). *The psychology of sex*. London: J. M. Dent & Sons.

Peterson, H. (1928). *Havelock Ellis: Philosopher of love*. London: George Allen & Unwin.

Emergency Contraception

Emergency contraception (EC) is an over-the-counter birth control that females can take after intercourse in order to prevent a possible pregnancy. It can be used in situations such as unprotected sex, unwanted sex, or failed birth control. The medication is available in both pill form and as an intrauterine device (IUD). For the pill form, women in the United States do not need a prescription to obtain it. However, the IUD requires a physician or nurse practitioner for insertion. There are no age restrictions or limits. EC will not terminate a preexisting pregnancy. Some types of EC can be effective for up to 5 days, or 120 hours, after sexual intercourse. Other types are effective for up to 3 days, or 72 hours, after sex. However, it is not as effective as other birth control methods used before sex, and therefore it should not be used or substituted as a form of regular birth control. Furthermore, EC only works to prevent pregnancy and does not prevent sexually transmitted infections.

EC prevents pregnancy mainly in two ways: through synthetic hormone pills and intrauterine devices. One of the most widely used synthetic hormones is called levonorgestrel, a form of progesterone. This hormone prevents pregnancy by delaying the release of an egg or preventing fertilization or implantation of the egg to the uterus. The level of levonorgestrel that is used in EC is higher than levels found in daily birth control pills. These pills are typically taken in one dose and do not have restrictions in order to purchase them. If taken within three days (seventy-two hours) as directed, these pills are 89 percent effective, and they are more effective the sooner they are taken after intercourse.

The newest one-pill form of EC contains ulipristal acetate. It works by temporarily delaying the release of an egg from the ovary and can be used for up to five days after unprotected sex or failed birth control. Unlike the levonorgestrel pills, ulipristal acetate's effectiveness remains consistent throughout the entire five days. It is currently only available by prescription and through online ordering. If taken as directed, it is 85 percent effective.

Another type of hormonal EC is combination daily birth control pills. Combination pills contain both synthetic estrogen and progesterone. Under the instruction of a physician, women can take between two and five daily birth control pills within three days of unprotected sex to prevent pregnancy. Different brands require different doses, and the doses are typically taken twelve hours apart. For this reason, consultation with a physician is often recommended to avoid overdosing or painful side effects.

Finally, copper IUDs are the most effective form of EC with an effectiveness rate of more than 99 percent. The copper causes an inflammatory reaction in the uterus to create a hostile environment for sperm. It can be inserted by a medical professional up to five days after sex and can remain in the uterus for up to ten years.

Lauren Wesley

See also: Conception; Contraception; Intrauterine Device (IUD); Pregnancy; Synthetic Hormones.

Further Reading

Bedsider. (2019). Emergency contraception. Retrieved from http://bedsider.org/methods/emergency_contraception#details_tab

National Institutes of Health. (2019). Emergency contraception. Retrieved from http://www.nlm.nih.gov/medlineplus/ency/article/007014.htm

Planned Parenthood. (2019). Emergency contraception. Retrieved from http://www.plannedparenthood.org/learn/morning-after-pill-emergency-contraception

World Health Organization. (2018). *Emergency contraception.* Retrieved from https://www.who.int/news-room/fact-sheets/detail/emergency-contraception

Endometriosis

Endometriosis occurs in women of reproductive age, and diagnosis occurs most often in the thirties and forties. Endometrium tissue grows outside of the uterus and often attaches to the reproductive organs, bladder, vagina, rectum, or peritoneum (lining of the abdominal and pelvic cavities). Like normal endometrium tissue, the tissue outside the uterus follows the pattern of the menstrual cycle and thickens, builds up, and bleeds with the passing of each month. However, this tissue outside the uterus has nowhere to go and so builds up more and more every month. Often during menstruation, women with endometriosis experience mild to severe abdominal and pelvic pain that is often associated with menstrual cramps. Women who come from families with a history of endometriosis have a higher chance of also having the condition. Often treatment is temporary and symptoms return.

There is no exact cause of endometriosis. Researchers believe that there is a hereditary component to the condition because women with a family history of endometriosis are five to seven times more likely to be diagnosed. For a while, many doctors and researchers thought that the cause was retrograde menstruation, which occurs when endometrial cells and tissue flow backward into the fallopian tubes during menstruation. However, endometriosis and retrograde menstruation are two separate conditions that could possibly be related. There is also a possibility that the condition may result from an immune system disorder in which endometrial cells outside the uterus are not killed and thus build upon one another.

The most common symptom of endometriosis is mild to severe abdominal and pelvic pain that sometimes extends into the lower back region. Pain may worsen or become unbearable during menstruation and is often associated with and mistaken for heavy cramping. Women with endometriosis may experience heavy periods and less often may experience more than one episode of menstrual bleeding within a month. Other symptoms of this condition include pain either during or after intercourse and infertility.

Laparoscopy is the most exact manner of diagnosing endometriosis. Laparoscopy is a surgery in which a laparoscope is inserted into a small incision made in the abdomen. The abdominal and pelvic organs are observed, and a small piece of tissue is removed for analysis. Doctors may also complete other tests such as pelvic examinations and ultrasounds.

There is no cure for endometriosis. However, there are treatments to help with severe pain and infertility. The most common treatment for younger women is hormonal contraceptives such as birth control pills and the noncopper intrauterine device. Other treatments include laparoscopic excision surgery. Laparoscopic excision surgery is the most effective treatment and removes the built-up tissue. However, more tissue may return every month following the procedure. Having a hysterectomy may be an option, but tissue buildup can still occur.

There are no preventative techniques for endometriosis. However, during menstruation using heating pads and taking anti-inflammatory drugs, such as ibuprofen, may aid with abdominal and pelvic pain.

Camilla Loggins

See also: Endometrium; Menstruation; Uterus.

Further Reading

American College of Obstetricians and Gynecologists. (2012). Endometriosis. Retrieved from http://www.acog.org/-/media/For-Patients/faq013.pdf?dmc=1&ts=20150930T0042200720

Endometriosis Foundation of America. (2015). What is endometriosis? Retrieved from http://www.endofound.org/endometriosis

Mayo Clinic. (2016). Endometriosis. Retrieved from http://www.mayoclinic.org/diseases-conditions/endometriosis/basics/definition/con-20013968

PubMed Health. (2014). Endometriosis: Overview. Retrieved from http://www.ncbi.nlm.nih.gov/pubmedhealth/PMH0072685/

Endometrium

The endometrium, also referred to as the uterine lining, is the mucosal lining inside a female's uterus. It plays a pivotal role in pregnancy as the site of implantation, where a young embryo attaches itself to the lining approximately six to seven days after fertilization. It serves as a source of nourishment for the developing embryo through the proteins and glycogen that are secreted by the uterine glands, which are located within the endometrium. The uterine lining also goes through cyclical changes as it prepares for a pregnancy, or menstruation in the event that a pregnancy does not occur.

The endometrium goes through a monthly cycle of physical changes that occur in four phases, called the menstrual, proliferative, secretory, and ischemic phases. During these phases, the endometrium thickens to prepare itself for implantation, and if an embryo is not present to implant, it then sheds itself. These phases are concurrent with the ovarian cycle when eggs are matured and released for fertilization. Estrogen and progesterone contribute to the stimulation of the endometrium as it prepares itself to receive an embryo.

In the menstrual phase, during approximately the first five days of the cycle, the endometrium, containing a mixture of blood and debris, sheds itself, and this constitutes the menstrual flow. The second phase, known as the proliferative phase, occurs between days six and fourteen of the cycle. At this time, the endometrium rebuilds after shedding from the previous phase. Proliferation takes place as estrogen stimulates the formation of thick mucosa and uterine glands. This phase occurs along with ovulation (typically around day fourteen), when the egg is released from the ovary. The increase in progesterone that is released during ovulation leads to the secretion of uterine fluid by the endometrial glands, which marks the beginning of the secretory phase. This phase occurs between days fourteen and twenty-eight. The secretions released during this phase are necessary for embryonic implantation and development. Finally, in the absence of fertilization, the ischemic phase begins as estrogen and progesterone decline, oxygen reduces, and the endometrial blood flow diminishes, causing the endometrium to shed. This occurs between days twenty-seven and twenty-eight of a typical twenty-eight-day cycle.

Abnormalities of the endometrium can indicate a number of conditions that affect thousands of women each year. One of the most common is endometriosis, a condition where the tissues of the endometrium grow outside the uterus. In severe cases, the endometrium can encase the surrounding organs, causing other tissues to develop into adhesions that bind organs together. Another condition, adenomyosis, occurs when the endometrial lining grows into the muscular wall of the uterus, which can cause an enlarged uterus and painful menstrual cycles.

Endometrial cancer, also referred to as uterine cancer, develops when cancer cells form in the endometrium. One of the first symptoms of endometrial cancer is vaginal bleeding, which is why this type of cancer is often diagnosed early. In the United States, endometrial cancer is the most common type of female reproductive cancer.

Lauren Wesley

See also: Endometriosis; Menstruation; Pregnancy; Uterine Cancer; Uterus.

Further Reading

American Cancer Society. (2015). *Endometrial (uterine) cancer.* Retrieved from http://www.cancer.org/cancer/endometrialcancer/detailedguide/endometrial-uterine-cancer-key-statistics

Aria Health. (2015). *Endometrial conditions.* Retrieved from https://www.ariahealth.org/programs-and-services/centers-of-excellence/women-s-health/endometrial-onditions

Mayo Clinic. (2015). *Adenomyosis.* Retrieved from http://www.mayoclinic.org/diseases-conditions/adenomyosis/basics/definition/con-20024740

Mayo Clinic. (2015). *Endometrial cancer.* Retrieved from http://www.mayoclinic.org/diseases-conditions/endometrial-cancer/basics/definition/con-20033696

WebMD. (2015). *Endometrium and cervix.* Retrieved from http://www.webmd.com/women/the-endometrium-and-cervix

Epididymis

The epididymis is a structure of the male reproductive system. It is located on each testicle and is often referred to as the housing center for sperm. The epididymis is made up of tightly coiled tubes that create a pathway for sperm. It is crescent shaped and has three parts: a tail, head, and body. The head is located on the top of the testes and is considered the widest region of the epididymis. This is where sperm are stored until they are matured and sent to the body of the epididymis. The body is narrow and moves sperm from the head to the tail of the epididymis. The tail of the epididymis is located on the bottom of the testes and connects to the vas deferens. All these parts combined help ensure the safe travel of sperm until they reach their next destination.

Prior to entering the epididymis, sperm develop in the seminiferous tubules, which are a large set of condensed tubes inside the testicles. After sperm is produced, is it usually nonmotile and requires a large amount of liquid to be transferred to the next location—the epididymis. The immature sperm make their way to the epididymis, where they usually spend about a week finding their way through the largely coiled tubes. During this time, they begin to mature and develop a slow swimming forward motion. When the matured sperm finish passing through the epididymis, they travel into the vas deferens upon sexual stimulation, leading to possible ejaculation. When the sperm is transferred from the epididymis to the vas deferens, it has a paste-like consistency. Through muscular contractions, the vas deferens transfers the mature sperm to the ejaculatory duct. This sperm is then combined with fluids secreted from the prostate gland, which gives semen its texture and odor, and the seminal vesicles, which give sperm fructose for energy. Finally, this fluid travels down the ejaculatory duct and into the urethra, where it will be propelled out of the penis.

The epididymis contains stereocilia inside each of its structures. Stereocilia are long projections that are nonmotile. The point of stereocilia is to take 90 percent of the fluid used to transfer the sperm to the epididymis and only leave mature mobile sperm. The epididymis can store matured sperm for up to a month until it expires and the stereocilia begin to absorb it completely. When this happens, expired sperm are then replaced with younger, immature sperm.

The epididymis is very important for sperm and fertility. If something damages the epididymis, such as trauma, sperm production and reproduction can be hindered. While sperm can still be produced, they cannot be stored and, therefore, will not be viable. A possible injury to the epididymis could come from a urinary infection that develops due to bacteria like *Escherichia coli* (*E. coli*). This is most common in older men because of an increase in restriction or obstruction of urine flow. Another example of a complication would be epididymitis, which occurs when the epididymis tube swells, resulting in testicle pain and inflammation. This is most commonly caused by a bacterial infection or sexually transmitted infection (STI). Most of the time, epididymitis can be treated with antibiotics, ice, and rest. However, if not properly treated, chronic epididymitis or continuous pain and swelling in the testicles may occur, possibly requiring surgery.

In order for epididymitis to be diagnosed, doctors will examine the groin and swollen testicles to assess for enlarged lymph nodes. Rarely doctors may perform a rectal exam to determine if the prostate is also swollen. Some tests to diagnose epididymitis include STI screenings, urine and blood tests, and ultrasounds. Screenings may include a small swab that is inserted into the penis to test the discharge inside of the urethra as well as urine and blood tests. Ultrasounds can be used to assess the level of blood flow in the testicles. If there is less blood flow than average, the pain and swelling could be due to another possible condition of the testicles. However, if the flow of blood is higher than average, the doctor may request further testing and possibly confirm the diagnosis of epididymitis.

It is known that temperature influences the function of the epididymis. For sperm to be produced, the body requires the testicles to be at a specific temperature, slightly below core body temperature. If the testicles are exposed to higher or lower temperatures for long periods of time, sperm count may decrease, possibly leading to decreased fertility. With significant temperature changes, the life span of the sperm being stored inside the epididymis can be shortened.

Casey T. Tobin

See also: Semen; Seminiferous Tubules; Sperm; Testicles; Vas Deferens.

Further Reading

Lehmiller, J. (2013). *The psychology of human sexuality.* Hoboken, NJ: John Wiley & Sons.

Maier, T. (2009). *Masters of sex.* New York: Basic Books.

Sullivan, R., & Mieusset, R. (2016). The human epididymis: Its function in sperm maturation. *Human Reproduction, 22*, 574–587.

Erectile Dysfunction

People with penises may experience erectile dysfunction. Erectile disorder may be diagnosed if an individual reports repeatedly being unable to have or maintain an erection during sexual activity with a partner. People who are experiencing erectile dysfunction may also experience low self-esteem, a lack or reduction in self-confidence, depressed mood, and a decrease in their sense of masculinity. Because of the difficulty with experiencing an erection and the associated negative feelings, some people with erectile dysfunction may avoid sexual activities and may experience less sexual satisfaction and lower sexual desire. An individual's partner or partners may also experience some of these same feelings as a result of their partner's erectile dysfunction.

Approximately 8 percent of men report experiencing erectile problems the first time they have sex, and this may be related to using drugs or alcohol or to various psychological factors, such as not wanting to have sex or feeling peer pressure. The majority of these cases will resolve on their own. When erectile dysfunction occurs later in life, it is often associated with medical factors such as diabetes, cardiovascular disease, or other diseases that affect how the body functions. In these cases, erectile dysfunction can be persistent for many people. Other psychological factors, such as neuroticism, depression, anxiety, and posttraumatic stress disorder, can also be linked with erectile dysfunction. Other risk factors include smoking, lack of exercise, and decreased sexual desire. There are often both medical and psychological causes for erectile dysfunction, and it can also co-occur with other sexual disorders, including premature (early) ejaculation and male hypoactive sexual desire disorder.

According to the *Diagnostic and Statistical Manual of Mental Disorders, Fifth Edition* (*DSM-V*), in order for a diagnosis of erectile disorder to be made, an individual must experience at least one of the following symptoms during almost all or all (75–100%) occasions of sexual activity: (1) marked difficulty in obtaining an erection during sexual activity, (2) marked difficulty in maintaining an erection until the completion of sexual activity, or (3) marked decrease in erectile rigidity. To meet criteria for diagnosis, symptoms need to have occurred for a minimum of around six months, and they need to cause clinically significant distress to the individual. Finally, the erectile difficulties should not be better explained by a nonsexual mental disorder or as a consequence of severe relationship distress or other significant stressors, and they should not be a side effect of substance or medication use or another medical condition.

In addition, the *DSM-V* recognizes that erectile disorder can occur in specific identified situations or in all contexts. It can also be lifelong or acquired, meaning that it begins after a period of relatively normal sexual function, such as in later life. Severity of distress associated with symptoms of erectile disorder can be mild, moderate, or severe.

Erectile dysfunction becomes more common with age, particularly over the age of fifty years. Approximately 13–21 percent of men aged forty to eighty years complain of occasional erectile difficulties; however, older men (ages sixty to seventy years) are increasingly likely to report significant erectile problems. Only

2 percent of men under the age of forty years report frequent erection difficulties. Age has been shown to be associated with erectile dysfunction in both heterosexual and sexual minority men.

Heather L. Armstrong

See also: Diagnostic and Statistical Manual of Mental Disorders (DSM); Erectile Dysfunction Drugs; Erection; Penis; Sexual Disorders, Male.

Further Reading

American Psychiatric Association. (2013). *Diagnostic and statistical manual of mental disorders* (5th ed.). Arlington, VA: Author.

Hart, T. A., Moskowitz, D., Cox, C., Li, X., Ostrow, D. G., Stall, R. D., ... Plankey, M. (2012). The cumulative effects of medication use, drug use, and smoking on erectile dysfunction among men who have sex with men. *Journal of Sexual Medicine, 9*, 1106–1113.

Hirshfield, S., Chiasson, M. A., Wagmiller, R. L., Remien, R. H., Humberstone, M., Scheinmann, R., & Grov, C. (2010). Sexual dysfunction in an internet sample of U.S. men who have sex with men. *Journal of Sexual Medicine, 7*, 3104–3114.

Ivanković, I., Šević, S., & Štulhofer, A. (2015). Distressing sexual difficulties in heterosexual and non-heterosexual Croatian men: Assessing the role of minority stress. *Journal of Sex Research, 52*(6), 647–658.

Laumann, E. O., Nicolosi, A., Glasser, D. B., Paik, A., Cingell, C., Moreira, E., & Wang, T. (2005). Sexual problems among women and men aged 40–80 y: Prevalence and correlated identified in the Global Study of Sexual Attitudes and Behaviors. *International Journal of Impotence Research, 17*, 39–57.

Shindel, A. W., Vittinghoff, E., & Breyer, B. N. (2012). Erectile dysfunction and premature ejaculation in men who have sex with men. *Journal of Sexual Medicine, 9*, 576–584.

Erectile Dysfunction Drugs

Erectile dysfunction drugs (EDD) are prescription medications used to treat men with erectile dysfunction (ED), the inability to obtain or maintain an erection. This condition, also known as impotence, affects, to some extent, as many as 50 percent of men over age forty.

Erectile dysfunction can have any of several causes, including low levels of testosterone, diseases affecting blood vessels, diabetes, pelvic injuries, and psychological problems. Whatever the cause, the end result is that the penis is prevented from growing hard and erect. For the penis to become erect, blood needs to flow into, and fill, two sponge-like regions called corpora cavernosa, which run the length of the penis.

Sildenafil citrate, one of the first and most common EDDs, works by relaxing the smooth muscles that surround the blood vessels in the penis, thereby widening the vessels and increasing blood flow into the corpora cavernosa. The drug is taken in the form of a blue pill, preferably thirty minutes to one hour before sexual activity, though it could remain effective as long as four hours. Dosage depends on the precise diagnosis of the individual's condition. The drug does not automatically produce an erection. Some form of sexual stimulation must occur for it to work, such as arousal prompted by a sex partner or by sexual images.

People with cardiovascular diseases who are using nitrate medications should not use sildenafil citrate because the drug combination increases the risk of heart attack and stroke during sexual activity. Consequently, the Food and Drug Administration (FDA) warns physicians to be cautious about prescribing sildenafil citrate to men with heart disease or high blood pressure.

Some people using EDDs experience prolonged, painful erections called priapism. Such erections can cause tissue damage to the penis, so medical attention is needed if an erection lasts more than two hours. Sildenafil citrate has also been linked to sudden vision loss in a small number of individuals. In such cases, the drug causes an unintended increase in the flow of blood to the optic nerve. Other adverse effects associated with EDDs include nausea, headache, dizziness, hearing problems, sweating, swelling in hands or feet, and shortness of breath.

Sildenafil citrate was developed based on the work of several scientists, including pharmacologists Robert F. Furchgott, Louis Joseph Ignarro, and Ferid Murad, who shared the 1998 Nobel Prize in Physiology or Medicine for their research into how a gas called nitric oxide causes muscle relaxation and blood vessel widening. Clinical trials by pharmaceutical scientists indicated that sildenafil citrate was effective in 70 percent of about 4,000 men in whom it was tested, leading to the patent of their medication in 1996.

The FDA approved sildenafil citrate in March 1998. The drug soon became a best-selling product, with 3.6 million prescriptions written in the first four months of its availability. In 2005, the FDA approved a version of sildenafil to improve exercise ability in adults with pulmonary arterial hypertension (high blood pressure in the lungs).

Other EDDs used to treat patients with erectile dysfunction, all of which work through mechanisms similar to those of sildenafil citrate, include tadalafil, vardenafil hydrochloride, and avanafil. The widespread use of these EDDs has had a few surprising social effects. For example, they have been linked to an increase in sexually transmitted infections among the residents of senior citizen facilities.

A. J. Smuskiewicz

See also: Arousal; Erectile Dysfunction; Erection; Male Sexuality; Penis; Priapism; Sexual Disorders, Male; Sexual Dysfunction, Treatment of; Sexuality among Older Adults.

Further Reading

Loe, M. (2006). *The rise of Viagra: How the little blue pill changed sex in America.* New York: New York University Press.

Morgentaler, A. (2003). *The Viagra myth: The surprising impact on love and relationships.* San Francisco: Jossey-Bass/Wiley.

Erection

Erections occur in both penises and clitorises, although they work differently, serve different functions, and look different. Penile erections are the result of a complex internal system activated by erectile tissue, vascular (blood flow) and cavernosal smooth muscle, brain function, complex nerve function, and neurotransmitters. Similarly, the clitoris engorges and arouses but is distinguished in that it does not become "hard" but rather full and swollen. While both penile and clitoral erections indicate the presence of physical arousal, neither are necessary for sexual pleasure, as pleasure is highly subjective.

The human penis is comprised of three cylindrical structures working in unison, along with muscles, nerves, arteries, and veins. There are two corpora cavernosa and one corpus spongiosum, which run the length of the penis. It is helpful to remember that cavernosa are full of caverns, tiny holes that function like cups that fill up with blood to enable the penis to engorge and create the erection. The cavernosa are supported at the base of the penis by the penis's crura (legs), which reach deep inside the body. These in turn are further supported by the ischiocavernosus muscles that run underneath the bones of the pelvis, which contract during an erection to keep the blood inside the penis. The spongiosum is padded tissue that wraps around the urethra. It is made of squishy tissue that swells to prevent restriction of the urethra during arousal. The urethra is the tube where both urine and ejaculate leave the body, although it is rare for urine to come out during an erection. The corpus spongiosum is surrounded by the bulbospongiosus muscle. This muscle is responsible for increasing pressure to sustain the erection as well as for contracting and providing the pulsing sensation during ejaculation. This muscle may also be felt during urination when squeezed to stop the flow of urine.

The three cylinders of the penis are bound together inside the skin by the tunica albuginea (TA), which acts like a sock that wraps around them and tightens to help keep the blood in during an erection. The TA is a dual-layered structure that wraps both lengthwise and circularly around the cylinders. It is made of collagen fibers to promote hardness and elastin to support flexibility.

Penile erections result from relaxation of cavernosal and vascular smooth muscles, which leads to dilation of the arteries, which allows blood in, and vein compression, which keeps the blood trapped inside. When the penis is flaccid, vascular and cavernosal smooth muscles are in a contracted state.

The clitoris is a similar though not identical anatomical structure that also contains erectile tissue. The clitoris is approximately four inches long and, like the penis, consists of two joined corpora cavernosa reaching down within the body as crura (legs). Each corpus cavernosum contains tiny blood vessels and is wrapped by the tunica albuginea. The TA in the clitoris, however, is only a single layer, unlike the dual structure found in the penis. As a result, there is no function for trapping blood, which results in engorgement but not hardness. The vestibular bulbs of the clitoris are analogous to the spongiosum in the penis except they are separate from the urethra and the crura of the clitoris. The clitoral glans (or head) is the part of the clitoris that protrudes from between the top of the inner labia of the vulva and can be seen externally. However, unlike the penis, the majority of the clitoris is internal and extends to deep within the body. Like the penis, the crura are comprised of erectile tissue and are adjacent to the vagina and urethra.

Penile erections are often required for penetrative sex but not for receiving pleasure. This means a penis may still enjoy touch whether erect or not. Likewise, clitoral erections indicate the presence of genital arousal but alone are not an indication of sexual pleasure nor satisfaction. The only way for a person to know if pleasure is happening is for them to talk about it with their partner(s).

Penile erections do not always happen on demand, and they are notoriously unreliable. There is a misconception (especially in Western culture) that erections occur readily and spontaneously, with no incentive, and that males are always ready for sex. This is not true. While some people experience penile erections without any sexual stimuli, others may have difficulty achieving or maintaining an erection even in the presence of stimuli they find sexually arousing. This can become more prominent with age.

Penile erection problems can stem from a variety of sources, including anxiety, trauma and injury, poor dietary choices, poor general health, diabetes, aging, and smoking, all of which can affect blood flow. Erectile dysfunction (ED) is a common experience estimated to affect 30 million people in the United States with up to 52 percent of men aged forty to seventy years experiencing mild to complete ED. The worldwide prevalence of ED is projected to increase to 322 million men by the year 2025. While treatment for ED can include pharmacology (pills) and psychosexual (talk therapy) treatment, often a simple change in routine can help if there are no underlying physiological factors. Despite controversy in popular media, there is no evidence that consumption of pornography alone is a direct cause of ED. It is hypothesized that high-intensity, frequent masturbation may reduce sexual incentive for partnered sex and potentially reduce the effectiveness of traditional sexual incentives. In other words, a lot of masturbation may potentially reduce a person's level of sexual interest or desire, potentially making it less likely they will get an erection on demand when they are with a partner. However, it is hard to say what a "normal" amount of masturbation is because each person is unique. Instead, highly frequent masturbation may become a behavioral choice people can manage by accessing better-quality sex education and reflecting on their sexual health values.

The same sexual function problems that cause erectile dysfunction in penises can also cause problems in clitorises and vulvas, although they may manifest differently. These include spinal cord injury or disease of the central or peripheral nervous system, including diabetes and motor neuron disease.

Cyndi Darnell

See also: Arousal; Clitoris; Erectile Dysfunction; Erectile Dysfunction Drugs; Penis; Sexual Dysfunction, Treatment of; Touching, Sexual Arousal and.

Further Reading

Berman, J. R., Berman, L. A., & Kanaly, K. A. (2003). Female sexual dysfunction: New perspectives on anatomy, physiology, evaluation and treatment. *EAU Update Series, 1*(3), 166–177.

Blechner, M. J. (2017). The clitoris: Anatomical and psychological issues. *Studies in Gender and Sexuality, 18*(3), 190–200.

Braun-Harvey, D., & Vigorito, M. A. (2016). *Treating out of control sexual behavior.* New York: Springer Publishing.

Darnell, C. (2019). *The atlas of erotic anatomy and arousal.* Retrieved from https://cyndidarnell.com/atlas-of-erotic-anatomy-arousal/

Yuh, L., & Shindel, A. (2017). Anatomy of penile erection. In S. Minhas & J. Mulhall (Eds.), *Male sexual dysfunction: A clinical guide* (22–29). Sacramento, CA: Wiley-Blackwell.

Zaid, U. B., Zhang, X., & Lue, T. F. (2017). Physiology of penile erection. In S. Minhas & J. Mulhall (Eds.), *Male sexual dysfunction: A clinical guide* (14–21). Sacramento, CA: Wiley-Blackwell.

Erogenous Zones

Erogenous zones are areas of the body with concentrated nerve endings that are highly sensitive to touch and, when stimulated through touch, allow an individual to experience sexual arousal. Erogenous zones may be split into two categories: nonspecific erogenous zones and specific erogenous zones. Nonspecific erogenous zones contain the typical density of dermal nerves. These are areas of the body that have "usual haired skin" such as the back and sides of the neck. Specific erogenous zones are found in mucocutaneous areas (where mucosa transitions to skin) of the body, specifically the genitals, perineum (area between the anus and scrotum or vulva), lips, and nipples. In these areas, nerve concentrations are raised higher in the dermis than in the typical haired skin mentioned above (Winkelmann, 1959). This nerve structure makes these areas extra sensitive to touch.

Sigmund Freud discussed erogenous zones when he theorized about the psychosexual development of humans. He stated that children have specific erogenous zones through which they seek and receive pleasure. During the "oral phase," children from birth to age 1.5 years are focused on their mouth to receive pleasure. From age 1.5 years to age three years, children are focused on their anus during their "anal stage." During the "phallic stage," which occurs between the ages of four and five years, children focus on their genitals. From age five to puberty, Freud believed children take a break from their sexual development to focus on other areas of growth and, therefore, he believed that during this "latency stage," they do not focus on a specific erogenous zone. However, from puberty on, during a stage called the "genital stage," the focus of sexual pleasure returns to the genital erogenous zone.

A 2014 study conducted in Canada sought to understand how female bodies reacted to various types of touch on various body parts. This study revealed that not all areas of the body respond similarly to sensory experiences. Different areas of the body were subjected to different sensory experiences: light touch, pressure, and vibration. The data showed that the neck, forearm, and vaginal margin were among the areas of the body most sensitive to light touching. The areola was the area of the female body least sensitive to light touch. With regard to pressure, the clitoris and nipples were most sensitive and the lateral breasts and abdomen were least sensitive to pressure. The clitoris and nipples were among the most sensitive to vibration.

In a Finnish study in 2016, 704 volunteer participants were given pictures of male and female bodies and were asked to indicate where on the male and female bodies they would expect touch to elicit sexual arousal. Researchers collected this data and created "erogenous zone maps" based on the body parts frequently indicated by the participants as being sexually arousing when touched. While the data showed that the entire body has the potential to be an erogenous zone, the "hotspots" or most frequently indicated body parts consisted of the breasts, genitals, and anus. On a whole, about 24 percent of the total body area was found to be capable of producing sexual arousal when touched. After the "hotspots" mentioned above, the next most common areas to be indicated as erogenous zones included the chest, neck, and mouth. Researchers were also surprised that the back, thighs, and shins ranked highly despite the fact that these areas have low tactile sensitivity.

Other results stemming from this study indicate that erogenous zones are perceived differently depending on the type of sex being had. When discussing partnered sex, participants were more generous in the number of body parts they considered to be erogenous zones. In partnered sex, the entire skin area could be considered sensitive and arousing. However, in the context of masturbation, participants were more selective in the body parts they considered erogenous zones, focusing mostly on the breasts, genitals, and inner thighs.

Gender differences were also highlighted in this research. On the pictures of female bodies, participants indicated a greater total area of erogenous zones than on the pictures of male bodies. It is important to note that this data was driven by participant perception and response.

Erogenous zones are frequently discussed in the media and popular culture. However, there is not an overwhelming amount of research on erogenous zones. It is agreed that erogenous zones are areas of the body that, when stimulated, lead to sexual arousal. However, the specific body parts are up for discussion and are often based on personal preference.

Amanda Manuel

See also: Arousal; Freud, Sigmund; Touching, Sexual Arousal and.

Further Reading

Cardeau, D., Belanger, M., Beaulieu-Prevost, D., & Courtois, F. (2014). The assessment of sensory detection threshold on the perineum and breast compared with control body sites. *Journal of Sexual Medicine, 11*(7), 1741–1748.

Freud, S., Strachey, J., & Richards, A. (1977). *On sexuality: Three essays on the theory of sexuality and other works*. Harmondsworth: Penguin Books.

Nummenmaa, L., Suvilehto, J. T., Glerean, E., Santtila, P., & Hietanen, J. K. (2016). Topography of human erogenous zones. *Archives of Sexual Behavior, 45*, 1207–1216.

Winkelmann, R. K. (1959). The erogenous zones: Their nerve supply and significance. *Mayo Clinic Proceedings, 34*(2), 39–47.

Erotophilia and Erotophobia

Erotophilia and erotophobia have been involved in many aspects of psychology, sex education, and even politics. Erotophobia can be described as an irrational fear of anything sexual in nature and is something that can be clinically diagnosed. However, it is also seen as a personality trait, being on the far end of a personality spectrum, opposite of erotophilia. Erotophilia refers to someone who thinks of sex as a positive part of life, often having a positive attitude and positive feelings toward sex. An erotophilic is not ashamed to discuss sex and sexuality and believes sex is an essential part of a healthy relationship.

The words "erotophilia" and "erotophobia" come from the Greek god of erotic love, Eros. "Eroto" means relating to eroticism, sexual arousal, or sexual excitement, and "philia" means a love of a specified thing. This means that erotophilia literally means a love of eroticism. A phobia, on the other hand, is an irrational fear of something, so erotophobia is an irrational fear of eroticism.

Looking at erotophobia as a clinical phobia, it is the irrational fear of anything pertaining to sex. "Erotophobia" is also an umbrella term that can include many different, more specific phobias, such as a fear of nudity, a fear of sexual images, a fear of sex education, a fear of sexual disclosure, and homophobia. The fear can be related to other psychological problems, such as social anxiety or body dysmorphic disorder, or it can be very specific only to something related to sex. A person with erotophobia can have a feeling of guilt about their own sexuality. Erotophobia can have several causes or underlying factors, including sexual abuse, other traumas, and religious beliefs. Symptoms of the phobia can vary from person to person but typically include anxiety, dread, and panic when exposed to anything that is sexual in nature. These symptoms and the phobia itself can be very debilitating, meaning that it can affect the person's sex life, sexuality, and their daily life in negative ways.

Although erotophobia is a clinical disorder, it is also seen in psychological research as a personality trait that determines how someone responds to sexual cues. A person can fall anywhere on the spectrum from erotophobia (negative feelings or a fear of sexual cues) to erotophilia (positive feelings toward sexual cues). In this sense, erotophobia is a more general aversion to sex rather than a debilitating disorder. Erotophobes are less likely to talk about sex, and they have more negative reactions to sexual material. They also tend to have more traditional sex roles, meaning that they may not experiment when it comes to sexual activity or explore their sexuality. They also tend to have sex less, fewer sexual partners, more sex guilt, and more negative feelings when it comes to masturbation and homosexuality. In a general sense, erotophobic people are more traditional with sexuality and are not comfortable talking about, learning about, or exploring their sexuality.

People on the opposite side of the spectrum are considered erotophilic and have positive feelings toward sexual aspects of life. They are more likely to masturbate, think about sex, and fantasize. They generally have sex for the first time earlier than do erotophobes and have more sexual partners. They are more open to exploring sexuality, less traditional, and more open to learning about sex and sexuality. There are online tests that people can take to see where they fall on the spectrum and if they are more erotophobic or erotophilic.

In addition to seeing how erotophilic and erotophobic people feel about sex and sexuality, these personality measurements are also very helpful when it comes to sexual health and relationships. For sexual health, these measurements are used to see how sexually healthy people are. Research has found that erotophilic people are more likely to protect against sexually transmitted infections, do breast self-examinations, and go to regular gynecologist appointments. People who are comfortable talking about their sexuality and learning more about it are more likely to use contraception. This openness to sexual aspects of life leads to having a safer sex life and a better understanding of sexual health. Having a fear of sexuality and a fear of learning more about how to engage in sex safely can be damaging to erotophobic people. Although they have a fear of or negative feelings toward sexual aspects of life, they are not asexual beings, meaning they still participate in sexual intercourse, just not in the safest or most pleasurable ways. In addition to sexual health, being an erotophobe may bring problems to relationship or marriage. Sex is a very important aspect of many people's relationships, so if one person has very negative feelings toward sex while the other person doesn't, this can cause a disconnect in the sexual aspect of their relationship. This disconnect may not allow for the couple to connect in other ways that are important to them, creating significant problems for their relationship.

Finally, erotophobia has also been used by activists in the political world. These antioppression activists use the word "erotophobia" to describe sex-negative attitudes as a form of oppression. They believe that people who wish not to talk about sex or engage in exploring their sexuality use their beliefs in a way that affects how they feel about other people. The activists believe that being erotophobic puts constraints on sexuality and that people use their erotophobic feelings to discriminate against those who are more open about their sexuality. Activists also believe that erotophobia is a particularly damaging phobia, comparing it to racism, sexism, homophobia, and other isms and phobias that are particularly relevant in our society today. Some even believe that erotophobia is intertwined with social inequality and politics, stating that overcoming the irrational fear of sexual aspects of life is one of the first steps one can take toward a democratic society. Activists are against erotophobia in general because they feel that this discomfort with sex and sexuality makes the subjects taboo, meaning that society is taking a step in the wrong direction. Activists wish for our society to become more open with sex and sexuality as it is a normal part of life, but erotophobia gets in the way of accomplishing that.

Casey T. Tobin

See also: Asexual; Communication, Sexual; Homophobia; Sex Guilt; Sexual Avoidance; Sexual Health.

Further Reading

Balzarini, R. N., Shumlich, E., Kohut, T., & Campbell, L. (2018). Sexual attitudes, erotophobia, and sociosexual orientation differ based on relationship orientation. *Journal of Sex Research.* Online ahead of print.

Fisher, W., White, L., Byrne, D., & Kelley, K. (2010). Erotophobia-erotophilia as a dimension of personality. *Journal of Sex Research, 25,* 123–151.

García-Vega, E., Rico, R., & Fernández, P. (2017). Sex, gender roles and sexual attitudes in university students. *Psicothema, 29*(2), 178–183.

LeVay, S., Baldwin, J., & Baldwin, J. (2018). *Discovering human sexuality* (4th ed.). Sunderland, MA: Sinauer Associates.

Essure Coil

The Essure coil was a permanent female birth control procedure and was touted as a nonsurgical alternative to tubal ligation. The procedure was approved by the Food and Drug Administration (FDA) in 2002 and was reported to be about 99 percent effective, with statistics showing that fewer than one out of one hundred women who have undergone successful Essure implantation procedures experience an unplanned pregnancy. Approximately 750,000 women around the world have been fitted with Essure coils. However, because of growing reports of serious adverse side effects, the production and use of Essure coils was stopped in 2018.

The Essure procedure involved inserting small, flexible metal and fiber coils inside the fallopian tubes, which carry the egg from the ovaries to the uterus. The coils were inserted through the natural openings in the vagina and cervix, so no surgical incision was required. Once the coils were in place, scar tissue began to build up around them. After a period of approximately three months, the tissue buildup created a barrier that blocked any sperm from reaching an egg, thus preventing conception. As the procedure was not surgical, it typically required a one-hour outpatient visit to a clinic, followed by one to two days of decreased physical activity. X-rays were taken at a follow-up appointment at three months to determine whether or not enough scarring had occurred to create a viable barrier. Until this barrier was fully formed, people were advised to use additional forms of birth control to prevent unwanted pregnancies.

Although the Essure procedure was considered to be a highly effective means of birth control, it was not without risk. If an accidental pregnancy occurred after receiving the Essure coil, it was more likely to be an ectopic pregnancy, meaning it had implanted somewhere outside the uterus (usually within the fallopian tube itself). Additional risks involved with the procedure include infection, rash or other allergic reaction to the nickel-titanium alloy in the coils, pain in the pelvic region, bleeding or spotting, perforations in the uterus or fallopian tube due to insertion of the coils, or only partial tubal blockage some six months or more after the procedure has taken place. In addition, Essure does not provide protection against sexually transmitted infections.

Although considered a permanent form of birth control, the Essure coil procedure is reversible and, once removed, should not prevent future planned pregnancies.

In recent years, complaints against Essure surged, with the FDA fielding some five hundred reports of "adverse events" related to the contraception device in 2013 alone. Because of the growing number of complaints, and product recalls and suspensions, the manufacturer of the Essure coil stopped producing and selling them in 2018.

Tamar Burris

See also: Contraception; Fallopian Tubes; Sterilization; Tubal Ligation.

Further Reading

Bullough, V. L. (2001). *Encyclopedia of birth control.* Santa Barbara, CA: ABC-CLIO.

Zorea, A. W. (2012). *Birth control.* Westport, CT: Greenwood.

Estrogen

Estrogens are the primary female sex hormones. They are produced in the ovaries, fat cells, and adrenal glands. Estrogens are essential for reproductive development and regulate the menstrual cycle. They are also produced synthetically for use in birth control medications and hormone replacement therapy.

In the female body, estrogens are instrumental in the onset of puberty and the development of secondary sex traits. These hormones are also important for proper functioning of the reproductive system, playing a role in triggering ovulation and preparing the uterus for implantation of a fertilized egg, which will develop into a fetus. During pregnancy, estrogen levels remain high and work with the hormone progesterone to stop ovulation. Natural estrogens are also essential for bone formation and condition, working with vitamin D and calcium to rebuild bone tissue. Postmenopausal women have significantly lower levels of estrogen, leading to bone tissue being broken down more than being built up, causing women to be more at risk of osteoporosis, a condition in which bones are weak and brittle and break easily. Johns Hopkins Medicine reports that estrogen also helps maintain the body's ability to clot blood and affects the condition of one's skin, hair, mucus membranes, and pelvic muscles. The hormone may also affect brain cells, with some studies finding that postmenopausal women with low estrogen levels have reduced memory and depressed mood.

Estrogens produced synthetically are a key component in oral birth control medicines. The synthetic hormones are identical to the ones produced in the human body and are made in the laboratory from the plant chemicals of yams and soybeans. The hormones work to keep estrogen levels high, essentially "tricking" the body into thinking it is pregnant and thereby preventing ovulation from occurring.

Hormone replacement therapy is also a major use of synthetic estrogens. Although most often used to relieve uncomfortable symptoms during and after menopause, they are also prescribed to younger women who do not produce enough estrogen in the body, which causes problems with the reproductive process. It is also given to adolescent girls who need higher estrogen levels in order to induce puberty. Estrogen therapy may also be used by trans women during their gender transition process.

Despite the benefits of estrogen replacement, research has shown that taking synthetic estrogen in this form for a prolonged period can pose serious health risks. Similar risk factors exist for those who take oral contraceptives over a long period. Estrogen causes an increased risk of endometrial cancer, ovarian cancer, and breast cancer and may also cause gallbladder disease. According to the National Institute of Health, people who took estrogen, especially along with progestin (synthetic progesterone), suffered a greater incidence of heart attack, stroke, blood clots in the lungs or legs, and dementia. For this reason, women should use estrogen hormone therapy only for short periods and at the lowest dose possible that will control symptoms. In addition, alternative forms of birth control may be recommended for those who find such risks undesirable.

Christina Girod

See also: Birth Control Pills, Estrogen-Progestin; Hormone Replacement Therapy; Progesterone; Puberty; Sex Hormones; Synthetic Hormones.

Further Reading

Lark, S. M. (2004). *The estrogen decision: Self-help book.* Berkeley, CA: Celestial Arts Publishing.

Watkins, E. S. (2007). *The estrogen elixir: A history of hormone replacement therapy in America.* Baltimore: Johns Hopkins University Press.

Evolutionary Perspectives on Gender and Sexual Behavior

Evolutionary theory is often associated with the phrase "survival of the fittest." According to evolutionary theory, environments are constantly changing, and those animals that are best able to adapt to their environment are the ones most likely to survive and reproduce. In this way, reproduction becomes the key component; at the heart of it, evolutionary theory is concerned with the transfer of useful (adaptive) genetic traits by parents to their offspring.

Because evolutionary theory is so biologically based, it may seem odd to consider the implications for social behavior. However, evolution does affect and has affected how animals, including humans, behave in social contexts, and an entire branch of science, called sociobiology, is devoted to its study. Sociobiology can be used to help explain and understand a wide variety of human behaviors, including gender roles and sexual behavior.

Gender roles are the socially constructed ways that people are expected to behave in any given context within a specified culture. For example, men are typically expected to be more physical and aggressive, while women are generally seen as being more emotional. Traditionally, men have been expected to be the providers for their families, while women have been expected to assume a caretaking role, often staying home from work, or ceasing to work outside the home entirely, in order to care for children. While these expectations have been shifting in recent years, their influence is still felt.

In dating and sex, many heterosexual people still believe that men should be the initiator—asking and then paying for a first date, leaning in for the first kiss, and initiating sexual contact. Women, on the other hand, are often encouraged to be more passive and let the guy "take the lead." Many people also believe that women should be more sexually conservative than men, and women who break this expectation may be shamed, both publicly and personally. Gender roles also influence what people find attractive. In general, tall, muscular, socially dominant, and successful men are seen as attractive, while attractiveness in women is often determined by slimness and breast size as well as a pleasing demeanor.

Even though gender roles are socially prescribed, male and female gender roles have been influenced by evolution because of the different roles that men and women play in reproduction and the subsequent strategies they have developed because of these differences. Biologically speaking, men play only a minor role in reproduction; they produce the necessary sperm and mate with a woman who may then become pregnant. Their contribution could last only a few minutes. Women, on the other hand, are the ones who become pregnant, and this nine-month commitment is only the beginning. Once the baby is born, the infant is entirely dependent on the mother for sustenance until weaned. In many cases, the mother remains the primary caregiver throughout the offspring's childhood. This difference in parental investment has been proposed as one of the primary reasons that people have evolved to have the gender roles they do.

In addition, because of these differences in required parental investment, evolutionary theorists have proposed that heterosexual men and women have developed different sexual strategies to deal with short-term and long-term mating situations. For men, because their parental investment is minimal, it may be in their best evolutionary interest to mate with numerous women in short-term scenarios in order to produce more offspring to carry their genetic material into the next generation. What this means is that men may be evolutionarily predisposed to prefer having many sexual partners and to be more inclined to engage in casual sex relationships such as one-night stands. For women, however, because of their longer parental investment, there is limited benefit to engage in short-term sexual relationships with partners who will not be around to help care for any children that should result. Therefore, it may be more evolutionary advantageous for women to find a mate that is willing to make a long-term, monogamous commitment to provide care and resources to the family to ensure the success of their children. Following this logic, it should also be more advantageous for women to be more sexually selective than men, and therefore have fewer sexual partners, since the potential pregnancy is theoretically more costly. If these differences are truly grounded in our evolutionary past, we would expect to find them in most cultures all over the world. David Schmitt (2003) sought to explore this assumption in a survey of 16,288 people from fifty-two nations on six continents; as expected, he found universal differences in the sexual strategies of men and women, suggesting that at least in part, human sexual behavior has evolutionary roots.

Evolutionary strategies also influence what people look for in a partner. Heterosexual men are more likely to seek youthful, physically attractive partners since youth and health are signals of high fertility. Heterosexual women, on the other hand, may be more attracted to older, well-established, and successful men who are able to provide them with the necessary resources for raising healthy children. Support for these "universally attractive" characteristics has also been found across numerous studies in varied cultures.

Ultimately, people are influenced by many factors, and no one theory can account for everything. In addition to evolutionary forces, people's attitudes toward gender roles, both personally and in a general sense, are influenced by family values, peer norms, social and cultural expectations, religious beliefs, and past experiences. Therefore, evolution is just one piece in the puzzle when it comes to explaining why people behave the way they do, especially when it comes to gender and sexuality.

Heather L. Armstrong

See also: Casual Sex; Gender Roles, Socialization and; Monogamy; Physical Attractiveness; Sexual Dimorphism; Stereotypes, Gender; Stereotypes, Sexual.

Further Reading

Buss, D. M. (1999). *Evolutionary psychology: The new science of the mind.* Boston: Allyn & Bacon.

Buss, D. M. (2003). *The evolution of desire: Strategies of human mating* (Rev. ed.). New York: Basic Books.

Buss, D. M., & Schmitt, D. P. (1993). Sexual strategies theory: An evolutionary perspective on human mating. *Psychological Review, 100,* 204–232.

Gangestad, S. W., & Simpson, J. A. (2000). The evolution of human mating: Trade-offs and strategic pluralism. *Behavioral and Brain Sciences, 23,* 573–644.

Schmitt, D. P. (2003). Universal sex differences in the desire for sexual variety: Tests from 52 nations, 6 continents, and 13 islands. *Journal of Personality and Social Psychology, 85,* 85–104. doi: 10.1037/0022-3514.85.1.85

Trivers, R. L. (1972). Parental investment and sexual selection. In B. Campbell (Ed.), *Sexual selection and the descent of man 1871–1971* (136–179). Chicago: Aldine Press.

Exhibitionism

Exhibitionism is considered a paraphilia and is characterized by sexual excitement experienced through genital or sexual exposure, usually to an unsuspecting, and therefore nonconsenting, person, usually a stranger. Some exhibitionists may also experience a strong desire to be observed by others during sexual activity. Exhibitionistic disorder is a paraphilic disorder. Exhibitionistic disorder is classified by the *Diagnostic and Statistical Manual of Mental Disorders.* In order for a diagnosis to be made, the person must experience ongoing and intense sexually arousing fantasies, urges, or sexual behaviors that involve exposing the genitals to an unsuspecting person, and the person has to have acted on these sexual urges with a nonconsenting person, or they must experience significant distress or difficulty in the workplace or in other social situations.

Exhibitionism involving unsuspecting, nonconsenting individuals is a sexual crime and is punishable by jail. Prevalence of exhibitionistic disorder is not known, although it is estimated to affect 2–4 percent of males; it is less common among females although the exact prevalence is unknown. Perpetrators of exhibitionism will often masturbate as part of their exposure to others. Many people who engage in this behavior are never arrested either due to lack of reporting or the ability to escape quickly before police arrive. While it is a noncontact sexual crime, it may still have a psychological impact on victims, who often feel violated.

Individuals who engage in exhibitionism may have difficulty controlling their impulses. Exhibitionism, when it involves an unsuspecting other, may be a threatening act as it displays a power dynamic where the perpetrator exercises control over another by shocking them. The motivation behind exposing the genitals may be to entice a potential sexual partner, or it may be to elicit a reaction from the unsuspecting victim. Looks of shock, disgust, and fear are often the desired reactions and may allow the exhibitionist to feel sexual arousal and pleasure. In interviews, some exhibitionists have reported feeling very disappointed if they do not elicit the reaction of fear, disgust, or shock, as this is desired for them to feel better emotionally and sexually.

Most exhibitionists feel a tremendous amount of guilt and shame after exposing themselves to unsuspecting others, and they often report feeling out of control. Many report they feel they are suffering by having to deal with this impulse-control issue and the emotional aftermath of exposing themselves.

Many exhibitionists start to display this behavior during adolescence; however, the causes of exhibitionism are not known. People with exhibitionistic disorder are also more likely to have other psychological problems. Among a nonclinical population sample, exhibitionism has been found to be associated with psychological problems, substance use, and sexual risk taking or novelty seeking.

Some people may seek treatment for exhibitionism on their own as they experience shame and distress as a result of this behavior. Others may be required to attend treatment due to arrest. Group therapy is a very common form of treatment for exhibitionism; individual therapy is also an option. In any therapy, the goal is for the patient or client to learn distress tolerance skills and behavioral and impulse control and then to implement them when confronted with emotions that would trigger an urge to engage in exhibitionism. During the process, the patient gains insight into their behavior and their motivation to engage in exhibitionism.

Amanda Manuel

See also: Diagnostic and Statistical Manual of Mental Disorders (DSM); Paraphilias; Sexual Consent; Voyeurism.

Further Reading

American Psychiatric Association. (2013). *Diagnostic and statistical manual of mental disorders* (5th ed.) Washington, DC: Author.

Balon, R. (2016). Exhibitionistic disorder. In R. Balon (Ed.), *Practical guide to paraphilic disorders* (77–91). New York: Springer.

Hayes, R. M., & Dragiewicz, M. (2018). Unsolicited dick pics: Erotica, exhibitionism or entitlement? *Women's Studies International Forum, 71*, 114–120.

Långström, N., & Seto, M. C. (2006). Exhibitionistic and voyeuristic behavior in a Swedish national population survey. *Archives of Sexual Behavior, 35*(4), 427–435.

Piemont, L. (2007). Fear of the empty self: The motivations for genital exhibitionism. *Modern Psychoanalysis, 32*(1), 79–93.

Swindell, S., Stroebel, S. S., O'Keefe, S. L., Beard, K. W., Robinett, S. S., & Kommor, M. J. (2011). Correlates of exhibitionism-like experiences in childhood and adolescence: A model for development of exhibitionism in heterosexual males. *Sexual Addictions & Compulsivity, 18*, 135–156.

Yarber, W., Sayad, B., & Strong, B. (2010). Variations in sexual behavior. In *Human sexuality diversity in contemporary America* (7th ed.). New York: McGraw-Hill.

Extramarital Sex

Extramarital sex (EMS) occurs when either one or both partners of a marriage engage in sexual acts with a person or people other than their spouse. The scenarios for what EMS looks like are widely varied and unique to every couple's understanding of their relational boundaries. EMS can be described in terms of behaviors that range from sexual intercourse to flirting. Other perspectives detail who is having EMS with whom, how often, and for what purpose. Finally, EMS within the context of the marriage can be permissive, tolerated, nonpermissive, and even punishable depending on the laws of the geographic location.

Permissive EMS, also known as consensual nonmonogamy, is when both partners agree that one or both are able to engage in sexual activities with people outside the marriage. This consensual arrangement can take many forms, such as an open marriage, swinging, or polyamory. In an open marriage, spouses remain committed to each other while allowing romantic or sexual relationships with outside partners. In polyamory, the individual(s) may have multiple romantic partnerships with all parties having an awareness of the others. Swinging is when the couple, either individually or together, engages in some form of sexual activity with other people. With each type of relationship or lifestyle, the couple usually creates boundaries and rules for communication, sexual behaviors, and emotional attachments.

Adultery and infidelity are often associated with nonpermissive EMS. Adultery addresses the legal aspect of having sex with someone who is not your spouse and is often cited as grounds for divorce. As marriage is a legally binding contract, adultery can have legal ramifications in many states. For example, in Massachusetts, an adulterer can be incarcerated for up to three years and have a fine up to $500. Infidelity is concerned with the breaking of the marital vows, or the promise to not have sex outside of the marriage. While many marriages in the United States are built on monogamy (having only one romantic or sexual partner), 34 percent of men and 24 percent of women report having engaged in extramarital sexual activities.

Though the descriptor "extramarital sex" has only been discussed in the context of marriage, the sentiment of the act, permissive or not, also applies to committed couples who are not legally bound. In these cases, it may be referred to as "extradyadic sex," or sex outside of the couple.

Darci Shinn

See also: Adultery; Cheating and Infidelity; Monogamy; Open Marriage; Polyamory; Swinging.

Further Reading

Edwards, J. N. (1973). Extramarital involvement: Fact and theory. *Journal of Sex Research, 9*, 210–224.

Hertlein, K. M., Weeks, G. R., & Gambescia, N. (2008). *Systemic sex therapy.* New York: Routledge.

Rhode, D. L. (2016). *Adultery: Infidelity and the law.* Cambridge, MA: Harvard University Press.

Tafoya, M. A., & Spitzberg, B. H. (2007). The dark side of infidelity: Its nature, prevalence, and communicative functions. In B. H. Spitzberg & W. R. Cupach (Eds.), *The dark side of interpersonal communication* (2nd ed., 201–242). Mahwah, NJ: Lawrence Erlbaum Associates.

Thompson, A. P. (1983). Extramarital sex: A review of the research literature. *Journal of Sex Research, 19*(1), 1–22.

F

Fallopian Tubes

The fallopian tubes, also called oviducts, are a pair of four-inch-long trumpet-shaped tubes located on each side of the uterus that connect the ovaries to the uterus. They are responsible for the transportation of a mature ovum, or egg, from the ovaries to the uterus. Each tube contains hairlike projections called cilia, which propel the ovum forward toward the uterus. The fallopian tubes are also the site where fertilization takes place when an ovum meets with sperm.

The fallopian tubes consist of four parts, including the isthmus, ampulla, infundibulum, and fimbriae. Beginning at the end of the tubes that attach to the uterus, the isthmus is the thick, walled region that constitutes the narrowest portion. The tubes expand into the ampulla, which makes up the largest section of the tubes, to extend beyond the isthmus and curve around to connect to the bell-shaped infundibulum. At the end of the infundibulum are the fimbriae, which are the fingerlike projections that surround the ovary to be in position to receive ova when released.

Triggered by the release of estrogen from the ovaries, the smooth muscle of the fimbriae begins a series of contractions to move the ovum into the fallopian tubes. Once the ovum has reached the inside of the infundibulum, the wavelike motions of the cilia create a current to keep the ovum moving along through the ampulla and isthmus toward the uterus. The process of ovulation typically takes three days as the ovum moves from ovary to the uterus. Fertilization usually takes place in the ampulla about twelve to twenty-four hours after the ovum is released.

There are several conditions that can damage the fallopian tubes, often resulting in scar tissue that interrupts ovulation and keeps the cilia from being able to transport an ovum or embryo to the uterus. These conditions can include pelvic inflammatory disease, endometriosis, uterine fibroids, and ectopic pregnancies, a pregnancy when implantation of the embryo occurs in the fallopian tube. Tubal blockage is a common symptom of these diseases where the fallopian tubes are blocked by various abnormal tissues. Depending on the location and the extent of the blockage, surgical removal of these tissues may be possible. Most surgical procedures involve the removal of the unhealthy tissue and fusion of the two healthy ends of the tubes to repair and re-create an unblocked tube. The success rates vary, and the likelihood of an ectopic pregnancy increases.

The fallopian tubes can be permanently blocked or cut through with various sterilization procedures if an individual decides they do not want children. The cutting, blocking, or tying of the tubes is called tubal ligation. Tubes can be cut, a small piece can be removed, or instruments such as clips, rings, or clamps can be applied. Although intended to be permanent, the ligation procedure can be reversed in some cases.

Lauren Wesley

See also: Conception; Endometriosis; Essure Coil; Ovaries; Pelvic Inflammatory Disease (PID); Tubal Ligation; Uterus.

Further Reading

Barclay, T. (2018). Fallopian tube. Retrieved from http://www.innerbody.com/image_repfov/repo03-new.html#full-description

Healthline. (2015). Uterine tube (fallopian tube). Retrieved from http://www.healthline.com/human-body-maps/fallopian-tubes

Planned Parenthood. (2019). Sterilization. Retrieved from https://www.plannedparenthood.org/learn/birth-control/sterilization

Rebar, R. W. (2019). Problems with the fallopian tubes and abnormalities in the pelvis. Retrieved from https://www.msdmanuals.com/en-gb/home/women-s-health-issues/infertility/problems-with-the-fallopian-tubes-and-abnormalities-in-the-pelvis

Family Planning Clinics

Family planning clinics are medical clinics that help people control the number of children that they have as well as the timing of pregnancies. At full-service clinics, people can obtain counseling services, birth control pills and other contraceptive methods, sterilization surgery, treatment for infertility, and abortions. Some clinics do not offer all such services, but they can refer patients to other clinics or health care providers. The services provided at family planning clinics, depending on the type of clinic and the patient's particular case, may be paid for by the patients themselves, by insurance companies, or by government programs, such as Medicaid in the United States.

Some family planning clinics offer other health care services in addition to family planning. These services may include screenings for breast and cervical cancer, testing for HIV and other sexually transmitted infections, counseling regarding menopause, advice on adoption, and general checkups and physical examinations. Many women use family planning clinics as their regular source of health care. Although most family planning services are designed for women, clinics also usually offer limited services for men, such as infertility treatment.

Family planning can have several benefits for women, their families, and society at large. Wise family planning can help people achieve or maintain their economic and social autonomy and independence. It can protect the health of adolescents and older women whose youth or advanced age puts them and their pregnancies at risk for problems or neonatal complications. Pregnancy prevention options, like contraception, avoids the need for abortion.

Preventing unintended pregnancies can save society money by avoiding the need for social services to raise children whose parents are unable to care for them. Because many single adolescent mothers drop out of school to raise their children, preventing those pregnancies would allow these individuals to stay in school and eventually get better jobs, which benefits the economy in the long term. Family planning can further benefit society by slowing population growth.

According to the U.S. Department of Health and Human Services, publicly funded—that is, government-funded—family planning clinics in the United States prevent about 1.94 million unintended pregnancies each year, including

400,000 teen pregnancies. These numbers do not include the hundreds of thousands of unintended pregnancies prevented by services obtained in private clinics.

African American and Hispanic women are less likely to have access to family planning services than white women. Other population segments that are less likely to have access to family planning are people with low incomes, without a high school diploma, and with a cohabiting relationship (as opposed to a married relationship). These people may not be able to afford the services because of a lack of health insurance or an inability to get public assistance; because clinic locations and hours are not convenient; or because they may not be aware of the services.

The services of family planning clinics have led to increased contraception use in many regions of the world, including developing countries, though the rate of contraception use remains low in sub-Saharan Africa. Throughout the world, modern contraception methods are used by approximately 57 percent of women aged fifteen to forty-nine. In Asia, this rate increased from 60.9 percent in 2008 to 61.9 percent in 2014. In Latin America, the rate rose from 66.7 percent in 2008 to 67.0 percent in 2014. During this period in Africa, the rate rose from 23.6 percent to 27.6 percent.

According to the World Health Organization (WHO), an estimated 225 million women in developing countries would like to delay or stop their pregnancies but do not have the means to do so. In those poor nations, WHO family planning advocates are working to increase access to a variety of contraception methods, to educate the public about contraception benefits, and to remove the cultural stigmas associated with birth control. However, certain segments of developing nations' populations have especially severe unmet family planning needs, including refugees from wars, migrants, urban slum dwellers, and adolescents.

Family planning clinics are often at the center of the abortion controversy—the debate over whether a woman has the right to terminate an unwanted pregnancy and, if so, under what conditions. In the United States, abortion during the first trimester (first three months) of pregnancy has been legal under any condition since the Supreme Court's *Roe v. Wade* ruling in 1973. Also, according to that ruling, individual states can regulate abortion as they deem appropriate beginning in the second trimester.

Despite the established legal right to have an abortion, various "pro-life" (or anti-abortion) groups that oppose abortion for religious or other reasons do not recognize this right. Some of these groups post members outside family planning clinics to try to prevent people from entering the clinics. Some of the more radical antiabortion groups have even vandalized, bombed, or set fire to clinics, and others have resorted to assassinating doctors or other people who work in the clinics. In response to such terrorist-like acts, as well as to various restrictions placed on abortions by some state governments, "pro-choice" groups have increased their efforts to defend the right to have abortions at safe medical clinics.

One of the largest operators of family planning clinics is an organization called Planned Parenthood Federation of America (PPFA), headquartered in New York City. This group operates clinics in some one thousand communities throughout the United States. It also helps to support family planning programs in other countries. PPFA's work—including providing abortions at some of its centers and dispending birth control advice to adolescents—is opposed by some.

A. J. Smuskiewicz

See also: Abortion, Elective; Abortion Legislation; Contraception; Fertility; Infertility; Planned Parenthood; *Roe v. Wade*; Sterilization; Teen Pregnancy.

Further Reading

Planned Parenthood Federation of America. (2019). Home page. Retrieved from http://www.plannedparenthood.org

World Health Organization. (2018). *Family planning: A global handbook for providers, 2018 edition.* Geneva: WHO. Retrieved from https://www.who.int/reproductivehealth/publications/fp-global-handbook/en/

Fantasy, Sexual and Erotic

Sexual fantasies, defined as mental images that a person finds to be sexually arousing, are one of the most common forms of sexual expression. In fact, most people, of all sexual orientations and gender identities, say they have fantasized before. Fantasy content is derived from many sources and varies widely from one person to the next, although there are some predictable gender differences in the nature of people's fantasies. Once thought to be revealing of psychopathology, fantasies are now typically viewed as a normal and healthy part of one's sexuality.

Put simply, a sexual fantasy is a conscious thought that turns one on. The "conscious" aspect is an essential element here because it distinguishes a sex fantasy from a sex dream. Within a fantasy, there is conscious control over the content and direction of the narrative, unlike in dreams. Studies have consistently found that almost everyone has sexual fantasies. In fact, most have reported prevalence rates of greater than 90 percent. However, men are more likely to report having sex fantasies, and they report having them more often than women.

Fantasies can occur at any time of day. For instance, people may fantasize while they are at work, exercising, watching television, engaged in conversation, or even at religious services. However, it is not uncommon for fantasies to coincide with sexual activity. Most people say that they have previously fantasized during both masturbation and sexual intercourse.

Given the range of settings in which fantasies can occur, it is clear that fantasies are designed to serve multiple purposes. For instance, fantasies are sometimes nothing more than a mental distraction or a way of relieving boredom. Other times, fantasies are used to plan out a future sexual event. And yet other times, fantasies might be called on during sex to enhance or maintain arousal, or perhaps to compensate for a less-than-satisfying sexual experience.

Fantasy content is incredibly varied and idiosyncratic. This means that one person's fantasies may bear no resemblance to another's. Further, a given fantasy theme might lead some people to experience sexual arousal, while others might respond to the same thought with disgust or revulsion.

The content of sexual fantasies is derived from multiple sources. For instance, some fantasies are inspired by past sexual events (e.g., reliving one's first or favorite sexual experience), while others may be inspired by pornography or other forms of media. However, while some fantasies may indeed have their roots in sexual histories, the origin of sexual fantasies is actually far more complex. Fantasies are a unique product of individual psychology (including our personality, attachment style, and learned experiences), culture, and evolutionary history.

Survey research on sexual fantasy has revealed that the most popular themes revolve around novelty (e.g., trying a new sexual position or having sex in a new and exciting location, such as on a beach or under a waterfall), love and romance, sex with someone other than one's current partner (e.g., celebrities, acquaintances, strangers), sex with multiple partners, as well as dominance and submission.

Fantasies about so-called paraphilic (i.e., unusual or uncommon) sexual interests were once thought to be rare but are actually more popular than previously believed. For instance, a large number of men and women fantasize about things like voyeurism (i.e., watching other people have sex) and sadomasochism (i.e., deriving sexual pleasure from giving or receiving pain). Research suggests that very few fantasies are statistically rare. These include fantasies about sex with animals (zoophilia) and sex with prepubescent children (pedophilia).

There are several important differences between men and women when it comes to the nature of their sexual fantasies. For one thing, men's fantasies tend to be more sexually explicit and are more likely to involve themes of group sex (e.g., threesomes, orgies) compared to women's. In addition, whereas men are more likely to fantasize about dominance, women are more likely to fantasize about submission. Finally, women's fantasies are more likely to contain emotional and romantic imagery than are men's.

Few differences in fantasy content have been noted based on sexual orientation. The primary difference for gay and lesbian persons compared to heterosexuals is the gender of the person(s) about whom they are fantasizing. Interestingly, studies suggest that most asexual persons have sexual fantasies too; however, research has not yet systematically explored how the content of asexuals' fantasies compares to persons of other sexual orientations.

Historically, sexual fantasies were viewed as problematic, a view attributable to none other than Sigmund Freud, who famously argued that happy people do not fantasize and that sexual fantasies tend to reflect unresolved psychological issues. Today, however, psychologists have largely rejected this Freudian notion and believe that sexual fantasies are part of a healthy sex life. Indeed, research has found that the people who have the most sexual fantasies tend to be the most sexually satisfied.

That said, specific kinds of fantasies can be problematic, such as when people fantasize about nonconsensual sexual activities (e.g., sex with children or nonconsenting adults). Persistent fantasies about activities that pose a serious risk of harm to others may warrant treatment to the extent that they become personally distressing or one feels a strong urge to act on them.

Justin J. Lehmiller

See also: Arousal; Desire; Freud, Sigmund; Masturbation; Paraphilias.

Further Reading

Kahr, B. (2008). *Who's been sleeping in your head?: The secret world of sexual fantasies.* New York: Basic Books.

Joyal, C. C., Cossette, A., & Lapierre, V. (2015). What exactly is an unusual sexual fantasy? *The Journal of Sexual Medicine, 12*, 328–340.

Lehmiller, J. J. (2018). *Tell me what you want: The science of sexual desire and how it can help you improve your sex life.* Boston: Da Capo Lifelong Books.

Leitenberg, H., & Henning, K. (1995). Sexual fantasy. *Psychological Bulletin, 117*, 469–496.

Wilson, G. D. (2010). Measurement of sex fantasy. *Sexual and Relationship Therapy, 25*, 57–67.

Zurbriggen, E. L., & Yost, M. R. (2004). Power, desire, and pleasure in sexual fantasies. *Journal of Sex Research, 41*, 288–300.

Fausto-Sterling, Anne

Anne Fausto-Sterling (1944–) is a scientist, researcher, and professor of biology and gender studies at Brown University in Providence, Rhode Island. She is well known for her research on sex, gender roles, gender identity, sexuality, intersexuality, and other topics in the field of sexology. Fausto-Sterling has a bachelor's degree in zoology from the University of Wisconsin (1965) and a PhD in developmental genetics from Brown University (1970). While she has many publications in peer-reviewed journals, her most well-known writings are two of her earlier books: *Myths of Gender: Biological Theories about Women and Men* (1992, second edition) and *Sexing the Body: Gender Politics and the Construction of Sexuality* (2000), as well as the article "The Five Sexes," which appeared in *The Sciences*, a peer-reviewed academic journal (1993). She has dozens of other academic publications and has given lectures around the world on topics regarding sex, gender, intersexuality, and nature versus nurture. Her current work utilizes dynamic systems theory to better understand how difference from a cultural perspective becomes bodily difference.

In approaching the fields of sexology and feminist and gender studies from a biological perspective, Fausto-Sterling delved into the constructs of sex and gender and focused on how much of these concepts are biological imperative and how much are socially constructed. Moreover, her work suggests that there are more than two biological sexes (commonly identified as only male and female) and that society is doing a disservice to individuals by not recognizing the more biologically diverse variation of sexes that are present in humans. She feels doctors and other medical professionals may be unethical in their practices of assigning a sex to intersex infants only a few hours after birth without more information about how those children may identify their gender in the future. An advocate for better understanding of intersexuality, she views the concept of and need for sexing bodies as a social creation and not part of our biology.

In addition to her thoughts and writings on genetics, she also engages in dialogue and theoretical discussion on gender roles, sexual orientation, and gender identity, positing that nurture of a sexual or gendered variety has a much larger impact on gender and sexual orientation than any component of either nature or biology. Fausto-Sterling's research and writings encourage society to expand its definitions of what it means to be male and female, not only from a biological framework but also in how gender roles and activities are viewed as men's work and women's work.

By working at the intersection of biology and sexuality, Fausto-Sterling brings a unique lens to the studies of sex and gender, engaging in interdisciplinary conversations. While much of her work focuses on children and individuals with intersex conditions, her theoretical frameworks for reexamining how society views, creates, and reinforces gender have cemented her in the canon of feminist literature and gender studies as one of the first people to approach gender diversity from a genetic perspective.

Shanna K. Kattari

See also: Binary Gender System; Feminist Theory; Gender; Gender Diversity; Gender Roles, Socialization and; Intersexuality; Sexology; Sexual Orientation; Stereotypes, Gender; Stereotypes, Sexual; Transgender.

Further Reading

Biography. (n.d.). Anne Fausto-Sterling. Retrieved from http://www.annefaustosterling.com/biography/

Brown University. (2017). Anne Fausto-Sterling. Retrieved from https://vivo.brown.edu/display/afaustos

Fausto-Sterling, A. (1992). *Myths of gender: Biological theories about women and men.* New York: Basic Books.

Fausto-Sterling, A. (1993). The five sexes. *The Sciences, 33*(2), 20–24.

Fausto-Sterling, A. (2000). *Sexing the body: Gender politics and the construction of sexuality.* New York: Basic Books.

Fausto-Sterling, A. (2012). *Sex/gender: Biology in a social world.* New York: Routledge.

Feinberg, Leslie

Leslie Feinberg (1949–2014) was a grassroots activist and journalist who was born September 1, 1949, in Kansas City, Missouri. Feinberg later moved to Buffalo, New York, in the 1960s and considered hirself a young butch lesbian. Feinberg preferred to use gender-neutral pronouns like "zie" or "ze" (pronounced like "see") and "hir" (pronounced like "here"). Feinberg described hirself as "an anti-racist white, working class, secular Jewish, transgender, lesbian, female, revolutionary communist." Zie was married to Minnie Bruce Pratt, a lesbian poet-activist.

Feinberg's experiences with medical professionals led hir to advocate for a better understanding of trans health issues and needs among health care providers and medical professionals. From December 1995 to December 1996, Feinberg was dying of endocarditis, a bacterial infection that lodges and proliferates in the valves of the heart. Doctors refused to treat Feinberg, hospitals told hir to leave, and zie was called a freak, troubled, and other derogatory names. Feinberg was also diagnosed with other serious infections and health disorders such as late-stage Lyme disease; these health conditions ultimately led to hir death in 2014.

Feinberg's novel *Stone Butch Blues* was published on March 1, 1993, by Firebrand Books. It won the prestigious American Library Association Award Gay and Lesbian Book Award and was a finalist for the LAMBDA Literary Award. Feinberg also wrote nonfiction work including *Transgender Warriors: Making History from Joan of Arc to RuPaul*, which was the first to analyze the historical roots of transgender oppression. *Transgender Warriors* won the 1996 Firecracker Alternative Book Award for Non-Fiction. Another of hir nonfiction books, *Trans Liberation: Beyond Pink or Blue*, contains speeches and essays written by the author and other trans activists. Hir second novel, *Drag King Dreams*, was published in March 2006.

Feinberg was a well-known activist in the United States and other parts of the world who worked to help build a strong bond between the LGBT communities. Ze was a political activist and a national leader of the Workers World Party and was a managing editor of its newspaper, *Workers World*. Feinberg was a trade unionist, antiracist, and socialist, and ze helped to build connections of unity between these movements and others that were advocating for those oppressed by their nationalities, sex, disabilities, and class or socioeconomic status as a whole. For more than three decades, Feinberg advocated for the treaty rights and freedom of Native nations and for the freedom of political prisoners in the United States. Finally, Feinberg was also known for touring around the United States speaking at pride rallies, protests, and on college and university campuses.

Lauren Ewaniuk

See also: Gay Rights Movement; Pronoun Usage; Transgender.

Further Reading

Feinberg, L. (1993). *Stone butch blues*. Ann Arbor, MI: Firebrand Books.

Feinberg, L. (1998). *Transliberation: Beyond pink or blue*. Boston: Beacon Press.

Transgender Warrior. (n.d.). Home page. Retrieved from http://www.transgenderwarrior.org/

Female Ejaculation

Also known as "squirting" or "gushing," "female ejaculation" refers to the release of fluid from what is likely the paraurethral ducts during sexual arousal or orgasm. These ducts, called Skene's glands, are located on both sides of the vaginal opening and seem to act in a similar manner to the prostate (which provides the fluid for male ejaculate or semen). The expelled fluid is often described as somewhat "milky" in appearance, sweet tasting, without odor, and ranging widely in volume. Female ejaculation is considered a normal part of sexuality and, as far as researchers have discovered, there is nothing unhealthy about this experience.

The phenomenon of female ejaculation has actually been described for many years, possibly dating back to the days of Aristotle. Popular cultural discussion of female ejaculation, however, is relatively recent. The book *The G Spot, and Other Recent Discoveries about Human Sexuality* is often credited with helping female ejaculation reemerge into the public consciousness as well as sparking renewed discussion about this phenomenon within the medical community. Research on female ejaculation, however, is still relatively sparse and quite incomplete. It remains unclear what percentage of women experience female ejaculation, with estimates ranging anywhere from 10 percent to 69 percent, depending on the definitions and methods utilized by researchers. The purpose of the fluid release is also unknown, though suggestions have included an antimicrobial function to protect females from vulvo-vaginal infections following sexual activity. In addition, the exact source and makeup of the fluid continues to be a topic of debate among medical professionals and researchers and is related to controversy surrounding the existence of the "G-spot" in women.

The term "female ejaculation" is considered a misnomer by many health care professionals, as the fluid itself is not the same as male ejaculate (semen). That said, however, a major controversy surrounding female ejaculation has involved the composition of the expulsed fluid. Specifically, much of the existing research has focused on determining whether female ejaculate is, or contains, urine. In a recent review of the literature, researchers concluded that female ejaculation may present as whitish secretions from the "female prostate" (i.e., Skene's glands) or coital incontinence in which diluted urine is released. Indeed it is argued that both may occur simultaneously, making it difficult to parse "true" female ejaculation from symptoms of urinary incontinence. According to researchers who have conducted chemical analyses of female ejaculation, however, the fluid may be similar but is not the same as urine. Such studies have revealed that female ejaculate includes creatinine, prostate-specific antigen, glucose, and fructose, among other substances. Of note, the undetermined makeup of female ejaculate has resulted in specific social implications around censorship. For example, following the argument that female ejaculate is simply urine, the United Kingdom's British Board of Film Classification has banned films that allegedly show female ejaculation, as portraying urination during sex is considered to be obscenity under U.K. law (Rosen, 2014).

Often debates about female ejaculation are tied to the existence of the Grafenberg spot, or "G-spot," a sensitive area on the anterior wall of the vagina, which, when stimulated, is reported to variably result in orgasm and ejaculation. The G-spot was named for Dr. Ernst Grafenberg, a German-born obstetrician and gynecologist. In 1950, Grafenberg described that stimulation of this area of the vagina seemed to cause the female urethra to enlarge and swell. He also noted a fluid emerging from the urethra that he believed to be distinct from urine. It has been argued that, due to its location, stimulation of the G-spot also involves simultaneous stimulation of the paraurethral tissue in which the Skene's glands are located and, in which, it has been argued that the ejaculate fluid is stored. As such, many believe that having a G-spot-induced orgasm increases the likelihood of female ejaculation.

Related to disagreements about the composition of female ejaculate and G-spot involvement is a third controversy. Specifically, where is female ejaculate stored prior to squirting? As noted, many point to the Skene's glands, located in the paraurethral tissue, as the source of female ejaculation. Others have argued that the paraurethral tissue cannot hold the volume of fluid reportedly ejaculated by some women and instead point to the bladder as the largest potential source of female ejaculate located in the pelvis. Overall, health care professionals and researchers continue to debate the major points of female ejaculation—what it is, where it comes from, and why it exists.

Jennifer A. Vencill

See also: Arousal; Ejaculation; Grafenberg Spot (G-Spot); Orgasm; Vaginal Lubrication.

Further Reading

Grafenberg, E. (1950). The role of the urethra in female orgasm. *International Journal of Sexology, 3,* 145–148.

Ladas, A. K., Whipple, B., & Perry, J. D. (1982). *The G spot, and other recent discoveries about human sexuality.* New York: Holt, Rinehart, and Winston.

Pastor, Z. (2013). Female ejaculation orgasm vs. coital incontinence: A systemic review. *Journal of Sexual Medicine, 10,* 1682–1691.

Rosen, R. (2014, December). No female ejaculation, please, we're British: A history of porn and censorship. *The Independent.* Retrieved from https://www.independent.co.uk/life-style/health-and-families/features/no-female-ejaculation-please-we-re-british-a-history-of-porn-and-censorship-9903054.html

Whipple, B. (2015). Female ejaculation, G spot, A spot, and should we be looking for spots? *Current Sexual Health Reports, 7,* 59–62.

Wimpissinger, F., Stifter, K., Grin, W., & Stackl, W. (2007). The female prostate revisited: Perineal ultrasound and biochemical studies of female ejaculate. *Journal of Sexual Medicine, 4,* 1388–1393.

Female Genital Cutting

Female genital cutting (FGC), often referred to as female genital mutilation or female circumcision, is a procedure that intentionally alters, injures, or removes female genitalia or organs for nonmedical purposes. FGC can be classified into four major categories: type 1, clitoridectomy (partial or total removal of the clitoris); type 2, excision (partial or total removal of the clitoris and labia minora, with or without removal of the labia majora); type 3, infibulation (sealing the vaginal opening with or without clitoridectomy); and type 4, all other harmful procedures to female genitalia. More than 200 million girls and women today have undergone FGC, and 3 million girls are at risk of undergoing FGC every year. Young girls (younger than fifteen years of age) are most likely to experience FCC, specifically if located in one of the thirty African, Middle Eastern, or Asian countries where FGC is most concentrated. FGC is performed by community members (mostly women, although in some communities it may be performed by men) who range from non-medically trained religious leaders or circumcisers to trained health professionals. The environment is generally unsterile, and the procedure is most often completed without anesthetic. A variety of instruments are used in performing FGC, such as razor blades, knives, scissors, glass, sharpened rocks, and fingernails. FGC has been found to provide no benefit to the health of young girls and women and, contrarily, has been linked to several negative physical, psychological, and psychosexual health outcomes.

The practice of FGC is deeply rooted in societal norms and cultural traditions that have persisted for generations. FGC is traditionally a ceremonial event that prepares girls for marriage and adulthood under the belief that FGC protects the virginity and virtue of young girls, increases male and female sexual pleasure, and maintains feminine hygiene and cleanliness. The ceremonies also provide economic benefit because they are accompanied by community spending (such as food and gifts), are a form of income for circumcisers or practitioners, and can improve the status and worth for young girls or women when it is time for marriage. In most cases, only women are present at the ceremony and, therefore, mothers and grandmothers largely maintain the tradition of FGC. Men, however, also contribute to upholding the tradition as they prefer to marry women who have been "cut," believing their virginity has been preserved and they are more suitable for marriage.

Today, FGC is a widely condemned practice that is recognized as a human rights violation of girls and women. The prevalence and support of FGC has decreased in many countries over the last three decades; however, decline has occurred more rapidly in some countries than others, with some countries experiencing nominal change. There are currently laws prohibiting FGC in twenty-six African and Middle Eastern countries, in addition to thirty-three countries with large populations that practice FGC. The legislation and penalty for violating legislation varies from country to country, and it has been argued that to increase success, legislation needs to be accompanied by programming and strategies that influence a sociocultural shift toward ending FGC.

Nicole C. Doria and Matthew Numer

See also: Circumcision; Clitoris; Female Sexuality; Labia; Virginity; Vulva.

Further Reading

Jiménez Ruiz, I., Almansa Martínez, P., & Alcón Belchí, C. (2017). Dismantling the man-made myths upholding female genital mutilation. *Health Care for Women International, 38*(5), 478–491.

Klein, E., Helzner, E., Shayowitz, M., Kohlhoff, S., & Smith-Norowitz, T. (2018). Female genital mutilation: Health consequences and complications—A short literature review. *Obstetrics and Gynecology International, 2018*, 1–7.

Lewnes, A., & UNICEF Innocenti Research Centre. (2005). *Changing a harmful social convention, female genital mutilation/cutting* (Innocenti digest). Florence, Italy: UNICEF Innocenti Research Center.

Odukogbe, A., Afolabi, B., Bello, O., & Adeyanju, A. (2017). Female genital mutilation/cutting in Africa. *Translational Andrology and Urology, 6*(2), 138–148.

UNICEF. (2013). Female genital mutilation/cutting: A statistical overview and exploration of the dynamics of change. Retrieved from https://data.unicef.org/wp-content/uploads/2015/12/FGMC_Brochure_Lo_res_1613.pdf

UNICEF. (2016). Female genital mutilation/cutting: A global concern. Retrieved from https://data.unicef.org/wp-content/uploads/2016/04/FGMC-2016-brochure_250.pdf

World Health Organization. (2018). Female genital mutilation. Retrieved from http://www.who.int/news-room/fact-sheets/detail/female-genital-mutilation

Female Sexuality

"Female sexuality" refers to everything that distinguishes an individual as female rather than male or another gender. It may also be thought of as femaleness or being female. "Female sexuality" can refer to biological factors, such as physical sexual characteristics and reproductive organs; psychological factors, such as attitudes, emotions, and ideas; and cultural factors, such as the ways in which social expectations influence dressing styles and other behaviors.

The biological factors that distinguish a female from a male are present at birth in the form of female genitals. These include a clitoris, vulva, vagina, uterus, and ovaries. A female is born with each of her ovaries containing approximately 400,000 immature eggs. Only about 400 of these eggs will eventually mature.

At puberty, which usually begins between the ages of ten and twelve in females, the ovaries start producing increased amounts of estrogen—the hormone that triggers body changes that characterize a sexually mature female. The breasts grow, hips become wider, and the monthly menstrual cycle begins. In a menstrual cycle, an egg matures and is released by an ovary, and the uterine wall develops a special lining. If the egg is fertilized by sperm, it will implant itself in the uterine wall, resulting in pregnancy. If the egg is not fertilized, the uterine lining is shed and passes out of the vagina in menstrual bleeding. Usually, the ovaries decline in functioning between the ages of forty-five and fifty-five, a period known as perimenopause.

Sexual pleasure for many woman is associated with physical stimulation of the clitoris, which is filled with sensitive nerve endings. Stimulation of the clitoris by a penis, sex toy, fingers, tongue, or other means can feel very pleasurable and may lead to orgasm. Some people can experience multiple orgasms in a brief period of time if pleasurable stimulation, often involving the clitoris, is continued. However, others may have difficulty experiencing orgasm. If experiencing orgasm is difficult, this may be related to improper or insufficient clitoral or other sexual stimulation, stress, the use of certain medications, or other physical or psychological conditions. Lack of awareness of the important role the clitoris plays in sexual pleasure, as well as a general lack of awareness of the body and sexuality, are also associated with difficulties with orgasm. Fortunately, in most cases, exploration and communication, both on one's own and with a partner, can help increase the likelihood of orgasm.

There are numerous psychological factors associated with female sexuality. A woman has certain attitudes, emotions, ideas, and behaviors that constitute her self-identity as a female. These may consist of the ways in which she walks, talks, dresses, and wears her hair and makeup. They may also include her concepts of what it means to have a good job or to be a good wife or mother.

According to many biologists, psychologists, and sociologists, some of these "female" attitudes and ideas are the result of complex genetic and hormonal influences—the biological aspects of being female. However, others are the result of cultural influences regarding expectations of what a woman should act like in any given society.

Not all people conform in their sexuality to their biological sex. Some people who are born with male bodies have a psychological sexuality or gender identity that is female. Conversely, some people who are born with female bodies have a psychological sexuality or gender identity that is male.

Much of a female's concept of her sexuality is derived from the diverse experiences she has while growing up as a girl and while living as a woman. Influencing her ideas of her own femininity and sexuality are such things as the types of toys, clothes, and chores given to her by her parents; the ways in which her peers act regarding their sexuality; the ways in which prominent women are portrayed by teachers in school; and the ways in which women in popular culture are portrayed on television shows, in movies, and in the music industry.

For example, one girl might be exposed to experiences that lead her to believe that an essential part of being female is focusing on an ideal outer beauty, involving constant dieting to stay slim, spending money on expensive clothes, and wearing elaborate makeup. Another girl's experiences might lead her to believe that such concerns are frivolous and that it is much more important to get a good education and to have a successful career. Yet another girl might come to expect that her main role as a female is to be a good wife and mother.

Since the sexual revolution of the 1960s and 1970s, liberal cultural influences have allowed many women in the United States and other Western nations to pursue their dreams of accomplishing anything they choose to accomplish. By contrast, many conservative, traditional cultures, such as those in Islamic nations of the Middle East, enforce extremely limited roles for women in society. Despite the improved opportunities for women in modern society, a frequent criticism of popular portrayals of women in the United States is that too much emphasis is placed on the overtly sexual aspects of being female, giving girls a shallow concept of their own sexuality.

A. J. Smuskiewicz

See also: Black Sexuality; Gender Identity; Gender Roles, Socialization and; Male Sexuality; Media and Sexuality; Puberty; Religion, Diversity of Human Sexuality and; Social Learning Theory, Gender and.

Further Reading

Bergner, D. (2014). *What do women want? Adventures in the science of female desire.* New York: Ecco Press.

Eckert, K. G. (2014). *Things your mother never told you: A woman's guide to sexuality.* Downers Grove, IL: IVP Books.

Hite, S. (1976). *The Hite report: A national study of female sexuality.* New York: Seven Stories Press.

Femininity

Femininity is the set of attributes, behaviors, roles, expectations, social norms, and qualities associated with the female sex. Femininity is both biologically and socially constructed based on biological factors (i.e., being born with a vagina).

Some traits often associated with femininity include being gentle, empathetic, caring, conflict and anger avoidant, tolerant, submissive, relationship focused, meeting expectations of beauty, and being sexually passive or uninterested. Femininity as a concept is inherently white and includes "traditional" Western beauty standards (e.g., height, body size, breast size, weight, hair color). Media portrayal of the "ideal" woman can lead to poor self and body image, which can in turn lead to the acceptance and practice of more traditionally gendered roles. Just being born female is not enough to be considered feminine; one also needs to show others that they are feminine through their behavior, their appearance, and other aspects related to the traditional gender role.

Judith Butler defined gender as "an identity instituted through a stylized repetition of acts . . . instituted through stylization of the body . . . [in] which the body gestures, movements, and enactments . . . constitute the illusion of . . . a gendered self" (Butler, 1998). Like the description of femininity above, this definition of gender also describes how one must not only look the part of female but also act feminine in order to maintain the idea of one's femininity through a repeated performance. Media also plays a role in how femininity and masculinity are performed by not only repeating what is socially acceptable but also by creating caricatures of sexualized responsibility, which can lead to hyperfemininity and hypermasculinity, which can create problems for individuals as well as societies.

The idea of how to be feminine and how to be a woman has been historically performed and repeated, a lifelong "project" or "strategy" defined and shaped by social norms that can change across time and across cultures. Women who do not conform to these social norms can be subject to bullying and other forms of negative social consequences. Because of the importance of social interactions in people's lives, if people face prejudice and discrimination from others because of their gender, or the way they present themselves as female through, for example, their behavior, speech, and clothing, this can lead to feeling bad about oneself and can cause lower self-esteem and self-worth. Likewise, those who do conform to these norms of femininity are often seen as "beautiful" and may be socially rewarded. This can be problematic as it may lead some women to engage in "beauty practices" like dieting, coloring their hair, or having plastic surgery that they would otherwise not want to do in order to seem "attractive."

Femininity is also racialized. Because social norms of femininity and masculinity are traditionally based on Western ideals, typically white characteristics (e.g., white skin, blonde hair, blue eyes) are often seen as the most beautiful and the most feminine. Black women, for example, are at an intersection of being both the minority sex and race. Physically, black women often do not meet the Eurocentric ideals of beauty, simply by being born with different skin color and hair texture. While the "right" body frame can sometimes be achieved, there are still supposed "black sexual characteristics" that would need to be overcome to meet white femininity standards. Black women's sexuality, which is often portrayed and viewed in stereotypical ways, does not lend itself to traditional notions of femininity. Different stereotypes of black female sexuality lend themselves to masculine traits by way of being the head of a household, not being docile and compliant, and being considered overly sexual or having too many sexual partners. Many women manipulate features that can be changed to meet the standard of white feminine beauty. Women of color, both inside and outside the United States, use bleaching creams to lighten their skin as a way to achieve whiteness. Many women also use chemicals in their hair to achieve either the correct texture or color in order to conform to these beauty ideals. Cosmetic surgery has also been a way, for those with financial means, to achieve the "ideal" female form of larger busts and smaller waists. Worldwide, eyelid surgery, foot binding, girdles, and the other aforementioned means are also used to achieve the purported "ideal" look.

Donna Oriowo

See also: Black Sexuality; Double Standards, Sexual; Female Sexuality; Gender Roles, Socialization and; Masculinity.

Further Reading

Butler, J. (1998). Performative acts and gender constitution: An essay in phenomenology and feminist theory. *Theatre Journal, 40*(4), 519–531.

Collins, P. H. (2005). *Black sexual politics: African Americans, gender, and the new racism.* New York: Routledge.

Deliovsky, K. (2008). Normative white femininity: Race, gender, and the politics of beauty. *Atlantis, 33*, 49–59.

Dittmar, J. (2009). How do "body perfect" ideals in the media have a negative impact on body image and behaviors? Factors and processes related to self and identity. *Journal of Social and Clinical Psychology, 28*(1), 1–8.

Oriowo, D. O. (2016). *Is it easier for her? Afro-textured hair and its effects on black female sexuality: A mixed methods approach* (Order No. 10120152). Retrieved from Dissertations & Theses @ Widener University; ProQuest Dissertations & Theses A&I. (1805610606).

Stephens, D., & Few, A. L. (2007). The effects of images of African American in hip hop on early adolescents' attitudes toward physical attractiveness and interpersonal relationships. *Sex Roles, 56*, 251–264.

Feminist Theory

Feminist theory is the system of ideas used to study, analyze, and understand gender inequality and consists of academic principles used to illustrate feminism. Colloquially, feminism represents the belief that individuals of all genders should have equal political, economic, social, and basic rights. According to bell hooks (2015), feminism is "a movement to end sexism, sexist exploitation, and oppression." This definition directly indicates that sexism, inequality, and oppression underlie gender inequity and addresses the misconception that feminism is "antimale." The feminism definition offered by bell hooks acknowledges that sexist thinking and behavior can be perpetuated by people of any gender and age and, thus, conceptualizing feminism as "anti-male . . . reflects the reality that most folks learn about feminism from patriarchal mass media" (hooks, 2015). That is, the misconception that feminism is "antimale" is, in and of itself, a result of inequity and is not in line with feminist theory. Adopting a feminist perspective is relevant to persons of all genders and, thus, many cisgender (those whose birth-assigned sex and gender identity align) men advocate for feminist theory and identify as feminists. Moreover, individuals of all genders who work within feminism and feminist theory often share the common goal of shifting attention from exclusively focusing on the perspective of cisgender men to focusing on how systems of power and oppression interact to maintain inequality, oppression, and injustice.

Feminist theory posits that power and oppression maintain imbalances in equity and opportunity that affect all areas of existence, including economics (e.g., unequal pay), politics (e.g., leaders are typically cisgender men), religion and family systems (e.g., traditional gender roles), and psychology (individuals' beliefs about what one is capable of achieving). To understand how power and oppression lead to gender inequity, feminist theory focuses on various gender-related constructs, such as gender roles and stereotypes, media depictions of gender and sex, social hierarchies, and sexual objectification. In particular, feminist theory aims to understand the nature of gender inequity and argues that societal gender roles play a large part in how we come to think about others, the larger community, and ourselves.

Importantly, many disciplines of feminist thought inform and shape feminist theory. For example, intersectionality is one discipline that provides critical perspectives on how social identities like gender, race, and class interconnect and inform, disrupt, and expand our understanding of behavior and culture. Feminist theory considers the myriad biases shaped by sociocultural contexts. As such, feminist theory has critiqued "objective" methods of data collection and interpretation by calling into question an "objective truth" to human behavior that can be observed outside of its sociocultural context. Nonetheless, feminist theory has garnered subjective and empirical support. Moreover, the principles underlying gender inequity (i.e., feminist theory) explain many sexual and gender-related phenomenon, including, but not limited to, sexual violence, sexual consent, discrimination against women and the LGBTQ+ community, the lack of women in science, and economic injustice. Ultimately, the goal of feminism and feminist theory is to promote and strive for equity and justice.

G. Nic Rider and Janna A. Dickenson

See also: Female Sexuality; Gender; Gender Roles, Socialization and; Sexism; Stereotypes, Gender; Stereotypes, Sexual.

Further Reading

Allen, A. (2018). *The power of feminist theory.* New York: Routledge.

hooks, b. (2015). *Feminism is for everybody: Passionate politics.* New York: Routledge.

Tolman, D. L. (2012). Female adolescents, sexual empowerment and desire: A missing discourse of gender inequity. *Sex Roles, 66*(11–12), 746–757.

Fertility

Fertility is the quality or state of being fertile, where being fertile is the natural ability to produce offspring, not including stillbirths. Like all body systems, the reproductive tract does not exist in isolation and can change in response to other events in the body. Thus, fertility is dependent not only on reproductive organs but also on the brain, hormones, adipose tissue (fat cells), and glands. The human body is very complex, so it is important to be mindful that, while not necessarily discussed here, other body systems potentially affect fertility as well. Other factors that influence fertility for both partners are age, weight, diet, history of infection, exposure to environmental toxins, genetics, exercise, and consumption of alcohol, tobacco, and other substances.

Female fertility is rooted in the menstrual cycle. At birth, the ovaries contain approximately one million oocytes (eggs) in an immature state. Over time, some of the oocytes die due to lack of stimulation in a normal process called atresia. During puberty, which usually occurs between the ages of nine and fourteen years, an egg begins to mature in its follicle. At maturity, it bursts out and is picked up by the fallopian tube in a process called ovulation. If there are no sperm to fertilize the egg, it is expelled from the body, along with the uterine lining, in a process called menstruation. The whole cycle is called the menstrual cycle (period) and typically runs twenty-five to thirty days. It is important to note that the onset of menstruation, also called menarche, does not mean a female is fertile. Oftentimes a female's first ovulation occurs several months to two years after menarche.

The fertility window (FW) is the time during a female's cycle when pregnancy is possible and is based on when ovulation occurs, usually fourteen days before the start of menstruation. The FW is different for every woman and includes the five days before ovulation, since sperm can survive for up to five days in the female body, and the day of ovulation itself. Fertility drops off sharply twelve to twenty-four hours after the oocyte is released, since the oocyte is only viable for about twenty-four hours.

Many women use fertility calendars to track their cycles and then calculate their FW. Day one is the first day of menstruation, while the last day is the day before the next period starts. For individuals with inconsistent cycles and who are trying to conceive, it is recommended that they have sexual intercourse every two to three days to optimize chances of pregnancy.

If, during the ovulation phase, a sperm is available to fertilize the egg and fertilization occurs, the resulting zygote will float from the fallopian tube into the uterus. Approximately five to six days after fertilization, the zygote has become a blastocyst and is now ready for implantation into the uterine wall. Roughly 50 percent of fertilized blastocysts do not implant or stop developing; if this occurs, the female will menstruate as usual. However, if successful implantation and development occur, a woman may experience a missed period and become aware that she is pregnant.

Sometimes the menstrual cycle can be irregular, meaning it arrives sooner than twenty-five days, later than thirty days, or not at all, despite not being pregnant. Having an occasional irregular cycle may be caused by stress, illness, diet, exercise, or variance in routine. Consistently irregular periods can be indicative of larger problems with the reproductive system. For example, periods occurring too closely together may mean that the eggs are not reaching maturity before ovulation. Periods that are too far apart can mean that ovulation is not regular, which could be caused by polycystic ovarian syndrome.

The quality and quantity of fertilizable eggs are also dependent on the female's age. Women ages nineteen to twenty-six years are typically the most fertile and have a 50 percent chance of conceiving during the peak of the FW. Chances of conceiving decline by 10 percent from ages twenty-seven to thirty-four and then decline more rapidly from age thirty-five to thirty-nine. According to the American Society for Reproductive Medicine, a woman's chance of becoming pregnant is less than 5 percent per month at age forty.

Oocyte quality is synonymous with its ability to implant into the uterus once it has been fertilized. One explanation for this is that energy-producing mechanisms within the egg do not function as well as they did when they were younger and therefore are unable to sustain the energy needed to keep growing until implantation. In addition, research shows that between the ages of thirty and thirty-five years, the rate of chromosomal abnormalities increases from 1 in 526 (under thirty years) to 1 in 385. By age forty-five, the rate of chromosomal abnormalities jumps to 1 in 66.

Males generally become fertile between ages twelve and sixteen years with the onset of puberty. In the seminiferous tubules located in the testes, many new sperm cells are generated daily, roughly one thousand per second. However, the full process of creating sperm (spermatogenesis and spermiogenesis) takes sixty-five to seventy-five days.

Male fertility is dependent on the characteristics of the semen, which includes ejaculate volume, total number and concentration of sperm present, sperm morphology (normal shape), percentage and total motility (progressive and nonprogressive movement), presence of antibodies, and viability. Fertility in males is often evaluated using a semen analysis. Some conditions that can alter semen and sperm quality are the presence of varicoceles (enlarged veins that cause testicles to overheat), diabetes, paralysis, cystic fibrosis, infection, testicular failure, exposure to environmental toxins like pesticides and lead, and substance use.

By contrast, infertility is the inability to conceive offspring. Medically, infertility in women under thirty-five years old is described as the desire to have a baby with the inability to become pregnant after one year of sex without contraception with the same partner, or the inability to carry a pregnancy to term. If a woman is age thirty-five or older, the time criteria to be diagnosed with infertility is reduced to six months. Between 10 percent and 15 percent of couples living in the United States are affected by infertility. In roughly a third of cases, infertility can be traced to male causes, and likewise, in an additional third of cases, infertility can be traced to female causes. For the remaining third, the infertility is either linked to both male and female factors or considered unexplained. Infertility may be treated in several ways, including medication, surgery, intrauterine insemination, or assisted reproductive technology (ART).

Although infertility is a medical condition, it can cause high levels of psychological distress. Some people grow up with the expectation that they will become parents and that it is a biological imperative as well as significant life role. One study found that women feel guilt, blame themselves, and wonder what they may have done to deserve having trouble with fertility. Sometimes women have a hidden and prolonged sense of loss and may feel that they are missing out on the pregnancy and birth experiences, passing on of their genetics, and fulfilling their ideal of family; they may also feel as though they are disappointing others and may experience diminished self-worth and self-esteem. Reactions to infertility are similar to any loss and include shock, grief, depression, anger, frustration, and a feeling of having no control over one's future.

Sterility, which is relatively rare, is the complete inability to conceive offspring. Some conditions that cause sterility are Klinefelter syndrome (a chromosomal pattern of XXY), androgen insensitivity syndrome (being unable to process male hormones), hypogonadism (inadequate production of testosterone), and Turner syndrome (genetic disorder in females). Other causes of infertility include radiation therapy, trauma to the reproductive tract, repeated incidence of sexually transmitted infections, or exposure to some diseases (e.g., mumps), among others.

People may also choose to become sterile as a means of birth control. Males may undergo a vasectomy, a procedure that purposefully blocks the sperm cells from mixing with the seminal fluid and inhibits them from becoming part of the ejaculate. Females may choose to have a tubal ligation, which blocks sperm from entering the fallopian tubes, preventing it from fertilizing the oocyte.

While some choose to suspend fertility via contraception, others attempt to prolong it. Many people are choosing to delay having children until they are older, possibly because of education, career, or prioritizing other life goals. Over 20 percent of new mothers are over thirty-five years, and one in seven children are born to them. Technology has proposed a solution to the aging gamete factor as cryopreservation (freezing eggs or sperm) is increasingly used for a variety of situations. Like many decisions in life, it is important to weigh the pros and cons before making a decision. Gamete freezing does not guarantee that a baby will result as there are the general risks involved when using ART procedures as well as other overall risks involved in the freezing process.

Darci Shinn

See also: Assisted Reproductive Technology; Conception; Contraception; Fertility Awareness Methods of Contraception; Fertility Drugs; Infertility; Menarche; Menstruation; Ovulation; Pregnancy; Puberty; Sperm.

Further Reading

Alter, C. (2015, July 27). Buying time. *Time*, 41–45.

American Society for Reproductive Medicine. (2012). *Optimizing natural fertility*. Retrieved from https://www.reproductivefacts.org/news-and-publications/patient-fact-sheets-and-booklets/documents/fact-sheets-and-info-booklets/optimizing-natural-fertility/

Centers for Disease Control and Prevention. (2019). *Infertility FAQs*. Retrieved from http://www.cdc.gov/reproductivehealth/infertility/index.htm

Chandra, A., Copen, C. E., & Stephen, E. H. (2013). *Infertility and impaired fecundity in the United States, 1982–2010: Data from the National Survey of Family Growth*. Centers for Disease Control: National Health Statistics Reports, 62, 571–577.

Fertility Coalition (2019). *Getting the timing right*. Retrieved from http://yourfertility.org.au/for-women/timing-and-conception

Jones, R. E., & Lopez, K. (2006). *Human reproductive biology* (3rd ed.). New York: Academic Press.

Levine, H. (2016). *9 things every woman must know about her fertility*. Retrieved from http://www.health.com/health/gallery/0,,20987648,00.html

Lindsey, R., & Driskill, C. (2013). The psychology of infertility. *International Journal of Childbirth Education, 28*(3), 41–47.

Mneimneh, A. S., Boulet, S. L., Sunderam, S., Zhang, Y., Jamieson, D. J., ... Kissin, D. M. (2013). States monitoring assisted reproductive technology (SMART) collaborative: Data collection, linkage, dissemination, and use. *Journal of Women's Health, 22*(7), 571–577.

Perkins, S., & Meyers-Thompson, J. (2007). *Infertility for dummies.* Indianapolis: Wiley Publishing.

Resolve. (2016). *What is infertility?* Retrieved from http://www.resolve.org/about-infertility/what-is-infertility/

USC Fertility. (2016). *Female egg quality is synonymous with the probability of embryo implantation.* Retrieved from http://uscfertility.org/fertility-treatments/female-egg-quality/

Fertility Awareness Methods of Contraception

Although they may be derided as old-fashioned in industrialized countries, fertility awareness methods (FAMs) of birth control can meet the needs of many individuals. Some people use FAMs because they limit the risk of pregnancy while respecting cultural and religious norms. Others like the fact that no hormones or other chemical agents are involved, or that they are low-cost, ecological solutions. FAMs, also called "natural family planning" or "the rhythm method," have the advantage of allowing a better understanding of the menstrual cycle and the reproductive system. However, it should be noted that these methods have limited effectiveness and require considerable discipline to be put into practice. Furthermore, both partners must commit to abstain from penile-vaginal intercourse on the "unsafe" days. This restriction of sexual activity for fear of unwanted pregnancy means that sexual relations are associated with procreation, which has followed a downward trend as more "modern" contraceptive methods become available.

FAMs are ways to identify the fertile days of the menstrual cycle by monitoring the signs and symptoms of ovulation or by tracking the fertile days. They include the calendar method, the temperature method, the cervical mucus method, and the symptothermal method (i.e., the previous three methods combined), among others. A recent advance is the personal fertility monitor, which allows tracking the menstrual cycle via an app on a smartphone. FAMs generally require the partners to collaborate and to exercise discipline. Partners must commit to abstain from penile-vaginal sex during fertile days, or they must use an alternative contraceptive method during this time. In addition, determining the fertile period requires knowledge, an adjustment period, and daily attention. Therefore, users of these methods should be well informed beforehand, for instance, by reading pamphlets and other publications. This helps them make informed decisions about the potential risks of these methods.

The methods based on tracking the fertile days are not the most effective. The effectiveness varies across individuals and depends greatly on the partners' motivation to prevent pregnancy. Several additional factors may come into play, such as the health care provider's knowledge and the quality of the information that is provided, the frequency of penile-vaginal sex, the contraceptive method used during the fertility window (e.g., abstinence versus withdrawal method versus barrier methods), as well as origin from a country where FAMs are more widespread. With typical use, the limited data available indicate that FAMs have about a 75 percent effectiveness rate overall. With perfect use, the effectiveness rates are 91 percent for the calendar method, 97 percent for the cervical mucus method, and 98 percent for the symptothermal method.

Like other contraceptive methods, FAMs come with both advantages and disadvantages. Notably, there are no side effects or health risks. FAMs also help individuals to understand their body and menstrual cycle better, and they are very useful for identifying the fertile days if an individual wishes to get pregnant. Moreover, FAMs allow individuals to respect certain religious and cultural norms concerning contraception. In addition, FAMs require both partners to collaborate, which means that both partners have to participate in decisions about contraception. On the other hand, FAMs require good knowledge of the menstrual cycle and the different birth control strategies available to use on fertile days as well as an adjustment period that can last several months. Abstinence from penile-vaginal sex is required on certain days, and users must be alert to the signs and symptoms of fertility on a daily basis. Numerous factors, including stress, illness, medications, vaginal infections, adolescence, and perimenopause, can modify the menstrual cycle, making it harder to accurately observe and interpret fertility signals. FAMs are also less suitable for those who are uncomfortable about exploring their body or who find it difficult to negotiate conception issues (e.g., in an intimate relationship where domestic violence is present). Furthermore, FAMs provide no protection from sexually transmitted infections.

Sylvie Lévesque

See also: Cervical Mucus Method; Contraception; Fertility; Ovulation.

Further Reading

Black, A., Guilbert, E., Costescu, D., Dunn, S., Fisher, W., Kives, S., . . . Todd, N. (2015). Canadian contraception consensus (Part 2 of 4). *Journal of Obstetrics and Gynaecology Canada, 37*(11), 1036–1039.

Glasier, A., & Gebbie, A. E. (2008). *Handbook of family planning and reproductive healthcare* (5th ed.). London: Churchill Livingstone.

McVeigh, E., Guillebaud, J., & Homburg, R. (2013). *Oxford handbook of reproductive medicine and family planning.* Oxford: Oxford University Press.

Planned Parenthood. (2019). Fertility awareness. Retrieved from https://www.plannedparenthood.org/learn/birth-control/fertility-awareness

Serena. (2019). Home page. Retrieved from www.serena.ca

World Health Organization. (2018). *Family planning: A global handbook for providers.* Retrieved from https://www.who.int/reproductivehealth/publications/fp-global-handbook/en/

Fertility Drugs

Fertility drugs are prescribed medications used to treat infertility in women due to a variety of causes. The majority of fertility drugs are used to stimulate or regulate ovulation in women who do not ovulate regularly each month. Although about

50 percent of women who use fertility drugs achieve pregnancy, certain risks are present with many of these medical treatments.

The most common fertility drug used by women is clomiphene citrate. Clomiphene is a synthetic hormone that is used to induce ovulation or to help the body maintain a regular ovulation cycle. It works by stimulating the pituitary gland to release follicle-stimulating hormone (FSH), which directs the ovaries to develop egg-producing follicles. Clomiphene is taken orally in fifty-milligram tablets for three to five days at the beginning of a menstrual cycle. It is estimated that 85 percent of women treated with clomiphene will ovulate, and of these about half will become pregnant within four to five cycles.

Although it has been used for over thirty years, there remain some side effects and risks from the use of clomiphene. The American Society for Reproductive Medicine recommends that clomiphene be used for no more than three to six cycles based on preliminary studies that show there may be an increased risk of ovarian cancer in women who use it for more than twelve cycles. However, this risk has yet to be proven. Common side effects from the use of clomiphene include hot flashes, anxiety, headaches, nausea, and ovarian cysts.

In the case that clomiphene is not successful in inducing ovulation, alternative drugs may be tried. Letrozole is an aromatase inhibitor that stimulates the release of FSH by suppressing the body's production of estrogen. Although it has fewer side effects than clomiphene, its success in stimulating ovulation appears to be slightly lower. Metformin works by lowering the body's insulin level in order to improve ovulation in women with polycystic ovary syndrome. Side effects from metformin use include nausea, abdominal pain, and allergic reactions.

Other fertility drug treatments that are used in the event clomiphene is unsuccessful include injections of FSH, luteinizing hormone (LH), and human menopausal gonadotropin. Each bypasses the pituitary gland to directly stimulate the ovaries to produce multiple eggs. Once follicles are matured, a woman may be given an injection of human chorionic gonadotropin hormone in order to trigger release of the eggs. A serious complication that sometimes occurs with these drugs is known as ovarian hyperstimulation syndrome (OHSS), in which the ovaries become enlarged and fluid builds up in the abdomen, resulting in a swollen stomach, nausea and vomiting, and severe abdominal pain. Women who experience symptoms of OHSS should seek emergency treatment as the condition can be life-threatening.

In some women, the pituitary gland produces excess amounts of the hormone prolactin. This overproduction causes problems with the release of FSH and LH, which interfere with normal ovulation. Two oral medications that reduce prolactin levels are bromocriptine and cabergoline. Side effects with these drugs include nausea, dizziness, headache, and decreased blood pressure.

Once the ovaries develop follicles, ovulation must be regulated to control the release of eggs in preparation for assisted reproductive technology procedures such as in vitro fertilization. Leuprorelin and nafarelin are gonadotropin-releasing hormone agonists that hyperstimulate the ovaries to produce multiple eggs.

Certain drugs are used to enhance other fertility treatments. Methylprednisolone is a steroid that is taken to improve the uterine lining in preparation for embryo implantation. Progesterone is a natural hormone injected once ovulation has occurred that also improves the uterine lining to increase the chances of a successful embryo implantation following fertilization of the egg or eggs.

With all fertility drug use, the greatest risk is increased incidence of multiple births. With clomiphene use, the chance of having twins is 10 percent, while the chance of having triplets is only 1 percent; higher-order multiples are very rare. According to a study published in the *American Journal of Epidemiology*, 22.8 percent of multiples are conceived using fertility drugs. Health risks to infants include increased chance of premature birth and low birth weight. Some 60 percent of twins and more than 90 percent of all other multiples are born prematurely. Premature birth carries the risk of intellectual disability, cerebral palsy, developmental delays, vision and hearing problems, and death.

For many women, fertility drugs have made the possibility of becoming pregnant a reality. Although the drugs do carry certain side effects and risks, the success rate of fertility drugs is sufficient for many women to attempt these treatments. In all, over 190,000 infants are conceived each year with the intervention of fertility drugs.

Christina Girod

See also: Artificial Insemination; Assisted Reproductive Technology; Fertility; Follicle-Stimulating Hormone; Infertility; Ovulation; Pregnancy.

Further Reading

Aboulghar, M., & Rizk, B. (Eds.). (2011). *Ovarian stimulation*. Cambridge: Cambridge University Press.

March of Dimes Foundation. (2010, January). Fertility drugs contribute heavily to multiple births. *ScienceDaily*. Retrieved from www.sciencedaily.com/releases/2010/01/100120104002.htm

Fetishism

"Fetishism" refers to an obsessive fascination with, and sexual arousal from, inanimate objects or body parts not normally associated with sex. Objects might include high-heeled shoes, skirts, pantyhose, panties, or purses. Body parts might include feet, armpits, hair, or other nongenital parts. Most people have some degree of sexual fetishism, and that is considered a normal, healthy part of human sexuality. However, if the sexual fetish is ongoing and interferes with normal social functioning and conventional sexual practices, causes significant distress, or if sexual arousal is impossible without the fetish object, it may be diagnosed as fetishistic disorder, as specified by the *Diagnostic and Statistical Manual of Mental Disorders* (*DSM-5*).

Fetishistic disorder is classified as a type of paraphilic disorder, a group of conditions that involve atypical sexual desires and extreme behaviors. In fetishistic disorder, the affected individual must look at, hold, rub, smell, taste, or wear the fetish object, or have their partner do so, in order to achieve sexual arousal and orgasm. In most cases, the individual performs these acts alone while masturbating. Men who practice fetishism by wearing women's clothes, typically masturbating while wearing the clothes, are said to have transvestic fetishism.

Psychologists classify fetish objects as form fetishes or media fetishes. Form fetishes prompt arousal primarily by their perceived-to-be-appealing shapes, such as a stiletto-heel shoe, a strappy purse, or a delicate bracelet. Media fetishes prompt arousal by their perceived sensual feel and texture, such as lacy panties and bras, silky nylons, leather skirts, and fur coats. In some cases, it is mainly the smell or sound of an object or body part that causes arousal, such as the odor of an armpit or foot, the sound of heels on the floor while walking, or the sound of a zipper on a dress. For some people, merely looking at photographs of the fetish objects is enough to arouse them, though they are likely to prefer possessing the objects.

Fetishists typically make collections of their preferred fetish objects. Some people with fetishistic disorder may even resort to stealing these objects from stores or homes or assaulting other people to get the objects. Compulsive thoughts of the object and powerful urges regarding the object can become so psychologically dominant that the individual becomes unable to focus on anything else, including work, family relationships, and other personal responsibilities. It is not uncommon for people with fetishistic disorder to take a job at a particular business to facilitate their fetish behavior, such as a clothing or shoe store.

Although individuals with fetishistic disorder may experience intense sexual excitement and pleasure while engaged in the practice, afterward they may have feelings of mental anguish, distress, shame, or guilt regarding the behavior.

Fetishistic disorder is much more common in men than women. In fact, clinical data suggest that it is extremely rare in women and is almost exclusively a male condition. However, the prevalence of this condition within the general population cannot be stated with certainty. That is because the distinction between "normal" fetishism and fetishistic disorder is not always clear. Furthermore, many individuals who engage in fetishistic behavior do so in private and do not seek treatment. Thus, they are never tabulated in medical statistics.

Psychologists do not fully understand the causes of sexual fetishism, and most studies on the topic have focused on males. This research suggests that fetishistic behavior is associated with certain social experiences. Men who are socially isolated, lack confidence in their masculinity and sexual attractiveness, and fear rejection from women are more likely to report sexual fetishes, although it is impossible to determine if their social experiences contribute to, or are the result of, their fetish. It may be that their feelings of sexual inadequacy and their inabilities to develop intimacy with other people are compensated for by exercising control over the fetish objects and by other fetishistic practices.

Research also indicates that the roots of fetishism may begin in childhood and adolescence, when certain objects become mentally associated with feelings of sexual excitement or gratification, especially during masturbation. Such associations tend to develop through an unconscious learning process called conditioning, in which the mind forms new associations between certain stimuli and certain responses that were not previously associated. For example, and adolescent male may see an attractive woman in high-heeled shoes and become aroused and experience sexual urges, leading him to masturbate so that he experiences sexual gratification. In the future, if the shoes have become paired with arousal, they will be arousing on their own, even without the presence of the attractive woman.

Most experiences of fetishism do not require treatment. However, if the fetish is significantly impairing social or sexual functioning or causing significant distress, the individual may seek treatment to decrease their compulsive thoughts and urges. Treatment typically involves a combination of psychotherapy or other forms of counseling and drug therapy. To be successful, these therapies usually have to be performed on a continuous, long-term basis.

One of the main forms of psychotherapy used to treat fetishistic disorder is cognitive behavioral therapy, which seeks to change destructive conditioned thoughts into useful productive thoughts and, consequently, into useful productive behaviors. Thought stopping is an example of a technique used in cognitive behavioral therapy. In this technique, the individual learns to stop any developing thoughts related to the fetish and immediately substitute other thoughts about less harmful fantasies. Biofeedback is another technique that might be useful for helping the individual control harmful thoughts.

Among the drugs that are commonly used in treatment are antiandrogens, which temporarily reduce testosterone levels and the frequency of sexually arousing mental imagery and sexual fantasies in men. Other drugs that may be incorporated into treatment are antidepressants, such as selective serotonin reuptake inhibitors, which help to decrease sex drive.

While some types of fetish objects are fairly common (e.g., shoes, feet, leather, latex), there are many other—though much more rare—forms of sexual fetishes and arousal. These include agalmatophilia (arousal from statues), apotemnophilia (arousal from thoughts of oneself as an amputee), coprophilia (arousal from feces), psychrophilia (arousal from being cold or watching others who are cold), and xylophila (arousal from wood or bark).

A. J. Smuskiewicz

See also: Arousal; Kink; Paraphilias.

Further Reading

Bering, J. (2014). *Perv: The sexual deviant in all of us.* New York: Doubleday.

Bressert, S. (2019). Fetishistic disorder symptoms. Retrieved from http://psychcentral.com/disorders/fetishism-symptoms

Huffington Post. (2013). 46 sexual fetishes you've never heard of. Retrieved from https://www.huffpost.com/entry/sexual-fetish_n_4144418

Scorolli, C., Ghirlanda, S., Enquist, M., Zattoni, S., & Jannini, E. A. (2007). Relative prevalence of different fetishes. *International Journal of Impotence Research, 19,* 432–437.

5-Alpha-Reductase Deficiency

5-alpha-reductase deficiency is one of a group of congenital disorders characterized as causing disorders or differences of sexual development (DSDs). Individuals with 5-alpha-reductase deficiency have X and Y chromosomes, but at the time of birth they appear to have female or ambiguous genitalia. This is because 5-alpha-reductase is an enzyme that converts testosterone into dihydrotestosterone or DHT. A lack of DHT during gestation means that the external genitalia of these XY infants develop more like they would in an XX or typical female child.

Although testosterone is often described as the main hormone responsible for masculinization, dihydrotestosterone is a more active version of testosterone that causes many of the physiological changes associated with a male-typed body. DHT is particularly important in the development of the external reproductive structures of the body prior to birth. When DHT is absent in an XY fetus, several structures follow stereotypical female instead of male development. Specifically, the clitoris is formed instead of the penile glans, the labia minora instead of the shaft of the penis, and the labia majora instead of the scrotum.

Without surgical intervention to remove the testes, individuals with 5-alpha-reductase deficiency will make normal male amounts of testosterone at the time of puberty. At this time, their bodies may suddenly masculinize. Their clitoris can lengthen into a penis, their testicles descend into the scrotum, and they can have other male pattern physical development. The degree to which this happens depends on the specific mutations that have caused their 5-alpha-reductase deficiency.

5-alpha-reductase deficiency has been documented around the world. However, because it is a genetic condition, it is more common in certain populations, including in the Dominican Republic, Papua New Guinea, Turkey, and Egypt. In the Dominican Republic, 5-alpha-reductase deficiency is common enough in certain villages that individuals with this condition are known as *guevedoces*, which means "penis at twelve." These individuals are generally encouraged to embrace their male gender identity. The response to the sudden masculinization of 5-alpha-reductase deficiency children at puberty has been met with different responses in other cultures.

Gender assignment for infants born with 5-alpha-reductase deficiency is challenging—medically, ethically, and culturally. Research suggests that, regardless of the appearance of their genitals at the time of birth, a slight majority of these children will go on to develop a male gender identity. This is thought to be because, unlike individuals with complete androgen insensitivity syndrome, children with 5-alpha-reductase are exposed to normal levels of testosterone during fetal development. Prenatal testosterone exposure has been linked to gender identity formation in several conditions characterized as DSDs. The formation of a male gender identity may also be because of the changes in their bodies that these individuals experience at the time of puberty, if their testes are not removed during childhood.

Historically, many parents have chosen to assign children with 5-alpha-reductase deficiency as female because of the appearance of their genitalia. This choice has become more controversial over time, in part because of data suggesting that many children with 5-alpha-reductase deficiency will develop a male gender identity. As such, a growing percentage of these children are now being assigned male at birth rather than female.

There are some parents who still choose to assign children with 5-alpha-reductase deficiency as female at birth. In the United States and in states where doing so is legal, these parents may also choose to remove the child's testes with the goal of trying to maintain the child's female identity rather than risking that exposure to increased levels of testosterone at puberty could encourage male gender identity development. It is possible that removal of the testes can be beneficial to those individuals who maintain a female gender identity at puberty, who might be harmed by masculinization of their bodies. However, gonadectomy can be traumatic or problematic for individuals with a male gender identity.

A growing number of activists and medical professionals have begun to argue against genital "normalization" surgeries for infants with differences of sexual development, including 5-alpha-reductase deficiency, except in cases where those surgeries have a clear benefit for the child's health. They advocate for surgery to be postponed until children are old enough to make their own decisions about what they want to happen to their bodies. In contrast, proponents of genital surgery during childhood argue that asking a young person to make this decision is beyond their emotional or intellectual capacity and that therefore it is more appropriate for the choice to be made by parents and professionals.

Elizabeth R. Boskey

See also: Androgen Insensitivity Syndrome; Androgens; Chromosomal Sex; Congenital Adrenal Hyperplasia; Gender Identity Development; Intersexuality; Sex Reassignment Surgery; X Chromosome; Y Chromosome.

Further Reading

Byers, H. M., Mohnach, L. H., Fechner, P. Y., Chen, M., Thomas, I. H., Ramsdell, L. A., ... Keegan, C. E. (2017). Unexpected ethical dilemmas in sex assignment in 46,XY DSD due to 5-alpha reductase type 2 deficiency. *American Journal of Medical Genetics Part C: Seminars in Medical Genetics, 175*(2), 260–267.

Cohen-Kettenis, P. T. (2005). Gender change in 46,XY persons with 5alpha-reductase-2 deficiency and 17beta-hydroxysteroid dehydrogenase-3 deficiency. *Archives of Sexual Behavior, 34*(4), 399–410.

Imperato-McGinley, J., Guerrero, L., Gautier, T., & Peterson, R. E. (1974). Steroid 5alpha-reductase deficiency in man: An inherited form of male pseudohermaphroditism. *Science, 186*(4170), 1213–1215.

Kolesinska, Z., Ahmed, S. F., Niedziela, M., Bryce, J., Molinska-Glura, M., Rodie, M., ... Weintrob N. (2014). Changes over time in sex assignment for disorders of sex development. *Pediatrics, 134*(3), e710–e715.

Reis-Dennis, S., & Reis, E. (2017). Are physicians blameworthy for iatrogenic harm resulting from unnecessary genital surgeries? *American Medical Association Journal of Ethics, 19*(8), 825–833.

Fluidity, Gender

"Gender fluidity," sometimes also known as "multigender," "pangender," and "gender flexible," is a term describing an individual whose gender identity or gender expression fluctuates over time or in different situational contexts. The term "fluidity" suggests the tendency to change shape and form. This term was initially applied to sexuality to describe sexual fluidity—the notion that sexual attractions, desires, and behaviors can change over time and across situations and may lead to a shift in sexual identity. Thus, gender fluidity is the idea that gender identities and expressions may shift across contexts, situations, and over time. As such, gender fluidity suggests that some people can feel that they are in between, neither, outside of, or both man and woman, and that self and social perceptions can and do shift.

Gender fluidity challenges the idea that people must have a single, stable gender identity. Cisgender individuals experience their gender as congruent with their sex assigned at birth, and some transgender individuals may endorse a singular, stable gender that differs from their sex assigned at birth. Gender fluidity, on the other hand, suggests a tendency to oscillate between and combine attributes of masculinity and femininity. People who identify as gender fluid may describe their gender identity as changing from mood to mood, day to day, or situation to situation. Also, gender-fluid people may identify with others of all different genders along a spectrum of gender identity and expression. For example, one study found that gender-fluid participants described the ability to "understand people better" as a result of experiencing both masculine and feminine socialization.

Sometimes gender fluidity can be frustrating or confusing to gender-fluid individuals and others. Gender-fluid people may feel like their gender identity is unpredictable. The ambiguity and instability of gender identity may lead to personal and social distress due to transgressing social forces that regulate gender identity and expression. For example, Wilchins (2002) said, "Looking gender normative is vital to social acceptance . . . few things are more uncomfortable than seeing someone whose gender you can't discern," meaning that appearing in a way that is consistent with masculine and feminine gender norms is generally more socially accepted than gender presentations that deviate from gender ideals.

However, many people find their gender fluidity to be a source of strength and positivity. When they understand and accept the validity of their experience, people often feel that gender fluidity empowers them to self-identify or "disidentify" in whatever way is appropriate. For instance, author and activist Jeffery Marsh (2015) said gender fluidity means "you don't need to decide your gender." Individuals who are gender fluid have described their ability to deconstruct gender binaries, the authority to self-define, and the aptitude to identify as and empathize with a broad spectrum of genders.

Jory M. Catalpa, Nova J. Bradford, Janna A. Dickenson, and G. Nic Rider

See also: Agender; Bigender; Binary Gender System; Fluidity, Sexual; Gender; Gender Diversity; Gender Expression; Gender Identity; Gender Roles, Socialization and; Gender Transition; Genderqueer; Nonbinary Gender Identities.

Further Reading

Bauman, Z. (2000). *Liquid modernity.* Malden, MA: Polity Press.

Bradford, N. J., Rider, G. N., Catalpa, J. M., Morrow, Q. J., Berg, D. R., Spencer, K. G., & McGuire, J. K. (2018). Creating gender: A thematic analysis of genderqueer narratives. *International Journal of Transgenderism, 20*(2–3), 155–168.

Butler, J. (1990). *Gender trouble.* London: Routledge.

Diamond, L., & Butterworth, M. (2008). Questioning gender and sexual identity: Dynamic links over time. *Sex Roles, 59*, 365–376.

Diamond, L. M., Pardo, S. T., & Butterworth, M. R. (2011). Transgender experience and identity. In S. J. Schwartz, K. Luyckx, & V. L. Vignoles (Eds.), *Handbook of identity theory and research* (629–647). New York: Springer.

Marsh, J. (2015, August 19). What is gender fluid? Retrieved from https://www.youtube.com/watch?v=3Hj1Dm4sob4

Muñoz, J. E. (1999). *Disidentifications: Queers of color and the performance of politics.* Minneapolis: University of Minnesota Press.

Wilchins, R. (2002). Deconstructing trans. In J. Nestle, C. Howell, & R. A. Wilchins (Eds.), *GenderQueer: Voices from beyond the sexual binary* (56). Los Angeles, CA: Alyson Books.

Fluidity, Sexual

Historically, sexual orientation has been defined as an enduring pattern of sexual attractions, desires, fantasies, and behaviors for people of a specific gender or sex that differs and/or is similar to their own. Whereas this definition characterizes the experiences of many individuals, unexpected changes in sexual attractions, identities, and behaviors can also occur. Over the past several decades, Lisa Diamond, PhD, and other researchers have shown that some individuals experience changes in their same-sex (or same-gender, hereafter denoted same-sex/gender) and other-sex (or other-gender, hereafter denoted other-sex/gender) desires. Such shifts may be transient or lead to a lasting change in their overall pattern of attractions, desires, fantasies, and behaviors.

Sexual fluidity is defined as the capacity for one's attractions, desires, fantasies, and behaviors to be flexible and change across time, situations, and contexts. Like sexual orientation, sexual fluidity is a trait that varies from person to person. Some individuals tend to show stable patterns of sexual attractions, desires, and behaviors, whereas others show variation in their overall pattern of attractions, desires, and behaviors. For example, some gay men and lesbians may experience occasional other-sex/gender attractions whereas others do not, just as some heterosexuals experience occasional same-sex/gender attractions whereas others do not.

Furthermore, sexual fluidity differs from bisexuality and other nonexclusive sexual orientations. One difference is that sexual fluidity does not denote the direction of your attractions, nor does it imply sexual orientation, whereas bisexuality does. Bisexuality and other nonexclusive sexual orientations imply stable, enduring predispositions toward a pattern of mixed sexual attractions, desires, and behaviors. In contrast, sexual fluidity represents a situation-dependent capacity for change in attractions, desires, and behaviors and does not specify the direction of this change (you can be a fluid lesbian, a fluid heterosexual, etc.). Because both fluidity and bisexuality may look similar (both show a nonexclusive pattern of attractions), it is difficult for researchers to know whether nonexclusive patterns of attractions, desires, and behaviors arise from a nonexclusive sexual orientation or sexual fluidity. Nonetheless, research has repeatedly demonstrated that individuals have the capacity to have flexible erotic responses over time.

Researchers believe that female sexuality is more fluid than male sexuality. Several studies have shown that more cisgender (individuals whose gender identity and birth-assigned sex align) women than cisgender men show patterns of nonexclusive sexual attractions. In fact, many studies examining the percentage of exclusive and nonexclusive attractions among lesbian, gay, bisexual, and other nonheterosexual sexual orientations (LGB+) individuals demonstrate that more than half of cisgender LGB+ men show an exclusive pattern of same-sex sexual attractions. Yet, the majority of cisgender LGB+ women show nonexclusive patterns of attractions. In addition, cisgender women are more likely than cisgender men to show change in their desires, attractions, and behaviors over time (from year to year). This pattern is also evident at the population level. For example, the percentage of people reporting same-sex/gender sexual behavior across the past several decades has been relatively stable for men, whereas the percentage of women reporting same-sex/gender sexuality has increased linearly over the past several decades.

The reasons as to why female sexuality is more likely to be fluid than male sexuality are unclear. However, some researchers believe that social factors are relevant. For example, one study examining the percentage of people reporting same-sex/gender sexual behavior in the United States demonstrated that the changes in same-sex/gender sexuality across the population years were driven by increases in bisexual patterns of behavior. That is, rates of nonexclusive same-sex/gender sexual behavior changed, whereas exclusive same-sex/gender sexual behavior did not change. This study also found that such population-wide increases in same-sex/gender behavior were partially attributable to increases in social acceptance of same-sex/gender sexuality.

Some researchers suggest that social and cultural factors may explain gender differences in sexual fluidity. It is well documented that female sexuality is more strongly shaped by social factors than is the case for male sexuality. One possibility is related to a historical context in the United States, in which female sexuality has been subjected to far greater control than male sexuality. As this social control lessens, perhaps there is an increase in women's willingness to act on predispositions for bisexuality that went unexpressed in previous (and more restrictive) decades. Another possibility that some have posited is that there may be more cultural homophobia directed toward men's same-sex/gender sexuality than women's same-sex/gender sexuality. If social acceptance of same-sex/gender sexuality continues to increase, might men eventually be just as fluid as women? Although the answer to this question is as of yet unknown, more research will likely illuminate a greater understanding of these potential gender differences. Like all forms of human behavior, multiple factors (genetic, endocrinological, biological, social, cultural, emotional, cognitive) likely influence sexual fluidity.

Finally, capacity for a flexible erotic response does *not* mean that individuals who are sexually fluid can choose their sexual responsiveness. Research has demonstrated that effortful attempts to change one's sexual attractions, desires, and behaviors are not effective and are potentially harmful. Rather, sexual fluidity denotes unintentional, noneffortful change. As Lisa Diamond has eloquently stated in a recent article, "Whereas observational studies of 'naturally occurring' change can reveal important information about the expression of sexuality of the life course, studies on effortful therapeutic change are primarily relevant for understanding the psychological consequences of the social privileging of heterosexuality over same-sex sexuality."

Janna A. Dickenson and G. Nic Rider

See also: Bisexuality; Fluidity, Gender; Same-Sex Attraction and Behavior; Sexual Identity; Sexual Orientation.

Further Reading

Baumeister, R. F., & Twenge, J. M. (2002). Cultural suppression of female sexuality. *Review of General Psychology, 6*(2), 166.

Diamond, L. M. (2008). *Sexual fluidity: Understanding women's love and desire.* Cambridge, MA: Harvard University Press.

Diamond, L. M. (2016). Sexual fluidity in male and females. *Current Sexual Health Reports, 8*(4), 249–256.

Twenge, J. M., Sherman, R. A., & Wells, B. E. (2016). Changes in American adults' reported same-sex sexual experiences and attitudes, 1973–2014. *Archives of Sexual Behavior, 45*(7), 1713–1730.

Follicle-Stimulating Hormone

Follicle-stimulating hormone (FSH) is a hormone produced by the pituitary gland that plays an essential role in regulating the menstrual cycle by helping to trigger ovulation. It is also present in males and is essential to the production of sperm.

In the female body, the level of FSH changes according to the phase of the menstrual cycle. FSH peaks right before ovulation, as the hormone plays a role in selecting the most mature follicle in the ovaries for releasing an egg. Once ovulation occurs, the level of FSH decreases. If pregnancy does not occur, FSH begins to build up again after the menstruation period ends as the female body prepares for the next cycle of ovulation. It is also responsible for the onset of puberty regarding the maturation of the ovaries.

In the male body, FSH levels remain mostly constant because there is no cyclic process to the male reproductive system. FSH works with other hormones to maintain healthy sperm cell production. The hormone also plays a role in the onset of puberty and the development of testicular function.

Monitoring of FSH levels can help to diagnose and often resolve problems with infertility. In women, measuring the amount of FSH in the blood can tell doctors if a woman is ovulating normally and, if she is not, to determine what may be the problem. An FSH blood test can indicate the presence of ovarian cysts (benign fluid-filled growths on the ovaries) or polycystic ovary syndrome, in which a hormone imbalance causes follicles to fail to release eggs and to develop into small cysts instead.

Higher FSH levels can also indicate the onset or completion of menopause (the ending of monthly menstrual periods) and is especially helpful in diagnosing premature menopause. Abnormally high FSH levels can also indicate the presence of a tumor in the pituitary gland. Finally, high levels of FSH can also be a sign of

Turner syndrome, in which an individual has only one X chromosome (a normal female chromosome pair is XX). Low amounts of the hormone may also be caused by abnormally low body weight and malfunction of the pituitary gland.

In men, the FSH test can determine if the testicles are producing sperm of normal quantity and quality. Higher than normal FSH levels in men may be caused by advanced age; genetic abnormalities such as Klinefelter syndrome, in which a man has an extra X chromosome resulting in an XXY genotype (normal males have an XY chromosome pair); and damage to testicles due to alcohol abuse, chemotherapy, or radiation. It may also indicate a tumor in the pituitary gland.

In children, the FSH test is given to determine if higher or lower levels of the hormone than normal are present. Higher than normal amounts of FSH can result in the early development (younger than age ten) of secondary sex characteristics, while lower than normal amounts can tell doctors why some adolescents have a delay in the onset of puberty (later than age fifteen).

Synthetic FSH is sometimes given to women in combination with luteinizing hormone to treat infertility. This combination is called menotropins and is most often used when other types of fertility treatments have failed, such as clomiphene. It is administered as a subcutaneous injection immediately prior to ovulation. It may also be given to men to promote better sperm production. However, menotropins are usually used to stimulate a greater number of follicles to ovulate in preparation for intrauterine insemination, gamete intrafallopian transfer, or in vitro fertilization.

Although menotropins can successfully result in pregnancy, there are several risk factors involved in their use. Due to the fact that more than one follicle is being developed, the risk of ovarian hyperstimulation syndrome (OHSS) is higher. It is a painful condition and can be life-threatening if not treated. Symptoms of OHSS include severe abdominal pain, nausea and vomiting, weight gain, diarrhea, shortness of breath, and decreased urine output. The maturation of more than one follicle also increases the chance of becoming pregnant with multiple babies. Using menotropins is also associated with increased risk of blood clots, stroke, or heart attack, as well as a higher incidence of ovarian cancer.

Christina Girod

See also: Fertility Drugs; Infertility; Menstruation; Ovulation; Sex Hormones.

Further Reading

Goldberg, J., & Krause, L. (2016). What is a follicle-stimulating hormone level test? Retrieved from https://www.healthline.com/health/fsh

National Institutes of Health. (2019). Follicle-stimulating hormone (FSH) levels test. Retrieved from https://medlineplus.gov/lab-tests/follicle-stimulating-hormone-fsh-levels-test/

Stewart, S. C. (1996). *The American Medical Women's Association guide to fertility and reproductive health.* New York: Dell Publishing.

Foreplay

"Foreplay" usually refers to various intimate activities that people engage in before sexual intercourse or before some other sexual act. Foreplay activities, such as kissing and caressing, typically have the effects of increasing sexual desire and arousal in both partners and often lead to some form of sexual act in which one or both partners experience orgasm.

Importantly, however, foreplay does not have to lead to an orgasmic sexual act. People also sometimes engage in foreplay activities just to enjoy the pleasurable feelings generated by those activities. Foreplay is important if all participants are to thoroughly enjoy the sexual experience, including both the physical sensations and the emotional feelings. Foreplay helps ensure that partners are in a similar sensual and erotic mood and that they want the same thing—to share sexual pleasure with each other.

It is commonly believed that women enjoy foreplay more than men. However, foreplay "works" as a result of biochemical reactions that all people experience. Foreplay helps all people obtain more enjoyment out of the sexual experience by increasing levels of oxytocin, dopamine, and other biochemical hormones that lead to feelings of pleasure in the brain. Foreplay further increases blood flow to the skin, which makes nerves in the skin more sensitive to touch. The nerves relay sensations to the brain, which interprets them as pleasurable.

Any act meant to increase sexual interest, desire, or arousal can be considered foreplay. Verbal aspects of foreplay may include flirtatious chatting or teasing, suggestive whispering, compliments, or even an intelligent conversation that engages both individuals. Text messaging or phone calls with flirtatious comments might also be considered verbal foreplay. Visual aspects of foreplay may include the wearing of sexy clothes in front of an intended partner, such as a woman showing off her legs in a miniskirt and stiletto heels to a man in whom she is interested. The gradual removal of clothes—either by the person wearing them or by that person's partner—can also be an effective form of foreplay. Certain body postures, such as a suggestive crossing of the legs, may be considered foreplay. Visual foreplay can be as simple as the wink of an eye or a prolonged gaze. Atmospheric aspects of foreplay may involve dim lights, candles, and romantic music. Some people consider an entire date, such as a movie and dinner, an extended form of foreplay if it leads to sexual intercourse.

When most people think of foreplay, however, they think of intimate acts that involve physical contact, usually in the privacy of a bedroom, living room, or other place away from other people. Physical foreplay might begin with a soft kiss on the neck, an intermingling of fingers, or a gentle stroke of an arm or leg. This may progress to more passionate kissing and the removal of clothing. Foreplay usually reaches its height with various forms of touching, rubbing, caressing, hugging, kissing, licking, nibbling, or sucking of body parts that have extra nerve sensitivity or special sensual connotations—so-called erogenous zones. These parts include the breasts and nipples, the shoulders, the stomach, the inner thighs, the buttocks, and the genitals. Any part of the body may be touched in foreplay to help elicit erotic feelings.

Some people engage in certain kinds of "games" as part of foreplay. They might enjoy role-playing or fantasy games in which they dress in erotic, sexually stimulating clothing. For example, a man might cross-dress in women's lingerie, or a woman might dress like a leather-clad dominatrix, playfully enforcing acts of discipline on her partner. Some partners get excited by playing bondage games, involving such equipment as handcuffs, chains, and ropes. Other partners may get "turned on" by watching pornographic videos as part of foreplay. Sex toys, such as vibrators and dildos, are common objects used in foreplay, though they may also be used in the sexual act itself. Foreplay games are limited only by the imagination of the people involved as well as by whatever the partners find acceptable.

Some people use alcohol, cannabis, or other mind-altering substances to enhance the sensual feelings of foreplay. Whatever acts, games, or substances are used in foreplay, it is ethically important that both partners feel comfortable and safe in using them. If one partner objects to any form of foreplay, the other partner should respect that objection.

A. J. Smuskiewicz

See also: Afterplay; Arousal; Erogenous Zones; Kissing; Oxytocin; Touching, Sexual Arousal and.

Further Reading

Ross, L. (2010). *The secrets to sensational foreplay: The hottest ways to touch your lover for incredible pleasure, stronger orgasms, and longer, better sex.* Minneapolis: Quiver/Quarto Publishing.

Spurr, P. (2008). *Fabulous foreplay: The sex doctor's guide to teasing and pleasing your lover.* New York: St. Martin's Griffin.

Foreskin

In the human male, the foreskin is a double-layered fold of skin, smooth muscle, and nerves that covers the glans and the urinary meatus at the tip of the penis. The role of the foreskin remains somewhat unclear. Some believe it protects the glans and increases the pleasure of sexual intercourse by increasing sensitivity. The foreskin also provides natural lubricant for the glans, making intercourse more enjoyable for both partners. For others, the role of the foreskin is minor. Its removal through circumcision is a method of improving hygiene and preventing medical issues with the penis. Circumcision also plays an important religious role in certain faiths, such as Judaism.

The foreskin is also sometimes referred to as the "prepuce," which is a broader technical term that includes the clitoral hood in women. The outer skin of the foreskin is an extension of the penis's skin and covers almost, if not all, of the penis when in a flaccid state. However, when the penis is erect, the foreskin is drawn back. The tip of the foreskin includes a band of skin with many nerve endings that respond to fine touch. The inner skin is also exposed, and it includes many nerve endings. During intercourse or masturbation, the sensitivity of these areas increases the pleasurable experience of the male. The foreskin also keeps the glans moist, acting as a natural lubricant. Some research indicates that the loss of the foreskin decreases the sensitivity of the glans. It may also reduce the likelihood of ejaculation.

The foreskin normally cannot be retracted until males reach a certain age. Forcing it can cause pain and injury. Other medical conditions related to the foreskin include phimosis, in which the foreskin cannot be pulled back from the glans. The resulting inability to make sure the area under the foreskin is kept clean may lead to a painful infection called balanitis. A more serious problem is paraphimosis. In this case, the foreskin is pulled back but swells and cannot return to its position covering the glans. This situation is a medical emergency and requires quick action to prevent the loss of blood flow to the glans. Paraphimosis may require immediate circumcision in some cases.

Tim J. Watts

See also: Circumcision; Penis; Phimosis; Religion, Diversity of Human Sexuality and.

Further Reading

Better Health Channel. (2014). Foreskin care. Retrieved from https://www.betterhealth.vic.gov.au/health/conditionsandtreatments/foreskin-care

NHS. (2018). Tight foreskin (phimosis and paraphimosis). Retrieved from https://www.nhs.uk/conditions/phimosis/

Foucault, Michel

Significantly challenging contemporary assumptions surrounding the concept of sexuality, Michel Foucault (1926–1984) was a renowned French philosopher of the late twentieth century. Most famous in the realm of sexology for his innovative assertion that the overall concept of "sexuality" is not only subject to the influence of cultural relevance but is actually a social construct in and of itself has revolutionized many areas in the field of study. His deconstructive analyses comparing modern and historical contexts of sexual behavior support the notion of present-day sexuality as a venture only as recent as the eighteenth century. More specifically, he argued that the tendency to classify people according to categories based on particular sexual behaviors, such as the operations of sexual orientation, is uniquely modern in that sexual behaviors had been previously understood as descriptive components of a person and are now essentially fashioned into prescriptive models to claim as one's sexual identity (Clark, 2008).

While recognizing the obvious advantages to organizing in the name of civil liberties, Foucault did not agree with invalidating the whole of our personhood by sexualizing ourselves and commodifying our interests. Foucault hoped society, as a whole, could ultimately surpass the need to advance sexual minority politics by developing a more universalized understanding of queerness that might assume a multifaceted spectrum of diversity as the new norm. He saw transgression of established mores as sanctioning them the default, thus fundamentally depending on them. For this, and various other social commentaries, Foucault has had a tremendous influence on queer and feminist theory, especially in regard to sexual identity politics. While often critiqued for an overall lack of consideration for the female experience in his social analyses, his suggested alternatives were ultimately inclusive substitutions for the current alienating systems.

Educated in Paris at the elite École Normale Supérieure, Foucault had the luxury of studying with distinguished existential-phenomenologist Maurice Merleau-Ponty. This is where he also met philosopher historian George Canguilhem, who would later assist with his doctoral thesis *Folie et déraison: Histoire de la folie à l'âge classique* (Madness and Insanity: History of Madness in the Classical Age).

With degrees in philosophy, psychology, and eventually a diploma from the Institut de Psychologie at Paris for psychopathology, Foucault went on to teach in Paris, Sweden, Tunisia, and Germany in the 1950s and 1960s. His first major publication *Folie et déraison: Histoire de la folie à l'âge classique* (Madness and Civilization: A History of Insanity in the Age of Reason, 1961), was quickly followed by *Naissance de la clinique: Une archéologie du regard médical* (The Birth of the Clinic: An Archaeology of Medical Perception, 1963), and *Les mots et les choses: Une archéologie des sciences humaines* (The Order of Things: An Archeology of the Human Sciences, 1966). In 1968, he was sought out to establish a philosophy department at Le Centre Expérimental de Vincennes outside of Paris. He left there soon after, in 1969, when he was elected to join Collège de France as the newly named chair, "history of systems of thought."

As a very involved political advocate in the 1960s and 1970s, Foucault worked closely with antiracist campaigns and efforts toward institutional penal reform, among others, while he lectured at various universities and worked on his publications. The first of his *Histoire de la sexualité* (History of Sexuality) series, *La volonté de savoir* (The Will to Knowledge), was released in 1976. His original plans to compose a six-volume series would never come to fruition, as he would only publish another two before his death: *L'usage des plaisirs* (The Use of Pleasure) and the unfinished *Le souci de soi* (The Care of the Self).

In the time Foucault directed toward sexuality and sexual identity, he took particular interest scrutinizing the influence of Western medicine and the Roman Catholic Church. His perspective of institutionalized sexuality as a means to control a given culture was refreshingly contrary to that of his colleagues. Adamantly refusing the notion that the twentieth century had "liberated" the modern world from the confines of the Victorian era, he proposed that stringent religious prohibitions of sex did not necessarily indicate a lack of its presence. Coining the term "repressive hypothesis," Foucault did not believe such a theory realistically accounted for the lived experience of sex as part of human socialization. He was less concerned with any allowances afforded and more focused on what new form sexual regulation had espoused. When dictated solely by Christian traditions and sexuality beliefs, acceptable sexual behavior was simply a matter of refraining from condemned acts. With the introduction of the pathological model, medical recognition of same-sex attraction shifted public opinion from what is "evil" to who may be "sick," removing the action of choice. When further exploration of homosexuality as an ailment exposed it simply as a natural inclination, Foucault remarked that such validation of "homosexuality" essentially alienated the homosexual as another species. Historically used for matters of convenience, he now saw classification reducing many to their sexual orientation, subsequently discounting all other attributes as secondary to this main aspect of identity. Foucault found this incredibly limiting in the shaping of one's self and the surrounding discourse. For this, he praised the ancient Greeks in their concern for themselves as works of art. To "know thyself" outside of any preconceived archetypes would be the inspiration for his last published work before dying of AIDS-related complications in 1984.

Ilyssa Boseski

See also: Homosexuality; Queer; Religion, Diversity of Human Sexuality and; Sexual Identity; Sexual Orientation; Sexual Revolution; Sexualization; Stereotypes, Sexual; Victorian Era.

Further Reading

Bullough, V. L., & Brundage, J. A. (1996). *Handbook of medieval sexuality.* New York: Routledge Taylor & Francis Group.

Clark, A. (2008). *Desire: A history of European sexuality.* New York: Routledge Taylor & Francis Group.

Foucault, M. (1978). *The history of sexuality* (Vols. 1–3, R. Hurley, Trans.). New York: Random House. (Original work published 1976)

Karras, R. M. (2005). *Sexuality in medieval Europe: Doing unto others* (2nd ed.). New York: Routledge Taylor & Francis Group.

Siedman, S., Fischer, N., & Meeks, C. (2011). *Introducing the new sexuality studies* (2nd ed.). New York: Routledge Taylor & Francis Group.

Freud, Sigmund

Sigmund Freud was a doctor in Austria who specialized in treating mental illnesses during the late 1800s and early 1900s. He developed a treatment method called psychoanalysis that is still used today. This "talking treatment" involves getting patients to talk openly about their feelings and personal history. Freud believed that many anxieties and emotional problems stem from traumatic events, unresolved conflicts, or unfulfilled wishes from a person's past, particularly childhood. He wrote and lectured about his theories concerning the conscious and unconscious mind, the importance of dreams, and sex-based desires. His ideas about sexuality were considered shockingly indecent at the time and remain controversial.

Sigismund Schlomo Freud was born on May 6, 1856, in Freiberg, Moravia, later part of the Czech Republic. Because of their Jewish heritage, his family endured anti-Semitic sentiments. They moved to Vienna, Austria, in 1860. Freud was extremely smart and learned multiple languages before he was a teenager. He wanted to become a research scientist but was not allowed by authorities to do so because of his Jewish background. Instead he went to medical school at the University of Vienna and studied neurology. He graduated in 1881.

Following graduation, Freud worked at a psychiatric clinic and became a proponent of a new drug called cocaine. He used it recreationally and enthusiastically recommended it to others. In that era, doctors did not know that cocaine was addictive. Freud did not become addicted to the drug, but this did happen to some of his colleagues. He did become a habitual cigar smoker, eventually smoking up to twenty-four cigars daily.

Freud focused on a condition called hysteria. It was characterized by anxiety or personality disorders along with physical symptoms with no apparent biological cause. Freud's friend, Dr. Josef Breuer, treated a young woman who had fits of confusion and delirium and episodes of muscle paralysis and other physical problems. Breuer encouraged her to talk openly about her past. He found that she temporarily felt better when she recalled her experiences around the time her symptoms first began. Freud became convinced that hysteria develops in people who have suffered some traumatic event in the past and then deeply buried their memories of it. The idea of repressed memories would become a cornerstone of psychoanalysis.

In 1895, Breuer and Freud published their findings in *Studies in Hysteria.* By this time, Freud had a thriving private practice. He had his patients recline on a couch in a soothing environment while they talked about their personal histories. Freud counseled them to remember and acknowledge forgotten traumas or unresolved problems from thc past. Then these issues were examined and discussed openly in an attempt to relieve the anxiety they had caused.

Freud considered dreams as peeks into the unconscious mind. His book *The Interpretation of Dreams* (1900) explained his early theories on this subject. It was followed by *The Psychopathology of Everyday Life* (1901), in which Freud said that slips of the tongue can have hidden meanings. For example, accidentally saying goodbye rather than hello when meeting a person could indicate buried unfriendly feelings about that person. Such slips of the tongue became known as "Freudian slips."

During Freud's lifetime, sexuality was not discussed openly. He broke this taboo with publication in 1905 of *Three Essays on the Theory of Sexuality.* Freud argued that the sex drive plays a huge role in human behaviors, not only for adults but also for children. His theories on childhood psychosexual development were considered scandalous and are still controversial today. For example, he theorized that young boys go through a stage in which they develop a sexual attraction to their mothers and hate-tinged jealousy of their fathers. This became known as the Oedipus complex, named after a character in an ancient Greek play.

In 1923, Freud published *The Ego and the Id*, which describes the three parts of the psyche (the mental processes, emotions, and drivers of behaviors). The id encompasses deeply selfish desires and is present at birth. As a child develops so does another part of the psyche called the ego. It functions both in the unconscious and conscious mind and creates realistic strategies to satisfy id-based desires. Last to develop is the superego. It consciously considers the social limits on behavior and the ramifications for violating them. Freud's theory is considered a revolutionary way of looking at the competing needs that drive human emotions and behavior.

Also in 1923, Freud was diagnosed with oral cancer, a consequence of his long addiction to cigar smoking. He underwent dozens of surgeries and painful procedures even as he continued to see patients. In 1938, Nazi Germany invaded Austria. Freud's Jewish background put him in danger; however, he was allowed to flee the country. His cancer worsened and caused him great pain. Finally, he asked his physician to administer him a lethal dose of morphine. He died on September 23, 1939, in London. He was eighty-three years old.

Although many of Freud's theories—particularly those relating to dreams and sexuality—have been heavily criticized and are no longer considered part of mainstream psychology, he has nevertheless made a lasting contribution to the fields of both psychology and sexology.

Kim Masters Evans

See also: Ellis, Henry Havelock; Oedipus Complex; Psychosexual Therapy.

Further Reading

Jacobs, M. (2003). *Sigmund Freud.* London: SAGE.

Loftus, E. F. (1993). The reality of repressed memories. *American Psychologist, 48,* 518–537.

PBS. (1998). Sigmund Freud. Retrieved from http://www.pbs.org/wgbh/aso/databank/entries/bhfreu.html

Friends with Benefits

Friends with benefits (FWB) relationships are a type of ongoing casual sex relationship in which two (or more) people agree to have sex with each other without the expectation of a committed romantic relationship. FWB relationships combine characteristics of friendship relationships with aspects of sexual relationships, and they are very common; around half of first-year university students report having had at least one FWB relationship.

While casual sex is not a new phenomenon, the way people describe and experience casual sex varies by time and by culture. In Western culture, social norms have shifted so that there is greater acceptance of premarital sex than in past decades. In addition, many people are waiting until they are older to get married, as compared to previous generations. There are many factors that contribute to this, including more acceptance of casual sex, as mentioned, but also because of advances in contraception and because more people are attending university or other postsecondary education. As a result of prolonged education, many young adults incur debt or live with minimal income; consequently, many choose to live at home longer and may delay marriage until they are more stable, both financially and in their careers. Prior to having a long-term committed relationship or marriage, some people may choose to engage in casual sexual relationships, including having one or more FWB relationship(s).

FWB relationships have been defined as "sex between two people who have an existing friendship, these two may or may not engage in sexual activity when they hang out with each other, they are usually not under the influence of alcohol or drugs, these two engage in sex with each other regularly" (Wentland & Reissing, 2014). Research suggests that FWB relationships differ from other types of casual sex relationships because FWB relationships include formal discussions about engaging in sexual activity, whether or not the relationship is exclusive or monogamous, and when to end sexual activity. People who engage in an FWB are also more likely to continue to have contact with each other after the sexual component of the relationship has ended. The increased level of communication between people in an FWB relationship is unique to this type of casual sex relationship. Further, research indicates that people in an FWB relationship have higher levels of respect and care for their FWB, and it is important to them that all partners agree to their negotiated rules about the relationship.

People begin FWB relationships for a variety of reasons. Among a sample of people in an FWB relationship, sex was the most commonly reported motivation for beginning the relationship, and wanting an emotional connection was second. Other motivations for FWB relationships included relationship avoidance and relationship simplicity as well as simply wanting an FWB relationship. Finally, some participants in this study also noted that sometimes there was no specific motivation to begin the relationship and that it spontaneously developed. FWB relationships are typically ongoing and usually end when one of the partners enters into a new dating relationship with another person.

Heather L. Armstrong

See also: Casual Sex; Dating; Hookup Culture; Online Dating.

Further Reading

Bisson, M. A., & Levine, T. R. (2009). Negotiating a friends with benefits relationship. *Archives of Sexual Behavior, 38*(1), 66–73.

Mongeau, P. A., Knight, K., Williams, J., Eden, J., & Shaw, C. (2013). Identifying and explicating variation among friends with benefits relationships. *Journal of Sex Research, 50*(1), 37–47.

Stein, J. B., Mongeau, P., Posteher, K., & Veluscek, A. (2019). Netflix and chill?: Exploring and refining differing motivations in friends with benefits relationships. *Canadian Journal of Human Sexuality, 28*(3), 317–327.

Wentland, J. J., & Reissing, E. D. (2011). Taking casual sex not too casually: Exploring definitions of casual sexual relationships. *Canadian Journal of Human Sexuality, 20*(3), 75–91.

Wentland, J. J., & Reissing, E. D. (2014). Casual sexual relationships: Identifying definitions for one night stands, booty calls, fuck buddies, and friends with benefits. *Canadian Journal of Human Sexuality, 23*(3), 167–177.

Frotteurism

Frotteurism involves a person gaining arousal from rubbing a body part against someone else without consent. A person who engages in frotteurism is a "frotteur." Academics reference the behavior as "frottage," a French word meaning "rubbing." The first scholar on record to explore the behavior is Richard Freiherr von Krafft-Ebing, who wrote about it in *Psychopathia Sexualis* (1886). Frotteurism first appeared as a paraphilia in the American Psychiatric Association's *Diagnostic and Statistical Manual of Mental Disorders* (*DSM*) in 1980. In the current version of the *DSM*, frotteurism involves repetitive, intense sexual arousal from nonconsenting touching or rubbing that impairs social functioning and lasts at least six months.

Frotteurs are typically middle-class young males with high IQs. They target women in crowded public places, where the likelihood of bodily contact is great. Research implies this includes locations such as elevators, buses, subways, concerts, and churches. The goal involves deliberately bringing a clothed part of the body into contact with the target. Some frotteurs desire contact involving any part of the body, but the height of frotteurism involves areas directly related to sexual arousal. This includes the genitals but also the buttocks and breasts. Traditionally interpreted as a voluntary action, researchers are now considering the likelihood of impulsive frotteurism, which involves a hypersexual person with severe psychiatric illness. Research shows as many as 10 percent of males have engaged in frotteurism. Samples of males who claim to have coerced a female into sex have frotteurism participation rates up to 77 percent.

Victims are typically attractive to the frotteur, wear tight clothing, and fail to recognize victimization. Female college students self-report high rates of victimization. People are often unsure if they are victims with cultural norms typically allowing a limited amount of touching in crowded environments. Some frotteurs target multiple victims in one situation. Others target one person, who is typically the object of their sexual fantasies. After contact, some frotteurs retreat to a private location to masturbate. The occurrence of an orgasm may take place when contact occurs if the frotteur is extremely aroused.

Consensual-based behaviors associated with frotteurism may unintentionally support actions associated with it. This includes lap dances given by exotic dancers, dancing while using themes of sex simulation, and abstinence-related "dry humping."

There is limited literature on frotteurism. What does exist typically uses small samples derived from convenience. Moreover, previous research inconsistently applies diagnostic criteria cited in the literature. More studies to legitimize existing research, and generate new information, are necessary.

Jason S. Ulsperger

See also: Arousal; *Diagnostic and Statistical Manual of Mental Disorders* (*DSM*); Krafft-Ebing, Richard von; Paraphilias.

Further Reading

Clark, S. K., Jeglic, E. L., Calkins, C., & Tater, J. R. (2016). More than a nuisance: The prevalence and consequences of frotteurism and exhibitionism. *Sex Abuse: A Journal of Research and Treatment, 28*(1), 3–19.

Johnson, R. S., Ostermeyer, B., Sikes, K. A., Nelsen, A. J., & Coverdale, J. H. (2014). Presence and treatment of frotteurism in the community: A systematic review. *Journal of the American Academy of Psychiatric Law, 42*(4), 478–483.

Langstrom, N. (2010). The DSM diagnostic criteria for exhibitionism, voyeurism, and frotteurism. *Archives of Sexual Behavior, 39*(2), 317–324.

FTMInternational

Female to Male International (FTMI), also known as FTMInternational, was founded in 1986 by Lou Sullivan in San Francisco, California. With the mission "FTMInternational builds and strengthens FTM lives," FTMI is the first known organization specifically to support and connect transgender men worldwide.

FTMInternational has provided hundreds of educational presentations, panels, and workshops and has been featured in numerous documentaries on television, film, and radio as well as in major magazines and newspapers. FTMI also provides extensive public education on the transgender community.

Sullivan began holding support group meetings in December 1986 and started publishing the FTMI quarterly newsletter in 1987. He got the idea for FTMI from a Los Angeles group known as Under Construction, founded in 1983 by Jeff Shevlowitz.

In 1992, FTMI published the first edition of *The FTMI Yellow Pages*, a resource guide for transgender men. As the community grew, it became too time-consuming to continue updating the resource guide. The eighth and final printed edition in 2005 was 108 pages in length.

FTMI has a long list of accomplishments and community "firsts," such as organizing one of the first conventions specifically for transgender men. A Vision of Community: The First All-FTM Conference of the Americas was held August 1–20, 1995, in San Francisco and continued annually for three years. FTMI also provided support for other FTM gatherings in North America in the early 2000s, including True Spirit, FORGE Forward, and the Malibu Men's Retreat, among others. A popular fund-raising project titled Calendar: The Men of FTMI was published in 2005 and featured photos of transgender men in classic "beefcake" poses.

Another important service provided by FTMI was developing and maintaining a network of support groups for transgender men to connect with each other and share experiences and resources. During the most active period in the 2000s, FTMI had about 5,000 members around the world, with chapters or affiliated groups in more than a dozen U.S. cities as well as other countries.

In addition to his community-building work, founder Lou Sullivan was also a writer and researcher who published several books and papers about the transgender experience. He was one of the first FTMs to openly identify as a gay man. Like a number of other young gay men of his generation, Sullivan became HIV-positive and died in 1991 of complications from AIDS. FTMI developed the Lou Sullivan Award in his name; it has been awarded to approximately fifteen trans men since its inception, beginning with Jamison Green, who became president of FTMI after Lou's death.

FTMI received designation as a 501(c)(3) nonprofit organization in 1996. Chapters continue operations around the globe. The quarterly newsletter is available via email subscription, and a listing of professionals and clinics for gender dysphoria is available online at www.ftmi.org or by phone at (877) 267-1440.

C. Michael Woodward

See also: Gender Expression; Gender Identity; Gender Transition; Green, Jamison; Transgender; Transsexual.

Further Reading

FTMInternational. (2019). Home page. Retrieved from www.ftmi.org

Smith, B. D. (2017). *Lou Sullivan: Daring to be a man among men.* Oakland, CA: Transgress Press.

G

Galactorrhea

Galactorrhea is a spontaneous discharge of milky fluid from the nipples. It is not related to breastfeeding and can occur in adults of any gender, as well as in infants, although it is most commonly seen in women. Galactorrhea itself is not a disease but rather is a symptom of an underlying condition. Research suggests that somewhere between 5 percent and 32 percent of all women are affected by this issue.

There are many possible causes of galactorrhea, including chronic kidney disease, hypothyroidism (an underactive thyroid), an injured spinal cord, use of sedatives or other medications, chronic emotional stress, and use of birth control pills. The most common cause has been identified as overproduction of prolactin, which is the hormone that stimulates milk production after giving birth. As the pituitary gland is in charge of producing prolactin, prolactin-secreting tumors in the pituitary gland are largely to blame for this problem. In males, galactorrhea is also typically associated with decreased testosterone levels. When the condition occurs in infants, it is usually a result of high estrogen levels in the mother, which cross the placenta and create enlarged breast tissue and a possible milky discharge in the baby. At times, however, galactorrhea presents without any known cause. When this happens, it is usually attributed to prolactin sensitivity, meaning that even normal levels of prolactin in the body can trigger nipple discharge.

In addition to a milky secretion, galactorrhea may also have other symptoms, including an abnormal menstrual cycle, increase or decrease in appetite or body weight, loss of sex drive, headaches, vision problems, and abnormal hair growth. In order to test for the condition, a medical professional will conduct a physical exam and run laboratory tests on a fluid sample from the discharge. Blood tests to check for hormone levels, a pregnancy test, and imaging tests to check for tumors and suspicious breast tissue are also usually required. After a diagnosis is made, a course of treatment will be decided. In very mild cases, it is not unusual to recommend no medical treatment and allow the condition to clear on its own. When treatment is required, it is usually focused on the underlying cause of the problem. For example, if a pituitary tumor is found to be the cause, medication may be prescribed to shrink the tumor, or surgery may be performed to remove it. In addition, in the case of hypothyroidism, medication to counteract the low thyroid activity will most likely be prescribed.

Reports suggest that the earliest known cases of galactorrhea occurred in the mid-1800s, but correlation between the condition and problems with the pituitary gland was not made until the 1950s. The development of computed tomography and magnetic resonance imaging in the 1970s helped to confirm this connection by allowing doctors to readily identify pituitary tumors. Since this time, much research related to galactorrhea has been devoted to determining how prolactin secretion is regulated and developing medications that can help control this function as well as the growth of pituitary tumors.

Tamar Burris

See also: Breast, Female; Breastfeeding.

Further Reading

Javadpour, N. (1987). *Tumor markers: Biology and clinical applications.* Westport, CT: Praeger.

Mayo Clinic. (2019). Galactorrhea. Retrieved from https://www.mayoclinic.org/diseases-conditions/galactorrhea/symptoms-causes/syc-20350431

Gay Affirmative Therapy

Gay affirmative therapy is a form of psychotherapy for people who experience same-sex attraction that encourages them to accept their sexual orientation. This is in contrast to other unethical forms of therapy that try to diminish same-sex sexual behaviors or to "convert" these behaviors to heterosexual (so-called gay conversion therapy). Many therapists who practice gay affirmative therapy expand the coverage of such therapy to bisexual, transgender, and "queer" (challenging traditional norms of sexuality and gender) or "questioning" (exploring different sexualities and genders) patients, in which case it is referred to as LGBTQ+ (lesbian, gay, bisexual, transgender, queer/questioning, and more) therapy. To simplify the present discussion, this article refers to "gay affirmative therapy," though the principles discussed could also apply to other LGBTQ+ individuals.

The main guiding principle of gay affirmative therapy is that the patient needs to feel comfortable, happy, and proud about their sexuality—not ashamed or worried about it. Patients are helped to embrace their sexuality in a positive (affirmative) way, despite whatever negative reactions they may encounter from other people.

Several guidelines for gay affirmative therapy are provided by the American Psychological Association (APA), the American Association for Marriage and Family Therapy (AAMFT), and other professional associations of therapists. Many guidelines seek to overcome previous ideas about homosexuality being a mental illness. Many guidelines also seek to educate professional therapists about how to help patients successfully deal with antigay stigmas that remain in some segments of society as well as antigay teachings that remain in some religions. Therapists are encouraged to educate themselves as much as possible about LGBTQ+ issues and to become involved with the LGBTQ+ community—even to become advocates on behalf of the community.

The APA and AAMFT guidelines note that many people with same-sex attraction encounter opposition not only from society in general but also specifically from family members and friends who do not understand their sexuality. For many people, that kind of personal opposition is the most difficult, complex aspect of their sexual orientation. In some cases, it may be possible for the family or friends to eventually learn about and accept the individual's sexual orientation.

Therapy may be able to help the patient talk openly to family and friends about the issue, and family members might even participate in the therapy sessions. In other cases, however, overcoming rejection from family or friends is not possible, and the patient might be encouraged to find emotional support elsewhere, such as with LGBTQ+ support groups, both in the local community (if available) and online.

Some mental health professionals who provide gay affirmative therapy are clinical psychologists with PhD degrees. Others are licensed clinical professional counselors. Still others may have other academic credentials. Some may specialize in LGBTQ+ issues, while others may have more generalist backgrounds. When looking for an affirmative therapist, the patient should be sure to feel comfortable with, and confident in, the therapist of their choice.

Not all therapists who perform gay affirmative therapy agree with or follow all the AAMFT or APA guidelines. Nevertheless, their therapy may still be effective for their clients. Scientific research suggests that, as a whole, gay affirmative therapy can be effective at helping patients live happy, fulfilled lives.

A. J. Smuskiewicz

See also: Heterosexism; Homophobia, Internalized; Homosexuality; Psychosexual Therapy; Same-Sex Attraction and Behavior; Sexual Orientation.

Further Reading

Johnson, S. D. (2012). Gay affirmative psychotherapy with lesbian, gay, and bisexual individuals: Implications for contemporary psychotherapy research. *American Journal of Orthopsychiatry, 82*(4), 516–522.

Kort, J. (2008). *Gay affirmative therapy for the straight clinician: The essential guide.* New York: W. W. Norton & Company.

Gay Rights Movement

The gay rights movement refers to the social, legal, and political activities conducted to advance the civil rights of gay and lesbian people. The U.S. movement dates to the 1950s, when homosexuality was illegal and considered to be a psychological disorder and dangerously immoral. Gay people regularly faced harassment from police and discrimination in employment and other areas of their lives. Over the decades, gay rights advocates have worked to change laws and social attitudes toward gay and lesbian individuals. Significant reforms have occurred. Homosexuality is no longer illegal or branded a psychological disorder. Many laws and policies have been amended to prohibit discrimination based on sexual orientation. For example, gay and lesbian individuals can now openly serve in the U.S. military and legally marry in all states.

The roots of the U.S. gay rights movement lie in the early 1950s. Many gay people of that era referred to themselves as homophiles. The prefix "homo-" means "same," and the suffix "–philes" means "lovers of." All states had longstanding sodomy laws that prohibited oral and anal sex, even between consenting adults in private. Thus, sexual activities between homophiles were illegal by definition. The American Psychiatric Association (APA) publishes the *Diagnostic and Statistical Manual of Mental Disorders* (*DSM*), a listing of mental disorders. The

1952 *DSM* classified homosexuality as a "sociopathic personality disturbance." A sociopath is someone who disregards social moral conventions for selfish reasons and can be so antisocial as to be violent.

The criminality, immorality, and psychological sickness associated with homosexuality were used to justify all kinds of discriminatory practices. People known or suspected of being gay were refused housing and employment and fired from their jobs. This was particularly true in occupations that involved children, such as teaching, and in government and military positions. As a result, many gay professionals tried to "stay in the closet"—that is, to keep their sexual orientation a secret.

A subculture is a group of people with shared beliefs or interests that are different from the larger society to which they belong. By the early 1950s, gay subcultures had emerged, particularly in large cities. Homophiles began forming local organizations to provide a forum to discuss and tackle various civil rights concerns. For example, the Mattachine Foundation (later the Mattachine Society) was founded by Henry Hay in Los Angeles. Numerous chapters eventually sprang up around the country.

Within gay subcultures, there were neighborhood restaurants, bars, and clubs that became favorite hangouts. These establishments were often targeted by local officials, who viewed them as hotbeds of immoral behavior. Police raids on so-called gay bars were common during the 1950s and 1960s. Numerous people were arrested on charges such as public indecency and disorderly conduct; however, few convictions resulted. The purpose seemed to be harassment. Newspapers of that era typically listed the names, addresses, and occupations of arrested individuals.

By the mid-1960s, local homophile groups had banded together under umbrella organizations such as the East Coast Homophile Organizations and the North American Conference of Homophile Organizations. Activists staged protests and picketed in major cities to draw attention to discrimination against gay people. On June 28, 1969, a popular gay bar called the Stonewall Inn was raided by police in New York City. The crowd grew angry and began throwing bricks and bottles at police. The incident sparked several days of protest that attracted thousands of people.

The Stonewall riot garnered little public attention at the time. It was a tumultuous era with protests raging across the country over the Vietnam War and various social causes. However, on the one-year anniversary of the Stonewall riot, thousands of gay activists met and marched through New York City. It was likely the first gay pride parade. In 1973, the APA decided to remove homosexuality from the *DSM*. The decision followed intense lobbying by gay rights groups and protests at APA conventions and meetings. By this time, activists were much more vocal and public than in the past. Many referred to their cause as the gay liberation movement.

Gay individuals began making inroads in political circles. A handful of openly gay men and women were elected to local public office. Perhaps the best known of them was Harvey Milk, who won a seat on the San Francisco Board of Supervisors in 1977. He was murdered a year later by a former colleague on the board. In

1979, gay activists staged a national march in Washington, D.C., and rallied for federal laws to protect the civil rights of gay people. Such protections were slowly being implemented on the local and state level. For example, some cities modified their housing codes and other ordinances to prohibit discrimination based on sexual orientation. In 1982, Wisconsin became the first state to do likewise.

The gay rights movement faced considerable challenges during the 1980s. Conservative politicians, such as President Ronald Reagan, were elected to office with strong backing from the religious right (chiefly Christian groups favoring traditional moral values). There was strong resistance and outright resentment against gay rights activists and causes. Meanwhile, a new and deadly virus emerged that spread rapidly among men who had sex with men. First called gay-related immune deficiency disorder, its name was soon changed to acquired immune deficiency syndrome (AIDS). It was found to be caused by the human immunodeficiency virus, which is transmitted via bodily fluids, such as semen and blood. Initially, gay men were the chief victims of AIDS, and thousands of them became sick and died from it. However, it was soon detected in nongay people and became a public health priority.

Politicians and religious leaders who thought homosexuality immoral expressed little to no sympathy for the gay victims of AIDS. A 1987 march on Washington, D.C., included hundreds of thousands of gay activists demanding action from the federal government. Although the disease could not be transmitted through casual contact, public paranoia resulted in harassment and discrimination against gay and nongay sufferers. By the mid-1990s, the number of new AIDS cases was down, as was the death rate. The improvement came due to safer sex practices—for example, greater use of condoms—and powerful new AIDS treatments.

Throughout U.S. history, many tens of thousands of men (and some women) have been ousted from the military for being (or suspected of being) gay. It is an issue that has long occupied the gay rights movement. In 1993, the Pentagon implemented a new "Don't Ask, Don't Tell" policy. This provided some level of employment security for gay service members. However, it still meant that homosexuality had to be kept secret. The policy was finally repealed in 2010. Since that time, openly gay people have been allowed to serve in the U.S. military.

In the early years of the twenty-first century, the gay rights movement achieved two major milestones. In 2003, the U.S. Supreme Court ruled in *Lawrence v. Texas* that the handful of state laws that still prohibited sodomy were unconstitutional. A year later, Massachusetts became the first state to allow same-sex couples to legally marry. More states followed suit, but others resisted, even passing laws specifically banning gay marriage. In 2015, the U.S. Supreme Court ruled in *Obergefell v. Hodges* that laws banning same-sex marriage were unconstitutional.

Kim Masters Evans

See also: Don't Ask, Don't Tell; Homosexuality; LGBTQ+; Mattachine Society; Same-Sex Marriage; Sexual Orientation; Sexual Rights; Sodomy Laws; Stonewall Riots.

Further Reading

Clendinen, D., & Nagourney, A. (2013). *Out for good: The struggle to build a gay rights movement in America.* New York: Touchstone/Simon and Schuster.

Heredia, C. (2002, October). Henry "Harry" Hay—gay rights pioneer. *San Francisco Chronicle.*

PBS. (2019). Stonewall Inn: Through the years. Retrieved from http://www.pbs.org/wgbh/americanexperience/features/stonewall-inn-through-years/

Philipps, D. (2015, September). Ousted as gay, aging veterans are battling again for honorable discharges. *New York Times.*

Gay-Straight Alliance (GSA)

A gay-straight alliance (GSA) is any of numerous student-led clubs in high schools, colleges, and universities designed to make the schools safe, supportive learning and social environments for lesbian, gay, bisexual, transgender, and queer/questioning (LGBTQ+) students. ("Queer" refers to individuals who challenge traditional norms of sexuality and gender. "Questioning" refers to individuals who are exploring different sexualities and genders.) GSA groups are more common and widespread in the United States than in any other country, though they exist in several other nations.

The thousands of GSA groups in the United States can maintain connections with each other and with similar groups through the Gay-Straight Alliance Network, a national youth leadership organization based in San Francisco, California, and the Gay, Lesbian, and Straight Education Network (GLSEN), an organization of students, parents, and teachers based in New York City. Some GSA groups use alternative names to better reflect their particular membership or ideas, such as Gender-Sexuality Alliance, Queer-Straight Alliance, Pride Alliance, and Project Rainbow.

Many LGBTQ+ students suffer harassment, bullying, and violence at school, making school not only a dangerous place for them but also a difficult place to learn their academic material and to form friendships. Because of these serious problems, the main focus of most GSAs is raising student awareness of LGBTQ+ issues and enhancing the safety and acceptance of LGBTQ+ students.

GSA groups organize awareness-raising events at their schools and in their communities. They also usually take part in national LGBTQ+ campaigns, such as National Coming Out Day, Transgender Day of Remembrance, and GSA Day. Typical activities at a GSA event, such as National Coming Out Day (October 11), include meetings in which participants share their personal stories, panel discussions, painting of murals, writing workshops, poetry presentations, concerts, wine and cheese receptions, and other opportunities for expanding social contacts. For some events, these activities are spread out over several days.

After their origin in Massachusetts in the late 1980s, GSAs began to spread throughout the United States in the 1990s. The spread of these organizations accelerated after the October 1999 federal court ruling in Utah—*East High Gay/Straight Alliance v. Board of Education of Salt Lake City School District.* That case began in 1996, when the Salt Lake City School District tried to prevent a GSA at East High School from meeting. The American Civil Liberties Union and other organizations filed a lawsuit on behalf of the East High GSA. U.S. district judge Bruce Jenkins ruled that the school district violated the Equal Access Act, which gives all students the right to use school facilities for extracurricular activities at any school that receives public funds. That ruling removed all legal obstacles to the establishment of GSAs.

GSAs are proud of their accomplishments in both raising public awareness of LGBTQ+ issues and in improving the safety of schools for LGBTQ+ students. A report issued in 2007 by the GLSEN, titled *Gay-Straight Alliances: Creating Safer Schools for LGBT Students and Their Allies*, described several findings regarding GSAs and their accomplishments up to that time. The following are some of these findings, as they are worded in the report:

- Students in schools with GSAs are less likely to hear homophobic remarks in school on a daily basis than students in schools without a GSA (57% compared to 75%).
- LGBT students who attend schools with a GSA are less likely than those at schools without a GSA to report feeling unsafe in school because of their sexual orientation (61% vs. 68%) or because of the way in which they express their gender (38% vs. 43%).
- Sexual minority youth (youth who identify as lesbian, gay, or bisexual as well as youth who have same-sex romantic attractions or engage in same-sex sexual behavior) in Massachusetts schools with GSAs were half as likely as those in schools without a GSA to report experiencing dating violence, being threatened or injured at school, or missing school because they were afraid to go.
- LGBT students in schools with GSAs are less likely to miss school because they feel unsafe compared to other students: a quarter (26%) of students in schools with GSAs missed school in the past month because they felt unsafe compared to a third (32%) of students at schools without GSAs.
- Students in schools with GSAs or similar student clubs are two times more likely than students without such clubs to say they hear teachers at their school make supportive or positive remarks about lesbian and gay people (24% compared to 12%).
- LGBT students in schools with a GSA are significantly more likely than students in schools without a GSA to be aware of a supportive adult at school (84% compared to 56%). LGBT students who report having supportive faculty and other school staff report higher grade point averages and are more likely to say they plan to pursue post-secondary education than LGBT students who do not have supportive school staff.
- LGBT students in schools with a GSA have a greater sense of belonging to their school community than students without a GSA.

Since the release of this detailed report by the GLSEN, academic, safety, and social conditions have continued to improve for LGBTQ+ students in the United States, according to most GSA leaders. Nevertheless, incidents of intolerance and violence against LGBTQ+ students still occur at many schools.

A. J. Smuskiewicz

See also: Adolescent Sexuality; Antigay Prejudice; GLSEN (Gay, Lesbian and Straight Education Network); LGBTQ+.

Further Reading

Gay, Lesbian & Straight Education Network. (2007). *Gay-straight alliances: Creating safer schools for LGBT students and their allies.* New York: Gay, Lesbian & Straight Education Network.

Gay, Lesbian & Straight Education Network. (2019). 10 steps to start your GSA. Retrieved from https://www.glsen.org/activity/10-steps-start-your-gsa

Gay-Straight Alliance Network. (2019). Home page. Retrieved from http://www.gsanetwork.org

Gender

Gender is the assigned, assumed, or chosen social category encompassing the social and cultural characteristics representative of one's gender identity. "Gender" is a socially constructed word, where the meaning of gender is ever changing with research and growth in social, emotional, and developmental views. The definition of gender is often confused with sex. Sex is biologically determined from birth and is a representation of the combination of one's genetics, chromosomes, and hormones. An individual's sex is typically labeled and addressed as male, female, or intersex. The sex of a body does not bear any necessary or deterministic relationship to the social category, or gender, of that body.

Most individuals identify with their gender assigned at birth, typically boy or man or girl or woman. Other individuals (intersex) may be born with varied genitals or chromosomal mutations that make gender difficult to assign at birth. There is currently a heated debate on the appropriate standards of care for intersex infants. However, not all individuals may identify with the preconceived notions of their gender identity. Some individuals may identify as a gender other than the one assigned at birth, which may include, but is not limited to, man, woman, transgender, gender nonconforming, genderqueer, and agender. Gender can be broken down further to evaluate physical differences between genders, presentation, expression, and socialization. These aspects of gender are highlighted dependent on the theoretical lens that people use to look at and discuss gender.

The assumption of gender is typically associated with particular characteristics of a body associated with maleness or femaleness. These characteristics are associated with specific body morphology, or the shape and structure of one's body, or secondary sex characteristics. One of the physical qualifiers of gender is based on a hip to waist ratio; women typically have a smaller hip to waist ratio, while men have a more equal ratio. Another differential morphological assumption between men and women is the breadth of shoulders relative to height. Men have broader shoulders in relationship to their height, while women have a smaller shoulder breadth. Lastly, men and women tend to have differences between the thickness of limbs, with men typically having denser limbs than women.

Gender can also be assumed by secondary sex characteristics, which are physical traits associated with genetic sex or reproductive potential. Some of these secondary sex characteristics may include skin texture, body fat distribution, and patterns of hair growth. Based on these secondary sexual characteristics, individuals are typically assumed into certain gender categories. Men typically have a rougher skin texture, even body fat distribution, and thicker hair on legs, arms, and face. Women typically have a softer skin texture, body fat distribution toward the waist and hips, and thinner hair on legs, arms, and face.

Gender comportment is defined as the performance or presentation of one's gender, often based on gender assigned at birth. The performance of gender is a subtlety taught to children and youth both through direct observation as well as the redirection of gender-incongruent behaviors. Direct observation could be seeing a gender-typical behavior, such as a little girl watching her mom put on makeup, and interpreting this as a gender-typical behavior. That same little girl could be redirected toward more gender-congruent behaviors when she is yelled at for playing in the dirt with other children. Children can get these messages from family, friends, teachers, the media, or from people in any social situation. Gender and youth can be taught gender-typical bodily actions such as the ways that one is supposed to speak, tone of voice, ways of holding their body, and desirable ways of dressing.

Gender expression is the way that people communicate gender to others via clothing, mannerisms, hairstyle, and ways of speaking. Gender expression is not necessarily synonymous with one's gender assigned at birth or gender identity but is the way one presents their gender to others. People can express their gender as feminine, masculine, androgynous, or queer, among others. Gender expression is fluid and can change and develop across one's life span. Other people typically misinterpret one's gender expression as equivalent to their gender identity, which can cause problems for those whose gender is fluid or undefined.

Gender roles are the prescribed thoughts, actions, and feelings that one is supposed to experience, typically thought to be congruent with their gender assigned at birth. Children learn gender roles from family, friends, school, and teachers through modeling, observing, or redirection from someone else verbally or nonverbally to more gender-stereotypical behavior. Gender roles can be present from youth through adulthood, which can often become convoluted when that person is not interested in fitting that prescribed gender role. Some gender roles can be assumed, especially in the functioning and allocating of responsibility in relationships.

Gender theories critically analyze the development and makeup of gender through a multitude of lenses. Gender theories consider the biological, social, and cultural aspects of gender.

Biological theory focuses on the influences of genes and hormones on the development and expression of gender. Biological theory proposes no distinction between sex and gender but instead focuses on the creation of gendered behavior through biological sex. This theory is supported by research on brain hemisphere usage for language tasks. This research has indicated a difference between men's and women's use of their brain for language tasks. Men tend to use the left side of their brain independently in carrying out language tasks, while women tend to use both hemispheres of their brain. This difference between brain usage between genders was found to be facilitated by the higher levels of testosterone found in men.

Biosocial theory is an intersectional viewpoint of gender whereby nature and nurture have roles in gender development. In biosocial theory, people are born as a male or a female; however, social labeling, interaction, and treatment of boys and girls interact with their biological factors. Prenatally, infants are exposed to levels of hormones determined by chromosomes that develop the infant into their biological sex. Postnatal parents react and label their children based on their genitals and socialize the child to the gender they are assigned at birth.

Another more recently developed theory of gender is the enculturated lens theory, combining all former theories of gender and examining gender through the lenses of gender polarization androcentrism and biological essentialism. There are two key enculturation processes that are constantly linked and work together. The first process of enculturation focuses on the historical and institutional preprogramming of gender based on biology, era, and culture. The second process of enculturated lens theory focuses on the transmission of implicit lessons, or metamessages, about the present culture's lenses organizing social reality. Metamessages can be gathered culturally or socially based on one's interactions with the world.

Kimberly A. Fuller

See also: Agender; Androgyny; Bigender; Binary Gender System; Biological Sex; Childhood Gender Nonconformity; Cisgender; Evolutionary Perspectives on Gender and Sexual Behavior; Fluidity, Gender; Gender Diversity; Gender Dysphoria; Gender Expression; Gender Identity; Gender Identity Development; Gender Roles, Socialization and; Gender Transition; Genderqueer; Intersexuality; Nonbinary Gender Identities; Sexual Identity; Social Learning Theory, Gender and; Stereotypes, Gender; Transgender.

Further Reading

Feder, H. H., Phoenix, C. H., & Young, W. C. (1966). Suppression of feminine behaviour by administration of testosterone propionate to neonatal rats. *Journal of Endocrinology, 34*(1), 131–132.

Money, J., & Ehrhardt, A. A. (1972). *Man and woman, boy and girl: Differentiation and dimorphism of gender identity from conception to maturity.* Baltimore: Johns Hopkins University Press.

Quadagno, D. M., Briscoe, R., & Quadagno, J. S. (1977). Effect of perinatal gonadal hormones on selected nonsexual behavior patterns: A critical assessment of the nonhuman and human literature. *Psychological Bulletin, 84*(1), 62.

Shaywitz, B. A., Shaywltz, S. E., Pugh, K. R., Constable, R. T., Skudlarski, P., Fulbright, R. K., ... Gore, J. C. (1995). Sex differences in the functional organization of the brain for language. *Nature, 373*(6516), 607.

Gender Diversity

As gender is being deconstructed and expanded, the labels used to describe the diversity of gender identities are also growing and evolving. Historically, "transgender" has been an umbrella term for all gender identities that do not align with the assigned sex at birth; however, some gender minorities do not identify as transgender, feeling it reinforces the gender binary (a conceptualization of gender as only exclusively male or female). Alternatively, some individuals who do not identify on the gender binary prefer nonbinary or genderqueer labels. Previous terms for gender diversity include gender variant and gender deviant, both of which have received criticisms for othering (treating anything or anyone outside of the status quo as alien) and are used less frequently. Currently, "gender diverse" is a broad term that encompasses transgender and nonbinary identities. According to current national estimates, between 0.6 percent and 5.0 percent of Americans identify as transgender. When gender diversity is conceptualized more broadly (e.g., including nonbinary identities), it is anticipated that these numbers will increase notably. Growth in prevalence has been attributed to expanding gender identity language, availability of information about gender identity, online community support, and increased representation and acceptance.

"Gender diverse" encompasses an extensive collection of gender identities without one representation of gender diversity; however, gender-diverse individuals may have shared experiences of stigma, marginalization, and discrimination based on their gender identity. In particular, nonconforming gender expression including physical appearance and interpersonal factors (e.g., voice, pronouns, chosen name) can be a risk factor for discrimination. A series of bathroom bills that began with the North Carolina HB2 in March 2016 restricted the use of bathrooms to those that align with an individual's sex assigned at birth, with individuals singled out by appearance. A national study on discrimination found that gender-diverse individuals reported facing suspicion and hostility in bathrooms on a daily basis, including being verbally harassed, physically attacked, and denied access to facilities. In addition, some individuals reported that fear of these negative experiences contributing to limiting their food and water intake to minimize the need to use the bathroom, with these actions sometimes leading to health issues such as urinary tract infections.

Access to health care is another shared challenge for many gender-diverse individuals despite the fact that the 2010 Affordable Care Act provided gender-diverse individuals increased access to services and protections against gender-based discrimination. Gender-diverse individuals have reported experiences of gatekeeping (e.g., required professional letters to access gender-affirming treatment) and mistreatment by health care providers ranging from rough handling to refusal of services. For many gender-diverse individuals, chosen names and pronouns are an essential part of gender expression but can also be a source of frequent microaggressions. Using the correct pronoun for gender-diverse individuals can be as important as using a correct name. Misgendering (identifying someone by the wrong gender through incorrect pronouns) is a microaggression that can occur frequently and be a stigmatizing experience. Additional microaggressions include others' use of former names rather than chosen names, lack of representation on forms and identification, being tokenized (e.g., being expected to represent their gender), and being asked to explain their gender.

Gender diversity has been argued to be the next human rights movement. Cisnormativity (the general assumption that most people are cisgender and that cisgender is "normal") can create an environment where gender-diverse individuals experience microaggressions and barriers to basic needs. Despite these challenges, gender-diverse individuals demonstrate resilience, which can be bolstered when individuals feel free to explore their gender identity and expression and when they see themselves positively represented in others and their environment. In addition to personal resilience, social support is one of the strongest predictors of health outcomes for gender-diverse individuals, supporting the need for creating spaces that welcome and represent gender diversity.

M. Killian Kinney

See also: Agender; Bigender; Binary Gender System; Fluidity, Gender; Gender; Gender Expression; Gender Identity; Gender Identity Development; International Foundation for Gender Education (IFGE); Nonbinary Gender Identities; Queer; Questioning; Transgender.

Further Reading

Barker, M.-J. (2014, February 15). 57 genders (and none for me)? Reflections on the new Facebook gender categories. *Rewriting the rules.* Retrieved from https://www.rewriting-the-rules.com/gender/57-genders-and-none-for-me-reflections-on-the-new-facebook-gender-categories/

Brown, M. E., & Burill, D. (2018). *Challenging genders: Non-binary experiences of those assigned female at birth.* Miami, FL: Boundless Endeavors.

Budge, S. L., Rossman, H. K., & Howard, K. A. (2014). Coping and psychological distress among genderqueer individuals: The moderating effect of social support. *Journal of LGBT Issues in Counseling, 8*(1), 95–117.

Collazo, A., Austin, A., & Craig, S. L. (2013). Facilitating transition among transgender clients: Components of effective clinical practice. *Clinical Social Work Journal, 41*(3), 228–237.

Flores, A. R., Herman, J. L., Gates, G. J., & Brown, T. N. T. (2016, June). *How many adults identify as transgender in the United States?* Los Angeles, CA: The Williams Institute.

Grossman, A. H., Park, J. Y., & Russell, S. T. (2016). Transgender youth and suicidal behaviors: Applying the interpersonal psychological theory of suicide. *Journal of Gay & Lesbian Mental Health, 20*(4), 329–349.

Herman, J. L., Flores, A. R., Brown, T. N. T., Wilson, B. D. M., & Conron, K. J. (2017). *Age of individuals who identify as transgender in the United States.* Los Angeles, CA: The Williams Institute.

James, S. E., Herman, J. L., Rankin, S., Keisling, M., Mottet, L., & Anafi, M. (2016). *The report of the 2015 U.S. transgender survey.* Washington, DC: National Center for Transgender Equality.

Lewis, J. (2008). *Resilience among transgender adults who identify as genderqueer: Implications for health and mental health treatment* (Doctoral dissertation). Retrieved from ProQuest Information & Learning. (Accession number 57395)

McLemore, K. A. (2015). Experiences with misgendering: Identity misclassification of transgender spectrum individuals. *Self and Identity, 14*(1), 51–74.

Poteat, V. P., Sinclair, K. O., DiGiovanni, C. D., Koenig, B. W., & Russell, S. T. (2013b). Gay-straight alliances are associated with student health: A multischool comparison of LGBTQ and heterosexual youth. *Journal of Research on Adolescence, 23*(2), 319–330.

Richards, C., Bouman, W. P., Seal, L., Barker, M. J., Nieder, T. O., & T'Sjoen, G. (2016). Non-binary or genderqueer genders. *International Review of Psychiatry, 28*(1), 95–102.

Singh, A. A., Meng, S. E., & Hansen, A. W. (2014). "I am my own gender": Resilience strategies of trans youth. *Journal of Counseling & Development, 92*(2), 208–218.

Transgender Law and Policy Institute. (n.d.). *Transgender issues: A fact sheet.* Retrieved from http://www.transgenderlaw.org/resources/transfactsheet.pdf

Gender Dysphoria

Gender dysphoria is classified in the fifth edition of the *Diagnostic and Statistical Manual* published by the American Psychiatric Association. The diagnosis of gender dysphoria is used to indicate that individuals are experiencing dysphoria, or unease or dissatisfaction, with the sex they were assigned at birth because they identify with a different gender. In common language, individuals with gender dysphoria are often referred to as transgender, though individuals meeting the diagnostic criteria for gender dysphoria may identify with any gender identity and do not necessarily identify as transgender. Further, it is not necessary for individuals to be diagnosed as having gender dysphoria to consider themselves transgender.

Symptoms of gender dysphoria vary but often involve individuals feeling as if their body does not represent their true gender, feelings of unease or disgust toward their genitalia or bodily representations of their sex assigned at birth (secondary sex characteristics such as body hair, breast development, Adam's apple, wide hips, etc.), anger or unease when others refer to them using pronouns used to represent their sex assigned at birth, anger or unease when feeling pressured to wear clothing generally worn by individuals of the sex they were assigned at birth, and general discomfort regarding their physical body presentation. Individuals with gender dysphoria often struggle socially due to being bullied, harassed, assaulted, or ostracized. These situations may occur within family, school, employment, and other social environments and often lead to depression, anxiety, low self-esteem, social isolation, and, if severe, suicidal thoughts or attempts. It should be noted that in many cases, the dysphoria experienced as well as mental and social effects are more related to social responses to the individuals' gender identities rather than a direct consequence of those gender identities.

Among youth with gender dysphoria there is generally a stated desire to be of the gender with which they identify, a desire to present socially as the gender with which they identify, preferences for types of activities that are stereotypically associated with the gender with which they identify, and a taking on of the gender role with which they identify within role-plays. Post puberty, while the aforementioned continue, individuals' focus often turns more directly toward desiring to remove or modify physical characteristics of their sex assigned at birth and to obtain those of the gender with which they identify. For those who were assigned male at birth, this could include a desire to have body hair removed, breast augmentation, reduction of their Adam's apple, hip augmentation, and, in some cases, removal of their penis. Among those assigned female at birth, there may be a desire for stopping menses, removal of breast tissue, growth of body hair, and, for some, the surgical construction of a penis.

Per the World Professional Association for Transgender Health's Standard of Care Version 7, a diagnosis of gender dysphoria is required before individuals receive medical treatment such as gender-affirming hormones or gender-affirming surgeries. Treatment of gender dysphoria encompasses two areas: one social or emotional and the other physical. Within the social and emotional realm, treatment focuses on resolving internal concerns regarding the individual's gender identity; reducing depression, anxiety, substance use, and other mental health concerns; using family therapy to address conflicts related to the individual's gender identity and help others within their family understand them and their identity; and increasing the individual's ability to cope with negative social messaging related to their gender identity. Psychotropic medications are not used to treat gender dysphoria but may be used to treat accompanying depression, anxiety, or other psychosocial concerns.

Physical treatment involves the introduction of gender-affirming hormones or surgical procedures designed to produce the desired physical changes. For those assigned female at birth, treatment can include menses suppression or introduction of testosterone via injection or topical application. Testosterone supplementation will produce many male secondary sex characteristics, such as hair growth, lowering of the voice, and redistribution of body fat. Among those assigned male at birth, an antiandrogen may be used to reduce the impact of naturally occurring testosterone, and estrogen may be introduced. Supplementation of estrogen will result in breast growth, fat redistribution, thinning of body hair, and feminization of the facial structure. Various surgical procedures are also available to remove or recreate both male and female genitalia. Desires regarding physical changes are highly individualized, with some individuals with gender dysphoria wanting little to no changes to their bodies and others wanting to undergo extensive gender-affirming surgical procedures.

In previous editions of the *Diagnostic and Statistical Manual*, gender dysphoria was known as gender identity disorder and was classified within the section of sexual and gender identity disorders. This classification raised concerns that it conflated gender and sexuality, pathologized identifying as transgender or as a gender other than that which corresponds to the sex assigned at birth, and reinforced beliefs that people whose gender does not match their sex assigned at birth are mentally ill. Within the fifth edition of the *Diagnostic and Statistical Manual*, gender identity disorder was moved into its own chapter and the name changed to gender dysphoria to emphasize the dysphoria associated with individuals' experiences.

In the new edition, the diagnostic criteria were also divided into two sections—one for children and the other for adolescents and adults. This separation was done to reflect the aforementioned age-based differences in how gender dysphoria is experienced. While the diagnosis of gender dysphoria is still controversial among mental health professionals due to concerns about people receiving a mental health diagnosis based on their identities, the current diagnostic criteria represent a more positive understanding of how individuals experience conflicts between their gender identity and their sex assigned at birth.

Richard A. Brandon-Friedman

See also: Binary Gender System; Childhood Gender Nonconformity; *Diagnostic and Statistical Manual of Mental Disorders* (*DSM*); Gender; Gender Diversity; Gender Expression; Gender Identity; Gender Identity Development; Gender Transition; Nonbinary Gender Identities; Pronoun Usage; Testosterone Replacement Therapy; Transgender.

Further Reading

American Psychiatric Association. (2013). Gender dysphoria. In American Psychiatric Association, *Diagnostic and statistical manual of mental disorders* (5th ed., 451–460). Arlington, VA: American Psychiatric Publishing.

Coleman, E., Bockting, W., Botzer, M., Cohen-Kettenis, P., DeCuypere, G., Feldman, J., ... Lev, A. I. (2011–2012). Standards of care for the health of transsexual, transgender, and gender-nonconforming people, version 7. *International Journal of Transgenderism, 13*(4), 165–232.

Curtis, R., Levy, A., Martin, J., Playdon, Z.-J., Wylie, K., Reed, T., & Reed, B. (2007). *A guide to hormone therapy for trans people.* London: Department of Health.

Dhejne, C., Van Vlerken, R., Heylens, G., & Arcelus, J. (2016). Mental health and gender dysphoria: A review of the literature. *International Review of Psychiatry, 28*(1), 44–57.

Moolchaem, P., Liamputtong, P., O'Halloran, P., & Muhamad, R. (2015). The lived experiences of transgender persons: A meta-synthesis. *Journal of Gay & Lesbian Social Services, 27*(2), 143–171.

Orr, A., Baum, J., Brown, J., Gill, E., Kahn, E., & Salem, A. (n.d.) *Schools in transition: A guide for supporting transgender students in K–12 schools.* San Francisco, CA: National Center for Lesbian Rights.

Wylie, K., Knudson, G., Khan, S. I., Bonierbale, M., Watanyusakul, S., & Baral, S. (2016). Serving transgender people: Clinical care considerations and service delivery models in transgender health. *The Lancet, 388*(10042), 401–411.

Gender Expression

Gender expression is the way in which someone demonstrates or communicates their gender identity. This may be through a variety of outlets, including clothing, speech, posture, nonverbal communication, interests, and self-reference (pronouns that are used). Various forms of expression may present on a masculine or feminine spectrum. Often, gender expression is influenced by one's culture. Some people may also express their gender outside of masculine and feminine spectrums that are defined by their culture, and expression can fluctuate. In addition, gender expression may not necessarily fit in with cultural expectations or norms, which may lead to potential discrimination and stigma. Gender expression may or may not reflect someone's gender identity.

Rachel Snedecor

See also: Binary Gender System; Femininity; Fluidity, Gender; Gender; Gender Diversity; Gender Identity; Gender Transition; Masculinity; Pronoun Usage.

Further Reading

APA Task Force on Gender Identity and Gender Variance. (2008). *Report of the Task Force on Gender Identity and Gender Variance.* Washington, DC: American Psychological Association.

Gutierrez, N. (2004). Resisting fragmentation, living whole: Four female transgender students of color speak about school. *Journal of Gay & Lesbian Social Services, 16*(3–4), 69–79.

Hidalgo, M. A., Kuhns, L. M., Kwon, S., Mustanski, B., & Garofalo, R. (2015). The impact of childhood gender expression on childhood sexual abuse and psychopathology among young men who have sex with men. *Child Abuse & Neglect, 46*, 103–112.

Leibowitz, S., & de Vries, A. L. C. (2016). Gender dysphoria in adolescence. *International Review of Psychiatry, 28*(1), 21–35.

Masequesmay, G. (2003). Negotiating multiple identities in a queer Vietnamese support group. *Journal of Homosexuality, 45*(2–4), 193–215.

Mathy, R. M. (2001). A nonclinical comparison of transgender identity and sexual orientation: A framework for multicultural competence. *Journal of Psychology and Human Sexuality, 13*(1), 21–54.

Gender Identity

Gender identity cannot be adequately understood without a fundamental discussion of gender and gender norms. Gender is an abstract concept of masculinity, femininity, and, more recently, additional genders that are each constructed by society and reinforced through social systems (e.g., gender norms). While the terms "gender" and "sex" are often used interchangeably, this is inaccurate, as sex is a biological category based on chromosomes and physical attributes rather than a social construct, and conflating the two excludes a diverse range of gender identities. Gender identity is an individual's internal sense of their gender and may be static or fluid. Unlike social constructions of gender, gender identity is self-identified. In other words, one's gender identity can only be identified by the individual. The term "cisgender" refers to those whose gender identity is congruent with their sex assigned at birth (i.e., assigned female at birth and identifies as female). "Transgender" refers to someone whose gender identity is different from their sex assigned at birth (i.e., assigned male at birth and identifies as female). In the last decade, recognition of additional genders continues to increase including nonbinary identities, which refer to genders that are not exclusively male or female (e.g., genderqueer, genderfluid, trigender).

Conceptualizations of gender change with shifts in culture, which influence the concepts and language used to describe gender identity. Cultural expectations of gender such as gender norms of roles and expression are based on expectations of femininity, masculinity, and androgyny as it is currently socially constructed. The color pink, for example, was associated with masculinity and worn by boys until the 1950s, when the current blue for boys and pink for girls became dominant. In Western society, the dominant conceptualization of gender is grounded in the gender binary or an understanding of gender as either male or female and no other genders. This gender binary is evidenced by checkboxes in formal documents, gender markers on government identification, and men's or women's bathrooms. Recent social and legal changes have indicated a shift in the conceptualization of gender with fill-in gender options on forms, a third-gender marker on birth certificates and driver's licenses, and all-gender bathrooms.

Gender conceptualization has undergone several iterations and continues to evolve. Starting with the gender binary, gender then began to be understood on a single spectrum with some individuals fitting at some degree between entirely masculine and entirely feminine. Multiple spectrums followed that allowed for an individual's gender to be conceptualized as a degree of masculinity and degree of femininity from none to entirely. Then, gender-expansive models were created with multifaceted continuums of biological sex, gender identity, gender expression, and sexual orientation, including the Genderbread Person versions, then the Gender Unicorn. Finally, a multidimensional nonlinear galaxy of numerous possibilities (gender galaxy) is considered to be the most inclusive conceptualization of gender.

Gender has been described as performativity or an ongoing process of creating and re-creating gender through exchanges such as language and expression. While influenced by gender norms, how one expresses their gender identity can be as unique as their gender identity. An individual's gender expression may or may not align with expectations of gender norms. In addition to physical appearance, some individuals may express their gender identity through a chosen name or pronouns. For some, activism toward gender equality and representation of gender diversity is a part of gender identity. Gender expression plays a significant role in how one's gender identity is seen and, consequently, how one is gendered by those around them.

As understanding and acceptance of gender diversity increases, a growing number of people are openly identifying as transgender and nonbinary. This trend is especially evident among youth, particularly those in progressive countries and regions where many youth describe their gender expression as nonconforming or androgynous. As such, gender identities and related language continue to expand to represent this community. In addition to increasing awareness of gender diversity, language for gender identities can provide validation of individuals' gender identity as well as create a common label to unite people with shared experiences.

M. Killian Kinney

See also: Agender; Bigender; Binary Gender System; Cisgender; Fluidity, Gender; Gender; Gender Diversity; Gender Dysphoria; Gender Expression; Gender Identity Development; Gender Roles, Socialization and; Gender Transition; Genderqueer; Nonbinary Gender Identities; Queer; Transgender.

Further Reading

Beemyn, G., & Rankin, S. (2011). *The lives of transgender people.* New York: Columbia University Press.

Butler, J. (1990). *Gender trouble: Feminism and the subversion of identity.* New York: Routledge.

Kinney, M. K. (2018). *Carving your own path: Exploring non-binary identities.* Manuscript in preparation.

Paoletti, J. B. (2012). *Pink and blue: Telling the boys from the girls in America.* Bloomington: Indiana University Press.

Russel, E. B., & Viggiani, P. A. (2018). Understanding differences and definitions: From oppression to sexual health and practice. In M. P. Dentato (Ed.), *Social work practice with the LGBTQ community* (26–48). New York: Oxford University Press.

Vade, D. (2005). Expanding gender and expanding the law: Toward a social and legal conceptualization of gender that is more inclusive of transgender people. *Michigan Journal of Gender & Law, 11*(2), 253–316.

Wilson, B. D. M., Choi, S. K., Herman, J. L., Becker, R., & Conron, K. J. (2017). *Characteristics and mental health of gender nonconforming adolescents in California: Findings from the 2015–2016 California health interview survey.* Los Angeles, CA: The Williams Institute and UCLA Center for Health Policy Research.

Gender Identity Development

Gender identity is an internal sense of self that develops as an ongoing process and is influenced by the social construction of gender. As the social construction of gender changes, so too can the conceptualization of one's gender identity and expression change in comparison to social norms and expectations. Furthermore, gender identity is unique to each person whether their gender aligns with their sex assigned at birth (cisgender) or whether they are gender diverse. While gender norms can facilitate gender identity development for many individuals, transgender and nonbinary individuals are not typically represented in cultural norms of gender. Several models for sexual orientation identity development exist; however, gender identity development has received less attention. Currently, a model for cisgender identity development has not been created, but several models for gender identity development have been proposed.

The most frequently used gender identity model is Devor's (2004) stages of transgender identity formation. Devor's model included fourteen stages:

1. Abiding anxiety
2. Identity confusion about originally assigned gender and sex
3. Identity comparison about originally assigned gender and sex
4. Discovery of transgenderism
5. Identity confusion about transgenderism
6. Identity comparisons about transgenderism
7. Tolerance of transgender identity
8. Delay before acceptance of transgender identity
9. Acceptance of transgender identity
10. Delay before transition
11. Transition
12. Acceptance of posttransition gender and sex identities
13. Integration
14. Pride

As described by Devor in 2004, transitioning can vary among individuals from social transitioning (e.g., chosen name, pronouns) to physical transitioning (e.g., hormone replacement therapy, gender-affirming surgeries). Similar to other models, integration of gender identity and pride are the goals of identity development. In 2018, Kinney introduced a nonbinary gender identity development model. This model consists of eight stages:

1. Early freedom
2. Gender identity confusion
3. Language acquisition
4. Reconciling repression
5. Gender experimentation
6. Envisioning an ideal self
7. Disclosing gender identity
8. Gender identity integration

The importance of language acquisition is noteworthy in that language for nonbinary identities in Western culture has only recently emerged over the last decade. Similarly, envisioning an ideal self presents a challenge stage as nonbinary expression can vary broadly with little modeling in mainstream media.

Several key elements across gender identity development models include socialization about gender, isolation, language acquisition, and eventual acceptance of gender identity. Gender is a social construction and, as such, is taught and reinforced through interpersonal exchanges and social systems, including education, media, and policy. Throughout their lives, individuals are taught different gender norms for boys, men, girls, and women from toys to clothing to careers. Even before birth, gender norms begin with gender reveal parties for fetuses in utero with color-coded balloons and cakes (blue for boy and pink for girl). These subtle and not-so-subtle reinforcements of gender norms may not be as apparent to individuals whose gender aligns with such norms. However, gender-diverse individuals who do not see themselves represented or affirmed in gender norms can feel misunderstood and isolated. Acquiring language about gender can be a pivotal point in gender identity development marked by validation of gender. Language can also be a means to facilitate community building through shared gender identities and experiences, which may reduce feelings of isolation. Even once an individual understands their gender identity, cisnormativity (the assumption that most people are cisgender and that is "normal") and internalized stigma (e.g., accepted negative messages about gender-diverse individuals) may inhibit an individual from accepting their gender identity. Due to hostile environments, some individuals may repress or choose to conceal their gender identity as a strategic coping mechanism. An accumulative effect of invalidating experiences can lead to a deterioration of mental health among transgender and nonbinary individuals. Conversely, representation and affirmation of gender have been shown to ameliorate negative health implications for gender-diverse individuals, stressing the importance of building resilience among transgender and nonbinary individuals. Increasing the understanding of how gender is created, learned, self-identified, and affirmed can aid in learning ways to support healthy gender identity development across gender identities.

M. Killian Kinney

See also: Cisgender; Gender; Gender Diversity; Gender Dysphoria; Gender Expression; Gender Identity; Gender Roles, Socialization and; Gender Transition; Nonbinary Gender Identities; Questioning; Transgender.

Further Reading

Beemyn, G., & Rankin, S. (2011). *The lives of transgender people.* New York: Columbia University Press.

Cass, V. C. (1984). Homosexual identity formation: Testing a theoretical model. *Journal of Sex Research, 20*, 143–167.

Davis, C. (2009). Introduction to practice with transgender and gender variant youth. In G. P. Mallon (Ed.), *Social work practice with transgender and gender variant youth* (2nd ed., 15–35). London: Routledge.

Devor, A. H. (2004). Witnessing and mirroring: A fourteen stage model of transsexual identity formation. *Journal of Gay and Lesbian Psychiatry, 8*(1–2), 41–67.

Eliason, M. J. (1996). An inclusive model of lesbian identity assumption. *Journal of Gay Lesbian and Bisexual Identity, 1*(1), 3–19.

Fox, R. C. (1995). Bisexual identities. In A. R. D'Augelli & C. J. Patterson (Eds.), *Lesbian, gay, and bisexual identities over the lifespan: Psychological perspectives* (48–86). New York: Oxford University Press.

Kinney, M. K. (2018). *Carving your own path: A nonbinary gender identity development model.* Manuscript in preparation.

Levitt, H. M., & Ippolito, M. R. (2014). Being transgender: The experience of transgender identity development. *Journal of Homosexuality, 61*(12), 1727–1758.

Troiden, R. R. (1988). *Gay and lesbian identity: A sociological analysis.* Dix Hills, NY: General Hall.

Gender Roles, Socialization and

Gender roles are the beliefs, rights, attitudes, and behaviors that are associated with a particular sex and gender. Expectations of a person's gender role are assigned to people even before birth, for example, when someone asks a person who is pregnant if they are having a boy or a girl. Physical, emotional, and psychological aspects of how a child should act depend on societal standards. For example, in Western culture, the color pink, gentleness, and fragility are associated with girls, while the color blue, being tough, and having no tolerance for showing emotion is associated with boys. These ideas are typically based on female-identified or male-identified genitals, and there is a social expectation of appropriate associated behavior. It is important to note that these binary gender roles usually leave out people who are born with genitalia that is not typically male or female, and consequently, many parents of babies born with intersex conditions feel the need to raise their children as either boys or girls, and some may seek surgery for their infants in order to change the appearance of their genitals.

According to Longres (2000), socialization is "the process through which individual participation is defined and refined as individuals learn to function as a system member. Included are the processes by which people become aware of the expectations of others and learn the attitudes, knowledge, and abilities necessary to comply with those expectations." In order for infants and children to function within a certain system, there are roles that need to be met in the dichotomy of male and female. This is usually regardless of how those individual people feel about themselves. Two theories that are instrumental in explaining socialization's influence on gender roles are social learning theory and cognitive developmental theory. Social learning theory was developed by Albert Bandura in the 1970s. He theorized that through cognition, we have the ability to "use language, anticipate consequences, and make observations" through the socialization of our environment. For example, if a girl observes that only boys are allowed to speak in loud volumes without being reprimanded by adults and that girls who speak too loudly are punished, she will model her behavior in order to avoid the consequences.

Cognitive developmental theory, on the other hand, takes notice of how children correct their behaviors within the environment according to what other children and adults are doing. By taking the cues from the environment and paying close attention to what other girls and boys do, it informs the behavior of the individual. This gives a particular boy or girl the opportunity to "independently strive to act like proper girls or boys" (Yarber et al., 2010).

Larger societal institutions also play a part in shaping children's behavior. Teachers in school play an important role in reinforcing societal, cultural, and gender expectations among the students they teach. For example, boys may be encouraged to participate in more aggressive sports such as football, whereas girls may be steered away from football and encouraged into sports with less contact like gymnastics due to them being seen as fragile or unable to take care of themselves. Religious teachings and traditions are also ways to further perpetuate gender roles within the households and communities that practice them. If the religion of the family pushes for the dominance of females by males, and if all the people in leadership roles in that institution are also male, then it again reinforces the stereotype that girls are not granted top spots in these structured settings. Finally, the messages taken in by children through cartoons, advertisements, and TV shows give various favored examples of how girls and boys should behave in society. It is also important to note that as time goes along and systems change, the expectations for genders change as well.

Shane'a Thomas

See also: Binary Gender System; Gender; Gender Identity; Gender Identity Development; Sexual Learning; Social Learning Theory, Gender and; Stereotypes, Gender; Stereotypes, Sexual.

Further Reading

Lehmiller, J. J. (2014). *The psychology of human sexuality.* Hoboken, NJ: Wiley-Blackwell.

Longres, J. (2000). *Human behavior in the social environment* (3rd ed.). Belmont, CA: Wadsworth/Thomson Learning.

Yarber, W. L., Sayad, B. W., & Strong, B. (2010). *Human sexuality: Diversity in contemporary America* (7th ed.). New York: McGraw Hill.

Gender Transition

"Sex" and "gender" are often conflated into one idea in mainstream culture; that is, they are used interchangeably to mean the same thing. However, feminist scholarship over the past four decades has shown how sex and gender are two different constructs. Gender is here defined as the set of social, cultural, and linguistic norms that can be attributed to someone's identity, expression, or role as masculine, feminine, androgynous, or nonbinary. Whereas someone's sex is assigned at birth by medical professionals based on the appearance of genitalia, and related assumptions about chromosomal makeup, gender identity, expressions, and roles emerge over the life span, sometimes changing over time.

"Gender transition" can refer to some of those change processes. This term is generally used to indicate changes undergone by transgender people in relation to their identities. There are different forms of gender transition that people might undertake. Legal gender transition refers to the process of changing gender markers on legal documentations, which might include birth certificates, school transcripts, identification documents, marriage certificates, social security information, and so on. People who change their gender marker legally usually also change their name at the same time to ensure coherence between their name, appearance, and legal documentations. Requirements for changing gender markers legally vary from country to country and, within the United States, from state to state. Some states and countries require transgender people to have undergone some form of surgical intervention to modify their bodies to reflect the legal gender marker change sought, whereas others only require proof that the person is socially aligned with the change they are seeking.

Some people seek body modification through medical intervention and surgery as part of their process of gender transition. This could take the form of hormonal treatment to masculinize or feminize their bodies, or, in the case of prepubescent and pubescent transgender youth, it could mean seeking hormone blockers to stop physical changes that increase distress and gender dysphoria for the person undergoing treatment. As well as hormone treatment, some people seek surgical interventions, such as chest, genital, and facial reconstruction. The types and extent of those interventions depend on the person's identity and expression as well as the level of dysphoria—that is, incongruence between their bodies and identities—that they might experience. The surgical interventions chosen can also be dependent on physical limitations, financial access, and available medical techniques. For example, trans feminine people tend to seek genital reconstruction more frequently than trans masculine people given that this is more successful, and medically advanced, for the former than the latter group. These interventions are often referred to as being part of someone's medical gender transition process.

Finally, most transgender people undertake a process of social gender transition, which can include name and pronoun changes among family, friends, coworkers, or social networks, as well as changes in clothing, appearance, and sometimes mannerisms. Transgender people seeking legal and medical transition usually need to be supported by health providers in their transition efforts. Decisions made by health providers in relation to supporting people's gender transition decisions are usually based on the latest standards of care issued by the World Professional Association for Transgender Health.

Alex Iantaffi

See also: Gender; Gender Diversity; Gender Dysphoria; Gender Expression; Gender Identity; Hormone Replacement Therapy; Pronoun Usage; Sex Reassignment Surgery; Testosterone Replacement Therapy; Transgender; World Professional Association for Transgender Health (WPATH).

Further Reading

Brill, S., & Pepper, R. (2013). *The transgender child: A handbook for families and professionals.* San Francisco, CA: Cleis Press.

Coleman, E., Bockting, W., Botzer, M., Cohen-Kettenis, P., DeCuypere, G., Feldman, J., ... Monstrey, S. (2012). Standards of care for the health of transsexual, transgender, and gender-nonconforming people, version 7. *International Journal of Transgenderism, 13*(4), 165–232.

Guss, C., Shumer, D., & Katz-Wise, S. L. (2015). Transgender and gender nonconforming adolescent care: Psychosocial and medical considerations. *Current Opinion in Pediatrics, 26*(4), 421–426.

Iantaffi, A. (2015). Gender and sexual legitimacy. *Current Sexual Health Reports, 7*(2), 103–107.

Iantaffi, A., & Barker, M. J. (2017). *How to understand your gender: A practical guide for exploring who you are.* London: Jessica Kingsley Publishers.

Lev, A. I. (2013). *Transgender emergence: Therapeutic guidelines for working with gender-variant people and their families.* London: Routledge.

Richards, C., & Barker, M. J. (Eds.). (2015). *The Palgrave handbook of the psychology of sexuality and gender.* New York: Palgrave Macmillan.

GenderPAC

GenderPAC (Gender Public Advocacy Coalition) was a political advocacy organization that worked to further the rights of lesbian, gay, bisexual, and transgender (LGBT) people. It was headquartered in Washington, D.C. Like other political action committees (PACs), it lobbied Congress on behalf of legislation it supported, and it contributed money to candidates whom it supported. The organization was active from 1995 to 2009.

Transgender people (people who identify with a gender other than their sex or gender at birth or who express another gender by the way they dress and behave) constituted the primary focus of GenderPAC. However, it also dealt with matters of concern to other people with other diverse forms of gender or sexual orientation. The organization maintained a number of programs intended to educate the public and politicians about gender identity and expression and to promote its positions on these and other LGBT issues. The primary matters addressed by these programs were discrimination and violence against LGBT people in the workplace, schools, and communities. GenderPAC also developed networks to help LGBT youth and parents of these youth find support and assistance.

Transgender activist Riki Anne Wilchins founded GenderPAC in 1995 to fill the gap left by existing gay and lesbian organizations, which failed to address transgender issues in any substantial way. She continued to lead the group throughout its existence.

GenderPAC achieved a number of important accomplishments in its relatively brief existence. It developed the Congressional Non-Discrimination Pledge, in which approximately 200 members of Congress promised to support nondiscrimination against transgender people in their own offices. Besides lobbying Congress on such issues, GenderPAC also worked with several private corporations to convince them to protect gender identity and expression as part of their employment nondiscrimination policies.

GenderPAC's GenderYOUTH program was designed to assist college students in organizing chapters on campus to work for transgender rights. Schools were ranked according to their nondiscrimination policies regarding transgender students in GenderPAC's *Gender Equality National Index for Universities and Schools*. The organization also published the *National Survey of TransViolence* and *50 under 30: Masculinity and the War on America's Youth*, both of which featured reports of violent attacks against transgender people. Most of the documented attacks were against young African American or Hispanic trans women. These reports helped lead to congressional passage of the Matthew Shepard Act, which, among other things, extended federal hate crimes protections to transgender people. President Barack Obama signed the act into law in 2009.

Certain other transgender organizations criticized GenderPAC for not focusing exclusively on issues concerning transgender individuals. For example, GenderPAC worked to publicize violence and discrimination against some "gender-variant" individuals who were not transgender, such as a self-identified "butch lesbian" who was harassed at her workplace and later fired for appearing "too masculine." Wilchins defended the group against such criticism by stating that GenderPAC's mission was to move beyond the strict "identity form of organizing" and work toward true diversity.

In 2009, GenderPAC ceased to exist when its board determined that it had achieved many of its goals and that other organizations now existed to carry on advocacy for gender-related issues.

A. J. Smuskiewicz

See also: Gender; Gender Diversity; Gender Expression; Gender Identity; LGBTQ+; Shepard, Matthew; Transgender.

Further Reading

Theophano, T. (2015). Gender public advocacy coalition (GenderPAC). GLBTQ Archives. Retrieved from http://www.glbtqarchive.com/ssh/gender_public_advocacy_S.pdf

TrueChild. (2017). Home page. Retrieved from https://www.truechild.org

Genderqueer

Arguments against binary models of gender—those that understand male and female or man and woman, as exclusive and exhaustive possibilities—have increased over time as binary models fail to accommodate the diversity and fluidity of all gender identities. Binary views of gender exclude and erase individuals who identify as genderqueer, an identity that can be understood as neither exclusively male nor female. Genderqueer individuals often hold such gender identities as "bigender," "trigender," "pangender," "agender," "gender neutral," "nongendered," "genderless," "neuter," or "neutrois." The term "nonbinary" is often used interchangeably with "genderqueer," though some individuals may identify with one term and not the other. Many gender-fluid individuals, whose gender identity or gender expression fluctuates over time or in different situational contexts, identify as genderqueer or nonbinary. However, not all genderqueer individuals identify as gender fluid and thus experience a sense of consistency in their genderqueer identity across time and context.

The experience of genderqueer individuals is extremely diverse; some may identify as neither male nor female, whereas others may identify as both male and female. Some people may identify as genderqueer but do not consider themselves transgender, whereas other genderqueer individuals do identify as members of the transgender community. In fact, 29 percent of respondents to the 2015 United States Transgender Survey used the term "genderqueer" to describe their gender identity. Furthermore, genderqueer individuals may hold multiple gender identities simultaneously. Some genderqueer individuals, for example, also hold identities of "trans man" or "trans woman." However, many trans men and trans women identify exclusively as men and women, respectively, and thus do not consider themselves genderqueer.

Some genderqueer individuals will choose to pursue medical interventions for gender transition, including hormone therapy and surgical interventions. On the other hand, a subset of genderqueer individuals consider themselves "nontransitioning" (i.e., they do not pursue medical interventions and may not even pursue social transition options such as changing their name or appearance). It is important to keep in mind the distinctions between gender identity and gender expression, such that genderqueer individuals may or may not be gender nonconforming in their physical appearance. Genderqueer individuals may pursue certain options for gender transition that are appropriate for their own desires and experiences, and thus their choices in this area are very diverse.

Though sometimes misunderstood, genderqueer identities represent a normal and natural manifestation of human diversity and can provide an important source of strength and positivity when individuals accept the validity of their experience. Many individuals describe a sense of freedom from the constraints of the gender binary after adopting a genderqueer identity because they are able to define the meaning and significance of their gender for themselves.

Nova J. Bradford, Jory M. Catalpa, and G. Nic Rider

See also: Agender; Bigender; Binary Gender System; Fluidity, Gender; Gender; Gender Diversity; Gender Expression; Gender Identity; Gender Transition; Nonbinary Gender Identities; Queer; Transgender.

Further Reading

American Psychological Association & National Association of School Psychologists. (2015). *Resolution on gender and sexual orientation diversity in children and adolescents in schools.* Retrieved from http://www.apa.org/about/policy/orientation-diversity

Bilodeau, B. L. (2005). Beyond the gender binary: A case study of two transgender students at a midwestern research university. *Journal of Gay & Lesbian Issues in Education, 3*(1), 29–44.

Bornstein, K. (1994). *Gender outlaw: On men, women, and the rest of us.* New York: Vintage.

Bradford, N. J., Rider, G. N., Catalpa, J. M., Morrow, Q. J., Berg, D. R., Spencer, K. G., & McGuire, J. K. (2018). Creating gender: A thematic analysis of genderqueer narratives. *International Journal of Transgenderism, 20*(2–3), 155–168.

Gates, T. G. (2010). Combating problem and pathology: A genderqueer primer for the human service educator. *Journal of Human Services, 30*(1), 54–64.

James, S. E., Herman, J. L., Rankin, S., Keisling, M., Mottet, L., & Anafi, M. (2016). *The report of the 2015 US Transgender Survey.* Washington, DC: National Center for Transgender Equality. Retrieved from http://www.transequality.org/sites/default/files/docs/USTS-Full-Report-FINAL.PDF

Muñoz, J. E. (1999). *Disidentifications: Queers of color and the performance of politics.* Minneapolis: University of Minnesota Press.

Puckett, J. A., Cleary, P., Rossman, K., Mustanski, B., & Newcomb, M. E. (2018). Barriers to gender-affirming care for transgender and gender nonconforming individuals. *Sexuality Research and Social Policy, 15*(1), 48–59.

Richards, C., Bouman, W. P., Seal, L., Barker, M. J., Nieder, T. O., & Tsjoen, G. (2016). Non-binary or genderqueer genders. *International Review of Psychiatry, 28*(1), 95–102.

Roen, K. (2002). "Either/Or" and "Both/Neither": Discursive tensions in transgender politics. *Signs: Journal of Women in Culture and Society, 27*(2), 501–522.

Genital Dysphoria

"Genital dysphoria" is a relatively new term with no comprehensive scientific definition. "Genital" refers to the sexual organs one has. "Dysphoria" is defined as a state of unease, unhappiness, or dissatisfaction. Combined, the term "genital dysphoria" describes a person who is very unhappy or uncomfortable with the genitals they have. The basic idea of this term is confusion or discomfort with the genital region, which can also include misconception of the genitals. Feeling as though you are not in the body you feel you belong in can cause severe stress, anxiety, and depression. Symptoms can cause a disruption in a person's everyday life, from work to school or engaging in social activities.

Genital dysphoria is extreme discomfort with one's genital region, often leading to feelings of being ashamed or embarrassed by their genitalia. Those with genital dysphoria may also have dysphoria for certain parts of their genitals, an example being their testicles. A lack of sexual desire could be associated with genital dysphoria, as individuals often do not want anyone to be sexually attracted to their genitals or to use them during sex. Masturbation fits into this realm, as those who experience genital dysphoria and masturbate may experience a sense of disconnect with their body and pleasure. In addition, many who do experience genital dysphoria may not masturbate due to their own disgust with their genitals, and this could be detrimental to one's healthy sexuality.

Genital dysphoria is associated with gender dysphoria and a transgender identity. Unlike genital dysphoria, gender dysphoria does have a concrete definition: it is when a person has a conflict with the sex they were born with and the gender they identify as, which causes distress. Gender dysphoria is labeled as a mental health condition and appears in the *Diagnostic and Statistical Manual of Mental Disorders, Fifth Edition*, whereas genital dysphoria does not. Transgender people identify as a different gender from the gender assigned at birth, and it is important to note that transgender people may suffer from gender dysphoria, but not all do. Though people with gender dysphoria may not particularly like the body they have, it does not always mean they are distressed by their genitals. Those with gender dysphoria may not hate their genitals but would choose the other set of genitals if possible. In addition, those with gender dysphoria may experience other dysphorias as well, such as their shoulders being too broad, their voice being too high, or not having enough curvature to their body. Considering the lack of research on the topic, it is hard to say how many people experiencing gender dysphoria also experience genital dysphoria.

Depression and anxiety can result from genital dysphoria, which can have negative mental and physical health consequences. Everyone who experiences genital dysphoria handles it uniquely. Some individuals experiencing genital dysphoria may employ a technique termed "tucking." Tucking is when a male puts their genitals between or behind their legs so that they are not visible. This process often involves taping the penis back between the legs toward the anus and then taping everything up, so there is no sign of a penis or testicles. This allows for the wearing of tight-fitting or more feminine clothes without revealing male genitalia. There are health concerns with tucking, though. First, it does not permit urinating. This could increase the risk for urinary tract infections if one holds their urine for an extended amount of time. Ripping off the tape could also irritate the skin over time. Along with that, where people tuck is typically a warm and moist area, which could result in fungal infections. Regardless, tucking is a method by which people make themselves feel more secure with the body they were born with.

Some individuals have also reported the feeling of a "phantom" genital. People may see their genitals as being of the opposite sex, or they may describe their genitals differently. This could include people labeling their penis as a clitoris, or a clitoris as a penis. Again, research in this area is extremely lacking, although this seems to occur more in individuals who are transitioning.

While genital dysphoria may not be currently recognized by the psychiatric society, given all the discussion about it, it seems likely that it will soon be classified and defined. This term clearly needs to be researched more in order to further understanding and knowledge on how to support those experiencing this dysphoria. Genital dysphoria can be incredibly distressing to some, so the more support they have, the greater the chance of improving their mental health.

Casey T. Tobin

See also: Gender Dysphoria; Gender Transition.

Further Reading

Blakeslee, S. (2008, April 13). Gender identity and phantom genital. *San Francisco Chronicle.* Retrieved from https://www.sfgate.com/opinion/article/GENDER-IDENTITY-AND-PHANTOM-GENITALIA-3219560.php

Drescher, J., & Pula, J. (2013). *Expert Q & A: Gender dysphoria.* Retrieved from https://www.psychiatry.org/patients-families/gender-dysphoria/expert-qa

Merriam-Webster. (2019). Dysphoria. Retrieved from https://www.merriam-webster.com/dictionary/dysphoria

Ramachandran, V., & McGeogh, P. (2007). Occurrence of phantom genitalia after gender reassignment surgery. *Medical Hypotheses, 69*(5), 1001–1003.

Samantharz. (2012, August 23). *Gender dysphoria and genital dysphoria.* Retrieved from http://transcoward.blogspot.com/2012/08/gender-dysphoria.html

Genital Warts

Genital warts (also commonly referred to as condyloma, condylomata acuminata, and venereal warts) are soft wart-like growths that occur along the external genitalia, including the penis, vulva, urethra, vagina, cervix, and around the anus. Genital warts are caused by the sexually transmitted virus known as the human papillomavirus (HPV). Currently there are more than 100 types of HPV, with approximately 40 types that can infect the genital tract. Genital HPV is the most common sexually transmitted infection (STI), with HPV types 6 and 11 now known to be the cause of more than 90 percent of genital warts. HPV is commonly passed via sexual contact, and therefore genital warts are considered to be an STI.

Almost all cases of genital warts are caused by HPV. Genital warts are spread through direct skin-to-skin contact, and this can occur during oral, vaginal, or anal sex. The majority of genital warts are caused by two specific types of HPV—HPV types 6 and 11. The virus can penetrate the skin or mucosal membranes (the lining of certain organs, such as the vagina, mouth, and anus) through microscopic abrasions in the genital area, which primarily occur during sexual activity.

HPV types 6 and 11 are considered to be low risk, which means that although they can cause a growth along the external genitalia, these growths tend to be benign and have a low risk of causing cancer. There are other HPV types, most commonly types 16 and 18, which are known as high-risk types because this subset causes cancer of the cervix, anus, and oropharynx (mouth). Fortunately, the majority of people infected with HPV have no symptoms because the body's immune system is able to suppress the virus, so there is no outward sign of infection. However, being asymptomatic can often be misleading because a person infected with the virus may not know they are infected and unknowingly pass the virus to a partner.

Following infection with HPV, it may take weeks, months, or even years before the warts can be detected, and not everyone who comes in contact with the virus will develop them. It is also possible (and common) to be infected by more than one type of HPV at the same time, so a person could get genital warts and have a low-risk HPV type and yet still be exposed to a high-risk HPV type that can cause cancer. If a person has genital warts or may have been exposed to genital warts, it is extremely important to let their health care provider know so that regular exams and Pap smears can be performed. There are certain risk factors that make it more likely to get genital warts or to spread them, including having unprotected sex, having multiple sexual partners, becoming sexually active at an early age, using alcohol and tobacco, being pregnant, and having a weakened immune system because of illness (such as HIV) or medication (such as immunosuppressants that are taken following an organ transplant).

Not all types of HPV cause genital warts. Several types of HPV have been found to be the cause of warts that occur on other parts of the skin, including the hands and feet. The warts that occur on the hands are commonly referred to as common warts, while those that occur on the feet are referred to as plantar warts.

Genital warts tend to be flesh-colored soft growths that occur along the surface of the genital tract. This includes the penis, scrotum, vagina, cervix, rectum, and anus; they can also occur in and around the mouth. These growths commonly look like a tiny cauliflower and can grow as a single wart or in clusters and range in size from very small to a large mass. Genital warts are typically asymptomatic, but depending on their size and location, they can cause pain or itching. They can also cause an increase in vaginal discharge or dampness in the genital area near the warts or vaginal bleeding either during or after sex.

The diagnosis of genital warts is typically a clinical diagnosis made at the time of a physical exam by a health care provider. The warts can be directly visualized with the naked eye but oftentimes are so small or flat in appearance that magnification is required. The magnification is done using a special scope, called a colposcope, which resembles a pair of binoculars. A dilute solution of vinegar, known as acetic acid, can be applied to the affected area to aid in better visualization of the warts. If HPV changes are present, the infected area will turn a whitish color. The colposcope is also used to look for any of these abnormal changes in the vaginal canal or on the cervix. A medical provider may not feel confident regarding the diagnosis of genital warts if the lesions do not have a classic appearance. At times the lesions may take on a different shape, color, or texture than is typical. If there is any clinical doubt as to whether or not a growth in the genital area is indeed a genital wart, the lesion should be biopsied (removed by the clinician) and sent to a lab so a pathologist can do the diagnosis with certainty.

Genital warts tend to grow for about six months, and then the growth of the wart stabilizes. Since the warts can still be emerging during this time, immediate treatment is not recommended since additional treatment may be required. Genital warts may also go away spontaneously without any treatment. When treatment is indicated, there are several options available, including medicines, freezing, laser, or surgery. Medical treatment options include a prescription cream applied by the patient at home. These creams tend to work either by destroying the wart tissue or by boosting the body's immune system so it is able to suppress the virus.

Other treatment options include those done by the health care provider and can be done in either the doctor's office or in an operating room. Treatment options done in an office setting include cryotherapy or freezing of the wart with liquid nitrogen, and application of a chemical called trichloroacetic acid, which is applied directly to the surface of the wart. Medicines applied by the health care provider are those that tend to have a greater risk of damaging the skin surrounding the wart and must be applied with caution. Surgical treatment options include excision of the warts using a scalpel (surgical knife); electrocautery, which burns off the wart using an electric current; or laser, which is a light amplified by the stimulated emission of photons that is used to vaporize or excise the warts. In general, smaller warts tend to respond more favorably to treatment than larger warts, and warts that are on a moist surface respond better to topical treatments when compared with warts on a drier surface. If the warts have not resolved after three treatments by a health care provider or after six prescription treatments, then treatment options should be reevaluated and surgical options for the treatment of the warts considered.

It is easier to prevent an STI than to treat an infection after it has occurred. To reduce the risk of becoming infected with HPV, it is important to practice safer sex and communicate with a partner about any STIs or potential exposure to one before beginning a sexual relationship. To help reduce the risk of becoming infected with HPV, condom use is recommended. It is important that condoms are used consistently and correctly before any sexual contact. Accurate condom use can significantly decrease the transmission of HPV. However, because HPV can be spread outside of the area covered by a condom, even perfect condom use is not a guaranteed way to prevent catching or spreading genital warts.

There is a vaccine currently available to prevent infection by the most common strains of HPV, including several of the high-risk types that cause cancer and several of the most common low-risk types that can cause warts. The vaccine is typically given as a series of shots over a period of about six months. HPV vaccination is recommended for all people, especially those age nine to twenty-six. Ideally, the vaccine should be given before the commencement of sexual activity due to potential exposure to HPV which can occur during any sexual act. However, even if individuals have previously had sexual experience, the vaccine is still recommended as it can help prevent future infection.

Lori Apffel Smith

See also: Cervical Cancer; Human Papillomavirus (HPV); Pap Smear; Sexually Transmitted Infections (STIs).

Further Reading

Grimes, J. A., Smith, L. A., & Fagerberg, K. (2013). *Sexually transmitted disease: An encyclopedia of diseases, prevention, treatment, and issues.* Santa Barbara, CA: Greenwood.

McAnulty, R. D., & Burnette, M. M. (Eds.). (2006). *Sex and sexuality.* Santa Barbara, CA: Praeger.

Newton, D. E. (2009). *Sexual health: A reference handbook.* Santa Barbara, CA: ABC-CLIO.

GLAAD

GLAAD is a nonprofit organization that advocates for more accurate portrayals of lesbian, gay, bisexual, transgender, and queer/questioning (LGBTQ) people in the U.S. media, as well as greater inclusion of the LGBTQ community in general. Formerly known as the Gay and Lesbian Alliance Against Defamation, the group dropped this name in 2013 and began to use only its acronym, GLAAD—a move meant to emphasize the expansion of its mission to include bisexual, transgender, and queer/questioning people.

Gay and lesbian advocates founded GLAAD in 1985 in response to what GLAAD now deems "defamatory and sensationalized" media coverage of gays and lesbians at the beginning of the HIV/AIDS epidemic. The group initially targeted the *New York Post* and the *New York Times* for reporting seen by the gay and lesbian community as discriminatory. Soon, however, it was actively monitoring all media outlets for any misrepresentation of gays and lesbians.

During the 1980s and 1990s, GLAAD convinced the *New York Times*, the Associated Press, and other prominent news outlets to officially change the terms they use to refer to gays and lesbians; it also pressured television networks to increase positive representations of gays and lesbians in their programming. GLAAD's efforts began to expand with the 1998 murder of Matthew Shepard, when the group not only led a media outreach campaign but also became part of a nationwide dialogue on antigay hate crimes.

GLAAD widened its mission in the early 2000s, first to include bisexual and transgender people and later when it reached out to Spanish-language television networks to encourage them to include the LGBTQ community in their programming. In 2006, GLAAD launched the "Be an Ally and a Friend" campaign, which asked straight people to work for positive LGBTQ representation as well.

As part of its work, GLAAD created an annual media awards program, meant to highlight positive portrayals of the LGBTQ community, and an annual Spirit Day, in which LGBTQ supporters wear purple to show support for LGBTQ youth and to denounce bullying. More recently, GLAAD has worked with the National Basketball Association, Boy Scouts of America, Facebook, and other social media to reduce discrimination against LGBTQ people within these forums.

Over the course of GLAAD's existence, positive portrayals of LGBTQ people in the media and elsewhere have skyrocketed, leading some media observers to question whether GLAAD may have rendered itself obsolete. Journalist James Kirchick, a fellow with the Foundation for Defense of Democracies, wrote in 2013, "The best thing the organization could do is dissolve—not because it is actively harmful, but rather because it is a victim of its own success." Others have made similar statements, criticizing GLAAD for being hypersensitive and too "politically correct" for an age of growing LGBTQ mainstreaming.

Some GLAAD critics also argue that the organization has moved too far away from its original mission and has instead developed a liberal bias. They point out that the organization has heavily criticized Fox News for discriminatory comments made about LGBTQ people on its shows but has failed to do so when the more liberal MSNBC has aired similar statements. GLAAD also was criticized after its former president Jarrett Barrios wrote a letter to the Federal Communications Commission in support of AT&T's purchase of rival T-Mobile—after AT&T had donated large sums of money to GLAAD.

Barrios was forced to resign from GLAAD in 2011, and the organization has since worked to improve its image across the political spectrum, working with religious leaders and other traditionally conservative groups. GLAAD leaders and supporters maintain that the organization remains relevant and important, especially in the areas of bisexual and transgender rights and representation, which lag behind those of gays and lesbians.

Terri Nichols

See also: Gay Rights Movement; LGBTQ+; Media and Sexuality; Shepard, Matthew.

Further Reading

GLAAD. (n.d.). Home page. Retrieved from http://www.glaad.org/

Kirchick, J. (2013, May). How GLAAD won the culture war and lost its reason to exist. *The Atlantic*. Retrieved from https://www.theatlantic.com/politics/archive/2013/05/how-glaad-won-the-culture-war-and-lost-its-reason-to-exist/275533/

GLMA: Health Professionals Advancing LGBTQ Equality

GLMA: Health Professionals Advancing LGBTQ Equality, or simply GLMA, is the newest name of the "world's largest and oldest association of lesbian, gay, bisexual, transgender, and queer (LGBTQ) healthcare professionals." Their mission is "ensuring health equity for lesbian, gay, bisexual, transgender, queer (LGBTQ) and all sexual and gender minority (SGM) individuals, and equality for LGBTQ/SGM health professionals in their work and learning environments. To achieve this mission, GLMA utilizes the scientific expertise of its diverse multidisciplinary membership to inform and drive advocacy, education, and research" (GLMA, 2018).

GLMA was founded in 1981, a time when community organizations' names tended to be less obvious about their mission in order to avoid harassment. The group was originally known as American Association of Physicians for Human Rights. Membership was initially open only to physicians, residents, and medical students. As the LGBTQIA+ movement has matured and become more visible and inclusive, the organization's identity and scope has evolved accordingly. The organization "came out" in 1994 and changed its name to Gay and Lesbian Medical Association (GLMA). In the years that followed, the group struggled between maintaining their established brand identity as GLMA and the perception as an organization exclusive of anyone not gay and lesbian. In 2012, the official name of the organization became GLMA: Health Professionals Advancing LGBT Equality. In 2018, the Q was added in LGBTQ to further broaden the outreach to queer-identified providers and individuals.

Despite the many shifts in name, GLMA has had a significant impact on public policy, clinical practice, and social perspective regarding sexual orientation and gender identity and expression, both for patients and providers.

A few examples of GLMA's accomplishments:

- Since 1982, GLMA's Annual Conference on LGBT Health has been the largest of its kind in the world.
- In 2007, GLMA codeveloped the Healthcare Equality Index with the Human Rights Campaign.
- In 2008, GLMS supported the quest for marriage equality by publishing a landmark research report, "Same-Sex Marriage and Health," which showed significant health disparities among families denied the right to marry.
- In 2010, GLMA initiated what became federal joint commission policy changes on hospital visitation and nondiscrimination.
- In 2012, GLMA filed an amicus brief supporting successful defense of the Affordable Care Act.

- In 2012, GLMA submitted a letter to Centers for Medicare and Medicaid in support of including sexual orientation and gender identity in electronic health records.

GLMA also provides several important resources for LGBTQ patients and providers, including an online directory to help patients locate LGBTQ-friendly providers in their area; an educational webinar series; and the biweekly *LGBT Health Digest*, which serves more than 6,000 subscribers. GLMA is also the parent organization to the Lesbian Health Fund (LHF), which supports research aimed at "improving the health of lesbians and other sexual minority women and their families" (GLMA, 2018). The total amount of funding LHF has awarded since its founding in 1992 is nearly $1 million.

C. Michael Woodward

See also: Gay Rights Movement; LGBTQ+; Same-Sex Marriage; World Professional Association for Transgender Health (WPATH).

Further Reading

GLMA. (2018). About GLMA. Retrieved from http://www.glma.org

GLMA. (n.d.). GLMA's impact. Retrieved from glma.org: http://www.glma.org/_data/n_0001/resources/live/Our%20Impact.pdf

GLSEN (Gay, Lesbian, and Straight Education Network)

GLSEN (Gay, Lesbian, and Straight Education Network) was formed in 1990 by teachers from Massachusetts who recognized that their LGBTQ+ students were often bullied and discriminated against, and so they wanted to improve the education system to make it better for those students. Since 1999, GLSEN has also been conducting research on LGBTQ+ issues in primary, middle, and high school. GLSEN's research staff are recognized throughout the country as trusted experts. Their research has been used to improve legislation and policy for LGBTQ+ students and has advocated for the presence of gay-straight alliances and other policies and resources in schools to build safe and respectful spaces. In addition, they also educate students and school staff about bullying and harassment, and they help to develop best practices and resources in order to create safe and affirming schools. Today, GLSEN is the leading national educational organization focused on ensuring safe schools for all students.

GLSEN works to change the pervasive problem of LGBTQ+ students being harassed at school because of who they are. One of the goals of GLSEN is to ensure that every student is valued and treated with respect in school, regardless of their sexual orientation, gender identity, or gender expression. They believe that a safe and positive school environment can help support and develop a positive sense of self, which in turn can lead to education achievement and personal growth. In order to accomplish this, GLSEN works with government, including Congress and the Department of Education, individual schools, and school districts to improve school environments and advocate for LGBTQ+ student issues, especially highlighting the negative effects that homophobia and heterosexism can have on students and schools. They also advocate for government funding to support all students in K-12 public school, including support for antiharassment policies, factual and evidence-based inclusive learning, and inclusive cocurricular and extracurricular activities.

GLSEN also creates school programs to help support the LGBTQ+ community. One example, the National Day of Silence, is a day when students from all across the country call attention to LGBT bullying and harassment in schools and the effects that this has on LGBTQ+ students. Another program, No Name-Calling Week, was inspired by *The Misfits*, a novel where students created a No Name-Calling Day at their school. GLSEN created this program to celebrate and promote kindness to create safe schools without name-calling, bullying, and discrimination. There are lessons and activities for grades K-12. Finally, Ally Week is a week for students of all sexual orientations to discuss and plan for how to become better allies to LGBTQ+ youth.

GLSEN welcomes all individuals who are committed to improving school climates and who value diversity within schools as members, regardless of sexual orientation, gender identity, gender expression, or occupation. GLSEN is governed by a national board of directors that establishes their mission, strategic aims, and public policy platform. The executive director and other delegates work together to develop and implement programs in line with the goals and mission of GLSEN.

Lauren Ewaniuk

See also: Gay-Straight Alliance (GSA); Sex Education.

Further Reading

GLSEN. (2017). Championing LGBTQ issues in K–12 education since 1990. Retrieved from https://www.glsen.org/

True Tolerance. (2017). Backgrounder: What parents should know about GLSEN. Retrieved from http://www.truetolerance.org/2011/what-parents-should-know-about-glsen/

Welcoming Schools. (2017). Creating safe and welcoming schools for all children & families. Retrieved from http://www.welcomingschools.org/

Gonorrhea

Gonorrhea is a sexually transmitted infection (STI) caused by the gram-negative bacterium *Neisseria gonorrhoeae*. It is a very common multistrain bacterial infection that can infect the penis, vagina, uterus, cervix, anus, urethra, eyes, or throat. The Centers for Disease Control and Prevention (CDC) estimate that nearly 820,000 new gonorrheal infections occur in the United States each year. The infection may be referred to colloquially as "the clap" or "the drip."

Gonorrhea bacteria live in the moist membranes of the urogenital tract as well as in the mouth and throat, eyes, and anus. It is typically transmitted through sexual contact by an infected partner. On rare occasions, touching the eye after touching an infected body part can cause transmission.

Ejaculation does not have to occur for the infection to be transmitted or contracted. Once a person has been infected by the bacteria, the typical incubation period is between two and five days, but the full range can be anywhere between one and eight days. It is also possible for gonorrhea to be passed from an infected pregnant female to the fetus during a vaginal birth. This can result in blindness, joint infection, or a blood infection in the newborn.

Many people with gonorrhea do not experience symptoms. Males with the infection are more likely to experience symptoms than females. Even when people do exhibit symptoms associated with gonorrhea, they are often mild and may be easily confused for a different vaginal or bladder infection.

Females with symptoms may experience painful or frequent urination, increased discharge that might turn yellow or green in color, vaginal bleeding between menstrual periods, painful intercourse, fever, vomiting, urethritis, and swelling of the vulva. Left untreated, the infection may cause cervicitis, and if the bacteria reach the bladder, it can cause cystitis.

Most males infected with gonorrhea develop symptoms, but they are typically mild. Initial symptoms often include a pus-like discharge from the urethra, reddening of the glans of the penis, and painful or frequent urination. Other common symptoms include painful erections, swelling and pain in the scrotum, and a low fever. If left untreated, the infection can spread to the urinary bladder, prostate gland, and epididymis.

People with an oral infection may experience a sore throat and itchiness. Anal infections can cause anal discharge, itching, soreness, bleeding, painful bowel movements, and potentially proctitis. If left untreated, the bacteria can enter the bloodstream, potentially inflaming the heart, brain, eyes, skin, spinal cord membranes, and joints.

Gonorrhea can be diagnosed by a health care professional in several ways. Discharge produced from the urethra, vagina, or anus may be tested, or cell samples collected from swabs may be taken from the penis, cervix, urethra, anus, or throat. These tests usually take about twenty-four to forty-eight hours. It is also possible to detect the infection through a urine test.

It is important to treat gonorrhea, as it can result in severe complications. In females, untreated gonorrhea can lead to pelvic inflammatory disease, which can affect a person's ability to get pregnant. In males, untreated gonorrhea can lead to epididymitis, which may cause infertility. In rare cases, people with untreated gonorrhea may develop disseminated gonococcal infection, which can cause arthritis and skin sores and potentially permanently damage joints.

Treatment for gonorrhea has changed as different strains of the infection have combatted commonly used antibiotics. For example, penicillin was the standard treatment until resistant forms dubbed "super gonorrhea" appeared in the 1990s. Fluoroquinolones may also be used, but a fluoroquinolone-resistant gonorrhea was discovered in Asia, the Pacific Islands, and California in the early 2000s. More recently, the CDC has recommended cephalosporin antibiotics; however, cephalosporin-resistant strains of gonorrhea have now also been found. Often, people with gonorrhea may also be infected with chlamydia, so many doctors prescribe dual antibiotics. Persons treated for gonorrhea should also be retested in six months.

Several measures can be taken to prevent contracting or transmitting gonorrhea. Abstaining from sexual intercourse will ensure no spread of the infection.

For sexually active individuals, using condoms and other barriers can greatly reduce the risk of transmission. Getting regularly tested for STIs can also help prevent the spread of the infection.

If someone has gonorrhea, treatment and partner notification can help prevent complications from the infection as well as transmission to others. Also, abstaining from sexual intercourse during treatment will ensure no spread of the infection or risk reinfection. According to the CDC, persons diagnosed or being treated with gonorrhea should tell all sexual partners within sixty days of the diagnosis or onset of symptoms.

Sarah Gannon

See also: Pelvic Inflammatory Disease (PID); Safer Sex; Sexually Transmitted Infections (STIs); Testing, STI.

Further Reading

Centers for Disease Control and Prevention. (2019). *Gonorrhea: CDC fact sheet (detailed version).* Retrieved from http://www.cdc.gov/std/gonorrhea/stdfact-gonorrhea-detailed.htm

Jones, R. E., & Lopez, K. H. (2014). *Human reproductive biology* (4th ed.). San Diego, CA: Academic Press.

Mayo Clinic. (2019). Gonorrhea. Retrieved from https://www.mayoclinic.org/diseases-conditions/gonorrhea/symptoms-causes/syc-20351774

Planned Parenthood. (2019). Gonorrhea. Retrieved from https://www.plannedparenthood.org/learn/stds-hiv-safer-sex/gonorrhea

Grafenberg Spot (G-Spot)

The G-spot, or Grafenberg spot, was named after Dr. Ernest Grafenberg (1881–1957), a gynecologist who described the "sensual potential" of this part of the anatomy during the 1950s. The G-spot was named in the 1980s and popularized by Beverly Whipple and John Perry in their book *The G Spot and Other Discoveries about Human Sexuality.* The G-spot is a very sensitive, erotic spot, located on the front wall of the vagina. It may be better described as a general area rather than as a specific spot. There is a lot of controversy over the existence of the G-spot.

The G-spot is located on the front wall of the vagina about one to three inches inside the vagina. It is a small, textured area that may be felt by the fingers and stimulated by fingers utilizing a "come hither" motion. Researchers hypothesize that this area is sensitive because the internal parts of the clitoris and the erectile tissue that surrounds the urethra meet in this area.

Another theory in regards to what makes this spot sensitive is that when the female body is aroused, the clitoris rises. This changes the angle of the stems of the clitoris inside the body, which may expose more nerve endings. Another theory offered is that the area is actually the area corresponding to the trigone of the bladder. Support for this theory comes from the fact that many people experience greater sensation in this area when the bladder is full. Many sex toys have been created specifically for the G-spot. While many people enjoy having this area stimulated, many others do not.

There is not a great deal of research on the G-spot in general, however, Beverly Whipple is most closely associated with researching this area. Many researchers question the existence of such a spot. In fact, in 2009, there was a *Journal of Sexual Medicine* debate on the topic held during the International Society for the Study of Women's Sexual Health Congress. During this debate, experts in the field of female sexuality were asked by researchers to form an opinion on the topic of the G-spot after given data to review. Some experts agreed the G-spot exists but note that it is not a consistent spot and may vary from person to person. Other scholars note the G-spot shows dynamic changes during stimulation and even allude to this spot being the source of stimulation that leads to female ejaculation, or "squirting." However, other scholars argue against the G-spot by discussing many contrasting findings on the topic.

In the past, most research about the G-spot was done on cadavers. Newer technology allows more thorough research to be done on living people; however, much more research is needed in order to understand more about this sometimes elusive spot.

Amanda Manuel

See also: Arousal; Clitoris; Erogenous Zones; Female Ejaculation; Orgasm; Sex Toys; Vagina.

Further Reading

Herbenick, D. (2012). *Sex made easy.* Philadelphia: Running Press Book Publishers.

Herbenick, D., & Stoddard, G. (2012). *Great in bed.* New York: DK Publishing.

Jannini, E. A., Whipple, B., Kingsberg, S. A., Buisson, O., Foldes, P., & Vardi, Y. (2010). Who's afraid of the G-spot? *Journal of Sexual Medicine, 7*(1), 25–34.

Joannides, P. (2012). What's inside a girl? *Guide to Getting It On* (6th ed., 77–105). Waldport, OR: Goofy Foot Press.

Whipple, B. (2015). Female ejaculation, G spot, A spot, and should we be looking for spots? *Current Sexual Health Reports, 7*, 59–62.

Green, Jamison

Jamison Green, PhD, is a well-known leader in the transgender rights movement. Since the early 1990s, Green has been an influential advocate for the transgender community through his publications, speaking engagements, consultation services, and membership on the board of multiple transgender and LGBT organizations of national and international renown. For nearly three decades, Green, who himself identifies as a transgender man, has made significant contributions to the field of transgender health and LGBTQ workplace equality.

Jamison Green was born female-bodied on November 8, 1948, in Oakland, California. He was adopted at one month old by a couple who wanted to raise a daughter, but he began showing signs of atypical gender development early in his life. In his website, Green recalled that he started refusing typical young girls' clothing before age two and, by the time he reached grade school, it became clear to him that he was different than other girls and boys. As a baby, Green was given female first and middle names, but in 1964, at the age of fifteen, he adopted the name Jamison and started going by the gender-neutral nickname Jamie. Although Green knew by his early twenties that he was transsexual, the social climate and stigma surrounding gender variance in the early 1970s prevented him from seeking out care from gender specialists and from pursuing legal gender change. It was then in his late twenties that he began living openly as lesbian and began a long-term relationship with a woman who would later become the mother of his two children. Although not legally male at the time, Green was listed as the father on both children's birth certificates. Green's romantic relationship with the mother of his children ended in 1989, but they remained close, as coparents, until her death in 2008. Other significant events in Green's life were his legal name change in 1991 and his marriage to Heidi A. Bruins (now Heidi B. Green), an instructional design consultant and political activist, in 2003.

Green received a bachelor degree in English in 1970 and a master of fine arts in English/creative writing in 1972, both from the University of Oregon, Eugene. He went on to pursue a career in technical writing, whereby he managed publications for various technology manufacturing companies and ultimately worked his way up to the level of vice president at a publicly held software publishing firm. His accomplishments as a professional writer extended to the fields of medical and legal writing as well—an experience that equipped him with valuable knowledge and skills he later applied to his work as an advocate for transgender people's rights. It was not until the early 1990s that Green began his earliest advocacy efforts, working with attorneys, legislators, and other policy makers to develop language regarding gender identity and expression as it relates to employment, housing, and public accommodation laws. In the 1990s, among other distinctions, he served as leader of FTMInternational—the world's largest advocacy organization for female-to-male individuals and their families—for eight years (1991–1999) and was influential in the establishment of the Transgender Protection Ordinance in San Francisco. In 1994, working alongside the San Francisco Human Rights Commission, he authored the *Report on Discrimination against Transgendered People*, which provided a comprehensive public evaluation of the experiences of transsexual and transgender individuals living in San Francisco. This report helped motivate city supervisors to pass legislation that added gender identity to the list of protected classes and led the Human Rights Commission to organize a group of volunteers from the transgender community to assist in providing sensitivity training to various social service agencies. Expanding his reach beyond social services, Green eventually became known as an expert on workplace gender nondiscrimination policies and practices and provided consultation services to various organizations, including major corporations and governmental agencies seeking to ensure compliance with state and local laws concerning gender identity.

The 2000s and beyond helped consolidate Green's visibility and influence as an advocate for transgender people's rights. His efforts helped establish new models for transinclusive workplace benefits and policies, which ultimately had effects on a national level, becoming adopted in 2002 as benchmarks by the Corporate Equality Index—a tool used to rate workplaces on LGBTQ equality. In 2004, Green published *Becoming a Visible Man*, an autobiographical analysis of the emerging transgender community, describing his own transition from living as a lesbian woman to affirming his identity as a bisexual trans man; and that same year, his book received the Sylvia Rivera Award for best book in Transgender Studies from the Center for Lesbian and Gay Studies and was a finalist for the Lambda Literary Award. In 2011, Green earned his doctorate (PhD) in equalities law from the Manchester Metropolitan University in England and became president-elect of the World Professional Association for Transgender Health (WPATH), an international and interdisciplinary professional organization that he had served as an elected board member since 2003. From June 2016 to the time of this writing, Green has served as president of the WPATH Executive Committee as well as chairperson and board of directors liaison of their ethics committee. He has also served on the boards of various other organizations, including Gender Education and Advocacy, the Transgender Law and Policy Institute, the Equality Project, and Trans Youth Family Allies.

Cristina L. Magalhães and Marissa A. Worth

See also: FTMInternational; Gender Identity; LGBTQ+; Transgender; Transsexual; World Professional Association for Transgender Health (WPATH).

Further Reading

Denny, D. (Ed.). (1998). *Current concepts in transgender identity.* New York: Garland Publishing.

FTMInternational. (2009). FTMInternational facts. Retrieved from https://www.ftmi.org

GLSEN. (2018). *Jamison Green: Transgender activist.* Retrieved from https://www.glsen.org/sites/default/files/Jamison%20Green%20Backgrounder.pdf

Green, J. (2004). *Becoming a visible man.* Nashville, TN: Vanderbilt University Press.

Green, J. (2008). *Jamison Green & associates: Education and policy consulting on transgender and transsexual issues.* Retrieved from http://jamisongreen.com

World Professional Association for Transgender Health. (2013). Home page. Retrieved from https://www.wpath.org/about/EC-BOD

Gynecomastia

Gynecomastia is an endocrine disorder that creates abnormal male breast tissue growth. It can affect one or both breasts and typically is seen in pubescent boys and older adult men as they undergo hormonal changes. Statistics show that the benign condition is quite common—some 50–60 percent of boys experience gynecomastia, and around 70 percent of men age fifty and older are also affected by this disorder. In addition, an estimated 60–90 percent of all male infants are born with gynecomastia; however, many of these children will never present any symptoms.

Although gynecomastia is typically more of an uncomfortable or embarrassing problem than a truly dangerous one, in some cases it can signal a more serious underlying issue. Some of these issues include kidney failure, liver failure, or malnutrition. More commonly, gynecomastia is caused by natural hormone changes that decrease the amount of testosterone in the system while at the same time increasing estrogen levels. In other instances, factors such as illicit drug and alcohol use, anabolic steroid use, and side effects from certain medications can trigger gynecomastia. Tumors in the pituitary or adrenal glands, or an overactive thyroid, may also cause the condition. And, in about 2 percent of gynecomastia cases, the disorder is caused by a testicular tumor.

A person affected by gynecomastia may be wholly asymptomatic, or they may experience swelling and tenderness in the breasts. Some people may notice that one breast is larger than the other. To diagnose the condition, a medical practitioner will conduct a physical exam and may recommend certain laboratory tests, including tissue biopsies or a magnetic resonance imaging exam. In some cases, blood tests will be conducted to check the blood hormone levels, or a doctor will advise studies of the liver and kidneys to look for underlying problems creating the gynecomastia. If the condition is caused by natural hormone changes, the body will most likely return to normal without medical intervention, and treatment is usually contained to ice packs and over-the-counter pain medications to relieve tenderness and swelling. Gynecomastia caused by puberty usually disappears within six months to two years without treatment, and gynecomastia in infants (due to higher estrogen levels in the mother) will generally go away in one to two weeks. If the condition does not improve on its own or if another underlying cause is determined, there may be further treatment required. Possible courses of action include hormone treatment to reduce estrogen levels, medication or surgery to shrink or remove a tumor, and surgery to remove excess breast tissue.

Gynecomastia has been a recognized disorder since the time of ancient Greece. It is thought that Galen of Pergamon, a second-century Greek physician and philosopher, was the first to introduce the term "gynecomastia" in medical references. Several different medical and surgical treatments of the condition were recorded throughout the 1800s, and treatment continues to evolve as new advances in medicine are made.

Tamar Burris

See also: Breast, Female; Estrogen; Testosterone.

Further Reading

Meletis, C. D., & Woods, S. G. (2009). *His change of life: Male menopause and healthy aging with testosterone.* Westport, CT: Praeger.

Watson, S., & Miller, K. (2004). *The endocrine system.* Westport, CT: Greenwood.

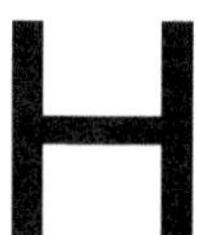

Hepatitis

Hepatitis is a virus that infects the liver. There are three common types: hepatitis A (HAV), hepatitis B (HBV), and hepatitis C (HCV). According to the Centers for Disease Control and Prevention (CDC), although the different strains may cause similar symptoms, they can affect the liver differently and have different modes of transmission. HBV is most likely to be transmitted through sexual contact and is the focus of this article. While HAV and HCV can be transmitted through sexual contact, it is rare, especially for HCV. According to the CDC, there are nearly 20,000 new HBV infections reported in the United States each year, but the actual number of infected individuals is expected to be much higher.

The virus lives in semen, vaginal fluid, blood, and urine and can be transmitted during sexual intercourse. It can also be spread by an infected pregnant person to their infant at birth. According to the CDC, nearly two-thirds of HBV cases are acquired through unprotected sexual intercourse. HBV can also be transmitted by sharing needles or syringes.

There are two types of HBV infection: acute and chronic. Acute HBV lasts less than six months. When it lasts longer, it becomes chronic. Chronic HBV can lead to severe liver infections. According to the Mayo Clinic, adults are more likely to develop acute HBV, while infants and children are more likely to develop chronic HBV. The CDC estimates that between 700,000 and 1.4 million individuals have chronic HBV in the United States. Globally, the number of persons infected with HBV is estimated to be approximately 240 million.

According to the CDC, approximately 70 percent of adults develop symptoms from HBV. Symptoms of acute HBV may appear between six weeks and six months after exposure. These symptoms typically last for a few weeks, but some people may have them for up to six months. Symptoms include extreme fatigue, fever, nausea, vomiting, loss of appetite, abdominal pain, headache, jaundice, joint pain, and dark urine or feces.

Individuals infected with chronic HBV may experience long-term health issues such as liver damage, liver failure, or liver cancer. The CDC estimates that 15–20 percent of people with chronic HBV develop serious liver conditions. They also estimate that approximately 2,000–4,000 people die each year from a HBV-related liver disease in the United States. Globally, this number is estimated to be about 786,000 deaths each year.

According to the CDC, there are different blood tests to diagnose HBV, and they may be ordered as a single test or multiple tests. These tests are designed to find antibodies or antigens in the body and may determine whether or not a person has an acute or chronic infection, has recovered from the infection, is immune to

HBV, is currently a carrier of the virus, or if they would be a good candidate for a vaccination.

The Mayo Clinic states that a doctor might also test samples from the liver to assess whether or not there is liver damage. This test involves the insertion of a thin needle under the skin and into the liver to remove a tissue sample. The sample is then taken to a laboratory for analysis.

There is no cure for HBV. However, most adults' immune systems clear the virus and develop immunity to it. When someone is diagnosed with acute HBV, rest, healthy nutrition, and fluids are often recommended. For those diagnosed with chronic HBV, there are several medications that have been developed to treat the virus and help slow down the process of liver damage.

For those who want to prevent contracting HBV, a vaccine for the virus has been available since 1981. It usually involves three to five shots over six months. The vaccination is more than 90 percent effective in all persons immunized before exposure to HBV. If a pregnant person has HBV, they can prevent passing the infection to the infant at birth through a series of vaccinations and hepatitis B immune globulin (HBIG) injections.

According to the Mayo Clinic, if someone thinks they have been exposed to the virus and have not been vaccinated, they can receive an injection of HBIG within twelve hours of exposure. This can help prevent development of HBV. For those who are not vaccinated, either abstaining from or using condoms during sexual intercourse can reduce the risk of transmission. Individuals should also refrain from using or sharing unclean needles or syringes. Partner notification can contain the spread of the virus.

Sarah Gannon

See also: Pregnancy; Safer Sex; Sexual Health; Sexually Transmitted Infections (STIs); Testing, STI.

Further Reading

Centers for Disease Control. (2019). *Viral hepatitis: Hepatitis B information.* Retrieved from http://www.cdc.gov/hepatitis/hbv/index.htm

Jones, R. E., & Lopez, K. H. (2014). *Human reproductive biology* (4th ed.) San Diego, CA: Academic Press.

Mayo Clinic. (2019). *Hepatitis B.* Retrieved from https://www.mayoclinic.org/diseases-conditions/hepatitis-b/symptoms-causes/syc-20366802

Planned Parenthood. (2019). *Hepatitis B.* Retrieved from https://www.plannedparenthood.org/learn/stds-hiv-safer-sex/hepatitis-b

Herpes

The human herpes virus (HHV) is commonly associated with sores or blisters on the lips and genitals. When these sores appear on the lips, they are generally called cold sores. There are eight types of herpes viruses: herpes simplex viruses (HSV) 1 and 2, HHV 3 (chicken pox/shingles), HHV 4 (mononucleosis or mono), HHV 5 (cytomegalo virus), HHV 6 (roseola virus), HHV 7, and HHV 8

(Karposi's sarcoma-associated herpes virus). HSV 1 and 2 are most commonly noted in sexual health classes as sexually transmitted infections because they can infect the mucoepithelial tissue (tender skin that is not mucus membrane). Herpes sores can appear on the lips and around the mouth, genitals, anus, and buttocks. It is commonly said that HSV 1 is oral herpes and HSV 2 is genital. However, either HSV strain can infect either area.

HSV 1 and 2 are contracted through skin-to-skin contact or contact with moist areas that may contain the virus (e.g., saliva or lip balm). When the virus comes in contact with mucoepithelial tissue, the virus travels down the nerve endings to the bundle of nerves called a ganglion. Oral herpes infections live in the trigeminal ganglia (by the temple on either side of the head), and genital herpes infections reside in the sacral ganglia (at the sacrum or base of the spine). It is possible to transmit the herpes virus through oral-genital or genital-genital contact when one of the partners is infected with the herpes virus.

During an outbreak, sores appear on or around the mouth, genitals, anus, or buttocks. Outbreaks can be caused by sunlight, trauma (being hit), irritation, stress, illness, hormones, or menstruation. The likelihood of an outbreak increases during illness because herpes is an opportunistic infection—it takes the opportunity to break out when the immune system is suppressed. The virus is able to be transmitted from a herpes sore during an outbreak. Transmission can also occur before a sore is present, when the skin feels tingly or a dull pain is present with no visible sore. Only about 10 percent of outbreaks are severe blisters. The majority of herpes sores are classified as small, itchy ulcers.

Many people have some form of the herpes virus. One estimate from 1999–2004 suggests that 60 percent of people have HSV 1, and about 20 percent of people have HSV 2. It is common for oral herpes infections to be transmitted in childhood. Family members with oral herpetic sores may kiss younger family members and transmit the virus unknowingly.

Because herpes is a chronic condition, herpes outbreaks are usually treated with suppressive drug therapy. Acyclovir, valacyclovir, and famciclovir are antiviral drugs that suppress the virus and prevent outbreaks. These drugs can be taken proactively (before an outbreak) or reactively (at the onset of pain or a sore). Taking the drugs proactively is the best way to limit transmission.

Despite the common prevalence of herpes and the relative ease of treatment, stigma about herpes still persists. The common belief that an individual's sex life is over once they contract herpes in the genitals can contribute to strong negative feelings upon diagnosis. The false belief that herpes ends a person's sex life is perpetuated by the lack of knowledge around how herpes works and treatment efficacy. As a reaction to herpes stigma, people who have been diagnosed with herpes have formed support groups and dating sites. Confronting social stigma with little-known facts about herpes can contribute to a better understanding of how herpes exists in our society and end harmful narratives that contribute to herpes misinformation.

Mark A. Levand

See also: Sexual Health; Sexually Transmitted Infections (STIs); Testing, STI.

Further Reading

Bradley, H., Markowitz, L. E., Gibson, T., & McQuillan, G. M. (2014). Seroprevalence of herpes simplex virus types 1 and 2—United States, 1999–2010. *Journal of Infectious Diseases, 209*(3), 325–333.

Hunt, R. (2005). Herpes viruses. In P. R. Murray, K. S. Rosenthal, & M. A. Pfaller (Eds.), *Medical microbiology* (5th ed.) New York: Elsevier Mosby.

Jones, R. E., & Lopez, K. H. (2006). *Human reproductive biology* (3rd ed.) Burlington, MA: Academic Press.

Margolis, T. P., Imai, Y., Yang, L., Vallas, V., & Krause, P. R. (2007). Herpes simplex virus type 2 (HSV-2) establishes latent infection in a different population of ganglionic neurons than HSV-1: Role of latency-associated transcripts. *Journal of Virology, 81*(4), 1872–1878.

Mertz, G. J. (2008). Asymptomatic shedding of herpes simplex virus 1 and 2: Implications for prevention of transmission. *Journal of Infectious Diseases, 198*(8), 1098–1100. doi: 10.1086/591914

Heterosexism

Heterosexism describes a behavioral system that denies, denigrates, and stigmatizes any nonheterosexual form of behavior, identity, relationship, or community. Heterosexism is often misused as synonymous with homophobia. However, heterosexism is the systemic display of homophobia within societal institutions, created through the assumption that the world is heterosexual and that heterosexuality is superior and normative. In the 1990s, queer scholars began referring to this as normative heterosexuality or heteronormativity. Heteronormativity illustrates the cultural dichotomy that exists between heterosexuality and homosexuality.

Heterosexism is analogous to sexism and racism, with similar parallels in the way it approaches issues in mainstream culture. Heterosexism uses the invisibility of homosexuality to minimize its existence while attacking it personally and institutionally when it becomes more visible. Historically, heterosexism has been found in large societal institutions like religion and law.

While sexuality has been a topic of conversation for centuries, terms such as "homosexuality" and "heterosexuality" are more recent. The term "heterosexism" was coined around 1972, coinciding with the publication of *Society and the Healthy Homosexual.* Two separate letters to the editor in the July 10 edition of an Atlanta newspaper, *The Grey Speckled Bird*, used the term to parallel the treatment and denigration of lesbian and gay individuals as similar to the treatments of other individuals based on their gender and race.

Development of this term continued throughout the 1970s and 1980s through lesbian-feminist writers who often focused on the layers of homophobic oppression through the prevalence of patriarchy, gender roles, and power relations. The original analysis of homosexuality derived through the lens of psychopathology, focused on homophobia as an attitude instead of focusing on systems' and institutions' treatment of LGBTQ+ people. Three of the most significant institutions that have exemplified heterosexism throughout history are (1) religion, (2) law, and (3) psychology and psychiatry.

Religion was one of the first institutions that perpetuated heterosexism through its views and teachings on sexuality. Throughout history, Christianity has long been one of the most dominant religions, and it has been verbal about its teaching on sexuality. Christian law has expressed antipathy toward three major aspects of sexuality: (1) nonprocreative sexual conduct (e.g., masturbation, contraception use), (2) marital sex only for sensual gratification (e.g., all intercourse positions beyond missionary), (3) and sex not sanctioned by (heterosexual) marriage (e.g., adultery, premarital sex). Sex that gay men engage in, historically known as sodomy, can be categorized underneath all three of these problematic areas.

Historically, Christianity commonly focused on the differences between *being* homosexual versus *acting* on homosexual desires. An individual could identify as homosexual, but acting on these desires or engaging in a relationship with a person of the same gender would be considered a sin. This viewpoint on homosexuality falls within the view of "love the sinner, hate the sin." Certain groups, such as white American Evangelical Protestant Christians, believe that those who openly identify as LGBTQ+ need to be helped to reach salvation or risk deprivation of civil liberties. Some white Evangelical Protestant Christians may participate in extreme antigay activist groups that attempt to disallow LGBTQ+ individuals from adopting, fostering, and working in certain child-centered careers.

The second major heterosexist institution is within law and criminalization. For centuries, many aspects of sexual deviance were considered a crime, including participation in homosexual behaviors. Originally, there were three forms of stigma surrounding sexuality-related concerns: laws prohibiting or restricting private sexual acts between consenting adults, laws specifically denying civil liberties to gay and lesbian individuals, and laws that reinforce power differentials (i.e., adult-child relationships). Laws prosecuting sodomy can be found as far back as the thirteenth century in France and Spain. After the colonization of the United States, legislation across the United States was created in the 1700s and 1800s and existed until 2003 in some parts of the country; some of these laws still remain on the books in some states. Statutes on sodomy were often written in Latin or described using phrases such as "the unmentionable vice" or "wickedness not to be named," insinuating the negative stigma associated with homosexuality.

Laws about sodomy have typically applied exclusively to men. Historically, if people were assumed or found to be participating in homosexual acts, they were imprisoned until cured, resulting in a loss of employment and ostracization from their families. Some exceptions to the poor treatment of homosexual men were allowed when it would benefit the country, as in American drafts for World War I. In the initial onset of World War I, homosexual men were allowed to participate as service men but were often asked not to share their sexual orientation. However, during World War II, stigma toward homosexuality increased, and, as the war dwindled and fewer people were needed for active duty, the country's view of homosexuality shifted from criminal or sinner to more of sexual deviant or psychopath. Homosexuality became an acceptable medical rationale for exclusion from service.

Heterosexism still exists within the U.S. legal system but to a lesser degree than before. Marriage equality was voted on in the United States Supreme Court in June 2015 and was approved with a 5–4 vote. Other legislation is still ongoing, especially legislation about workplace discrimination, rights for transgender individuals, and helping LGBTQ+ youth homelessness. There is still a lot of development that needs to happen to further assist LGBTQ+ individuals on a legal front. However, with views shifting away from criminality and illness, there has been a plethora of progress in passing new LGBTQ+-positive legislation.

During the nineteenth and early twentieth century, views of homosexuality changed from homosexuality as criminal activity to homosexuality as a pathology. Homosexuality was defined through the actions of the person, or "the homosexual," and was created to describe the opposition of normalcy. The focus of homosexuality as a pathology did not become solidified until the twentieth century. Researchers such as Havelock Ellis and Richard Krafft-Ebing were instrumental in making homosexuality a diagnosis in the *Diagnostic and Statistical Manual*, which reduced the amount of imprisonment of homosexuals but resulted in increased stigma around homosexuality as an illness. A comparison study between heterosexual and homosexual men, which found that there were no significant differences in the mental health status between the two groups, conducted by Evelyn Hooker in 1971, led to the removal of homosexuality as a clinical diagnosis in the *DSM-III* in 1973. Some level of heterosexism still exists among some therapists who attempt to perform conversion therapy, a type of therapy that seeks to change the sexual orientation of lesbian, gay, and bisexual people. Most therapeutic practices ban this type of treatment.

Kimberly A. Fuller

See also: Gay Rights Movement; Heterosexuality; Homophobia; Homosexuality; Religion, Diversity of Human Sexuality and; Sodomy Laws.

Future Reading

Herek, G. M. (2004). Beyond "homophobia": Thinking about sexual prejudice and stigma in the twenty-first century. *Sexuality Research & Social Policy, 1*(2), 6–24.

Herek, G. M., Chopp, R., & Strohl, D. (2007). Sexual stigma: Putting sexual minority health issues in context. In *The health of sexual minorities* (171–208). New York: Springer.

Heterosexuality

Heterosexuality is one of several sexual orientation categories used in popular media, mainstream culture, medicine, health, and research. The term "heterosexual" often refers to persons who report sexual attraction and affection toward persons belonging to "the other biological sex" or gender. Often used synonymously with the term "straight," heterosexuality denotes a sexual orientation identity in which a man is attracted to a woman or a woman is attracted to a man. Heterosexuality is an encompassing term that includes identity, identity management, sexual behavior, physiological arousal, and fantasies that one has toward a member of a different gender or biological sex. Given the various facets that construct heterosexuality, identifying exclusively as heterosexual does not preclude someone from having a same-sex experience or encounter. Relatedly, having a same-sex encounter does not necessarily mean someone identifies as gay, lesbian, bisexual, or queer. Recent research indicates that heterosexuality is typically a stable sexual orientation identity and tends to be more stable over time for heterosexual-identified men than for heterosexual-identified women. Heterosexual-identified individuals might also engage in heterosexual identity management practices, including conforming to gender norms and public displays of affection with members of the other sex.

Heterosexuality has been conceptualized using various philosophical paradigms, including essentialism, social constructivism, poststructuralism, and feminism, but the term "heterosexual" only entered into popular mainstream arenas during the late nineteenth and early twentieth century. Prior to the writings of Richard von Krafft-Ebing, Albert von Schrenk-Notzing, and Sigmund Freud, the term "heterosexuality" was not part of modern everyday vernacular, especially not as an identifying characteristic of one's sexual orientation. Furthermore, in Katz's (1995) historical review of the construct, heterosexuality was initially used to denote perverse and deviant sexual behaviors (i.e., sex for pleasure) versus behavior exclusively for procreative purposes. It was not until Freud normalized sexual identity development, and helped influence the ideology, that heterosexuality became the sociocultural and sexual "norm." To date, the "norm of heterosexuality" has been challenged, and many scholars agree that sexual orientation is fluid and resides more on a continuum than as a binary.

Similar to lesbian, gay, and bisexual identity development models, there have been recent attempts to articulate a model of heterosexual identity development. One such model contends that heterosexual identity is made up of both individual and social identity development processes. Both processes occur within the context of biology, gender norm socialization, culture, religion, sexual prejudice and stigma, privilege, and microsocial mandates (e.g., family, church). This model of heterosexual identity development also consists of five statuses: unexplored commitment (social mandates for acceptable gender and sexual roles), active exploration (intentional examination of one's own sexual needs, values, expression), diffusion (absence of examining one's own sexuality), deepening and commitment (entrusting to one's sexual needs, values, and expression), and synthesis (coming to a state of congruence). The model has yet to be empirically validated.

Franco Dispenza

See also: Biological Theories of Sexual Orientation; Fluidity, Sexual; Heterosexism; Kinsey's Continuum of Sexual Orientation; Sexual Identity; Sexual Orientation; Storms's Model of Sexual Orientation.

Further Reading

Davis-Delano, L. R., & Morgan, E. M. (2016). Heterosexual identity management: How social context affects heterosexual marking practices. *Identity, 16*(4), 299–318.

Katz, J. N. (1995). *The invention of heterosexuality.* Chicago: University of Chicago Press.

Mock, S. E., & Eibach, R. P. (2012). Stability and change in sexual orientation identity over a 10-year period in adulthood. *Archives of Sexual Behavior, 41*, 641–648.

Worthington, R. L., & Mohr, J. J. (2002). Theorizing heterosexual identity development. *The Counseling Psychologist, 30*, 491–495.

Worthington, R. L., Savoy, H. B., Dillon, F. R., & Vernaglia, E. R. (2002). Heterosexual identity development: A multidimensional model of individual and social identity. *The Counseling Psychologist, 30*, 496–531.

Hirschfeld, Magnus

Known fondly as the "Einstein of sex," Magnus Hirschfeld (1868–1935) was one of the most revolutionary sexologists of the early twentieth century. Alongside Havelock Ellis and Sigmund Freud, Hirschfeld paved the way for modern scientific sexuality studies. While most notable for his overabundant data collections, Hirschfeld contributed to the field in a plethora of ways. Prior to his work, most sexual research was essentially theoretical or based on considerably limited case samples. In an attempt to substantiate homosexuality as a natural variance of human behavior, his scientific explorations and social politics fashioned him the founding father of modern LGBTQ+ advocacy. As a gay cross-dressing man himself, his empirical research on LGBTQ+ prevalence afforded remarkably accurate statistics and pioneered Western interest in cross-gender behavior. Albeit modernly controversial, his original contrivance of the word "transvestite" was tailored to differentiate between cross-dressing persons and persons who were homosexual, as these concepts were widely misinterpreted as one and the same. Regardless of contemporary interpretation or notoriety, Magnus Hirschfeld's contributions to the field of sexology were undeniably revolutionary.

Having studied medicine at distinguished universities across Germany, Hirschfeld began his career in human sexuality by opening his very own medical practice for obstetrician sciences in Magdeburg, Germany, in 1894. Releasing activist publications under the pen name Ramien Hirschfeld, his earlier writings include a thirty-four-page pamphlet entitled *Sappho und Sokrates, Wie erklärt sich die Liebe der Mannër und Frauen zu Personen des eigenen Geschlechts?* (Sappho and Socrates, How Can One Explain the Love of Men and Women for Individuals of Their Own Sex?). He went on to publish a variety of influential materials and founded numerous renowned academic journals, conferences, and committees, including the world's first homosexual rights organization, *Wissenschaftlich-Humanitäre Komitee* (The Scientific-Humanitarian Committee), 1897; the first scholarly journal for scientific sexology, *Zeitschrift für Sexualwissenschaft* (Journal of Sexology), 1908; the provocative book unveiling his innovative terminology, *Die Transvestiten* (The Transvestite), 1910; his first comprehensive sexological work, *Naturgesetze der Liebe* (Natural Laws of Love), 1912; the compelling text *Die Homosexualität des Mannes und des Weibes* (Male and Female Homosexuality), 1914; the brilliant but prejudicially invalidated medical resource, *Sexualpathologie* (Sexual Pathology), 1917–1920 (Vol. 1–3); the illustrious *Institut für Sexualwissenschaft* (Institute for Sexual Research), 1919; and the wholly progressive and substantiating contribution of *The International Conference of Sexual Reform Based on Sexual Science*, 1921.

As a politically minded scientist, Hirschfeld worked endlessly to publicly validate sexuality as innate and not a deliberate choice. His introduction of the word "transvestite" sought to outline the essential differences between cross-dressing, homosexuality, and fetishism for uninformed outsiders, attributing diversity to the inspirational focus of each and not simply any observed comparable behaviors. Today, the word "transgender" would best represent the conceptual framework the term attempted to illustrate. Regardless, the word itself was quite ineffectual as it was not used again for decades until the works of Harry Benjamin, who is often mistaken as the original author. While Hirschfeld's theories expanded for years, he initially proposed homosexuals as a "third sex" (sexual intermediaries) in a way that might be better understood today as a form of transgender expression combined with same-sex attraction. He himself also believed that all persons were originally born bisexual, eventually losing interest in either sex over the course of one's life experiences. His efforts to depathologize atypical sexual behavior broadened to other prominent objections of natural expression, such as childhood sexuality and the curious explorations of adolescence. Hirschfeld reproached the condemnation of masturbation, believing the irrational fear of it to be far more dangerous than the act itself.

Although faulted with his own biases, such as a general lack of inherent objectivity in the conviction that homosexual persons were fundamentally more altruistic than their heterosexual counterparts, Hirschfeld dedicated his life to sexual reform in the name of equality. His Institute for Sexual Research alone was home to over 20,000 sexological books and journals; over 35,000 images and artifacts; and the first contraceptive clinic of Berlin, Germany. Ultimately, Nazi rioters destroyed the renowned institute in May 1933 when Hirschfeld was traveling to Paris for the latest newsreel. It was there that he watched the ghastly footage. Stripping the walls of his legacy bare, Nazi book burnings erased much of Hirschfeld's work. Seen as a "Jewish science," the Nazi party sought to prevent the corruption of a new Aryan nation from the "perverted" ideals of sexology. Such opposition would halt European sexological research for two decades, never salvaging lost chronicles. Fleeing for his life, Hirschfeld spent the next two years in France before he died at the age of sixty-seven on his birthday, May 14, 1935.

Ilyssa Boseski

See also: Antigay Prejudice; Benjamin, Harry; Bisexuality; Ellis, Henry Havelock; Freud, Sigmund; Gender; Gender Diversity; Heterosexuality; Homosexuality; LGBTQ+; Masturbation; Sexology; Sexual Orientation; Transgender; Transsexual; Transvestite.

Further Reading

Bullough, V. L. (1994). *Science in the bedroom: A history of sex research.* New York: BasicBooks.

Dose, R. (2014). *Magnus Hirschfeld: The origins of the gay liberation movement.* New York: Monthly Review Press.

Hooper, A., & Holford, J. (2004). *Anne Hooper's Sexology 101: From Victorian transvestites to '70's swingers and Internet Viagra.* Berkeley, CA: Ulysses Press.

Mancini, E. (2010). *Magnus Hirschfeld and the quest for sexual freedom: A history of the First International Sexual Freedom Movement.* London: Palgrave Macmillan.

Wolff, C. (1986). *Magnus Hirschfeld: A portrait of a pioneer in sexology.* London: Quartet Books.

Homophobia

Homophobia is considered to be the fear of gay, lesbian, bisexual, or queer people or same-gender sexual behaviors. Homophobia is believed to result from learning and reinforcement over the life span; tolerance and acceptance of sexual minorities are also considered learned behaviors. The development of negative attitudes is often the result of both explicit teachings in an individual's family, educational, or social setting (including some cultural and religious teachings) and implicit messages about the worth or characteristics of sexual minorities. Silence about sexual minorities' experiences and the invisibility of sexual minority role models may also contribute to the development of homophobia.

Homophobia may be externalized in the forms of negative words or actions expressed toward others or internalized by sexual minorities, primarily in the form of negative thoughts about one's identity or sexual behaviors. Homophobia has historically been considered one of the causes of antigay prejudice, and it has sometimes been assumed that those who express the highest levels of homophobia may be compensating for same-gender attractions. However, there is little empirical evidence to substantiate this assertion.

The study of homophobia is closely related to the study of antigay prejudice and discrimination. Over time, many researchers have shifted their paradigms and language from the concept of *homophobia* to that of *homonegativity*, negative attitudes toward sexual minorities that may or may not arise from fear. Thus, a person may experience or express homonegativity without experiencing a sense of fear (phobia), anxiety, or threat from sexual minorities. Emerging research on homophobia or homonegativity has also made distinctions among types of homonegativity. In traditional or classical homonegativity, individuals tend to express more explicitly negative sentiments or misperceptions of sexual minorities (e.g., "gay men can't be trusted around children"). Modern measures of homonegativity are designed to measure more subtle forms of negativity, such as the belief that sexual minorities make unreasonable demands on society (Morrison & Morrison, 2003).

Homophobia and homonegativity are often based on inaccurate or incorrect assumptions about sexual minorities, such as the misconception that sexual minorities may try to recruit others to same-sex behaviors, or a faulty assumption that sexual minorities are more likely than heterosexual-identified individuals to sexually abuse children. Neither of these assumptions is supported by research.

Researchers measure homophobia or homonegativity in the forms of attitude statements (e.g., "gay men are sick"), behaviors such as discrimination in employment and housing, or desire for social distance from sexual minorities (a preference to have a lesbian friend or family member or to have sexual minorities live outside one's community, for example). Homophobia and homonegativity are, however, difficult for social scientists to measure accurately, as researchers must often rely on self-report. Participants' responses to measures of homophobia often vary by the context in which the research is conducted (e.g., a conservative religious environment rather than a gay and lesbian community center), and research participants often respond in socially desirable ways to studies of this type. Further, it is difficult to rely on observational studies of homophobia, as it may be impossible to discern the motivations behind an individual's actions.

Overall, studies of homophobia and homonegativity show some cultural differences in attitudes, with several studies noting higher levels of homonegativity among African American adults than their European American peers. However, the two groups report similar levels of intent to discriminate (or to refrain from discrimination) against sexual minorities. Many studies have also reported gender differences in this area, with men reporting higher levels of homonegativity, particularly against gay men, than their female peers.

Very little research exists on the impact on heterosexual individuals in maintaining homophobic or homonegative attitudes. However, research on sexual minorities indicates that both homonegative statements and actions received from others and internalized homophobia can be damaging to mental health and increase the risk of depression, anxiety, substance abuse, sexual compulsivity, and partner violence.

Over time, homophobic and homonegative attitudes are becoming less common and less socially acceptable in many communities. Generational differences are often evident in studies of homonegativity, with adolescents and younger adults reporting more neutral or favorable attitudes toward sexual minorities than older adults.

Elizabeth A. Maynard

See also: Antigay Prejudice; Biphobia; Bisexuality; Heterosexism; Homophobia, Internalized; Homosexuality; Queer; Transgender; Transphobia.

Further Reading

Bieschke, K. J., Perez, R. M., & DeBord, K. A. (Eds.). (2007). *Handbook of counseling and psychotherapy with lesbian, gay, bisexual, and transgender clients* (2nd ed.) Washington, DC: American Psychological Association.

Dworkin, S. H., & Pope, M. (Eds.). (2012). *Casebook for counseling lesbian, gay, bisexual, and transgender persons and their families.* Alexandria, VA: American Counseling Association.

Morrison, M. A., & Morrison, T. G. (2003). Development and validation of a scale measuring modern prejudice toward gay men and lesbian women. *Journal of Homosexuality, 43*(2), 15–37.

Homophobia, Internalized

Homophobia is considered to be a fear of lesbian, gay, bisexual, and queer people or same-sex sexual behaviors. Internalized homophobia is the experience of this fear by a sexual minority person. The term suggests that the individual has taken in (internalized) a fear of sexual minorities from their environment, and they may hold negative beliefs and sentiments both toward the self and toward other sexual minorities. Mental health professionals have noted that internalized homophobia is widespread and may be a significant contributor to mental health problems among sexual minority clients.

Internalized homophobia is generally assumed to be the product of learning, both in childhood and across the life span. Homonegative statements and formal teachings are common across many cultural and religious groups, and most children and adolescents are exposed to these negative messages. Further, homonegativity may be reinforced by stereotyped portrayals of gay, lesbian, bisexual, and queer individuals; silence about sexual minorities in many communities; and an absence of positive role models. Misinformation about sexual minorities may also contribute to internalized homophobia/homonegativity. For example, generalizations of gay men as promiscuous, flamboyant, or pedophilic may increase an individual's negative sentiments.

While the term "homophobia" has been used for several decades to describe negative attitudes toward sexual minorities, the concept of homonegativity has been gaining wider acceptance among researchers and mental health professionals. While homophobia assumes that a person's negative sentiments or attitudes are based in fear, homonegativity describes negative sentiments and attitudes that may arise from any source. Thus, a person may be homonegative but not homophobic.

Research on internalized homophobia and homonegativity is less extensive than research on externalized homonegativity. This is due in part to difficulties creating reliable and valid measures of internalized homophobia. Further, most early studies of homonegativity focused on the attitudes and behaviors of participants who were presumed to be heterosexual. Thus, these studies measured attitudes toward members of a group perceived to be different from the self. Other studies have focused more on sexual minorities' experiences responding to others' prejudice and/or negative statements rather than on the phenomenon of negativity toward oneself.

Internalized homophobia/homonegativity may be difficult to detect. At the most explicit level, individuals may express disgust, unhappiness, or rejection of themselves due to their sexual orientation or sexual behaviors. Internalized homophobia may also be present in more subtle forms, such as not caring well for one's general or sexual health or not advocating for one's needs or rights in relationships. Some studies have noted correlations between internalized homophobia/homonegativity and depression, anxiety, substance abuse, partner violence, and compulsive sexuality. These studies suggest that sexual minorities who hold more positive and accepting views of themselves may be at lower risk for these and related mental health concerns.

Interventions to reduce or eliminate internalized homophobia/homonegativity may occur at both the individual and systems level. Many individuals find that individual or group counseling may promote greater levels of self-acceptance and self-care. Further, seeking out positive role models and critiquing stereotyped presentations of sexual minorities may also reduce internalized homophobia. Both sexual minority and majority members may engage in advocacy to address homonegative language and discriminatory policies and practices.

Recent research suggests generational differences in antigay prejudice, homophobia, and homonegativity, with adolescents and young adults expressing lower levels of homonegativity than older adults. Further, over the last thirty years, many cultural and religious groups have demonstrated increasing tolerance, acceptance, or celebration of sexual minorities and same-gender romantic and sexual relationships. Thus, more positive messages and welcoming communities are available than in the past. As overall levels of homonegativity decline in the United States and many other countries, internalized homophobia and homonegativity may also be expected to decline.

Elizabeth A. Maynard

See also: Antigay Prejudice; Biphobia; Bisexuality; Gay Affirmative Therapy; Heterosexism; Homophobia; Queer; Transphobia.

Further Reading

Bieschke, K. J., Perez, R. M., & DeBord, K. A. (Eds.). (2007). *Handbook of counseling and psychotherapy with lesbian, gay, bisexual, and transgender clients* (2nd ed.) Washington, DC: American Psychological Association.

Dworkin, S. H., & Pope, M. (Eds.). (2012). *Casebook for counseling lesbian, gay, bisexual, and transgender persons and their families.* Alexandria, VA: American Counseling Association.

Homosexuality

Homosexuality refers to a sexual orientation in which the individual is sexually attracted to other individuals of the same sex. The word "homosexuality" has a history of pathologization, and, as such, many people with a homosexual sexual orientation prefer to be referred to as gay or lesbian. Individuals who are sexually attracted to both people of the same sex and people of the other sex are referred to as bisexual.

Estimates of the prevalence of gay and lesbian sexual orientations generally range from about 2–15 percent of the population. The estimates vary widely, partly because surveys may use different criteria for describing same-sex behavior, attraction, or identity and partly because respondents may think of their own sexuality in different ways.

Many people have occasional sexual experiences with other individuals of the same sex—or they previously had such experiences—but they do not consider themselves to be gay or lesbian. For example, it is common for teenagers to experiment with same-sex activities, though most of these people are primarily or exclusively heterosexual as adults. In another example, some prison inmates report engaging in same-sex behavior because their preferred partners of the other sex are unavailable. However, when they are released from prison, many return to their previous heterosexual lifestyle.

Such facts about human behavior reveal that sexuality consists of an extremely complex and dynamic set of behaviors. A large U.S. survey (consisting of 13,500 men and women) published by the National Center for Health Statistics in March 2011 attempted to distinguish between various homosexual and bisexual behaviors and identities. According to the survey results, 2–4 percent of men and 1–2 percent of women reported their sexual identity as gay or lesbian. A bisexual sexual identity was reported by 1–3 percent of men and 2–5 percent of women. From 4–6 percent of men and 4–12 percent of women reported that they have had some same-sex sexual contact. (The ranges in percentages are due to the different ways in which the researchers classified the data, such as by age, race, year of response, and other factors.)

Although the causes of homosexuality are not fully understood, the general scientific consensus is that it is primarily congenital—people are born that way. A team of American and British researchers reported in 2014, based on their genetic analysis of 409 pairs of homosexual brothers, that sexual orientation may be influenced by certain kinds of genetic mutations (changes) on two chromosomes—chromosome 8 and the X chromosome. Exactly how these genetic factors may influence sexual orientation is not known.

Other research has indicated that part of a brain region called the hypothalamus is smaller in gay men than in straight men. This part, called the sexually dimorphic nucleus, seems to be a similarly small size in gay men and in women compared with its relatively larger size in straight men.

Among the most important functions of the hypothalamus is to receive signals from the nervous system that prompt it to secrete substances called neurohormones, which, in turn, regulate the secretion of hormones by the pituitary gland. Thus, if the hypothalamus is associated with sexual orientation, it is possible that the brains of gay people may regulate hormone activity differently than the brains of straight people. The physical development of the hypothalamus itself is affected by hormonal chemical reactions as the fetus grows inside the womb. However, much more research is needed to understand how (and if) this process occurs.

Some psychologists believe that an individual's social experiences, upbringing, and other environmental factors may influence sexual orientation or expression. If true, that could mean that complex combinations of both environmental and biological processes influence an individual's sexual orientation.

When considering the causes of homosexuality, it is important to keep in mind that same-sex behavior is not exclusive to the human species. Same-sex behavior has also been observed in a wide array of animal species, including apes, monkeys, dolphins, sheep, albatrosses, geese, and certain insects.

The gay and lesbian populations have certain health care issues that are of special concern compared with the heterosexual population. Gay and lesbian people often experience social and political violence and discrimination, which can contribute to symptoms of anxiety and depression. They may also be more likely to have problems with substances. A major health concern among gay, bisexual, and other men who have sex with men is the human immunodeficiency virus (HIV), which, if left untreated, can progress to acquired immunodeficiency syndrome (AIDS). When first discovered in the 1980s, HIV/AIDS was almost always fatal. However, since then, much progress has been made in treatment and prevention, and many individuals living with HIV today live long and happy lives with the use of highly active antiretroviral medications.

In the past, homosexuality has been viewed as a form of mental illness, both by the public and by mental health experts. That view began to change during the early twentieth century as psychiatric experts, including Sigmund Freud and Havelock Ellis, argued that homosexual people did not have a pathological condition. (Freud actually proposed that all people were innately bisexual.) In the 1940s and 1950s, the pioneering sexuality researcher Alfred Kinsey revealed that homosexual and bisexual activities were much more common than previously thought—including among supposedly heterosexual people.

Despite the advances in scientific and medical knowledge, the idea of homosexuality as an illness to be cured remains ingrained in more conservative and traditional parts of society. In so-called gay conversion therapy, people unethically attempt to convert the homosexual orientation of a patient to a heterosexual orientation. Some individuals claim that this therapy helped them to become "straight." However, most psychiatric experts condemn this type of therapy as useless and dangerous to the mental health of patients. Instead of trying to convert gay and lesbian people, most therapists try to help those struggling to accept their sexual orientation through gay affirmative therapy.

Throughout world history, different cultures have held varying views on homosexuality. In ancient Greece, male same-sex relations, particularly between a young man and an older man, were apparently favored over heterosexual relations—though they did not supplant heterosexual relations. Similar attitudes existed in ancient Rome, where many older men had younger male lovers. These men, however, were not strictly "homosexual." Most were married to women and had children. Rather, ancient societies simply accepted same-sex activities along with heterosexual activities as part of the spectrum of human sexuality. In addition to Greece and Rome, a number of other ancient "pagan" societies also either encouraged, or at least widely accepted, same-sex behavior.

In Western societies, those liberal, broad-minded sexual attitudes changed as Christianity cemented its power throughout Europe during the Middle Ages. Traditional Judeo-Christian teachings condemn homosexuality as immoral, sinful, and unnatural, as do traditional Islamic teachings. In those intolerant times, homosexuals had to hide their sexual orientation or be subject to severe punishment, even death. Such antigay attitudes persisted for many centuries and became institutionalized into laws.

Although social attitudes and laws were harsh, those ideas could not eliminate same-sex behavior and orientations. Homosexuality is simply a part of the mosaic of human nature—it always has been, and it always will be. Over time, gay and lesbian people became more forceful in fighting for their rights through various political and advocacy organizations—and eventually a cultural shift was affected.

During the late twentieth and early twenty-first century, homosexuality became increasingly accepted into the "social mainstream" in most developed nations in Europe, parts of Asia, and the Americas, including the United States. This cultural shift can be attributed partly to continued advances in scientific knowledge about human sexuality. It can further be attributed to the widespread recognition of gay rights as a form of civil rights, somewhat akin to the U.S. civil rights movement for African Americans in the 1950s and 1960s and the women's liberation movement in the 1960s and 1970s.

In the United States, Canada, many European and South American countries, as well as other socioeconomically advanced nations, laws have been passed to ban discrimination against gay and lesbian people in employment, housing, and other activities. Furthermore, in many of these countries, same-sex marriages or civil unions (with legal rights similar to marriage) have been legalized. Sadly, gay and lesbian people continue to be subject to social discrimination and legal punishment, and in some extreme countries, this can still include the death penalty.

A. J. Smuskiewicz

See also: Antigay Prejudice; Asexuality; Bisexuality; Ellis, Henry Havelock; Freud, Sigmund; Gay Affirmative Therapy; Gay Rights Movement; Heterosexuality; Homophobia; Homophobia, Internalized; Kinsey, Alfred; LGBTQ+; Same-Sex Attraction and Behavior; Sexual Orientation; Ulrichs, Karl.

Further Reading

American Psychological Association. (2019). Sexual orientation & homosexuality. Retrieved from https://www.apa.org/topics/lgbt/orientation

Chandra, A., Mosher, W. D., Copen, C., & Sionean, C. (2011). Sexual behavior, sexual attraction, and sexual identity in the United States: Data from the 2006–2008 National Survey of Family Growth. *National Health Statistics Reports, 36*, 1–36. Retrieved from http://www.cdc.gov/nchs/data/nhsr/nhsr036.pdf

Herek, G. M. (2012). Facts about homosexuality and mental health. Retrieved from https://psychology.ucdavis.edu/rainbow/html/facts_mental_health.html

LeVay, S. (2011). *Gay, straight, and the reason why: The science of sexual orientation.* New York: Oxford University Press.

Norton, E. (2012). Homosexuality may start in the womb. *Science.* Retrieved from http://news.sciencemag.org/evolution/2012/12/homosexuality-may-start-womb

Hooker, Evelyn

Evelyn Gentry Hooker (1907–1996) was a psychologist who overcame many obstacles to earn a doctorate in psychology and work in the field when women were not welcomed in academia. Evelyn was one of nine children born into a poor Nebraskan family. She grew up in Colorado, and her mother encouraged her to get an education, as she had not been able to do so herself. Evelyn did well in school, despite some social ostracism due to her nearly six-foot height, and earned a scholarship to the University of Colorado Boulder. In 1924, she began her studies there and earned a living by working as a maid. She majored in psychology and became passionate about her study of the subject.

After completing her undergraduate degree, she was offered an instructorship at the university, which enabled her to continue her studies and earn a master's degree. When she completed her degree, her mentor, Karl Muenzinger, encouraged her to apply for a doctoral program at an eastern university. The psychology department at Yale turned her down, as they did not want a woman in the program. Instead, she attended Johns Hopkins University in Baltimore, where she earned her doctorate in 1932. After which, she was offered a teaching position at a small women's college near Baltimore and worked there for two years. At that point, she contracted tuberculosis, and friends supported her to recuperate at a sanitarium in California. As she recovered, she took a part-time position teaching psychology at Whittier College. She then received an anonymous fellowship to study clinical psychology in Europe. This was just before World War II, and Evelyn witnessed some of the extreme forms of oppression coming from totalitarian regimes in Germany and Russia. The experience in Europe deepened her concern to work for social justice.

After her return to California, she applied for a position at UCLA. They turned her down because, as the chairman of the psychology department said, they already had three women who were "cordially disliked." Instead, she was offered a job as research associate in the psychology department of the extension division at UCLA. She remained there doing research until 1970. Of special significance is the groundbreaking work she did with gay males. In 1945, one of her students,

Sam From, met with her after class and told her that he was homosexual and that he very much enjoyed her class. Over time, Evelyn and her first husband socialized with Sam and his friends. Evelyn spent time with more homosexual people in social settings, enjoying conversations and discussing world events. After some time, Sam challenged her to scientifically study "people like him."

At the time, homosexuality was classified as a mental illness in the *Diagnostic and Statistical Manual* (*DSM*) of the American Psychiatric Association. Gay men were not allowed to work in government jobs or in the military, and homosexual behavior was illegal. Most research on gay men was based on those who had been in treatment with a mental health professional, not on gay men who were living their lives without mental illness. Sam's challenge to Evelyn was to find out if homosexuality really was an illness. She was intrigued by the question and felt compelled by her experience witnessing the effects of persecution in Europe in the 1930s and discrimination in her own personal and professional life. Her proposed research program was especially risky as she applied in 1953 for the National Institute of Mental Health (NIMH) grant during the height of the extremely conservative McCarthy era. There were simply no scientific data about nonimprisoned, nonpatient homosexuals. By this time, Evelyn had divorced her first husband and married Edward Hooker, a professor of English at UCLA, and taken his surname.

Against the odds, Evelyn was given the six-month NIMH grant, and to ensure confidentiality, she conducted the research out of her home. She found thirty gay men through the network of Sam's friends and through the Mattachine Society, one of the first organizations of gay men in the United States. She also recruited thirty heterosexual men for comparison. The groups were matched in age and IQ and were equal in educational levels. Evelyn administered three standard personality tests to the two groups. She took all the identifying information off each participant's score sheets and had three expert clinicians examine her results. Unaware of the subjects' sexual orientation, the three men could not distinguish between the two groups based on the test results. And they found no apparent pathology among the gay participants.

Her research, "The Adjustment of the Male Overt Homosexual," was published in 1957. This landmark study showed that homosexuals were not inherently abnormal and that there was no difference between the pathologies of homosexual and heterosexual men. When it was published, it was controversial, but it was validated soon thereafter by other investigators. She continued to study homosexuality through the 1960s and was asked to lead the NIMH Task Force on Homosexuality. The Task Force produced a report in 1969 that said that homosexuality should be considered neither pathological nor criminal. The report and her earlier studies became a crucial element in the decision to have homosexuality removed from the *DSM-III* in 1973. This meant that homosexuality was no longer classified a mental illness.

At the age of sixty-three, Evelyn retired from research and started a private practice in Santa Monica. Most of her clients were gay men and lesbian women. In her later life, she would be awarded the Distinguished Contribution in the Public Interest Award by the American Psychological Association. The University of

Chicago opened the Evelyn Hooker Center for Gay and Lesbian Studies in her honor. She died at her home in Santa Monica, California, in 1996, at the age of eighty-nine.

Michael J. McGee

See also: Diagnostic and Statistical Manual of Mental Disorders (*DSM*); Homosexuality; Mattachine Society; Sexology.

Futher Reading

Floyd, J. Q., & Szymanski, L. A. (2007). Evelyn Gentry Hooker: The "hopelessly heterosexual" psychologist who normalized homosexuality. In E. A. Gavin, A. Clamar, & M. A. Siderits (Eds.), *Women of vision: Their psychology, circumstances, and success* (177–188). New York: Springer.

Kimmel, D. C., & Garnets, L. D. (2000). What a light it shed: The life of Evelyn Hooker. In G. Kimble & M. Wertheimer (Eds.), *Portraits of pioneers in psychology* (Vol. 4, 252–267). Washington, DC: American Psychological Association.

Sears, B., Hunter, N., & Mallory, C. (2009). *Documenting discrimination on the basis of sexual orientation & gender identity in state employment.* Los Angeles: The Williams Institute.

Hookup Culture

Hooking up is a form of noncommitted sexual activity, prominent in sexuality literature since 2000, with much research characterizing it as confined to young adulthood. The college atmosphere fosters hooking up, establishing a "hookup culture" where hooking up is the dominant way people experience intimacy. Not only are hookups a common way to establish intimate relationships but students are unlikely to recognize other alternatives, which powerfully underlies the commonness of hooking up.

Describing the ubiquity of the hookup culture, researchers Wade and Heldman (2012) refer to hooking up as hegemonic, which means that the practice of hooking up seems inescapable: many individuals will partake because they see no alternative, even though hooking up may not be their personal preference. Wade and Heldman also describe elements of the hookup scene that have become normalized, such as the expectation of college as a place to seek out sexual exploration and the anticipation of male partners putting pressure on females. The popularity of these beliefs among college students makes these behaviors seem common and unproblematic, which encourages hooking up. Situating this within larger cultural changes, such as more liberal university policies regarding dormitories as well as the "pornification" of the culture and its resulting increase in self-objectification, it can be seen that these elements combine to promote hooking up.

Hookups have been defined differently throughout both the academic literature and mainstream publications, yet most characterize hookups as noncommitted intimate interactions. Some scholars refer to hookups as a casual sexual encounter that occurs only one time, between strangers, without the expectation of a long-term relationship. Others define hookups more broadly, as a sexual experience ranging from kissing to intercourse between people not in a committed relationship.

In college, gendered expectations frame choices for males and females differently. Modern women are expected to want and enjoy sex, but the sexual double standard persists and shapes the enactment of sexuality for young women. The vagueness of the term "hooking up" can thus protect the woman's reputation. The "strategic ambiguity" of the term allows men to earn status by emulating hegemonic masculinity and women to perform emphasized femininity as a way of living up to gender ideals.

Within hookup culture, men have a wider range of behaviors that are considered appropriate. Women are assumed to be more relationship-oriented and emotional, they are often seen as the object of pleasure, and they are judged more harshly for their sexual choices. Notions of masculinity, especially in college, tell men that they are expected to want sex, seek sex, and engage in it without emotional consequence. These views characterize women as a vehicle for male pleasure devoid of subjectivity. This complicates things for young men who seek an emotional connection to a sex partner or who desire a committed relationship and for women, who may doubt the sincerity of a young man's desire for a relationship. Perceptions that "all men" want sex and "all women" want relationships shape the sexual double standard and may operate in hookup culture.

Hookup culture research centers on heterosexual college students. Future studies should include bisexual, gay, and transgender voices. In addition, investigations of sexuality outside college and among older adults are needed to gain a full understanding of the extent of hookup culture.

Rachel Kalish

See also: Casual Sex; Dating; Double Standards, Sexual; Friends with Benefits; Intimacy, Sexual and Relational; Online Dating.

Further Reading

Bogle, K. A. (2008). *Hooking up: Sex, dating and relationships on campus.* New York: New York University Press.

Crawford, M., & Popp, D. (2003). Sexual double standards: A review and methodological critique of two decades of research. *Journal of Sex Research, 40,* 13–27.

Currier, D. M. (2013). Protecting emphasized femininity and hegemonic masculinity in the hookup culture. *Gender & Society, 27,* 704–727.

Heldman, C., & Wade, L. (2010). Hookup culture: Setting a new research agenda. *Sex Research and Social Policy, 7,* 323–333.

Wade, L., & Heldman, C. (2012). Hooking up and opting out: Negotiating sex in the first year of college. In L. M. Carpenter & J. DeLamater (Eds.), *Sex for life: From virginity to Viagra, how sexuality changes throughout our lives.* New York: New York University Press.

Hormone Replacement Therapy

Hormone replacement therapy (HRT), sometimes called hormone treatment, usually refers to the restoration of the female sex hormones estrogen and progesterone in women whose ovaries have stopped producing these chemical substances. In most cases, the therapy is meant to relieve unpleasant symptoms that many middle-aged women experience before, during, and after menopause, the time when menstrual periods stop and the natural production of these hormones lessens. The final menstrual period typically happens sometime between age forty-five and fifty-five.

In the years leading up to menopause, levels of estrogen start to decrease in the body. In approximately 75 percent of women, the falling estrogen levels lead to recurring hot flashes, characterized by feelings of heat spreading over the face and body and by sweating. Sudden chills may follow the hot flashes. These feelings often occur at night, making it difficult to sleep. Falling estrogen levels also commonly lead to dryness and irritation of the vagina, causing much discomfort, especially during sexual intercourse. The dryness makes the vagina more prone to infection. Still other changes that commonly occur during and after menopause are frequent shifts in mood, weakening of the bones (known as osteoporosis), and increased risk for cardiovascular disease.

The gradual changes associated with menopause typically happen over a period of seven to ten years. Some women are able to deal with these changes on their own, considering them to be a natural part of the aging process, and they do not seek HRT. However, other women find the changes so unpleasant that they seek HRT to help relieve the symptoms.

Estrogen is the main hormone that needs to be replaced to relieve the worst symptoms of menopause. However, studies have shown that the use of estrogen alone in HRT increases the risk of uterine cancer. The addition of progesterone or progestin, a synthetic form of progesterone, reduces this risk, so women who still have their uterus are usually prescribed both hormones. Women who have had a hysterectomy (surgical removal of the uterus) may receive only estrogen in HRT. The hormones used in HRT can be administered in different ways, including pills, skin patches, gels and sprays applied to the skin, vaginal rings (devices inserted into the vagina), and intrauterine devices (which are inserted into the uterus).

Many physicians had previously believed that long-term HRT could help prevent several diseases in postmenopausal women, including osteoporosis, heart disease, Alzheimer disease and other forms of dementia, and certain cancers. Those beliefs were contradicted in 2002 by a comprehensive study reported by the U.S. National Institutes of Health (NIH), which found that neither estrogen-only HRT nor estrogen-and-progesterone HRT were effective at preventing most of these diseases—except for osteoporosis, colon cancer, and (with estrogen-only HRT) breast cancer. The NIH study further revealed that HRT might actually raise the risks of gallbladder disease, liver disease, blood clots, stroke, heart attack, and (with combined HRT) breast cancer—especially if the therapy is extended over several years. Risks were found to be greatest the later in life that women started HRT.

Because of these health risks, many physicians now discourage the use of HRT or urge only limited, short-term use of HRT for managing hot flashes and other menopausal symptoms. These doctors recommend limiting HRT to the lowest possible doses for the shortest possible time period—a few months to a few years. Any woman taking HRT should receive regular checkups and screenings for breast cancer and other potential diseases associated with the therapy.

There are a number of alternatives to HRT for managing the symptoms of menopause. Antidepressant medications can help reduce the severity and frequency of hot flashes. Lubricants can relieve vaginal dryness. Medications called bisphosphonates, together with a regular exercise regimen, can reduce the bone-loss effects of osteoporosis.

Some people believe that certain kinds of phytoestrogens (estrogen-like compounds derived from plants) and synthetic estrogen-like compounds may offer some of the advantages of HRT without the disadvantages of real estrogen. These estrogen-like compounds are often referred to as bioidentical hormones. However, there is little scientific evidence to support the effectiveness or safety of these products.

In addition to HRT given to women to counter the effects of menopause, HRT may also be used by transgender people during their gender transition process. Trans women are given forms of estrogen to make their bodies develop female characteristics, such as breasts and smooth, hairless skin. By contrast, trans men are given testosterone, the male sex hormone, to make their bodies develop male characteristics, such as facial hair. Various forms of hormone treatments are also used to treat people with certain types of cancer. For example, some people with prostate cancer are given both estrogen- and testosterone-blocking hormones as part of their treatment.

A. J. Smuskiewicz

See also: Estrogen; Gender Transition; Menopause; Progesterone; Sex Hormones; Synthetic Hormones; Testosterone; Testosterone Replacement Therapy.

Further Reading

American College of Obstetricians and Gynecologists. (2018). The menopause years. Retrieved from https://www.acog.org/-/media/For-Patients/faq047.pdf?dmc=1&ts=20191114T1611432976

Hormone replacement therapy. (2019). Retrieved from https://www.nhs.uk/conditions/hormone-replacement-therapy-hrt/alternatives/

Mayo Clinic. (2018). Hormone therapy: Is it right for you? Retrieved from http://www.mayoclinic.org/diseases-conditions/menopause/in-depth/hormone-therapy/art-20046372

Hot Flashes

Hot flashes are brief feelings of intense warmth in the body. They can also be accompanied by redness or blotching of the skin, perspiration, and increased heart rate. On their own, hot flashes are not an illness. Rather, they are typically a symptom of hormonal conditions and are most commonly due to menopause, the time in a female's life when levels of estrogen decrease and menstrual periods stop. Around 70 percent of menopausal women experience hot flashes.

The exact cause of hot flashes is not yet understood, but it is believed that they occur due to combined factors that include changes in the reproductive hormonal system along with increased sensitivity in the hypothalamus, which regulates the temperature of the body. Hot flashes can last anywhere from a few seconds to several minutes and usually begin with an uncomfortable warmth that spreads from the head or chest area throughout the rest of the body. They are most common at night but can occur at any time of day. Some people experience up to ten or more hot flashes in a twenty-four-hour period.

Although they are often viewed as a hallmark characteristic of menopause, hot flashes can also occur in males. In older men, the decline in reproductive hormones (testosterone) is more gradual than in women, which prevents many from experiencing hot flashes. However, some men, particularly those with prostate cancer, are more susceptible to hormonal imbalances and hot flashes. Research conducted at Harvard University showed that 70–80 percent of men with prostate cancer who have received a specific type of treatment called androgen deprivation therapy suffer from hot flashes. Hot flashes can also be a side effect of certain medications and other illnesses, such as tumors in the endocrine system.

Hot flashes are typically diagnosed through a physical exam and discussion with a medical practitioner. If there are other symptoms along with the hot flashes or the cause seems unclear, a doctor may recommend blood tests to check for hormonal imbalances and other conditions. There are a wide variety of treatments for hot flashes, including taking estrogen through hormone replacement therapy (HRT), acupuncture, and supplementing with botanical herbal remedies like black cohosh. For many years, different derivatives of HRT were the only treatments approved by the Food and Drug Administration (FDA); however, in June 2013, the FDA approved the first nonhormonal treatment in the form of paroxetine, a pharmaceutical antidepressant. Around the same time, findings in a new study suggested that scientists think they have pinpointed the exact locations in the brain where menopausal hot flashes begin, which may lead to more advanced treatment down the road. At this time, none of the known treatments cure hot flashes, but they can be useful in diminishing the frequency and intensity of the warm spells. Most who experience menopausal hot flashes will see this symptom gradually disappear after a few years even without medication or treatment; in males, the symptom takes longer to subside.

Tamar Burris

See also: Estrogen; Hormone Replacement Therapy; Menopause; Perimenopause; Sex Hormones.

Further Reading

Gannon, L. R. (1985). *Menstrual disorders and menopause: Biological, psychological, and cultural research.* Westport, CT: Praeger.

Gillespie, C. (1989). *Hormones, hot flashes, and mood swings: Living through the ups and downs of menopause.* New York: Harper Perennial.

Lerner-Geva, L., Boyko, V., Blumstein, T., & Benyamini, Y. (2010). The impact of education, cultural background, and lifestyle on symptoms of the menopausal transition: The Woman's Health at Midlife study. *The Journal of Women's Health, 19,* 975–985.

McCain, M. V. E. (1991). *Transformation through menopause.* Westport, CT: Praeger.

National Institutes of Health. (2016). *Menopausal hormone therapy information.* Retrieved from www.nih.gov/health-information/menopausal-hormone-therapy-information

North American Menopause Society. (2019). Menopause 101: A primer for the perimenopausal. Retrieved from https://www.menopause.org/for-women/menopauseflashes/menopause-symptoms-and-treatments/menopause-101-a-primer-for-the-perimenopausal

Human Immunodeficiency Virus (HIV)

The human immunodeficiency virus (HIV) is a virus that attacks and weakens the body's immune system, making it difficult for people to fight everyday infections and diseases. If left untreated, HIV can progress to acquired immune deficiency syndrome (AIDS); however, it is important to distinguish that HIV is not AIDS and that most people living with HIV who have access to HIV medication will never develop AIDS.

Globally, HIV is a serious public health epidemic. In 2018, there were approximately 38 million people living with HIV, and approximately 1.7 million new cases were diagnosed. Anyone can get HIV regardless of age, sex, gender, or sexual orientation. HIV can be passed through contact with bodily fluids that contain the virus, including blood, semen and preejaculate fluid, rectal fluid, vaginal fluid, and breast milk. As such, HIV can be sexually transmitted. It can also be transmitted through sharing needles or other substance use equipment used to inject drugs; sharing needles used for tattooing, body piercing, or acupuncture; or during pregnancy, birth, or breastfeeding. HIV cannot be passed by shaking hands, hugging or kissing, coughing or sneezing, or by using swimming pools, toilet seats, or water fountains.

There is currently no cure for HIV; however, there are very effective medications called highly active antiretroviral therapy (HAART) that allow people living with HIV to live long and healthy lives and prevent the virus from being passed to others. In order to best treat HIV, early diagnosis is important. Everyone should have an HIV test performed, and those who engage in behaviors that may expose them to HIV, such as having new or multiple sexual partners or sharing substance use equipment, should test more regularly.

There are several ways to prevent passing or acquiring HIV sexually. Condoms remain an important tool as they prevent the transmission of the virus. A new condom must be used for every new sexual experience. In addition, people who are living with HIV and who take their medication as prescribed cannot pass on the virus. New research has shown that when people living with HIV take their medication, the virus becomes undetectable in their blood and so cannot be passed on to anyone else (Undetectable=Untransmittable, U=U).

New medications have also been developed for people who are not living with HIV to take in order to protect themselves from acquiring the virus. Preexposure prophylaxis (PrEP) is a medication that when taken daily, or for several days ahead of a potential exposure to HIV (for example before having condomless anal sex with an unknown sexual partner), is highly effective at preventing HIV acquisition. Unfortunately, this mediation is not yet available in all areas, and if it is available, it may be very expensive. Because of the potential for this new medication to eliminate the spread of HIV, public health agencies are calling on governments and other organizations to make this medication freely and widely available to everyone who may be at risk for HIV.

In addition, if someone is not taking PrEP and they suspect that they may have been exposed to the virus, they should go immediately to their doctor in order to begin a course of postexposure prophylaxis. This involves taking an HIV medication every day for twenty-eight days in order to help prevent HIV acquisition.

Given advances in HIV treatment and prevention, the end of the global HIV epidemic should be in sight. However, essential medications and prevention techniques are not available in all places and, if available, can be very expensive. Also, because of HIV stigma and discrimination, many people fear being tested and so may unknowingly be living with HIV. This is problematic for the individual as they will not be receiving treatment that can improve their health and well-being, and it is problematic for any of their sexual partners who may be unknowingly exposed to the virus. Using condoms, taking HIV medication as prescribed if living with HIV, and using prevention techniques like PrEP are the key to eliminating HIV around the world.

Heather L. Armstrong

See also: Acquired Immunodeficiency Syndrome (AIDS); Safer Sex; Sexually Transmitted Infections (STIs); Testing, STI.

Further Reading

CATIE. (2019). The basics. Retrieved from https://www.catie.ca/en/basics

Centers for Disease Control and Prevention. (2019). HIV. Retrieved from https://www.cdc.gov/hiv/default.html

Eisinger, R. W., Dieffenbach, C. W., & Fauci, A. S. (2019). HIV viral load and transmissibility of HIV infection: Undetectable equals untransmittable. *Journal of the American Medical Association, 321*(5), 451–452.

National Health Service. (2018). Overview: HIV and AIDS. Retrieved from https://www.nhs.uk/conditions/hiv-and-aids/

UNAIDS. (2019). 90-90-90: Treatment for all. Retrieved from https://www.unaids.org/en/resources/909090

Human Papillomavirus (HPV)

Human papillomavirus (HPV) is the most common sexually transmitted infection (STI) in the United States. Approximately 20 million Americans are currently infected with HPV, and there are six million new cases diagnosed each year. HPV is so common that at least 50 percent of sexually active people will be infected with the virus during their lifetime, with some estimates as high as 75–80 percent, or three out of every four people.

HPV is a virus that belongs to the papillomavirus family. There are almost two hundred known types of HPV, with the majority causing no symptoms in most people. However, several types can cause warty growths on the surface of the skin known as common warts, which tend to occur on the hands, or plantar warts, which occur most often on the feet. In addition to these types of HPV, there are approximately forty HPV types, known as genital HPV, that can be passed through sexual contact and infect the genital areas, which includes the vulva, vagina, cervix, rectum, anus, penis, or scrotum. Fortunately, in up to 90 percent of cases of HPV infection, the body's immune system is able to naturally clear the HPV infection within two years, and as a result, most people infected with HPV are asymptomatic and never know they were infected. It is the HPV infections that are persistent and not able to be cleared that are the ones that typically can lead to problems, including genital warts and cervical, penile, anal, or oropharyngeal (mouth and throat) cancer, depending on the type and location of the virus.

Genital HPV infections are often classified as either low risk or high risk, depending on their ability to cause cancer. The low-risk HPV types can cause genital warts, which are also known as condyloma, and include types 6 and 11. Genital warts can grow inside and around the opening of the vagina, the vulva, cervix, penis, scrotum, thigh or groin, and in or around the anus. Rarely, these warts can grow in the mouth or throat of a person who has had oral sex with an infected partner or in a child exposed to the virus in the birth canal at the time of delivery. The size of the warts may vary from being so small that they are not visible with the naked eye and are often flat and flesh colored, to large clusters or groups of bumpy, raised, cauliflower-like growths. Symptoms may include itching, burning, and discomfort.

The high-risk HPV types are the ones that cause cancer, most commonly cervical cancer. The types of virus that most commonly cause cervical cancer in the United States include types 16 and 18, which cause 70 percent of the cases of cervical cancer each year. HPV types 31 and 45 also cause cervical cancer but are much less common. It is important to understand that having high-risk HPV does not mean that an individual has cancer but rather that it can lead to cancer. This is why it is so important to have regular follow-up visits with a doctor (usually a gynecologist or urologist), so any changes on the cervix, or anus, can be detected on a Papanicolaou (Pap) smear, which is used to screen for cervical and anal cancer in developed countries.

Other types of HPV that are considered to be high risk include those types linked to other types of cancer, including cancers of the penis, vulva, vagina, anus, and throat and mouth cancers (known as oropharyngeal cancer, which includes the back of the throat, tonsils, and base of the tongue). Those who smoke are at a higher risk of developing cervical cancer.

Of the two hundred types of HPV that are known, approximately forty are transmitted through the anogenital tract (the vulva, vagina, cervix, anus, and penis). The virus is normally transmitted through sexual activity, including genital-genital contact (intercourse), oral-genital contact (oral sex), and anal-genital contact (anal sex). Transmission by routes other than sexual intercourse is much less common for genital HPV (such as finger-genital contact) but is a possible source of transmission. Sharing contaminated objects, like sex toys, may also be another source of transmission, as the virus is capable of living on an inert object for extended periods of time.

In order to understand how HPV causes infection, it is important to understand the types of cells the HPV virus infects. These cells are called keratinocytes, and they make up 95 percent of the cells located on the epidermis, or outer layer of the skin. The major function of the epidermis is to act as a barrier against environmental damage from things like bacteria, viruses, fungi, parasites, heat, ultraviolet radiation, and loss of water. If a pathogen does invade the outer layers of the epidermis, the keratinocytes react by producing various substances that help the immune system fight the offending pathogen. Keratin, which is a protein that is produced by the keratinocytes, helps to thicken the keratinocyte, forming more of a physical barrier. This process is known as cornification, and once the keratinocytes become fully cornified, they are shed and replaced by new cells. The average turnover time for this to occur is twenty-one days.

Keratinocytes are also located along the surface of certain mucous membranes, which are responsible for absorbing various nutrients and secreting certain chemicals. These keratinocytes occur along the outermost layer of these mucous membranes, which is known as the squamous layer, and are found in the mucosa of the mouth, throat, esophagus, and anus of the digestive tract; the cornea and conjunctiva of the eye; the cervix and vagina of the genital tract; and the urethra of the urinary tract.

Because genital HPV is passed by skin-to-skin and genital contact, it is most often spread during vaginal and anal sex. The virus cannot bind to live tissue, instead infecting epithelial tissues through microabrasions (tiny cuts or tears in the skin) or other skin trauma. The infectious process can take as long as twelve to twenty-four hours, and it can take weeks, months, or even years following the initial contact with a person who has HPV to develop warts or abnormal changes of the cervix. The virus can survive for many months and at low temperatures without a host, making it even more difficult to determine when the exposure occurred. It is possible to be infected with more than one strain of HPV, and this risk increases with a greater number of sexual partners.

Perhaps the most challenging aspect of HPV infection is that the vast majority is silent, meaning there are no symptoms. Most people have no idea they are infected with HPV until they develop warts or cancerous changes, and even these signs are often noticed only by a clinician performing an exam. Cervical cancer frequently has no symptoms but may cause an abnormal vaginal discharge or bleeding after intercourse. This is one reason the regular Pap smear is so important. The primary screening tool for detecting cervical HPV infection is done in conjunction with the Pap smear. People who have receptive anal sex should also have regular anal Pap smears. Certain changes occur in the outer layer of the cells of the cervix and anus (known as squamous epithelial cells) when these cells are infected by HPV, and they become known as koilocytes. Cellular changes include things like a large nucleus that stains darker and a halo or light area around the nucleus.

In addition to these microscopic changes, there is also an FDA-approved test that can be done to test for HPV DNA and is known as a hybrid-capture test. This test can be done at the same time as a Pap smear using a liquid-based cytology, where, instead of smearing the cervical or anal cells directly onto a slide at the time of collection, the cells are placed in a liquid-based medium and then transported to the lab where they are processed and then placed onto the slide for review. This allows the person reviewing the slide, known as a cytologist, a better, clearer view of the cells and also allows for HPV testing to be done. HPV testing can detect the DNA of the eighteen HPV types that most commonly affect the genitals and can distinguish between the low-risk and high-risk HPV types but is unable to determine the specific HPV type. HPV testing is recommended for those patients who are aged thirty and older and for those patients needing a follow-up to an abnormal Pap smear to help determine who is considered to be at greatest risk for developing cancer before there are any visible changes to the cells. Those patients who have a negative HPV test and a negative Pap smear are at very low risk of developing cancer and therefore can have less frequent screenings. HPV testing is currently not recommended for those younger than thirty since HPV infection is so common and usually resolves on its own. This helps to prevent any unnecessary procedures from being done to the patient that may lead to problems later in life, including pregnancy-related complications due to cervical incompetence and possible miscarriage or preterm delivery.

HPV cannot be directly treated with antiviral medicines. However, conditions caused by HPV can be treated. Treatment depends on which subset of HPV disease is present—genital warts or precancerous (or cancerous) changes.

For genital warts, there are two broad types of treatment: self-applied creams or gels and physician-based treatment. Treatments done by a physician include cryotherapy, or freezing off the wart; application of an acid that helps to burn off the wart; electrocautery, which destroys the wart using an electrical current; laser therapy, which vaporizes the wart; and surgical removal.

Treatment of cervical or anal dysplasia (abnormal cell growth) depends on the type of dysplasia present. An abnormal Pap result does not mean the patient has cancer but only that some abnormal cells have been found. It often takes years before abnormal cells can become cancer, and cells that are only mildly abnormal may go away on their own. Additional testing is usually necessary to follow an abnormal Pap smear, which may include a repeat Pap smear in six to twelve months, an HPV test, or a more detailed exam of the cervix, called a colposcopy, with or without a biopsy. If the follow-up results confirm the presence of high-risk HPV, whether through HPV testing or if moderate to severe dysplasia or greater is confirmed on biopsy, then treatment may be necessary. This involves removing the abnormal cells, either by ablation (vaporizing the abnormal cells with either laser therapy or cryotherapy, which freezes the abnormal cells) or excision (cutting out the abnormal cells using either a scalpel or cold knife, using a laser or a hot knife, or a procedure known as a loop electrosurgical excision procedure, which uses a fine wire loop with an electrical current to excise the abnormal portion of the cells.

As there is no medical cure for HPV, it is best to prevent the infection. There are currently HPV vaccines available to protect against the types of HPV that are the cause of most cancer and warts. The vaccines are made up of virus particles, not live or attenuated, so it is not possible to acquire any HPV-related infections at the time of vaccination. The HPV vaccines are recommended for all people ages nine to twenty-six, as the vaccine is most effective if it is given before any sexual activity, and consequently potential HPV exposure, has occurred. The vaccine can also be given in later adulthood to prevent future infection. The vaccines are typically given as a series of shots over approximately six months. Vaccine side effects are minimal and include pain and redness at the injection site, nausea, headache, and dizziness. It is important to know that the vaccine does not replace the need to wear condoms to lower the risk of getting another type of HPV that is not included in the vaccination or another STI. Condoms cannot fully protect against HPV infection, as a condom may not cover all of the infected area. The vaccine has not been proven to be effective against HPV infections that are already present from past exposure. It is important to know that those who receive the HPV vaccine should continue to have routine cervical or rectal screenings, since 30 percent of HPV-related cancers are caused by HPV types other than type 16 or 18.

During pregnancy, genital warts may grow in number and size due to the suppression of the immune system, which naturally occurs during pregnancy. Treatment is usually delayed until after childbirth to see if the warts will go away on their own. The majority of the time, the warts do not become problematic during pregnancy and thus do not tend to cause any complications. Most children born to someone with an HPV infection also tend not to have any complications due to HPV. Rarely, warty growths occur in an infant's throat following an exposure to a large amount of the virus, so a C-section might be recommended in the event that there is a very large amount of the virus present due to an extreme number or size of warts. This is done both to help minimize exposure to the baby and to help minimize trauma to the birth canal, as this tissue can be very difficult to repair in the event of a cut or tear, which can occur at the time of delivery.

Lori Apffel Smith

See also: Cervical Cancer; Genital Warts; Penile Cancer; Sexually Transmitted Infections (STIs); Testing, STI.

Further Reading

The American College of Obstetricians and Gynecologists. (2019). Pap smear (Pap test): Resource overview. Retrieved from https://www.acog.org/Womens-Health/Pap-Smear-Pap-Test

The Anal Cancer Foundation. (2019). About HPV/HPV & cancer. Retrieved from https://www.analcancerfoundation.org/about-hpv/hpv-cancer/

Centers for Disease Control and Prevention. (2019). Human papillomavirus (HPV). Retrieved from https://www.cdc.gov/hpv/

Centers for Disease Control and Prevention. (2019). HPV vaccine schedule and dosing. Retrieved from https://www.cdc.gov/hpv/hcp/schedules-recommendations.html

Office on Women's Health. (2019). Human papillomavirus. Retrieved from https://www.womenshealth.gov/a-z-topics/human-papillomavirus

Hyde Amendment

The Hyde Amendment banned the use of certain federal funds to pay for abortion. Currently, the only exceptions to the rule are if the pregnancy is the result of rape or incest or if the mother's life is in danger. The Hyde Amendment is a provisional "rider" rather than a permanent law, meaning that it must be renewed yearly as part of the annual Department of Labor or Department of Health and Human Services appropriations bill. With that, the language of the amendment is liable to change each time it is adopted, and there have been several years in which the amendment has either failed to pass or has gotten close to failing.

Antiabortion advocate Rep. Henry Hyde (R–Ill.) sponsored the original Hyde Amendment in response to the landmark 1973 *Roe v. Wade* decision legalizing abortion. It passed the House of Representatives with a vote of 207–167 on September 30, 1976, but due to controversy surrounding the constitutionality of such a ban, the Hyde Amendment did not actually go into effect until 1980. Although the language in the original amendment did not allow for any exceptions, arguments in Congress eventually led to a compromise and the possibility of funding in cases of rape, incest, and life-threatening situations was added to the provision in the late 1970s; however, between 1981 and 1989, the exceptions of rape and incest were temporarily removed from the legislation. With the possibility of changes annually, these exceptions were then reinstated in the 1990s with the understanding that they may once again be vetoed in any annual review.

Because the Hyde Amendment mostly affects abortions funded by Medicaid and is thought to be the only such medical procedure ever to have been fully banned from the comprehensive health care program, opponents of the provision argue that it unfairly targets low-income people who are unable to pay for abortions out of pocket. As a result of the legislation, it has been stated that one in four low-income women who would choose abortion are forced to carry a baby to term due to their financial situation. The lack of federal funding for abortions created by the amendment has also resulted in many state governments allocating precious state resources to abortion services instead of other services, either voluntarily or through court-ordered requirements.

Although the Hyde Amendment itself affects only funding through the Department of Health and Human Services, by the 1980s it had become a model for other, similar amendments to legislation governing funding through several government programs. For example, health programs through the U.S. Armed Forces no longer fund abortions, and programs for Peace Corps volunteers and Native American health care services also do not fund abortion services.

Tamar Burris

See also: Abortion Legislation; *Roe v. Wade*.

Further Reading

Haney, J. (2009). *The abortion debate: Understanding the issues*. Berkeley Heights, NJ: Enslow Publishing, LLC.

McBride, D. E., & Keys, J. L. (2018). *Abortion in the United States: A reference handbook*. Santa Barbara, CA: ABC-CLIO.

Rubin, E. R. (1998). *The abortion controversy: A documentary history*. Westport, CT: Praeger.

Yarnold, B. M. (1995). *Abortion politics in the federal courts: Right versus right*. Westport, CT: Praeger.

Hymen

The hymen is a thin membrane that partially covers the opening of the vagina. It is present in most—but not all—human females at birth. If it is present, it might be torn during the first sexual intercourse. However, the hymen can also be torn prior to sexual intercourse. Thus, contrary to popular belief, the presence or absence of a hymen is not necessarily associated with virginity.

The hymen, which is named after the ancient Greek god of marriage, has no known biological function. It varies in size, shape, and thickness between people. One common shape is the form of a half-moon along the rear edges of the vagina, leaving a vaginal opening about the width of a finger—wide enough for the monthly menstrual fluids to leave the body. Other hymens may be attached to the front or side edges of the vagina in ways that form other shapes. As long as the opening is sufficiently large to allow menstrual bleeding and tampon use, the hymen is considered "normal."

If the hymen is present during the first sexual intercourse, it typically separates from the vaginal walls and is torn during insertion of fingers, penis, or sex toy into the vagina. The tearing of tissue may lead to temporary minor pain and bleeding, which is no cause for concern. The hymen can also separate from the vaginal walls as a result of strenuous physical exercise that causes the tissue to stretch excessively, such as riding a bicycle or horse. Other ways in which the tissue can be perforated include the insertion of a tampon and masturbation. In some cases, the hymen tears for unknown reasons.

As the absence of a hymen is not proof of the lack of virginity, the presence of a hymen is not necessarily evidence of virginity. Some women have a hymen that is so flexible or small that it remains intact after sexual intercourse. An intact hymen may need to be surgically removed if still present during pregnancy so that it does not block the passage of the baby through the vagina.

Some people have hymens with excess tissue that causes problems with inserting or removing tampons or may obstruct menstrual bleeding. For example, an imperforate hymen completely covers the vaginal opening, blocking the release of menstrual fluid. The blocked fluid builds up inside the vagina, leading to the development of an abnormal mass and pain in the abdomen or back. Individuals with this condition may also experience pain or discomfort when they urinate or defecate.

A microperforate hymen has only one, or perhaps a few, tiny openings in its tissue. The openings may not be large enough to allow normal menstrual bleeding. An individual with this condition may be unable to insert a tampon, or, if it can inserted, it may be difficult to remove. A septate hymen has one or more bands of tissue running across the vagina to create two or more small vaginal openings rather than one. Such conditions also make it difficult to insert and remove a tampon.

Minor surgery can correct all these problematic conditions by removing the excess tissue to create a larger vaginal opening.

The mistaken belief that the absence of a hymen is proof of sexual intercourse can have serious social consequences for a woman. In cultures that place a high value on female virginity prior to marriage, such as those in strict Islamic countries, the discovery that a woman who is expected to be a virgin lacks a hymen could lead to divorce, public humiliation, or even execution. To avoid such consequences, some women resort to a surgical procedure called hymenoplasty, in which hymen tissue is restored or created.

A. J. Smuskiewicz

See also: Hymenoplasty; Vagina; Virginity.

Further Reading

Center for Young Women's Health. (2019). Types of hymens. Retrieved from http://youngwomenshealth.org/2013/07/10/hymens

Roye, C. (2008, December). Hymen mystique remains intact in bare-all culture. *Women's eNews.* Retrieved from http://womensenews.org/story/media-stories/081203/hymen-mystique-remains-intact-in-bare-all-culture#.VAiUXl6Viu4

Hymenoplasty

Hymenoplasty, also known as hymenorrhaphy, is a cosmetic, surgical repair of the hymen, otherwise known as reconstruction surgery for the hymen. The hymen is a layer of tissue that covers the vagina. The membrane typically has one or more openings that allow for the use of tampons and for menstrual blood to flow. This opening will get larger during sexual intercourse or childbirth; however, the hymen can also tear or rip during intense physical activity, masturbation, or tampon use. Some women are also born without a hymen. The hymenoplasty procedure involves repair and reconstruction of the hymen so that it appears to be back to a pretorn, "virgin-like" state. There is minimal recovery time where a woman must refrain from certain activities that might interfere with the healing process. Such activities include riding a bike, swimming, and engaging in intercourse. There are many different motivations why a woman would elect to have this surgery. Some women might want to have a hymenoplasty in order to appear as a virgin with a partner, to help recover from sexual abuse or trauma, or to enhance sex with a partner. Despite the reasoning for the surgery, it is elective and not covered by insurance, meaning the cost would have to come out of pocket.

The actual hymenoplasty procedure is fairly simple, and patients should experience little to no surgical complications. To begin the process to see if a patient is a potential candidate for the procedure, consultations and gynecological exams are required. Potential hymenoplasty patients must be at least eighteen years old and cannot have any sexually transmitted infections or genital cancers. Before surgery begins, the patient is given a local anesthesia. During surgery, a plastic surgeon sews up torn skin from the hymen to appear as though it is still intact. The procedure takes less than an hour to complete. Some common side effects are swelling, bruising, pain, bleeding, or numbness. The recovery time is minimal, and a typical patient is able to return to normal activities within a few days; however, it is not recommended to engage in strenuous activities while the incision is healing. Strenuous activities include things like riding a bike or intense cardio. Dissolvable stitches are commonly used when undergoing a hymenoplasty, and there should be little to no scarring from the procedure if there are no complications. A patient may engage in sexual intercourse eight weeks after the surgery.

Even though a hymenoplasty may seem like an unnecessary or superficial procedure, there are a few reasons why the procedure can help ensure a woman's safety and improve self-image. One reason why a woman may wish to undergo a hymenoplasty is because she is required to be a virgin until her wedding night, often because of religious or family beliefs. In many cultures, the viability of the hymen determines whether the woman is a virgin prior to being wed. After the consummation of the marriage, the mother of the bride will check to see if the sheets have blood on them, to prove that the bride has refrained from sexual activities prior to the wedding night. If it is determined that the tissue was previously torn and not intact prior to the night of the wedding, many cultures will shame the bride and consider her impure. Because of this disgrace, an individual may seek out the assistance of a doctor to surgically repair her hymen. Normal pain and bleeding will occur once the hymen is torn again during intercourse, so her partner will not know that she is not a virgin. If a woman is not a virgin on her wedding night in some cultures she might be isolated, beaten, exiled, or killed. In these cases, having a hymenoplasty can be life-saving. In countries where it is widely believed that a woman must be a virgin until her wedding night, there are many plastic surgeons that specialize in doing hymenoplasty procedures. There is debate about whether hymenoplasty procedures are considered ethical when deception is involved, such as if a woman is having the surgery to deceive a partner into thinking she is still a virgin. Whether someone thinks that this intent is wrong or not, it is still ultimately the woman's and the doctor's decision whether the procedure will happen. Feminist activists have spoken publicly about the need for hymenoplasty procedures because of the safety and sexual freedom aspects. There is a need for this type of surgery in many cultures for a multitude of situations that range from safety to trust.

It is also important to note that bleeding or lack thereof does not mean that the hymen is or is not intact. As individuals are becoming more educated on the hymen, the views on virginity and hymens are changing. Although it is difficult to change traditions, many have expressed that using the hymen as an indicator of virginity should be a thing of the past.

There have also been testimonials from women who have undergone a hymenoplasty to spice up the relationship with their significant other. The procedure can make a woman feel "revirginized," which can add a layer of excitement to a relationship. Some women have expressed that they get this procedure because they want to lose their virginity to their current partner instead of the person they originally lost it to, or because their hymen was previously torn by vigorous exercise, masturbation, or even tampon use. Finally, this procedure can be done to increase sexual pleasure. By tightening the hymen, many have claimed that the sexual experience is much more enjoyable than prior to the surgery.

Another reason why a woman may choose to have a hymenoplasty is because of rape or abuse. If a woman's hymen is torn from being raped or abused, it can be very traumatic and a constant reminder of the trauma. Having a hymenoplasty after experiencing such trauma can help a woman during the healing process, which can help when recovering from the abuse. Sexual abuse survivors who have their hymens repaired may feel as though they have a fresh start to sexual independence and freedom.

There are other alternatives to a hymenoplasty. Those who cannot afford the high price of this procedure can buy an artificial hymen. This cheaper alternative comes with fake blood within a prosthetic membrane. The membrane is inserted into the vagina twenty minutes before sexual intercourse, and when it is penetrated it will start to bleed, giving the illusion that the original hymen has been broken. This mock hymen can be purchased online and discretely shipped. If one is looking to improve sexual experiences, there are other surgeries that tighten vaginal muscles. Laser vaginal rejuvenation is a treatment that uses lasers to heat the inside of the vaginal walls, thus tightening the entire vaginal cavity, including the hymen. It is important to note that the hymen will not return to its virgin-like state; however, it appears to tighten up. Another alternative is vaginoplasy, plastic surgery of the vagina. During a vaginoplasty, the surgeon will tighten the vaginal muscles, which also brings in the hymen. Similar to laser vaginal rejuvenation, the vaginoplasty will not completely repair the hymen, only bring it closer together, which may help to improve the overall sex life of an individual.

Casey T. Tobin

See also: Double Standards, Sexual; Hymen; Vagina; Virginity.

Further Reading

Aquirre Specialty Care. (2019). Hymenoplasty. Retrieved from https://www.ascdenver.com/aguirre-specialty-care-services/cosmetic-gynecology/hymenoplasty/

Center for Young Women's Health. (2013). What can make the hymen break? Retrieved from https://youngwomenshealth.org/2013/07/31/hymenbreak/

Chozick, A. (2015, December 15). Virgin territory: U.S. women seek a second first time. *The Wall Street Journal.*

Lybrate. (2019). Hymenoplasty: Procedure, cost, risk, recovery and hymenoplasty surgery side effects. Retrieved from https://www.lybrate.com/topic/hymenoplasty

Zikalala, Z. (2018, April 21). Why women are opting to get their virginity restored through hymenoplasty. *Health 24.* Retrieved from https://www.health24.com/Lifestyle/Woman/Your-body/why-women-are-opting-to-get-their-virginity-restored-through-hymenoplasty-20180416

Hypersexuality

Hypersexuality may also be referred to as compulsive sexual behavior, out-of-control sexual behavior, hypersexual disorder, sexual addiction, or historically when applied to women, nymphomania. It is characterized by an often distressing obsession with sexual thoughts, urges, or behaviors. The obsession may be so consuming that it causes much distress for the individual and can adversely affect their self-esteem, health, relationships, career, and other aspects of life.

Various types of thoughts and acts may be part of hypersexuality, including masturbation, looking at pornographic photos and videos, having affairs or engaging in sexual relationships outside of a primary monogamous partnership, and paying for sex. For many people, some of these thoughts and acts are very enjoyable, and they may not pose a serious problem. However, for the individual with hypersexual disorder, the thoughts and acts become highly disruptive and harmful to themselves and, in some cases, to others.

Knowing the difference between "normal," unproblematic sexual urges and acts and those that constitute a serious, compulsive disorder means recognizing certain symptoms. Symptoms that suggest a disorder include the following:

- feeling that the sexual impulses are so intense that they are beyond control
- feeling strongly compelled to do certain sexual activities even if they do not bring pleasure or satisfaction
- engaging in sexual behaviors as an escape from problems such as stress, boredom, depression, and loneliness
- continuing to engage in the behaviors despite the risk of serious consequences, such as the loss of a job, the loss of a spouse or partner, legal problems, and sexually transmitted infections
- having a compulsive state of mind that causes trouble establishing or maintaining close, emotional relationships with people

If these symptoms are present, it is best to seek help from a sexual therapist, doctor, psychiatrist, or other mental health professional as soon as possible. Compulsive sexual behaviors tend to escalate and expand over time—similar to drug use—as the individual seeks to maintain the "high." Although feelings of guilt, shame, and low self-esteem may haunt the individual, the compulsive behaviors continue, often leading to financial debt (if paying for sex or pornography), drug and alcohol abuse, serious mental health concerns, and arrests for sexual or substance abuse offenses.

The causes of hypersexuality are not fully understood, but experts believe that several factors may play a role. One factor may be abnormally high levels of neurotransmitters in the brain. These chemicals, such as serotonin, dopamine, and norepinephrine, transmit biochemical signals among the neurons (nerve cells) of the brain, leading to rewarding feelings of pleasure, desires to seek more pleasure, and other altered moods. High levels of testosterone, the male sex hormone, prompt some men to become unusually sexually obsessive and aggressive.

For some individuals, a tendency toward hypersexuality has been related to certain other diseases, including epilepsy, dementia, Huntington disease, and Parkinson disease. In addition, some people with histories of physical or sexual abuse; addictions to alcohol, drugs, or gambling; or bipolar disorder or other mental health disorders may develop hypersexuality. However, doctors warn that hypersexuality can affect anyone.

The first step in getting treatment is to be professionally evaluated for hypersexuality or compulsive sexual behavior disorder. To make a diagnosis of this condition, a mental health professional may conduct examinations of both physical and mental health. Part of this examination may include asking the patient numerous questions about their health; emotions, thoughts, and behaviors related to sex; relationships with family and friends; and use of drugs and alcohol.

Different doctors and other health professionals may diagnose hypersexuality according to different criteria. Diagnosis is complicated by the fact that the American Psychiatric Association's *Diagnostic and Statistical Manual of Mental Disorders*—the main guide for diagnosis of mental disorders—does not include a specific category for hypersexuality or compulsive sexual behavior. Thus, a patient's condition may be diagnosed as a form of impulse control disorder or some other disorder, like paraphilic disorder. However, in its newest edition, the World Health Organization's *International Classification of Diseases, Eleventh Revision*, included compulsive sexual behavior disorder as an impulse control disorder.

Once a diagnosis is made, typical treatment for a patient struggling with hypersexuality includes a combination of psychotherapy, medications, and participation in "self-help" groups (such as Sexaholics Anonymous, similar to Alcoholics Anonymous). The treatment is designed to help the patient control and limit their excessive sexual urges and behaviors while maintaining a healthy level of sexual activity. Some patients may need to receive treatment for additional, associated disorders, such as drug or alcohol addictions, obsessive-compulsive behaviors, anxiety, or depression.

Psychotherapy involves talking with a therapist, who ideally helps the patient learn how to better manage compulsions and urges. A patient undergoing psychotherapy should become increasingly aware of unconscious thoughts and develop insights into factors responsible for problematic urges and motivations. The patient should also learn how to replace unhealthy thoughts and acts with healthy ones. Depending on the patient's particular case, some psychotherapy sessions may include spouses or other family members. A strong support system of family and friends can be crucial to successful treatment.

A variety of medications are available to help treat patients with hypersexuality. Many of the available medications act on neurotransmitters to reduce the feelings of reward and pleasure derived from the compulsive, problematic acts, thereby reducing the urges that lead to the acts. Such drugs include lithium and naltrexone. Other medications reduce the depression that leads to the need to find escape, such as fluoxetine and sertraline. Still other medications reduce the effects of testosterone, such as medroxyprogesterone and luteinizing hormone–releasing hormone agonists.

A. J. Smuskiewicz

See also: Compulsivity, Sexual; *International Classification of Diseases, Eleventh Revision (ICD-11)*; Out-of-Control Sexual Behavior; Pornography Addiction; Sexaholics Anonymous.

Further Reading

Mayo Clinic. (2019). Compulsive sexual disorder. Retrieved from http://www.mayoclinic.org/diseases-conditions/compulsive-sexual-behavior/basics/definition/con-20020126

Weiss, R. (2014). Nymphomaniac—A realistic look at female hypersexuality? Retrieved from http://www.psychologytoday.com/blog/love-and-sex-in-the-digital-age/201404/nymphomaniac-realistic-look-female-hypersexuality

Weiss, R. (2018). Hypersexuality: Symptoms of sexual addiction. Retrieved from http://psychcentral.com/lib/hypersexuality-symptoms-of-sexual-addiction/00011488

Hypogonadism

Hypogonadism is a medical condition that produces insufficient levels of sex hormones in both males and females. There are two types of hypogonadism, primary and secondary, that are characterized by the causes of the lack of hormone production. Primary means the gonads (i.e., testes and ovaries) cannot make enough sex hormones. The gonads still receive messages from the brain to produce the hormones but are simply unable to respond accurately. Secondary hypogonadism occurs when one's brain cannot send messages to the gonads to produce sex hormones. There are many diseases and syndromes that are linked to causing secondary hypogonadism, such as cancer treatments, hereditary diseases, medications, or injury.

The symptoms of hypogonadism vary slightly between males and females, with the list of possible symptoms for males being longer than that of females. Males can experience loss of body hair, muscle loss, abnormal breast growth, reduced growth of the penis and/or testicles, erectile dysfunction, a low or absent sex drive, infertility, osteoporosis, fatigue, hot flashes, and difficulty concentrating. Symptoms of secondary hypogonadism do not usually present until after puberty. According to some, a poor sense of smell is also a symptom in the case of secondary hypogonadism in males. Although hypogonadism is generally less common in females, symptoms in females include low or absent sex drive, slow or absent breast growth, difficulty conceiving, an abnormal menstrual cycle, hot flashes, and milky discharge from the breasts.

Predominately affecting men, hypogonadism results in decreased sperm and testosterone production. Men who have a decrease in testosterone levels may experience less sexual desire. In most cases, this can be treated with testosterone replacement therapy. Hypogonadism can be caused by Klinefelter syndrome, where an individual has one Y chromosome and more than one X chromosome. This extra X chromosome disturbs the development of the testicles, which in turn obstructs the proper production of hormones. Male hypogonadism can also be caused by undescended testicles—when the testicles stay inside the abdominal cavity instead of dropping down into the scrotum. This normally occurs after birth and can be corrected with surgery but if left untreated can cause damage to the testicles and interrupt hormone production. Hypogonadism can also be caused by too much iron, which affects both the testicles themselves and the pituitary gland, meaning both the signal to produce hormones and the actual production of hormones is dysfunctional. Other possible causes include infections such as the mumps, traumatic injury, and aging.

In women, hypogonadism can be caused by Turner syndrome, which is characterized by only having one X chromosome. Turner syndrome leads to abnormal development of the ovaries and therefore the abnormal releasing of sex hormones. Female hypogonadism may also be due to ovarian cysts or polycystic ovarian syndrome, as cysts on the ovaries prevent the release of hormones. Other possible causes of hypogonadism among females include trauma, drug interactions, radiation, tumors, and excess iron.

For both sexes, hormone production associated with the brain can be affected in many ways. Genetically, an abnormal development of the hypothalamus known as Kallmann syndrome (delayed or absent puberty) can affect the release of hormones from the gonads. The hypothalamus controls the pituitary gland, which tells the gonads when to release hormones. Diseases such as tuberculosis or sarcoidosis are inflammatory to the hypothalamus and pituitary and consequently can disrupt communication. Lower release of hormones is also associated with opioid medications, hormone therapy, and obesity. Stress and recurring illnesses can also affect the brain's ability to send signals to the gonads to release hormones.

Symptoms of hypogonadism are seen in the secondary sex characteristics first. In men, this includes decreased muscle growth, decreased body hair production, low libido, and breast enlargement. In females, this includes either failing to start menstruation or stopping menstruation, decrease in breast development, hot flashes, mood changes, low libido, and abnormal hair growth.

To diagnose hypogonadism, one must test the levels of hormones, including luteinizing hormone and follicle-stimulating hormone. In addition, in women the test will examine estrogen levels, and in men testosterone levels will be assessed. Besides hormones, other tests will include iron level, sperm count in men, and thyroid tests. An ultrasound of the ovaries can be done to determine if there are cysts. Other scans that may be needed include brain scans to find tumors or abnormalities in the hypothalamus or pituitary gland.

Treatment for hypogonadism depends on the cause of the problem. The most likely course of action will be hormone therapy. In women, this usually includes estrogen and progesterone. In men, this is testosterone therapy. Women may also be prescribed testosterone to help with low libido, which is a common symptom. These hormones can be delivered in a patch or pill form for women, or through injection, patch, gel, or solution for men. If the problem is in the hypothalamus or pituitary, surgery to remove growths may be necessary, as well as radiation therapy or other interventions. If the problem is genetic, then hypogonadism cannot be cured and must just be managed. Other causes, like cysts or tumors, can be removed and may return the gonads to their normal functioning.

Hypogonadism can lead to many complications besides the visible side effects like abnormal body hair or loss of muscle growth. It can lead to infertility and early menopause in women. Estrogen therapy can lead to blood clots, endometrial cancer, and breast cancer. In men, hypogonadism can cause osteoporosis, infertility, and weakness. The complications from treatment include the risks of radiation and the possibility of excess testosterone.

Casey T. Tobin

See also: Androgen Insensitivity Syndrome; Androgens; Congenital Adrenal Hyperplasia; 5-Alpha-Reductase Deficiency; Hormone Replacement Therapy; Klinefelter Syndrome; Polycystic Ovary Syndrome (PCOS); Sex Hormones; Turner Syndrome.

Further Reading

Hyde, J., & Delamater, J. (2017). *Understanding human sexuality* (13th ed.) New York: McGraw-Hill.

Lehmiller, J. (2013). *The psychology of human sexuality*. Hoboken, NJ: John Wiley & Sons.

Mayo Clinic. (2019). Male hypogonadism. Retrieved from https://www.mayoclinic.org/diseases-conditions/malehypogonadism/symptoms-causes/syc-20354881

Hysterectomy

Hysterectomy is the surgical removal of the uterus, the organ in which fetal development takes place. Thus, after undergoing a hysterectomy, a person no longer has the ability to become pregnant.

Hysterectomies are performed for several different reasons. The most common reason is the removal of large fibroids, which are abnormal, noncancerous growths of muscle and connective tissue in the wall of the uterus. Fibroids often cause a great deal of pain as well as excessively heavy menstrual bleeding. If the fibroids are small enough, physicians might be able to eliminate them with hormone-based treatments or remove each of them individually in surgery. However, large fibroids, in most cases, can be removed only by removing the entire uterus.

Hysterectomies may also be performed as treatment for cancers of the female reproductive organs (mainly the uterus, cervix, or ovaries), treatment for endometriosis (a condition in which cells from the uterine lining grow outside the uterus, such as on the ovaries or in the abdominal cavity), and treatment for pelvic inflammatory disease (an infection of the reproductive organs). Some people have a uterus that slides into an abnormal position within the vaginal canal—a condition called uterine prolapse—requiring hysterectomy. Still other conditions that may require hysterectomy are adenomyosis (thickening of the uterine wall) and abnormal vaginal bleeding or chronic pain in the pelvic region not necessarily related to fibroids. Finally, hysterectomy may also be performed as part of the gender transition process for trans men.

Depending on the goal of treatment, the type of hysterectomy may vary. In a total hysterectomy, the entire uterus, including the cervix, is removed. In a subtotal, or supracervical, hysterectomy, all of the uterus except the cervix is removed. In a radical hysterectomy, the uterus and cervix, the upper part of the vagina, and surrounding lymphatic tissue and ligaments are removed. One or both of the fallopian tubes and ovaries may also be removed in some hysterectomies. The more radical and extensive forms of surgery are usually associated with cancer treatments.

Different surgical techniques can be used to perform a hysterectomy. The surgeon may remove the uterus and associated organs through a large open incision in the abdominal wall or in any of various minimally invasive procedures (MIPs). Abdominal hysterectomies, in which the surgeon makes a horizontal or vertical incision 5–7 inches (13–18 centimeters) long in the abdomen, account for about 65 percent of all hysterectomies. This kind of procedure generally requires a hospital stay of two to three days, and it leaves a visible scar on the abdomen. Full recovery may require as long as six weeks.

In one type of MIP hysterectomy, the surgeon removes the uterus through a small incision in the vagina, leaving no visible scar. In another type of MIP hysterectomy, one or more small incisions are made in the abdomen, through which a laparoscope (a tube with a camera at the end) and surgical tools are inserted. Then, while viewing the inside of the body on a video screen, the surgeon makes the necessary cuts to remove the uterus through the small incisions. Some forms of laparoscopic hysterectomy may involve the use of a robotic system of surgical tools, which the surgeon can manipulate with remote controls outside the body.

All these MIP procedures allow the patient to spend less time in the hospital and have shorter recovery times compared with traditional abdominal hysterectomies. Those who have had an MIP hysterectomy may be able to resume their normal daily activities in three to four weeks. Those who are obese or who have certain other health problems are not good candidates for MIP hysterectomy.

Hysterectomy is considered a low-risk form of surgery. However, a small percentage of patients may experience complications after surgery such as chronic pain, blood clots, infection, urinary incontinence, vaginal prolapse (in which part of the vagina protrudes from the body), or formation of a fistula (an abnormal connection between the vagina and bladder). Hysterectomy may cause earlier-than-normal menopause. Some also experience feelings of sadness and depression after a hysterectomy.

A. J. Smuskiewicz

See also: Cervical Cancer; Endometriosis; Gender Transition; Ovarian Cancer; Pelvic Inflammatory Disease (PID); Uterine Cancer; Uterus.

Further Reading

Kelley, K. (2012). *What 250,000 women know about hysterectomy.* Seattle, WA: Amazon Digital Services, Inc.

Mayo Clinic. (2019). Abdominal hysterectomy. Retrieved from https://www.mayoclinic.org/tests-procedures/abdominal-hysterectomy/about/pac-20384559

Streicher, L. F. (2013). *The essential guide to hysterectomy: Advice from a gynecologist on your choices before, during, and after surgery.* Lanham, MD: M. Evans & Company.

I

Incest

The word "incest" comes from the Latin word "incestus," meaning impure. Incest refers to sexual contact of any kind between relatives, and approximately 34 percent of child sexual abuse cases are committed by family members. Incest is illegal in the United States, and each state has their own legal definition of what constitutes incest. The reasoning behind incest being illegal is that children born from incestuous relationships have a higher probability of being born with physical or intellectual disabilities. As such, many states used to require blood tests prior to issuing marriage licenses. Incest can occur in many different forms, such as sexual contact between siblings, a child and parent, child and grandparent or aunt or uncle. Incest also refers to adult relationships where the individuals are consenting but are too closely related to marry; this is also considered a crime but not necessarily sexual abuse. Incest that is sexual abuse can have long-lasting effects on the survivor as family members are seen as caretakers and are supposed to keep the child safe. Oftentimes, the victims do not recognize that what has occurred is abuse.

In many cases of incest between siblings, the event or events may have occurred out of curiosity and as such are more along the lines of sex play, which is a healthy part of childhood sexuality. The determinants of whether the incident is sexual play include if the siblings are near in age; if coercion, threats, and aggression were not involved; and if the participants gave consent. This type of play can be seen as typical development and part of being a curious child. However, when the above characteristics are not in play and there is a larger age gap, if coercion is involved, or if there is a lack of consent between siblings, this type of victimization can have a lasting effect on the individuals and does not fall within harmless experiences. While this type of incest can occur between any formation of siblings, the most common is that of older brothers and younger sisters.

Another form of incest is parent-child incest in which a parent takes advantage of their child. Research indicates that stepfathers are more likely to sexually abuse their stepdaughters than their biological children. Mothers can also sexually abuse children, biological or step, but this is either much less common or much less reported. Parent-child incest can be very hard to disclose because the parent figure will covertly groom the child and explain to them, in many cases, that the behavior is normal and how it is supposed to be. The nonoffending parent is often either unaware or in denial. Also, it is common that the victim of the abuse will still care for or love their abuser and be very confused about the feelings they are experiencing. Victims may also be concerned about the reactions of other relatives and be worried that people will not believe them. Sexual abuse by a parent breaks the bond of trust that children have with most adults and can leave them feeling alone.

The effects of incest are similar to those of other forms of child sexual abuse; however, research has shown that the effects tend to be more severe when the abuser is a family member. Many survivors deal with guilt, shame, and blame throughout their life. They may also struggle with low self-esteem and low self-worth, and they may experience other unhealthy relationships as they grow into adulthood. They may also deal with sexual dysfunctions or unhealthy sexual behavior. All these symptoms may lessen over time with the help of therapy and gaining understanding that what happened to them is not their fault. Children who are raised in incestuous homes also may not realize that what happened to them was abnormal, and they may continue the pattern of abuse in their own families.

Amanda Baker

See also: Child Sexual Abuse; Childhood Sexuality; Pedophilia; Rape; Rape, Abuse and Incest National Network (RAINN); Sexual Abuse.

Further Readings

Davis, L. (1988). *The courage to heal: A guide for women survivors of child sexual abuse.* New York: Perennial Library.

Herman, J. L. (1997). *Trauma and recovery.* New York: Basic Books.

O'Keefe, S. L., Beard, K. W., Swindell, S., Stroebel, S. S., Griffee, K., & Young, D. H. (2014). Sister-brother incest: Data from anonymous computer assisted self interviews. *Sexual Addiction & Compulsivity, 21*(1), 1–38.

RAINN. (2019). Incest. Retrieved from https://www.rainn.org/get-information/types-of-sexual-assault/incest

Stroebel, S. S., Kuo, S.-Y., O'Keefe, S. L., Beard, K. W., Swindell, S., & Kommor, M. J. (2013). Risk factors for father-daughter incest: Data from an anonymous computerized survey. *Sexual Abuse: A Journal of Research and Treatment, 25*(6), 583–605.

Infertility

Infertility is the inability to conceive or carry a pregnancy to term after twelve consecutive months of unprotected intercourse for mixed-sex couples under the age of thirty-five. The timespan is reduced to a period of six months for mixed-sex couples who are age thirty-five and over. The Centers for Disease Control and Prevention (CDC) reports that more than one in eight mixed-sex couples deal with infertility. Some national and international health organizations, such as the World Health Organization, the American Society for Reproductive Medicine, and the American College of Obstetricians and Gynecologists, recognize infertility as a disease. Many factors, conditions, and diseases contribute to infertility for both males and females, including cancers, lifestyle habits, sexually transmitted infections (STIs), age, and reproductive disorders. Contrary to popular belief, infertility is not solely a female problem. The National Survey of Family Growth, a study conducted by the CDC in 2002, found that 7.5 percent of all sexually experienced men under the age of forty-five sought medical help for infertility-related problems.

Age is a major factor in fertility for females since the production of ovum ceases during menopause. Unlike males, females are born with all the primary oocytes they will ever have. This means that female oocytes are as old as the person to whom they belong. Primary oocytes are the immature eggs that eventually go through meiotic cellular division to form mature ova. During the embryotic stage, females have approximately three million oocytes in each ovary. By birth, this number is reduced to about one million, and by puberty, the average female has roughly 100,000 oocytes in each ovary. This loss of eggs is called atresia and accounts for the loss of 95 percent of primary follicles by puberty. Atresia continues throughout adulthood until the average female is left with just 1,000 primary follicles at around age forty and no follicles by around age fifty. Once females reach the age of menopause, usually around age fifty, this marks the end of fertility, menstrual cycles, and ovulation. It should be noted that some people begin menopause before age fifty, while others will enter menopause after the age of fifty.

As the quantity of eggs diminishes, so does their quality, which also contributes to infertility with age. Up to 90 percent of ova have abnormal chromosomes by age forty. At the age of thirty-five, a healthy female has about a 78 percent chance of conceiving within one year if they are having monthly, unprotected intercourse. Approximately 30 percent of females at this age will take longer than a year to conceive. By the age of forty, fertility drastically declines. As much as 90 percent of the ova can be chromosomally abnormal, and the endometrial lining becomes thinner as the blood supply to it is reduced. In any given month for a healthy forty-year-old, the chance of conception is approximately 5 percent. This percentage drops to 3 percent over age forty-five.

Lifestyle factors such as weight, smoking, consumption of alcohol, and stress also greatly affect fertility. Being underweight or overweight can interrupt ovulation due to hormonal imbalances that can result from excessive weight gain or loss. The absence of ovulation will result in infertility, which can be corrected once a more healthy weight is reached. Since the sex hormone estrogen is accumulated in body fat, those who are underweight do not have enough body fat to store the appropriate levels of estrogen in order to maintain menstruation and ovulation, leading to infertility. In addition, those who are underweight tend to produce an antiestrogen, which essentially causes a cessation of the menstrual cycle. Conversely, those who are overweight store too much body fat, which has an adverse effect on the production of estrogen. Instead of estradiol, the principal female hormone, those who are overweight metabolize estradiol into estrone and estriol, two weaker forms of estrogen, which leads to the cessation of ovulation. In both cases, infertility is the end result when weight gain or loss is too extreme.

Lifestyle habits such as excessive drinking, smoking, and stress can lead to infertility as well. Alcohol interrupts the hypothalamic-pituitary regulation of the sex hormones estrogen and progesterone, which interferes with menstruation cycles and ovulation. Cessation of ovulation and menstrual cycles is more common in heavy drinkers and alcoholic women; however, studies have found this same effect on female social drinkers who drank as few as three alcoholic beverages a day. Smoking also has drastic effects on the reproductive system due to the toxic chemicals present in cigarettes, such as nicotine, cyanide, and carbon monoxide. These chemicals can lead to increased loss of ova, as they damage the genetic material in the ovum, which implicates not only infertility but also premature menopause. Female smokers tend to experience menopause one to four years earlier than nonsmokers. Also, infertility rates among smoking women are twice that of nonsmokers.

Another lifestyle habit that greatly affects fertility and increases the chance for infertility is stress. Stress may account for up to 40 percent of unexplained fertility. Scientists are unsure of exactly how stress affects fertility, but studies have shown that ovulation occurs less frequently among those who are stressed compared with those who are not under stress. Excessive levels of stress can lead to functional hypothalamic amenorrhea, where there is a complete absence of the menstrual cycle.

One of the most severe symptoms of infections, diseases, and conditions of the female reproductive organs is infertility. In many cases, STIs such as chlamydia and gonorrhea can lead to infertility if these infections develop into pelvic inflammatory disease (PID), which can result in damage, scarring, and blockage of the fallopian tubes. The National Institute of Child Health and Human Development reported in 2017 that 10–20 percent of chlamydia and gonorrhea cases result in PID. This could mean that more than 24,000 women become infertile each year in the United States from PID.

Several other conditions can also lead to infertility, often due to their interference with the uterus, cervix, or fallopian tubes. Endometriosis, a disease that causes the endometrial tissue to grow outside the uterus, can affect the fallopian tubes and ovaries by obstructing them and preventing fertilization. Polycystic ovary syndrome (PCOS) is one of the leading causes of infertility in women. PCOS is when the presence of multiple cysts on the ovaries leads to a hormone imbalance. The cysts cause an overproduction of androgens, or male sex hormones, which can stop ovulation and menstruation. Other conditions involve abnormalities of the uterus. Uterine fibroids, which are benign tumors that grow on the uterus, can interfere with the implantation of a fertilized ovum. In less common cases, the uterus or cervix can have abnormalities in the size, shape, or structure, which can render females infertile due to the inability of sperm to reach the ovum or obstruction in the implantation of a fertilized ovum.

While males do not encounter the same level of reproductive aging as females, sperm is very susceptible to environmental and biological factors. There are several factors that contribute to the quality and quantity of sperm needed for fertilization. Sperm count is a major factor in fertility for males, as the average ejaculate contains approximately three hundred million sperm. Those males who produce 20 percent below this amount are considered infertile. Frequency of ejaculation also contributes to sperm count since sperm is produced at a constant rate of about two hundred million per day. When males ejaculate too often, it can reduce the number of sperm in the ejaculate. In addition, in the average healthy young male, approximately 20 percent of sperm are abnormal with different structural deformities such as a missing tail, two tails, coiled tails, two heads, no head, or small heads. This percentage increases as men age, which can also leave older men with lower levels of fertility.

In the same way lifestyle factors affect females, these behaviors also impact male fertility. Excessive alcohol consumption, smoking, drugs, poor diet, and stress all reduce sperm count and fertility. Alcohol decreases testosterone levels in males, which affects sperm production. Smoking directly affects sperm quality by damaging a specific protein, protamine 2, contained in sperm. Sperm are not able to fertilize an egg in the absence of this protein, rendering males infertile. Other factors such as poor diet and excessive weight gain can reduce testosterone levels and increase estrogen, affecting both quality and quantity of sperm.

Certain infections, conditions, and diseases adversely affect the male reproductive system often through tubal blockage, which prevents sperm from moving out of the male body and into the female vagina. STIs, such as chlamydia and gonorrhea, if left untreated can lead to scarring and blockage of the epididymis, the tubes where sperm mature. The development of varicoceles, a condition that leads to infertility, occurs when the veins on the testicles are too large and cause the testes to overheat from the increased blood supply. The testicles are maintained at five degrees below normal body temperature for optimal sperm production. When a varicocele is present, sperm production and quality can be reduced. Another condition, cystic fibrosis, causes a blockage of the vas deferens, the tube that carries sperm to the urethra. In some cases of cystic fibrosis, the vas deferens is completely missing from the reproductive system.

Transgender and gender-variant people may also deal with infertility. In addition to the considerations noted above, hormones and surgeries that may be pursued during the gender transition process can result in infertility. Consequently, trans people who wish to have biological children may need to consider sperm or ova freezing and storage prior to transition, or may need to delay or stop some biological aspects of transition until after they have children.

Lauren Wesley

See also: Artificial Insemination; Assisted Reproductive Technology; Endometriosis; Fertility; Intracytoplasmic Sperm Injection; Menopause; Menstruation; Ova Donation; Ovulation; Pelvic Inflammatory Disease (PID); Polycystic Ovary Syndrome (PCOS); Pregnancy; Sperm; Surrogate Mothers.

Further Reading

Centers for Disease Control and Prevention. (2002). National survey of family growth. Retrieved from http://www.cdc.gov/nchs/nsfg.htm

Centers for Disease Control and Prevention. (2019). Infertility. Retrieved from http://www.cdc.gov/reproductivehealth/Infertility/Index.htm

National Fertility Association. (2019). Medical conditions. Retrieved from https://resolve.org/infertility-101/medical-conditions/

National Institute of Child Health and Human Development. (2017). What is the link between sexually transmitted diseases or sexually transmitted infections (STDs/STIs) and infertility? Retrieved from https://www.nichd.nih.gov/health/topics/stds/conditioninfo/infertility

National Institute on Alcohol Abuse and Alcoholism. (1994). Alcohol alert. Retrieved from http://pubs.niaaa.nih.gov/publications/aa26.htm

Stillman, R. J. (2017). Smoking and infertility. Retrieved from https://www.asrm.org/globalassets/asrm/asrm-content/learning--resources/patient-resources/protect-your-fertility3/smoking_infertility.pdf

Intercourse

"Intercourse" is a word that describes specific sexual acts. Usually "intercourse" describes one specific sexual act, the penis entering the vagina and thrusting until the penis ejaculates. The word "intercourse" can also include the thrusting of the penis into and out of the vagina, with the vagina meeting each thrust, so that it is a two-person activity. Traditionally, intercourse is seen as the primary sex act, largely for the purpose of procreation, since sexual intercourse is the way the sperm and the egg can join together. In that case, intercourse continues until ejaculation occurs, spurting forth semen and sperm as they travel along their path to meet a single egg in the fallopian tube.

Aside from the reproductive model, there is also the recreational model, where couples have sexual intercourse for pleasure. In a mixed-sex couple, this includes penis insertion into a vagina, as well as thrusting usually until ejaculation and orgasm, with the release of sperm and semen into the vagina. Of course, intercourse is often accompanied by loving gestures, tenderness, kissing, holding, cuddling, touching, fondling, quiet talking, soft sounds, and pleasurable touching and sharing. In a same-sex couple, insertive intercourse may also take the role of a penis inserted into an anus or a sex toy or fingers inserted into an anus or vagina. Also, more than two partners may be involved.

In addition, sexual intercourse can include oral intercourse, often called oral sex, and anal sex, which is sex using the anus. Oral sex includes kissing, sucking, or licking a partner's genitals. Oral sex can also include fingers and toys for additional stimulation or pleasure. For protection from sexually transmitted infections (STIs), some couples use either condoms or dams to cover the genitals.

During anal sex, a partner uses their fingers, penis, hands, mouth, lips, tongue, or toys for penetration, pleasure, and stimulation of the anus. If there is penetration during anal intercourse, it is important to use a water-based lubricant. The anus and rectum do not produce lubrication. If lubrication is not used, irritations or tiny scratches and scrapes can result from the stimulation. In addition, it is important, to use either insertive or receptive condoms. Receptive condoms (sometimes also called female condoms) can be used for protection during anal sex without the internal ring as it can be removed easily, but it's important to use water-based or silicone-based lubricant.

Some individuals see intercourse as the sole purpose of sex. However, in reality, it is just one of the many ways people can feel and give pleasure. Some see the tenderness, passion, and expressions of sensuality as "less than" or not "the real thing." Those with narrow views about intercourse as only the penis and the vagina fail to see the entire body as a means for giving and receiving pleasure. For example, if a man is worried about not having an erection, the partners can pleasure each other without having penetrative intercourse, without judgment or feeling as though they are lacking something. When there is illness or aging, it should not matter if age affects traditional intercourse as other activities can be explored that will also bring pleasure and connection. If the point of a sexual experience is pleasure, people can use the bodies they have without narrowly defining intercourse as the main event or without feeling like a failure if it is not a part of their experience. So, while intercourse is one way to have sex, it is not and does not need to be the goal or the "best part" of sex with another. It is just one of the many ways to be intimate with someone else.

Judith Steinhart

See also: Anal Intercourse; Ejaculation; Oral Sex; Orgasm; Penis; Safer Sex; Vagina.

Further Reading

Byers, E. S., Henderson, J., & Hobson, K. M. (2009). University students' definitions of sexual abstinence and having sex. *Archives of Sexual Behavior, 38*(5), 665–674.

Gillibrand, R., & Turner, K. (2013). "Let's talk about sex": A post-structuralist discourse analysis into the meanings and experiences of anal sex for gay men. *Psychology of Sexualities Review, 4*, 54–67.

Herbenick, D., Reece, M., Schick, V., Sanders, S. A., Dodge, B., & Fortenberry, J. D. (2010). Sexual behaviour in United States: Results from a national probability sample of men and women ages 14–94. *Journal of Sexual Medicine, 7*, 255–265.

International Classification of Diseases, Eleventh Revision (ICD-11)

The *International Classification of Diseases for Mortality and Morbidity Statistics, Eleventh Revision* (*ICD-11*) is "the foundation for the identification of health trends and statistics globally, and the international standard for reporting diseases and health conditions" (World Health Organization [WHO], 2018). The *ICD* provides definitions and diagnostic criteria for diseases, disorders, injuries, and other health conditions and can be used for research and clinical purposes. It is maintained and published by the World Health Organization.

The *ICD* was first published by the WHO in 1948. However, it evolved out of the *International List of Causes of Death*, which had been used and maintained by the International Statistical Institute since 1893. There were five versions of the *International List of Causes of Death*, and so, when the *ICD* was published in 1948, it was known as *ICD-6*. Since then, additional versions have been published, culminating in the most recent version, *ICD-11*, which was released on June 18, 2018. Member states of the United Nations will begin to use *ICD-11* for their morbidity reporting on January 1, 2022.

With respect to sexuality, *ICD-11* has a dedicated chapter (chapter 17) titled "Conditions Related to Sexual Health." *ICD-11* has additional categories for changes in male or female genital anatomy, paraphilic disorders, adrenogenital disorders, infections that can be transmitted sexually, and contact with health services for contraceptive management.

The previous version, *ICD-10*, was approved in 1990. Because of significant advances in research and clinical practice, as well as major shifts in social attitudes, policies, laws, and human rights standards, many changes were included in *ICD-11* that were not recognized in previous versions.

Importantly, in the new *ICD-11*, all trans-related categories were deleted from the chapter "Mental and Behavioral Disorders." As such, the WHO has now officially recognized that being transgender and gender diverse are not mental health conditions. Instead, new trans-related categories such as "Gender Incongruence of Adolescence and Adulthood" and "Gender Incongruence of Childhood" have been developed in the chapter "Conditions Related to Sexual Health."

Sexual dysfunctions are also classified by the *ICD-11* in the chapter "Conditions Related to Sexual Health." There are four main groupings of sexual dysfunctions: (1) sexual desire and arousal dysfunctions, (2) orgasmic dysfunctions, (3) ejaculatory dysfunctions, and (4) other specified sexual dysfunctions. There is also a separate grouping of sexual pain disorders.

While *ICD-11* has substantial overlap with the *Diagnostic and Statistical Manual of Mental Disorders, Fifth Edition* (*DSM-5*), there are some notable differences. In *ICD-11*, a diagnosis of hypoactive sexual desire dysfunction can be applied to both men and women, while in *DSM-5*, it is separated into female sexual interest/arousal disorder and male hypoactive sexual desire disorder (Reed et al., 2016). In addition, in *ICD-11*, there are separate categories for men and women for genital arousal: female sexual arousal dysfunction and erectile dysfunction. For women, this differs from how sexual interest/arousal disorder is classified in *DSM-5*. In *ICD-11*, sexual arousal is considered separately from sexual desire. For men, *ICD-11* distinguishes between the subjective experience of orgasm (orgasmic dysfunction) and ejaculation (delayed ejaculation); this distinction is not recognized in *DSM-5* (Reed et al., 2016). Finally, *ICD-11* has a category for early ejaculation as opposed to "premature (early) ejaculation" as classified in *DSM-5*.

Heather L. Armstrong

See also: Desire Disorders; *Diagnostic and Statistical Manual of Mental Disorders* (*DSM*); Dyspareunia; Sexual Disorders, Female; Sexual Disorders, Male; Sexual Dysfunction, Treatment of.

Further Reading

Reed, G. M., Drescher, J., Krueger, R. B., Atalla, E., Cochran, S. D., First, M. B., … Saxena, S. (2016). Disorders related to sexuality and gender identity in the ICD-11: Revising the ICD-10 classification based on current scientific evidence, best clinical practices, and human rights considerations. *World Psychology, 15*(3), 205–221.

World Health Organization. (2018). *International classification of diseases for mortality and morbidity statistics* (11th Rev.). Geneva: Author. Retrieved from https://icd.who.int/en

International Foundation for Gender Education (IFGE)

The International Foundation for Gender Education (IFGE), a nonprofit organization, was founded in 1986 to promote acceptance of transgender people. Founder Merissa Sherrill Lynn wrote in regard to its need:

> The cross-dressing and transsexual phenomena have been an integral part of the human experience as long as there has been a human experience. These phenomena have manifested themselves in every society and in every walk of life throughout history and continue to affect the lives of vast numbers of people. Yet, as common as they are, ignorance of them, and the resulting intolerance and fear, continues to cost good people their happiness, their jobs, their families, and their lives. It costs society its neighbors, its friends, and its productive citizens. The International Foundation for Gender Education is dedicated to overcoming this devastating ignorance. (International Foundation for Gender Education, 1996)

IFGE's original headquarters was located at 123 Moody Street in Waltham, Massachusetts. IFGE operated a bookstore featuring books on transgender topics and issues. The office included a reading room that was open to the public. During office hours, IFGE would also provide information and referrals by phone.

IFGE held the first of its many annual conferences in 1987, entitled Coming Together—Working Together, dedicated to "education, planning, and strategizing about gender-related issues." The convention was held in a different city each year to provide support and exposure for local transgender communities. The final conference was held in 2012 in conjunction with the annual Gold Rush convention in Colorado.

Another major project was assuming publication of a full-color quarterly magazine. The magazine began publishing in the late 1970s as *The TV-TS Tapestry*, by the Tiffany Club in Boston, and covered a wide range of topics of interest to the community. It became *Transgender Tapestry* in 1995. IFGE took over the magazine and continued publication until the early 2000s. For many years, *Tapestry* enjoyed the largest circulation for any magazine of its kind. IFGE also provided training and education to professional service providers and organizations, such as the American Psychiatric Association and the American Association of Sex Education Counselors and Therapists, and produced video, audio, and printed materials in support of education about issues of gender. In addition, IFGE maintained the mailing list for the Congress of Transgender Organizations, a loose network of groups and organizations, mostly small grassroots clubs, across North America dedicated to the transgender community.

Finally, IFGE oversaw the Winslow Street Fund, a permanent endowment for grants and scholarships for transgender community members. The fund was managed by an independent board of trustees and grew to an estimated $100,000. The TSELF scholarship fund gave about $5,000 annually to community.

Denise LeClair became the executive director in 2000. Over time, the organization's presence in Massachusetts closed, and the office moved to the Washington, D.C., area. IFGE appears to have ceased operations at the end of 2012. As of 2018, the status of the Winslow Street Fund is unknown along with any of the organization's remaining assets, if any.

C. Michael Woodward

See also: American Association of Sexuality Educators, Counselors and Therapists (AASECT); Gender Expression; Gender Identity; GLSEN (Gay, Lesbian and Straight Education Network); Nonbinary Gender Identities; Transgender; World Professional Association for Transgender Health (WPATH).

Further Reading

GenderWiki. (2014, September 13). *IFGE*. Retrieved from http://www.geekbabe.com/dlv/mydlv/wiki/index.php/IFGE

International Foundation for Gender Education. (1996). *What is IFGE?* Retrieved from https://www.digitaltransgenderarchive.net/files/vh53wv85s

LinkedIn. (2018). *Denise LeClair*. Retrieved from https://www.linkedin.com/in/dcleclair/

Intersexuality

According to the Intersex Society of North America, "intersex" is a general term used for a variety of conditions in which a person is born with a reproductive or sexual anatomy that does not seem to fit the typical definitions of female or male. A baby may be born with genitals that appear to be in between the usual male and female, or a baby may have external genitalia that resemble typical female genitals but also have mostly male-typical anatomy on the inside. The individual may not know of this internal anatomy until puberty, when the flood of hormones causes multiple changes within their body. Clearly, human bodies do not come in the neat packages that a gender binary assumes.

Intersex is a socially constructed category that reflects real biological variation. Though it is difficult to say exactly how prevalent intersex conditions may be, statistics show that 1 in every 1,500 to 1 in every 2,000 babies are born with atypical genitalia; however, that does not include all people with intersex conditions because of the many hormonal and chromosomal variations that are not usually noticeable at birth. Male people typically have XY sex chromosomes, and female people typically have XX chromosomes. However, chromosomal mix-ups occur in various ways. People can have additional X or Y chromosomes, such as XXY, XXXY, XXX, or XYY. They may also be lacking a chromosome and so have only an X chromosome. All these conditions are the result of abnormalities that occur during cell division when producing eggs and sperm. Klinefelter syndrome is the most common atypical sex chromosome pattern, and somewhere between 1 in 500 and 1 in 1,000 males born have one or more extra X chromosomes. People with Klinefelter syndrome have some variation of extra chromosomes, such as 47,XXY or 48,XXYY. Most of these gender-identify as men and are never diagnosed; they may not find out until they undergo sterility testing later in life during attempts to conceive children. Those with Klinefelter syndrome tend to be especially tall and have broader hips, less body hair, and less muscle control and coordination.

Another chromosomal variation is Turner syndrome (45,X), which occurs when an individual is born with only one X chromosome. This occurs when an X egg or sperm merges with an egg or sperm without a sex chromosome. These individuals usually gender-identify as women, and they tend to be short with distinctive features such as a webbed neck, low-set ears, arched or "shield" chests, and a higher likelihood of obesity; most are infertile and at higher risk for certain health problems. Research suggests that Turner syndrome appears in 0.8 percent of zygotes, making it the most common human chromosomal anomaly, but only 3 percent of these fetuses survive to term. In the end, about 1 in 2,700 live newborns has Turner syndrome. For people with Turner syndrome, the external genitalia, vagina, and uterus develop normally, but the ovaries do not. In place of ovaries, 45,X people have only streaks of tissue called streak gonads/ovaries, and these do not produce typical levels of hormones.

Intersex conditions can also be caused by hormonal variations. Congenital adrenal hyperplasia (CSH) occurs when a fetus has a hyperactive adrenal gland that produces masculinizing hormones. If the fetus is XX, then the baby will be born with masculinized genitals, most notably an enlarged clitoris that resembles a small to medium-sized penis. Most XX babies born with CSH identify as female when they grow older. Androgen insensitivity syndrome (AIS) is caused by the inability of cells to recognize androgens released by the testes both before and after birth. AIS occurs in the bodies of people with XY chromosomes; these individuals develop testes that produce testosterone and other androgens; however, their testes remain in their abdomens. Because their bodies do not recognize androgens, as fetuses, their external genitalia development followed the female body plan. Again, they may be unaware of their internal anatomy development until puberty hits and unexpected changes begin to occur.

Babies born with external genitalia that varies from the typical male or female genitalia have been "corrected" by doctors' surgeries for years; however, more recently there is greater acceptance and understanding of people with intersex conditions. In 2018, the American Academy of Family Physicians issued a policy opposing medically unnecessary surgeries on children with intersex conditions. In the 1960s, surgeons popularized "normalizing" cosmetic operations, but no data has ever demonstrated that these operations help children "fit in" or "function in society." Dr. Alice Dreger has studied sexual development disorders and the people affected by these experiences. Dreger has noted that "the thing that people with intersex suffer from most is shame, it's not surgery. The surgeries are motivated by shame" (Callahan, 2009). Dreger believes people with intersex conditions need a positive message about love and acceptance as well as social recognition. A recent European consensus statement on intersex surgery "advises that the intervention be postponed until the individual is old enough to be actively involved in the decision whenever possible." Dreger also recommends that the parents and child work with a multidisciplinary team of pediatricians, surgeons, psychologists, geneticists, and social workers to make an informed decision on surgery.

Numerous adults with intersex conditions have voiced their distrust of medical professionals due to childhood surgeries. Some people who underwent surgeries as children have begun to speak out against them as human rights violations. As the result of surgeries, some individuals were assigned the wrong gender, while others suffer from sexual dysfunction and infertility. Because of this, three U.S. surgeons general, the United Nations, the World Health Organization, Physicians for Human Rights, the American Academy of Family Physicians, Human Rights Watch, and Amnesty International have condemned medically unnecessary surgery on children with intersex conditions. In August 2018, California became the first state to pass a resolution condemning the operations.

While the gender binary continues to exist, the discourse of intersex rights challenges the notions of solely two genders and sexes. Large-scale changes are beginning to happen; intersex individuals in New York City obtained medically accurate birth certificates, and Colorado issued its first intersex birth certificate in 2018. Germany became the first EU country to offer a third gender option on birth certificates, and this was hailed as a "small revolution" by intersex activists. These small victories for the human rights of people with intersex conditions are encouraging; however, governmental plans to define sex based on "genitalia at birth" threatens this progress.

Martha Goldstein-Schultz

See also: Androgen Insensitivity Syndrome; Binary Gender System; Biological Sex; Chromosomal Sex; Congenital Adrenal Hyperplasia; 5-Alpha-Reductase Deficiency; Fluidity, Gender; Klinefelter Syndrome; Nonbinary Gender Identities; Sex Chromosomes; Sex Hormones; Sex Reassignment Surgery; Transgender; Turner Syndrome, X Chromosome; Y Chromosome.

Further Reading

Callahan, G. N. (2009). *Between XX and XY: Intersexuality and the myth of two sexes.* Chicago: Chicago Review Press.

Compton, J. (2018). *"You can't undo surgery": More parents of intersex babies are rejecting operations.* Retrieved from https://www.nbcnews.com/feature/nbc-out/you-can-t-undo-surgery-more-parents-intersex-babies-are-n923271

Fausto-Sterling, A. (2018, October). Why sex is not binary. *New York Times.* Retrieved from https://www.nytimes.com/2018/10/25/opinion/sex-biology-binary.html

Intersex Society of North America. (2019). What is intersex? Retrieved from http://www.isna.org/faq/what_is_intersex

Knight, K. (2018). *US Medical Association stands against unnecessary intersex surgeries.* Retrieved from https://www.hrw.org/news/2018/09/17/us-medical-association-stands-against-unnecessary-intersex-surgeries

O'Hara, M. E. (2018). *Colorado is the first US state to issue an intersex birth certificate.* Retrieved from https://www.them.us/story/colorado-intersex-birth-certificate

Wade, L., & Ferree, M. M. (2015). *Gender: Ideas, interactions, institutions.* New York: W. W. Norton & Company.

Intimacy, Sexual and Relational

Sexual and relational intimacy are aspects of a close interpersonal relationship. Intimacy, in its most general sense, is the feeling of being close or connected to someone and belonging together. Intimacy is not a thing but a process that changes over time, that can wax and wane according to the individuals in the relationship. Intimacy is thought to be an essential part of long-term love relationships.

There are many forms of intimacy, some existing specifically in a relationship and others not. Within the context of a relationship, a person may experience emotional, intellectual, physical, sexual, spiritual, or experiential intimacy. While each of these forms of intimacy is valuable, every person will seek out the type of intimacy that helps them to feel close and connected to another person or their partner. Broadly speaking, relational intimacy occurs when two people have developed a relationship of safety, trust, and openness where they are able to connect through physical touch (i.e., hand holding or bodily closeness), emotional openness (sharing of one's feelings), consensual sexual engagement (from kissing to intercourse), or in-depth discussion of shared interests. In order for any form of intimacy to occur, there must be reciprocal trust, emotional closeness, and self-disclosure. The presence of relational intimacy is important because it validates individuals' self-worth by providing them a chance to feel understood and accepted for who they are, and it is a buffer against mental health issues such as anxiety and depression.

Sexual intimacy most often occurs in the context of a romantic relationship. Sexual intimacy is a yearning for a sexual connection that may or may not include intercourse. Often, sexual intimacy can be described as "making love," because there is a simultaneous emotional and physical connection. In more recent years, however, sexual intimacy has been blurred due to the shifting experiences of sexual engagement. For instance, sexual interactions exist in various relationship forms, such as friends with benefits or in hookup culture. In these scenarios, two people consent to a primarily sexual relationship that is mutually beneficial. Most often, the sexual interactions in these more casual situations lack sexual intimacy and are based on the mutual desire for sexual pleasure. In contrast, sexual intimacy involves the combining of sexual expression with the desire to feel close and connected to another person.

In addition to sexual intimacy, one of the defining features of relational intimacy is the presence of, or desire for, emotional intimacy. Emotional intimacy exists in a relationship where there is an emotional bond or connection to another person. When two partners engage in an emotionally intimate relationship, they crave openness, trust, closeness, and vulnerability. In essence, an individual is able to feel seen, understood, and accepted. Emotional intimacy fosters closeness and commitment and is only possible through communication.

Emotional intimacy plays a large role in maintaining sexual desire and relationship satisfaction, which in turn predicts more sexual frequency and satisfaction. In general, higher levels of intimacy, both sexual and emotional, are related to greater satisfaction and well-being and more effective communication.

Abby Girard

See also: Companionate Love; Consummate Love; Dating; Friends with Benefits; Hookup Culture; Love; Marriage; Romantic Attraction and Orientation; Sternberg's Triangular Theory of Love.

Further Reading

Timmerman, G. (1991). A concept analysis of intimacy. *Issues in Mental Health Nursing, 12*, 19–30.

van Lankveld, J., Jacobs, N., Thewissen, V., Dewitte, M., & Verboon, P. (2018). The associations of intimacy and sexuality in daily life: Temporal dynamics and gender effects within romantic relationships. *Journal of Social and Personal Relationships, 35*(4), 557–576.

Yoo, H., Bartle-Haring, S., Day, R. D., & Gangamma, R. (2014). Couple communication, emotional and sexual intimacy, and relationship satisfaction. *Journal of Sex and Marital Therapy, 40*, 275–293.

Intracytoplasmic Sperm Injection

Intracytoplasmic sperm injection (ICSI) is the process of injecting a single sperm cell into an oocyte (egg) for the purpose of fertilization. Conventional in vitro fertilization (IVF) requires many sperm to facilitate fertilization, while ICSI allows it to occur when minimal sperm are available. ICSI is typically used in situations where sperm count is very low, sperm motility (ability to move) or morphology (shape of head, neck, and tail) is poor, sperm are unable to attach to the oocyte, traditional IVF failed to produced fertilized oocytes, sperm is surgically collected, sperm is frozen and of poor quality, and when embryos require genetic testing.

Similar to IVF, fertility drugs will be administered to the female partner to stimulate her ovaries to produce many mature oocytes. Sperm are collected via masturbation, thawing, or surgically, if required. The ICSI procedure is done in a sterile environment and is completed in several basic steps. First, a mature oocyte is retained with a specialized pipette. Next, a surgical needle is used to pick up a sperm cell. The needle is used to puncture the membrane of the oocyte, and the sperm cell is released into the egg's cytoplasm. Once oocytes and sperm are merged, the remaining culturing (assisted growing) and embryo transfer processes are the same as traditional IVF.

While ICSI is recommended for male factor infertility, many couples choose the procedure to optimize chances for fertilization. In the United States, of the more than one million IVF cycles that utilized fresh oocytes (nonfrozen) from 1996–2012, 65.1 percent used ICSI, and, of those, only 35.8 percent reported male factor infertility. ICSI outcome is typically dependent on oocyte and sperm quality and the maternal age of the female partner. According to the American Society of Reproductive Medicine, approximately 50– 80 percent of ICSI procedures produce an embryo (fertilized egg).

Problems associated with ICSI can include damaging the oocyte(s), the oocyte not becoming fertilized, and suspended embryo growth. If any of these occur, the merging of the two cells will not result in a pregnancy. Several analyses have shown that compared to traditional IVF, ICSI has been linked to higher incidents of autism, chromosomal abnormalities, birth defects, imprinting disorders, and intellectual disabilities. It has been hypothesized that, unlike IVF and spontaneous in vivo conception, ICSI bypasses normal impediments to fertilization and therefore increases the transmission rate of genetic defects. These genetic defects are potentially related to the cause of infertility, other medical conditions the patients may have, or the ICSI procedure itself.

Darci Shinn

See also: Artificial Insemination; Assisted Reproductive Technology; Fertility; Fertility Drugs; Infertility; Pregnancy; Sperm.

Further Reading

American Society of Reproductive Medicine. (2014). *What is intracytoplasmic sperm injection (ICSI)?* Retrieved from https://www.reproductivefacts.org/globalassets/rf/news-and-publications/bookletsfact-sheets/english-fact-sheets-and-info-booklets/what_is_intracytoplasmic_sperm_injection_icsi_factsheet.pdf

Boulet, S. L., Mehta, A., Kissin, D. M., Warner, L., Kawwass, J. F., & Jamieson, D. J. (2015). Trends in use of and reproductive outcomes associated with intracytoplasmic sperm injection. *Journal of the American Medical Association, 313*(3), 255–263.

Jain, J., & Gupta, R. S. (2007). Trends in the use of intracytoplasmic sperm injection in the United States. *New England Journal of Medicine, 357*(3), 251–257.

Intrauterine Device (IUD)

An intrauterine device, also known as an IUD, is a long-acting, reversible contraceptive. It is a small T-shaped device that fits inside a person's uterus. IUDs have the highest user satisfaction among all types of reversible birth control in North America and are the leading form of contraception worldwide. Their popularity is unsurprising due to the effectiveness and hassle-free quality of IUDs. It is important to note that an IUD does not prevent sexually transmitted infections or HIV transmission. An IUD is inserted into the uterus by a doctor or trained practitioner and may last between three and ten years with over 99 percent effectiveness at preventing pregnancy. After insertion, there is no need to remember to take daily pills, change patches or rings, or otherwise think about one's primary form of birth control. Though initially expensive, it is the most cost-effective birth control option due to the one-time cost and longevity of the device.

In addition to being the most effective form of reversible birth control, an IUD does not require a long period of abstinence following its removal. Return to fertility is usually very quick, and pregnancy may occur as soon as a week after having an IUD removed.

There are two types of IUDs: hormonal or copper. The T-shaped structure of the IUD alters the lining of the uterus so that implantation cannot occur, therefore preventing pregnancy. An IUD prevents fertilization from occurring and therefore is not an abortifacient or device that causes abortion.

Hormonal IUDs release levonorgestrel, a form of the hormone progestin. The hormones in these IUDs thicken cervical mucus, making it more difficult for sperm to get through the cervix and meet with an egg. The hormones also prevent ovulation. In addition to effectively preventing pregnancy, a hormonal IUD may help shrink fibroids and lessen the painful effects of endometriosis. It may also help to prevent endometrial cancer. People who have very heavy menstrual periods or painful cramps may benefit from a hormonal IUD, which helps to reduce cramping and lightens bleeding or halts the period altogether.

A copper IUD does not release any hormones. This IUD lasts a few years longer than a hormonal IUD. It is an option for women who do not want hormones or who would like to have a regular period as the copper IUD does not interrupt periods. Menstrual periods may even be heavier with this type of IUD. The copper IUD releases copper ions, which prevent the sperm and egg from meeting and destroy sperm once it enters the cervix.

A doctor or trained practitioner must insert an IUD through the cervical opening. It cannot be inserted if the person is already pregnant or has a pelvic infection. Insertion may be uncomfortable, though many describe the discomfort as mild. Ibuprofen may be taken prior to insertion to aid in pain management. It is important to find a doctor who inserts IUDs regularly as experience aids in inserting the device quickly and with minimal discomfort. Once the IUD is inserted, two nylon strings will hang from the cervical os so it may be removed at a later time. When it is time to remove an IUD, another may be inserted immediately if desired. Some cramping and bleeding may be expected for a few days to few weeks following insertion. After this subsides, the IUD should not be noticeable in the uterus.

There is a small chance that an IUD may be expelled after it has been placed. Between 2 and 10 percent of people with an IUD may experience this, and it is more likely in those who have not had children. Expulsion is most likely to occur within the first three months of the IUD being placed and is most common during the first period.

In 2012, the American College of Obstetrics and Gynecology recommended that the IUD should be considered as a first-line contraceptive method for female adolescents. Recent research has confirmed young women find this form of birth control effective and report a desire for continued use of IUDs for pregnancy prevention.

Amanda Manuel

See also: Cervix; Contraception; Endometriosis; Menstruation; Pregnancy; Synthetic Hormones; Uterus.

Further Reading

Friedman, J. O. (2015). Factors associated with contraceptive satisfaction in adolescent women using the IUD. *Journal of Pediatric and Adolescent Gynecology, 28*(10), 38–42.

Joannides, P. (2012). Birth control: Sperm v. egg. In P. Joannides (Ed.), *Guide to getting it on* (6th ed., 713–173). Waldport, OR: Goofy Foot Press.

Yarber, W., Sayad, B., & Strong, B. (2010). Contraception, birth control, and abortion. In *Human sexuality: Diversity in contemporary America* (7th ed.). New York: McGraw-Hill.

J

Jealousy

Jealousy can be described as a series of interrelated emotional, cognitive, and behavioral processes. Jealousy is based on the fear that one could have something they deem valuable taken away from them via an external source.

Jealousy as an emotion arises out of social comparison. Jealousy is a complex emotion that combines the primary emotions of fear, sadness, and anger. The feeling of jealousy is associated with unpleasant judgments of inadequacy, scarcity, or diminished value. This connects jealousy to self-critical feelings like grief, humiliation, and shame. When present in relationships, jealousy also creates dissatisfaction and suspicion. Routinely cited physiological reactions include a racing heart, feelings of nausea, or a "sinking" feeling in one's chest. This emotion can become overwhelming and cause those experiencing it to develop more aggressive emotional positions. Examples of these are rage, anxiety, and resentment.

Jealousy is widely understood as a different emotion than envy, although people often use the terms interchangeably. Envy is commonly understood as desiring a trait, possession, or the status of someone else. Envy also arises out of social comparisons and feelings of inadequacy, like jealousy, which would explain why the two terms are seen as synonymous. Jealousy is different because it is rooted in the fear that someone will take something away from you. For example, Arnold is jealous that his girlfriend hangs out with another guy because he fears that she is cheating on him. Arnold is feeling jealous because he does not want to lose his girlfriend's attention. Arnold could start feeling resentful toward his girlfriend and begin to feel insecure in this relationship.

Emotions influence cognitive processes. Jealousy as a cognitive construct is rooted in one's belief that they have a right to possess something they desire, whether it be a physical possession like money or experiences of intrinsic value, such as status or recognition. Jealousy is intensified by how much value is placed on the item or experience and the depth of belief in its scarcity. Jealousy usually involves a rival, so the thoughts associated with jealousy tend to lead to unfavorable hierarchy judgments and critical judgments of others, including deeming them as being undeserving.

It is natural that, as a result of comparisons, jealousy will diminish one's self-esteem and cause the person feeling jealous to reevaluate their social status. Jealousy causes us to focus on the negative and can create negative self-judgments, such as thoughts that one is not good enough or deserves to lose what is important to them. It would be expected that feelings of jealousy would first arise from the thought that someone has something desirable, followed by a perception of loss, and culminating in a sense of inadequacy. It is important to note that these threats may be real or imagined. Thoughts based on jealousy can be unconsciously motivated; people are not always explicitly aware that this emotion is a driving force behind their thought processes. Negative self-judgments can lower a person's self-esteem and hold them back from pursuing their goals. If jealousy is coupled with beliefs of unfairness, thoughts about revenge or retribution may arise.

As with other emotions, feelings of jealousy often have behavioral outcomes. The results of romantic jealousy are the most discussed in research. Given that jealousy is the third leading motive in spousal homicide and the fourth leading cause of domestic abuse, it is clearly an emotion worthy of investigation. Overtly aggressive behaviors associated with jealousy are violence, belittling, stonewalling, arguing, surveillance, and blaming. Jealousy can show up in covert ways in social interactions, which also harm vital connections. Jealousy can be expressed passive-aggressively through reactive attention-seeking, consistent bids for reassurance, sarcasm, and emotional distancing. Sibling rivalry is also a well-researched context of jealous behavior. Older siblings tend to be jealous of their younger siblings because of the changes in their guardians' time and attention. This could cause the siblings to fight or argue frequently or prompt the older sibling to overcompensate in order to attain more of their parents' attention. When perceived as ineffective, children withdraw from the imagined competition altogether and begin distancing themselves from family members.

Often, people cope with jealousy by practicing destructive solutions. Instead of peacefully confronting the situation, people can bottle up this negative emotion and begin emotionally or physically distancing themselves, creating disputes, or making bids for reassurance. Moving through jealousy in a healthy, productive manner can be difficult and requires one to become more self-aware. Talk therapy is one of the most effective ways to resolve jealousy because the therapist helps the client to analyze their cognitive processes and behaviors. Recognizing that jealousy is a negative emotion rooted in fear is the first step in resolving this issue. Once one can acknowledge what they are afraid to lose, then they can focus on how this has been affecting their behavior and take productive steps to getting what they desire. Every situation is multifaceted and requires one to be honest with themselves about their true motives.

Shadeen Francis and Nicole Williams

See also: Cheating and Infidelity; Intimacy, Sexual and Relational.

Further Reading

Castiglia, P. T. (1992). Jealousy. *Journal of Pediatric Health Care, 6*(4), 212–213.

Harris, C. R. (2002). Sexual and romantic jealousy in heterosexual and homosexual adults. *Psychological Science, 13*(1), 7–12.

Salovey, P. (Ed.). (1991). *The psychology of jealousy and envy*. New York: Guilford Press.

Stearns, P. N. (2012). Jealousy. In V. Ramachandran (Ed.), *Encyclopedia of human behavior* (2nd ed., 479–489). San Diego, CA: Elsevier.

White, G. L. (1981). A model of romantic jealousy. *Motivation and Emotion, 5*(4), 295–310.

Johnson, Virginia

Virginia E. Johnson was a pioneering American sexologist. She was the partner of researcher William H. Masters, and the two helped bring the discussion of sex into mainstream American society during the 1960s and 1970s. The pair was the first to apply rigorous scientific techniques to study sex and enjoyed success helping those who were suffering dysfunction. Johnson began as a research assistant but worked her way into an equal relationship with Masters. She supplied many of the ideas that helped make their work more acceptable to the general public and brought a more personable touch to balance Masters's sometimes dry scientific approach.

Mary Virginia Eshelman (later Johnson) was born on February 11, 1925, in Springfield, Missouri. She was the elder of two children. When Johnson was five, her family moved to Palo Alto, California, where her father worked as a groundskeeper for a hospital. She proved to be a gifted student. When the family returned to Missouri in 1933, Johnson skipped several grades. She also displayed a musical talent and studied piano and voice. In 1941, Johnson enrolled at Drury College in Springfield. After completing one year, she took a job at the state's insurance office. Johnson's mother was a Republican state committeewoman and arranged for Johnson to sing at many party functions. She sang country songs on a local radio station under the name of Virginia Gibson. In 1947, Johnson took a job as a business writer for the *St. Louis Daily Record.*

Johnson married a Missouri politician in the early 1940s, but the marriage ended after two days. She also had a brief marriage to a much older lawyer. On June 13, 1950, Johnson married George V. Johnson, the leader of a dance band. She sang with the band until their two children, a boy and a girl, were born. In 1956, Johnson's third marriage ended in divorce.

In 1956, Johnson decided to return to college at Washington University to earn a sociology degree. Looking for a job, she was hired by Masters, professor of clinical obstetrics and gynecology, as a research assistant. Masters was beginning a study of human sexuality and believed he needed a mature woman who was intelligent and outgoing to put his female subjects at ease. Johnson fit the bill, but she soon proved to be much more capable than Masters realized.

Masters's research was the first study of human sexuality that applied scientific research standards. He had cutting-edge equipment that measured heart rates and brain activity of volunteers as they masturbated or had sex. Color film captured the action. A total of 382 men and 312 women eventually took part in the study. Johnson helped Masters to understand the women's point of view and offered important advice about the study. The pair published their findings in 1966 in *Human Sexual Response*. Although written in clinical language for a professional audience, the book quickly captured the country's attention. Johnson convinced Masters to appear on popular talk shows and discuss their findings, making them more accessible to everyone.

In 1964, Masters and Johnson opened the Reproductive Biology Research Foundation in St. Louis and began treating couples with sexual problems. Johnson became the assistant director in 1969 and codirector in 1973. The foundation became the Masters and Johnson Institute in 1973. Using a unique "couples therapy" method, the institute claimed a success rate of 80 percent when treating dysfunctional couples. They also worked with same-sex couples. Masters and Johnson controversially expanded their practice to include reparative therapy, or the practice of trying to change a person's sexual orientation from gay to straight.

In 1971, the two were married after Masters divorced his first wife. Additional books followed, including *Human Sexual Inadequacy* in 1970 and *The Pleasure Bond: A New Look at Sexuality and Commitment* in 1975. Many awards followed, and Masters and Johnson became a household name in sexuality.

Masters and Johnson divorced in 1992 but continued to collaborate professionally. In the late 1990s, Johnson opened the Virginia Johnson Masters Learning Center. She died of heart disease on July 24, 2013, in St. Louis.

Tim J. Watts

See also: Masters, William H.; Masters and Johnson Four-Stage Model of Sexual Response; Sexology.

Further Reading

Fox, M. (2013, July). Virginia Johnson, widely published collaborator in sex research, dies at 88. *New York Times*. Retrieved from http://www.nytimes.com/2013/07/26/us/virginia-johnson-masterss-collaborator-in-sex-research-dies-at-88.html?pagewanted=all&_r=0

Masters, W. H., & Johnson, V. E. (1966). *Human sexual response*. New York: Bantam Books.

Jorgenson, Christine

Christine Jorgensen is considered the first American trans celebrity. She was born George William Jorgensen Jr. on May 30, 1926, in Bronx, New York. Her father was a carpenter and her mother a housewife; she was close with her older sister, Dorothy. Jorgensen described herself as an ashamed and fearful child who knew she was unlike other boys. This difference was observable as a physical, emotional, and sexual immaturity. Specifically, Jorgensen spoke of her genitals as underdeveloped and abnormal.

Standing five feet, six inches fully grown, Jorgensen was drafted into the army and served as a clerk for over a year; afterward, she moved to Hollywood, where she first discussed her feminine emotions with close confidants. Using her slight frame and effeminate behavior as evidence for physiological causality, Jorgensen pursued a medical explanation for her problem by enrolling in a training program for medical technicians. In July 1950, Dr. Christian Hamburger, an endocrinologist in Copenhagen, agreed to provide Jorgensen with experimental hormone treatment at no cost. After noticing subtle physical changes and significant psychological changes from hormone therapy—her testicles atrophied, her libido decreased, her capacity to become erect diminished, her nipple and genital regions experienced the darkening of skin pigmentation, and her mood dramatically improved, Jorgensen underwent surgery to remove her testicles in September 1951. Her scrotum was removed and shaped into labia in November 1952, shortly after the U.S. State Department approved the name change on her passport. In the midst of these surgeries, Christine's facial hair was removed via electrolysis, hormones continued to enlarge her breasts, and she underwent plastic surgery on her ears. Though she was treated with great respect in Denmark, Christine decided to return home to the United States.

The *New York Daily News* broke her story on December 1, 1952; the front-page headline read "Ex-GI Becomes Blonde Beauty," and Christine Jorgensen became an overnight celebrity. Speculation remains regarding the identity of the tipster. Jorgensen reported an initial feeling of great shock that anyone paid attention to her transition. She sold the rights to her story to *American Weekly* to be serialized and distributed globally; the five-part narrative went beyond her feminine appearance and behavior, introducing the world to a sympathetic human being tortured by a glandular imbalance. At a time when postwar America wanted to reaffirm rigid sex roles (in what was referred to as the "crisis of masculinity"), Jorgensen highlighted ambiguity. She endorsed the European theories of human bisexuality, stating that she was more woman than man; she and her doctors believed female organs had always existed within her, comparing her postoperative body to a woman who had undergone a hysterectomy (able to have sexual relations while unable to have children). She clarified her stance on sex by stating that all human beings are psychologically, hormonally, and genetically intersexed but that pseudo-hermaphrodites have the genitals of both sexes. Becoming a voice for many, Jorgensen noted her cultural impact as an American individualist during the increasingly conformist Cold War era. Questions arose regarding the "normality" of Jorgensen's sexuality: was her attraction to men prior to her operations diagnostic for a homosexual mental disorder, or was she always a heterosexual woman?

When further details of Jorgensen's case became a matter of public record, American society rejected her as a woman. Because her anatomy was considered completely male before her operation, she was, in the eyes of the American scientific community, a cross-dresser and not an intersexed person who required surgical and hormonal intervention. Though the controversy upset Jorgensen, it maintained curiosity about her and allowed for nonintersexed individuals to explore the possibility of transition.

After the initial surge of fame, during which she received over twenty thousand letters, Jorgensen booked speaking and performance engagements throughout the United States. She stated that her stage work generally drew heterosexual couples of middle age. Jorgensen believed that she would never live to see the day that she was not viewed first as a transsexual, noting the pressure to perform femininity with precision and perfection. As a stigmatized celebrity under intense scrutiny, Christine was the butt of many cruel jokes in popular culture. Counter to her project on individualism, she wanted to be accepted as "normal," and being the subject of ridicule felt torturous and isolating. In 1953, a feature-length cult film, *Glen or Glenda* or *I Changed My Sex*, allegedly inspired by Christine's story, was released without Christine's consent. Finding it insulting, Christine refused to act in it, though the production company still used her name and photos to promote the release.

By 1954, press in the United States began to differentiate between people who were transsexual versus intersexed. Throughout the 1950s, the prevalence of stories that included people of trans experience grew dramatically due to the fame of Christine Jorgensen. In 1959, Jorgensen's request for a marriage license in the state of New York was denied. The sex listed on her passport with a supporting letter from her doctor did not suffice, because her birth certificate still read "male." She later decided not to marry. Christine presented herself as an independent woman who wanted to marry but cared about having a life (especially friendships and a career) of her own.

Jorgensen continued receiving medical treatment to support her transition until her death. In 1954, she had a vagina constructed from skin grafts that were removed from her thighs. There is speculation over whether or not she underwent reconstructive surgery of the vagina in the late 1960s and in 1980. Jorgensen released an autobiography, *Christine Jorgensen: A Personal Biography*, in 1967; the text sold nearly half a million copies and was loosely adapted to film in 1970. Life as an entertainer, lecturer, author, and public figure continued until her death. She recognized the significance of her story for the worlds of science and American culture; she understood her individuality and candor as catalysts for the sexual revolution of the 1960s.

In 1989, Jorgensen died from lung and bladder cancer at the age of sixty-two. Her obituary in the *New York Times* featured photographs of her as George and shortly after her 1952 return from Denmark to the United States (McQuiston, 1989).

Chrissandra Andrae

See also: Gender; Gender Identity; Gender Transition; Intersexuality; Sex Reassignment Surgery; Transgender; Transsexual.

Further Reading

Jorgensen, C. (1957). *Christine Jorgensen reveals*. J Records.

McQuiston, J. (1989, May). Christine Jorgensen, 62, is dead; Was first to have a sex change. *New York Times*, p. D22. Retrieved from https://www.nytimes.com/1989/05/04/obituaries/christine-jorgensen-62-is-dead-was-first-to-have-a-sex-change.html

Meyerowitz, J. J. (2002). *How sex changed: A history of transsexuality in the United States*. Cambridge, MA: Harvard University Press.

Sopelsa, B. (2019). #Pride50: Christine Jorgensen—World's first trans celebrity. Retrieved from https://www.nbcnews.com/feature/nbc-out/pride50-christine-jorgensen-world-s-first-trans-celebrity-n1006131

Joy of Sex, The

First published in 1972, Alex Comfort's *The Joy of Sex: A Gourmet Guide to Lovemaking* was the first illustrated sex manual released by a major publisher in the United States. It sold 3.8 million copies in its first two years and became the best-selling sex manual of the 1970s. Repeatedly updated and revised, the latest edition is *The New Joy of Sex* (2008) by Alex Comfort and Susan Quilliam.

The author, Alexander Comfort (1920–2000), was a British biochemist and physician. The author of fifty-one books and numerous scientific papers, he specialized in gerontology but also wrote novels, plays, poetry, and song lyrics (for Pete Seeger), and became a noted peace activist and cofounder of the Campaign for Nuclear Disarmament. For a time, he taught at the London Hospital Medical College. It was his students' shocking ignorance of many sexual matters that first encouraged Comfort to write *The Joy of Sex*, which he originally conceived as a medical textbook. He later taught at Stanford University and UCLA's Institute for Neuroscience and Human Behavior. While in the United States, Comfort visited the Sandstone Retreat, a California resort that catered to swingers.

The Joy of Sex presented sex as fun and encouraged experimentation. Organized into sections labeled "Starters," "Sauces," "Main Courses," and "Problems," and sorted alphabetically within these sections, it presented definitions, suggestions, and advice on sexual practices ranging from anal intercourse and bondage to voyeurism and the "X position." Uninhibited, lighthearted, and witty, it lacked the moralizing tone of past marriage manuals and was accompanied by pencil drawings of a loving couple enjoying the activities the book described. Comfort's advice often mixed the practical with humor, noting, for example, that coin-operated vibrating hotel beds "are apt to run out at a critical moment, or make you ill."

The runaway success of *Joy of Sex* led to a sequel, *More Joy of Sex* (1973), as well as *The Joy of Gay Sex* (1977) by Charles Silverstein and *The Joy of Lesbian Sex* (1977) by Emily L. Sisley and Bertha Harris. Along with the original, all these went through several print runs and updates, which included information on HIV and other sexually transmitted infections as well additional sex advice. The later editions of *Joy of Sex* eliminated, qualified, or revised Comfort's sometimes questionable humor, preachy tone, and overstated preferences and opinions (including his declaration that "vibrators are no substitute for a penis"), his fondness for body hair, abhorrence of deodorants, and encouragement of orgies.

The success of *The Joy of Sex* opened the gates to what became a flood of sex manuals in the 1970s, few of which matched Comfort's gentle humor and genuine interest in improving the sex lives of readers.

Stephen K. Stein

See also: Sex Education; Sexual Revolution.

Further Reading

Allyn, D. (2001). *Make love, not war. The sexual revolution: An unfettered history*. New York: Routledge.

Comfort, A., & Quilliam, S. (2008). *The new joy of sex*. London: Mitchell Beazley.

Hebblethwaite, C. (2011, October). How the Joy of Sex was illustrated. *BBC News Magazine*. Retrieved from http://www.bbc.com/news/magazine-15309357

Martin, D. (2000, March). Alex Comfort, 80, dies; a multifaceted man best known for writing "The Joy of Sex." *New York Times*. Retrieved from https://www.nytimes.com/2000/03/29/us/alex-comfort-80-dies-a-multifaceted-man-best-known-for-writing-the-joy-of-sex.html

Talese, G. (1980). *Thy neighbor's wife*. New York: Doubleday.

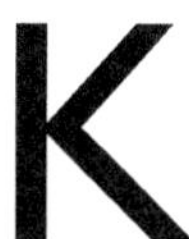

Kama Sutra

The *Kama Sutra*, sometimes called *Kama Sutra—A Guide to the Art of Pleasure*, is a compilation of advice about sensuality, sexual pleasure, and social expectations. The book was written in India sometime around the first century BCE by a Hindu man named Vatsyayana. There is some mystery surrounding the origins of the *Kama Sutra*. The word "kama" means "the life of the senses." A "sutra" is a manual or scripture. Therefore, *Kama Sutra* is a manual of the life of the senses and focuses heavily on sensual pleasures and the importance of celebrating sexual pleasure. The *Kama Sutra* contains many sutras that are unable to be traced back to their origin.

The *Kama Sutra* has shaped culture in many ways as it has been a leader in the world of sex manuals. It challenges some concepts of patriarchy, sexism, and heteronormativity as it explores and celebrates various aspects of female sexuality, pleasure, and nontraditional sex practices. The *Kama Sutra* is also a reflection of culture as it encourages "kama" and acknowledges sexual pleasure as an important aspect of living a good life.

There are seven sections of the *Kama Sutra*. The first section is about society and social norms. This text was intended for wealthy men. As such, it outlines how to fill the role of a wealthy gentleman. The second section explores sexual union. Sexual acts, body parts, and nonmarital sex, among other topics, are discussed. The third section details how a gentleman acquires a wife, while the fourth section discusses the role of the wife. As this is a cultural and sexual manual, the fifth section discusses the proper way to interact with the wives of other men. In a similar fashion, the sixth section discusses "courtesans," more commonly known as prostitutes. The final section discusses the means of attracting others. Altogether, this instructional guide influenced wealthy young men in the art of pleasure, their role in society, and the social norms of their culture and relationships.

The Kama Sh'astra Society of London and Benares first published the *Kama Sutra* in 1883 in London. The publication was largely secret and was only put in circulation for a private audience. The text was republished in the United States in 1961. It was met with some resistance due to its content. However, the United States was also dealing with the release of Alfred Kinsey's sex research, which helped guide this "risqué" text into society's awareness. The *Kama Sutra* itself is a very difficult text to read as it was originally intended for the highly educated men of India. As such, the *Kama Sutra* has been made into a commodity and may now be seen in condensed versions that focus more on sexual positions and sexual pleasures than on social and societal norms and expectations. The *Kama Sutra* has been made into movies, pop-up books, shortened texts, and plays.

Amanda Manuel

See also: Tantric Intercourse.

Further Reading

Grant, B. (2005). Translating The Kama Sutra. *Third World Quarterly, 26*(3), 509–516.

Kureishi, H. (2011). It's a sin: The Kama Sutra and the search for pleasure. *Critical Quarterly, 53*(1), 1–5.

Peterson, V. (2002). Text as cultural antagonist: The Kama Sutra of Vatsyayana. *Journal of Communication Inquiry, 26*(2), 133–154.

Kaplan, Helen Singer

Dr. Helen Singer Kaplan was a twentieth-century leader in the field of sex therapy. She established the first-ever sexual disorders clinic at a U.S. medical school and published numerous works on the treatment of sexual disorders. Because Kaplan believed that sexual disorders might indicate deeper emotional issues, her approach to treating sexual problems was deemed psychosexual therapy. Her frankness about the subject of sex and her very vocal support of the sexual revolution of the 1960s earned her the nickname "Sex Queen."

Kaplan was born Helen Singer in Vienna, Austria, on February 6, 1929, the daughter of a wealthy Austrian couple who owned a jewelry business. As World War II heated up in Europe, the family immigrated to the United States in 1940, losing their fortune in the process; Kaplan gained citizenship seven years later. A budding artist as a child, she studied painting at Syracuse University, receiving her undergraduate degree with honors in 1951. From there, she went on to receive a master's degree in psychology from Columbia University in 1952 and, three years later, completed her doctorate in psychology at the same school. Then, in 1959, she became a full-fledged medical doctor, earning her medical degree from New York Medical College, a medical school that is part of the New York Medical College–Metropolitan Hospital Center. As she began her career, she also continued her studies, completing an extended course in psychoanalysis in 1970.

After interning at several hospitals and clinics in New York, Kaplan worked as a psychiatrist at the same time as she embarked on a professional teaching career. She first developed and taught a behavioral sciences program for psychiatric residents at her alma mater, along with teaching basic psychiatric courses for freshman medical students at the school. She later worked as a psychiatrist at three hospitals, all the while continuing to hold multiple teaching and directorship positions in the behavioral sciences department at New York Medical College–Metropolitan Hospital Center. In her role at the center, she also created trainings in human sexuality for both the psychiatric and the obstetrics-gynecology staff.

In 1970, Kaplan became a professor of psychiatry at New York Medical College–Metropolitan Hospital Center and began a six-year stint with the school's undergraduate psychiatry department. That same year, she also established the human sexuality program at the Payne Whitney Clinic, which is part of the New York Hospital–Cornell Medical Center organization. As part of the program, Kaplan founded the first outpatient facility for the treatment of psychosexual disorders. In her job as program director, she oversaw the training and coursework in the field of human sexuality for Cornell University medical students and the center's psychiatric residents.

The work done at the Payne Whitney Clinic generated extensive research into the treatment of sexual dysfunctions. In part because of this clinical research, Kaplan developed cutting-edge theories on sexual disorders and produced some 110 different publications on human sexuality and sexual dysfunctions. She also gave lectures and presentations around the world and mentored some of the most well-known sex therapists of the late twentieth century, including Dr. Ruth Westheimer (more commonly known as Dr. Ruth). At the time of her death on August 17, 1995, in New York City, Kaplan remained at the helm of the prestigious human sexuality program she founded. Her work is still considered highly relevant today, and several of her books remain in print.

Tamar Burris

See also: Desire; Kaplan's Triphasic Model; Psychosexual Therapy; Sexual Disorders, Female; Sexual Disorders, Male; Sexual Revolution.

Further Reading

Greene, J. R. (2010). *America in the sixties.* Syracuse, NY: Syracuse University Press.

Kaplan, H. S. (1979). *Disorders of sexual desire and other new concepts and techniques in sex therapy* (Vol. 2). New York: Simon & Schuster.

Kaplan, H. S. (2013). *New sex therapy: Active treatment of sexual dysfunctions.* New York: Routledge.

Schroeder, E., & Kuriansky, J. (2009). *Sexuality education: Past, present, and future.* Santa Barbara, CA: Praeger.

Kaplan's Triphasic Model

The triphasic model is a model of sexual response developed by noted sex therapist Helen Singer Kaplan in 1970. Kaplan's aim in creating this theory was to revision the human sexual response cycle as created by her predecessors William Masters and Virginia Johnson. The model views sexual responsiveness as both a cognitive and physiological phenomenon resulting in three independent but interrelated phases: desire, arousal, and orgasm.

The Kaplan triphasic model was developed following Masters and Johnson's 1960s theory of the sexual response cycle. In their theory, Masters and Johnson described four phases of human sexual response: an excitement phase, plateau phase, orgasm phase, and a resolution phase. Kaplan believed sexual desire to be a separate clinical entity from excitement (arousal) and subsequently reconceptualized and condensed the model.

The characterizing feature of Kaplan's sexual response model is the desire phase. Sexual desire is an innate drive for sexual satisfaction, often referred to as "lust." Before Kaplan's model, sexual desire had been overlooked as a necessary stage in sexual response. However, Kaplan recognized that sexual experiences did not necessarily contain an element of desire, such as in partnerships that lacked passion or attraction but were consummated apathetically, reluctantly, or merely out of obligation. Kaplan introduced desire as a catalyst for sexual experiences.

She described desire as a carnal hunger preceding physical interaction, a psychological hunger that led to an interest in sexual activity and orgasm seeking. Desire was a key mechanism in the sexual response process as it functioned to allow for the arousal process to begin.

The excitement or arousal phase represents the second phase of Kaplan's triphasic model. While it is the starting place of Masters and Johnson's theory, Kaplan believed sexual response to start in the mind and then transition to the body. In this stage, physical stimulation begins in response to psychological desire. Sexual excitement is a series of physiological changes that prime an organism for sexual activity. Characteristics of sexual excitement include increased heart rate, increased breathing, and increased blood flow to the penis, testes, vulva, clitoris, and nipples (also referred to as vasocongestion). Dilation of the pupils and increased color in the cheeks and genitals may also occur. During this excitatory process, erections may occur and vaginas may begin to lubricate in preparation for sexual activity. The excitement phase may last for minutes or hours.

The resolution phase literally represents the climax of the triphasic model. During this phase, individuals are predicted to reach orgasm after acting on their desire and excitement. An orgasm is seen as the highest point of sexual arousal, during which a series of rhythmic, involuntary reflex muscle contractions of the genitals and anus occur. Physically and emotionally, an orgasm produces highly pleasurable feelings. Orgasms may result from a number of activities including but not limited to oral sex, intercourse, manual stimulation, masturbation, intimate massages, fantasies, and sex toys. The average orgasm only lasts a few seconds and is typically accompanied by ejaculation for most men and often for some women as well. As this is the final stage of sexual response proposed by Kaplan, once orgasm is experienced the cycle returns to the prearoused state. Multiorgasmic individuals may not spend much time in prearousal before reentering the cycle at the desire phase.

While the triphasic model was created to describe healthy sexual response, it has also been used to address and assess sexual dysfunction. Kaplan believed that all sexual dysfunction fell into one of the three categories and could be distinctly classified as a disorder belonging to a discrete stage. Because each of the categories was separate and distinct, the thought was that an individual could properly function in two of the phases but might find a problem in the third. In her book *The Evaluation of Sexual Disorders: Psychological and Medical Aspect*, Kaplan describes psychosexual dysfunctions as being among the most prevalent, worrying, and distressing medical complaints of that time. She believed that if a disorder could be correctly diagnosed into a stage, there was a good chance that it could be properly resolved. Each stage-based disorder was associated with a different set of causes and was therefore believed to respond to different and specific therapeutic interventions. For example, Kaplan understood orgasmic problems to be dependent on an individual's level of distress; these problems were not seen as sexual but instead as problems of pain or fear of pain. Effective treatments of orgasmic problems would then address these underlying issues and allow for the pleasurable experience of orgasm.

Kaplan focused specifically on desire disorders within the clinical population and found that 38 percent of 5,580 patients diagnosed with sexual disorders also met the criteria for sexual desire disorders. Finding the root of desire disorders, such as hypoactive sexual desire disorder, proved to be incredibly complex as they involved both immediate factors and historical factors that blocked desire. Kaplan concluded that desire-phase disorders were not only distressing for couples but were also the most difficult to treat as they were associated with deep-seated psychological difficulties. Kaplan's work on sexual dysfunction contributed a new perspective to the field of sexual dysfunction, as it introduced the idea that intrapsychic causes can be influenced by culture, development, and conflict. Kaplan's qualitative research resulted in the discovery that relationships with a lack of trust, power struggles, contractual disappointments, sexual sabotage, and partner rejection were all more likely to also include some form of sexual dysfunction, especially disordered desire. She placed a strong emphasis on social learning theory as a base for understanding the etiology and treatment of sexual dysfunction. Kaplan's treatments emphasized the use of erotic techniques and a concern with the unconscious conflicts, fears, and desires that are involved in sexuality. It was Kaplan's belief that "it is possible to treat the symptom, even if it's deep rooted" (Kaplan, 1983).

While Kaplan's model was generally well received for its attention to the psychological aspects of sexual response, her framework also received some criticism. The primary reason the triphasic model was called into question by the psychological community was because it assumed that men and women have similar sexual responses. Following research done by prominent sexologist and biologist Alfred Kinsey and the differences in sexual behavior between men and women, a genderless response cycle made many concerned that the model pathologized normal behavior in women. For example, many women reported pleasurable sexual experiences that did not include desire at the onset but that grew gradually throughout the experience. Others reported feeling desire and yet having no interest in acting on it, or not feeling desire at all and being concerned that they could not have satisfying sex without it. Of course, these situations proved problematic in light of the proposed model.

Further, many women do not move progressively or sequentially through the phases Kaplan described. Sex educator and researcher Beverly Whipple argues that women may not even experience all the phases—they may reach orgasm and satisfaction without experiencing sexual desire, or they can experience desire, arousal, and satisfaction but not orgasm. This thinking was echoed by Rosemary Basson, who later created a model of female sexual response that differentiated between spontaneous desire and "responsive desire," which was in reaction to a partner's sexual interest rather than a spontaneous stirring of her own libido. This distinction initially helped explain the assumed difference between men's typical, seemingly instantaneous sexual interest and women's more circular desire, although more recent research suggests there are potentially more similarities between the sexes than previously assumed.

Another critique came from feminist scholars after the pleasure revolution. As a largely biologic model, Kaplan's triphasic model has been criticized for failing to take into account nonbiologic experiences of sex, particularly pleasure and satisfaction. It also does not consider the role that sexuality and libido play in the progression of the cycle. As such, critics of the theory feel the model is overly simplistic and limited in scope.

Shadeen Francis

See also: Arousal; Basson, Rosemary; Desire; Desire Disorders; Kaplan, Helen Singer; Kinsey, Alfred; Masters and Johnson Four-Stage Model of Sexual Response; Orgasm; Sexual Dysfunction, Treatment of; Sexual Satisfaction.

Further Reading

Kaplan, H. S. (1980). The new sex therapy. In J. Marmor & S. M. Woods (Eds.), *The interface between the psychodynamic and behavioral therapies* (363–377). New York: Springer.

Kaplan, H. S. (1983). *The evaluation of sexual disorders: Psychological and medical aspects*. London: Psychology Press.

Masters, W. H., & Johnson, V. E. (1966). *Human sexual response*. Boston: Little, Brown, & Co.

Sachs, B. D. (2007). A contextual definition of male sexual arousal. *Hormones and Behavior, 51*(5), 569–578.

Whipple, B., & Brash-McGreer, K. (1997). Management of female sexual dysfunction. In M. L. Sipski & C. J. Alexander (Eds.), *Sexual function in people with disability and chronic illness. A health professional's guide* (509–534). Gaithersburg, MD: Aspen Publishers, Inc.

Wood, J. M., Koch, P. B., & Mansfield, P. K. (2006). Women's sexual desire: A feminist critique. *Journal of Sex Research, 43*(3), 236–244.

Kegel Exercises

Kegel exercises are a type of exercise for the pelvic floor muscles. The pelvic floor muscles support the bladder, reproductive organs, and rectum in both men and women. These muscles may become either too tight (hypertonic) or too loose (hypotonic). In either case, this muscle dysfunction, known as pelvic floor dysfunction, can lead to urinary incontinence (resulting in the leaking of urine), fecal incontinence (resulting in the leaking of stool or gas), or pelvic pain.

The pelvic floor muscles may be located by pretending to stop the flow of urine, as the muscles that contract with this motion are some of the pelvic floor muscles. A Kegel exercise involves the contraction and release of these muscles, with the aim of strengthening the muscles. Kegels should not be done during urination as this can lead to bladder dysfunction.

Popular advice suggests that all women should perform Kegel exercises to maintain vaginal tightness, treat or prevent urinary incontinence, treat pain during intercourse (dyspareunia), and improve orgasm. Men are told less often about Kegels in popular sources, although some do recommend Kegel exercises for men as a way of addressing urinary and fecal incontinence. Kegel exercises may also be recommended for the treatment of erectile disorder, although the effect of Kegels depends on the cause of the erectile disorder.

Since incontinence and pain with intercourse may be caused by either hypertonicity or hypotonicity of the pelvic floor, Kegel exercises may not help and can actually worsen the problem. For women and men with pelvic floor muscles that are too tight, Kegel exercises encourage them to hold the muscles even tighter, which may cause symptoms to worsen, resulting in an increase in pain or incontinence. It is important not to perform Kegel exercises without proper assessment and instruction (many people perform Kegels incorrectly or when they are not advised).

Kegel exercises are particularly recommended for women with vaginismus, a condition in which the muscles of the outer third of the vagina contract involuntarily, causing penetration to be painful or impossible. However, as is the case with pain and incontinence, Kegel exercises may worsen this condition. Women with vaginismus may have underlying pelvic floor dysfunction with pelvic muscles that are hypertonic. Kegel exercises can cause women to tighten their muscles even more, thereby increasing muscle spasm and pain with penetration.

Instead of attempting Kegel exercises on their own, men and women with pelvic pain or incontinence symptoms can seek the services of a pelvic floor physical therapist, a physical therapist that is specially trained to work with the pelvic floor. The physical therapist can assess whether the pelvic floor is too tight or too loose, perform manual muscle release, and instruct the patient in the proper Kegel exercise technique if these exercises are indicated. Rather than traditional Kegel exercises, the physical therapist may recommend reverse Kegels, or pelvic floor relaxation.

Adrienne M. Bairstow

See also: Dyspareunia; Pelvic Floor Muscles; Vaginismus.

Further Reading

Pelvic Health Solutions. (2019). Reverse Kegels/pelvic floor drops. Retrieved from http://pelvichealthsolutions.ca/for-the-patient/persistent-pelvic-pain/pelvic-floor-muscle-tightness/reverse-kegelspelvic-floor-drops/

Pelvic Health Solutions. (2019). What is pelvic floor physiotherapy? Retrieved from http://pelvichealthsolutions.ca/for-the-patient/what-is-pelvic-floor-physiotherapy/

Kellogg, John Harvey

John Harvey Kellogg (1852–1943) was a physician and skilled surgeon who was avidly dedicated to health reform, including that related to sexuality. He emphasized the importance of a healthy diet, regular physical exercise, preventative medicine, and natural remedies. He was also something of an inventor; among his many creations were the breakfast cereals granola and corn flakes. Kellogg wrote extensively and lectured widely on health topics. In 1879, Kellogg published *Plain Facts about Sexual Life*, which was subsequently released in many revised editions, during which the name was changed to *Plain Facts for Old and Young*. It was one of the earliest texts that directly addressed sexual matters, and it sold over half a million copies. He also advocated enemas, hydrotherapy, and vegetarianism.

In 1876, Kellogg took over as superintendent of the Western Health Reform Institute, which had been started a decade earlier in Battle Creek, Michigan, by Seventh-Day Adventists to promote natural remedies consistent with their religious beliefs. He renamed it the Battle Creek Sanitarium, which became known as The San, and greatly expanded its offerings. The San catered to a celebrity clientele. Kellogg took no salary for running The San, but profits from his cereal and book sales made him extremely wealthy.

Sexual activity, or rather abstinence from such activities, was a cornerstone of Kellogg's approach to hygiene. He felt that sexual activity was potentially hazardous to one's emotional, physical, and spiritual health and wellness. Kellogg suggested that many diseases were caused by sexual intercourse and avidly advocated for sexual abstinence. Interestingly, Kellogg and his wife, Ella Ervilla Eaton, are thought to have never consummated their marriage; they had no biological children but adopted and raised eight. Likewise, he was a staunch opponent of masturbation and listed nearly forty problems he said masturbation caused, including acne, bad posture, bashfulness, boldness, defective development, epilepsy, fickleness, mood swings, and heart palpitations. A healthy diet, according to Kellogg, was essential to controlling sexual desires. He believed that a simple, plain diet, particularly one built around cereals and nuts, like the ones he developed and forced on patients at The San, was helpful for controlling sexual urges. He recommended avoiding stimulating food and drink, since he believed things like meat and spiced foods were to blame for increasing one's sex drive.

Victor B. Stolberg

See also: Abstinence; Masturbation.

Further Reading:

Hunnicutt, B. K. (1996). *Kellogg's six-hour day.* Philadelphia: Temple University Press.

Kellogg, J. H. (1882). *Plain facts for old and young.* Burlington, IA: I. F. Segner.

Kellogg, J. H. (1902). *Ladies' guide in health and disease: Girlhood, maidenhood, wifehood, motherhood.* Battle Creek, MI: Modern Medicine Publishing.

Kellogg, J. H. (1918). *Rational hydrotherapy: A manual of the physiological and therapeutic effects of hydriatric procedures, and the technique of their application in the treatment of diseases.* Battle Creek, MI: Modern Medicine Publishing.

Wilson, B. C. (2014). *Dr. John Harvey Kellogg and the religion of biologic living.* Indianapolis: Indiana University Press.

Kink

In the late nineteenth century, "kinky" developed as a slang term that referred to illicit or stolen goods. By the late 1950s, people in the United States and Britain used "kink" or "kinky" to refer to a host of atypical sexual practices, including cross-dressing, fetishism, group sex, role-playing, and a variety of sadomasochistic activities, labeled BDSM in the 1990s. The term combines the abbreviations for bondage and discipline (B&D), dominance and submission (D/S or D&S), and sadism and masochism (S&M or S/M). "Kinky" can also refer to specific exotic or fetishistic clothing, such as "kinky boots."

Ideas as to what activities are kinky vary from person to person and have changed over time, making exact definitions difficult. In Rick James's hit song

"Super Freak" (1981), kinky and freaky are synonyms for promiscuity and group sex. "Three's not a crowd" for the "very kinky girl." Sharon Crane Bakos opens her book *Kink* (1995) with a chapter on anal sex and notes, "twenty years ago, oral sex was considered kinky" (p. xvi). As sexual horizons expanded, the realm of kinky activities narrowed. By the late 1990s, kink had become virtually synonymous with fetishism and BDSM activities, and Bakos devotes most of her book to these topics.

Beginning with the Eulenspiegel Society in New York in 1971, clubs devoted to fetish, BDSM, and other kinky activities formed in cities across the United States. More than a hundred operated by 1986 when the National Leather Association (NLA), an educational, social, and advocacy organization, formed. The NLA's leaders hoped to unite kinky people of all genders, orientations, and interests across the United States and Canada. They organized Living in Leather, an annual conference of people with fetish and BDSM interests that offered a mix of educational seminars, entertainments, and parties. The NLA grew to almost 1,000 members, but kinky people proved too diverse to unite behind any single organization.

Instead, kinky organizations proliferated, as did events that catered to them, which by the late 1990s ranged from Boston's Fetish Fair Fleamarket devoted to shopping, kinky pageants like the International Mr. and Ms. Leather contests in Chicago and San Francisco, the Kink in the Caribbean couples' party at a tropical resort, and numerous local conferences that followed Living in Leather's model of presenting a mix of daytime educational seminars and evening sex parties. Cities that one might not ordinarily associate with kinky sex, including Columbus, Ohio; St. Louis, Missouri; Tulsa, Oklahoma, and many others have kinky organizations that host annual conferences.

Numerous surveys, both popular and academic, indicate that many Americans are interested in kinky activities, which helps explain the popularity of E. L. James's novel *Fifty Shades of Grey* (2011). People's changing interests, though, may well change what is considered kinky in the future.

Stephen K. Stein

See also: BDSM; Fetishism; Paraphilias; Sexual Expression.

Further Reading

Bakos, S. C. (1995). *Kink: The shocking hidden sex lives of Americans.* New York: St. Martin's Press.

Khan, U. (2014). *Vicarious kinks: S/m in the socio-legal imaginary.* Toronto: University of Toronto Press.

Schmall, T. (2018, January). Your partner probably wants a kinkier sex life. *New York Post.* Retrieved from https://nypost.com/2018/01/31/your-partner-probably-wants-a-kinkier-sex-life/

Shahbaz, C., & Chirinos, P. (2017). *Becoming a kink aware therapist.* New York: Routledge.

Stein, S. (2012). *Twenty-five years of Living in Leather: The National Leather Association, 1986–2011.* Daytona Beach, FL: Adynaton.

Wismeijer, A. A. J., & Van Assen, M. A. (2013). Psychological characteristics of BDSM practitioners. *Journal of Sexual Medicine, 10*(8), 1943–1952.

Kinsey, Alfred

Alfred Kinsey (1894–1956) is best known for his research in sex, gender, and reproduction. Among his writings were the hugely popular *Sexual Behavior in the Human Male* (1948) and *Sexual Behavior in the Human Female* (1953), together known as the Kinsey Report. He is also known for his measure of heterosexual and homosexual behavior, known as the Kinsey Scale. Kinsey was born June 23, 1894, in Hoboken, New Jersey, to Alfred Seguine Kinsey and Sarah (née Charles) Kinsey. He was the oldest of three children in a devout Methodist household. His father was very strict and had many rules. Kinsey's parents were poor during his childhood, and this may have led to him receiving inadequate medical treatment for a variety of diseases, including rickets. As a result, he developed a curvature of his spine that prevented him from being drafted in 1917 for World War I.

Kinsey attended Columbia High School, where he was a quiet but hard-working student, interested in biology, botany, and zoology. In 1912, Kinsey graduated as valedictorian of his high school class. Despite the fact that Kinsey wanted to study botany, his father insisted he study engineering at Stevens Institute of Technology. However, after two years, Kinsey left Stevens and transferred to Bowdoin College in Maine, where he studied biology. He graduated, magna cum laude, with a bachelor of science degree in biology and psychology in 1916.

Kinsey continued to study biology in graduate school at Harvard University's Bussey Institute, focusing his studies on gall wasps and amassing a collection of more than five million. Kinsey was granted his doctor of science degree in 1919 and published several papers in 1920 on the gall wasp.

After graduation, Kinsey accepted a job as an assistant professor in zoology at Indiana University in Bloomington, Indiana. A top expert on the gall wasp, in 1930 Kinsey published his findings in the paper *The Gall Wasp Genus Cynips: A Study in the Origin of the Species.*

In 1938, Kinsey agreed to teach a marriage course at Indiana University. His students wanted to learn a wide range of topics about marriage, and they wanted the course to have both male and female students. To learn more about his students, he required them to fill out a survey about their sexual histories. When his students starting asking him questions about sex, Kinsey realized there was very little scientific data on the matter. Members of the faculty at Indiana University disliked what Kinsey was teaching and petitioned the president of the university to remove him from the course. The president gave Kinsey a choice to keep his class or do research but not both. Kinsey chose the research and decided to apply the principles of scientific research toward the topic of sexual behavior, eventually with funding from the National Research Council and the Rockefeller Foundation's Medical Division.

Kinsey, together with his research team, collected more than 17,000 sexual histories between the years 1938 and 1956. Dr. Kinsey believed face-to-face interviews were the best way to get honest answers, and he required his team to memorize over 300 questions and response codes for each. Kinsey promised complete confidentiality to participants in order for them to share their deepest secrets with him. The results of these interviews form the basis for the Kinsey Report books.

In 1920, Kinsey met his future wife, Clara McMillan, at a zoology department picnic. Like Alfred, Clara had little experience dating and no experience with sex. In January 1921, Alfred proposed, and the couple was married on June 3, 1921. Because of their inexperience, Clara and Alfred struggled for almost a year before consummating their marriage. They even went to see a local doctor who determined that Clara had an "adherent clitoris," which required corrective surgery. Alfred and Clara had four children together: Donald, born in 1922, who died of diabetes at the age of four; Anne, born in 1924; Joan, born 1925; and Bruce, born in 1928. They had an open marriage, and Alfred, who was bisexual, had both male and female partners, including his student Clyde Martin. The couple was married from 1921 until Alfred's death in 1956.

In 1947, in order to guarantee absolute confidentiality to individuals interviewed and to provide a secure, permanent location for the growing collection of interview data and other materials Kinsey was collecting on human sexuality, he established the Institute for Sex Research, known today as the Kinsey Institute as a not-for-profit corporation affiliated with Indiana University. The Kinsey Institute is still in existence and advancing sexual health and knowledge worldwide.

In 1953, following the publication of Kinsey's report on female sexuality, a committee of the U.S. House of Representatives started investigating Kinsey and the Rockefeller Foundation for possible ties to the Communist Party. As a result, the foundation terminated Kinsey's funding. Kinsey was devastated, and though he spent the next two and a half years trying to secure funding from alternate sources, he never succeeded. Kinsey died disappointed that he had not persuaded the world that sex was good and that tolerance of the enormous variety of sexual behavior that existed was right. But his dream did not die with him. Kinsey lived just long enough to see the American Law Institute's Model Penal Code, published in 1955, which gives the right of consenting adults to engage in homosexual and anal sex. In 2004, Liam Neeson starred in *Kinsey*, a movie dedicated to portraying Alfred Kinsey's life and accomplishments.

Lauren Ewaniuk

See also: Kinsey's Continuum of Sexual Orientation; Sexology; *Sexual Behavior in the Human Male and Sexual Behavior in the Human Female.*

Further Reading

Christenson, C. V. (1971). *Kinsey: A biography.* Bloomington: Indiana University Press.

Kinsey Institute. (2012). *The Kinsey Institute for research in sex, gender, and reproduction.* Retrieved from http://www.kinseyinstitute.org

Public Broadcast Station. (2005, October 24). American experience: Kinsey. Retrieved from http://www.pbs.org

Kinsey's Continuum of Sexual Orientation

Dr. Alfred Kinsey (1894–1956) created the Kinsey Scale during his work as a professor and sex researcher at Indiana University in Bloomington, Indiana. The Kinsey Scale is a scale ranging from 0 to 6 that showcases a continuum of sexual orientation and debunks the idea that there are only two sexual orientations, homosexuality and heterosexuality. The scale only considers sexual behavior in its rating system and relies on self-report as the individual research participant or client is the one reporting the frequency of their sexual behaviors with same- and other-sex partners. Kinsey made some assumptions regarding gender and sex in his scale, as only two genders and sexes are included. As such, it follows a gender and sex binary, assuming people are male or female, man or woman (Yarber, Sayad, & Strong, 2010).

Dr. Kinsey did not believe that being heterosexual or homosexual was fixed. He also argued that, in accounting for one's sexual orientation, it is important to look at behavior and proportions of sexual behaviors. This led to the creation of a 7-point scale ranging from 0-6 that accounts for different proportions of sexual behaviors. On the scale, "0" indicates an individual has exclusively other-sex behavior. Thus, the designation of a "0" also means "exclusively heterosexual." A "1" indicates mostly other-sex behavior with some same-sex behavior. This may be thought of as "mostly heterosexual." The number "2" equates to mostly other-sex behavior with a good deal of same-sex behavior as well. This may be classified as "somewhat bisexual." A "3" on the rating scale indicates equal amounts of same-sex and other-sex behaviors and may be considered "equally bisexual." A "4" is also "somewhat bisexual" as it indicates the individual has some other-sex behavior but mostly same-sex behavior. A "5" is mostly same-sex behavior with occasional other-sex behavior. Exclusively homosexual is indicated by a number "6" on the scale and reveals sexual behavior is exclusive to same-sex partners.

Dr. Kinsey and his staff of researchers and interviewers utilized the Kinsey Scale during the interviews they conducted for data collection on sexual behavior. While today the scale is largely used as a self-report measure, in many cases, Kinsey or his colleagues conducting the interview assigned a number to the participant after the interview based on what the participant described as their sexual experiences. As such, the scale was not posed as a question to people unless they described significant homosexual experiences. If this were the case, the interviewer asked the participant to self-report on a scale from 0 to 6 where they fell on the continuum after the scale was described to them. However, it was possible for the interviewer to change the response if they did not believe it accurately reflected what had been described to them by the participant. In addition, some leniency was allowed in assigning a number to represent same- and other-sex sexual experiences. While rare, it was possible for intermediate values to be used, such as 2–3 or 4–5 instead of relying on just one number.

There is a clear assumption in this scale that individuals are sexual. However, Kinsey and his team of researchers occasionally came across individuals who did not engage in sexual behaviors and were not interested in engaging in sexual behaviors with persons of the same or other sex. Therefore, while not indicated on the scale, in this case the interviewer assigned the participant an "X." The "X" category was meant to represent individuals who did not experience sexual arousal or desire to either heterosexual or homosexual stimuli. This was always a category that was assigned, not self-reported, as the only people who were asked to self-report were people who described a certain level of homosexual experience, which, by default, excludes individuals who fell into the "X" category.

Prior to Kinsey's research about human sexuality and the development of the Kinsey Scale, it was widely believed that only two sexual orientations existed: heterosexuality and homosexuality. Bisexuality was not legitimized as a sexual orientation, as many people assumed if someone ever engaged in any homosexual behavior, they were homosexual. Kinsey argued against this narrow view of sexual orientation as his research unfolded and found that many people who gave their sexual histories had engaged in sexual behavior with both sexes regardless of identifying as heterosexual or homosexual.

Kinsey's research also revealed to him that sexual attraction might be fluid over the course of someone's life. As such, if someone has mostly other-sex interactions today and is rated as a "1" on the Kinsey Scale, the following year it is possible for them to be a "3" or "4" on the scale as attraction and behavior may change. To Kinsey, it was clear that bisexuality is a legitimate sexual orientation and that one does not have to conform to a heterosexual or homosexual identity. Kinsey's work on sexual orientation and the creation of the Kinsey Scale ushered in criticism of a dichotomous understanding of sexual orientation and has allowed there to be space for bisexuality to be acknowledged. Also, the scale brought to light the reality that, for many people, sexual orientation may be fluid, and sexual behaviors may change over time.

Kinsey and his work advocated for tolerance of sexual difference. His research revealed that many people explored their sexuality through varying behaviors and varying partners. As such, the distinction between what had been previously assumed to be "normal" and "abnormal" sexual behavior was rendered meaningless as many people behaved in ways that contradicted societal expectations of "normal" sexuality. The Kinsey Scale reflects this discovery by acknowledging various sexual behaviors.

There have been many researchers, educators, and therapists who have criticized the Kinsey Scale, arguing it is limiting in the understanding of sexual orientation. Critics state that factors other than just sexual behavior contribute to sexual identity. As this scale only considers sexual behavior, it provides limited insight into an individual's sexual attractions, feelings of love, fantasies, and desired behaviors that have not been acted on. The criticism of the scale has spurred other models to more fully account for a broader understanding of sexual orientation. For example, the Klein Sexual Orientation Grid considers sexual attraction, sexual behavior, sexual fantasy, emotional preference, social preference, heterosexual/homosexual lifestyle, and self-identification in the past, present, and ideal situation to expand on the understanding of sexual orientation spanning a continuum.

Researchers, therapists, and educators have used and continue to use the Kinsey Scale in their work and practice. The scale is a good way to begin discussing sexual orientation as a continuum and to steer away from a dichotomous view of sexual orientation. For researchers, therapists, and educators with a behavioral focus, the Kinsey Scale is a good tool for collecting data on sexual behavior.

Amanda Manuel

See also: Bisexuality; Fluidity, Sexual; Heterosexuality; Homosexuality; Kinsey, Alfred; Same-Sex Attraction and Behavior; *Sexual Behavior in the Human Male* and *Sexual Behavior in the Human Female*; Sexual Orientation; Storms's Model of Sexual Orientation.

Further Reading

Weinrich, J. D. (2014). Notes on the Kinsey scale. *Journal of Bisexuality, 14*(3–4), 333–340. doi: 10.1080/15299716.2014.951139

Yarber, W., Sayad, B., & Strong, B. (2010). *Human sexuality diversity in contemporary America* (7th ed.). New York: McGraw-Hill.

Kissing

Kissing is a low-risk sexual activity that many people engage in on a frequent basis. Kissing feels good because the lips and mouth are very sensitive to touch due to high concentrations of nerves in these areas. Kissing is a sensual experience because so many of the senses are actively involved in kissing, such as taste, touch, and smell.

Kissing serves an important function in mate selection. A French kiss, or kissing with tongue, allows genetic information to be exchanged during the kiss. This information allows partners to determine if their kissing partner is a genetically compatible partner. A 2008 study revealed that kissing allows many chemicals to flood the brain. Neural messages induce sexual excitement, feelings of euphoria, and partner bonding. A kiss is good for overall health as chemical reactions that occur during kissing reduce stress and increase motivation and social bonding.

A study at the University of Albany revealed that kissing allows partners to "know" their partner's chemical makeup by the taste of their mouth and lips. The study also showed that kissing promoted bonding by increasing levels of oxytocin in the body (oxytocin is the bonding hormone) and decreasing cortisol in the body (cortisol is the stress hormone). Finally, the study also concluded that kissing increases sexual arousal.

Since kissing serves such an important role in helping a person determine if their partner is a good fit chemically, it is not surprising that a "bad kiss" may be deemed a deal breaker for a relationship. Technique and the chemical reaction that occurs can determine a good kiss from a bad kiss. One study showed that 59 percent of men and 66 percent of women could be initially attracted to someone and then lose that feeling of attraction after a first kiss, if they deemed it to be a "bad kiss." Both men and women equally stated that a bad first kiss is a good reason to stop dating or hooking up with someone.

Men and women may have different expectations about kissing. In a study at the University of Albany, half of the male participants stated they would be comfortable having sex with someone without kissing them. The female participants, on the other hand, responded quite differently, with only 15 percent reporting they would be comfortable having sex with someone without kissing them. Studies have also indicated that women tend to place more significance on a kiss than men do in regard to foreplay. Women tend to experience kissing as very arousing and tend to be more excited to kiss for a longer period of time than men. Men tend to report that kissing is a step to more sexual activity and would prefer to spend less time focused on this activity than women would.

Studies have also revealed that women tend to enjoy kissing more than men do and may like to engage in this activity more frequently than men. Lesbian couples tend to engage in the most kissing, with heterosexual couples coming in second place; gay couples tend to spend the least amount of time kissing. However, men are more likely to want to engage in kissing with tongue than women. They are also more likely than women to believe that kissing will lead to sex. In one study, 50 percent of men reported that they believed kissing would lead to sex compared with 33 percent of women who stated they believed kissing would lead to sex.

In many cultures, kissing is an expression of love and intimacy. It is often highly acceptable as a sexual activity, and, in some cultures, it is appropriate to engage in kissing publicly. Persons of all genders, sexual orientations, and ages may enjoy various forms of kissing.

In American culture, many people think of kissing as a peck on the lips, a lip lock, a French kiss, or a long make-out session. However, these forms of kissing are not universal to all cultures. In some cultures, breath is considered to be highly intimate. Therefore, instead of necessarily touching lips or tongues together, people may exchange breath with one another. In other cultures, people may rub their noses together. Kissing styles vary across cultures in all types of relationships.

Amanda Manuel

See also: Afterplay; Arousal; Foreplay; Intimacy, Sexual and Relational; Oxytocin; Touching, Sexual Arousal and.

Further Reading

Herbenick, D., & Stoddard, G. (2012). *Great in bed: Thrill the body, blow the mind.* New York: DK Publishing.

Walter, C. (2008). Affairs of the lips. *Scientific American Mind, 19*(1), 24–29.

Yarber, W., Sayad, B., & Strong, B. (2010). *Human sexuality: Diversity in contemporary America* (7th ed.). New York: McGraw-Hill.

Klinefelter Syndrome

Klinefelter syndrome is a chromosomal disorder affecting males. Males with the syndrome are born with at least one extra X chromosome (one of two sex chromosomes), which can slow sexual development because of lowered testosterone and cause increased breast growth. Depending on its severity, the condition is treatable with testoterone replacement therapy, breast reduction, or counseling.

Occurring in approximately 1 in every 500–1,000 males, Klinefelter syndrome (named for Harry Klinefelter, an American physician who in 1942 described a set of symptoms that characterized the condition) is one of the most common chromosomal disorders affecting males. Typically, males have both an X and a Y chromosome. In the most common cases of Klinefelter syndrome, males are born with one extra X chromosome (XXY instead of XY). In rarer variants of the syndrome (occurring in approximately 1 in every 50,000 newborns), males are born with several extra X chromosomes or one extra X chromosome in some cells but not in others (known as mosaic Klinefelter syndrome). In any instance of the disorder, it is not an inherited condition but rather arises from a disruption occurring during production of the egg or sperm cells, which then meet to form the embryo.

The risk of health conditions increases with the number of extra X chromosomes. Men with generalized Klinefelter syndrome often have small testicles, weak bones, taller than average stature, enlarged breast tissue, decreased sex drive, and fertility issues. Often the condition remains undiagnosed until adulthood. In boys, the disorder may be suspected in the event of delayed, absent, or incomplete puberty. Variants of Klinefelter syndrome tend to cause more severe signs and symptoms than classic Klinefelter syndrome. In addition to affecting male sexual development, variants of Klinefelter syndrome are associated with intellectual disability, distinctive facial features, skeletal abnormalities, poor coordination, and severe problems with speech. Individuals with mosaic Klinefelter syndrome, on the other hand, may have milder signs and symptoms depending on how many cells have an additional X chromosome.

Researchers suspect that Klinefelter syndrome is underdiagnosed because the condition may be mild in many instances or the features of the condition may overlap with those of other conditions. The two main tests used to diagnose the disorder are hormone testing and chromosome (karyotype) analysis. In each case, blood samples can reveal abnormalities in hormone levels or the shape or number of chromosomes that characterize the presence of the disorder. Other tests involve an examination of the genital area as well as tests to check reflexes and mental function. Although the chromosomes cannot be repaired, one or more treatments may minimize problems once a diagnosis is made, such as testosterone replacement therapy (to improve bone density), breast tissue reduction, fertility treatments, or counseling.

Linda Tancs

See also: Chromosomal Sex; Gynecomastia; Intersexuality; Puberty, Delayed; Sex Chromosomes; Testosterone; Turner Syndrome; X Chromosome; Y Chromosome.

Further Reading

Wattendorf, D. J., & Muenke, M. (2005). Klinefelter syndrome. *American Family Physician, 72*(11), 2259–2262.

Weingarten, C. N., & Jefferson, S. E. (2009). *Sex chromosomes: Genetics, abnormalities, and disorders.* Hauppauge, NY: Nova Science Publishers.

Krafft-Ebing, Richard von

Richard von Krafft-Ebing was a German psychiatrist during the nineteenth century who became the first major researcher in sexual paraphilias and diversity. In his major work, *Psychopathia Sexualis*, he popularized or coined such terms as "heterosexual," "homosexual," "sadism," "masochism," and "pedophile." Although Krafft-Ebing saw people with differing sexual practices as deviants or morally corrupted individuals, he favored an approach stressing treatment and cure instead of criminal confinement. Krafft-Ebing's pragmatic liberalism was evident in his support for the decriminalization of homosexuality in Germany and the study of women's sexual desires.

Richard von Krafft-Ebing was born on August 14, 1840, in Mannheim, Germany, into a family of the minor nobility. He followed his maternal grandfather into medicine but was attracted to psychiatry as a specialty. Beginning in 1872, he taught psychiatry at the University of Strasbourg but soon took a position at the University of Graz. Besides his teaching duties, Krafft-Ebing also worked as superintendent of the Feldhof mental asylum. He was troubled by the fact that patients there were treated more like criminals than individuals needing treatment. In 1879, Krafft-Ebing published his first book, *Text-Book of Insanity*. It called for doctors to search for the cause of a patient's mental illness and offer therapy.

In 1886, Krafft-Ebing published his most important work, *Psychopathia Sexualis*. He attempted to classify various types of sexual deviance and to suggest their causes and methods of treatment. He illustrated each type of behavior with case studies of patients he had examined. Krafft-Ebing believed his book should be a reference source for doctors, psychiatrists, and judges. He realized the subject of his study would attract great attention. To reduce the access of the lay public to the lurid details, Krafft-Ebing wrote much of *Psychopathia Sexualis* in Latin. The work went through twelve editions during Krafft-Ebing's lifetime. In each edition, he added to the number of case studies. After the first edition of *Psychopathia Sexualis*, many individuals with sexual disorders contacted Krafft-Ebing. They spoke to him on condition of anonymity, often to discuss taboo behavior they had been unable to share with family or friends.

Krafft-Ebing's pioneering work greatly influenced later sexologists and psychologists, including Sigmund Freud and Carl Jung. The latter pair eclipsed him in the field, but his writings laid the groundwork on which they built. Krafft-Ebing helped to move sexual dysfunction from being ignored, dismissed as insanity, or a matter for religious authorities. For all his liberal attitudes about causes and treatment of sexual deviant behavior, however, Krafft-Ebing remained true to his Victorian culture. He believed that any sex act that was not committed in the context of marriage and for the purpose of procreation was morally wrong. Homosexuality was therefore wrong, even if it was not a crime. In 1871, the German Empire implemented a legal code, including Paragraph 175, that criminalized homosexuality. Krafft-Ebing raised eyebrows when he publicly opposed the statute. He also believed that normal, healthy women were sexually passive and had little or no interest in sex. Any exceptions were signs of mental illness.

Krafft-Ebing died in Graz, Austria-Hungary, on December 22, 1902.

Tim J. Watts

See also: BDSM; Freud, Sigmund; Paraphilias; Victorian Era.

Further Reading

Hunnicutt, A. (2015). Krafft-Ebing, Richard von (1840–1902). In *GLBTQ: An encyclopedia of gay, lesbian, bisexual, transgender & queer culture*. Retrieved from http://www.glbtqarchive.com/ssh/krafft_ebing_r_S.pdf

Krafft-Ebing, R. (1903). *Psychopathia sexualis* (12th ed., F. J. Rebman, Trans.). New York: Rebman Company. (Original work published 1886).

McFatridge, K. (n.d.). Richard von Krafft-Ebing (1840–1902). Retrieved from http://psychistofwomen.umwblogs.org/sexuality/pre-kinsey/krafft-ebing/

L

Labia

The labia are two pairs of folds of skin that are the visible portion of the vulva. The labia majora is the outer pair, which usually covers the inner labia minora. They help protect the urethra and vagina and can play an important role in sexual arousal and orgasm. Normal, healthy labia can vary widely in size and appearance. However, some women are concerned that their labia seem larger than they should be and so seek plastic surgery, known as labiaplasty, to reshape one or both sets of labia.

The word "labia" is derived from the Latin word for "lip." To a certain extent, both pairs of labia play the same role as the lips do for the mouth. The labia majora is the generally larger, outer pair. They begin just below the mons pubis and above the clitoris. The labia majora rejoin above the perineum. They are composed of skin and fatty tissue and are normally larger toward the front. During and after puberty, the skin may become darker than the rest of the body. At puberty, pubic hair also begins to emerge on the labia majora. The inner and outer surfaces have sebaceous (oil) glands as well as two types of sweat glands.

The labia minora is the inner and generally smaller pair. They are folds of soft, fat-free skin without any hair. The upper portions join at the clitoris hood and rejoin just below the vaginal opening. The inner surface is moist and contains many sebaceous glands.

The labia are one of the erogenous zones. Stimulation causes an increased flow of blood to the area, and the labia will increase in size. Orgasms and the accompanying contractions will help remove the blood, and the labia will return to their normal appearance.

Some women have larger labia, which may cause discomfort, especially when wearing tight clothing or when participating in some activities. Other women may be concerned that their labia's appearance is not "normal" because they are comparing themselves to unrealistic ideals, such as is seen in pornography. A controversial surgical procedure known as labiaplasty can be performed to change the labia's size or appearance. As with any surgery, there are dangers such as infection, scarring, or bleeding. Sexual intercourse may also be painful after a labiaplasty.

Tim J. Watts

See also: Erogenous Zones; Labiaplasty; Pubic Hair; Vulva.

Further Reading

Center for Young Women's Health. (2019). Labia. Retrieved from https://youngwomenshealth.org/2013/07/16/labia/

Women's Health Victoria. (2019). The labia library. Retrieved from http://www.labialibrary.org.au

Labiaplasty

Labiaplasty is a surgery that reduces or reshapes the labia majora or labia minora. The surgery may be medically necessary in cases where the size of the labia causes a person significant emotional distress or physical discomfort. Surgery can be warranted in cases of symptomatic structural abnormalities related to labial size or shape; in these cases, the labia create physical discomfort. Female genital cosmetic surgery strictly for aesthetics warrants careful consideration about the difference between medical need and trends in physical enhancements.

The labia minora are part of the female exterior genitalia commonly referred to as the inner lips. They are paired folds of non-hair-bearing smooth tissue within the labia majora. The labia majora are fatty, hair-bearing outer lips. The labia minora cover the urethral opening and the opening of the vagina except during sexual arousal, when the labia deepen in color, engorge, and flair slightly. This engorgement is part of the female sexual response cycle and is the result of increased pelvic blood flow. Because the labia minora are attached to the base of the clitoral glans, movement of the labia minora indirectly stimulates the clitoris.

Typically, the labia are of roughly equal dimension and are most visible when the legs are separated. Labia minora diagnosed as enlarged, or hypertrophic, may be greatly unequal in dimension or protrude beyond the cusp of the labia majora. Labia majora may be diagnosed if they are significantly asymmetrical or elongated.

The medical community has not reached consensus on what normal, functional labia look like. Defining normal labia minora as being hidden between labia majora is subjective, as normal female genitalia vary in their length, shape, and coloration.

Labial size is usually congenital; however, size can also be affected by exposure to exogenous androgens in infancy, hormonal changes, childbirth, manual stretching, and aging. Labial enlargement also may occur secondary to some medical conditions. The size of the labia minora is no indication of masturbation or partnered sexual activity, contrary to some common misconceptions.

Labia minora that protrude beyond the labia majora may be irritated by tight clothing, create hygiene problems during menstruation or toileting, interfere with sexual activities, and/or feel uncomfortable while a person is sitting or participating in exercise.

The goal of labiaplasty on the labia minora is to remove labial tissue a patient deems excessive and to create symmetrical, smaller labia. Several types of procedures are in use, but the data are limited on long-term outcomes. Patients should be aware of the options and discuss the risks and benefits of each with their surgeon.

One technique for labiaplasty involves a straight amputation of the tissue deemed excessive. This results in a scarred suture line along the new edge of the labia. The new edge is smoother and lighter pink than the natural edge was, which can give the labia a more youthful look; however, the scar line can lead to irritation and discomfort later on.

Another technique involves the amputation of V-shaped wedges of tissue. One cut is made from the midline of the labia to the outer edge; another cut is from the midline cut toward the end of the labia close to the vaginal opening. The tissue is sutured to close the gap created by the removal of the wedge to maintain the natural edge.

Sometimes, a second surgery is required to correct wound dehiscence, which occurs when a wound ruptures along surgical suture. Patients at greater risk for dehiscence tend to be either older or obese, or they may have diabetes. Poor knotting or grabbing of stitches, as well as trauma to the wound after surgery, may also lead to wound dehiscence.

Labia majora deemed excessively large can be reduced in size through liposuction or laser surgery. If age, weight loss, or pregnancy have caused the labia majora to lose fullness, or to appear to sag, the labia can be reduced through surgery. The labia majora can also be injected with fat transferred from elsewhere on the patient's body. Synthetic fillers can be used but generally have less desirable outcomes.

Labiaplasty carries the same risk of any surgery in terms of infection, bleeding, and wound healing issues. People who take blood thinners, smoke, or have immune suppressive disorders are at greater risk for surgical complications.

Problems specifically related to labiaplasty on the labia minora, which is more common than labia majora surgery, may include permanent changes in sensation, ongoing pain, asymmetry of the labia, scarring, and dyspareunia. These issues can interfere with sexual pleasure, which can, in turn, have an impact on sexual relationships. If the clitoral hood is also reduced in size, complications may occur in terms of damage to the clitoral glans and nerves responsible for sexual pleasure.

While cost is not a medical risk, it can be a personal financial risk. Labiaplasty for strictly cosmetic reasons is not covered by insurance. Another risk is that while someone may expect the surgery to resolve body image issues, there is no guarantee that the labia will look as expected or that any result would satisfy that psychological need.

It is not uncommon for adolescents to be concerned about their body looking attractive. As sexually explicit images have become increasingly accessible, physicians are seeing more young female patients who seek labiaplasty. Some surgeons have advocated that the minimum age for this procedure be set at eighteen years.

The risk of being unhappy with the surgical outcome will decrease if patients should seek out surgeons willing to share before and after photos of their surgeries. This will increase the odds that both surgeon and patient agree on the desired aesthetic outcome.

According to the American Society for Aesthetic Plastic Surgery, labiaplasty procedures increased 44 percent between 2012 and 2013. The tailoring of body parts to suit societal perceptions of beauty is not new, but most other cosmetic procedures do not require the resection (removal) of healthy, normal tissue related to sexual function.

The practice of female genital cosmetic surgery, specifically labiaplasty, has increased in popularity as images of female genitals in sexually explicit media have idealized small, symmetrical labia minora. The trend of pubic hair removal makes labia more visible and subject to critical assessment as well. While some people pressure themselves to match the idealized form, many patients seeking labiaplasty recall having heard specific negative comments about their labia from sexual partners and others. Another reason people seek out cosmetic labiaplasty is to satisfy their desire to have more youthful-looking genitalia.

Women who consider their labia minora to be unattractive or irritating may feel deformed or abnormal, and these feelings can result in embarrassment, negative body image, and low sexual self-esteem. Some of these concerns may be alleviated if health care providers and surgeons explain that variations in labial dimension are normal.

Many surgical websites promote postsurgical improvements in self-esteem, body image, and sexual relationships; however, no long-term studies evaluating the effects of such surgery have been done. What is known is that most women do not have female cosmetic genital surgery, and women with all shapes and sizes of labia can feel confident and sexually satisfied.

Melanie Davis

See also: Dyspareunia; Hymenoplasty; Labia; Pornography; Vulva.

Further Reading

Creighton, S. M., & Liao, L.-M. (2019). *Female genital cosmetic surgery: Solution to what problem?* Cambridge: Cambridge University Press.

Goodman, M. P. (2013). *You want to do what? Where? Everything you ever wanted to know about women's genital plastic & cosmetic surgery.* Davis, CA: author.

Lee's Theory of Love Styles

Lee's theory of love styles was developed by Canadian sociologist John Lee (1973). He proposed that there were six ways of loving or understating love, which he called love styles. The three primary love styles are eros, storge, and ludus. The three additional styles are pragma, mania, and agape. In general, people tend to have a fairly consistent love style throughout their life, but they can also express different styles within a romantic relationship, and they may experience different love styles in relationships with different partners.

Eros, named for the Greek god of love, encompasses erotic, powerful, physical, and passionate love. Experiencing erotic love is important for relationship and sexual satisfaction with a partner. The eros love style is associated with a sense that the individual and the partner were meant for one another and that they have the right physical chemistry between them.

The storge love style is love that is based on a strong sense of friendship and compatibility. It develops when people enjoy similar activities and starts as liking and friendship and then can build into affection and commitment. This style of love can be seen as love and affection between siblings and friends, but storgic love can also be seen in romantic relationships. In these relationships the friendship and long-term commitment are valued above short-term excitement, sexual gratification, or physical appearance.

Ludus, named for the Latin word for game or play, is a love style in which love is seen as a game to be played. Typically, people with a ludic love style tend to enjoy short-term sexual relationships with a variety of people, without commitment. A ludic love style tends to be associated with lower relationship satisfaction. Males may be more likely to report a ludic love style than females, and it may be more common among younger people and those who have never been married.

The pragma love style may be considered as having elements of both storge and ludus love styles. In this love style, compatibility is the ultimate goal. Someone with a pragmatic love style may have a list of qualities that they are looking for in a partner, and potential partners are then screened against this list to see how well they match up. Pragmatic love involves making rational decisions and prioritizing compatibility and other desired characteristics above emotion.

The mania love style has been described as the ludus style but "without the confidence." This style of love is possessive, jealous, and insecure. It is dependent and obsessive, and someone with a manic love style may have trouble concentrating on anything other than their partner. People with a manic love style may desire love, but they also tend to be mistrustful, jealous, and insecure.

The final love style is agape love. Agape love is selfless, giving, and altruistic love. This love may be characteristic of a parent's love of their child. Within a romantic relationship, a person with an agape love style tends to be compassionate and to place their partner's happiness above their own. This style of love is rare.

Heather L. Armstrong

See also: Attachment Theory of Love; Companionate Love; Consummate Love; Love; Sternberg's Triangular Theory of Love.

Further Reading

Hendrick, S. S. (2004). Close relationship research: A resource for couple and family therapists. *Journal of Marital and Family Therapy, 30*(1), 13–27.

Hendrick, S. S., & Hendrick, C. (1997). Love and satisfaction. In R. J. Sternberg & M. Hojjat (Eds.), *Satisfaction in close relationships* (56–78). New York: Guilford Press.

Lee, J. A. (1973). *Colours of love: An exploration of the ways of loving.* Toronto, ON: New Press.

Lee, J. A. (1988). Love-styles. In R. J. Sternberg & M. L. Barnes (Eds.), *The psychology of love* (38–67). New Haven, CT: Yale University Press.

Smith, K. B. (2017). Attraction, intimacy, and love. In C. F. Pukall (Ed.), *Human sexuality: A contemporary introduction* (2nd ed.). Don Mills, ON: Oxford University Press.

LeVay, Simon

Simon LeVay is a British neuroscientist who has practiced and lived in the United States since 1972. His early work involved investigations into the visual cortex of animals, but he is best known for his investigation into biological and anatomical causes of homosexuality. LeVay was motivated to start his research because of his own sexual orientation and a personal crisis. When he proposed in 1993 that gay and straight men had differences in their brains, scientists and the general public quickly responded. Although LeVay never claimed his work proved a biological cause of homosexuality, many observers treated it as if it had. LeVay has spent the rest of his life trying to educate the public about homosexuality and its roots.

LeVay was born on August 28, 1943, in Oxford, England. His father was an orthopedic surgeon, and his mother was a pathologist who stayed home to care for their five sons. The couple divorced when LeVay was eleven. He attended private schools as a child before enrolling at the University of Cambridge. His parents encouraged him to become a doctor, so he began focusing on the sciences. LeVay received a bachelor's degree in natural sciences in 1966 but later dropped out of medical school. He then entered the University of Gottingen in Germany and studied neuroanatomy. LeVay earned a PhD in 1971 and accepted a position as a postdoctoral research fellow at Harvard Medical School in 1972. He remained at Harvard until 1984, when he moved to the Salk Institute for Biological Studies in San Diego. Most of LeVay's early research centered on the visual cortex of animals.

LeVay had realized he was gay when he was thirteen and became comfortable with that fact. While studying in Germany, he began a long-term relationship with Richard Hersey, an American student. Hersey was one of the reasons LeVay moved to the United States. After twenty-one years together, Hersey died in 1990 of AIDS. Deeply affected, LeVay decided to direct his research toward something related to his gay identity. He was aware that researchers had discovered sex-related differences in the brains of men and women. The nerve bundles connecting the two halves of the brain were usually larger in women than in men, for example.

To determine if gay men's brains differed from those of straight men, LeVay autopsied the brains of forty-one people. Nineteen were homosexual men, sixteen were heterosexual men, and six were women. Special attention was paid to the third interstitial nucleus of the anterior hypothalamus (INAH3). The hypothalamus is a small part of the brain known to direct male sexual behavior, including attraction to women. The examination of the INAH3 could not be performed on living people. In 1991, LeVay published his findings in an article entitled "A Difference in Hypothalamic Structure between Heterosexual and Homosexual Men" in *Science*. He found that gay men had INAH3 clusters that were half the size of straight men's. The female brains had INAH3 clusters that were about the same size as those of gay men. LeVay concluded that his findings suggested sexual orientation has a biological basis.

The response to LeVay's article was swift. Some gay rights advocates believed that he had shown being gay was not a choice but biologically driven, like eye color. Others criticized his work, pointing out the small sample size and the failure to include lesbians. In addition, the very small size of the INAH3 clusters made relative differences very small. LeVay responded to the criticism by stating that he believed other factors helped determine a gay identity. He believed prenatal influences were very important, for example. LeVay's research helped encourage other researchers to explore if other physical differences based on sexual orientation could be found.

LeVay resigned his position at the Salk Institute in 1993 to devote himself to educating others about homosexuality. He helped found the Institute of Gay and Lesbian Education, an open institute for those who wanted to know more about gay and lesbian individuals in society. In 2003, LeVay became the director of human sexuality studies at Stanford University.

Tim J. Watts

See also: Biological Theories of Sexual Orientation; Homosexuality; Sex Differentiation of the Brain and Sexual Orientation; Sexual Orientation.

Further Reading

LeVay, S. (1991). A difference in hypothalamic structure between heterosexual and homosexual men. *Science, 253*(5023), 1034–1037.

LeVay, S. (2016). *Gay, straight, and the reason why: The science of sexual orientation.* New York: Oxford University Press.

LGBTQ+

"LGBTQ+" is an acronym used to refer to the community of individuals who identify as sexual and gender minorities. "L" stands for lesbian, "G" for gay, "B" for bisexual, "T" for transgender, "Q" for either questioning or queer, and "+" for those who identify within the community but are not represented by the first five letters. LGBTQ+ has generally replaced other acronyms such as GLBT or LGB that were previously used. Aside from the initials used in LGBTQ+, several others are used in various contexts. Other commonly used initials include a second "Q" to represent questioning or queer, "I" for intersex, "A" for asexual or ally, "P" for pansexual, "D" for demisexual, "2-S" or "2S" for two-spirit, "NB" or "N-B" for nonbinary, "S" for skoliosexual, "GNC" for gender nonconforming, "SGL" for same-gender loving, "C" for curious, and an additional "A" for either asexual or ally.

The term "gay" first became slang for men who were sexually attracted to men in the mid-1900s. As the gay rights movement gained momentum during the 1960s, some began using the term "gay" to refer to all sexual minorities. Within the early 1970s, the phrase "gay and lesbian" became more prominent as lesbians established a more public profile. During the 1980s, the acronym "GLB" was often used to refer to those who were gay, lesbian, or bisexual. During the 1990s, the acronym "GLBT" became more common as individuals who identified as transgender became a more prominent part of the sexual and gender minority community. Within the early 2000s, the G and L began switching places, with "LGBT" becoming the most commonly used acronym.

As individuals who identified as sexual or gender minorities but did not identify as lesbian, gay, bisexual, or transgender became more vocal within the later-2000s and early to mid-2010s, the acronym underwent several variations. Additional letters were added within different media in an attempt to incorporate the variety of identities included under the umbrella of sexual and gender minorities. The length and infinite variations of these acronyms became known as alphabet soup and led to some confusion. For example, there has been a great deal of disagreement about what the Q stands for. The 2016 GLAAD Media Reference Guide states that the preferred acronym is "LGBTQ," with the Q representing queer, but others suggest the Q should represent those who are questioning their sexual or gender identities. Also, some question using an A to stand for allies, as they feel allies, while important, are not part of the sexual and gender minority community. In order to limit the length of the acronym while remaining inclusive of individuals who identify as any sexual or gender minority, "LGBTQ+" has become the most commonly used acronym.

Aside from "LGBTQ+," several other acronyms are used in different contexts. Within the social and health sciences, "SGM" is often used to represent sexual and gender minorities. Alternatively, medical literature commonly uses the acronyms "MSM" (men who have sex with men) or "WSW" (women who have sex with women) as their research is more focused on sexual behaviors rather than the personal or social identities of those engaging in the behaviors. Within educational environments, the acronym "GSA" was originally used to stand for gay-straight alliance but has often also been described as gender and sexuality alliance.

Richard A. Brandon-Friedman

See also: Asexuality; Bisexuality; Gender Identity; Homosexuality; Queer; Sexual Identity; Sexual Orientation; Transgender.

Further Reading

Chauncey, G. (1994). *Gay New York.* Chicago: University of Chicago Press.

Faderman, L. (2015). *The gay revolution: The story of struggle.* New York: Simon & Schuster.

GLAAD. (2016). *GLAAD media reference guide* (10th ed.). New York: Author.

Love

Love tends to be considered as a powerful emotion that may be present within multiple types of relationships where one feels compassion and companionship. However, love as is usually conceptualized in Western cultures is a relatively new phenomenon and can take on many different roles within society. There are many different types of love, such as sexual love, familial love, friendly love, and passionate love. Each type of love has its role within our lives.

According to anthropologists, romantic love plays a primary role in Western cultures where the main focus tends to be on the individual. Consequently, romantic love is allowed and able to play a major role in an individual's life and can also become a part of their identity. In Eastern cultures, the focus tends to be more on collectivism, and, as such, romantic love is not seen as needed for individual identity. In Western cultures, romantic love is often seen as the primary reason to be in a relationship with someone and to marry. In Eastern cultures, because cultural values focus more on responsibilities toward family and society, romantic love is not seen as necessary for marriage, and the practice of arranged marriages is more common.

There are many types of love. Most often when discussing love, individuals think of romantic love, which is defined as the idealization of another. This is the strong emotional bond individuals feel toward a romantic partner. Individuals can also feel love toward family and friends. This is a different type of love, involving deep care and concern with the other's well-being. Some experiences of love may be considered as unconditional love, where the person is able to look past any negative traits or behaviors of the other and still love them, such as the love between parent and child.

In 1986, Dr. Robert Sternberg created the triangular theory of love. He theorized that there were three main components of love, just like there are three angles in a triangle. The three components are intimacy, passion, and commitment. Sternberg proposed that different types of love could be described based on the relative amount of each component present. He also proposed that the relative amount of each component, the therefore the style of love experienced, can also change over the course of a relationship. This theory consists of eight different types of love:

1. Consummate love, where passion, intimacy, and commitment are all present
2. Liking, where only intimacy is present
3. Infatuation, where only passion is present
4. Empty love, where only commitment is present
5. Romantic love, where intimacy and passion are present but commitment is absent
6. Companionate love, where intimacy and commitment are present but passion is absent.
7. Fatuous love, where passion and commitment are present but intimacy is absent
8. Nonlove, where commitment, intimacy, and passion are all absent

Attachment theory can also be used to describe love. In the 1960s, John Bowlby discussed how people develop expectations and understanding of relationships based on the attachment they form in childhood with their primary caregivers, typically their mother. According to attachment theory, these early experiences can have a significant impact on how people love and experience relationships as adults. As adults, there are four main types of attachment: secure, anxious-ambivalent (or preoccupied), fearful-avoidant, and dismissive-avoidant. Individuals with a secure attachment experienced positive, responsive relationships with their primary caregiver and as a result develop the expectation of positive, supportive relationships as adults. They have a positive view of self and of others. Individuals who experienced unsupportive or challenging relationships with their caregivers as children develop insecure attachment patterns as adults. Individuals with an anxious-ambivalent attachment have a negative self-view but a positive view of others. As adults, they may be overly dependent on others for self-worth and may be preoccupied and insecure with their relationships. Individuals with a fearful-avoidant attachment style have negative feelings of others and a negative self-view. Consequently, they often fear letting others get close to them and report high levels of fear of rejection. Finally, adults with a dismissive-avoidant attachment experience a positive self-view but a negative view of others. Consequently, they are self-reliant and report a low need for intimacy. In a relationship, they are often distant and may downplay the importance of intimacy.

Amanda Baker

See also: Attachment Theory of Love; Companionate Love; Consummate Love; Intimacy, Sexual and Relational; Lee's Theory of Love Styles; Sternberg's Triangular Theory of Love.

Further Reading

Perel, E. (2006). *Mating in captivity.* New York: HarperCollins.

Psychologist World. (2019). Attachment theory. Retrieved from https://www.psychologistworld.com/developmental/attachment-theory

Robert, J. S. (n.d.). Triangular theory of love. Retrieved from http://www.robertjsternberg.com/love

Lubricants

Lubricants are substances, either organic or manufactured, that assist in the reduction of friction between surfaces that come in contact with one another. Lubricants are useful in many sexual situations. Men produce a natural lubricant that is clear and colorless and is emitted from the urethra of the penis during sexual arousal. This is often called preejaculate or precum. Preejaculate helps neutralize the urethra area, as urine is acidic, creating a more favorable environment for the passage of sperm. Women naturally produce their own lubrication in the vagina during sexual arousal to reduce friction and irritation from penetration and to enhance sexual arousal. External lubricants can also be used to enhance the sexual experience.

The production of lubrication varies from woman to woman. Some women may produce large amounts of lubrication, while others may be unable to create enough lubrication to reduce friction. Lubrication production will also vary over time and in different contexts. Lubrication production is influenced by hormone levels. As an example, a woman may have less lubrication during menopause as the result of lower estrogen levels. In addition to changes in hormones, other reasons that cause low levels of vaginal lubrication may be breastfeeding, chemotherapy, other treatments for breast cancer, dehydration, and depression medication (Obos Sexuality & Relationship Contributors, 2014). When this is the case, external lubricants can be useful during sexual activity.

External lubricants are a liquid or gel-type substance that can be applied during sex to make the vulva, vagina, or anal areas wetter. Lubrication can also be applied to a penis to reduce friction from penetration. To choose lubricants, one must be aware of their own comfort and safety, and sometimes people may have to try different types of lubricants to find the one that works best for them.

There are three different types of lubrication: water based, silicone based, and oil based. The most common type is water-based lubrication. Most water-based lubricants contain synthetic glycerin, a lipid, oil, or fat that is used to moisturize and soften skin, to create the effect of natural lubrication. Water-based lubricants are safe to use with latex condoms, easy to find, and low cost. Lubricants that contain synthetic glycerin may dry out quickly and can trigger yeast infections in women who are prone to them. Water-based lubricants that do not contain glycerin tend to last longer than lubricants that do. These lubricants are also safe to use with latex condoms but are usually thicker than ones with glycerin. These lubricants are not as easily found in a drugstore and so are usually found online or at sex stores.

Silicone lubricants last three times longer than water-based lubricants but can cause irritation if not immediately rinsed off after sex. These lubricants also contain glycerin, and they can be expensive and cannot be used with other silicone sex toys. They are safe to use with latex condoms. Silicone lubricants are not as easily accessible as water-based lubricants and may be purchased online or in sex stores.

Oil-based lubricants may be natural or synthetic oil based. These types of lubricants are fairly easy to find as they can already be in your kitchen or bathroom. Natural oil-based lubricants work well for sexual arousal and foreplay, are usually very safe to use, and are low cost and easily accessible. Coconut oil is one example. Synthetic oil-based lubricants may irritate the vulva, vagina, and anus and so should be used only for external play like massages or masturbation. One major drawback of oil-based lubricants is that they destroy latex condoms, making them much more prone to breaking during intercourse. Because of this, if condoms are being used during the sexual experience, a water- or silicone-based lubrication should be used.

Casey T. Tobin

See also: Condoms, Female (Receptive); Condoms, Male (Insertive); Vaginal Lubrication.

Further Reading

Herbenik, D., Reece, M., Schick, V., Sanders, S., & Fortenberry, D. (2014). Women's use and perceptions of commercial lubricants: Prevalence and characteristics in a nationally representative sample of American adults. *The Journal of Sexual Medicine, 11*(3), 642–652.

Jozkowski, K. N., Herbenik, D., Schick, V., Reece, M., Sanders S., & Fortenberry D. (2013). Women's perceptions about lubricant use and vaginal wetness during sexual activities. *The Journal of Sexual Medicine, 10*(2), 484–492.

Obos Sexuality & Relationship Contributors. (2014). How to choose a lubricant for pleasure and safety. Retrieved from https://www.ourbodiesourselves.org/book-excerpts/health-article/how-to-choose-lubricant/

Luteinizing Hormone

Luteinizing hormone (LH) is one of several hormones secreted by the anterior lobe of the pituitary gland, located beneath the brain near the skull's center. LH, along with follicle-stimulating hormone (FSH, another pituitary secretion), regulates the activity of the gonads (ovaries and testes). These hormones are crucial to the reproductive process for all people.

In women of childbearing age, LH and FSH trigger a monthly increase in production of estrogen by the ovaries, leading, in turn, to ovulation. These hormones also prompt the monthly development of the corpus luteum, a structure in the ovaries that secretes a hormone called progesterone, which leads to the growth and maintenance of the endometrium, an extra lining of cells and blood vessels in the walls of the uterus. The endometrium is necessary for pregnancy—that is, the implantation of the embryo in the uterine wall and its subsequent growth into a fetus.

The monthly increase in a woman's LH secretion, known as the "LH surge," lasts from about twenty-four to forty-eight hours, during which time the hormone produces its main effects. If pregnancy does not occur, LH levels decline as menstruation happens. Levels of LH also decline if pregnancy does occur. As an embryo develops in the uterus, its placenta secretes an LH-like hormone called human chorionic gonadotropin, which takes over LH's role in maintaining the function of the corpus luteum.

The LH surge can be used to predict ovulation and, thus, the time when sexual intercourse is most likely to result in pregnancy. Levels of LH can be easily measured in urine samples at home with urinary ovulation predictor kits, also called LH kits. Used daily at the expected approximate time of ovulation, a change from a negative to positive reading on a test strip indicates that ovulation will occur within twenty-four to forty-eight hours.

In men, LH and FSH stimulate Leydig cells in the testes to produce testosterone. This hormone prompts the development of male sexual characteristics, including the maturing of the testes so that they produce healthy, viable sperm.

Levels of LH (which can be measured in either blood or urine samples) normally change throughout an individual's life. They typically rise in women after menopause because of the loss of a biochemical feedback mechanism that helps to regulate LH levels during childbearing years. This rise is normal in older women and poses no special health risks. Normal LH levels for women before menopause range from five to twenty-five international units (IU) per liter (L). These levels peak during the middle of menstrual cycles. Normal levels after menopause range from fourteen to fifty-two IU/L. Normal LH levels in men older than age eighteen range from about two to nine IU/L.

High or low LH levels can be signs of certain disease conditions. In younger women, persistently elevated LH levels (lasting longer than the LH surge) might suggest premature menopause, polycystic ovary syndrome (ovary abnormalities that include cysts, menstrual cycle problems, and a hormone imbalance), Swyer syndrome (the absence of functional gonads), Turner syndrome (a chromosomal abnormality that causes physical and mental disabilities), or other conditions.

In men, higher-than-normal levels of LH are usually associated with testicular problems. Such problems may be related to any of several conditions, including injury, cancer, or Klinefelter syndrome (a chromosomal abnormality).

Lower-than-normal levels of LH may be signs of hypogonadism (failure of the ovaries or testes), hypopituitarism (failure of the pituitary gland), hyperprolactinemia (excess amounts of prolactin hormone, leading to sexual problems),

Kallman syndrome (failure of puberty to begin or to be completed), anorexia nervosa (an eating disorder), stress, or other conditions.

A. J. Smuskiewicz

See also: Follicle-Stimulating Hormone; Hypogonadism; Menstruation; Ovulation; Pregnancy; Sex Hormones; Testosterone.

Further Reading

Endocrine Society. (2018). What is luteinizing hormone? Retrieved from https://www.hormone.org/your-health-and-hormones/glands-and-hormones-a-to-z/hormones/luteinizing-hormone

Society for Endocrinology. (2018). Luteinizing hormone. Retrieved from https://www.yourhormones.info/hormones/luteinising-hormone/

Lymphogranuloma Venereum

Lymphogranuloma venereum (LGV) is a sexually transmitted infection (STI) caused by specific strains of *Chlamydia trachomatis* that can cause genital ulcer disease (GUD) and other complications depending on where in the body the infection is located. Like many other STIs, LGV can be present in a person without causing signs or symptoms of disease. Similar to the other bacterial causes of GUD, there are tests available for diagnosis, and it can be treated with antibiotics. LGV can be effectively prevented by the use of condoms for sexual intercourse.

While syphilis and herpes are commonly transmitted with oral sex as well as anal and vaginal intercourse, it is less common for LGV to be transmitted orally, although it is possible, and there are occasional reports of oral transmission in men who have sex with men. More commonly, penile-anal or penile-vaginal condomless sex is the means of transmission.

Unlike other more common forms of *Chlamydia trachomatis*, LGV can cause a lesion at the site of infection during the first stage of the disease process. The lesion is usually small and painless, although in the past few years there have been medical reports of some LGV lesions being somewhat tender; this may be because of coinfection with HIV or other STIs. Sites of infection can be the penis, vulva, vagina, cervix, anus, rectum, mouth, or throat. Infection can happen when a person has sex with a person who has LGV and condoms are not used. The person with LGV usually does not know they have it because the lesion may be hidden, small, and not painful. LGV may be diagnosed at the same time as another STI, including HIV.

LGV is seen more often in men, and, since the early 2000s, LGV has been more common in men who have sex with men. Prior to this time, LGV was more commonly seen with heterosexual activity in tropical countries such as in parts of Asia, the Caribbean, and Africa, and in men who have multiple sexual partners, such as soldiers, sailors, and tourists returning to their home country after being in tropical countries where LGV is more common. LGV may be harder to detect if the lesion is located internally in the vagina or rectum.

LGV can progress through three stages of disease if left untreated. Between three and twenty-one days after exposure, a small, painless sore appears at the site of infection. If the lesion is missed and not treated, it usually heals up within a week by itself; however, if the infection was acquired anally, it can cause anorectal pain, bleeding, and pus. After the lesion heals, the bacteria remains in the lymph tissues, leading to the second stage of LGV, two to four weeks later. Symptoms of the second stage depend on where the bacteria entered the body. If the lesion was deep in the vagina or cervix, the lymph nodes in the pelvis become painful and inflamed, so the woman might experience fevers and back and pelvic pain. If the lesion was in the anus or rectum, then inflammation and infection of the rectum can occur with pain, blood, and discharge. If the bacteria entered the body via the vulva or penis, then the second stage appears as painful swollen lymph nodes in the groin, which may rupture if not treated. If the lesion was on the lips or the throat, then the symptoms will appear in that area. If LGV is left untreated after the second stage, symptoms can become more severe in stage three. There can be extreme swelling of the lymph glands and genitals, which can cause long-term damage, including scarring, chronic swelling, pain, and sexual dysfunction.

LGV can be prevented by using condoms. People who are sexually active should be tested regularly for STIs, and if they have any STI symptoms, they should visit their doctor or an STI clinic for diagnoses and treatment as prescribed.

Antibiotic resistance is becoming an increasing concern globally. Several STIs have become resistant to the antibiotics used for treatment, thus creating the need for newer and more expensive antibiotics to effectively treat the disease. Resistance to some antibiotics used to treat LGV has been found in some infections, but the majority of cases remain treatable with azithromycin or doxycycline. If these treatments fail, sexual health physicians may prescribe moxifloxacin.

Kelwyn Browne

See also: Safer Sex; Sexually Transmitted Infections (STIs).

Further Reading

Centers for Disease Control. (2015). 2015 sexually transmitted diseases treatment guidelines: Lymphogranuloma venereum (LGV). Retrieved from https://www.cdc.gov/std/tg2015/lgv.htm

Ceovic, R., & Gulin, S. J. (2015). Lymphogranuloma venereum: Diagnostic and treatment challenges. *Infection and Drug Resistance, 8*, 39–47.

World Health Organization. (2016). *Global health sector strategy on sexually transmitted infections, 2016–2021*. Geneva: World Health Organization.

Wylie, K. R. (Ed.). (2015). *ABC of sexual health* (3rd ed.). Chichester, UK: Wiley-Blackwell.

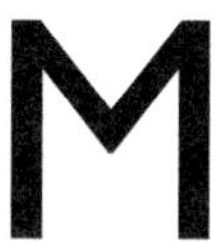

Madonna-Whore Dichotomy

Historically, female sexuality has been seen as passive, which is in direct opposition of male sexuality, which is perceived as aggressive. Social conditioning begins early for all people. Young girls are often taught and rewarded for being passive "good girls." A "good girl" is one who adheres to the double standards imposed on her by society. A "good girl" does not have sex often, she does not have sex early on in a relationship, and she does not sleep with a lot of men. These standards are quite different for men, who are viewed as hypermasculine when they have frequent sex with many women. Women who "behave like men" by having and enjoying lots of sex, when they want and with whomever they want, are a threat to the traditional standards set forth by men. This type of woman is labeled as a "whore," while a "good girl" is labeled as a "Madonna." Researchers have argued that these Western ideas about female sexuality are shaped by Christian teachings and that women are categorized and judged based on the degree to which they have carnal knowledge and their degree of submission to authority. A Madonna is virginal, sweet, and nurturing, while a whore is a woman who has sex outside of marriage and exudes sexuality. These labels act as a way to limit and control women's behavior and keep men in a position of power. The two boxes women fall into encapsulate the Madonna-whore dichotomy. The Madonna-whore complex arises when men seek loving and committed relationships with women.

Sigmund Freud (1856–1939), considered by some to be the father of psychology, first began using the term "Madonna-whore dichotomy" or "Madonna-whore complex" in order to explain issues that arise for men in relationships with women they love. Freud suggested that men place women into one of two categories: that of "Madonna" or that of "whore." He postulated that men do this in order to understand the discomfort they experience due to the polarization of both desiring and fearing women.

Men seek nurturing, virginal, maternal women as wives and mothers of their children. However, they also want women who they can have sex with. It is difficult for men to see a woman as both sexual and sweet, nurturing, and maternal. As such, the Madonna-whore dichotomy and Madonna-whore complex can be quite problematic for men and their relationships with women.

The Madonna-whore dichotomy sees a woman's goodness and her sexuality as mutually exclusive. Love is good and wholesome; sex is dirty and shameful. When a man loves a woman, he can admire and respect her. However, if she has sex with him, she must be dirty and not worthy of respect. This may cause sexual issues within a relationship as a man tries to reconcile how to see his partner as both a good woman and a sexual person. In an effort to maintain the Madonna view of this partner, he may seek an outside affair to satisfy his need for sex without debasing his Madonna partner. His outside affair would be with a woman labeled a "whore."

Researchers argue that while many of Freud's theories are antiquated, the Madonna-whore complex is still visible in society. The media constantly highlights female sexuality and encourages women to purchase products to appear attractive and desirable to men—thus engaging the "whore" label. However, women are also endlessly shamed for being sexual as exemplified by insults such as "slut" used to curtail overtly sexual behavior or suggestion. Therefore, women are expected to be both Madonnas and whores and yet are vilified for not fitting neatly into one of those two boxes. Likewise, men continue to want both a woman they can bring home to their family and a woman to be sexual with. As such, Freud's description of the Madonna-whore dichotomy as a way to describe this dialectical conundrum is still relevant today.

Amanda Manuel

See also: Double Standards, Sexual; Female Sexuality; Feminist Theory; Freud, Sigmund; Gender Roles, Socialization and; Male Sexuality; Religion, Diversity of Human Sexuality and; Slut Shaming; Social Learning Theory, Gender and.

Further Reading

Conrad, B. K. (2006). Neo-institutionalism, social movements, and the cultural reproduction of a mentalité: Promise Keepers reconstruct the Madonna/whore complex. *The Sociological Quarterly, 47*, 305–331.

Hartman, U. (2009). Sigmund Freud and his impact on our understanding of male sexual dysfunction. *Journal of Sexual Medicine, 6*(8), 2332–2339.

Landau, M. J., Goldenberg, J. L., Greenberg, J., Gillath, O., Solomon, S., Cox, C., Martens, A., & Pyszczynski, T. (2006). The siren's call: Terror management and the threat of men's sexual attraction to women. *Journal of Personality and Social Psychology, 90*(1), 129–146.

Male Sexuality

The descriptive term "male" in the phrase "male sexuality" implies that this type of sexuality is different than the sexualities of those with female or intersex genitalia and the socialization that accompanies a person's gender identity. Male sexuality is often understood to mean cisgender (i.e., when a person's assigned sex is aligned with their gender identity; commonly abbreviated as "cis") male sexuality. When the prefix "cis" is left off of a term related to assigned sex or gender, the default assumption by most people is that the person being referred to is cisgender. This is due to the influence of heteronormative and heterosexist beliefs associated with assigned sex, gender, and sexuality. However, as with many default assumptions, this is not always the case. For example, "male sexuality" can also refer to trans men or trans males (i.e., men who were assigned female at birth but identify as men, as opposed to men who were assigned male at birth and identify as cis males or men). In these cases, the term "male sexuality" expands to include sexual experiences of people who have a penis and testicles but also of those who have a clitoris, vulva, and vagina. It is important to remember that while words like "male" and "sexuality" seem easily definable, they can have widely varying meanings to different people.

As mentioned above, male sexuality is typically understood to refer to the experience of cisgender males due to the influence of heteronormativity and heterosexism on the way people think about masculinity and sexuality. While the constructs of heteronormativity and masculinity are slowly expanding to be more inclusive and less heterosexist, the fear of stigma associated with not being masculine or heteronormative enough continues to be widespread. While it seems clear that male sexuality is expanding to accommodate what were previously considered nonconforming sexual and gender expressions, it is also clear that beliefs around heteronormative masculinity and sexuality continue to get in the way of self-awareness and repress sexuality by reinforcing privilege and shaming sexual exploration.

This phenomenon tends to be particularly true for males and masculine people, who are generally expected to express their sexuality in a more heteronormative way as compared to the expectations on females or feminine people. Males and masculine people can get caught in a cycle of never feeling they are masculine enough, leading to fear of exposure that they are not masculine enough, leading to feeling shame about this fear, which loops back into fearing not being masculine enough, and so on. Shame around the fear of never being masculine enough leads to self-censorship, and shameful silence is the glue that holds up the mask of heteronormative masculinity.

Research on male sexuality indicates that sexual shame is created and maintained by the social constructs of heteronormativity, heterosexism, and phallocentric and hegemonic masculinity. Heteronormativity leads to stigma in those with nonconforming sexual preferences, which can result in sexual shame and mental health issues associated with internalized stigma, including depression and detachment from one's identity. While today there is a variety of attitudes toward sexual pleasure, Victorian-era sex, negativity dating back nearly two centuries, has instilled and driven a need to control nonconforming sexuality.

Sexual shame does not originate within the individual but is created within an individual through the internalization of social and cultural messages (via media, academia, language, etc.) that devalue people because of who they are or who they are not. Some people (i.e., the less privileged) are more susceptible to internalizing stigma and experiencing the resulting shame than others (i.e., the more privileged). People with less privileged identities (e.g., individuals who are assigned female at birth but identify as men or those who are gender nonconforming, nonstraight, and nonwhite) tend to be on the receiving end of social stigma more frequently and consistently than are people with more privileged identities (e.g., those who are cisgender males, heterosexual, and white). It follows that those with less privileged identities tend to experience stigma more frequently beginning at an earlier age than those who are more privileged, and therefore they tend to suffer more from the mental health issues associated with shame than those who are more privileged. Those with more privileged identities who have not been affected by stigma, or who have experienced stigma less frequently, have been protected by their privileged identities and insulated from experiencing the sexual shame that might otherwise result from internalizing the stigma related to an atypical sexual practice.

Research on privileged status and sexual expression shows that white males with higher socioeconomic status (SES) can "risk" sexual expression that is considered less masculine according to heteronormative standards, because privileges associated with having a higher SES can offset stigma associated with being perceived as less masculine. Conversely, black men face stereotypes of being hypersexual and hypermasculine, so the social cost to black men with atypical sexualities can be higher given that they face racism and potential stigma on multiple levels. This is an example of hegemonic masculinity, which has been described as a set of normative practices exemplified by hypermasculine authority figures (e.g., sports and entertainment industry icons) that allow for and promote male dominance over females and white male dominance over black males. Though only a minority of men might want to or be able to enact these practices, hegemonic masculinity puts men who do not comply at odds with those who do, reinforcing a power structure among men with different social locations and between men and other genders.

Contrary to the idea of hegemonic masculinity, male sexuality is actually more fluid and functions as a shifting set of practices that are relative depending on context (like social, cultural, and political location and identification). The authors support the idea that male sexuality can and does change, given that challenges to hegemonic masculinity (e.g., feminist resistance to patriarchy and men with atypical sexual expressions and preferences) and adjustments to those challenges are common. The authors state that because of these challenges, hegemonic masculinity takes substantial effort to maintain and requires the policing of male sexuality. Along these lines, some argue that the deterioration of hegemonic masculinity gives males the freedom to act in ways that have traditionally been considered nonnormative for male sexuality. It is promising that masculinity is being examined in this way and seems to be exhibiting signs of change. However, the fear of stigma associated with not being "masculine enough" continues to be widespread and slow to dissipate. Some believe there is a cultural balancing of power taking place in the subsiding of male social dominance, though it is difficult to say what effect this will have on male sexuality.

Even though heteronormativity and heterosexism still have influence, male sexuality has been expanding to include social interactions with different sexual orientations, behaviors previously considered more feminine (e.g., sexual passivity, emotional intimacy, and physical affection), and a decreased tolerance of violence. Research examining online sexual culture has found that people are gaining a more expansive, nuanced, and multifaceted understanding of their identities, taking factors into account like skin color, atypical sexual preferences and expressions, and different types of interactions, like friendships, romantic relationships, and hookups. The authors state that heteronormative male sexuality no longer provides the roadmap it once did for sexual relationships or lifestyle, and a broader understanding of identity is needed to embrace a more accurate, expanded concept of male sexuality. While this growing inclusivity is promising, both obvious and hidden forms of heteronormativity and heterosexism persist in the sociopolitical privileging of heterosexuality and masculinity.

Dulcinea Pitagora

See also: Binary Gender System; Black Sexuality; Female Sexuality; Femininity; Gender Identity; Gender Roles, Socialization and; Heterosexism; Masculinity; Sexual Disorders, Male; Sexual Expression.

Further Reading

Anderson, E. (2012). Shifting masculinities in Anglo-American countries. *Masculinities and Social Change, 1*(1), 40–60.

Anderson, E., & McCormack, M. (2016). Inclusive masculinity theory: Overview, reflection and refinement. *Journal of Gender Studies.* Published online October 23, 2016.

Beasley, C. (2015). Introduction to special issue of men and masculinities: Heterodox hetero-masculinities. *Men and Masculinities, 18*(2), 135–139.

Blashill, A. J., & Powlishta, K. K. (2012). Effects of gender-related domain violations and sexual orientation on perceptions of male and female targets: An analogue study. *Archives of Sexual Behavior, 41*(5), 1293–1302.

Branfman, B. A. (2015). "(Un)Covering" in the classroom: Managing stigma beyond the closet. *Feminist Teacher, 26*(1), 72–82.

Connell, R. W., & Messerschmidt, J. W. (2005). Hegemonic masculinity: Rethinking the concept. *Gender & Society, 19*, 829–859.

Dean, J. J. (2014). Heterosexual masculinities, anti-homophobias, and shifts in hegemonic masculinity: The identity practices of black and white heterosexual men. *The Sociological Quarterly, 54*(4), 534–560.

Dowsett, G. W., Williams, H., Ventuneac, A., & Carballo-Diéguez, A. (2008). "Taking it like a man": Masculinity and barebacking online. *Sexualities, 11*(1–2), 121–141.

Foucault, M. (1990). *The history of sexuality, volume 1: An introduction.* New York: Vintage Books.

Hunter, A. (1993). Different door, same closet: A heterosexual sissy's coming out party. In S. Wilkinson & C. Kitzinger (Eds.), *Heterosexuality: A feminism and psychology reader* (367–385). London: SAGE Publications.

Kimmel, M. S. (1997). Masculinity as homophobia. In M. M. Gergen & S. N. Oavis (Eds.), *Toward a new psychology of gender.* London: Routledge.

Kippax, K., & Smith, G. (2001). Anal intercourse and power in sex between men. *Sexualities, 4*(4), 413–434.

Lehmiller, J. (2018). *Tell me what you want: The science of sexual desire and how it can help you improve your sex life.* Boston: De Capo Lifelong Books.

Li, G., Pollitt, A. M., & Russell, S. T. (2015). Depression and sexual orientation during young adulthood: Diversity among sexual minority subgroups and the role of gender nonconformity. *Archives of Sexual Behavior, 4*(2), 1–15.

McCormack, M., & Anderson, E. (2014). Homohysteria: Definitions, context and intersectionality. *Sex Roles, 71*(3–4), 152–158.

Pachankis, J. E. (2007). The psychological implications of concealing a stigma: A cognitive–affective–behavioral model. *Psychological Bulletin, 133*(2), 328–345.

Quinn, D. M., & Chaudoir, S. R. (2009). Living with a concealable stigmatized identity: The impact of anticipated stigma, centrality, salience, and cultural stigma on psychological distress and health. *Journal of Personal and Social Psychology, 97*(4), 634–651.

Schlicter, A. (2004). Queer at last? Straight intellectuals and the desire for transgression. *GLQ: A Journal of Lesbian and Gay Studies, 10*(4), 543–564.

Maltz Hierarchy

Wendy Maltz introduced the hierarchy of sexual interaction in 1995 as a framework for evaluating sexual behavior in an interpersonal context to be used in sex education, sex addiction recovery work, and sex therapy. The model contains two parts. The first part describes the two directions in which sexual energy can be channeled: positive or negative. The positive direction leads toward feelings of integration and connectedness, whereas the negative direction leads to disintegration and disconnection. The second part describes different levels of positive and negative sexual interactions and the effects they generate on both individuals.

The Maltz Hierarchy defines sexual energy as a benign, natural force that is influenced by innate drives and hormones. Maltz asserts that this sexual energy is inherently neutral and describes it as a sort of hotel lobby, in that it is at ground zero. It can be channeled in a positive direction (the "above ground" levels), leading to increased intimacy and connection, or a negative direction (the "below ground" levels), leading to disconnection and disintegration. In both the negative and positive direction, there are three levels that describe either increasingly harmful or beneficial sexual interaction.

In the negative levels, sex is an upsetting or traumatic ordeal imposed on one person by another rather than a journey that partners take together. The underground levels become increasingly constricted in terms of interpersonal options, and the negative consequences of the behavior become more intense. Disconnection and disintegration of both the perpetrator and victim increase as the levels move more "below ground," and victims may suffer from serious damage to their self-image or sense of sexuality.

Level -1 is known as "impersonal interaction." This level describes sexual energy that is channeled in a way that leaves partners feeling misused and misunderstood. This level involves legal but coercive sexual interaction and failures of communication that lead to regret, sexual shame, or physical harm. Partners may be depersonalized or treated as sexual objects. This is often due to belief in societal myths (e.g., that sex is uncontrollable, that women should be sexually subservient). Both partners may engage in dishonest or unsafe behavior, such as failing to communicate about using protection or failing to ensure consent and enjoyment of both partners, leading to at least one partner feeling used.

Level -2 is known as "abusive interaction." This level describes sexual energy and communication that is intentionally abusive and exploitative. One person acts to control the other using psychological pressure, manipulation, or other means of control. Examples are often illegal, such as nonviolent acquaintance rape, spousal rape, and incest. Victims are seen as subservient and not as agents who can change or control the sexual experience. The perpetrator of this damaging behavior uses humiliation, degradation, or threats as weapons to control the sexual encounter. Perpetrators often feel entitled to sexual contact and use distorted thinking and beliefs to rationalize the harm they are causing to victims.

Level -3 is known as "violent interaction." At this level, which is the most disintegrated and disconnected in the hierarchy, the perpetrator uses all the tools of manipulation and coercion seen in the previous level but also asserts absolute control over the victim's body. Sexual energy is channeled into expressing rage and hate. Perpetrators at this level see sex organs as weapons and targets and often victimize others in a mechanical and ritualistic way. In the most extreme cases, this involves sexual torture and serial killings.

On the upper levels, sexual energy is channeled in a way that results in mutual choice, caring, respect, and a sense of safety. As in the negative levels, these positive traits and the feelings of intimacy increase with each level.

Level +1 is known as "role fulfillment." This level describes sexual energy that adheres to social norms regarding role fulfillment. This is typically based on well-defined gender roles, where partners are following rules as to how sex is initiated and performed and who is subservient and who is dominant. Those in the subservient role may agree to sex to please the other out of a sense of duty. This is distinct from the negative levels because the subservient partner does not feel coerced, and the dominant partner does not intentionally coerce them. Both gain a positive sense of self as a result of fulfilling a duty or role. Staying at this level is ultimately limiting as sex lacks creativity or passion. There is little room for enhancing sexual pleasure or deepening emotional intimacy.

Level +2 is known as "making love." This level describes sexual energy that is focused on mutual pleasure and communication. There is permission and allowance for both partners to experiment with what feels good and right, and both partners share a view that sex is special and should be improved and enhanced for both. Sex becomes a celebration of the body. At this level, both partners feel able to reveal their true selves and feel more intimately connected. They create a bond through sexual relating that leads to increased feelings of specialness and caring. However, while both partners have broken free from prescribed roles, this level can still be limiting due to the subtle pressure felt to be a "good lover." Sexual pleasure and orgasm may be seen as an ultimate goal.

Level +3 is known as "authentic sexual intimacy." This level results in a shared sense of deep connection and respect for both the other person and their body. Both partners have an authentic and conscious intention of expressing love for the other person through sex (rather than simply focusing on enhancing sexual pleasure). This level of relating can open up new dimensions in the relationship, leading to a true spiritual connection and a sense of deep safety and security. Both know that they can stop to negotiate the sexual experience at any time without shame or guilt. Emotional honesty and true intimacy are seen as more important than whether both partners climax or how long the sexual encounter lasts.

The Maltz Hierarchy is a valuable tool for examining sexual interactions. It is useful for sex education as it teaches that sexual behavior and the consequences it creates are based on choices of individuals and couples. In sex therapy work, it can help victims of sexual violence understand the damage caused by these events.

It does not judge specific sexual acts. Spanking, for example, can be seen as either a positive or negative behavior depending on the context in which it is performed and the intent. Further, the levels are fluid in that partners can move between them, even within the same sexual encounter.

While Maltz explicitly states that the model is intended to apply to individuals from all sexual orientations, there is explicit use of binary gender language, leaving it unclear if the model can accurately represent the sexual experiences of nonbinary or trans individuals.

On an important note, there is currently no empirical research to support the Maltz Hierarchy, and yet there are several potentially fruitful paths here. Researchers might investigate the model's claims regarding motivations, cognitions, and psychosocial effects that exist at each level. This model will only be sustained if research is conducted to support its claims and to expand its use.

Ed de St. Aubin, Lucas Mirabito, and Juan Pablo Zapata

See also: Intimacy, Sexual and Relational; Psychosexual Therapy; Sex Education; Sexual Abuse.

Further Reading

Maltz, W. (1995). The Maltz Hierarchy of sexual interaction. *Sexual Addiction and Compulsivity, 2*, 5–18.

Marriage

Marriage is present in most cultures in one form or another. It may be religious or political and may take on many different structures, but some form of joining people together has been present for much of history. Marriage can be defined in legal or religious structures and may mean different things. For example, marriage in a Christian context denotes a partnership between two people, traditionally a man and a woman, based on a conclusion reached from interpretations of natural law. These definitions will stem from the context in which marriage is believed to exist (i.e., spiritual, social, or legal).

In most societies, many evolutionary biologists conclude that marriages developed as a structure in which to have children. Marriages are often viewed as permanent in most cultures and can take on many different structures in relation to society.

The structure of marriage can largely be grouped into two categories: monogamy and polygamy. Monogamy ("mono" meaning "one," "gamos" meaning "marriage") traditionally refers to a marriage with one partner. As society's use of these words developed, monogamy became used to describe a sexual relationship in which two partners only have sexual experiences with each other. However, in terms of a contractual marriage, it means that there is only one contract between two people. Polygamy ("poly" meaning "many," "gamos" meaning "marriage") refers to a marriage structure containing many marital contracts. This group can further be broken down into polyandry ("andros" meaning "men") in which a woman is married to multiple men, or polygyny ("gyne" meaning "woman"), in which a man is married to multiple wives. These terms were developed in a traditional gender binary and leave little room for definitions of marriages including trans, intersex, and genderqueer individuals. Less common marital structures include group marriages (many people living together, considering themselves married) or common-law marriages (a legal default of long-term couples cohabitating). While common-law marriage is a common experience, not all states in the United States recognize it, and thus it is less often considered in the marriage discussion.

Some psychologists and sociologists will further clarify marriages into marital typologies. The nature of the typology may depend on the particular focus of the scholar making the distinction. For example, whether a wife is considered property of the husband (despotic marriage type) or if husband and wife are viewed as equals (democratic marriage type) can be a marital type based on the role of the wife and power. The distinction of a marriage based on a wife and political power is a more economic distinction, while relationship dynamics between the couple guide most of the marital typology today. More recent marriage and relationship scholars like John Gottman identify types of stable marriages and what makes a couple work. Through his studies, Gottman found five marriage types: validating, volatile, conflict-minimizing, hostile, and hostile-detached. The validating, volatile, and conflict-minimizing couples were most stable and least likely to divorce, while the hostile and hostile-detached couples were more likely to divorce.

Many cultures and religions observe marital ceremonies differently. Some religious ceremonies involve expressing love before a divine being or deity, accompanied with some rituals meaningful to that particular community. Whether the ritual involves a hand wrapping, gifting of a symbolic token to the marital parties, the giving of a dowry, a sacrifice, or a donation, the meaning of such a ritual exists in nearly every type of culture and society. The underlying theme from all these ceremonies is the expressed new status of members being wed. Many ceremonies involve a change in appearance, such as clothing, which can also have a symbolic meaning. There is often a change in social status and living situation of the individuals being married (often called a bride and groom).

Marriage ceremonies also have a familial component. Whether the burden is financial or symbolic, it is a common cultural tradition that the families of the bride and groom are involved in a certain way. Even religious ceremonies of the same denomination can change based on geographic location of the families or simply family traditions.

In the United States, the legal structure of marriage is based on the Christian tradition, often requiring an official (of the state or religious clergy member recognized by the state) and at least two witnesses to be present. All states require that a couple obtain a marriage license, and the requirements for this may vary. Some states require sexually transmitted infection tests for couples about to wed or have regulations on who can marry whom (i.e., the closeness of relatives may affect their ability to marry depending on the state).

In many cultures, sex and sexuality are tied to marital contracts. The production of children can be seen as part of this marital contract. The conception of children outside of this contract may be seen as "infidelity" or a breach of this contract. Consequently, many monogamous marriages see sexual activity with other people who are not part of the marriage as sexually immoral. This experience is often termed "extramarital sex." In the United States, marriage may be seen as the only socially acceptable platform for sexual activity by some groups and people.

In most cultures, there are sexual components built into the expectation of marriage. Components of virginity, fertility, children, frequency of sexual activity, sexual satisfaction, or sexual taboos are often present in subtle or overt discussions of marriage. For example, in some Mediterranean cultures, it is appropriate to display a bloody sheet after the marital sexual encounter (often called the consummation of a marriage) to show the breaking of a hymen and prove the virginity of a wife. Other Christian cultures have expectations of children and may even mandate that a couple procreate. Other cultures, such as Hinduism and Judaism, may have specific guidelines on how sexual pleasure can be given or how often it should be sought.

Not only are these components present in the expectation of marriage, but they are also an integral part of the language we use to discuss marriage. For example, "gamos," the Greek word for marriage, is also the root of the word "gamete," another name for the reproductive cells (sperm and egg). This gives us an idea of the intersection of the naming of cells and the role of sex and marriage in society.

As mentioned above, virginity is often closely tied to marriage during discussion of sexuality. Virginity can be defined in many different ways. Research has looked for a consensus, but a specific and consistent definition among various groups has not been identified. While varying definitions exist, the theme revolves around vaginal-penile intercourse. This reality, however, may create a social stigma based on the inferiority of women. In one qualitative study, researchers asked midwives about virginity control and hymen reconstruction (a process by which a female-bodied person may seek surgical measures to rebuild a hymen to portray virginity) and identified three themes. These themes included the recognition of misogynistic practices that reinforce the gendered order, the desire to raise awareness of these practices that demean women based on this order, and the idea of promoting autonomy in women and providing culturally sensitive care. The study concluded that the concept of virginity is closely tied to the concept of the patriarchy. The article suggests various types of activism, such as international debates and interdisciplinary cooperation, may assist in increased gender equality. An important note is that the hymen can break from various other activities, such as intense exercise or riding a bicycle, and it is not indicative of one's virginity status. Though it has been long believed to be related to sexual purity, current research claims otherwise.

Mark A. Levand

See also: Adultery; Extramarital Sex; Fertility; Intercourse; Marriage, Cross-Cultural Comparison of; Monogamy; Open Marriage; Polygamy; Polygyny; Premarital Sex; Religion, Diversity of Human Sexuality and; Unconsummated Marriage; Virginity.

Further Reading

Adams, J. A., Botash, A. S., & Kellogg, N. (2004). Differences in hymenal morphology between adolescent girls with and without a history of consensual sexual intercourse. *Archives of Pediatrics & Adolescent Medicine, 158*(3), 280–285.

Bersamin, M. M., Fisher, D. A., Walker, S., Hill, D. L., & Grube, J. W. (2007). Defining virginity and abstinence: Adolescents' interpretations of sexual behaviors. *Journal of Adolescent Health, 41*(2), 182–188. doi: 10.1016/j.jadohealth.2007.03.011

Christianson, M., & Eriksson, C. (2015). Promoting women's human rights: A qualitative analysis of midwives' perceptions about virginity control and hymen "reconstruction." *European Journal of Contraception & Reproductive Health Care, 20*(3), 181–192. doi: 10.3109/13625187.2014.977435

Gottman, J. M. (1993). The roles of conflict engagement, escalation, and avoidance in marital interaction: A longitudinal view of five types of couples. *Journal of Consulting and Clinical Psychology, 61*(1), 6.

Gottman, J. M. (1999). *The marriage clinic: A scientifically-based marital therapy.* New York: W. W. Norton & Company.

Hans, J. D., & Kimberly, C. (2011). Abstinence, sex, and virginity: Do they mean what we think they mean? *American Journal of Sexuality Education, 6*(4), 329–342. doi: 10.1080/15546128.2011.624475

Hegazy, A. A., & Al-Rukban, M. O. (2012). Hymen: Facts and conceptions. *The Health, 3*(4), 109–115.

Marriage, Cross-Cultural Comparison of

Marriage is the union of two people in a socially or formally recognized manner, establishing legal rights and obligations between them. In many cultures, marriage requires a legal contract; in others, a marriage can be recognized socially without the involvement of a legal document or ceremony. Throughout the twentieth century, marriage laws have changed around the world to allow people of different races or religions to marry and to limit or forbid child marriages, forced marriages, and polygamy. Most recently, the definition of marriage in some cultures has shifted to include same-sex couples—notably in the United States, where the U.S. Supreme Court ruled on June 26, 2015, that same-sex couples have a constitutional right to marry.

The purpose of marriage has changed significantly over the course of recent centuries. In ancient and medieval times, throughout much of the world, marriage was used to form alliances between families, accumulating property and skills to strengthen a family's position and to perpetuate their well-being. As wealth and prosperity became elements of power within civilizations, marriages were arranged to form unions between wealthy families, accumulating resources and effectively keeping out those who were "beneath their station." Marriage became a strategy rather than an act of love, even to the point of creating political capital by matching a man and a woman from powerful families.

In predominantly rural, preindustrial societies in Europe and Asia, most young people married before they were out of their teens, becoming part of extended families that shared responsibility for tending the land and livestock. From the Middle Ages until the 1700s, families in many European countries required a potential wife to buy her husband with a dowry—a collection of money, property, and other goods that added to the man's wealth and influence. People in the lower classes also considered these issues, even if there was no official dowry—marrying to merge adjoining tracts of land, bring goodwill to their homes from other families, or gain skills from which the combined families could benefit. Marriage was viewed as a business transaction or a negotiated contract.

The modern cultural view of marriage for love did not emerge until the late eighteenth century, when it took hold in the United States and western Europe. The concept rose from a desire to find personal satisfaction and fulfillment from the choice of a mate rather than basing the decision to marry solely on financial and social gain.

In the 1950s and 1960s, marriage in the United States became idealized as a union between a male breadwinner and a female homemaker, a structure that emerged in earnest after World War II. With the advent of the women's liberation movement of the 1970s and 1980s, two-income families became the new norm, and women even emerged as family breadwinners in the 1990s. By 2002, according to the U.S. Bureau of Labor Statistics, one in three married women in America earned more money than her husband.

Marriage practices around the world have been defined first by traditional religious values and more recently by the realities of everyday life, especially as rural communities have been replaced by cities and industry. Many countries have passed laws in the twentieth and twenty-first centuries that limit or forbid traditions that violate basic human rights.

In the Middle East and North Africa, for example, the common practice of marrying early—especially for women in their teens—has given way in recent years as the population in these countries moves to the cities. The Population Reference Bureau reports that women are marrying later, in their twenties and thirties, and only 1–4 percent of women ages fifteen to nineteen are married in Tunisia, Algeria, and Lebanon, countries that promoted teenaged marriage in the twentieth century. Families in Egypt and other Middle Eastern countries require a dowry from the groom in many cases, half of which is held in reserve to use in a settlement if the couple should seek divorce.

In China, passage of the 1980 New Marriage Law gave people the freedom to choose their own marriage partner rather than relying on parents and others to choose a spouse for them. The law forbids coercion into marriage by third parties, establishes gender equality between a husband and wife, and prohibits abuse and desertion by either spouse. Until 2015, China also exercised a policy of one child per marriage (with many exceptions) and two children if the first one is a girl. As a result of this devaluation of female children, some couples aborted their female babies once they discovered the gender of the fetus. This practice, exercised since the law's passage in 1979, created a significant shortage of women to marry the eligible men—with unmarried men outnumbering unmarried women by million in 2013. Since 2016, China has changed the policy to a two children per marriage policy.

In Latin American countries, many young couples have opted to live in consensual unions with their partners rather than formalizing their relationship with marriage. In Colombia, El Salvador, Honduras, and Ecuador, as much as 20 percent of the population age fifteen and over lives in consensual unions as opposed to less than 5 percent in the United States, according to the United Nations

Statistics Division's Demographic Yearbook. This predominantly Roman Catholic region of the world does not view divorce as an option for ending a marriage, so divorce was illegal in countries including Brazil and Argentina until as recently as 1987. Fewer than one in one thousand people are divorced in most Latin American countries.

The complexities of marriage in India date back to before the evolution of Hinduism, but the modern era has brought the subjugation of women and the practice of teenage marriage largely to an end in South Asia. Arranged marriages are still prevalent, but both people must consent to the marriage, and they have the right to refuse the match. Many couples meet on their own and decide that they will marry and then go through the rituals of arranged marriage to create lasting bonds between their extended families. The actual rituals and traditions vary by region throughout the country, but they often involve a "sponsor," a relative who may bring in a professional matchmaker to help identify the best candidates for marriage. While this system may seem archaic, it does result in one of the lowest national divorce rates in the world: only 1.1 percent of marriages in India end in divorce. (Compare this with 45.8 percent in the United States.)

Marriage traditions in Africa differ distinctively from one group of people or region to the next, but some themes can be found throughout the continent. African brides are considered the link between the ancestors and the children yet to be born, so they are trained from a young age to prepare for the responsibilities of marriage. The marriages themselves are often negotiated between families, and in some cultures the bride and groom have never met before the wedding day arrives. In Sudan, the woman must bear two children before the marriage is considered completed, while the Wodabee of Niger choose their own cousins for marriage. In Ethiopia, the Amhara people permit a temporary marriage, in which the bride moves in with the groom and receives a housekeeper's wages while she performs the duties of a wife—including bearing children. This form of marriage can move to permanent status by agreement between the spouses.

Randi Minetor

See also: Civil Union; Dating, Cross-Cultural Comparison of; Marriage; Monogamy; Open Marriage; Polyamory; Same-Sex Marriage.

Further Reading

Coontz, S. (2006). *Marriage, a history: How love conquered marriage.* New York: Penguin.

Stockard, J. E. (2002). *Marriage in culture: Practice and meaning across diverse societies.* Belmont, CA: Wadsworth Publishing Company.

Masculinity

Masculinity is the set of traits, attributes, behaviors, and roles traditionally associated with men or manhood of a given culture; however, these qualities are distinct from biological sex and therefore can be exhibited by persons of any sex or gender. Traditional Western forms of masculinity surround notions of stoicism, independence, and virility. Some visions of model manhood also include culturally specific milestones (e.g., the onset of facial hair, loss of virginity, tribal warrior rituals, bar mitzvahs) as well as more universal notions, such as producing and providing for offspring.

During the late 1980s and early 1990s, social theory exploring the context of masculinity gained substantial attention. Particularly, feminist and gender theorists examined the conventional expectations and roles associated with gender identities. Theorists such as Michel Foucault, Kate Bornstein, John Money, Anne Fausto-Sterling, and Leslie Feinberg explored various parts of gender identity development including biological, psychological, sociological, and philosophical considerations. Although their respective opinions may vary on the significance of biological predisposition, it is generally accepted that rigid masculine social scripts are upheld by both implicit and explicit guidelines imposed to replicate a socially constructed cultural ideal of manhood. In other words, masculinity is not inherent or established by a single milestone but contingent on ongoing displays of masculinity, whatever they may be according to any given culture.

While many cultures have historically acknowledged varying forms of gender expression, traditional Western views generally promote the notion of a binary gender system (i.e., "man" or "woman"). This is where the idea of femininity as the complete opposite of masculinity stems from. Systems divided into two categories such as this imply a polarized "opposition," which means that to be one is to not be the other. Incidentally, rigid social scripts (of any kind) that are more focused on exclusionary criteria ultimately limit the potential for adequate script fulfillment by way of creating more room for criticism and failure than success. Modern examples regarding masculinity often include "real men do not cry," "real men are aggressive," "real men are the head of their household," and many other similar narratives. An overemphasis of exclusion as fundamental criteria promotes an inflexible and uniform expression of masculinity known as "hegemonic masculinity." When these strict "masculine" traits are overidealized and assumed to be a complete opposite to "feminine" traits, a hierarchy of social measure is established that devalues feminine expression and female persons, such as exhibited in patriarchal societies. In Latin America, the term "machismo" is used to describe the phenomena of a patriarchal masculine pride that denigrates femininity, particularly in Latino communities. Like many other forms of hegemonic masculinity, machismo explicitly deems feminine traits as undesirable and a direct deviation from masculine performance. It can easily be seen how these social constructs would be problematic to the social position of women in any given culture where they may be present. That is not to say men do not face alienation or injustice under patriarchal authority or that healthier and more flexible expressions of masculinity do not (and cannot) exist; in fact, academic exploration of masculinity studies support that they do indeed.

Preoccupation with a singular version of manhood ignores the great variance of masculine expression both cross-culturally and cross-historically. Normative Westernized models of masculine ideals tend to overlook or actively invalidate experiences of those who do not meet all the expectations of hegemonic masculinity, such as male persons who are not heterosexual, able-bodied, cisgender, or of heritage other than the predominant race. This can be seen in typical models of masculinity that do not include homosexual men (due to heterosexist and homophobic assertions of gay men as feminine), disabled men (according to expectations of physical prowess and exceptional fertility), transgender men (due to their assigned sex at birth), as well as people of color often navigating additional and/or conflicting masculine scripts. Specifically, people of color are often subject to ill-fitting or contradictory masculine scripts and prejudices that their white counterparts are not. Such can be seen among American stereotypes that emasculate Asian and East Asian men, who may adhere to masculine expressions more traditional to their own cultural heritage, and the stereotypes that hypersexualize black and Latino men, painting them as dangerously masculine. Therefore, modern Westernized interpretations of masculinity are often innately exclusionary and/or unattainable for many. Historically speaking, these modern constraints remain suspect even when limited to the experience of white males. Although the nineteenth century white European "dandy," a docile and educated man of the upper class, would be deemed effeminate by modern standards, it was the ideal of masculine sophistication in its day. While several historical models of masculinity may have remained somewhat preserved, such as "the warrior" and "the family man," there are apparent limitations regarding who can "be a man" and how they may do it.

Ultimately, the definition of "masculinity" is subject to the culture in which it exists as well as direct circumstance. Although typically associated with men, social constructionism recognizes the essence of masculinity to be rooted in performance and not biology. Once again, this indicates that it is not inherently related to the male sex or gender but contingent on the active expression of culturally designated attributes. Just as one must commit acts of kindness to be deemed kind, one must act under the scripts of masculinity to be deemed masculine.

Ilyssa Boseski

See also: Binary Gender System; Black Sexuality; Bornstein, Kate; Cisgender; Fausto-Sterling, Anne; Feinberg, Leslie; Femininity; Feminist Theory; Foucault, Michel; Gender; Gender Identity; Gender Roles, Socialization and; Heterosexism; Heterosexuality; Homophobia; Homophobia, Internalized; Homosexuality; Male Sexuality; Money, John; Sexism; Stereotypes, Sexual; Transgender.

Further Reading

Butler, J. (2004). *Undoing gender.* New York: Routledge.

Cortes, J. (2014). *Macho ethics: Masculinity and self-representation in Latino-Caribbean narrative (Bucknell studies in Latin American literature and theory).* Lewisburg, PA: Bucknell University Press.

Fausto-Sterling, A. (2012). *Sex/gender: Biology in a social world.* New York: Routledge Taylor & Francis Group.

Foucault, M. (1978). *The history of sexuality: An introduction.* New York: Pantheon Books.

Kimmel, M. S., & Messner, M. A. (2012). *Men's lives* (9th ed.). New York: Pearson.

Plante, R. F., & Maurer, L. M. (2010). *Doing gender diversity: Readings in theory and real-world experience.* Boulder, CO: Westview Press.

Mastectomy

Mastectomy is the surgical removal of a breast. The main reason that this procedure is performed is to treat people who have breast cancer by removing breast tissue and, thereby, preventing the cancer from spreading to other tissues and organs in the body. Some people get a mastectomy to prevent the development of breast cancer. Those individuals usually know that they have certain gene mutations that raise the risk of breast cancer development, or they know that other women in their family have had breast cancer. Such procedures are known as prophylactic mastectomies.

There are different types of mastectomies that can be performed after a cancerous tumor is discovered in the breast. Such discoveries are usually made with an x-ray procedure called a mammogram. The type of mastectomy performed in any case depends on the size and location of the tumor, the extent to which the cancer might have spread, and the age and general health of the patient. A simple, or total, mastectomy involves removal of the entire affected breast, often including the overlying skin. A double mastectomy involves removal of both breasts. In a subcutaneous mastectomy, the underlying breast tissue is removed, but the skin and nipple are preserved. In a conventional radical mastectomy, the breast is removed along with the lymph nodes under the arm and the muscles in the chest wall. In a modified radical mastectomy, the breast and the underarm lymph nodes are removed, but the muscles of the chest wall are left intact.

Modified radical mastectomies have been the most common type of breast cancer surgery since the 1970s. Before that, conventional radical mastectomies were more common. However, the conventional type of surgery leaves the body severely disfigured as a result of the removal of chest muscle. Furthermore, the individual may be unable to use their arm after the surgery. Modified radical mastectomies have been shown to be just as effective at removing cancer as the conventional procedure, and the person keeps the use of the arm and can have the breast more easily reconstructed. A typical modified radical mastectomy lasts two to three hours, during which time the patient is under general anesthesia. The patient is typically in the hospital for no more than three days.

Breast reconstruction is a surgical procedure in which the removed breast tissue is replaced with natural tissue taken from other parts of the body or with an artificial implant. The implant consists of a soft silicone shell filled with either silicone gel or saline (salt water). It is positioned beneath the chest muscle. Some people choose to have breast reconstruction during the same operation in which the breast is removed. However, doctors may recommend waiting several months to undergo reconstruction. Healing from immediate reconstruction could lead to delays in radiation treatment or chemotherapy for those who would benefit from such therapies after surgery. Those who do not wish to undergo breast reconstruction can wear a breast prosthesis, which is an artificial breast placed inside a bra.

In some cases, breast cancer may not need to be treated with a full mastectomy for successful treatment. If the mammogram reveals only a limited area of cancer inside the breast, the tumor, along with a small amount of surrounding tissue and the underarm lymph nodes, can be removed in a procedure called a lumpectomy, or partial mastectomy. The rest of the breast is preserved and treated with radiation to kill any cancer cells that might remain inside. Lumpectomy is usually considered only if the tumor is smaller than two inches (five centimeters). Cancer may return after some lumpectomies—and even after some mastectomies. Some people who are good candidates for lumpectomy because of their small tumor size may still choose to undergo a full mastectomy because it provides a greater chance that all the cancer will be removed.

There are several additional reasons that a mastectomy may be performed. Trans men may choose to have a double mastectomy as part of their gender transition process. Boys or men may also choose to undergo mastectomy if they have a condition called gynecomastia, in which male breast tissue swells to resemble female breasts. This condition is caused by a hormone imbalance or the use of certain drugs.

Many well-known women have had mastectomies. Actress Angelina Jolie chose to have a double mastectomy, followed by reconstructive surgery, in 2013. Jolie did not have breast cancer at the time; however, she feared that such cancer would eventually develop, because she had a close family history of breast cancer, and genetic tests showed that she had the BRCA1 gene mutation, which is known to increase risk. Mutations in the BRCA2 gene are also associated with breast cancer.

A. J. Smuskiewicz

See also: Breast, Female; Breast Cancer; Gender Transition.

Further Reading

Breastcancer.org. (2019). Mastectomy. Retrieved from http://www.breastcancer.org/treatment/surgery/mastectomy

Lesh, M. (2013). *Let me get this off my chest: A breast cancer survivor over-shares.* West Covina, CA: StoryRhyme.com Publishing.

Lucas, G. (2005). *Why I wore lipstick to my mastectomy.* New York: St. Martin's Griffin.

Masters, William H.

William Howell Masters (1915–2001) was a world-renowned gynecologist who devoted his career to the sexual function of humans. Dr. Masters was born on December 7, 1915, in Cleveland, Ohio. Along with his research partner, Virginia Johnson, he helped revision sex therapy and sex education in the United States. He pioneered research into the nature of the human sexual response and the diagnosis and treatment of sexual disorders and dysfunctions.

Dr. Masters attended Lawrenceville School in New Jersey and afterward went to Hamilton College in Clinton, New York, where he graduated in 1938 with his bachelor's degree. He then enrolled at the University of Rochester Medical School. During medical school, he worked under his mentor, Dr. George Washington Corner, who introduced Masters to reproductive research. Once he graduated with his medical degree, he opted to focus on studying the physiology of sex in humans due to this being an under researched area at the time and one he felt would be challenging.

After graduation, Dr. Masters moved to St. Louis to start a career in obstetrics and gynecology at St. Louis Maternity Hospital and Barnes Hospital. In 1944, he also began studying pathology at Washington University School of Medicine. Then, in 1947, he joined the faculty of the Washington University School of Medicine, where he became a specialist on hormone replacement therapy for aging women.

In 1954, Dr. Masters started his research into human sexuality. In 1956, he added his coresearcher, Virginia Johnson. Their research was extremely controversial for the time. Masters and Johnson would watch clients who presented with sexual dysfunctions have sex. They also used cameras and electronic devices to gain even more data from their research. For example, they were able to place cameras inside a plastic phallus to see the physiological responses of the vagina during stimulation. As a result of directly observing anatomical and physiological sexual responses, they were able to develop a different method for the treatment of sexual dysfunctions. In 1959, the duo started to counsel individuals with sexual difficulties, and they formed a specific approach to sex therapy, which they later taught to other clinicians at the Masters and Johnson Institute. They developed the therapy technique of sensate focus and showed that 80 percent of clients they treated with their approach experienced a long-term resolution of sexual dysfunction. Masters' research focused on the mechanics of sex and the moral reasoning behind it, which often led him down controversial paths. However, with this, Masters and Johnson were able to help make sex therapy popular in the United States.

Masters and Johnson published their first research on the human sexual response cycle in a book aptly named *Human Sexual Response* in 1966. In this book, they described a four-stage model of the sexual response cycle: (1) excitement, (2) plateau, (3) orgasm, and (4) resolution. In 1970, they published *Human Sexual Inadequacy*, which discussed treatment for premature ejaculation, erectile dysfunction (impotence), and the inability to experience orgasm. Both books were aimed at a medical audience but became best sellers among the general public as well.

Dr. Masters retired in 1994 and closed down the Masters and Johnson Institute. Dr. Masters was married three times, including once to his research partner, Virginia Johnson. In his first marriage, he had two children. Dr. Masters passed away on February 16, 2001, in Tucson, Arizona, from Parkinson disease at the age of eighty-five.

Amanda Baker

See also: Hormone Replacement Therapy; Johnson, Virginia; Masters and Johnson Four-Stage Model of Sexual Response; Sensate Focus; Sexology; Sexual Dysfunction, Treatment of; Start-Stop Technique.

Further Reading

Bullough, V. L. (1994). *Science in the bedroom: A history of sex research.* New York: Basic Books.

Kinsey Institute, Indiana University. (2019). *Masters and Johnson collection.* Retrieved from https://kinseyinstitute.org/collections/archival/masters-and-johnson.php

Masters, W. H., & Johnson, V. E. (1966). *Human sexual response.* New York: Bantam Books.

Masters, W. H., & Johnson, V. E. (1970). *Human sexual inadequacy.* New York: Bantam Books.

Masters, W. H., & Johnson, V. E. (1974). *The pleasure bond.* New York: Bantam Books.

Masters, W. H., & Johnson, V. E. (1979). *Homosexuality in perspective.* New York: Bantam Books.

Masters, W. H., Johnson, V. E., & Kolodny, R. C. (1977). *Ethical issues in sex therapy and research.* Boston: Little, Brown and Company.

Masters, W. H., Johnson, V. E., & Kolodny, R. C. (1986). *Masters and Johnson on sex and human loving.* Boston: Little, Brown and Company.

Masters, W. H., Johnson, V. E., & Kolodny, R. C. (1994). *Heterosexuality.* New York: Gramercy Book.

Severo, R. (2001, February). William H. Masters, a pioneer in studying and demystifying sex, dies 85. *New York Times*, p. B7. Retrieved from https://www.nytimes.com/2001/02/19/us/william-h-masters-a-pioneer-in-studying-and-demystifying-sex-dies-at-85.html

Masters and Johnson Four-Stage Model of Sexual Response

In 1957, William H. Masters and Virginia E. Johnson as a team began researching human sexual response, dysfunction, and disorders at the Department of Obstetrics and Gynecology at Washington University in St. Louis. They were influenced by growing public and educational support that medicine should consider sexuality. In their words, "if the problems in the complex field of human sexual behavior are to be attacked successfully, psychologic theory and sociologic concept must at times find support in physiologic fact" (Masters & Johnson, 1966). To do this, they used direct observation of anatomical and physiological sexual responses of humans. Their earliest research culminated in 1966 with the publication of their book *Human Sexual Response*.

Masters and Johnson owed some of their interest in sexology to Alfred Kinsey. Between 1930 and 1952, Kinsey compiled statistics reflecting patterns of sexual behavior in the United States. This work was of great sociological value, but it could not be used to interpret physiological or psychological response to sexual stimulation. Realizing this, two basic questions formed the basis for Masters and Johnson's research program: (1) What physical reactions develop as people respond to effective sexual stimulation? (2) Why do people behave as they do when responding to effective sexual stimulation? In other words, the intent of the questions was to create a foundation of basic scientific information. They were not trying to answer why men and women respond as they do. Furthermore, they realized that their lab and clinical research populations were insufficient representations of the general population for drawing definitive conclusions.

Their 1966 work was based on the observations of 10,000 sexual response cycles. The observations were not limited to intercourse with a partner. Three-quarters of the cycles observed were of heterosexual women, while 2,500 were of heterosexual men. In their 1979 work, *Homosexuality in Perspective*, Masters and Johnson reported observations of 1,200 response cycles of eighty-two homosexual women and ninety-four homosexual men. Through their research, they determined that a more concise picture of physiological reactions to sexual stimuli could be accomplished by dividing the human male and female cycles of sexual response into four separate phases. These phrases are (1) excitement, (2) plateau, (3) orgasm, and (4) resolution. The phases were intended to be a framework for a detailed description of physiological variations in sexual reactions. They were not built as a finalized theory but as a basis for categorization and developing scientific theory.

With this framework in place, they identified many variations in male sexual response. Those variations primarily differed in terms of duration rather than intensity. As a result, they found only one general sexual response pattern for males. For females, intensity and duration mattered. Specifically, three sexual response patterns were identified for females. These responses were not affected by sexual orientation or the nature of the sexual activity (e.g., masturbation, partnered activity). The source of sexual stimulation (e.g., tactile or psychological) also did not matter (Masters & Johnson, 1966).

The sexual response cycle has the same four phases for all people. In the first phase, the excitement phase, sexual response develops from any source of tactile or psychological stimulation. The pelvic region fills with an increased supply of blood and other fluids; breathing, heart rate, and blood pressure increase; and the skin may flush. Myotonia (increased muscle tension) and vasocongestion (engorgement of blood vessels) also occurs. In females, the vagina produces a lubricant, the clitoris swells, breasts enlarge, and the cervix and uterus move upward. In males, the testes swell, the penis grows erect, and the scrotum tightens. If there is enough stimulation for an individual, the intensity of response increases rapidly. This allows the excitement phase to be lengthened or shortened. If the stimulation is physically or psychologically objectionable, or interrupted, the phase may lengthen or even end.

If effective simulation continues, the person enters the plateau phase. Sexual tensions are intensified and eventually reach an extreme level just before an orgasm. Muscle spasms may begin in the feet, face, and hands. The tip of the penis may increase in size and darken in color, and the Cowper's gland may secrete lubricating fluid. The outer labia darken as well and the outer passageway of the vagina narrows. In addition, testes withdraw into the scrotum in males, and the clitoris retracts under its hood in females. The length of this phase depends largely on the effectiveness of the stimuli combined with individual drive for sexual tension to increase. If either the stimuli or the drive is inadequate, the individual will fall into a prolonged resolution phase.

If sufficient stimulation is present, the subsequent phase is the orgasmic phase. This phase is limited to the few seconds when the vasocongestion and myotonia from sexual stimuli are released. These contractions occur at the base of the penis for men, while in females, the vaginal muscles and uterus contract. This rate slows down after five to twelve contractions in females and after three to four in males. Such an involuntary climax represents the maximum sexual tension of a particular encounter. Contractions occur at a rate of one every 0.8 seconds. Sensual awareness of an orgasm is focused on the pelvis. For females, the focus is concentrated on the clitoris, vagina, and uterus. For males, the focus is concentrated on the penis, prostate, and seminal vesicles. The female orgasmic experience varies greatly in terms of intensity and duration, while the male experience tends to follow the pattern of ejaculation with less individual variation. Total body involvement is experienced depending on the individual's reaction pattern.

After the orgasm is the resolution phase. In simple terms, the resolution phase is an involuntary reverse reaction pattern that returns an individual through the plateau and excitement levels of stimulation into an unstimulated state. Muscles begin to relax. Females have the potential to reach the orgasmic phase from any point in the resolution phase as long as there is effective stimulation again. Males have a refractory period, which might extend the resolution phase in terms of lower excitement levels. Only after the refractory period can a male reach higher levels of sexual tension. A male's physiological ability to respond to stimulation again is much slower than a female's, with only a few exceptions. Sexual tension only completely dissipates when all sexual stimuli have stopped.

Masters and Johnson made sure to emphasize that individual variation in the duration and intensity of every physiological response is wide. They went as far as to say that their four-phase model is not able to evaluate psychological aspects of elevated sexual tension. However, they also said that the model provides a structure for investigation and ensures the correct placement of physiological responses within a sequential continuum. Some researchers have said that such a linear model primarily reflects a male response cycle, while a nonlinear model may better reflect a female response cycle.

To be sure, there are clear differences of anatomy between the sexes as well as the already stated differences in duration and intensity patterns. Yet, in Masters and Johnson's book, they recognize a number of direct parallels in sexual response between the sexes and emphasize the similarities between the sexes more than the differences. That is, the mechanisms of arousal for males and females are similar: vasocongestion and myotonia, engorgement of blood vessels, and increased blood flow into tissue.

Masters and Johnson's work helped dispel widely held beliefs of the time: that women experience different sorts of orgasms and that only men seek sexual satisfaction. They also dispelled the belief that homosexual and heterosexual satisfaction are fundamentally different, because orgasmic frequency was comparable for both.

The four-phase model of sexual response had a major impact on sexology research, yet it was only the beginning. For Masters and Johnson, definitive data on sex would only "become available as the mores of our society come to accept objective research in human sexuality" (Masters & Johnson, 1966). Complete and definitive data is perhaps growing today, while pharmaceutical companies and psychiatric and mental clinicians use their model to define sexual health and sexual problems.

Louis Varilias

See also: Afterplay; Arousal; Foreplay; Johnson, Virginia; Kaplan's Triphasic Model; Kinsey, Alfred; Masters, William H.; Orgasm; Sexual Desire Model; Sexual Satisfaction.

Further Reading

Kinsey Institute. (2018). Masters and Johnson collection. Retrieved from https://kinseyinstitute.org/collections/archival/masters-and-johnson.php

Masters, W. H., & Johnson, V. E. (1966). *Human sexual response.* Boston: Little, Brown.

Masters, W. H., & Johnson, V. E. (1970). *Homosexuality in perspective.* Philadelphia: Lippincott, Williams & Wilkins.

Our Bodies Our Selves. (2011). Models of sexual response. Retrieved from https://www.ourbodiesourselves.org/book-excerpts/health-article/models-sexual-response/

USBC SexInfo. (2019). The sexual response cycle. Retrieved from http://www.soc.ucsb.edu/sexinfo/article/sexual-response-cycle

Masturbation

Masturbation is the touching and stimulation of one's own genitals and other body parts for the purpose of sexual pleasure. Fingers as well as sex toys, such as vibrators and dildos, may be used in masturbation. Masturbation may or may not include orgasm or ejaculation. According to most physicians and psychiatrists, masturbation is a common, natural, generally harmless, and potentially beneficial activity. However, many people feel guilt and shame over the practice as a result of religious beliefs or other ideas regarding morals and ethics. In some cultures and societies, masturbation is strongly condemned as sinful and immoral.

Masturbation is somewhat more common among men than women. In one major U.S. study, 95 percent of men said that they have masturbated at least once compared with 89 percent of women. The percentages of adults who masturbate on a regular basis are estimated to be about 70 percent for men and 50 percent for women.

Children and adolescents also masturbate. Although masturbation is usually associated with sexual self-satisfaction, children may begin masturbating long before they reach puberty. If this occurs, motivation is likely to be curiosity, self-exploration, and self-soothing rather than sexual in nature. Masturbation typically increases greatly in frequency after puberty before leveling out—in many, but not all, people—during the twenties or thirties.

People may masturbate for different reasons. It is a way to experience sexual pleasure when a partner is not available—though some statistics suggest that people who do have regular sex partners masturbate more often than those who do not have partners. Masturbation is also a way to relieve stress and tension and to relax.

To help them masturbate, people usually think of or look at erotic, sexual imagery, such as pornographic photographs or videos or memories of a previous sexual encounter. People with penises often stimulate the penis, scrotum, perineum (the area between the genitals and anus), or anus. People with vulvas often stimulate the clitoris, labia, vaginal opening, perineum, or anus. Other sensitive body parts, such as the breasts, nipples, and thighs, may also be touched.

Masturbation has many benefits. Stress relief is one of the most common psychological benefits. Other potential psychological benefits could include a sense of peace and well-being; improved sleep; and enhanced understanding of, confidence in, and comfort with one's own sexuality.

Potential physical benefits include help with sexual dysfunctions, such as erectile dysfunction and difficulty with orgasm. This enhanced sexual function could result from improved knowledge about sexual stimulation obtained through masturbation. Better sexual function might also be related to strengthened muscle tone in the pelvic, genital, and anal areas obtained from masturbation. For some people, masturbation might help to relieve menstrual cramps and might help to decrease the risk of urine leakage and uterine prolapse.

Some partners engage in mutual masturbation, in which they masturbate in the presence of each other. They may also help each other masturbate with their fingers or sex toys. Benefits of mutual masturbation could include greater understanding of what "turns each other on," both physically and emotionally, resulting in a stronger, healthier relationship. In addition, mutual masturbation is safer than sexual intercourse because there is less risk of sexually transmitted infections and no risk of pregnancy.

There are some risks associated with masturbation. The main physical risk of frequent masturbation is skin irritation, unless adequate lubrication is used. If an erect penis is forcefully bent during masturbation, there is a risk of rupturing the blood-filled chambers inside the penis—a condition that requires surgery to repair.

Psychological risks of masturbation are potentially more serious. For some people, masturbation may become compulsive to the point that it interferes with their social relationships, sexual relationships, work activities, or other daily functioning. Some individuals who frequently masturbate may eventually experience difficulties having an orgasm through conventional intercourse because they are so used to the experience during masturbation.

Contrary to certain popular myths, masturbation does not lead to blindness, unusual hair growth, shrinking sex organs, or stunted growth, and it cannot deplete sperm cells in men.

A. J. Smuskiewicz

See also: Adolescent Sexuality; Childhood Sexuality; Mutual Masturbation; Orgasm; Religion, Diversity of Human Sexuality and; Sex Toys; Touching, Sexual Arousal and.

Further Reading

National Health Service. (2018). Masturbation Q&A. Retrieved from https://www.nhs.uk/live-well/sexual-health/masturbation-faqs/

Planned Parenthood. (2019). Masturbation. Retrieved from https://www.plannedparenthood.org/learn/sex-and-relationships/masturbation

Mattachine Society

The Mattachine Society was one of the earliest homophile organizations in the United States. Harry Hay was one of the key founders of Mattachine. Hay was a communist organizer in Los Angeles and a sought-after teacher of communist theory. In 1950, he assembled a group of his friends, including Rudi Gerenreich, Bob Hull, Chuck Rowland, and Dale Jennings, to organize the International Bachelors Fraternal Order for Peace and Social Dignity (sometimes referred to as Bachelors Anonymous). Steeped in communist strategy, the organization was structured as a secret society with underground guilds that were separated so that no one person could reveal the identities of other members. Within a year, the group reorganized along a more conventional form and filed as a California nonprofit corporation, renamed the Mattachine Society, in 1951. At the same time, they set up the Mattachine Foundation for legal purposes. The name was inspired by the Société Mattachine, a secret fraternal organization in thirteenth- and fourteenth-century France and Spain of unmarried townsmen who performed music, dance, and rituals while wearing masks to hide their identities. Mattachine Society wanted to educate people about gay issues.

In 1952, Dale Jennings, one of the Mattachine board members, was arrested and charged with lewd conduct. Most people charged in the 1950s with lewd conduct would plead guilty and pay a fine so as to avoid publicity that could destroy their marriages or employment. Jennings felt that the police had set him up and that it was a case of entrapment. He sought and received help from the Mattachine to fight the charges. Jennings stood up in court and admitted to being gay and educated the jury about police entrapment and how police routinely targeted gay people for abuse. The jury was hung (eleven wanted acquittal), and the judge dismissed the case. Although this was the first successful defense against police entrapment of gay individuals, none of the mainstream press carried the story.

In 1953, some of the members of the Mattachine wanted to publish a monthly newsletter. To that end, the Mattachine formed a new organization, ONE, Incorporated. It began publishing in January 1953 and became the voice of the gay rights movement. Immediately, the U.S. postmaster general seized copies of ONE, claiming the publication was obscene, lewd, lascivious, and filthy, and refused to deliver it. ONE sued and eventually won a Supreme Court Case, *ONE, Inc. v. Olesen*. The court ruled that material on homosexuality was not automatically obscene and could be distributed through the postal system. This was probably the most important court decision in the gay rights movement, as it allowed gay men and lesbian women to educate society to reduce hatred and discrimination.

Also, in 1953, Fred M. Snyder, legal adviser to the Mattachine Foundation, was called by Joseph McCarthy to testify before the House Un-American Activities Committee. Snyder was unabashedly open about being gay. This confused McCarthy since the committee and other government organizations were used to people trying to hide their homosexuality. At the same time, a convention was held in Los Angeles with more than 500 representatives from other chapters of Mattachine and homophile organizations attending. At that time, it was the largest such gathering of gay people in U.S. history. A power struggle occurred between those who wanted Mattachine to become more politically active and those who wanted a more moderate, education-based organization. The moderates won, and the old Mattachine Foundation board resigned, including the founders and the old communist influences.

Over the next forty years, the Mattachine Society and ONE evolved, changed names a number of times, floundered, regrouped, merged, but survived. Now, the ONE Institute is primarily a library and archive collection located on the campus of the University of Southern California. It contains the largest collection of books, magazines, articles, paintings, and memorabilia on homosexuality in the world, with more than 1 million items catalogued.

Chuck Stewart

See also: Gay Rights Movement; Sexual Orientation; Sexual Rights.

Further Reading

Kaczorowski, C. (2015). Mattachine Society. Retrieved from http://www.glbtqarchive.com/ssh/mattachine_society_S.pdf

Martin, K. (2018). The Mattachine Society & LGBTQ history. Retrieved from https://www.magellantv.com/articles/the-mattachine-society-lgbtq-history

Media and Sexuality

The media are communication tools used for sharing information in a variety of ways. We most often think of "the media" as mass media, meaning those channels of communication that reach a large audience: radio, television, motion pictures, books, newspapers, magazines, the internet, and so on. Sexuality has been present in media since the beginning of time. Many of the earliest drawings, paintings, and sculptures are representations of naked bodies or sexual behaviors.

While sexual content has always been present in the media, its existence has also been cause for concern. Various people have criticized the media's depictions of sexuality for promoting immoral behavior, perpetuating sexism, corrupting youth, and demeaning human beings. Within a hundred years of the invention of the printing press, the first illustrated pornographic book, *I Modi* by Pietro Arretino and Marcantonio Raimondi, was printed in Rome (and destroyed by the Vatican).

In the mid-nineteenth century, photography became generally available to the public, and by 1873, the U.S. Congress passed the nation's first obscenity law, banning some photos. Soldiers in the Civil War had acquired through the mail large numbers of photographs of naked women, and the new law made them illegal. A couple decades later, when Thomas Edison popularized the moving picture, one of the first films seen by the masses was "The Kiss." It caused a sensation in 1896, and newspapers and the Catholic Church called for censorship. A major concern was that motion pictures were morally problematic for youth. Critics said that children would so desire to see the movies that they would steal the price of admission, and once inside the theater, they would watch scenes of immoral behavior and then imitate what they saw in the films.

In the early to mid-twentieth century, radio and television started out relatively tame. However, more recently, with the proliferation of cable television and internet radio channels, more and more sexual content is broadcast. Cable television programs may include full frontal nudity, a broad range of sexual behaviors, and depictions of sexual violence. Some radio stations regularly play sexually suggestive music and feature on-air personalities who discuss sexuality in ways that would have been impossible twenty years ago. Research into the content of prime-time television programs shows that more than 75 percent of them contain sexual content. However, only 14 percent of sexual references address the risks or responsibilities of sexual behavior. Television shows targeting teenagers actually have more sexual content than programs targeting adults.

Researchers who have investigated popular music have found that 37 percent of the most popular songs in a given year have sexual content. Of these songs,

65 percent had references to degrading sex, which is characterized by one person having an insatiable sexual appetite, the other person being objectified, and sexual value being based only on physical attributes. Most of these sexually degrading songs were rap music. Other research suggests that young people who listen to a lot of this music are more likely to engage in sexual activity than those who do not listen to it as much.

Americans access the internet more and more, with continuous opportunities to view sexual content, whether it is intentional or inadvertent. The internet offers many websites with information on sexual health and education and access to a wide array of sexually explicit material. Data from 2014 show that the average American is online for nearly five hours daily, between their use of computers and cell phones (not voice calls). Virtually all (92 percent) young people use the internet daily. People go online to connect with friends and to meet people in chatrooms, newsgroups, bulletin boards, social networking sites, online dating or "hookup" sites, in multiplayer games, and so on (Bonebrake, 2002). Sexual content is available in all these online spaces and certainly on sites that offer explicit scenes of every kind of sexual behavior.

With so much sexual content in the media, some individuals are particularly concerned with its impact on young people. Adolescents are developing their ideas about sexual identity, gender role and expression, body image, and sexual behavior. Many adults worry that the messages that youth receive are irresponsible or inaccurate. In the absence of effective, comprehensive sexuality education in schools, the media have become the United States' most persistent sexuality educators. Unfortunately, much of the sexual content in the media does not contribute to young people's healthy sexual development.

Teenagers spend seven and a half hours a day with media, more time than is spent doing anything else but sleep, so the influence of the media on teens' development cannot be overestimated. Adolescents often use more than one media source at a time, for example, reading while listening to music or texting while watching television. Their exposure to media is therefore often more intense than if they were using just one form of media at a time.

In one study, 51 percent of teenagers said they had actively looked for sexual content in the media. Males were more likely to look for this kind of content (63%) than females (40%), and movies were the most often used source, followed by television, music, online pornography, and magazines.

Some analysts have pointed out media portrayals that normalize gender stereotypes may encourage youth to emulate narrow and sexist behaviors. The images of ideal bodies in advertising, television, and movies can lead to shame, poor self-esteem, or disordered eating among young people who do not resemble the ideal. The volume of sexual behaviors that are shown or implied is enormous when compared to the amount of time devoted to discussions of safer sex, contraception, or the challenges of an unplanned pregnancy. The ultimate message conveyed in mass media is that sex is fun, that everyone is doing it, and that there are few negative outcomes. Researchers debate the impact this has on youth, but the facts are that teenagers in the United States have significantly higher rates of unintended pregnancy and sexually transmitted infections than teens in other developed nations.

Some researchers suggest that a heavy diet of sexual content in the media leads to earlier sexual intercourse. Others contend that adolescents who are more interested in sex are both more likely to view sexual media *and* to initiate sexual behaviors but that there is no cause-and-effect relationship between the two. In an analysis of twenty-one longitudinal studies, Wright found a doubled risk for early sexual intercourse among teens who are exposed to more sexual content. He suggested that the effect of media on sexual behavior is driven by the acquisition and activation of sexual scripts. Script theory has been applied to sexual behaviors since the 1960s and posits that scripts give behavioral options in daily life, including those that can lead to sexual behavior. One of the ways that individuals are exposed to sexual scripts is through the media.

Some cultural analysts have suggested that mass media portrayals of gender are problematic. They cite examples of male characters in action and adventure movies and television shows where the only emotion they typically display is anger. Often when a female character displays anger, other characters' response to her is that she is crazy or out of control. When characters are sad, the male may have a single tear but otherwise remain stoic, while the female is portrayed as vulnerable and actually cries emotionally. Gender stereotypes like these and many others are pervasive in the media and suggest to people who are exposed to them that this is normal, desirable behavior rather than emotionally limiting and dehumanizing.

The appeal of sexual content in the media helps to make media producers profitable. People are naturally interested in sexual imagery and messages, and various media outlets use that interest to entertain and sometimes exploit. Some media producers are interested in promoting products, and others are interested in providing helpful information and services to support sexual health. Whatever their goals, media producers have a profound influence on how we learn about sexuality, help to shape our values about sexuality, and contribute to public discussions and policies about sex, gender, and relationships.

While some people might seek to censor sexual content in the media, there is no way to escape exposure to it. Various groups advocate for media literacy to help young people think critically about the media environment in which we live. Key points to consider are that all media messages are constructed, and they each have their own creative ways of making their story effective. Each user of media will interpret the message through the lens of their own experience. Media have embedded values and points of view. The *National Enquirer* will tell a story differently than the *New York Times* because they have different points of view. Finally, most media messages are developed to gain profit or to influence the consumer. Media literacy helps people to recognize fantasy and constructively integrate it with reality.

Michael J. McGee

See also: Advertising, Sex in; Gender; Pornography; Sex Education; Sexual Health; Sexual Identity; Sexual Script; Sexualization.

Further Reading

Bleakley, A., Hennessy, M., & Fishbein, M. (2011). A model of adolescents' seeking of sexual content in their media choices. *Journal of Sex Research, 48*(4), 309–315.

Bonebrake, K. (2002). College students' Internet use, relationship formation, and personality correlates. *CyberPsychology & Behavior, 5*, 551–557.

Brown, J. D., L'Engle, K. L., Pardun, C. J., Guo, G., Kenneavy, K., & Jackson, C. (2006). Sexy media matter: Exposure to sexual content in music, movies, television, and magazines predicts black and white adolescents' sexual behavior. *Pediatrics, 117*(4), 1018–1027.

Butters, G. R. (2007). *Banned in Kansas: Motion picture censorship 1915–1966*. Columbia: University of Missouri Press.

Collins, R. L., Martino, S. C., Elliott, M. N., & Miu, A. (2011). Relationships between adolescent sexual outcomes and exposure to sex in media: Robustness to propensity-based analysis. *Developmental Psychology, 47*(2), 585.

Gray, F. (2003). The Kiss in the Tunnel (1899): G. A. Smith and the emergence of the edited film in England. In L. Grieveson & P. Kramer (Eds.), *The silent cinema reader*. London: Routledge.

Kunkel, D., Eyal, K., Finnerty, K., Biely, E., & Donnerstein, E. (2005). *Sex on TV 4: A biennial report to the Kaiser Family Foundation*. Menlo Park, CA: Kaiser Family Foundation.

Lenhart, A. (2015, April 9). Pew Research Center. *Teens, social media & technology overview 2015*. Retrieved from http://www.pewinternet.org/2015/04/09/teens-social-media-technology-2015/

McGarry, M. (2000). Spectral sexualities: Nineteenth-century spiritualism, moral panics, and the making of US obscenity law. *Journal of Women's History, 12*(2), 8–29.

Primack, B. A., Gold, M. A., Schwarz, E. B., & Dalton, M. A. (2008). Degrading and non-degrading sex in popular music: A content analysis. *Public Health Reports, 123*(5), 593.

Rideout, V. J., Foehr, U. G., & Roberts, D. F. (2010). *Generation M^2: Media in the lives of 8- to 18-year-olds*. Menlo Park, CA: Henry J. Kaiser Family Foundation.

Steinberg, L., & Monahan, K. C. (2011). Adolescents' exposure to sexy media does not hasten the initiation of sexual intercourse. *Developmental Psychology, 47*(2), 562.

Strasburger, V. C. (2012). Adolescents, sex, and the media. *Adolescent Medicine-State of the Art Reviews, 23*(1), 15.

Talvacchia, B. (2001). *Taking positions: On the erotic in Renaissance culture*. Princeton, NJ: Princeton University Press.

Thoman, E., & Jolls, T. (2008). *Literacy for the 21st Century: An overview and orientation guide to media literacy education*. Malibu, CA: Center for Media Literacy.

Wright, P. J. (2011). Mass media effects on youth sexual behavior assessing the claim for causality. *Communication Yearbook, 35*, 343–385.

Medical Treatment of Sex Offenders

The use of pharmaceutical interventions in the management of adult sex offenders is typically used in conjunction with psychological interventions. Unfortunately, to date there has been relatively little empirical research conducted on the use of pharmacological agents to help control deviant sexual arousal among convicted sex offenders. The research that has been conducted on antilibidinal drugs relates primarily to three medications: medroxyprogesterone acetate (MPA), cyproterone acetate (CPA), and leuprolide acetate. Interest in sex drive–reducing medications has increased over the last two decades primarily based on the theoretical assumption that a reduction in sex drive or elimination of the ability to achieve erections will subsequently lead to a reduction in deviant sexual behavior.

Research on the effectiveness of MPA in sex offender treatment has shown that MPA decreases testosterone to castration levels and decreases both the frequency and intensity of deviant sexual urges. Bradford and Pawlak (1993) conducted a double-blind crossover study examining the effects of CPA in nineteen sex offenders who met diagnostic criteria for a paraphilia (i.e., sexual deviation). Results indicated that CPA was associated with reductions in sexual fantasies and some decrease in sexual arousal as measured by self-report.

Several researchers have commented on the negative side effects that may accompany the use of such medications. Side effects can include weight gain, depression, liver damage, difficulty breathing, gynaecomastia, nausea, and diabetes. Given the range of side effects associated with these medications, compliance has become an issue both within clinical settings and for the purpose of completing research studies.

Leuprolide acetate, although prescribed for a variety of conditions that are not forensic in nature (e.g., fertility problems in women and in the treatment of prostate cancer) began to be used with sex offenders in the early 1990s. This medication was associated with reductions in sex drive as well as having relative tolerability with reference to side effects. Unfortunately, only one controlled study using long-term rates of recidivism as a dependent measure has been conducted with sex offenders. Previous research on leuprolide acetate administration with sex offenders has been limited to case studies. Although limited in nature, the case study approach has resulted in findings supportive of the use of leuprolide acetate with sex offenders. For example, Kreuger and Kaplan (2001) presented twelve case reports of men suffering from various paraphilic disorders who received leuprolide acetate. Self-report data from these clients indicated that leuprolide acetate administration was associated with suppression of deviant sexual interests and behavior.

One study compared a group of sex offenders receiving both leuprolide acetate and cognitive behavioral treatment (CBT) directed at sex offending, with two comparison groups: a group of sex offenders who received only CBT and a group of violent non-sex offenders who received no treatment. As the vast majority of sex offenders also presented with a history of nonsexual offenses, the second comparison group was considered appropriate. Results indicated that the group of sex offenders receiving both leuprolide acetate and CBT were significantly less likely to reoffend than the violent non-sex offenders, using any violent recidivism as the criterion outcome measure and using Cox regression analyses to control for differences between groups on actuarial risk assessment data.

Jan Looman, Jeffrey Abracen, and Alessandra Gallo

See also: Androgens; Castration; Compulsivity, Sexual; Out-of-Control Sexual Behavior.

Further Reading

Bradford, J. M., & Pawlak, A. (1993). Double blind placebo crossover study of cyproterone acetate in the treatment of the paraphilias. *Archives of Sexual Behavior, 22*(5), 383–402.

Dickey, R. (1992). The management of a case of treatment resistant paraphilia with a long acting LHRH agonist. *Canadian Journal of Psychiatry, 37*(8), 567–569.

Gallo, A., Abracen, J., Looman, J., Jeglic, E. L., & Dickey, R. (2019). The use of leuprolide acetate in the management of high-risk sexual offenders. *Sexual Abuse, 31*(8), 930–951.

Harrison, K. (Ed.). (2010). *Managing high-risk sex offenders in the community.* Portland, OR: Willan Publishing.

Krueger, R. B., & Kaplan, M. S. (2001). Depot-leuprolide acetate for treatment of paraphilias: A report of twelve cases. *Archives of Sexual Behavior, 30*(4), 409–422.

Raymond, N., Robinson, B., Kraft, C., Rittberg, B., & Coleman, E. (2001). Treatment of pedophilia with leuprolide acetate: A case study. *Journal of Psychology & Human Sexuality, 13*(3–4), 79–88.

Rosler, A., & Witzum, E. (2000). Pharmacotherapy of paraphilias in the new millennium. *Behavioral Sciences and the Law, 18*, 43–56.

Saleh, F., & Berlin, F. (2003). Sex hormones, neurotransmitters, and psychopharmacological treatments in men with paraphilic disorders. *Journal of Child Sexual Abuse, 12*(3–4), 233–253.

Megan's Law

Megan's Law was created in response to the rape and murder of seven-year-old Megan Kanka on July 29, 1994, in Mercer County, New Jersey, by her neighbor Jesse Timmendequas. Timmendequas had two previous convictions for sexually assaulting young girls. The murder attracted national attention and led to the introduction of Megan's Law, which requires law enforcement authorities to make information available to the public regarding registered sex offenders. Individual states decide what information will be made available and how it should be disseminated. Information can include the offender's name, picture, address, incarceration date, and nature of their crime. The information is often displayed on free public websites but can be published in newspapers or distributed in pamphlets or through various other means. The federal law requires all fifty states to release information to the public about known convicted sex offenders. If a state fails to comply with minimal release of information standards established by the federal government, then that state risks losing federal law enforcement funding.

Before Megan's Law, the Jacob Wetterling Crimes Against Children and Sexually Violent Offender Registration Act of 1993 required states to have a sex offender and crimes against children registry. It is named for Jacob Wetterling, who was abducted near his home and murdered in 1989. Investigators later learned that, unbeknownst to local law enforcement, sex offenders were being sent to live in halfway houses nearby. This was amended with Megan's Law in 1996.

After Megan's Law, the Adam Walsh Child Protection and Safety Act (2006) supplements the law with new registration requirements and a three-tier system for classifying sex offenders according to their risk to the community. This act significantly strengthens registration and notification laws across the nation by increasing the duration of registration for sex offenders, increasing in-person verifications, requiring active sex offender notification programs, requiring certain juveniles to register, requiring registration for adults convicted of an instant offense that may not be a sex crime if they have a prior sex crime conviction that predates Megan's Law, requiring registration for sex offenders entering the country, creating a federal felony for sex offenders failing to register (maximum penalty of up to ten years), and providing funding to the U.S. marshals to track down those offenders.

Lauren Ewaniuk

See also: Child Sexual Abuse; Rape; Sexual Assault.

Further Reading

Crime Victims Center. (n.d.). Megan's Law & The Adam Walsh Child Protection Act. Retrieved from https://www.parentsformeganslaw.org/public/meganFederal.html

Zgoba, K., Dalessandro, M., Veysey, B., & Witt, P. (2008). Megan's Law: Assessing the practical and monetary efficacy. Washington, DC: United States Department of Justice.

Menarche

Menarche is a person's first menstrual period, which occurs in the later stages of puberty, usually between the ages of nine and fifteen, with most people who have a uterus having their first menstrual period around the age of twelve or thirteen. The largest determining factors of the age at which most adolescents will experience menarche are heredity, weight, racial background, and other factors.

Many young people have concerns over the timing of menarche. Some worry that they will be the last of their peers to experience this milestone, while others are concerned about being the first of their friends. There is clearly a lot of worry, fear, and uncertainty that comes with menarche—when and where it will happen (in school, at a friend's house, while swimming at a pool party), what it will be like, and whether anyone will notice or somehow be able to tell.

One factor that appears to have a great impact on how a young person will view their menarche experience is whether, and to what degree, they felt prepared for the experience. This includes knowing what to expect, being informed that menarche is a normal experience that all folks with uteruses go through, and having information about menstrual hygiene, such as using pads, tampons, and menstrual cups. Research has shown that the more prepared a young person is, the more positively they will view their experience with menarche. Many folks in the United States experience their first period without knowing what is happening to them, which can understandably be a very frightening experience. This helps to highlight the importance of reproductive health education both from school and at home.

Along with all this concern, many young people are also very excited and eager about getting their first menstrual period. Some see it as an important milestone, a step toward womanhood and maturity. Others may just be curious to know what all the fuss is about or desire to be like their peers who have already experienced menarche. Some choose to celebrate this milestone with their close family and friends by having a menarche party (also called a first moon party or period party), though this is still fairly uncommon as much of American society, like many other societies, still often view menstruation with great stigma and secrecy and largely consider it to be a very private matter that should be kept hidden from others.

The event of menarche is responded to in a variety of ways in other cultures. In many Indigenous/Native American societies, women are considered powerful life-givers; therefore, a young person's first menstruation is held in high reverence and celebrated with several days of honored rituals. Conversely, in other cultures, such as in some areas of Nepal, menstruation is viewed with extreme stigma and superstition. In cultures such as these, it is believed that menstruating women are unclean and thought to be so toxic that their touch alone could cause crops to die, spoil their cow's milk, or cause men to become seriously ill. These girls and women are often sent to live outdoors in a hut away from the family (a practice that was recently criminalized, but still occurs illegally), and they must adhere to very strict rules and prohibitions until they are no longer menstruating.

Lyndsay Mercier

See also: Menstruation; Puberty; Sex Education.

Further Reading

Boston Women's Health Book Collective. (2005). *Our bodies, ourselves*. New York: Scribner.

Harris, R. H. (2018). *It's perfectly normal: Changing bodies, growing up, sex, and sexual health*. Somerville, MA: Candlewick Press.

Nalebuff, R. K. (2009). *My little red book*. New York: Twelve.

Menopause

Menopause is the time in a woman's or other female-bodied person's life when they stop having periods and are no longer able to become pregnant without medical intervention. In North America, this is roughly around the age of fifty-one years but can vary between about age forty-five and fifty-five. During this time, hormone levels change, and the ovaries decline in function and stop releasing eggs. Menopause is considered to have occurred when a person has not had a menstrual period for one year.

Perimenopause is the period of development prior to menopause; for most, this begins in their mid-thirties or forties. During this time, hormones levels begin to drop, and fertility decreases; many also experience irregular menstrual cycles. At perimenopause, an individual's brain begins to change due to hormonal shifts in the body, and these differences in the levels of estrogen and progesterone can cause individuals to experience mood swings, irritability, anxiety, and depression. Other symptoms associated with menopause include lower sexual desire, difficulty sleeping, hot flashes, and loss of bone density. During menopause, many people also experience a reduction in their natural vaginal lubrication, which causes the tissue of the vagina to become thinner and drier. This may make sex uncomfortable or painful, although for some, this is helped by the use of commercial lubricants. It is important to note that not all individuals experience symptoms, and a person's expectations of menopause, as well as their overall general health, can greatly influence their experience.

Hormonal treatments, often called hormone replacement therapy (HRT), are available to those experiencing menopausal changes to help alleviate some of the symptoms. HRT contains female hormones, typically estrogen and progesterone, and can come in pill, cream, or patch form. If these medications are taken, it is recommended to use the lowest dose possible for a short period of time as research from the Women's Health Initiative (2016) found that using HRT can lead to an increased risk for breast cancer, heart disease, stroke, blood clots, and urinary incontinence. Menopausal and postmenopausal individuals may introduce or continue self-care regimens in their lives, such as yoga, meditation, physical exercise, social support, and other practices to support the whole self.

The experiences associated with menopause differ widely from one person to the next, and a psychosocial lens is necessary to analyze the biological changes and the cultural attitudes toward menopause. In cultures that reward women for reaching the end of the fertile period, menopause is associated with fewer physiological symptoms. According to one researcher, women in India described menopause as being associated with increased social status, and more recent studies also support the view that women from different cultural groups have diverse attitudes about menopause that reflect a more or less positive context for this life stage. A woman's personal attitudes about aging and her multiple roles in life may influence the ease or difficulty with which she experiences menopause.

The North American Menopause Society (NAMS) provides a variety of resources on health-related issues, such as sexual changes, osteoporosis, and sleep disturbances associated with the hormonal changes of menopause. NAMS advises women to see this transition as a stimulus for new beginnings, to take a closer look at one's own health, relationships, and satisfying activities. Menopause is a significant event in an individual's life, with biological, social, and psychological changes reflecting their personal and cultural values of motherhood, fertility, and aging.

Martha Goldstein-Schultz

See also: Andropause; Estrogen; Female Sexuality; Fertility; Hormone Replacement Therapy; Infertility; Menstruation; Perimenopause; Progesterone; Sex Hormones; Sexuality among Older Adults.

Further Reading

Costanian, C., McCague, H., & Tamin, H. (2018). Age at natural menopause and its associated factors in Canada: Cross-sectional analysis from the Canadian Longitudinal Study on Aging. *Menopause, 25*(3), 265–272.

Devi, N. J. (2007). *The secret power of yoga: A woman's guide to the heart and spirit of the Yoga Sutras*. New York: Three Rivers Press.

Erikson, E. H. (1963). *Childhood and society* (2nd ed.). New York: Norton.

Gillespie, C. (1989). *Hormones, hot flashes, and mood swings: Living through the ups and downs of menopause*. New York: Harper Perennial.

Lerner-Geva, L., Boyko, V., Blumstein, T., & Benyamini, Y. (2010). The impact of education, cultural background, and lifestyle on symptoms of the menopausal transition: The Woman's Health at Midlife study. *The Journal of Women's Health, 19*, 975–985.

National Institutes of Health. (2016). *Menopausal hormone therapy information*. Retrieved from www.nih.gov/health-information/menopausal-hormone-therapy-information

Newman, B. M., & Newman, P. R. (2015). *Development through life: A psychosocial approach*. Stamford, CT: Cengage Learning.

North American Menopause Society. (2019). Retrieved from www.menopause.org

Northrup, C. (2012). *The wisdom of menopause: Creating physical and emotional health during the change*. New York: Bantam Books.

U.S. Department of Health and Human Services Women's Health Office. (2018). *Menopause and sexuality*. Retrieved from www.womenshealth.gov/menopause/menopause-and-sexuality

Menstruation

Menstruation is the monthly fluctuation of hormones that controls the female body's production and release of an egg from the ovaries into the uterus for fertilization. It culminates with the discharge of the uterine lining if a fertilized egg fails to implant in the uterus. The hormones typically fluctuate on a twenty-eight-day cycle; however, each body has its own rhythm, so some people experience cycles that are longer or shorter. The menstrual cycle is a cooperative act between the ovaries, uterus, and the hormones that control them.

There are several hormones involved in the menstrual cycle, and they are all important to the overall process. Hormones act as regulators of communication between various parts of the body. In this case, these hormones communicate between the hypothalamus in the brain and the reproductive organs. Follicle-stimulating hormone (FSH) acts on different areas depending on the sex of a person. In females, follicle-stimulating hormone is responsible for promoting the growth of the egg cell. The next hormone, luteinizing hormone (LH), is responsible for triggering ovulation as well as maintaining the corpus luteum, which develops from the follicle after ovulation. In short, FSH matures the egg cell, and LH controls the ovulation process. Estrogen is the main female hormone and has many important uses throughout the body, both in men and women. In the menstrual cycle, estrogen is responsible for both the growth of the uterine lining and the regulation of FSH. Progesterone is also important during menstruation. It is secreted by the corpus luteum in the ovary in order to support blood flow to the endometrium. Progesterone's role also varies in later stages of the menstrual cycle depending on if there is an embryo to maintain.

The ovarian process begins at the beginning of the menstrual cycle. There are two phases in this process: the follicular phase and the luteal phase. The follicular phase occurs first. This is when FSH stimulates the ovary to develop and mature an egg cell. This begins after the cessation of the previous menstrual flow (menses). Many cells begin to develop during this time; however, typically only one reaches full maturation as once a cell becomes dominant, the others regress. After an egg cell reaches its full maturation, there is a spike in LH, which causes the next step, ovulation. Ovulation is when the mature egg cell breaks from its casing, pushes out through the ovarian wall, and travels down the fallopian tube into the uterus. A person is most fertile during the few days before and after ovulation. This is because as the egg travels down the fallopian tube, it is possible for fertilization to occur if sperm cells are present.

Just after menses, while the ovaries are in the follicular stage, the uterus is in the proliferative phase. This is when estrogen is at its highest production. While glands in the uterine wall grow, the tissue that lines the inner wall of the uterus (endometrium) thickens. The endometrium is at its thickest when ovulation occurs. This timing is important because the thickened wall is where the fertilized egg will be implanted. Implantation is when the fertilized egg burrows into the endometrium and begins to grow. It is also possible to have an egg that is fertilized but does not implant.

The second half of the ovarian process is called the luteal phase. After the release of the egg out of the casing to the fallopian tubes, the casing remains in the ovaries and is known as the corpus luteum. LH promotes the extended life of the corpus luteum while it secretes progesterone. These levels peak in the week after ovulation. There are two possibilities after this point. If fertilization and implantation take place, the implanted embryo will produce its own hormones, causing the corpus luteum to grow and secrete even more progesterone to maintain the pregnancy. If fertilization and implantation do not occur, then the corpus luteum will disintegrate over the remaining time of the cycle.

If there is implantation and an embryo starts to form, the increased progesterone will help maintain the endometrium and increase blood flow, and the endometrium will continue to thicken in order to better maintain the embryo. If there is no pregnancy, the degeneration of the corpus luteum will cause progesterone levels to drop. When the hormone levels drop, the endometrium loses its blood supply and sheds itself during menses. Both the endometrium tissue and blood from the tissues detach and flow down the cervix and out of the vagina.

Rebecca Polly

See also: Endometrium; Estrogen; Fallopian Tubes; Fertility; Follicle-Stimulating Hormone; Luteinizing Hormone; Menarche; Menopause; Ovaries; Ovulation; Pregnancy; Progesterone; Sex Hormones; Uterus.

Further Reading

Bobel, C. (2010). *Third-wave feminism and the politics of menstruation.* New Brunswick, NJ: Rutgers University Press.

Boston Women's Health Book Collective. (2005). *Our bodies, ourselves.* New York: Scribner.

Harris, R. H. (2018). *It's perfectly normal: Changing bodies, growing up, sex, and sexual health.* Somerville, MA: Candlewick Press.

Hope, S., & Ravnikar, V. (2005). *The abnormal menstrual cycle.* Abingdon, UK: Taylor & Francis.

Nalebuff, R. K. (2009). *My little red book.* New York: Twelve.

Shail, A., & Howie, G. (2005). *Menstruation: A cultural history.* New York: Palgrave Macmillan.

Miller v. California

Miller v. California is a landmark Supreme Court decision made in 1973. It is currently the settled law used by U.S. courts to determine if something is obscene. In the Supreme Court's decision, it was determined that there were three criteria that must be met in order to determine if something is obscene:

1. Whether "the average person, applying contemporary community standards" would find that the work, taken as a whole, appeals to the prurient interest
2. Whether the work depicts or describes, in a patently offensive way, sexual conduct specifically defined by the applicable state law
3. Whether the work, taken as a whole, lacks serious literary, artistic, political, or scientific value (*Miller v. California*, 1973).

It is important to note that in order for something to be considered obscene, it must meet all three of these criteria. However, it is common for people to focus on the third criterion, which is sometimes referred to as the LAPS test, for lacking literary, artistic, political, or scientific value. The ruling is also notable in that the court stated that things that were found to be obscene were not protected by the First Amendment right to free speech.

The case originated in 1968, when Marvin Miller used the United States Postal Service to mail brochures advertising the sale of books and a movie with a sexual theme. Miller was convicted on charges of distributing obscenity, a decision that he then appealed. The appeal was eventually heard by the U.S. Supreme Court. Part of Miller's defense was based on an earlier decision made by the Supreme Court in the 1966 *Memoirs v. Massachusetts* case, in which the court deemed that if something had any literary value, it was protected under the freedom of speech. The *Miller v. California* decision reversed this, and the conviction of Mr. Miller was upheld. While there have been other cases that have attempted to redefine obscenity in the United States, the three-pronged test established by the *Miller v. California* decision remains the standard used to decide if something is obscene.

There are many critiques and criticisms of this decision, one of which is that the criteria are too vague. In the *Miller v. California* decision, the court addresses the fact that it is not possible to set one definition of obscenity for the entire country. The use of the term "contemporary community standards" in the first criterion was an attempt made by the court to allow the individual states to make their own decisions as to what was to be considered obscene. Since there is no clear definition of what community standards are, it is possible for a person to commit a crime and not realize that they have done so until a jury of their peers tells them they have.

In addition, the concept of focusing on local standards may have been easier to apply in the 1970s than it is today. Since the advent of the internet, the majority of pornography is distributed digitally. In a situation where an attempt is made to determine if something distributed online is obscene, it is difficult to identify what "community" means and therefore what that community's standards are.

Susan Milstein

See also: Commission on Obscenity and Pornography; Media and Sexuality; Pornography.

Further Reading

Adams, R. (2012). An objective approach to obscenity in the digital age. *St. John's Law Review, 86*(1), 211–247.

Gelber, K., & Stone, A. (2017). Constitutions, gender and freedom of expression: The legal regulation of pornography. In H. Irving (Ed.), *Constitutions and gender* (463–481). Cheltenham, UK: Edward Elgar Publishing.

Miller v. California. (1973). Retrieved from https://www.oyez.org/cases/1971/70-73

Walters, L. G., & DeWitt, C. (2005). Obscenity in the digital age: The re-evaluation of community standards. *NEXUS, 10*, 59.

Molluscum Contagiosum

Molluscum contagiosum is a common harmless viral skin infection that appears as small smooth spherical lumps the same color as the skin. The growths often have a dimple in the middle and occasionally can become itchy. As the name suggests, it is infectious and easily transmitted through skin-to-skin contact, including sexual activity, as well as by sharing contaminated objects like towels, toys, or clothes. A person with molluscum contagiosum can also spread the virus to other parts of their body via their hands and touch.

Molluscum contagiosum is caused by a poxvirus, molluscum contagiosum virus. The only symptom of molluscum contagiosum is the small bumps on the skin, which can range in size from a pinhead to as large as a pencil eraser. Most people will get about ten to twenty bumps, although people with a weakened immune system can have one hundred or more.

Molluscum contagiosum can be problematic for people with weakened immune systems, such as those living with HIV. Before the availability and use of antiretroviral therapy (ART) for the treatment of HIV, infection with molluscum contagiosum could be widespread on the body and face and not limited to the ano-genital areas. Management of the infection was also more challenging since the immune system was not strong enough to fight the virus. However, among people living with HIV who are on ART, treatment of molluscum contagiosum is the same for those who are not living with HIV.

Treatment for molluscum contagiosum is generally not recommended because the infection usually clears up on its own and does not normally cause any symptoms other than the spots. However, if the spots are affecting quality of life, or if people have a weakened immune system, treatment may be offered. Treatment may include topical medication or destruction of the papule in a clinic setting. This is recommended for lesions on the face and on the genitals and can easily be achieved by freezing each lesion with a small amount of liquid nitrogen, or through laser therapy, in a doctor's office. A more time-consuming and low-tech solution is to "de-roof" each spot using a needle to pop the papule, removing the contents with a swab, and then applying medication to the base of the papule. Over-the-counter topical creams are also available, such as medications to treat skin warts—for example, podophyllotoxin (0.5 percent). For small children who are fearful of creams or needles, oral cimetidine medication can be used.

Kelwyn Browne

See also: Human Immunodeficiency Virus (HIV); Sexually Transmitted Infections (STIs).

Further Reading

American Academy of Dermatology. (2018). Molluscum contagiosum. Retrieved from https://www.aad.org/public/diseases/contagious-skin-diseases/molluscum-contagiosum

Centers for Disease Control. (2015). Molluscum contagiosum. Retrieved from https://www.cdc.gov/poxvirus/molluscum-contagiosum/index.html

National Health Service. (2019). Molluscum contagiosum. Retrieved from https://www.nhs.uk/conditions/molluscum-contagiosum/#

Money, John

John Money (1921–2006) was born on July 8, 1921, in Morrinsville, New Zealand. Money was a well-known psychologist and sex researcher whose specialty was rooted in sexual and gender development. Money coined the terms "gender identity" and "gender role" and was the first to start the debate on the distinction between gender and biological sex. He was also the creator of "lovemaps," an individual's internal preference and understanding of sexual and erotic desires based on their past.

Money completed high school at age sixteen and went on to get a double master's degree from Victoria University in Wellington. He then became a junior lecturer at the University of Otago in Dunedin in 1944. He immigrated to the United States in 1947 to pursue more education. He started working as a clinical psychologist in Pittsburg, Pennsylvania, at a psychiatric clinic. From there, he went on to complete his PhD in psychology from Harvard University. He graduated in 1952 and went on to pursue a career at Johns Hopkins University.

During Money's career, he published more than forty books and authored hundreds of academic papers. Most notable was his 1972 book *Man & Woman, Boy & Girl: Gender Identity from Conception to Maturity*, which he coauthored with Dr. Anke Ehrhardt. Money stayed with Johns Hopkins University throughout his entire career. In 1966, he helped establish the Johns Hopkins Gender Identity Clinic. At Johns Hopkins, Money focused his research on gender identity and gender roles, paraphilias, and lovemaps.

Money's most notable contribution to the world of sex research was his introduction of terminology for gender identity and gender role. Money helped establish the difference between these terms, biological sex assignment, and sexual functioning of an individual, and he considered that biological sex and gender were two different concepts.

Money also contributed to the understanding of paraphilias and was successful in changing the wording of *DSM-III* from "perversions" to "paraphilias." Money proposed that "paraphilia" was a less judgmental word for individuals who were dealing with sexual problems outside the norm. He also advocated for changing "sexual preference" to "sexual orientation" due to his belief that sexual attraction is not completely voluntary or chosen.

Money also created the term "lovemaps," which he identified as an individual's sexual and erotic desires that are played out within interpersonal relationships. Money also described "vandalized lovemaps," which can result from trauma in one's lovemap and can lead to sexualization or repression and sometimes to paraphilias.

Money was well known for his role in the David Reimer case, also known as the John/Joan case. After Mr. Reimer had a botched circumcision at eight months old, his parents consulted with Money, who recommended for David to be raised female and to undergo surgery to remove his testes. Money believed that gender roles were entirely socialized so believed that David would successfully be raised as a girl. However, this turned out not to be true, and David (who was renamed Brenda) experienced lifelong psychological and physical distress. This case made national news and brought much scrutiny to Money. Money stood by his recommendation, although he opted to not talk about this case later in his career.

Money continued his research and writing throughout his life. He passed on July 7, 2006, the day before his eighty-fifth birthday. He had one short marriage and no children. Money was a lover of art and donated his collection to the East Southerland Gallery in Gore, New Zealand. Money's own lifelong works are housed at the Kinsey Institute at the University of Indiana.

Amanda Baker

See also: Biological Sex; Gender; Gender Identity; Gender Identity Development; Gender Roles, Socialization and; Paraphilias; Reimer, David.

Further Reading

Ehrhardt, A. A. (2007). John Money, Ph.D. *Journal of Sex Research, 44*(3), 223–224.

Green, R. (2006). John Money, Ph.D. (July 8, 1921–July 7, 2006): A personal obituary. *Archives of Sexual Behavior, 35*(6), 629–632.

Kinsey Institute, Indiana University. (2016). John Money, Ph.D. Retrieved from https://www.kinseyinstitute.org/about/profiles/john-money.php

Money, J. (1994). *Sex errors of the body and related syndromes: A guide to counseling children, adolescents, and their families* (2nd ed.). Baltimore: P. H. Brooks Publishing Company.

Money, J. (1999). *The lovemap guidebook: A definitive statement.* New York: Continuum.

Money, J., & Ehrhardt, A. (1972). *Man & woman, boy & girl: Gender identity from conception to maturity.* Northvale, NJ: Jason Aronson.

Monogamy

Monogamy is a type of relationship in which both partners are exclusive with each other. Originally, monogamy meant having only one partner for life, but its understanding has evolved into being with only one person at a time (serial monogamy).

Monogamy is the most widely known relationship type and the one that is most socially acceptable by the majority of religions. Monogamy has also been heavily debated as to whether or not it is the natural state for humans.

From a scientific standpoint, monogamy can be viewed from two different perspectives: genetic monogamy and social monogamy. Genetic monogamy occurs where there is a mutually exclusive reproduction or mating arrangement between two partners. Humans are one of the few primates that participate in genetic monogamy. In the animal kingdom, genetic monogamy is rare, although some birds are also genetically monogamous. Social monogamy refers to pair bonding, where two partners are socially exclusive of other potential partners; however, reproduction is not necessarily the goal of the dyad.

More recently, serial monogamy has become more socially acceptable and refers to a relationship style in which an individual dates or partners with only one individual at a time. Serial monogamy is very common; individuals are in one monogamous relationship until the relationship ends, and then they form a new monogamous relationship with their next partner.

Historically, Greek and Roman men were only allowed to be married to one female at a time and were not allowed concubines during marriage. These rules were even applied to rulers, and this was the accepted norm of this society. Monogamy has also been shown to be the dominant form of relationships within the Egyptian and Babylonians societies. Monogamy continues to be the most commonly reported type of relationship in the United States, and individuals who engage in polyamorous relationships (with more than one partner) often experience judgment, stigma, and discrimination.

Amanda Baker

See also: Polyamory; Polyandry; Polygamy; Polygyny; Serial Monogamy.

Further Reading

Low, B. S. (2003). Ecological and social complexities in human monogamy. In U. H. Reichard & C. Boesch (Eds.), *Monogamy: Mating strategies and partnerships in birds, humans, and other mammals* (161–176). Cambridge: Cambridge University Press.

Perel, E. (2006). *Mating in captivity.* New York: HarperCollins.

Perel, E. (2017). *The state of affairs.* New York: HarperCollins.

Phillips, A. (1996). *Monogamy.* New York: Random House

Reichard, U. H. (2003). Monogamy: Past and present. In U. H. Reichard & C. Boesch (Eds.), *Monogamy: Mating strategies and partnerships in birds, humans, and other mammals* (3–25). Cambridge: Cambridge University Press.

Ryan, C., & Jethá, C. (2010). *Sex at dawn: The prehistoric origins of modern sexuality.* New York: Harper.

Mutual Masturbation

Mutual masturbation is a sexual activity that involves stimulating one's own genitals—masturbating—for sexual pleasure in the presence of another person who is also masturbating. It is a way of being sexually intimate with another person without the risk of sexually transmitted infection or pregnancy.

Mutual masturbation can be a good way for partners to teach each other the kind of touch they enjoy, both in terms of where and how they like to be touched. Mutual masturbation can be a highly arousing activity because it allows partners to see each other become aroused and, if they continue long enough, to experience orgasm.

Some people are embarrassed to suggest mutual masturbation to a partner due to cultural taboos about masturbation. Some religions teach that masturbation is sinful, and some cultural beliefs lead people to think that masturbation should not be necessary when people are involved in partnered sexual relationships. Individuals should use their judgment about whether to practice self-pleasure and mutual masturbation. There are no medical reasons not to masturbate; indeed, there are many benefits to learning how to pleasure one's own body, such as relaxation, stress reduction, and increased awareness of control over one's sexual responses. Mutual masturbation is simply the act of sharing a healthy form of sexual expression with another person.

Mutual masturbation is a form of nonpenetrative sex because it does not include penetration of the mouth, vagina, or anus by a partner, unless sex toys are used. This qualifies mutual masturbation as a form of outercourse. People enjoy outercourse for many reasons, including a desire to avoid sexually transmitted infections and pregnancy, a desire to avoid penetrative sexual activity, and as a form of arousing sex play.

People who practice abstinence typically avoid penetrative sexual activity. The reasons for practicing abstinence vary from person to person. Some people practicing abstinence accept mutual masturbation as a healthy option; others feel that the behavior does not fall within their understanding of abstinence.

Like other sexual activities, mutual masturbation should only be practiced when both partners participate willingly and enthusiastically. If either partner feels pressured into the behavior, it will be neither a positive nor healthy experience.

Another definition of mutual masturbation is when partners touch each other's genitals for the purposes of sexual pleasure. This activity is also often called heavy petting. Mutual masturbation may involve touching another person's genitals over or under their clothing. In this instance, a risk for sexually transmitted infection exists if one person's hand or sex toy touches both their own and another person's genitals.

If individuals participating in mutual masturbation only touch themselves, no safer sex techniques are required. However, people who engage in mutual masturbation involving contact with each other's bodies should practice safer sex. Depending on the bodies of the partners involved, safer sex techniques may require the use of condoms, dams, or only touching each other over their clothing.

Melanie Davis

See also: Abstinence; Arousal; Masturbation; Sex Toys; Touching, Sexual Arousal and.

Further Reading

Dodson, B. (2011). Hands and toys for orgasms at any age. In J. Price (Ed.), *Naked at our age* (143–144). Berkeley, CA: Seal Press.

Joannides, P. (2017). Hand jobs and genital massage for females. In P. Joannides (Ed.), *Guide to getting it on* (7th ed.). Waldport, OR: Goofy Foot Press.

Klein, M., & Robbins, R. (1998). *Let me count the ways*. New York: Tarcher Putnam.

Moon, A. (2014). *Girl sex 101*. San Francisco, CA: Lunatic Ink.

Planned Parenthood. (2019). Outercourse. Retrieved from http://www.plannedparenthood.org/learn/birth-control/outercourse

Encyclopedia of Sex and Sexuality

Encyclopedia of Sex and Sexuality

Understanding Biology, Psychology, and Culture

VOLUME II: N–Z

Heather L. Armstrong, Editor

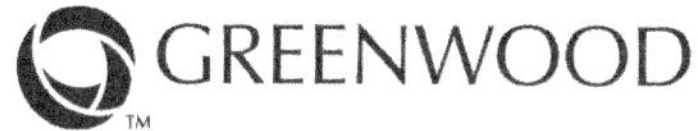

An Imprint of ABC-CLIO, LLC
Santa Barbara, California • Denver, Colorado

Library of Congress Cataloging-in-Publication Data

Names: Armstrong, Heather L., editor.
Title: Encyclopedia of sex and sexuality : understanding biology, psychology, and culture / Heather L. Armstrong, editor.
Description: Santa Barbara, California : Greenwood, [2021] | Includes bibliographical references and index. |
Identifiers: LCCN 2020024424 (print) | LCCN 2020024425 (ebook) | ISBN 9781440847684 (v. 1 ; hardcover ; alk. paper) | ISBN 9781440847691 (v. 2 ; hardcover ; alk. paper) | ISBN 9781610698740 (set ; hardcover ; alk. paper) | ISBN 9781610698757 (ebook)
Subjects: LCSH: Sex—Encyclopedias. | Sex (Biology)—Encyclopedias. | Sex (Psychology)—Encyclopedias.
Classification: LCC HQ21 .E647 2021 (print) | LCC HQ21 (ebook) | DDC 306.703—dc23
LC record available at https://lccn.loc.gov/2020024424
LC ebook record available at https://lccn.loc.gov/2020024425

ISBN: 978-1-61069-874-0 (set)
978-1-4408-4768-4 (vol. 1)
978-1-4408-4769-1 (vol. 2)
978-1-61069-875-7 (ebook)

25 24 23 22 21 1 2 3 4 5

This book is also available as an eBook.

Greenwood
An Imprint of ABC-CLIO, LLC

ABC-CLIO, LLC
147 Castilian Drive
Santa Barbara, California 93117
www.abc-clio.com

This book is printed on acid-free paper ∞

Manufactured in the United States of America

For the curious.

Contents

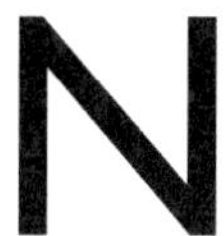

National Center for Transgender Equality

The National Center for Transgender Equality (NCTE) is a national organization dedicated to advocating for legal and social justice for transgender people. The NCTE mission is "By empowering transgender people and our allies to educate and influence policymakers and others, NCTE facilitates a strong and clear voice for transgender equality in our nation's capital and around the country" (National Center for Transgender Equality, 2019a).

The NCTE is a 501(c)(3) nonprofit organization founded in 2003 in Washington, D.C., by Mara Keisling, a native of Scranton, Pennsylvania. Keisling earned a bachelor of arts degree from Penn State University and studied American government at Harvard University as a graduate student. Prior to moving full time into transgender advocacy, she worked in public health marketing research and was an adjunct instructor in government at George Mason University and Marymount University.

In alignment with their mission, NCTE programs and projects address a very long list of issues that affect the transgender community, ranging from health, homelessness, military and veterans, immigration, voting rights, education, aging, and much more. In addition, NCTE works at all levels of government to improve related laws and legislation. The organization also educates the public about transgender issues, increases transgender people's awareness of their legal rights and the resources available to them, and encourages community engagement and civic participation. NCTE's first major achievement was leading the years-long effort to pass the Matthew Shepard and James Byrd Jr. Hate Crimes Prevention Act. Signed by President Barack Obama in 2009, it was the first federal law ever to explicitly protect transgender people. Also, the NCTE Privacy and Documentation program has significantly modernized national, state, and local policies related to identity documentation for transgender people, providing more people access to correctly updated drivers' licenses, birth certificates, and passports.

Of NCTE's many successes, however, the most impactful thus far may be the data collected from the national surveys NCTE has conducted. The 2011 National Transgender Discrimination Survey and the even larger 2015 U.S. Transgender Survey are the largest surveys ever specifically focused on the lives and experiences of transgender and nonbinary people (6,400 and 28,000, respectively). The results of these studies have helped policy makers and others to quantify and thus comprehend the epidemic of violence and discrimination transgender and nonbinary people experience.

In 2017, following the election of Donald Trump, the NCTE leadership launched a separate 501(c)(4) organization, the National Center for Transgender Equality

Action Fund. The action fund works more directly in the political process by mobilizing voters and engaging in electoral work supporting progressive, trans-inclusive candidates as well as transgender candidates running for office. The first three candidates endorsed by the NCTE Action Fund all won their races: Phillip Cunningham and Andrea Jenkins (Minneapolis City Council) and Danica Roem (Virginia House of Delegates).

As of 2018, NCTE had an annual budget of just over $2 million and more than twenty staff, fellows, and interns, with Keisling continuing to serve as founding executive director. Attorney Lisa Mottet, a close friend of the organization since its beginning, joined the staff as deputy executive director in 2013.

C. Michael Woodward

See also: Gender Expression; Gender Identity; National Transgender Advocacy Coalition (NTAC); Nonbinary Gender Identities; Shepard, Matthew; Transgender; Transsexual.

Further Reading

DiGuglielmo, J. (2011, November 17). Queery: Mara Keisling. Retrieved from http://www.washingtonblade.com/2011/11/17/queery-mara-keisling/

National Center for Transgender Equality. (2013, May 13). NCTE welcomes Lisa Mottet as deputy executive director. Retrieved from https://transequality.org/press/releases/ncte-welcomes-lisa-mottet-deputy-executive-director

National Center for Transgender Equality. (2018, April). Annual report 2017: Forward together. Retrieved from https://transequality.org/sites/default/files/docs/resources/annual report 2017 final.pdf

National Center for Transgender Equality. (2019a). National Center for Transgender Equality. Retrieved from https://transequality.org/

National Center for Transgender Equality. (2019b). National Transgender Discrimination Survey. Retrieved from https://transequality.org/issues/national-transgender-discrimination-survey

National Health and Social Life Survey

The National Health and Social Life Survey (NHSLS) was conducted in 1992 by the National Opinion Research Center at the University of Chicago. The study surveyed 3,432 women and men between the ages of eighteen and fifty-nine years who were living in the United States. It was designed to obtain information on a broad range of sexual activities and the social factors that might influence these behaviors. It separates itself from previous research in the field of sexuality in that it was one of the first large-scale studies conducted that used sound methodological research practices. It was hailed as "the most comprehensive representative survey to date of sexual behavior in the United States general population." The data were gathered utilizing both face-to-face interviews that lasted approximately ninety minutes as well as self-administered questionnaires.

The process of conducting the survey began in 1987, in part to try and gather more information about people's behaviors in response to the HIV epidemic. At that time, there was a lack of current information about people's sexual behaviors and their engagement in sexual practices that could spread HIV and other sexually transmitted infections (STIs). The funding for the original research project was supposed to be provided by the National Institutes of Health (NIH). However, due to some politicians' concerns that the government should not be supporting sex research, a bill was passed that included an amendment that prevented the NIH from funding the original study. Due to the lack of funding from government agencies, the survey had to be scaled down from its original intended size of over 10,000 participants to less than half that.

Findings from the NHSLS showed that those who were younger reported having more sexual partners than those of the older generations. While the age of engaging in first intercourse was lower in the younger respondents, they were also waiting longer to get married. The increase in sexual partners may therefore have been due to a longer time period between initiating sexual activity and getting married. The survey also found that the rate of cheating on a spouse was low, with less than 20 percent of women and 15–35 percent of men reporting being unfaithful while married.

The study also found that there were some behavior changes as a result of the HIV epidemic. Those who were considered most at risk of contracting HIV, the ones with multiple partners, were more likely to report that they had been tested for HIV and had changed their behaviors. These changes included using condoms more frequently, limiting their number of sexual partners, and being more aware of who their sexual partners were.

Since the NHSLS was conducted, it has not become substantially easier for researchers to receive government funding to investigate sexuality-related issues, despite the fact there is a public health concern regarding sexual behaviors and STIs. In 1989, one in twenty people between the ages of eighteen and twenty-four reported having had an STI in the last twelve months. Currently, the estimate is that half of all new STIs in the United States are in adolescents and young adults between the ages of fifteen and twenty-four.

Much has changed in the twenty-six years since the study was conducted. The NHSLS found that the majority of people had met their spouses and sexual partners through their social networks. The study was conducted before the internet, and researchers today are still trying to understand the impact that online dating and dating apps may have on people's sexual behaviors.

Susan Milstein

See also: Sexology; Sexuality across the Life Span; Sexually Transmitted Infections (STIs).

Further Reading

Laumann, E. O., Gagnon, J. H., Michael, R. T., & Michaels, S. (1992). National Health and Social Life Survey. Ann Arbor, MI: Inter-university Consortium for Political and Social Research [distributor].

Michael, R. T., Gagnon, J. H., Laumann, E. O., & Kolata, G. (1994). *Sex in America: A definitive survey*. Boston: Little, Brown and Company.

Michael, R. T., Isaacs, S., & Knickman, J. (1997). The National Health and Social Life Survey: Public health findings and their implications. In S. L. Isaacs & J. R. Knickman (Eds.), *To improve health and health care* (232–250). San Francisco: Jossey-Bass.

Miller, P. (1995). A review: They said it couldn't be done: The National Health and Social Life Survey. *The Public Opinion Quarterly, 59*(3), 404–419.

Satterwhite, C. L., Torrone, E., Meites, E., Dunne, E. F., Mahajan, R., Ocfemia, M. C. B., & Weinstock, H. (2013). Sexually transmitted infections among US women and men: Prevalence and incidence estimates, 2008. *Sexually Transmitted Diseases, 40*(3), 187–193.

Sociometrics. (2017). *National Health and Life Survey, 1992.* Retrieved from https://www.socio.com/products/aids-1213

National LGBTQ Task Force

The National Lesbian, Gay, Bisexual, Transgender, and Queer Task Force (National LGBTQ Task Force or the Task Force) was formed in 1973 and is the oldest still-active LGBTQ advocacy organization in the United States. When it started in 1973, it was known as the National Gay Task Force, which later changed to the National Gay and Lesbian Task Force, and most recently, in 2014, was renamed the National LGBTQ Task Force. These name changes were enacted in order to be more inclusive of a diversifying community that includes many different sexual orientations and gender identities.

The Task Force's official mission is to advance full freedom, justice, and equality for LGBTQ people. The vision and goal of the Task Force is to come together in building and strengthening grassroots movements, harnessing the power of the LGBTQ community. This is accomplished in a variety of ways, including providing training for activists and both state and local organizations working against anti-LGBTQ and for pro-LGBTQ legislations and referenda, helping to build capacity for creating social movements in the LGBTQ community. The Task Force also operates The Policy Institute, a progressive think tank offering policy analysis and doing research to further a pro-LGBTQ movement and to counter legislative and media attacks against LGBTQ individuals and communities.

Historically, the Task Force has been involved in many political issues tied to the LGBTQ community. From its inception in the 1970s, the Task Force has engaged regularly with women's and feminist movements, ensuring representation of lesbian women at the National Organization for Women's national conference and successfully getting an endorsement of gay and lesbian rights from the International Women's Year's conference in 1977. In the 1980s, the Task Force received some of the first federal funding dollars in order to offer community-based AIDS education and was very vocal on policies regarding national blood testing and the Federal Drug Administration's approval of a test for antibodies. The Task Force's work on monitoring how gay men and lesbian women were portrayed in the media and other venues of entertainment eventually led to the creation of the Gay Media Task Force, an organization that worked with television stations to improve the portrayal of gay men and lesbian women in their programming. A further political commitment of the Task Force is engaging with civil rights, including working against antisodomy laws, religious freedom laws that would legalize discrimination based on sexual orientation and gender identity, and now using a more intersectional lens to support issues of immigration and racism within and against the LGBTQ community.

Another large component of the Task Force is the creation and ongoing implementation of the national Creating Change Conference on a yearly basis. This conference is the largest gathering in the United States of LGBTQ organizers, leaders, and activists and is held in a different city each year in order to offer locations around the country. Creating Change 2019 was held in Detroit, Michigan, and provided attendees the opportunity to attend workshops about a variety of issues affecting the LGBTQ community, including immigration, sexuality, religion, disability, racial and ethnic identities, parenting, education, counseling/therapy, grassroots movements, activism, and more.

Shanna K. Kattari

See also: Acquired Immunodeficiency Syndrome (AIDS); GenderPAC; GLAAD; LGBTQ+; National Organization for Women (NOW); Sodomy Laws.

Further Reading

Creating Change Conference. (2019). Home page. Retrieved from http://www.creatingchange.org/

National Gay and Lesbian Task Force Records, 1973–2017. (n.d.). Retrieved from http://rmc.library.cornell.edu/EAD/htmldocs/RMM07301.html

National LGBTQ Task Force. (2019). About: Mission and history. Retrieved from http://www.thetaskforce.org/about/mission-history.html

National Organization for Women (NOW)

The National Organization for Women (NOW) is the largest organization of feminist activists in the United States. Since its founding in 1966, NOW's goal has been to ensure gender equality for women of all classes and backgrounds. In its conception, NOW focused especially on securing women's economic equality through an amendment to the U.S. Constitution. Other principal causes include women's reproductive rights, opposing racism and heterosexism, and ending violence against women.

NOW is regarded as the nonpartisan, grassroots wing of the women's rights movement. The organization communicates through collective action; they organize marches, rallies, nonviolent civil protests, public forums, and petitions. NOW's actions have established the organization as a major feminist force in the political arena. Their movements have promoted women into political positions; increased the academic and professional opportunities for women; and influenced tougher laws against domestic violence, sexual harassment, and racial discrimination.

The Civil Rights Act of 1964 was presented to Congress as a means to end discrimination on the basis of sex, race, nationality, and religion. Activists lobbied extensively for the inclusion of an amendment to outlaw sex discrimination in employment decisions. After much disagreement, this demand was realized through Title VII, a prohibition of discrimination in the workplace. To enforce and oversee national adherence to Title VII, the Equal Employment Opportunity

Commission (EEOC) was created. Despite their responsibilities to protect minorities in the workforce, the EEOC did not take a stance against gender-segregated job advertising. A few weeks after the legislation was passed, Yale law professor Dr. Pauli Murray publicly denounced the EEOC for its refusal to oppose sexist hiring practices. This caught the attention of author Betty Friedan, who immediately contacted Dr. Murray to discuss alternative strategies with other frustrated women's rights activists. More than twenty women assembled in Friedan's hotel room in solidarity. Friedan wrote the acronym NOW on a napkin, and out of the group's determination to create lasting institutional change, a new organization emerged.

In August 1967, NOW activists picketed wearing vintage clothing to make a statement against the *New York Times*' old-fashioned policies of gender-segregated advertising. Their demonstrations helped shift national advertising practices. Later that year, NOW drafted the "Bill of Rights for Women." This document pushed for the passage of the Equal Rights Amendment, the repeal of laws preventing abortion, and for the availability of publicly funded child care. NOW was the first national organization to support the decriminalization of abortion.

NOW made strides in the academic arena as well. In 1969, NOW chapters across the country laid the foundation for the first recognized women's studies courses in Michigan, California, and at Princeton. In 1973, NOW activists created the national march and vigil called Take Back the Night. This event was a protest of violence against women, with a highlight on sexual assault. Take Back the Night continues as an annual event across many countries, communities, and campuses.

On August 26, 1973, NOW's proposal for the memorialization of the passage of the suffrage amendment was accepted by Congress and the president, and the anniversary of the end of the suffrage movement became recognized as Women's Equality Day.

NOW has been criticized by various groups for their feminist and political views. NOW is often in opposition with fathers' rights groups and those who are against feminism as a movement, who experience the demand that women be treated equitably to be at their expense. NOW has also received the criticism that the organization focuses more on pursuing liberal politics rather than truly advocating for women's rights. Many political activists feel that NOW's scope is too narrow in focusing on American women and not using their power and privilege to support women internationally. Antiabortion activists take issue with NOW's discrediting of women who are not in support of abortion and consider the organization exclusionary. Also to the point of exclusion, in NOW's conception, several openly lesbian members of standing were expelled from the organization to make a point to the public that they were more than a gay rights group. There was significant pushback from over 400 feminists challenging NOW for heterosexism. After a public opposition at the 1970 Congress to Unite Women, NOW changed its stance on lesbian visibility, and in 1973 the NOW Task Force on Sexuality and Lesbianism was established. However, many feminists are still put off by the organization for the initial offense.

Shadeen Francis

See also: Abortion Legislation; Feminist Theory; Gender; Heterosexism; Sexual Assault; Sexual Rights.

Further Reading

National Archives and Records Administration. (1964). The civil rights act of 1964 and the Equal Employment Opportunity Commission. National Archives Identifier: 299891. Retrieved from https://www.archives.gov/education/lessons/civil-rights-act/

National Organization for Women. (1966). The National Organization for Women's 1966 statement of purpose. Retrieved from http://now.org/about/history/statement-of-purpose/

United States Equal Employment Opportunity Commission. (1964). Title VII of the civil rights act of 1964. Retrieved from https://www.eeoc.gov/laws/statutes/titlevii.cfm

National Transgender Advocacy Coalition (NTAC)

The National Transgender Advocacy Coalition (NTAC) was a 501(c)(4) civil rights organization "working to establish and maintain the right of all transgender, intersex, and gender-variant people to live and work without fear of violence or discrimination."

NTAC was the result of a dinner conversation on February 24, 1999, at La Panetteria restaurant in Bethesda, Maryland, during the GenderPAC Lobby Days event in Washington, D.C. The diners were all experienced community organizers and allies, mostly volunteers, from around the country who were engaged in GenderPAC's educational training and congressional lobbying event to build a national community voice, educate members of Congress about transgender people, and increase both national and municipal legislation protecting gender identity and expression. In the late 1990s, GenderPAC made a dramatic shift in its mission and strategy, moving away from advocacy specifically on behalf of transgender and gender-diverse people and toward a broader effort to decrease gender-based bias in society. Many leaders in the trans community disagreed with the political strategy and felt abandoned by the only visible national advocacy organization dedicated to their issues. Those at the dinner felt that a national voice for the community was still very much needed and agreed to work together toward this effort.

NTAC's primary function became educating transgender people about the political process and protocol and about how to have strategic conversations with representatives and their aides about the issues as a private citizen or constituent. The Lobby Days event provided community members and allies a day of training, preparation, and practice, then a full day on Capitol Hill meeting with said officials in both houses of Congress. The goal was not only to get transgender issues on the table nationally but also to empower those participating to continue lobbying and educating at the local level.

The seven founders from the dinner included Dawn Wilson (Lexington, Kentucky), Anne Casebeer (Louisville, Kentucky), Vanessa Edwards Foster (Houston, Texas), Jessica Redman (Houston, Texas), Sarah Fox (Columbus, Ohio), Cathy Platine (Delaware, Ohio), and award-winning journalist Monica Roberts (Houston,

Texas). Additional members joining the board shortly after its founding included Yosenio Lewis (first board president), Christine Stinson (first board treasurer), Transgender American Veterans Association (TAVA) cofounders Angela Brightfeather Sheedy and Monica Helms (who also designed the now-iconic transgender flag), and eighteen other activists from around the country.

NTAC was active from 1999 to 2009. In that time, it produced National Lobby Days five times in Washington, each time documenting in detail the conversations had by each citizen lobbyist. This provided a record of how legislators' knowledge and support of transgender issues changed over the years. The 2004 Lobby Days was captured by director Timothy Watts in the documentary film *Citizen Lobbyist.*

In addition to Lobby Days, NTAC helped expand the observation of the Transgender Day of Remembrance, a vigil honoring the lives of transgender people lost to violence each year, to cities worldwide. NTAC was also among the organizations that protested in Washington in 2007 after gender identity protections were again excluded from the Employment Nondiscrimination Act that was proposed (but never passed) by Congress.

C. Michael Woodward

See also: Gender Expression; Gender Identity; GenderPAC; National Center for Transgender Equality; Transgender; Transsexual.

Further Reading

GLAAD. (2019). Transgender resources. Retrieved from www.glaad.org/transgender/resources

Transgender Day of Remembrance. (2019). Retrieved from tdor.tgeu.org

Nocturnal Emissions

A nocturnal emission (also known as a wet dream) is the experience of ejaculation or orgasm during sleep for people assigned male at birth. This most often occurs during puberty when the testicles begin producing sperm, usually between the ages of twelve and fourteen years. Occasionally, there may be an overproduction of sperm, and if this happens, the body may naturally expel the sperm during sleep in the form of ejaculation. A sexual dream may or may not occur during the nocturnal emission. Since adolescents often initiate masturbation (resulting in ejaculation) around the time of puberty, a buildup of semen may not occur at all. Consequently, not all people who are assigned male at birth will experience a nocturnal emission, and it is estimated that only about half do. Once masturbation (or ejaculation due to other causes, such as sexual activity) is initiated, nocturnal emissions typically stop. Many girls and women (assigned female at birth) also experience orgasm during sleep, which is a similar yet distinct experience known as somnus orgasm.

It is possible, but rather rare, for adult males to experience ejaculation during sleep. This is likely because most adult males typically release semen through other means, such as masturbation or sexual activity. Some adults who have penises may experience a nocturnal emission after very long periods of abstaining from ejaculation or orgasm, though this may take months or even several years of abstinence. Other folks may still experience an occasional nocturnal emission for no apparent reason, though this is uncommon.

Experiencing ejaculation and orgasm during sleep is a normal and healthy event. It cannot be controlled, and it is not caused by any underlying medical, social, or psychological condition or behavior. Even though nocturnal emissions are perfectly normal, many people are unaware that they exist, and some cultures view the experience as very negative and harmful. One study found that boys who were not well informed about the experience of nocturnal emissions reported feeling frightened upon first ejaculating during sleep, comparable to many people's experiences of menarche. This highlights the importance of sexual health education both in schools and within the home so that young people are informed that nocturnal emissions are common and normal.

In some cultures, semen is often thought to be a very powerful and vital bodily fluid that contains supernatural qualities and ensures a man's health and longevity. Dhat syndrome is the belief held by some men in certain Indian cultures that nocturnal emissions are a serious threat to a man's health. This can result in a severe preoccupation due to fear of losing what is considered to be an extremely important bodily fluid necessary for mental, spiritual, and physical well-being. Receiving accurate sexual health education is reportedly the most effective treatment for Dhat syndrome, as it dispels some of the misconceptions surrounding nocturnal emissions and semen loss.

Lyndsay Mercier

See also: Ejaculation; Orgasm; Puberty; Semen; Sex Education; Somnus Orgasm.

Further Reading

Gaddis, A., & Brooks-Gunn, J. (1985). The male experience of pubertal change. *Journal of Youth and Adolescence, 14*, 61–69.

Harris, R. H. (2018). *It's perfectly normal: Changing bodies, growing up, sex, and sexual health.* Somerville, MA: Candlewick Press.

Malhotra, H. K., & Wig, N. N. (1975). Dhat syndrome: A culture-bound sex neurosis of the Orient. *Archives of Sexual Behavior, 4*(5), 519–528.

Nonbinary Gender Identities

Within Western societies, gender is often viewed as a binary with male on one side and female on the other (gender binary), but gender is more complex. As a social construct, gender has been understood to include other variations within other cultures and during other time periods. Many cultures traditionally referred to those who identified outside the gender binary as a third gender, but these individuals are commonly referred to as nonbinary within Western society. Nonbinary is an umbrella term to represent individuals who do not identify as exclusively female or male, including varying degrees of female and male, neither female nor male, another gender, or a combination of genders. The nonbinary umbrella includes genderqueer, genderfluid, bigender, trigender, among others as well as nonbinary as a gender, sometimes abbreviated as NB or enby.

Three cultural examples of nonbinary identities include the hijra of India, two-spirit people of First Nation tribal societies, and the māhū of Hawaii. Perhaps the most known is the hijra, who are individuals assigned male at birth but are recognized as neither male nor female and perform important cultural ceremonies. Despite legal recognition as a third gender and unique role in Indian society, the hijra continue to be seen as outcasts. Two-spirit people are individuals who embody both masculine and feminine spirits and have been revered since the seventeenth century. In First Nation societies, gender is not synonymous with biological sex but rather associated with roles within the society (e.g., caregiving, hunting). Finally, the māhū are free to equally express masculinity and femininity, similar to the Hawaiian god or goddess Laka, and they are respected for maintaining customs. Māhūs almost disappeared with Western colonization until a Hawaiian cultural renaissance in the 1970s. Similar to hijra, māhūs have been recognized as a third gender but face discrimination, with the name māhū sometimes used as a derogatory term. While facing discrimination, these culturally diverse identities have also been revered and admired—the hijra as sacred, two-spirit as healers, and the māhū as historical teachers.

Nonbinary individuals are inherently gender nonconforming as their gender by definition does not align with dominant gender norms. Gender nonconformity can increase the risk of experiencing microaggressions, particularly being misgendered (identifying someone by the wrong gender through incorrect pronouns). Stigmatizing experiences for nonbinary individuals can include being called by a former (often gendered) name rather than a chosen name; not seeing their gender represented on educational, medical, and legal forms; being tokenized (e.g., expected to be a representative their gender), and being asked to explain their gender.

Nonbinary gender expression varies and can include temporary, semipermanent, and permanent forms. Based on social norms, the expression of masculinity and femininity can be presented through hairstyles, body hair (removal or growth), and accessories. In addition, numerous prosthetics have been created, including breast forms, packers, and stand-to-pee devices. Youth may pursue puberty blockers to postpone puberty while postpubertal young adults and adults may use hormone replacement therapy. Permanent changes include top surgery (breast augmentation or removal of chest tissue) and gender affirmation surgery (genital surgery). Nonphysical expressions of gender include a chosen name and pronouns. They or them pronouns are the most often used gender-neutral pronouns by nonbinary individuals, although over one hundred gender pronouns have been proposed since the mid-nineteenth century. Correct use of pronouns has been found to be as important as the use of the correct name. Some nonbinary individuals describe political activism to be an expression of their gender identity and can include roles as a representative, a role model, and an educator.

A nonbinary gender identity development model was created to increase understanding of the unique experiences of nonbinary individuals. The eight stages of this model are (1) early freedom, (2) gender identity confusion, (3) language acquisition, (4) reconciling repression, (5) gender experimentation, (6) envisioning an ideal self, (7) disclosing gender identity, and (8) gender identity integration. In early freedom, gender is explored at a young age with few restrictions (e.g., tomboys).

Gender identity confusion follows due to a lack of language to describe nonbinary genders as well as enforcement of gender norms. Language acquisition is a pivotal point in nonbinary gender identity development, which is noteworthy as such language has only emerged in the last decade within Western culture. Along with affirmation from language comes the potential for building gender-based communities. For those who attempt to conform to gender norms, the model includes a stage for overcoming repression of a nonbinary gender identity and working toward acceptance that includes rejecting the gender binary (understanding of gender as exclusively male or female). During gender experimentation, gender is tried on in safe spaces to discover and self-identify one's gender and gender expression. The ability to envision an ideal self is associated with a greater comfort with gender identity and is challenged by the diversity of genders within the nonbinary umbrella and a lack of modeling of nonbinary identities in mainstream media. The decision to disclose nonbinary gender identities is dependent on the relationship to others and the environment with relevance, trust, and safety of concern. Finally, identity integration among nonbinary individuals is an acceptance of a nonbinary gender identity internally as well as an understanding of the strengths and limitations of the external environment.

As awareness and representation of nonbinary identities increases, a growing number of people are openly identifying as nonbinary, particularly among youth. Over a quarter of youth surveyed in California described their gender expression as nonconforming. Increasing numbers in gender diversity have been attributed to expanding language, labels, and information to describe gender diversity, and online support communities, as well as greater representation in media and growing acceptance. The multitude of gender identity options in social media reflects the expansion and growing acceptance of gender identity labels. In 2017, the first nonbinary character on television aired with Dillon on *Billions*, played by Asia Kate Dillon, who also identifies as nonbinary. In the same year, nonbinary identities received national news coverage with cover stories in *National Geographic* and *Time* magazine. Representation has increased with nonbinary role models and activists such as Alok Vaid-Menon, iO Tillet Wright, and Ruby Rose, who advocate for awareness of nonbinary experiences. Collectively, nonbinary activism has been described as a movement focused on the development of supportive communities, representation through documentation and research, and education to increase cultural awareness in media, social services, health care, and policies that affect nonbinary individuals.

M. Killian Kinney

See also: Agender; Bigender; Binary Gender System; Childhood Gender Nonconformity; Fluidity, Gender; Gender; Gender Expression; Gender Identity; Gender Identity Development; Genderqueer; Questioning; Two-Spirit.

Further Reading

Aulette, J. R., & Wittner, J. (2015). *Gendered worlds* (3rd ed.). New York: Oxford University Press.

Barker, M.-J. (2014, February 15). 57 genders (and none for me)? Reflections on the new Facebook gender categories. *Rewriting the rules.* Retrieved from https://www.rewriting-the-rules.com/gender/57-genders-and-none-for-me-reflections-on-the-new-facebook-gender-categories/

Baron, D. (2015, September 14). *Some notes on singular they* [web blog post]. Retrieved from https://blogs.illinois.edu/view/25/247504

Bergman, S. B., & Barker, M.-J. (2017). Non-binary activism. In C. Richards, W. P. Bouman, & M. J. Barker (Eds.), *Genderqueer and non-binary genders* (31–51). London: Palgrave Macmillan.

Brown, M. E., & Burill, D. (2018). *Challenging genders: Non-binary experiences of those assigned female at birth.* Miami, FL: Boundless Endeavors.

Flores, A. R., Herman, J. L., Gates, G. J., & Brown, T. N. (2016, June). *How many adults identify as transgender in the United States.* Los Angeles: The Williams Institute.

Fosco, M. (2015, October 24). Inequality within India's third gender community. *Seeker Global Issue.* Retrieved from http://www.seeker.com/inequality-within-indias-third-gender-community-1501537275.html?utm_source=facebook&utm_medium=seekersocial&utm_campaign=owned

Frohard-Dourlent, H., Dobson, S., Clark, B. A., Doull, M., & Saewyc, E. M. (2017). "I would have preferred more options": Accounting for non-binary youth in health research. *Nursing Inquiry, 24*(1), 1–9.

Kinney, M. K. (2018a). *Carving your own path: A nonbinary gender identity development model.* Manuscript in preparation.

Kinney, M. K. (2018b). *Carving your own path: Exploring non-binary identities.* Manuscript in preparation.

Lauria, E. (2017). Gender fluidity in Hawaiian culture. *The Gay & Lesbian Review Worldwide, 24*(1), 31–32.

McLemore, K. A. (2015). Experiences with misgendering: Identity misclassification of transgender spectrum individuals. *Self and Identity, 14*(1), 51–74.

McNabb, C. (2018). *Nonbinary gender identities: History, culture, resources.* Lanham, MD: Rowman & Littlefield.

Poteat, V. P., Sinclair, K. O., DiGiovanni, C. D., Koenig, B. W., & Russell, S. T. (2013). Gay-straight alliances are associated with student health: A multischool comparison of LGBTQ and heterosexual youth. *Journal of Research on Adolescence, 23*(2), 319–330.

Rankin, S., & Beemyn, G. (2012). Beyond a binary: The lives of gender-nonconforming youth. *About Campus, 17*(4), 2–10.

Richards, C., Bouman, W. P., & Barker, M. J. (Eds.). (2017). *Genderqueer and non-binary genders.* London: Palgrave Macmillan.

Wilson, B. D. M., Choi, S. K., Herman, J. L., Becker, R., & Conron, K. J. (2017). *Characteristics and mental health of gender nonconforming adolescents in California: Findings from the 2015–2016 California health interview survey.* Los Angeles: The Williams Institute and UCLA Center for Health Policy Research.

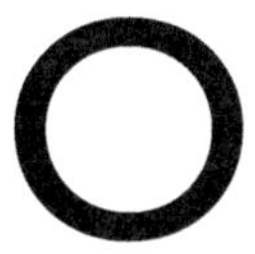

Obstetrics and Gynecology

Obstetrics and gynecology is the field of medicine concerned with pregnancy, childbirth, and the female reproductive organs. The term "obstetrics" refers to pregnancy, childbirth, and neonatal care (care of the baby during the first four to six weeks of life). "Gynecology" refers to the reproductive organs, including the ovaries, fallopian tubes, uterus, cervix, and vagina. Physicians who specialize in obstetrics are called obstetricians; those who specialize in gynecology are called gynecologists. However, many physicians specialize in both fields and are commonly referred to as OB/GYNs.

With respect to obstetrics, an OB/GYN cares for the health of both the pregnant person and the fetus throughout pregnancy. Responsibilities before delivery include providing advice to the mother on how to recognize signs of labor and perhaps deciding whether and when to induce labor. Then the OB/GYN may play a major medical role in the safe and healthy delivery of the baby. During delivery, the OB/GYN may help decide on the type of pain relief to provide while preserving the ability to use muscle movement for giving birth. The OB/GYN may also need to decide whether a vaginal birth or cesarean section (incisions made in abdomen and uterus for deliveries that would otherwise be problematic) is preferable or necessary. Furthermore, any complications that occur during delivery must be handled by the OB/GYN. In uncomplicated and unproblematic pregnancies, the pregnant person may choose not to use the services of an OB/GYN and may instead use a midwife.

In the weeks following delivery, the OB/GYN may provide postpartum care, including physical examinations to ensure that recovery is progressing appropriately from the physically demanding processes of pregnancy and childbirth. Care may involve the management of both physical problems (such as infections and blood clots) and psychological problems (such as postpartum depression). During this period, the OB/GYN also monitors the health of the newborn, addressing any problems that may develop.

Outside of their pregnancy and childbirth duties, OB/GYNs are involved in the treatment of female reproductive organ problems. Some of these gynecological problems are congenital, meaning that the individual was born with the conditions. Examples of congenital gynecological conditions include malformations of the vaginal tissues, cervix, and uterus. Other gynecological problems are caused by infections, such as vulvitis (inflammation of the folds of skin outside the vagina), vaginitis (inflammation of the vagina), cervicitis (inflammation of the cervix, often caused by sexually transmitted infections), pelvic inflammatory disease (infection of female reproductive organs, also often caused by sexually transmitted infections), and urinary tract infections.

Still other gynecological problems are the result of imbalances in hormone levels, resulting in such problems as menstrual irregularities, abnormal vaginal bleeding, infertility, and loss of sex drive.

Tumors of the female reproductive organs make up a substantial portion of conditions treated by OB/GYNs. In some cases, the tumors are benign (noncancerous); in other cases, the tumors are malignant (cancerous).

Some people also report to OB/GYNs with injuries to their reproductive organs as a result of trauma, such as that sustained in rape.

Yet another problem treated by OB/GYNs is endometriosis, a painful condition in which uterine tissue grows outside the uterus, such as on the ovaries or elsewhere in the pelvic region. This condition can have any of several causes, such as abnormal menstruation, immune system disorders, and surgical scars.

Besides handling health conditions involving the female reproductive organs, many OB/GYNs also treat disorders of the breasts, such as cancerous and benign tumors.

OB/GYNs can use many different techniques to diagnose their patients' medical problems. In addition to physical examinations and blood tests, diagnostic techniques include the following:

- Amniocentesis: examination of the amniotic fluid surrounding the fetus for signs of chromosomal abnormalities and birth defects
- Ultrasonography: an imaging technology for making prenatal diagnosis of birth defects, for general monitoring of the fetus's health, and for gynecological conditions
- Routine examinations of the vagina and cervix and their secretions to detect signs of cancer
- Pap smear: examination of cervical cells for signs of cancer
- Other biopsies of the reproductive organs to check for cancer
- Mammograms (X-rays of the breast) to check for cancer or other abnormalities
- Genetic tests to evaluate the risks of breast and ovarian cancer and other hereditary conditions

There is a vast variety of treatment methods provided by OB/GYNs, depending on the patient's particular needs.

Medications prescribed by OB/GYNs include contraceptive pills and other hormone-based drugs, antibiotics to fight infections, and drugs to kill cancer cells. Radiation therapy is also provided to fight cancer.

Some common obstetrical surgical procedures are cesarean section, episiotomy (incisions to enlarge the vaginal opening to make delivery easier), and abortion. Common gynecological surgical procedures include hysterectomy (removal of the uterus), repair of damage sustained as a result of childbirth or traumatic injuries, removal of benign or malignant tumors, and various other procedures involving the urinary and genital tracts.

OB/GYNs can provide all methods of birth control in addition to oral contraceptives, ranging from implanted devices (such as intrauterine devices) to permanent sterilization (tubal ligation). They can also provide any infertility treatment, such as in vitro fertilization and embryo implantation.

OB/GYNs sometimes have to address minor psychiatric problems that are associated with childbirth and other female reproductive issues. For patients struggling with severe psychiatric problems, referrals to psychiatrists or clinical psychologists are made.

To become an OB/GYN, a student must first earn an undergraduate degree, preferably one focusing on science and mathematics. They then apply to a medical school and upon passing the admission test attend the school for four years of basic medical education, laboratory work, and clinical rotations in hospitals and clinics under the supervision of a physician. Following graduation from medical school, the student undergoes an additional four years of residency training in reproductive and primary health care for women.

After this education and training, the individual must pass an examination to become licensed and legally able to practice. In the United States, the examination, which evaluates both knowledge and judgment, is called the United States Medical Licensing Examination (for MDs, or allopathic physicians) or the Comprehensive Osteopathic Medical Licensing Examination (for DOs, or osteopathic physicians).

Many OB/GYNs pursue subspecialties for which special certification is required. These subspecialties include maternal-fetal medicine (focusing on high-risk pregnancies), reproductive endocrinology (focusing on hormone and infertility issues), gynecologic oncology (dealing with cancer), urogynecology and reconstructive pelvic surgery (dealing with such abnormalities as pelvic organ prolapse and urinary tract disorders), and pediatric and adolescent gynecology (focusing on gynecological care for female children and teenagers).

To obtain these subspecialty certifications, OB/GYNs undergo about three years of fellowship training, and they must pass examinations administered by specialty boards, either the American Board of Obstetrics and Gynecology (for MDs) or the American Osteopathic Board of Obstetrics and Gynecology (for DOs). OB/GYNs must periodically renew their licenses and certifications to ensure that they remain up-to-date with medical advances.

OB/GYNs in the United States earned an average salary of approximately $212,500 in 2013. This profession is expected to see substantial job growth at least into the 2020s.

Before the dawn of the modern, scientific era of medicine in the early 1800s, women known as midwives were the main "professionals" who assisted during childbirth. Several medical advances shifted the responsibility of childbirth assistance from midwives to physicians and obstetricians. These advances included the development of delivery forceps, antiseptic delivery methods, anesthesia, and cesarean sections. However, midwives continue to practice today, and some women prefer their services to those of physicians.

The public acceptance of gynecological medical procedures was long held back by moral and religious objections to the examination of female genitalia. These public attitudes gradually changed as a result of some of the same scientific advances that furthered the practice of obstetrics—particularly the benefits of anesthesia and antiseptic methods of care.

During the mid- to late 1900s, there were many additional advances in obstetrics and gynecology. These included the widespread availability of effective birth control methods, increased knowledge regarding ways to prevent birth defects, technologies for monitoring the health of the baby in the womb (such as amniocentesis and ultrasonography), medicines for enhancing the health of newborns and mothers, and technologies for helping infertile couples achieve pregnancy (such as in vitro fertilization and embryo implantation).

A. J. Smuskiewicz

See also: Female Sexuality; Infertility; Pap Smear; Pregnancy; Sexual Disorders, Female.

Further Reading

American College of Obstetricians and Gynecologists. (2019). Home page. Retrieved from https://www.acog.org

American Journal of Obstetrics & Gynecology. (2019). Home page. Retrieved from http://www.ajog.org

Bowdler, N. C., & Elson, M. (2008). The gynecologic history and examination. *The global library of women's medicine.* Retrieved from http://www.glowm.com/section_view/heading/TheGynecologicHistoryandExamination/item/3

Oedipus Complex

The Oedipus complex is a concept in psychoanalytic theory, originally introduced by Sigmund Freud. It refers to a male child's unconscious sexual desire for his mother and fear and aggression toward his father. This psychodynamic conflict is usually resolved by the child identifying with his father and in adulthood seeking a sexual and romantic partner similar to his mother. Freud saw this as crucial for development of adult sexuality and personality (psychosexual development). Although originally formulated using material from men, Freud and later theorists have sought to apply this process to development in women as well.

Freud first described this concept in *Interpretation of Dreams*, and the name "Oedipus complex" was first used in *A Special Type of Choice of Object Made by Men*. In the former text, he describes how the idea arose from his own reactions and introspection from watching a performance of the play *Oedipus Rex* by Sophocles. The play is about the ancient Grecian myth of Oedipus, a man who fulfills an oracle's prophecy of killing his father and marrying his mother. Freud attributed the emotional impact of the play, which was very popular in his time, to a universal, repressed desire among men to slay their fathers and sexually possess their mothers. He noted the trope in other literary works, including Shakespeare's *Hamlet*. This is described as an example of a latent content in dreams and is of importance to dream interpretation during psychoanalysis. He further developed this dynamic and how it manifests in the development of male sexuality (as well as the ego) in the latter publication.

The Oedipus complex, like many of Freud's ideas, emphasized the role of libido. For Freud, libido meant an overarching energetic drive toward life, which includes sex but also other physical urges such as hunger. In his model, for an infant son, the most important focus of the libido at the start of life is the breast, and by extension, the mother (due to dependence on sustenance from breastfeeding). As a result of this libidinal drive, the son desires to become closer to the mother, the source of his life and survival. However, as he grows older, he becomes aware that he cannot be the sole possessor of his mother, as his father also has claim to her.

During the "phallic phase" of development (ages three to six years old), the son becomes more aware of his and others' bodies and begins to explore these bodies, and his libido shifts its focus to the penis. During this phase, he becomes aware that he cannot possess his mother through the use of his penis, as his mother sleeps with and has sex with his father. This leads to competition and jealousy directed at the father, and the child wishes to destroy the father. However, the developing ego, which operates based on the contingencies of reality, understands that he cannot directly aggress against the father, as the father is by far the more physically powerful of the two. This ambivalence results in significant distress and tension in the child, which is manifested as a fear of castration by his father (castration anxiety).

To resolve this tension, the child represses his desires for his mother and his aggression toward his father. Furthermore, the child identifies with (incorporates into his forming ego and superego) the traits and values of his father. This diminishes castration anxiety, as the child's similarity to his father protects him from the father's wrath. In this process, the child is able to individuate from the maternal care and identify with his same-sex parent. Eventually, this means growing up to be a man like his father, with the capacity to find a woman like his mother in order to gratify his adult libidinal urges.

This identification also means the child internalizes his father's adult sense of social morality. The child hence learns to obey societal laws and conventions as opposed to acting only through fear of punishment or anticipation of reward. If the child is unable to resolve this complex through identification with the father, it can lead to neurotic difficulties later in life. For example, maintaining a competitive stance with the father can lead to an adult man who is vain and aggressive. Freud also attributed some presentations of sexual promiscuity, paraphilic behaviors, and homosexuality to developmental difficulties in resolving the Oedipus complex.

Freud and later psychoanalytic authors have attempted to generalize the principles of the Oedipus complex to female psychosexual development as well. This includes the feminine Oedipus complex from Freud and the Electra complex from Carl Jung. However, these early models were not well developed, and understanding female sexuality appeared to have been a persistent area of difficulty for early psychoanalysts.

One recent model that seeks to elaborate on the feminine aspect of the Oedipus complex is the Persephone complex. This model takes its name from the ancient Grecian myth of Persephone, who oscillates between the shadowed underworld of her husband, Hades, and the sunny overworld of her mother, Demeter. The triangular conflict between child, mother, and father are seen as asymmetrical between boys and girls due to the biological role of the maternal care (e.g., breastfeeding) regardless of the sex of the child. Unlike for boys, competition between girls and their same-sex parent (mother) not only risks aggression from a more powerful adult but also the loss of life-giving maternal nurturance. Furthermore, girls must shift the focus of their libido to the father, someone who is relatively unfamiliar when compared to the mother. This results in ambivalence and conflicting loyalties to the mother and the father. To resolve this dynamic conflict, many girls often relinquish their sense of agency over their capacity both for sexuality and competitive aggression in order to protect their maternal relationship.

The Oedipus complex has remained controversial ever since its original publication. It has been criticized for being inapplicable to the experiences of women, pathologizing nonheterosexual (and noncisgender) sexuality, and for being exclusively focused on sexual motivations. Freud's approach emphasized repressed and transformed motivations and feelings as well as methods like introspection and free association. As such, the Oedipus complex, like many of Freud's models, has been difficult to operationalize and evaluate empirically outside of individual case studies. In contemporary research on the psychology of sexuality, other theories relating to child-parent relationships, such as attachment theory, have gained greater prominence. However, the Oedipus complex remains an important idea for psychoanalysis practitioners and theorists and in the study of literature and the humanities.

Silvain S. Dang

See also: Female Sexuality; Freud, Sigmund; Male Sexuality; Psychosexual Therapy.

Further Reading

Freud, S. (1953). The method of interpreting dreams: An analysis of a specimen dream. In J. Strachey (Ed. & Trans.), *The standard edition of the complete psychological works of Sigmund Freud* (Vol. 4, 96–121). London: Hogarth Press. (Original work published 1900).

Freud, S. (1953). A special type of choice of object made by men. (Contributions to the psychology of love I). In J. Strachey (Ed. & Trans.), *The standard edition of the complete psychological works of Sigmund Freud* (Vol. 9, 163–176). London: Hogarth Press. (Original work published 1910).

Holtzman, D., & Kulish, N. (2000). The feminization of the female oedipal complex, part I: A reconsideration of the significance of separation issues. *Journal of the American Psychoanalytic Association, 48*(4), 1413–1437.

Holtzman, D., & Kulish, N. (2002). The feminization of the female oedipal complex, part II: Aggression reconsidered. *Journal of the American Psychoanalytic Association, 51*(4), 1127–1151.

Scott, J. (2005). *Electra after Freud: Myth and culture.* Ithaca, NY: Cornell University Press.

Online Dating

Online dating is a method of arranging meetings between people—usually of a romantic or sexual nature—over the internet. This system of dating has exploded in popularity among a wide range of demographic groups during the twenty-first century, with tens of millions of people in the United States alone using online dating as a way to find partners. There are hundreds of dating websites catering to virtually every imaginable type of dating or sexual interest, including conventional two-person mixed-sex and same-sex relationships as well as less common relationships, interests, and lifestyles, such as swinging, polyamory, gender minority, dominatrixes/sadomasochism, and various fetishes. Some online dating sites specialize in particular age, ethnic, occupational, or religious groups, such as teenagers or middle-aged people, African Americans or Arabs, business people or farmers, and Christians or Jews.

Some online dating services are free to join; others charge fees to become a member. To participate, a user typically sets up a profile page by answering a series of questions about their appearance and interests and uploading personal photographs. The user also sets up search criteria for the type of partner they seek. When the user sees someone of interest, they can contact that individual through the online system and exchange messages, arranging an in-person meeting if so desired.

Dating apps for mobile phones facilitate the online dating process by making it easier and more convenient to browse through, find, and chat with potential partners who have similar interests and who live in the same area.

According to data compiled in 2015 by the highly respected Pew Research Center, approximately 15 percent of all adults (older than age eighteen) in the United States have arranged dates using online dating services, including dating websites (such as eHarmony, OkCupid, or Match.com), social networking websites (such as Facebook or Twitter), or mobile dating apps (such as Tinder). The most common adult age group that participates in online dating consists of individuals aged eighteen to twenty-four with about 27 percent reporting use; between 21–22 percent of adults age twenty-five to forty-four have arranged dates online. However, when the population size is narrowed to those adults who are "single and actively looking" for partners, this percentage increases to 38 percent (2013 data). Men use online dating slightly more often than women. Given that the popularity of online dating has continued to grow in recent years, it is expected that the actual percentage of users has now increased. In addition, 59 percent of adults surveyed in 2015 reported that online dating is a good way to meet people, indicating that attitudes are continuing to be more favorable toward online dating.

In 2013, Pew data revealed that about 23 percent of online daters either married or developed serious, long-term relationships with people they met online. Other data, however, suggest that romantic relationships originating online do not last as long as relationships between people who meet in traditional, offline ways.

Online dating carries some risk that the people being communicated with are not really what they seem to be or who they claim to be. This risk stems from the obvious fact that it is easier to lie about one's identity online than in person.

Many people are aware of the negative aspects of online dating—but that does not necessarily stop them from engaging in the practice. In 2013, 54 percent of online daters agreed that "someone else seriously misrepresented themselves in their profile." Furthermore, 28 percent of online daters said they were "contacted by someone through an online dating site or app in a way that made them feel harassed or uncomfortable." Among female online daters, 42 percent agreed with that statement, compared with 17 percent of males.

There have been numerous media reports of bad—even deadly—personal experiences when online daters meet in person. In one of the more extreme examples, a man who came to be known as the "Craigslist killer" was charged with robbing and killing a woman whom he met via an ad for "massage services" posted on the Craigslist website in 2009. He was also a suspect in at least two other robberies of women.

Critics of online dating argue that such dangers are inherently greater with online dating than traditional meetings, because online daters typically have never met before their initial romantic get-together. By contrast, traditional dates are more likely to be preceded by at least some informal, friendly get-togethers in which the individuals have a chance to get to know each other a bit before a formal date.

Some critics also blame online dating for making it too easy to participate in the "hookup culture," in which individuals meet purely for casual sex with no interest in pursuing a more meaningful relationship.

As such, if using online dating, it is important to be clear about one's expectations and desired outcomes and to ensure that steps are taken to ensure that any encounters occur safely.

A. J. Smuskiewicz

See also: Casual Sex; Dating; Dating, Cross-Cultural Comparison of; Hookup Culture; Online Sexual Activity; Sugar Daddies and Sugar Babies.

Further Reading

Smith, A., & Anderson, M. (2016, February). 5 facts about online dating. Retrieved from https://www.pewresearch.org/fact-tank/2016/02/29/5-facts-about-online-dating/

Smith, A., & Duggan, M. (2013, October). Online dating & relationships. Retrieved from http://www.pewinternet.org/2013/10/21/online-dating-relationships/

Wortham, J. (2013, February). Tinder, a dating app with a difference. *New York Times*. Retrieved from http://bits.blogs.nytimes.com/2013/02/26/tinder-a-dating-app-with-a-difference/?_r=0

Online Sexual Activity

Online sexual activity, also sometimes referred to as cybersex, refers to sexually arousing or satisfying internet-based computer activities. Online sexual activities include viewing or reading erotica; chatting with others about sex by using text or voice communication; sending or receiving sexually explicit emails; sharing sexual fantasies; participating in real-time cybersex in chatrooms, game spaces, or by using video streaming; contacting partners for real-time sexual encounters outside of cyberspace; chatting with others who share similar sexual interests; contacting others to pay for or to be paid for sex work; and seeking individuals to commit sex-related crimes. The scope and variety of online sexual activities continues to expand along with the scope of internet-facilitated activities.

Sexual subjects are the most searched-for topics on the internet. Early studies of cybersex in the 1990s suggested that up to one-third of internet users accessed some type of sexual content online, though many of these studies did not distinguish between sexual content designed to produce sexual arousal or gratification and those searches that were more educational. Technological advances and increased access to the internet, both at home and through smartphones, have made online sexual activities accessible to more individuals; researchers currently estimate that the percentage of the population who engages in online sexual activities is much higher than in earlier decades.

Research studies consistently indicate that the greatest levels of online sexual activity are reported by males, young people (adolescents and young adults), single individuals, and those living in urban areas. These data suggest that male college students may be among the highest users of online sexual activity and also the most at risk for problematic use. As a group, men are up to six times more likely to use internet pornography compared to women. Men report more interest in solitary online sexual activities such as viewing pornography and are more likely to pay for sexual images than women. Men are also more likely to report that their interest in online sexual activity decreases with age and is not problematic, and they are less likely to view online sexual activity as infidelity compared to women. In contrast, women report more personal problems with online sexual activity and are more likely to view it as cheating. Women also more often choose online sexual activities that involve a relational or romantic component, and some studies indicate that women are more likely than men to pursue real-life meetings with those they contact online. Interest in online sexual activity among women often remains stable across adulthood, with women ages thirty-five to forty-nine reporting more online sexual activity than similarly aged men.

Sexual orientation may also affect online sexual activity. Several studies suggest that gay men are more likely to engage in online sexual activity than heterosexual men, and cybersex and other online sexual activities may be part of the coming-out process for many individuals.

Studies suggest that online sexual activity may be related to loneliness, lack of a happy relationship, and a history of sexual problems. Cybersex has not been consistently or strongly related to sexual aggression, sensation seeking, dominance, hypermasculinity, or negative attitudes toward women. The relationship between online sexual activity and religion is a variable one; some highly religious people report lower levels of cybersex participation. However, several studies suggest that religious adults may engage in online sexual activities at rates similar to nonreligious peers.

Online sexual activities, including cybersex, present both benefits and drawbacks for users. These activities may provide sexual education and reproductive information, model safer sex behaviors, support relationship intimacy at a distance, and make sexual products more available to consumers. Distress related to cybersex and online sexual activities is often found in the forms of relationship isolation, impairment in sexual activities with a partner, perceptions of infidelity, superficial pseudo-intimacy with distant partners, exposure of youth to sexually explicit materials or sexual predators, impaired job performance and job loss, criminal convictions if illegal activities are pursued, financial strain from internet purchases, spiritual conflict, depression, anxiety, guilt, and an increased risk of sexually transmitted infections from partners met online.

Research suggests that the majority of cybersex users do not report problems related to cybersex activities. Some studies suggest that about 5 percent of cybersex users would be classified as having sexual compulsions, and another 10–20 percent may be at risk for other negative consequences from cybersex. However, no single cybersex behavior accurately predicts problematic use. Many problematic users of cybersex also report problems with other sexual compulsions, depression and bipolar disorder, anxiety, chemical dependency, and eating disorders.

Several brief assessments of online sexual activity problems are available, such as the Internet Sex Screening Test. A consultation with a mental health professional who specializes in sexual concerns is recommended before determining if an individual has an online sexual activity problem. Treatment for problematic online sexual activity often focuses on anxiety management, depression treatment, conflict resolution, and identifying face-to-face means of meeting sexual needs and interests. Treatment may be offered in inpatient hospital settings, outpatient counseling, twelve-step groups, and online programs.

Elizabeth A. Maynard

See also: Adultery; Fantasy, Sexual and Erotic; Online Dating; Pornography; Pornography Addiction; Sex Work.

Further Reading

Cooper, A. (Ed.). (2013). Cybersex: The dark side of the force (special issue). *Journal of Sexual Addiction and Compulsivity, 19*(1–2), 1–160.

Young, K. S., & Nabuco de Abreu, C. (2011). *Internet addiction: A handbook and guide to evaluation and treatment.* Hoboken, NJ: John Wiley & Sons.

Oophorectomy

An oophorectomy is the removal of the ovaries. The ovaries are almond-shaped organs that are responsible for the production of ova as well as the female sex hormones, and they are connected to the uterus via the fallopian tubes. An oophorectomy is a surgical procedure and can differ between individuals on the extent of the surgery required. For example, certain people may only require one ovary to be removed, while others may need the removal of both ovaries. This procedure is notable for its potential life-saving results for those who have or are at high risk for ovarian and breast cancer. As well as cancer risk reduction and removal, oophorectomies are performed for the reduction of ectopic pregnancies, endometriosis, noncancerous ovarian cysts, chronic pelvic pain, and pelvic inflammatory disease.

As previously mentioned, there are different types of oophorectomies. The individual's needs and the doctor's recommendation will determine which type of surgery is performed. The unilateral oophorectomy involves the removal of one ovary. Typically, a unilateral oophorectomy might be used to address and remove cancer that is housed in a single ovary. Usually if cancer is present, the adjacent fallopian tube will also be removed due to the shared blood supply between the cancerous ovary and the connecting fallopian tube. When both an ovary and a fallopian tube are removed, the procedure is referred to as a unilateral salpingo-oophorectomy.

Another type of oophorectomy involves the removal of both ovaries and is called a bilateral oophorectomy. This procedure is performed when an individual would like to reduce their risk for both ovarian and breast cancer. Removing both ovaries also removes the production of female sex hormones such as estrogen and progesterone, which then reduces the risk of cancer. In addition to cancer reduction, a bilateral oophorectomy may also be done to prevent the spread of already existing cancer cells in the ovaries. In some cases, both fallopian tubes may also be removed, rendering the procedure a bilateral salpingo-oophorectomy.

In addition, an oophorectomy can be either performed alone or with other procedures. As already mentioned, an oophorectomy paired with a salpingectomy is the removal of both the ovary and the connecting fallopian tube. An oophorectomy paired with a hysterectomy is called a complete hysterectomy and usually results in the removal of the ovaries, fallopian tubes, cervix, and uterus. When deciding whether a unilateral or bilateral oophorectomy needs to be performed, one issue that needs to be considered is if the individual still wants to become pregnant or carry a child. With both ovaries removed, ova are no longer released into the fallopian tubes, and, as such, internal fertilization of the egg is no longer possible. However, if both ovaries have been removed, pregnancy and birth may still be possible through alternative medical procedures like in vitro fertilization. However, if a hysterectomy is performed, pregnancy is no longer possible due to the complete removal of the uterus.

The actual oophorectomy surgical procedure can last anywhere from one to four hours, depending on the type of oophorectomy performed as well as the surgical route taken. There are two types of surgeries that can result in an oophorectomy. The first type of surgery is a laparoscopic surgery. This kind of surgery is ideal as it is the least invasive, and most patients can be out of the hospital soon after it is performed. During this surgery, four small incisions are made on the abdomen. Using these incisions, the doctor will use a small camera to see inside the body accompanied by small tools to remove the ovaries. In a typical procedure, the doctor will separate the ovary from its main blood supply and then pull the organ out from one of the small incisions.

The second option for surgery is referred to as a laparotomy. This surgery is typically not as preferred by doctors because of its invasive nature; however, in some cases, a laparotomy is the only option. During this operation, the doctor makes one large incision to remove the ovaries. Like the laparoscopic surgery, the doctor will then separate the ovary from its blood supply and subsequently remove the organ. Regardless of the procedural route taken, the patient will be put under general anesthesia during the operation.

Like any medical procedure involving surgery, potential complications may arise. For example, a surgery may start out with the laparoscopic approach, but after complications may result in the doctor performing a laparotomy instead. Other potential complications during the surgery may include bleeding, blood clots, and damage to other surrounding organs. In addition, proper aftercare is important to reduce the risk of potential infection of the surgical area and to make recovery as smooth as possible. Depending on the patient and the surgery, the recovery process may differ. Some individuals may stay in the hospital for hours or days after their oophorectomy. Those who received a laparoscopic surgery can usually make a full recovery within a few weeks. Contrastingly, those who received their oophorectomy via a laparotomy usually take six weeks to make a full recovery, and that recovery process can be extremely painful due to the invasive nature of the surgery. Similar to a laparotomy, a complete hysterectomy also takes a full six weeks to heal.

During the healing process, menopause may also be an experience that some will have to manage. Those who received a unilateral oophorectomy or a unilateral salpingo-oophorectomy should not experience any differences with their hormone levels or their menstrual cycle, if they are still menstruating. However, if an individual has not yet entered menopause and has a bilateral oophorectomy, a doctor might prescribe low doses of hormones to reduce menopause-related symptoms as the removal of both ovaries will affect sex hormone production, resulting in premature menopause for some women. Unfortunately, hormones prescribed might also have side effects such as headache, mood swings, and nausea.

Oophorectomies can differ in relation to how many ovaries are removed and whether or not the fallopian tubes are removed as well. In general, an oophorectomy may be used as a last-resort procedure because of its potentially invasive nature and the potential for the individual to enter early menopause. However, despite these drawbacks, an oophorectomy can still be beneficial and can be a lifesaving procedure for those who have been diagnosed with ovarian cancer and for those hoping to reduce their risk of ovarian and breast cancers.

Casey T. Tobin

See also: Breast Cancer; Endometriosis; Estrogen; Fallopian Tubes; Hormone Replacement Therapy; Hysterectomy; Menopause; Ovarian Cancer; Ovaries; Progesterone; Sex Hormones.

Further Reading

American Cancer Society. (2018). What is ovarian cancer? Retrieved from https://www.cancer.org/cancer/ovarian-cancer/about/what-is-ovarian-cancer.html

Boston Women's Health Book Collective. (2011). *Our bodies, ourselves.* New York: Simon & Schuster.

Rocca, W. A. (2017). Bilateral oophorectomy, accelerated aging: Late breaking news on a controversial issue. *Maturitas, 103,* 89.

Open Marriage

"Open marriage" is an umbrella term that includes different types of consensual nonmonogamous arrangements within a couple. Historically, the term was used to distinguish marriages where people had freely chosen each other. This was in opposition to closed marriages, where partnerships had been arranged by families or other systems, such as political alliances. In 1972, the publication of the book

Open Marriage by Nena and George O'Neill marked the transition of this term "open marriage" to indicate openness to consensual extramarital relationships within traditionally monogamous marriages. Other terms commonly used include "open relationships," "ethical nonmonogamy," and "responsible nonmonogamy."

There are several types of open marriages, including practices like swinging, polyamory, and ad hoc arrangements. For example, some couples might agree that it is acceptable for the other partner to have sex with someone else when traveling or if one of the partners becomes sick and sexually unavailable for a long period of time. Open marriage arrangements are only one type of nonmonogamy on a global scale, given that plural marriages of different kinds are not unusual in a range of places across the globe and in different religious traditions.

Open marriages have different norms and rules, which are very much dependent on the model adopted by the couple. Swingers, for example, usually view sex as a recreational activity to be pursued as a couple, usually with other swingers, and there is an understanding that romantic attachment is reserved for the couple and is not to be entered into with other people. On the other hand, polyamorous arrangements can include romantic as well as sexual attachments outside the marriage. Rules and norms in open marriages might also change as couples grow, come into contact with different ideas and communities, and broaden their own experiences and understanding of what they want their open marriage to be like. Sometimes marriages are open from the beginning and for the duration of the relationship; at other times couples might open their marriage for a period of time, then close it again. In addition, some marriages might be open only for specific partners and no other people in general. Within polyamorous practices, these are sometimes known as polyfidelitous arrangements, which can also be referred to as a closed group marriage.

Regardless of the type of open marriage, one of the common traits of an open marriage is the existence of ground rules and contracts within the couple. Those ground rules and contracts determine the rules of engagement for each partner. In some relationships, the rules might be different for each partner based on needs, comfort, and power dynamics. Even though ground rules and contracts in open marriages are usually freely entered into, couples are not immune from power dynamics that might influence the rules and contracts agreed. Power dynamics and communication are definitely issues to be carefully considered when negotiating ground rules or contracts in open marriages or when working with people who are considering opening up their marriage.

Communication is a key issue in open marriages, given that it is needed not only to negotiate ground rules and contracts but also to discuss new sexual encounters and relationships, negotiate safer sex, and manage emotions such as jealousy. The latter can be present to varying degrees in open marriages and needs to be carefully negotiated both when discussing opening a marriage and to maintain the relationship. Some couples might keep the status of their open marriage secret for fear of family or societal disapproval as well as because of potential legal repercussions. If couples have children, for example, they might fear that being visible as part of an open marriage might expose them to scrutiny from child protective services.

In recent years, some notable figures have been more public about their open marriages, and there has been more widespread media attention to ethical nonmonogamous practices in general, also reflected in a broader range of published resources and online networks. The prevalence of open marriages is not known, even though some scholars have tried to estimate it. However, given the range of relationships that might fall under this category, an accurate estimate has not been widely agreed on.

Alex Iantaffi

See also: Communication, Sexual; Extramarital Sex; Marriage; Marriage, Cross-Cultural Comparison of; Monogamy; Polyamory; Polyandry; Polygamy; Polygyny; Swinging.

Further Reading

Barker, M. (2018). *Rewriting the rules: An anti self-help guide to love, sex and relationships* (2nd ed.). New York: Routledge.

Barker, M., & Langdridge, D. (2010). Whatever happened to non-monogamies? Critical reflections on recent research and theory. *Sexualities, 13*(6), 748–772.

Bergstrand, C., & Williams, J. B. (2000). Today's alternative marriage styles: The case of swingers. *Electronic Journal of Human Sexuality, 3*(10), 1–10.

Block, J. (2009). *Open: Love, sex, and life in an open marriage.* Berkeley, CA: Seal Press.

Grunt-Mejer, K., & Campbell, C. (2016). Around consensual nonmonogamies: Assessing attitudes toward nonexclusive relationships. *The Journal of Sex Research, 53*(1), 45–53.

Munson, M., & Stelboum, J. (2013). *The lesbian polyamory reader: Open relationships, non-monogamy, and casual sex.* London: Routledge.

O'Neill, N., & O'Neill, G. (1972). *Open marriage: A new life style for couples.* New York: M. Evans and Company.

Rubin, R. H. (2001). Alternative lifestyles revisited, or whatever happened to swingers, group marriages, and communes? *Journal of Family Issues, 22*(6), 711–726.

Taormino, T. (2013). *Opening up: A guide to creating and sustaining open relationships.* San Francisco: Cleis Press.

Oral Sex

"Oral sex" is an umbrella term that encompasses both cunnilingus and fellatio. Cunnilingus is the stimulation of the vulva, vagina, and clitoris using one's mouth and tongue. Fellatio is the stimulation of the penis and testicles using one's mouth and tongue. Analingus, or the stimulation of the anus using one's mouth and tongue, also falls under the category of oral sex.

There are many terms used to describe oral sex. A common phrase to describe both fellatio and cunnilingus is "going down" on someone. Some popular terms used for fellatio are "giving head" and "blowjob." Cunnilingus may sometimes be referred to as "eating out." Many other euphemisms exist to describe oral sex in general, or fellatio or cunnilingus specifically. Oral sex is most often performed or received from a partner. However, when it comes to fellatio, some people are flexible enough to perform oral sex on their own penis, which is called autofellatio.

Oral sex, when performed simultaneously, is called "69." It is called "69" as the shape of that number is a visual representation of simultaneous oral sex.

Oral sex has become more popular and acceptable as a sexual practice over the past few decades. In a study of college students, 70–90 percent report engaging in oral sex at some point during their lives. A large majority of these study participants stated they had both performed and received oral sex. In this study, women reported giving oral sex more frequently than men gave oral sex.

Oral sex is a common sexual practice for persons of all genders and sexual orientations. It is most common among white middle-class Americans. It is most frequently performed and received during beginning stages of a sexual relationship and is most popular among high school and college-aged people.

In another national survey study conducted in 2002 of twenty-five- to forty-four-year-olds, 90 percent of men and 88 percent of women reported having engaged in oral sex with a partner. In participants aged fifteen to seventeen years, 13 percent of males and 11 percent of females had had oral sex but not penetrative sex. Among those aged eighteen and nineteen years, 11 percent of males and 9 percent of females had engaged in oral sex but not penetrative sex. In a college sample, just over 45 percent of both men and women reported engaging in oral sex with a partner within the last thirty days. Only one-fifth of study participants indicated they had never engaged in oral sex.

While oral sex has less risk of acquiring a sexually transmitted infection than penetrative sex, it still carries a chance of infection. Chlamydia, gonorrhea, herpes, HPV, and syphilis are all transmissible through oral sex. Although rare, HIV may also be transmitted through oral sex. As such, it is important to take precautions when engaging in oral sex, such as using condoms or dental dams. Open communication between partners about testing and sexual health is very important. Oral sex should be avoided when the person performing oral sex has a cold sore. In fact, anyone experiencing open sores in their mouth should take a break from oral sex until the mouth has healed, as these lacerations increase the risk of infection. However, even when cold sores are not present, herpes can still be transmitted from a partner who has ever had a cold sore, although the risk is less than when a sore is present.

More evidence is being collected about the transmission of HPV through oral sex, which may lead to cancers of the mouth, head, throat, or neck. This was brought into the spotlight in the media when actor Michael Douglas attributed his throat cancer to HPV he acquired through oral sex.

Fortunately, barrier methods of contraceptives are great for use during oral sex. Unfortunately, the use of protection during oral sex is quite uncommon. Condoms may be used for protection during fellatio. Many flavored condoms exist for the purpose of oral sex, and regular, unflavored condoms work just as well. Likewise, a dental dam, which is a thin piece of latex, may be used for protection during cunnilingus or analingus. If a dental dam is not available for use during cunnilingus or analingus, a condom may be used by cutting up the length of the condom and removing the ring. This will create a sheet of latex, which can then be spread over the vulva or anus. If using dental dams or unflavored condoms is unappealing due to the latex taste, flavored lubricants are available that can make it more palatable.

Oral sex is able to provide very direct stimulation to highly sensitive areas of the body. On a female body, the clitoris cannot always be directly stimulated during penetrative sex. However, during oral sex the clitoris is able to receive that stimulation, which is why orgasm may be more likely to occur during oral sex rather than penetrative sex.

Individuals who have a positive attitude toward their own body and genitals tend to be the most comfortable with oral sex. When looking at gender differences, men report feeling more pleasure in both giving and receiving oral sex than their female counterparts. Among both men and women, watching a partner receive pleasure is the biggest motivating factor in performing oral sex on someone.

Amanda Manuel

See also: Clitoris; Dental Dam; Penis; Safer Sex; Sexually Transmitted Infections (STIs); Testicles; Vagina; Vulva.

Further Reading

Herbenick, D. (2012). *Sex made easy: Your awkward questions answered for better, smarter, amazing sex.* Philadelphia: Running Press.

Seidman, S., Fischer, N., & Meeks, C. (2011). *Introducing the new sexuality studies* (2nd ed.). London: Routledge.

Yarber, W., Sayad, B., & Strong, B. (2010). *Human sexuality: Diversity in contemporary America* (7th ed.). New York: McGraw-Hill.

Orchiectomy

An orchiectomy (also known as an orchidectomy) is the surgical removal of one or both testicles. Reasons for an orchiectomy may include testicular cancer, infection in the testes, or gender or sex reassignment surgery. There are three main types of orchiectomy: simple, subcapsular, and inguinal; each of these is generally done under local anesthesia. While common today for health purposes, historically, the orchiectomy was used as a form of punishment.

A simple orchiectomy is commonly performed as part of sex reassignment surgery for transgender women. It may also be used as treatment for advanced cases of prostate cancer or in the event of a testicular injury. For this procedure, the patient lies flat on an operating table with the penis taped against the abdomen. The nurse then shaves a small area for the incision. After anesthetic has been administered, the surgeon makes an incision in the midpoint of the scrotum and cuts through the underlying tissue. The surgeon then removes the testicle(s) and parts of the spermatic cord through the incision. The incision is closed with two layers of sutures and covered with a surgical dressing. If the patient desires, a prosthetic testicle (or two) can be inserted before the incision is closed to mimic the look of the presurgery scrotum, which may help increase body image and self-esteem.

For transgender women, an orchiectomy may be used as a treatment for gender dysphoria as it will decrease the amount of male hormones in the body and change the external genital area to better match the individual's gender. It is commonly used alongside a penectomy, which is the surgical removal of the penis, and a vaginoplasty, which is the surgical creation of a vagina.

A subcapsular orchiectomy is also commonly performed for the treatment of prostate cancer. The operation is very similar to that of a simple orchiectomy, with the exception that just the glandular tissue that surrounds each testicle is removed rather than the entire gland itself. A subcapsular orchiectomy is done to remove the part of the testicle that produces testosterone. It assists in cases of prostate cancer and is an option available for men who do not want to undergo hormonal treatment while achieving the same outcome. The operation leaves the testicles in place, with a slightly smaller appearance than before. This type of orchiectomy is done primarily to keep the appearance of an ordinary scrotum, mainly to decrease the patient's chances of experiencing negative body image or feelings of demasculinization after surgery.

Inguinal orchiectomy, also called radical orchiectomy, is performed when the onset of testicular cancer is suspected and is completed to prevent a possible spread of cancer from the spermatic cord into the lymph nodes near the kidneys. An inguinal orchiectomy can be either unilateral or bilateral, meaning removing just one or both testicles. During this procedure, the surgeon makes an incision in the patient's groin area that is bigger and more invasive than the scrotal incision in the previously described methods. In addition to one or both testicles, the entire spermatic cord is also removed. A long, nonabsorbable suture may be left in the stump of the spermatic cord in the case that more surgery is deemed necessary in the future. After the cord and testicle(s) have been removed, the surgeon washes the area with saline solution and closes the various layers of tissues and skin with various types of sutures. The wound is then covered with sterile gauze and bandaged. This version of an orchiectomy is much more serious and invasive, and it carries a longer rate of postoperative healing, but is necessary to treat more advanced stages of testicular cancer.

Negative effects that a patient may experience after an orchiectomy include several different physical and psychological concerns, such as infertility and hypoandrogenism. Hypoandrogenism occurs when there is a lack of male hormones, called androgens, in the body. Because the testes produce much of the body's androgens, if they are removed, this production stops. Symptoms associated with hypoandrogenism include hot flashes, osteoporosis (a medical condition in which the bones become brittle and fragile from loss of tissue), feelings of demasculinization, sexual dysfunction, and depression, as well as gynecomastia (swelling of the breast tissue in males, caused by an imbalance of the hormones estrogen and testosterone). If a patient is able to retain one testicle, there are fewer side effects, and erectile function and sperm production may not be affected. With both testicles removed, however, the body is unable to make as much testosterone as it needs, which may result in a lower sex drive and make it challenging to have erections. A doctor can prescribe a testosterone gel, patch, or shot that may help ease these symptoms. Some patients may also require psychological counseling following an orchiectomy as part of their long-term aftercare. Many men have very strong feelings about issues involving their genitals and may feel depressed or anxious about their bodies or their relationships after genital surgery. In addition to individual psychotherapy, support groups are often helpful. There are active networks of prostate cancer support groups in Canada and the United States as well as support groups for men's issues in general.

While orchiectomies are now used as a surgical procedure for those seeking sex reassignment or as a treatment for cancer, they were historically used as punishment, similar to historical uses of castration. While the overall understanding of castration also includes the removal of the penis, removing the testicles alone was considered the true removal of "manhood" because the ability to reproduce was removed. Castration and removal of the testes would occur for things such as broken laws, rape, or for stepping out of social norms. It was also believed that castration had the ability to act as an anger management technique (Glass & Watkin, 1997).

However, historically, orchiectomy (or, at the time, castration) was not only used for punishment but also as a mark of leadership. Eunuchs existed in several early civilizations and would commonly work directly under the emperor or leader in power. These individuals were trusted and sought out for two main reasons. The first was the loyalty associated with choosing to be castrated as the act was believed to show a love and commitment toward a ruler as well as to show that the man was willing to devote his life to that work and not to marriage and a family. The second reason these men were sought out was because they were deemed trustworthy to have around the royal women, as it was assumed that they would not be tempted (Glass & Watkin, 1997). Historically, the use of orchiectomies has had many purposes. From punishment and leadership symbols to medical treatment and now sex reassignment, there are a plethora of reasons this procedure is relevant to sexuality today and in the future.

Casey T. Tobin

See also: Castration; Prostate Cancer; Sex Reassignment Surgery; Testicles; Testicular Cancer.

Further Reading

Delta Medix Urology. (2017). Radical & simple orchiectomy. Retrieved from https://www.deltamedix.com/urology/orchiectomy.php

Glass, J., & Watkin, N. (1997). From mutilation to medication: The history of orchidectomy. *BJU International, 80*(3), 373–378.

LeVay, S., Baldwin, J., & Baldwin, J. (2018). *Discovering human sexuality* (4th ed.). Sunderland, MA: Sinauer Associates.

Rosen, A., Jayram, G., Drazer, M., & Eggener, S. E. (2011). Global trends in testicular cancer incidence and mortality. *European Urology, 60*(2), 374–379.

Orgasm

An orgasm is a brief period of intense, pleasurable physical release after a buildup in sexual tension. The sexual tension builds as part of a sexual response cycle. There are several models of sexual response, one of which can be visualized as a circle, starting with seduction, when feelings of desire are triggered, before or while physiological arousal begins. Next the body experiences sensations, when arousal and excitement increase through sexual activity until a plateau is reached. Orgasm occurs if a person gives in to sexual release. During a period of reflection, the body rests or readies for more stimulation, and the mind interprets the experience.

It is normal for individuals to respond differently to sexual stimulation. For instance, some people experience orgasm very quickly, so the stages of sexual arousal seem to merge. Some people, usually women, are able to experience multiple orgasms. Most people require direct genital stimulation to build enough excitement to experience orgasm; however, some people can experience it through other means, such as nipple stimulation.

During an orgasm, most people experience similar sensations. Females commonly experience muscle contractions in the vagina, uterus, and pelvic region. Males commonly experience these same contractions in the penis, prostate, and pelvic regions. Other common characteristics include tension in the feet; increased blood pressure, heart rate, and breathing; decreased sensitivity to pain; and a sudden, forceful release of sexual tension. Flushing (blushing) may occur over the entire body before orgasm and disappear shortly afterward. Upon orgasm, males usually ejaculate, releasing seminal fluid through the urethra; some females ejaculate as well.

People can experience orgasm many ways, including for women through stimulation of the clitoris, labia, urethral opening, vaginal opening, and vagina. Other sensitive areas reach through the vagina, including the cervix; the G-spot, a sensitive area in the anterior wall (toward the lower abdomen); the clitoral crura; and the anterior fornix, located at the end of the anterior wall of the vagina. For men, orgasm may occur when stimulation is provided to the glans of the penis and frenulum (located where the glans and shaft meet), prostate, anus, and rectum. Some people are able to experience orgasm when other areas of the body, such as the nipples, are stimulated, as well as through imagination alone. Orgasms may involve the entire body or feel localized. The "right" orgasm is any kind a person enjoys.

Orgasms can provide a sense of comfort and well-being. They can help people feel either relaxed or energized. The contractions that accompany orgasm help tone the pubococcygeus muscle, which helps support the sexual organs and increase sexual pleasure. Orgasms may also bring partners physically and emotionally closer together.

The myth persists that orgasm comes naturally and easily to everyone who is sexually active; however, orgasm may be difficult to experience if people

- are unfamiliar with their sexual anatomy
- do not understand what an orgasm is
- do not feel free to express themselves sexually
- feel embarrassed by their sexual interest and responses
- have underlying emotional issues or cultural messages that impede sexual pleasure
- fear getting pregnant or getting a sexually transmitted infection

- focus only on a partner's needs
- spend too little time on arousal and stimulation
- are in an unhealthy or unsafe sexual relationship
- have a history of sexual abuse or intimate partner violence
- take medication that reduces desire, such as some blood pressure medications, antihistamines, and antidepressants
- have a medical condition that affects the sexual response cycle, such as diabetes or a neurological disease
- have had medical treatment affecting the sexual organs or nerves involved in orgasm
- have poor circulation throughout the body, particularly to the genitals
- experience hormonal changes that decrease sexual desire, increase time necessary for arousal, and may decrease the intensity of sexual response
- overindulge in alcohol and some nonprescription drugs

Humans have the physiological ability to experience orgasm from birth, but not everyone pursues it. Some very small children enjoy rubbing their genitals by hand or against pillows and other items. Others begin touching themselves—masturbating—during puberty, while others wait until they have sexual partners. Some people never experience orgasm due to psychological or cultural reasons or due to medical conditions or treatments that affect sexual arousal and orgasm.

The aging process can create changes in how people experience orgasm: more direct genital stimulation is usually needed as well as more time to build arousal. Older males and females often experience less strong physical sensations during orgasm; however, these changes need not indicate a decrease in sexual satisfaction overall.

For some people, orgasm is a spiritual, transcendent experience. For others, its benefits are more related to physical pleasure and comfort. Orgasm may be enjoyed by oneself or with a partner. While some people feel pressured to experience orgasm, intimacy and sexual activity can be enriching and satisfying regardless of whether orgasm is experienced. Indeed, many people find the sensuality of building arousal to be more emotionally rewarding than a few seconds of orgasm.

Melanie Davis

See also: Anorgasmia; Arousal; Ejaculation; Female Ejaculation; Masters and Johnson Four-Stage Model of Sexual Response; Sexual Disorders, Female; Sexual Disorders, Male; Somnus Orgasm.

Further Reading

Cass, V. (2004). *The elusive orgasm*. Bentley, Australia: Brightfire Press.

Joannides, P. (2017). *Guide to getting it on* (9th ed.). Waldport, OR: Goofy Foot Press.

Nagoski, E. (2015). *Come as you are*. New York: Simon & Schuster Paperbacks.

Whipple, B., & Brash-McGreer, K. (1997). Management of female sexual dysfunction. In M. L. Sipski & C. J. Alexander (Eds.), *Sexual function in people with disability and chronic illness: A health professional's guide* (509–534). Gaithersburg, MD: Aspen Publishers.

Outing

"Outing" refers to revealing an individual's sexual orientation or gender identity to other people. While individuals can "out" themselves, which is generally referred to as "coming out," "outing" occurs when someone other than the individual reveals the individual's sexual orientation or gender identity. Outing can occur with the individual's permission, but the phrase generally refers to informing others about the individual's sexual orientation or gender identity without the individual's permission. Outing has been used by some sexual minority rights activists as a political weapon by exposing public figures who are perceived to be anti-LGBTQ+ but are themselves LGBTQ+.

Outing can occur at any social level, from telling a peer, colleague, or family member about someone's sexual orientation or gender identity to making a public pronouncement about a public figure's sexual orientation or gender identity. While individuals coming out and being open about their sexual orientations or gender identities is generally associated with positive psychosocial outcomes, there are risks involved in doing so. Risks include social or familial rejection, social ostracization, harassment, and physical violence. These risks will also vary depending on an individual's country and culture. In some countries and cultures, sexual and gender minority individuals face severe legal and social consequences, including in some cases death. In Western cultures, these risks for youth may include being kicked out of their home; losing parental monetary and emotional support; and being subjected to considerable harassment, assault, and bullying within their social and educational environments.

When youth are able to choose the time, location, and to whom they will come out, they are able to judge the safety of the situation and to plan for various reactions. Youth generally evaluate the benefits and possible costs involved with coming out, making individualized decisions. When outed, however, youth are unable to control who learns about their sexual orientations and/or gender identities and may be unprepared for the negative responses that may occur. Many youth fear being outed so much that they do not report harassment or assault as doing so might out them to parents, peers, or others. Arguments in favor of outing youth include others feeling the youths' parents, school personnel, service providers, and so on deserve to know the youth's sexual orientations or gender identities; that youth need to be able to discuss their sexual orientations or gender identities with adults who can help guide them, and they cannot do this without those people knowing their sexual orientations or gender identities; and that letting others know the youth's sexual orientation or gender identities will aid in protecting the youth. Yet, the youth often also feel their privacy has been violated and may experience considerable distress, leading most mental health professionals to strongly recommend youth come out on their own terms and at their chosen time.

For adults, while problematic for many of the same reasons as noted for youth, outing may have less impact due to adults having more social and financial independence; being able to change their educational, occupational, or living environment with more ease; and having a more developed ability to control emotional responses. Even with that, adults who are outed may experience significant negative psychosocial outcomes, such as mental health and substance use concerns, loss of employment, social isolation, and many of the other noted difficulties for youth. As with youth, it is generally believed that adults should also be able to control to whom they come out and when and where that occurs.

Politically, outing can have significant repercussions. Starting in the later 1980s and becoming much more prevalent in the early 1990s, gay rights activists began publicly exposing public figures who they felt were being hypocritical by supporting legislation or policies that were harmful to LGBTQ+ individuals while either being LGBTQ+ themselves or engaging in same-sex sexual relationships. This practice was very controversial, with some viewing outing as a violation of individuals' privacy, while other prominent gay rights figures such as Michelangelo Signorile and Peter Tatchell defended the practice.

The politics of outing were heavily debated during the mid- and late 1990s and early 2000s by authors such as Larry Gross, Richard Mohr, Warren Johansson, and William Percy. Arguments made in favor of outing included exposing perceived hypocrisy, forcing individuals to publicly acknowledge their sexual orientations or gender identities and confront the possible repercussions of their political or public positions or statements to themselves and others like them, combating homophobia that may be linked to internalized homonegativity, helping others recognize that they know individuals who are sexual or gender minorities so that the others are forced to reconcile their assumptions about sexual or gender minorities and the reality of the people they know, and using it as a means of self-defense against those who threaten the LGBTQ+ community while secretly being a part of it. Opposing arguments generally focused on the invasion of privacy that occurs when individuals are outed, questions of mixing individuals' public and private identities, and the hypocrisy of LGBTQ+ rights activists promoting the rights of LGBTQ+ individuals to have private lives not subject to social or legal judgment from others while violating those rights for public figures. Other concerns were raised about possible mistaken outings and the effects that these could have on the careers of those erroneously exposed as LGBTQ+.

Outing has ended the careers of several politicians and led to the resignations of prominent religious leaders. In response to ethical concerns about these consequences, Johansson and Percy (1994) provided a matrix for making decisions about whether outing an individual was ethical, focusing on areas such as the motive for doing so, the source of the individual's public reputation, and the likely consequences of doing so on the individual's career, family life, and sexual life. Public discussion of the practices of political outing largely dissipated by the mid-2000s without any consensus about the propriety of the actions.

Richard A. Brandon-Friedman

See also: Coming Out; Gender Identity; LGBTQ+; Passing; Sexual Identity.

Further Reading

Gross, L. (1993). *Contested closets: The politics and ethics of outing.* Minneapolis: University of Minnesota Press.

Heatherington, L., & Lavner, J. A. (2008). Coming to terms with coming out: Review and recommendations for family systems-focused research. *Journal of Family Psychology, 22*(3), 329.

Johansson, M. A., & Percy, W. A. (1994). *Outing: Shattering the conspiracy of silence.* New York: Harrington Park Press.

Kosciw, J. G., Greytak, E. A., Giga, N. M., Villenas, C., & Danischewski, D. J. (2016). *The 2015 National School Climate Survey: The experiences of lesbian, gay, bisexual, transgender, and queer youth in our nation's schools.* New York: GLSEN.

Mohr, R. D. (1992). *Gay ideas: Outing and other controversies.* Boston: Beacon Press.

Orne, J. (2012). "You will always have to 'out' yourself": Reconsidering coming out through strategic outness. *Sexualities, 14*(6), 681–703. doi: 10.1177/1363460711420462

Schafer, A. (2015). Quiet sabotage of the queer child: Why the law must be reframed to appreciate the dangers of outing gay youth. *Howard Law Journal, 58*(2), 597–636.

Vaughan, M. D., & Waehler, C. A. (2010). Coming out growth: Conceptualizing and measuring stress-related growth associated with coming out to others as a sexual minority. *Journal of Adult Development, 17*(2), 94–109. doi: 10.1007/s10804-009-9084-9

Ziering, A. (Producer), & Dick, K. (Director). (2009). *Outrage* [Motion picture]. Magnolia Pictures.

Out-of-Control Sexual Behavior

The need to control our sexual urges, thoughts, and behaviors is human. Failing to successfully regulate one's sexual life can be distressing. Feeling sexually out of control involves excessive preoccupying sexual thoughts or repeating sexual behaviors that have shaming, hurtful, or damaging consequences. When a person concludes that their sexual urges, thoughts, and behaviors are beyond their control, they may call themselves a sex addict, pervert, scumbag, or cheater. Others may look on them with derision, contempt, fear, disgust, and punitive judgments.

After centuries of condemning out-of-control sexual behavior as rooted in devil possession, the last century medicalized this human behavior with diagnoses of nymphomania, Don Juanism, and hypersexuality. Each was eventually discarded, leaving the twenty-first century in a state of division and conflict among physicians, psychotherapists, sex therapists, sex researchers, and addiction counselors about whether sexual behavior on the extreme end of the normal range actually crosses a threshold from a behavior problem to a separate and distinct disease.

The World Health Organization's *International Classification of Diseases* (*ICD-11*) places compulsive sexual behavior disorder (CSBD) within the spectrum of impulse control disorders characterized by persistent failure over time to control intense, repetitive sexual impulses or urges, resulting in repetitive sexual behavior that leads to marked distress or impairment in personal, family, social, educational, occupational, or other important areas of functioning. Field testing will be conducted to determine if the *ICD-11* construct is cross-culturally generalizable. In the meantime, it remains unsettled how clinicians can distinguish normal variations in sexual behavior frequency, type, and consequences from CSBD.

Sexual imagery created for entertainment, sexual excitement, erotic arousal, and facilitating orgasm (almost universally called pornography) is portable and available 24/7 online and through mobile phone apps. Despite some people feeling deeply conflicted about their use and interest in sexual imagery, there remains no recognized diagnostic category of a disease of pornography addition in the medical, psychological, or other scientific literature. In some religious, moral, or cultural contexts, viewing sexual imagery for pleasure and porn-assisted orgasms pose existential moral threats (i.e., banishment, divorce, loss of everlasting life and salvation). Sex researchers have rigorously examined the notion of porn addiction. Their studies find that the perception of "porn addiction" is especially prevalent among highly religious individuals who have a relatively low frequency of actually viewing sexual imagery but who hold high levels of moral disapproval.

Out-of-control sexual behavior (OCSB) is defined as a sexual health problem in which a person's consensual sexual urges, thoughts, or behaviors feel out of their control. The term "OCSB" is not a diagnosis or conclusory label. It describes an individual's feelings and experiences about problematic consensual sexual behavior. OCSB does not include nonconsensual sexual behavior. Violating another person's body by using force, coercion, or exploitation in order to engage in a sexual act is not considered an out-of-control sexual behavior problem, and experts with specialized training in nonconsensual sex should be consulted if this occurs. An OCSB assessment for consensual sexual behavior first considers how drugs and alcohol, mental health, and medical conditions or medication-related side effects affect sexual behavior. OCSB assessment also screens for intimate partner violence.

OCSB treatment interventions emphasize changing both sexual and nonsexual self-regulation. Clients aim to improve their sexual health and regain control of their sexual lives through balancing safety and pleasure within their sex lives. Others may need to face their shame and secrecy about a specific sexual turn-on. Distinguishing sexual prejudice from a sexual behavior problem is a necessary treatment focus when conflicted or when rejecting one's own sexual orientation or erotic nature.

Saying that one has a sex addiction has become the common means to convey a real contradiction between one's sexual activity and their personal, relational, or spiritual values. It is also a way to ask for help. Self-diagnosing sexual behavior concerns can unfortunately lead to premature evaluation. If someone is experiencing OCSB, they should seek out a licensed therapist for professional help. It is also important to ask the clinician or therapist about their sexological training as well as the degree to which their religious beliefs influence their clinical assessment and treatment methods. Studies find that therapists who are more religiously influenced are more likely to label feeling sexually out of control as a sexual addiction disorder. A therapist certified by a national sex therapy association (e.g., American Association of Certified Sex Educators, Counselors, and Therapists) or a relationship therapist with advanced training in human sexuality will be prepared to explore a wide range of factors that can contribute to feeling sexually out of control. Out-of-control sexual behavior, while not a psychiatric disorder, is a real problem of sexual behavior regulation experienced by many people.

Douglas Braun-Harvey

See also: American Association of Sexuality Educators, Counselors, and Therapists (AASECT); Cheating and Infidelity; Compulsivity, Sexual; Hypersexuality; *International Classification of Diseases, Eleventh Revision* (*ICD-11*); Pornography Addiction; Sex Guilt.

Further Reading

Braun-Harvey, D., & Vigorito, M. (2016). *Treating out of control sexual behavior: Rethinking sex addiction*. New York: Springer Publishing.

Dickenson, J. A., Gleason, N., Coleman, E., & Miner, M. H. (2018). Prevalence of distress associated with difficulty controlling sexual urges, feelings, and behaviors in the United States. *JAMA Network Open, 1*(7), e184468.

Grubbs, J. B., Perry, S. L., Wilt, J. A., & Reid, R. C. (2018). Pornography problems due to moral incongruence: An integrative model with a systematic review and meta-analysis. *Archives of Sexual Behavior, 48*(20), 397–415.

Montgomery-Graham, S. (2017). Conceptualization and assessment of hypersexual disorder: A systematic review of the literature. *Sexual Medicine Reviews, 5*(2), 146–162.

Reed, G. M., First, M. B., Kogan, C. S., Hyman, S. E., Gureje, O., Gaebel, W., ... Claudino, A. (2019). Innovations and changes in the ICD-11 classification of mental, behavioural and neurodevelopmental disorders. *World Psychiatry, 18*(1), 3–19.

Ova

Ova, or eggs (singular ovum), are the round female sex cells that are stored in the ovaries. Human ova are very large cells and may be visible to the naked eye. Each ovum contains twenty-three chromosomes that are made up of half of the female's DNA or genes. During conception, the twenty-three chromosomes in the ovum pair with the twenty-three male chromosomes carried by a sperm, the male sex cell, in order to form the genetic material necessary to produce a baby.

Currently it is believed that an individual with ovaries has all the eggs they will ever have at birth. In other words, it does not appear that the body is able make eggs after birth. Typically, a female individual is born with approximately 800,000 eggs. However, by the time an individual reaches puberty, only about 300,000 eggs remain. Over time, the number of eggs an individual has continues to decrease, and so by menopause there are usually fewer than 10,000 eggs remaining. This is a very different process compared to sperm, which are continuously produced by male individuals, starting at puberty and lasting for the rest of their life. Because of this process, male individuals can potentially contribute to a pregnancy throughout their entire lives. Female individuals, however, can only become pregnant between puberty and menopause (roughly between the ages of eleven to fifty-one years).

At puberty, changes in hormones lead to the first ovulation. During this time, hormones begin to cause an egg to mature. During ovulation, hormones trigger the egg, causing it to emerge from its follicle in the ovary. It is then moved from the ovary into the fallopian tube and down toward the uterus. Between puberty and menopause, ovulation typically occurs every month, usually around day fourteen of the menstrual cycle. Usually, one egg emerges each month from alternating ovaries. Sometimes more than one egg is released; when this occurs, it is possible for each egg to be fertilized, which can result in having twins or triplets. Eggs can survive, and have the potential to be fertilized, for twelve to twenty-four hours after ovulation. If the egg is not fertilized, it moves into the uterus and dissolves. Ovulation becomes less frequent as individuals age and stops entirely at menopause.

As the result of penile-vaginal intercourse, an ovum may be fertilized by a sperm. In order for this to happen, the sperm needs to penetrate the outer layer of the egg cell. To do this, the sperm cell releases specific enzymes that break down the coating of the egg and allow the sperm to enter. If this occurs, the cells form a zygote, which may develop into an embryo. Fertilization typically occurs in the fallopian tubes. Some people experience difficulty becoming pregnant and so may seek out treatments in order to improve their fertility. For people who do not wish to become pregnant, contraceptive methods can be used. Most hormonal contraceptive methods act by preventing ovulation, by thickening the cervical mucus to prevent sperm from entering the female reproductive system, and/or by changing the environment in the uterus so that if fertilization of the egg does occur, implantation does not take place.

Because ova age at the same rate as the female individual, their quality decreases over time. This means that older individuals, those over the age of thirty-five, often have a harder time becoming pregnant. They also experience a higher rate of pregnancy loss or miscarriage, and there is a higher rate for chromosomal abnormalities in any offspring. Because of this, some people who know that they do not want to become pregnant until later in their life may freeze some of their eggs when they are younger in order to use them later. Some individuals may also choose to donate their eggs to others who are unable to become pregnant on their own, either because of infertility issues or because neither partner has their own eggs, such as with male same-sex couples.

Heather L. Armstrong

See also: Conception; Fertility; Menopause; Ova Donation; Ovaries; Ovulation; Sex Chromosomes; Sperm.

Further Reading

Boston Women's Health Book Collective. (2005). *Our bodies, ourselves*. New York: Scribner.

Cleveland Clinic. (2019). Female reproductive system. Retrieved from https://my.clevelandclinic.org/health/articles/9118-female-reproductive-system

Ova Donation

Ova donation is the act of one person giving their eggs to another who is having difficulty conceiving a child, or to scientists for stem cell research. Ova, or egg, donors must go through a long process of screening and medical procedures and are typically given several thousand dollars in compensation. All these factors and more have led to major ethical debates over the procedure.

Egg donations first became commercialized in 1978, after in vitro fertilization (IVF) produced the first successful "test tube baby" from an egg fertilized outside a woman's body. It was not until the 1990s, however, that use of donated eggs became a widely acceptable part of fertility treatments for women and couples who found it difficult or impossible to have children of their own. The market for eggs to be used in stem cell research grew up alongside IVF, with research initially being conducted on discarded eggs before some government agencies began paying women for their eggs directly. The latter practice remains rare, however, and the vast majority of ova donations still are used for IVF.

Today the market for donated eggs comes largely from women and couples who are willing to spend thousands, or even tens of thousands, of dollars to conceive a child. While some are simply seeking a healthy child, others pay top dollar for eggs from donors with very specific characteristics, such as high academic test scores, athletic abilities, or physical traits similar to themselves. Because the ova donation industry is largely unregulated, donor consent, screening, compensation, and follow-up care all can vary widely.

The American Society of Reproductive Medicine (ASRM) recommends that clinics purchasing eggs compensate the donor appropriately for the "time, inconvenience, and physical and emotional demands" associated with ova donation. According to ASRM guidelines, payments to ova donors should be limited to $5,000, and any payment above $10,000 is inappropriate. However, advertisements around college campuses commonly promise payments of $50,000 or more for donors with specific traits.

Although most egg donors surveyed said they chose to donate mainly to help others conceive a child, many also reported being motivated by other factors. These primarily include financial gain, and, to a lesser degree, a desire to learn about their own fertility or fertility treatment options or to "make up" for having had an abortion in the past. When unemployment rose sharply in 2007 and 2008, the *Wall Street Journal* reported a marked increase in women applying to donate eggs—a trend that worried ethicists, who cite research showing that women motivated primarily by financial gain are less able to give truly informed consent and are more likely to regret their decision.

There is particular controversy surrounding the practice of targeting college students for ova donation. Many medical ethicists also express concerns about putting a price tag on human body parts, the potential for exploiting women, and the inequalities of IVF in general, which allow only the wealthy to conceive a child in this way.

Prior to donating eggs, women must first apply and go through an initial screening process. Although IVF donor criteria vary, in general clinics require candidates to be between twenty and thirty years old and in excellent health. Candidates must disclose their full medical histories, as well as family medical history, and are nearly always disqualified for any incidence of sexually transmitted infections, cancer, diabetes, or mental illness, as well as for travel to certain foreign countries. Most candidates must also consent to a long list of medical tests for blood type, drug use, diseases, or potential genetic defects. They typically undergo a set of mental, psychological, and personality tests as well. Even those who qualify in theory may be put on a waiting list until a match is found for a woman or couple seeking the donor woman's particular characteristics.

If an ova donor is accepted, she then moves on to the next stage, the egg donation process itself, during which she must abstain from all smoking, alcohol, drugs, and sex for the duration of the procedure, which takes several weeks. Sex is typically banned because of the increased risk of unwanted pregnancy during fertility treatments.

Egg donation is composed of two separate phases: ovarian hyperstimulation, in which a series of hormonal drugs injected over several weeks prompt the ovaries to produce multiple mature eggs in just one menstrual cycle, and egg retrieval, which typically occurs just once. The first phase consists of three or sometimes four stages. Some donors may first take birth control pills so that their menstrual cycles and those of the egg recipient can sync up. The next three stages involve a series of drug injections that (1) suppress hormone levels, causing the donor's body to go through "artificial menopause"; (2) stimulate the production of multiple eggs; and (3) trigger the release of these matured eggs.

Between thirty-four and thirty-six hours after the final drug injection, the ova donor undergoes egg retrieval. Typically conducted while the donor is under general anesthesia, the surgical removal of eggs is performed by inserting an ultrasound probe with a suctioning needle attached. A physician guides the needle into each ovary and suctions out mature eggs. Following this procedure, donors typically spend an additional one to two hours at the clinic before returning home to recover. To ensure full recovery, donors usually return for a follow-up visit and ultrasound procedure after one week. In all, screening and medical procedures for ova donation take about sixty hours.

There has been little follow-up research on long-term side effects of ova donation, but some common risks of ovarian hyperstimulation include abdominal swelling, tension and pressure around the ovaries, mood swings, bruising at injection sites, vaginal dryness, and hot flashes. Severe side effects appear to be rare but may include ovarian hyperstimulation syndrome (OHSS), which leads to fluid buildup in the chest and abdomen and enlargement of the ovaries. Severe OHSS can cause permanent damage to ovaries, dehydration, blood clotting disorders, kidney damage, and even death.

Side effects of egg retrieval may include mild to moderate abdominal pain, damage to ovaries, vaginal bleeding, and infection. More serious risks include infertility and damage to adjacent organs, including the bladder, intestines, uterus, or blood vessels. Some doctors believe that repeatedly donating eggs may increase risk of cancer, leading some to call for a lifetime donation limit of three cycles.

Because of the risks involved, the ASRM and medical ethicists strongly recommend a lengthy process of informed consent for potential ova donors as well as insurance coverage for any future complications related to ova donation.

Terri Nichols

See also: Assisted Reproductive Technology; Infertility; Ova; Surrogate Mothers.

Further Reading

Almeling, R. (2011). *Sex cells: The medical market for eggs and sperm*. Berkeley: University of California Press.

American Society for Reproductive Medicine. (2012). Egg donation. Retrieved from https://www.reproductivefacts.org/globalassets/rf/news-and-publications/bookletsfact-sheets/english-fact-sheets-and-info-booklets/egg_donation_factsheet.pdf

Cohen, C. B. (1996). *New ways of making babies: The case of egg donation*. Bloomington: Indiana University Press.

Ovarian Cancer

Ovarian cancer is the abnormal, uncontrolled multiplication of cells within one or both of the ovaries. Most commonly, ovarian cancer originates in the epithelial tissue that covers the ovaries. In some cases, the cancer develops in other ovarian tissues.

Ovarian cancer is most prevalent in women who have experienced menopause, especially women who are older than age sixty. The disease is more prevalent among women in developed, Western nations than in the less developed nations of Asia and Africa. In 2014, there were about 22,000 newly diagnosed cases of ovarian cancer in the United States. Some 14,000 American women died from ovarian cancer that year.

The earlier a diagnosis for ovarian cancer is made and the earlier treatment is begun, the more successful the outcome is likely to be. Unfortunately, this cancer is typically diagnosed after it has spread beyond the ovaries, resulting in high mortality rates. On average, 45 percent of women are alive five years after diagnosis. If the cancer remains localized in the ovaries at the time of diagnosis, the five-year survival rate rises to about 92 percent. If the cancer has already metastasized to distant tissues of the body at the time of diagnosis, the five-year survival rate falls to about 22 percent.

A woman's risk for ovarian cancer is increased by the inheritance of mutations in either of two genes, known as BRCA1 and BRCA2. Approximately one in 200 women have at least one of these mutated genes, which also increase the risk of breast cancer (a much more common cancer than ovarian cancer). Blood tests can detect the presence of BRCA1 and BRCA2. A woman with either of these genes may choose to have her ovaries or breasts surgically removed to prevent the possible development of cancer.

Only 10 percent of ovarian cancer cases are associated with the BRCA1 and BRCA2 genes. Other cases have causes that are not fully understood. However, factors that are believed to increase the risk of ovarian cancer include a diet high in fat, never being pregnant, going through menopause relatively late in life (after age fifty), and having had a relatively early onset of menstruation (before age twelve). Some studies suggest that women who use hormone replacement therapy to relieve the symptoms of menopause are at an elevated risk for ovarian cancer.

Research indicates that certain factors may lower the risk of ovarian cancer. These factors include having given birth, having breastfed the infant, and having undergone a tubal ligation or hysterectomy. The use of oral contraceptives may also lower ovarian cancer risk, but such use may increase breast cancer risk.

People with ovarian cancer may notice chronic pain or cramps in the abdominal or pelvic areas as well as frequent nausea, bloating, abnormal vaginal bleeding, and an abnormally frequent need to urinate. Such symptoms can also be associated with less serious conditions. If the symptoms are noticed almost every day for two or three weeks, the person should see a doctor. The doctor is likely to perform a pelvic examination, looking for signs of abnormal lumps on the ovaries. Lumps may also be detected with an ultrasound examination.

A suspicion of ovarian cancer is usually followed up with a blood test and biopsy. The blood will be analyzed for elevated levels of a protein called cancer antigen 125 (CA-125). High levels of CA-125 could suggest any of various pathological conditions, including ovarian cancer, endometriosis, and uterine fibroids. To determine the precise condition, an ovarian tissue sample must be collected for biopsy. Additional tests, such as computed tomography, can be used to determine the stage of cancer development.

If the presence of cancer is confirmed, surgery is usually performed to remove one or both ovaries. In many cases, the uterus and fallopian tubes are also removed to try to ensure that all the cancer is gone. These procedures will make it impossible to have a future pregnancy, and they will cause immediate menopause if menopause had not yet occurred.

In the most advanced cases of ovarian cancer, additional tissues may be removed, including part of the intestines, the lining of the abdominal wall, and the spleen. Chemotherapy and radiation therapy may also be used in a patient's treatment. Follow-up therapy often includes routine blood tests to monitor levels of CA-125 and other substances that could indicate a recurrence of cancer.

As with breast cancer treatment, treatment for ovarian cancer sometimes results in emotional problems regarding a woman's perception of her body and her sexuality. Thus, psychological counseling may be incorporated into follow-up therapy.

A. J. Smuskiewicz

See also: Breast Cancer; Cervical Cancer; Oophorectomy; Ovaries; Uterine Cancer.

Further Reading

Friedman, S., Sutphen, R., Steligo, K., & Greene, M. H. (2012). *Confronting hereditary breast and ovarian cancer: Identify your risk, understand your options, change your destiny.* Baltimore: Johns Hopkins University Press.

National Cancer Institute. (n.d.). Cancer stat facts: Ovarian cancer. Retrieved from http://seer.cancer.gov/statfacts/html/ovary.html

Ovaries

The ovaries are two oval-shaped organs that are part of the female reproductive system. The ovaries store and release ova (egg cells) as well as the female sex hormones estrogen and progesterone. There is one ovary on each side of the uterus.

At birth, each of the ovaries contains approximately 400,000–800,000 immature eggs. The eggs begin to mature during puberty, usually between the ages of 10 and 12. Also at puberty, estrogen produced by the ovaries causes the development of female secondary sex characteristics, such as breasts and the accumulation of fat in the hips. One egg matures each month, from alternating ovaries, during the first half of each menstrual cycle. Eggs stop maturing as the ovaries stop functioning during perimenopause, which usually occurs between the ages of 45 and 55. After menopause, the ovaries shrink from the size of large grapes to the size of small peas.

Near the beginning of the monthly menstrual cycle, the ovaries increase their production of estrogen. This causes the walls of the uterus to begin building up an extra lining of cells and blood vessels in preparation for pregnancy. The release of an egg—ovulation—happens sometime in the middle of a menstrual cycle. Typically, the two ovaries alternate from one month to the next in performing ovulation. The ovary that releases the egg also releases progesterone, which maintains the thickened uterine lining.

Pregnancy occurs if the egg is fertilized by a sperm cell, which usually happens in a fallopian tube, one of two tubes that lead from the ovaries to the uterus. The fertilized egg implants itself into the uterine wall, where it develops into an embryo. If pregnancy does not occur, the ovary stops producing progesterone, leading to the discharge of the unfertilized egg and extra uterine lining through the vagina.

A number of diseases can affect the ovaries, including cancer, cysts, polycystic ovary syndrome, and premature ovarian failure. Ovarian cancer, which is most common in women older than sixty, is a serious sometimes hereditary disease that often goes undiagnosed until after it has spread to other parts of the body. Most women do not suspect the disease because of the lack of early symptoms or the resemblance of early symptoms to other conditions. Such symptoms include abdominal discomfort and bloating, loss of appetite, and frequent vaginal bleeding. A definitive diagnosis is obtained through the combination of a blood test, which reveals elevated levels of a protein called CA-125, and a biopsy, in which ovarian tissue is examined under a microscope. Treatment usually consists of chemotherapy (medications) and surgical removal of the ovaries and nearby tissues, sometimes including the uterus and fallopian tubes. Treatment for ovarian cancer is more successful the earlier it is diagnosed. If patients are diagnosed and treated before the cancer spreads beyond the ovaries, the five-year survival rate is about 90 percent. However, the average five-year survival rate for women with ovarian cancer is only about 44 percent.

Ovarian cysts are fluid-filled sacs that grow on the organs. They are common and usually harmless, often disappearing after a few menstrual cycles. However, large cysts may cause pain in the abdomen, lower back, and thighs and interfere with blood supply to the ovaries. Some cysts can develop into cancer. Problematic cysts can be surgically removed.

Polycystic ovary syndrome is a painful condition usually caused by an overproduction of testosterone by the ovaries or adrenal glands. This condition, which is most common in obese women, may include the growth of several ovarian cysts, hair growth on the face and body, irregular menstruation, and infertility. These symptoms can be managed and reduced with certain medications.

In premature ovarian failure, the ovaries stop functioning before the normal onset of menopause, causing infertility. Some cases are an adverse effect of medications, surgery, or radiation, while other cases are caused by certain diseases or other factors. Some whose ovaries have stopped functioning can still become pregnant through the use of donor eggs.

A. J. Smuskiewicz

See also: Fertility; Infertility; Menstruation; Oophorectomy; Ova; Ova Donation; Ovarian Cancer; Ovulation; Polycystic Ovary Syndrome (PCOS).

Further Reading

Friedman, S., Sutphen, R., Steligo, K., & Greene, M. H. (2012). *Confronting hereditary breast and ovarian cancer: Identify your risk, understand your options, change your destiny.* Baltimore: Johns Hopkins University Press.

Vliet, E. L. (2003). *It's my ovaries, stupid.* New York: Scribner.

Ovulation

Ovulation is the release of a mature ovum (egg cell) from an ovary. This release normally happens once a month during the middle of the menstrual cycle of a woman in her childbearing years, which typically last from approximately her early teens to her late forties.

The released egg travels down the fallopian tube, which connects the ovary to the uterus. If the egg is fertilized by a sperm cell, most often within the fallopian tube, pregnancy results, and the egg implants itself into the wall of the uterus, which has developed an extra lining of cells and blood vessels to support the growth of the embryo. Implantation usually occurs six to twelve days after ovulation. If the egg is not fertilized, it disintegrates into the thickened uterine lining, which is discharged through the vagina as menstrual bleeding (the "period").

At birth, the two ovaries contain a total of about eight hundred thousand immature eggs. At puberty, the eggs begin to mature. Ovulation tends to happen from one ovary one month and the other ovary the next month at roughly the same day each month, though the precise day of ovulation may vary over time. The monthly maturing of eggs is triggered by the release of follicle-stimulating hormone by the pituitary gland. That hormone activates cellular structures inside the ovary called follicles, which contain immature eggs. A few of these eggs begin to mature. Then, luteinizing hormone secreted by the pituitary gland causes one mature egg to move out of the ovary and into the fallopian tube.

Ovulation happens sometime between the eleventh and twenty-first day of the menstrual cycle (counting from the first day of the last period), with an average ovulation time at the fourteenth day of the cycle. An egg can survive—and be available for fertilization—for twelve to twenty-four hours after ovulation.

It is possible to track the likely time of ovulation in a number of ways, including using a basal thermometer and examining the cervical mucus. A basal thermometer is designed to measure tiny changes in body temperature inside the mouth at the same time every day. A temperature spike indicates that ovulation occurred two or three days earlier. Charting these spikes for a few months can help to create an accurate prediction of ovulation times. Cervical mucus—which can be checked by inserting a finger into the vagina—typically changes from a cloudy, sticky fluid to a clear, slippery fluid resembling raw egg white a few days before ovulation. The last day that the cervical fluid has such a clear appearance is usually the day that pregnancy is most likely to occur—the day before, or the day of, ovulation. There are also special kits and monitors that can be purchased to help track ovulation.

The regularity of the ovulation cycle—and of the menstrual period—can be upset by a number of factors, including illness, stress, excess exercise, alcohol or drug abuse, and even a change in normal daily routines. Ovulation problems are common causes of infertility and are sometimes related to malfunctions of the pituitary gland or other glands that result in abnormal hormone levels. For example, ovulation will not happen if the pituitary gland does not produce enough follicle-stimulating hormone or luteinizing hormone. Polycystic ovarian syndrome results in ovulation problems and infertility when the ovaries or adrenal glands produce too much testosterone.

Certain medications, such as clomiphene citrate, can be used to induce ovulation in women who experience irregularities with their cycles. However, some women with ovulation problems may need to use assisted reproductive technologies, such as in vitro fertilization or donor eggs, if they wish to become pregnant.

A. J. Smuskiewicz

See also: Cervical Mucus Method; Fallopian Tubes; Fertility; Fertility Drugs; Follicle-Stimulating Hormone; Infertility; Luteinizing Hormone; Menstruation; Ova; Ovaries.

Further Reading

American Pregnancy Association. (2019). Understanding ovulation. Retrieved from https://americanpregnancy.org/getting-pregnant/understanding-ovulation/

Rebar, R. W. (2019). Problems with ovulation. Retrieved from https://www.msdmanuals.com/en-gb/home/women-s-health-issues/infertility/problems-with-ovulation

Weschler, T. (2006). *Taking charge of your fertility: The definitive guide to natural birth control, pregnancy achievement, and reproductive health* (10th Anniversary Ed.). New York: HarperCollins.

Oxytocin

Oxytocin, also called alpha-hypophamine, is a hormone produced in the brain by the hypothalamus, especially the paraventricular nucleus, and by reproductive tissues. Hypothalamic oxytocin is stored and secreted by the posterior pituitary gland. Oxytocin circulates in the blood and binds to receptors in the amygdala and in reproductive tissues. It is associated with sexual, pair, and group bonding; identity formation; and parental and social behaviors. Synthetic oxytocin is an obstetric and psychiatric drug.

The corpus luteum, uterus, ovaries, and placenta in females, and the penis, epididymis, vas deferens, testes, and prostate in males, also produce and secrete oxytocin. Female receptors are concentrated in the uterus and breasts, multiply during pregnancy, and reach their greatest number during labor, even if preterm. Oxytocin production is a positive feedback cycle: rising levels stimulate further production and receptor growth. Oxytocin works in association with estrogen, progesterone, and prolactin.

Milk letdown is the only reproductive function that definitively requires oxytocin, but many functions are strongly associated with it, including orgasm, testosterone production, ejaculation, and sperm transport through the male reproductive tract, uterus, and fallopian tubes; corpus luteum shrinkage following ovulation; prostaglandin production, uterine contraction, and fetal and placental expulsion during birth; postbirth uterine shrinkage and hemorrhage prevention; and initiation of maternal nurturing following birth or upon encountering unfamiliar young. Oxytocin from the mother enters the fetal brain during labor, where it reduces cortical activity, lowering physical and neurological arousal. This may protect against perinatal hypoxia. Oxytocin in the infant is associated with recognition of and bonding to the mother and initiation of breastfeeding.

Maternal oxytocin levels during pregnancy and the postpartum period influence bonding behaviors by mothers with their infants. Levels in infancy influence later social responses and parental behaviors. Early-infancy deprivation of reciprocal affection changes oxytocin levels and is associated with trouble forming secure attachments in later childhood.

Oxytocin facilitates prosocial behaviors and responses, including pair bonding, sexual arousal and receptivity, trust, individual recognition, and recognition of and response to facial expressions and social cues. It reduces fear responses and threat reactions and may prevent fight-or-flight reactions during labor and birth. It is also associated with satiety, appetite suppression, and addictive behaviors.

Levels rise under both pleasant and stressful social conditions. High levels associated with isolation and partnership stress may motivate individuals to seek more pleasant interactions. Rises in association with cortisol may moderate stress-induced depression, anxiety, and cardiac response.

Oxytocin administration increases trusting behaviors but only in the absence of threatening social cues. Administration to persons in monogamous relationships increases physical distance between the pair-bonded individual and sexually attractive nonpartners. Genetic variation in oxytocin receptors is associated with differing individual responses to betrayal. Elevation in males is associated with empathy and protection of children. Oxytocin is also associated with group-favoring and cohesion behaviors, even when such behaviors are otherwise antisocial or unethical.

Pitocin, syntocinon, and carbetocin are pharmaceutical oxytocin. They are given by injection, intravenous drip, or nasal spray for labor induction, contraction stimulation, and uterine bleeding control and shrinkage. They also encourage lactation. Oxytocin treatment appears to enhance social cue, emotion, and facial expression recognition in autistic persons and in patients coping with depression, social anxiety, and schizophrenia.

Excess oxytocin in men is associated with benign prostate gland enlargement. Lack of oxytocin receptors in the brain is one feature of Prader-Willi syndrome.

Angela Libal

See also: Attachment Theory of Love; Benign Prostatic Hyperplasia; Intimacy, Sexual and Relational; Orgasm; Ovulation; Sex Hormones.

Further Reading

DeAngelis, T. (2008). The two faces of oxytocin. *American Psychological Association Monitor on Psychology, 39*(2). Retrieved from http://www.apa.org/monitor/feb08/oxytocin.aspx

Martin, R. D. (2015). Oxytocin: The multitasking love hormone. *Psychology Today.* Retrieved from https://www.psychologytoday.com/blog/how-we-do-it/201505/oxytocin-the-multitasking-love-hormone

P

Pansexuality

Pansexuality is a sexual orientation involving sexual or romantic attraction to all sexes and genders or sexual and romantic attraction to individuals that is not dependent on sex and gender. Other features, such as personality, intelligence, or physical appearance are still important in facilitating attraction to specific romantic or sexual partners. Pansexual people themselves may be of any gender or sex.

Pansexual individuals are heterogeneous and describe their sexuality in a variety of ways. One commonly reported experience is where the person's attraction is toward another person's features or traits regardless of the other person's gender or sex and that their sexual orientation transcends genders, sexes, and bodily features (such as male or female genitals). Another commonly reported experience is where the person can experience attraction toward men, women, and nonbinary genders and sexes and that the person can be attracted to all configurations of bodies (including genitals) and identities. A differentiation is sometimes made between being "panromantic" (romantic attraction regardless of gender and sex) and "pansexual" (physical attraction toward all sexes and genders). Individuals may report being romantically attracted to all genders and sexes but sexually attracted to only one or vice versa. Some pansexual individuals report a relative preference for one gender or sex over others despite experiencing attraction to all genders and sexes. Fluidity in sexual orientation, and nonidentification or rejection of existing labels and paradigms, are also commonly reported among pansexual individuals. Identification with a nonbinary gender identity (e.g., "agender") and identification with more than one gender identity are also common in some pansexual samples.

Pansexual individuals generally report that their ability and willingness to be attracted to all sexes and genders is the most important aspect of their identification with this sexual orientation. Previous sexual experiences and making a political statement (e.g., regarding the binary and nonbinary nature of gender) are reported as being much less important. Despite the capacity for attraction to any gender or sex, pansexual individuals are not uniformly attracted to everyone; qualities that are important for attraction in other orientations (e.g., personality, intelligence, physical appearance, shared experiences and values) are also important here. Pansexual individuals, like people of other orientations, vary in how choosy or selective they are about their partners and their interest in long-term committed relationships. Pansexuality also does not necessarily imply higher levels of sexual arousal or desire, greater promiscuity or interest in casual sex, or engagement in polygamy or polyamory.

Pansexuality is generally seen within the umbrella of plurisexuality or polysexuality, as it involves the capacity for attraction to more than one specific gender or sex. This is in contrast to monosexuality (e.g., gay, lesbian, straight, heterosexuality, homosexuality), where capacity for attraction is focused primarily on a single gender or sex. Bisexuality is the most well-known orientation within the broader plurisexuality category.

Pansexuality is often described as rejecting a binary understanding of sex or gender in contrast to bisexuality, which operates within that binary. However, it should be noted that bisexual individuals do not always see a binary understanding of gender as being important to their orientation. Some pansexual individuals also report bisexual as a suitable alternative description of their orientation. Other pansexual individuals report identifying as bisexual out of convenience in some contexts, such as where "pansexual" would not be easily understood by others or would require burdensome explanation. "Queer" and similar terms are also alternative ways some pansexual individuals identify themselves, often to capture both their sexual orientation and gender identity in one term.

Pansexual individuals may face discrimination outside and inside of LGBT communities. Pansexual individuals can experience prejudice from a position of heteronormativity (where heterosexuality is seen as the default or only acceptable form of sexual and romantic attraction for all individuals) due to having same-sex/gender attractions. Pansexual individuals can also experience ostracism from a position of homonormativity (where homosexuality is seen as the default or only acceptable form of sexual and romantic attraction for nonheterosexual individuals). Pansexual individuals report that they are often seen as gay or lesbian individuals who want to maintain straight privilege or are too scared to come out or as straight individuals who want to identify with LGBT groups or engage in indiscriminate sexual activity when intoxicated or disinhibited. Prejudice can also be targeted against promiscuity or polyamory and polygamy behaviors that may be (often inaccurately) ascribed to pansexual individuals.

Some researchers have used a "borderlands" model to understand pansexuality. Here, pansexuality is seen as one identity of many that emerge from the experiences of people who do not fall within the "borders" of traditional heteronormative and homonormative frameworks. Pansexuality, therefore, like all "borderlands" identities, is necessarily diverse, heterogeneous, and with fuzzy boundaries. It forms from individuals trying to construct personal meaning through adoption and rejection of elements from the multiple dominant paradigms that they are exposed to but do not fully identify with.

Nevertheless, a precise and empirically supported theory for the etiology and development of pansexuality specifically, or plurisexual orientations in general, remains to be established. Existing research into pansexual individuals has largely focused on young, postsecondary educated, and primarily Anglo, white, or European samples. Information collected using anonymous online self-report methods are most common. Further research is needed to understand if pansexual identities or experiences are applicable to individuals in other populations and settings.

Silvain S. Dang

See also: Binary Gender System; Bisexuality; Fluidity, Gender; Fluidity, Sexual; LGBTQ+; Nonbinary Gender Identities; Queer; Romantic Attraction and Orientation; Sexual Orientation.

Further Reading

Callis, A. S. (2014). Bisexual, pansexual, queer: Non-binary identities and the sexual borderlands. *Sexualities, 17*, 63–80.

Flanders, C. E., LeBreton, M. E., Robinson, M., Bian, J., & Caravaca-Morera, J. A. (2017). Defining bisexuality: Young bisexual and pansexual people's voices. *Journal of Bisexuality, 17*(1), 39–57.

Galupo, M. P., Ramirez, J. L., & Pulice-Farrow, L. (2017). "Regardless of their gender": Descriptions of sexual identity among bisexual, pansexual, and queer identified individuals. *Journal of Bisexuality, 17*(1), 108–124.

Gonel, A. H. (2013). Pansexual identification in online communities: Employing a collaborative queer method to study pansexuality. *Graduate Journal of Social Sciences, 10*(1), 36–59.

Pap Smear

The Pap test or Pap smear was developed by Dr. George Papanicolaou (for whom it was named, the official name being the Papanicolaou test) and is used today as a screening test for cervical and anal cancer caused by the sexually transmitted infection human papillomavirus (HPV).

The ideal timing for a cervical Pap smear is midcycle, between ten and twenty days after the first day of the previous period. Before the Pap smear, any intravaginal activity (sex, douching, medications, etc.) should be avoided for two days prior to the test. A metal or plastic speculum is inserted into the vagina in order to allow a good view of the cervix. A sample of cells is gently scraped from the inner and outer parts of the cervix using a thin wooden or plastic spatula or brush. An anal Pap test is similar in that a thin swab is inserted into the anus, which is then used to collect anal cells. These specimens are either placed on a slide and chemically fixed for examination under a microscope, or they are placed in a solution and transported to the lab for preparation there (this liquid-based method is currently much more common and felt to be more accurate). Using the liquid-based method also allows for testing for HPV if this is indicated. If the cells appear abnormal, further testing and treatment depends on the results of the HPV test and the degree and type of abnormality found.

Current American Cancer Society guidelines for screening recommend that a person with a cervix receive their first Pap test by age twenty-one, or within three years of becoming sexually active, whichever is first. A Pap test should be done at least every two years (depending on whether a liquid-based method or traditional slide method is used) through age thirty. Certain risks would require that a Pap test is done every year, including some previously abnormal results, human immunodeficiency virus infection, or decreased immunity. If there are no previous abnormal results, some may receive a Pap only every three years until age seventy. After that time, if there has not had an abnormal result within the previous ten years, it may be decided to stop doing Pap tests. However, if a hysterectomy has been done due to cervical cancer or dysplasia (abnormal Pap test results), a yearly Pap test is recommended as long as the person is in good health.

Currently, there is no consistent guidance on frequency or need for regular anal Pap tests. If someone is regularly engaging in receptive anal intercourse, they should speak with their health care provider about the possibility of HPV screening.

The Pap test has proven to be the most successful cancer screening and prevention test in modern medicine. According to the Centers for Disease Control and Prevention and National Institutes of Health, cervical cancer was the leading cause of cancer death in women in the United States during the early and mid-twentieth century. The Pap test became a part of routine health care in the United States during the 1950s. From 1955 to the early 1990s, cervical cancer deaths in the Unites States decreased by more than 60 percent, and it is now the fourteenth most frequent cancer in women. In 2009, slightly more than 11,000 cases of cervical cancer were diagnosed in the United States, with about 4,000 deaths annually. An additional 44,000 cases of high-grade cervical abnormality were diagnosed. However, it is important to note that more than 55 million Pap tests are performed in the United States every year, and roughly 3.5 million of these tests will require medical follow-up. Clearly, the vast majority of these abnormal Pap tests are not full-blown cancer, and many require only repeat Pap testing (without additional treatment).

In countries where the Pap test is not part of routine health screening, cervical cancer continues to be a significant public health crisis. Worldwide, cervical cancer continues to be the third most common cancer in women and the second most common cause of cancer-related deaths. Early diagnosis made possible by Papanicolaou's research has made prevention of cervical cancer a reality for women who have access to regular Pap tests. It has also provided a framework for cellular diagnosis of many types of cancer. Papanicolaou's test has saved the lives of countless women, but much work continues in order to provide this low-cost, life-saving test to women who have limited access to health care.

Anne M. Fogle

See also: Cervical Cancer; Genital Warts; Human Papillomavirus (HPV); Obstetrics and Gynecology.

Further Reading

American College of Obstetricians and Gynecologists. (2019). Pap smear (Pap test): Resource overview. Retrieved from https://www.acog.org/Womens-Health/Pap-Smear-Pap-Test

Anal Cancer Foundation. (2019). About HPV/HPV & cancer. Retrieved from https://www.analcancerfoundation.org/about-hpv/hpv-cancer/

Centers for Disease Control and Prevention. (2019). Human papillomavirus (HPV). Retrieved from https://www.cdc.gov/hpv/

Centers for Disease Control and Prevention. (2019). HPV vaccine schedule and dosing. Retrieved from https://www.cdc.gov/hpv/hcp/schedules-recommendations.html

Office on Women's Health. (2019). Human papillomavirus. Retrieved from https://www.womenshealth.gov/a-z-topics/human-papillomavirus

University of Wisconsin Hospitals and Clinics Authority. (2016). HPV and anal Pap testing. Retrieved from https://www.uwhealth.org/healthfacts/diagnostic-tests/7056.pdf

Paraphilias

In 1903, Friedrich Salomo Krauss (1859–1938) devised the term "paraphilias," derived from the Greek word "para" meaning "beside, aside" and "philos" meaning "loving." The term "paraphilia" was not commonly used, however, until the 1950s. Paraphilia replaced the terms "perversion" and "sexual deviation" in the third edition of the *Diagnostic and Statistical Manual of Mental Disorders* (*DSM*) in 1980. Today, paraphilias are described as sexual interests outside of interest in genital stimulation or foreplay with a mature consenting adult. Paraphilias are persistent and strong but not necessarily problematic. An important distinction was made in the fifth edition of *DSM* (*DSM-5*; 2013) between paraphilias and paraphilic disorder. For a paraphilia to be considered a disorder, it must cause distress or functional impairment to the individual or result in harm to the self or others. A paraphilia by itself does not equate to a mental health disorder, and many individuals have sexual preferences that can be considered paraphilic (e.g., foot fetish, lingerie, bondage). As long as the preferences do not cause distress or functional impairment, the individual and the practices should not be pathologized.

Paraphilias are classified as their own subset of disorders within the category of paraphilic disorders in the *DSM-5*. Dozens of paraphilias have been identified and linked to paraphilic disorders; however, the *DSM-5* only classifies the most commonly occurring and destructive in terms of legal ramifications. Eight paraphilic disorders are identified in the *DSM-5*, although "other specified paraphilic disorder" and "unspecified paraphilic disorder" are available for clinical use if one of the eight identified paraphilias is not appropriate. For an individual to meet criteria for a paraphilic disorder, the urges, desires, or behaviors must have been present for an estimated period of six months and must cause significant personal distress or cause harm to the self or others.

Paraphilias are divided into two subsets: erotic targets or erotic activities. Erotic targets refer to a sexual desire directed toward a specific group or subset. These targets may be human or other. Pedophilic disorder, or when an individual at least sixteen years old is attracted to a prepubescent child at least five years younger, is an example of a human erotic target. The individual may or may not have acted on their sexual urges and may or may not be attracted to both children and adults. Rates of pedophilic disorder are unknown in women but estimated at 3–5 percent among men. Nonhuman, or other, erotic targets may include fetishistic disorder or tranvestic disorder. Fetishistic disorder is diagnosed when an individual derives sexual pleasure from nonliving objects (e.g., socks, undergarments) or nongenital parts of the body (e.g., feet, hair) through urges, behaviors, or desires. This disorder occurs almost exclusively in men, although lifetime prevalence rates are unknown. Transvestic disorder is described as sexual arousal from dressing as the other gender. This disorder may be present with fetishistic disorder if the individual is sexually aroused by the specific clothing items. Transvestic disorder is specified to occur with autogynephilia if a male individual derives sexual pleasure from imaging himself as a female. This is different and should not be confused with gender dysphoria, or when an individual feels a continuous disconnect between their gender identity and biological sex. Transvestic disorder occurs more frequently in males than females and is estimated at 3 percent among men.

The second subset of paraphilic disorders is related to erotic activities, or when sexual desire is related to a sexual act from which an individual derives pleasure. This subset is divided into courtship disorders and algolagnic disorders. Courtship disorders describe paraphilic disorders with inaccurate and exaggerated aspects of human relationships. For example, voyeuristic disorder is when an individual at least eighteen years of age derives sexual arousal from watching an unknowing person who is naked, undressing, or participating in intimate acts. Estimated prevalence rates indicate that 12 percent of males experience this disorder, and it is less common in women. Exhibitionistic disorder is when an individual derives sexual pleasure from genital exposure to nonconsenting people. Lifetime estimated prevalence rate for exhibitionistic disorder in men is 2–4 percent and occurs less commonly in women. Frotteuristic disorders occur when an individual derives pleasure from touching a nonconsenting individual. Estimated population prevalence is unknown, but research indicates that approximately 30 percent of men will engage in at least one frotteuristic act in their lifetime.

Algolagnic disorders are paraphilic disorders related to pain and suffering of oneself or another person. Sexual masochism disorder is when an individual derives pleasure from enduring the infliction of pain from another. Sexual sadism disorder is when an individual derives sexual pleasure from inflicting suffering on another person. For it to be considered a paraphilic disorder, the individual must be distressed by the arousal or must inflict suffering on a nonconsenting individual.

Lauren G. Masuda and Stephen K. Trapp

See also: BDSM; Exhibitionism; Fetishism; Frotteurism; Kink; Pedophilia; Transvestite; Voyeurism.

Further Reading

American Psychiatric Association. (2013). *Diagnostic and statistical manual of mental disorders* (5th ed.). Washington, DC: Author.

Beech, A. R., Miner, M. H., & Thornton, D. (2016). Paraphilias in the DSM-5. *Annual Review of Clinical Psychology, 12*, 383–406.

Passing

The concept of "passing" has existed in transgender communities for decades, and the origin of the term is unclear. Generally, to "pass" means to be perceived as a cisgender (i.e., nontrans) person of the trans person's gender. *Trans Bodies, Trans Selves* also defines passing as "the ability to present our gender in such a way that we are consistently seen as our correct gender identity" (Erickson-Schroth, 2014).

That is, if a trans woman is perceived by others to be a cis woman, she can be understood to be passing. The politics of passing have shifted throughout time as the context in which trans individuals live has also shifted. For some, it might be a personal desire or choice to strive to "pass," while for others it might be necessary to live safely in their community.

Passing is a concept often applied to transgender individuals but can also be understood in other contexts—to be perceived as an identity one is not currently or has not always been. To "pass" as a (cis) man implies that one is not genuinely a man, for example. Passing may also be applied to a racial or disability context—to pass as white or able-bodied when one is not. In any of these contexts, passing might be something a person intentionally strives for, or it might be how they are unintentionally perceived by others.

Passing can be understood to be about one's gender expression and, more pointedly, the perception of one's gender rather than one's actual gender. Trans individuals whose gender expression does not align to societal expectations of their gender might be less likely to pass. This might include butch or masculine trans women, femme or feminine trans women, and androgynous trans people of all genders. If a trans man's gender expression does not fall into societal expectations of what a man "should" look like, he might be less likely to be perceived as a "real" or cis man. These individuals may also be referred to as "gender nonconforming".

Passing as a cis person is not the goal of every trans individual. For those who do strive to pass, it might be a choice made because that is how they can most authentically and fully live their lives *or* it might be a choice made for their own physical safety. Being spotted as a trans person (also called being "clocked" or "spooked") can be dangerous for trans individuals, whether it be at work, while on a date, or elsewhere. Trans people who are completely in the closet regarding being transgender, whether it is for safety, comfort, or other reasons, might be referred to as being "stealth" or simply remaining private about one's transgender status. Individuals who generally are regarded as passing may or may not also be stealth.

In the discussion of passing, nonbinary individuals are often left out. Some might also mistakenly assume that to "pass as nonbinary" means to have a completely androgynous gender expression. However, nonbinary individuals, like individuals of binary genders (i.e., men and women), can have any kind of gender expression—masculine, feminine, or other.

Some critique the concept of passing because of the implication of inauthenticity or deception. For trans women in particular, this can put their lives in danger if potential partners "discover" they are transgender, believe they have been deceived by the trans woman, and react violently. The concept of passing might also be seen as implying trans women are not "real" or authentic women, for example, as they are *merely passing* as women. Erickson-Schroth also points out that some "trans youth feel astounding pressure to prove [they] can fit into preexisting gender categories in our society and to prove [they] can live up to the standard of a 'real' man or woman, even among other trans youth."

Vern Harner

See also: Gender; Gender Expression; Gender Transition; Outing; Pronoun Usage; Transgender.

Further Reading

Erickson-Schroth, L. (2014). *Trans bodies, trans selves: A resource for the transgender community.* New York: Oxford University Press.

Pedophilia

Pedophilia is defined as a sexual attraction to children who are prepubescent, generally ages thirteen and younger, and is considered a paraphilia. For individuals who are sexually attracted to children who have started puberty, the term "hebephilia" should be used. It is also important to know that pedophilia labels the attraction and does not mean that a crime has been committed. If a crime has been committed, these individuals may be referred to as sex offenders, and while sex offenders can be diagnosed as pedophiles, not all pedophiles are sex offenders. Pedophilia means that people have thoughts and fantasies about and are sexually attracted to minors, but not all pedophiles have acted on these urges. It is estimated that 50 percent or less of the offender population are individuals with pedophilia.

"Pedophilia" was the diagnostic term previously used by the *Diagnostic and Statistical Manual of Mental Disorders* (*DSM*) published by American Psychiatric Association; however, in the latest version, *DSM-5*, it has been renamed as a pedophilic disorder and is classified under paraphilia disorders. Paraphilias are defined as "any intense and resistant sexual interest other than sexual interest in genital simulation or preparatory fondling with phenotypically normal, physiologically mature, consenting human partners" (American Psychiatric Association, 2013). Paraphilias may be experienced as recurrent urges, unusual fantasies, or atypical behaviors that are sexually arousing. In order for a paraphilia to be diagnosed as a paraphilic disorder, the individual must feel personal distress about their atypical sexual interest; have a sexual attraction that causes another psychological distress, injury, or death; or have sexual behaviors that involve an unwilling participant or a participant who is unable to give consent. The thoughts, behaviors, or urges must also be present for at least six months to be diagnosed, and in the case of pedophilic disorder, the individual must be at least sixteen years of age and more than five years older than the child(ren) in the fantasies. An individual with paraphilic disorder also has a higher rate of comorbidity with other mental health diagnoses, such as anxiety, depression, mood disorders, and substance abuse.

Individuals with pedophilic attraction usually suffer from extreme distress and have social impairments as well as difficulties holding a job. They typically have repeated strong sexual fantasies, urges, or behaviors and may have trouble finding satisfaction in relationships with other adults. They often suffer from low self-esteem, and their attraction to children may dominate their life and may lead them to live in fear and isolation.

There is no clear cause of pedophilia. Some research has suggested there may be biological factors associated with pedophilia, but this research is still new and not certain. There has also been research that shows that often individuals with pedophilic disorder have been sexually abused themselves during their childhood (*Psychology Today*, 2019), but this is not to be seen as a clear correlation. The majority of pedophiles are male, and it is very rare for females to be diagnosed with pedophilic disorder.

There are a few different types of treatment for pedophilia. Behavioral and cognitive therapy, either as outpatient or inpatient therapy, are often used and focus on empathy training and restructuring of distorted or deviant thought patterns. These types of therapy help individuals to focus on the feelings of the victims and to understand how their actions could harm their victims Therapy also helps individuals to understand why their thought processes could lead to personal trouble, and it tries to help them understand their deviant thoughts. Medications are also sometimes used in conjunction with therapy. Antiandrogens, medroxyprogesterone acetate, and leuprolide acetate can be used to help lower an individual's sex drive. A selective serotonin reuptake inhibitor may also be prescribed to treat compulsive sexual disorders and any comorbid mood disorders.

Amanda Baker

See also: Child Sexual Abuse; *Diagnostic and Statistical Manual of Mental Disorders* (*DSM*); Paraphilias; Sexual Abuse.

Further Reading

American Psychiatric Association. (2013). *Diagnostic and statistical manual of mental disorders: DSM-5*. Washington, DC: American Psychiatric Association.

Jahnke, S., & Hoyer, J. (2013). Stigmatization of people with pedophilia: A blind spot in stigma research. *International Journal of Sexual Health, 25*, 169–184.

Psychology Today. (2019). Pedophilia. Retrieved from https://www.psychologytoday.com/conditions/pedophilia

Virtuous Pedophiles. (2019). FAQ. Retrieved from http://www.virped.org/index.php/f-a-q

WebMD. (2012). What is pedophilia? Retrieved from http://www.webmd.com/mental-health/features/explaining-pedophilia

Pelvic Floor Muscles

The pelvic floor muscles are several muscles at the bottom of the pelvis that help support the organs of the pelvis. These organs include the large intestine, bladder, and uterus. The pelvic floor muscles also play an important role in control over urinary and bowel movements. Damage to the pelvic floor muscles, or a lack of muscle tone, can result in urinary or fecal incontinence and the prolapse of organs in the pelvis. The muscles can be strengthened by certain exercises or by surgery in extreme cases.

The major pelvic floor muscles include the levator ani and the coccygeus muscle. The associated fascia and connective tissue that help define the muscles are also usually considered part of the pelvic floor. The total group of muscles and tissues are sometimes called the "pelvic diaphragm," and the term may be used interchangeably with "pelvic floor." Small openings in the muscles allow the urethra, the anal canal, and the vagina to pass through the pelvic floor.

All people have pelvic floor muscles, and their main function is to support the organs located in the pelvic cavity. The muscles also play an important role in controlling the release of urine, feces, and flatulence. When the pelvic floor muscles tighten up, the internal organs are raised and sphincter muscles tighten the openings of the vagina, urethra, and anus. When the muscles relax, the sphincter muscles also relax, allowing urine and feces to pass through. The pelvic floor muscles also help to push these substances out of the body. Good muscle tone of these muscles can also improve sexual intercourse and satisfaction.

Pelvic floor muscles can suffer disorders when they become weak or damaged. The most important problems are urinary and fecal incontinence, in which a person loses control over their bladder and bowels, respectively. The other major problem associated with the pelvic floor muscles is pelvic organ prolapse, in which the organs drop down. In females, the organs may press against the vagina, while males more often suffer from pressure against the anal canal. In the latter case, the person can suffer from constipation as a result. If the pelvic floor muscles are very tight, sexual intercourse can be painful or even impossible.

Causes of pelvic floor muscle problems range from heavy lifting to high-impact exercise to other underlying medical conditions. Age, chronic coughing, and chronic constipation can also reduce muscle tone. Among women, the most common causes of problems are pregnancy and childbirth. Both events can cause damage to nerves controlling the pelvic floor muscles or even damage the muscles themselves.

Exercises can help strengthen the pelvic floor muscles. Known as Kegel exercises, the most common is a series of contracting and relaxing the muscles. Many people have difficulty isolating the pelvic floor muscles, so experts recommend working with a physical therapist and getting biofeedback to ensure that the exercises are being done correctly.

Tim J. Watts

See also: Dyspareunia; Kegel Exercises; Vaginismus; Vulvodynia.

Further Reading

National Institutes of Health. (2019). Pelvic floor muscle training exercises. Retrieved from http://www.nlm.nih.gov/medlineplus/ency/article/003975.htm

University of Chicago Medical Center. (2019). Pelvic floor disorders. Retrieved from https://www.uchicagomedicine.org/conditions-services/pelvic-health/pelvic-floor-disorders

Pelvic Inflammatory Disease (PID)

Pelvic inflammatory disease (PID) is an infection or inflammation in the upper genital area of a woman. This disease is received through the cavities of the cervix, uterus, fallopian tubes, and surrounding areas, ultimately affecting the endometrium, which is the lining of the uterus. During the 1960s, PID occurred more frequently in women who were infected with gonorrhea. In a twenty-year time frame, 20 percent of women who were diagnosed with gonorrhea developed PID. During the 1980s, an even larger development was discovered. Among women with PID, over 40 percent of cases were caused by chlamydia. In women under twenty-five years of age, the percentage was even higher, with 60–80 percent of cases being attributed to chlamydia. Among all women, more than half of PID cases are caused by *Chlamydia trachomatis* and *Neisseria gonorrhoeae*; in some cases, both these sexually transmitted infections are present

In 2001, more than 750,000 cases of PID were discovered in the United States. However, over the past two decades in North America and western Europe, PID has declined because of increased attempts to control *Chlamydia trachomatis* and *Neisseria gonorrhoeae*. Regardless of the progress, PID is still a poorly controlled disease.

The most commonly used outpatient method of treatment for PID is antibiotics that cover a broad spectrum of pathogens, as recommended by the guidelines of the Centers for Disease Control and Prevention. The antibiotics may include ofloxacin, levofloxacin, ceftriaxone plus doxycycline, or cefoxitin and probenecid plus doxycycline, all with optional chemical compounds for treating infections for full coverage against anaerobes and bacterial vaginosis.

Another efficient way to treat PID is to be admitted into a hospital for treatment by a doctor and other medical personnel. The "gold standard" for diagnosis is laparoscopy, which is costly, invasive, and impractical in a general practice setting. A laparoscopy is an internal abdominal examination. The outpatient method of treatment is the most commonly used method because the disease is often unnoticeable, and patients commonly treat themselves.

Some common symptoms associated with PID are discomfort and pain in the lower abdomen, vaginal bleeding, vaginal discharge, and painful intercourse. Some signs associated with PID are cervical lesions, tenderness in the abdominal area, high temperature, uterine masses, and uterine tenderness. There is no specific diagnosis, nor is there a laboratory test for PID. Women that delay seeking medical attention for PID are three times more likely to experience infertility or irregular pregnancy compared to women who sought immediate medical attention. Women with untreated PID are also more prone to developing other diseases, and PID may cause long-term reproductive disabilities.

The risk factors associated with PID are similar to those of other sexually transmitted infections. The most important risk factor is having chlamydia or gonorrhea. Other risks include smoking, sexual intercourse with numerous people, and not using barrier contraceptive methods like condoms.

Methods of preventing PID include practicing safer sex by using condoms, attending comprehensive sexual education classes, and being aware of sexually transmitted infections that lead to PID, especially chlamydia and gonorrhea. It is also possible to have multiple PID infections, as women who have previously had PID are more likely to be diagnosed with PID again if they have new sex partners and do not use condoms.

Reginald Barker

See also: Chlamydia; Gonorrhea; Infertility; Sexually Transmitted Infections (STIs).

Further Reading

Brunham, R. C., Gottlieb, S. L., & Paavonen, J. (2015). Pelvic inflammatory disease. *New England Journal of Medicine, 2015*(372), 2039–2048.

Haggerty, C. L., & Ness, R. B. (2007). Newest approaches to treatment of pelvic inflammatory disease: A review of recent randomized clinical trials. *Clinical Infectious Diseases, 44*(7), 953–960.

Hillis, S. D., Joesoef, R., Marchbanks, P. A., Wasserheit, J. N., Cates, W., & Westrom, L. (1993). Delayed care of pelvic inflammatory disease as a risk factor for impaired fertility. *American Journal of Obstetrics and Gynecology, 168*(5), 1503–1509.

McCormack, W. M. (1994). Pelvic inflammatory disease. *New England Journal of Medicine, 330*(2), 115–119.

Pearce, J. M. (1990). Pelvic inflammatory disease. *British Medical Journal, 300*(6732), 1090–1091.

Penile Cancer

Penile cancer is a cancer that can affect anyone who has a penis. It is relatively rare, especially among men in high-income countries like the United States. The prevalence of penile cancer is slightly higher among men from lower-income countries and can reach up to 10 percent of total cancer cases. Although it is a rare form of cancer, it has a high mortality. There are a variety of types of penile cancer and associated symptoms. There are also known risks associated with penile cancer and several strategies for prevention.

"Penile cancer" is an umbrella term used whenever cancer cells begin to develop on or in the penis. The most common type of penile cancer is squamous cell carcinoma (SCC) of the penis, which is present in 95 percent of penile cancer cases. Other types of penile cancer include melanoma, basal cell carcinoma, sarcoma, and adenocarcinoma; however, these types are even more rare. Thus, most of the research has been focused on the SCC cases. SCC cases can be categorized in four different ways: verrucous, papillary squamous, warty, and basaloid. The course of treatment is contingent on the type of penile cancer, size of the tumor, and the location of the tumor. Tumors can arise anywhere on the penis, meaning they can be on the surface of the skin (in situ) or invasive.

There are some common symptoms associated with penile cancer. Some of these symptoms include, but are not limited to, a lump on the penis, inflammation, a reddish rash, a sore that bleeds, small bumps, swelling, and flat growths. The previously listed symptoms can also be caused by infections or allergic reactions; thus, talking to a health care provider is recommended if any of these symptoms are present. Penile cancer is typically diagnosed after a health care provider conducts a diagnostic biopsy. Fortunately, there has recently been more attention drawn to these symptoms because the earlier the disease is found, the better. If the diagnosis is discovered at an early stage, there is a better chance of survival and recovery. There has also been work done to determine psychosocial factors that influence men's help-seeking behaviors when they identify symptoms.

Penile cancer is more prevalent among older men (typically sixty years and older), uncircumcised men, and men diagnosed with phimosis (when the foreskin cannot be pulled back). Some other recorded risks include poor penile hygiene, history of many sexual partners, and history of sexually transmitted infections. There have been several studies showing that human papillomavirus (HPV) and the human immunodeficiency virus have been associated with penile cancer. Lastly, tobacco use has been associated with penile cancer. Those who smoke cigarettes are at a higher risk of developing cancer, although how tobacco plays a role is still not clear. Although these are well-known risks, the disease may also be present in individuals who do not have these risks (i.e., circumcised, young, and nonsmokers).

As mentioned earlier, it is important to detect penile cancer as early as possible. If any symptoms are present, the individual must see a health care provider. The best way to prevent developing penile cancer is by practicing good genital hygiene, avoiding tobacco use, and avoiding sexually transmitted infections like HPV (i.e., having safer sex and using condoms). Research is still being conducted to learn more about penile cancer in hopes of lowering its prevalence and its morbidity rates.

Tori Peña

See also: Circumcision; Human Papillomavirus (HPV); Penis; Phimosis; Testicular Cancer.

Further Reading

Bleeker, M. C. G., Heideman, D. A. M., Snijders, P. J. F., Horenblas, S., Dillner, J., & Meijer, C. J. L. M. (2008). Penile cancer: Epidemiology, pathogenesis and prevention. *World Journal of Urology, 27*(2), 141.

Clark, P. E., Spiess, P. E., Agarwal, N., Biagioli, M. C., Eisenberger, M. A., Greenberg, R. E., … Ho, M. (2013). Penile cancer. *Journal of the National Comprehensive Cancer Network: JNCCN, 11*(5), 594–615.

Fish, J. A., Prichard, I., Ettridge, K., Grunfeld, E. A., & Wilson, C. (2015). Psychosocial factors that influence men's help-seeking for cancer symptoms: A systematic synthesis of mixed methods research. *Psycho-Oncology, 24*(10), 1222–1232.

Larke, N. L., Thomas, S. L., dos Santos Silva, I., & Weiss, H. A. (2011). Male circumcision and penile cancer: A systemic review and meta-analysis. *Cancer Causes & Control, 22*(8), 1097–1110.

Pizzocaro, G., Algaba, F., Horenblas, S., Solsona, E., Tana, S., Van Der Poel, H., & Watkin, N. A. (2010). EAU penile cancer guidelines 2009. *European Urology, 57*(6), 1002–1012.

Skeppner, E., Andersson, S.-O., Johansson, J.-E., & Windahl, T. (2012). Initial symptoms and delay in patients with penile carcinoma. *Scandinavian Journal of Urology and Nephrology, 46*(5), 319–325.

Tseng, H. F., Morgenstern, H., Mack, T., & Peters, R. K. (2001). Risk factors for penile cancer: Results of a population-based case-control study in Los Angeles County (United States). *Cancer Causes & Control, 12*(3), 267–277.

Penis

The penis is the primary male sex organ. Both urine and semen exit the body through the penis via the urethra. A number of medical conditions can affect the penis and may affect sexual function or the ability to urinate.

The head, or glans, of the penis is naturally covered with a foreskin, which may be surgically removed during circumcision. Two columns of tissue called the corpus cavernosa run along the sides of the penis. Blood vessels and small spaces in this tissue fill with blood to cause and maintain an erection. A column of tissue called the corpus spongiosum, running through the central region of the penis, houses the urethra. Nerves are spread throughout the penis. The nerves are highly sensitive, especially to stimulation during sexual experiences.

During puberty, the penis grows to its mature length and girth and becomes fully sexually functional. This growth coincides with the sexual maturity of the scrotum and testicles and the development of pubic hair. The male genitals typically become fully mature sometime between the ages of thirteen and eighteen. Penis size is the result of genetic factors and has no relation to the individual's masculinity or sexual abilities.

When sexually aroused—either through physical touching or thoughts—the arousal stimulates nerves to prompt the production of a substance called nitric oxide. This chemical compound, in turn, stimulates a cascade of enzyme activity that causes arterial muscles in the penis to relax. Blood then flows into and fills the spaces of the corpus cavernosa. As this happens, the penis becomes larger and firmer in preparation for sexual intercourse. Erections can happen outside of conscious awareness, particularly during sleep. Most young, sexually mature men have three to five erections during sleep. During a wet dream, an erection leads to ejaculation. Waking up with an erection is fairly common.

A number of structural and functional disorders can affect the penis. Erectile dysfunction is a relatively common condition that affects the function of the penis. In this condition, the penis is unable to produce or sustain an erection, usually because of insufficient blood flow resulting from arterial malfunction. The drug sildenafil and other phosphodiesterase inhibitors increase blood flow in the penis, allowing for a full and sustained erection. Testosterone injections may benefit some men with erectile dysfunction. Another structural condition, Peyronie's disease, is an abnormal curvature of the penis that may be caused by injury or other conditions during adulthood. Priapism is an abnormal, painful condition in which the penis remains erect for several hours—long after sexual arousal has ended. If this occurs, urgent medical attention is needed and injected drugs and various surgical procedures are options for correcting this condition.

Balanitis is inflammation of the glans, usually caused by an infection. Its symptoms include pain, tenderness, and redness. Urethritis is a painful inflammation and infection of the urethra, often associated with the sexually transmitted infections gonorrhea and chlamydia. Other sexually transmitted infections affecting the penis include syphilis, herpes, and penile warts. Most penile infections can be cured with antibiotics, though viral infections, such as herpes, require special antiviral medications to treat symptoms. Cancer of the penis is a rare condition, though it is more common in men who are uncircumcised.

Some males are born with defects of the penis. In hypospadias, the opening for urine elimination occurs on the underside of the penis instead of on the tip. In chordee, the end of the penis has an abnormal curvature, which may interfere with urinary or sexual function. Surgery is necessary to correct these birth defects.

Phimosis occurs if the foreskin covering an uncircumcised penis is too tight to allow for retraction during an erection. Depending on the severity of the condition, stretching, surgery, or circumcision may be required to restore proper functioning.

Another penile birth defect is micropenis, or microphallus, characterized by an atypically small penis. This is usually caused by a hormone imbalance. Testosterone injections during childhood can correct this condition.

A. J. Smuskiewicz

See also: Circumcision; Erection; Foreskin; Male Sexuality; Penile Cancer; Phimosis; Priapism; Pubic Hair; Sexual Disorders, Male.

Further Reading

Mayo Clinic. (2019). Penis health: Identify and prevent problems. Retrieved from https://www.mayoclinic.org/healthy-lifestyle/mens-health/in-depth/penis-health/art-20046175

National Health Service. (2018). 5 penis facts. Retrieved from https://www.nhs.uk/live-well/sexual-health/five-penis-facts/

Planned Parenthood. (2019). What are the parts of the male sexual anatomy? Retrieved from https://www.plannedparenthood.org/learn/health-and-wellness/sexual-and-reproductive-anatomy/what-are-parts-male-sexual-anatomy

Performance Anxiety

Sexual performance anxiety is the inability to experience a physical or emotional response to sexual activity due to either external or internal stressors. Sexual performance anxiety can affect people of all sexual experience levels and does not necessarily just occur among those who are sexually inexperienced. Even those who have much experience can be overcome by anxiety associated with sexual performance. The physical response of sexual performance can be affected by many internal factors, including poor body image, problems within the relationship, and concerns over premature or prolonged ejaculation. Sexual performance anxiety can affect people of any gender.

The physical responses, or lack thereof, that pertain to sexual performance anxiety come in many different forms. The most common of these is erectile dysfunction. Erectile dysfunction can occur when people with penises become stressed about what they think their partner will think of their sexual performance. This heightened stress level narrows the blood vessels, resulting in less blood flow to the penis, which makes it difficult to become physically aroused, even though erection is possible in other contexts. For people with vaginas, heightened levels of stress can result in lubrication difficulties, which can affect the ability to have pleasurable, comfortable sex. If sexual difficulties occur as the result of anxiety, this can create more anxiety, leading to more sexual difficulties, and, therefore, a cycle of anxiety and dysfunction can occur.

While the physical aspects of sexual performance anxiety are often similar across people, the effects of what is specifically causing the anxiety are more unique to the individual. Some aspects of sexual performance anxiety include problems within the relationship between the individual and their partner and concerns over prolonged or premature ejaculation. Poor body image, such as feeling that one's own body is unattractive and unappealing, is one of the leading causes of sexual performance anxiety (Lehmiller, 2013). This can be a self-fulfilling prophecy: if someone is lacking the confidence that they are "good enough," this attitude can lead to results that reflect their expectations.

There are numerous ways that people can overcome sexual performance anxiety. These might include behavioral techniques practiced either alone or with the partner, focusing on the nonpenetrative aspects of sex, being "present" in the moment (e.g., mindfulness), engaging in increased amounts of foreplay, and medications to treat sexual dysfunctions. Another important aspect of sex is communication. By communicating likes and dislikes, sexual partners can help to ensure that they and their partners are having sex that feels good and that leaves them physically and mentally satisfied. Finally, exercising is also an effective method to help reduce sexual performance anxiety. For example, exercising just twenty to thirty minutes a day can increase sexual stamina, which is one of the most prevalent causes of performance anxiety. Exercise can also improve physical health and body image, which is another frequently reported cause of sexual performance anxiety. Ultimately, exercise is a great way to both mentally and physically change the way people feel about themselves and perform in the bedroom.

If one experiences performance anxiety and the symptoms are frequent or seem to progress, it is best to seek professional advice. A doctor may be able to determine if there are complicating factors such as medication side effects or other physical ailments. Some medications that have an impact on sexual desire and sexual performance include antidepressants, anti-inflammatory medication, high blood pressure medications, and muscle relaxers. Speaking with a sex or relationship therapist may also be useful to learn techniques to manage performance anxiety and to address any underlying issues in the relationship.

Casey T. Tobin

See also: Psychosexual Therapy; Sensate Focus; Sexual Dysfunction, Treatment of.

Further Reading

Gunasekaran, K. (2018). *Sexual medicine.* New York: Springer.

Lehmiller, J. (2013). *The psychology of human sexuality.* Hoboken, NJ: Wiley Blackwell.

Maier, T. (2009). *Masters of sex.* New York: Basic Books.

McCabe, M., Althof, S. E., Assalian, P., Chevret-Measson, M., Leiblum, S. R., Simonelli, C., & Wylie, K. (2010). Psychological and interpersonal dimensions of sexual function and dysfunction. *The Journal of Sexual Medicine, 7*(1pt2), 327–336.

Perimenopause

During perimenopause, a female body transitions from its fertile, childbearing stage to its permanently infertile stage. Perimenopause means "around menopause" and lasts for several months to several years before the final menstrual period; it is considered over after twelve consecutive months without a menstrual period. At that point, the individual has entered menopause.

Perimenopause is caused primarily by fluctuating levels of estrogen and progesterone, the major female sex hormones. By the time menopause is reached, the levels of both of these hormones have substantially and permanently declined.

The timing of perimenopause varies, though most notice the first signs and symptoms sometime between their mid-thirties and their late forties. Certain genetic factors, smoking, radiation therapy or chemotherapy for cancer, and ovarian or uterine surgery (such as hysterectomy) may lower the age at which perimenopause starts. Symptoms typically become more severe as menopause grows nearer.

One common symptom of perimenopause is the development of irregularities in menstrual cycles. The cycles may become unusually long or short, the menstrual flows may become especially heavy or light, and some periods may be missed as ovulation fails to occur. A persistent change of seven or more days in menstrual cycle length is characteristic of an early phase of perimenopause. A time of sixty or more days between menstrual periods is characteristic of a late phase of perimenopause.

Vaginal dryness can occur as the vaginal tissues begin to lose their lubrication and flexibility. This symptom may be especially troubling during sexual intercourse and can cause pain or irritation that can be lessened with the use of commercial lubricants. The loss of tissue tone in this part of the body can also contribute to urinary incontinence. Another sexual problem that can develop during perimenopause is a reduction in sexual arousal and desire.

Some individuals may also experience hot flashes, night sweats, and associated sleeping problems during perimenopause, although the intensity and frequency of these problems will vary. Mood swings, including irritability and depression, may also be associated with perimenopause.

Disease-related physiological changes that worsen in many women as menopause approaches include the loss of bone density, the increase in low-density lipoprotein cholesterol, and the decrease in high-density lipoprotein cholesterol. The bone changes raise the risk of osteoporosis and fractures, and the cholesterol changes increase the risk of cardiovascular disease.

Some learn to tolerate the changes of perimenopause without seeking professional treatment. Others, however, find the need to consult physicians—especially those whose symptoms are unusually severe. In those cases, hormone replacement therapy and antidepressant drugs are among the treatment options. Some physicians also recommend physical exercise, dietary changes (including eating foods high in fiber, calcium, and vitamin D), and stress-reduction techniques (such as yoga or meditation).

A. J. Smuskiewicz

See also: Estrogen; Female Sexuality; Hormone Replacement Therapy; Hot Flashes; Lubricants; Menopause; Menstruation; Progesterone.

Further Reading

Mayo Clinic. (2019). Perimenopause. Retrieved from https://www.mayoclinic.org/diseases-conditions/perimenopause/symptoms-causes/syc-20354666

North American Menopause Society. (2019). Menopause 101: A primer for the perimenopausal. Retrieved from https://www.menopause.org/for-women/menopauseflashes/menopause-symptoms-and-treatments/menopause-101-a-primer-for-the-perimenopausal

Perineum

The perineum is a sensitive area of skin between the anus and the vulva or scrotum. This area lies below a set of muscles, called the pelvic floor muscles, that support the bladder and bowel. The perineum contains blood vessels and nerves that supply the urinary tract and genitals with nerve signals and blood signals.

The perineum benefits males and females in different ways. Perineal exercises can improve urinary and fecal problems. These exercises can also help those with erectile dysfunction and premature ejaculation as well as those with prostate problems. The best way to exercise the perineum is by attempting to stop the flow of urination. The perineum will contract when the exercise is performed right, and it should feel as though the muscles are moving up and down. A common way to strengthen the perineum is by doing Kegel exercises. Kegel exercises are easiest to perform when the bladder is empty and when sitting in a chair or standing with legs shoulder width apart. To do a Kegel exercise, the perineum is contracted for four seconds then released; this is known as one set. It is typically recommended that an individual repeats their Kegel exercises ten to fifteen times (or sets), two or three times a day. However, it is also important to speak with a doctor if experiencing any problems related to the pelvic floor.

Injury to the perineum can cause sexual and bladder issues. Nerves from the perineum carry signals from the bladder to the brain and spinal cord to let the brain know when the bladder is full. The same nerves also carry signals from the brain to the pelvic floor muscles to hold or release urine. Injury to these nerves can create bowel and bladder control issues. The perineum carries signals not only between the brain and the bladder or pelvic floor muscles but also between the brain and the genitals. As such, injury to these nerves can interfere with sexual function. During arousal, the brain directs the smooth muscles in the genitals to relax, which causes blood to flow to the genitals, including the penis. If these blood vessels are damaged, this can cause erectile dysfunction, which is the inability to have or maintain an erection firm enough to engage in penetrative sexual activity. Damage to the perineum can also cause damage to the penis and urethra because an internal part of the penis runs through the perineum and contains a section of the urethra.

The perineum also plays a significant role during childbirth. During vaginal delivery, the perineum stretches significantly to allow the baby to pass through the vaginal opening. This can result in a perineal tear. There is a greater risk of tearing when the baby is large, if a significant amount of weight was gained during pregnancy, or if having a baby at a younger or older age. Throughout pregnancy, people can work to stretch the perineum to help prevent tearing through regular perineal massages. The goal of perineal massaging is to relax the pelvic floor muscles and to stretch the vaginal opening. Often during childbirth, a doctor may perform an episiotomy to prevent tearing. An episiotomy is an incision in the perineum to make the vaginal opening larger for delivery. After an episiotomy, the perineum usually heals on its own with time, but it is important to limit physical activity and use ice packs to prevent swelling.

During pregnancy, Kegel exercises, also known as pelvic floor muscle training, are recommended to prevent urinary leakage. Kegel exercises are also recommended to improve sexual and digestive health, as these exercises can help to control urinary leakage while laughing, coughing, and sneezing and can decrease the urge to urinate and help control stool leakage. Kegel exercises also help to strengthen the muscles in and around the vagina. For some people, performing Kegel exercises during sexual intercourse can lead to stronger orgasms, more pleasure, and more arousal.

Although there are many functions of the perineum, everyone is at risk for perineal injury, which can be acute or chronic. The most common acute perineal injuries include perineal surgeries (such as during childbirth), straddle injuries (where a person's legs land on both sides of an object and the perineum forcefully strikes an object, such as a bike), sexual abuse, and impalement. Chronic perineal injuries, on the other hand, tend to be more severe and may result from a sport-related practice such as bike, horseback, or motorcycle riding. When bike riding, straddling a narrow, hard seat can pinch the blood vessels in the perineum, which can cause severe nerve damage. Research has shown that wider seats reduce perineal pressure. Constipation is also a cause of chronic perineal injury. The stool of people who are constipated is hard, dry, and difficult to pass, and straining by squeezing the perineum can cause damage to the blood vessels.

Most people do not often think about the perineum unless an injury has occurred. Perineal injuries are uncomfortable and can cause pain and irritation, but there are ways to prevent and reduce them, such as strengthening the muscles through Kegel exercises. A strong pelvic floor is beneficial for everyone. It is also important to keep the perineum clean and healthy to prevent irritation and infection.

Casey T. Tobin

See also: Kegel Exercises; Pelvic Floor Muscles; Premature Ejaculation; Sexual Dysfunction, Treatment of.

Further Reading

Galan, N. (2019). The importance of the perineum in childbirth. Retrieved from https://www.verywellhealth.com/the-perineum-2616422

Mayo Clinic. (2018). Kegel exercises: A how-to guide for women. Retrieved from https://www.mayoclinic.org/healthy-lifestyle/womens-health/in-depth/kegel-exercises/art-20045283

National Institutes of Health. (2014). Perineal injury in males. Retrieved from https://www.niddk.nih.gov/health-information/urologic-diseases/perineal-injury-males

Pfizer Global Study of Sexual Attitudes and Behaviors

The Global Study of Sexual Attitudes and Behaviors (GSSAB) was a large international study sponsored by Pfizer, a multinational pharmaceutical company headquartered in New York City. With a series of reports—the first published in 2004—the GSSAB investigated various aspects of sexual attitudes and behaviors among 27,500 men and women aged between forty and eighty years in twenty-nine countries on six continents. The study, which included a multinational team of researchers, was conducted in each country by interviewing people or asking them to fill out questionnaires and then analyzing the responses.

Much of the GSSAB analyzed the prevalence of different sexual problems, such as erectile dysfunction, lubrication difficulties, pain during intercourse, and lack of sexual interest. The study's sponsor, Pfizer, manufactures one of the most popular drugs for erectile dysfunction.

Findings from the study indicated that more than 80 percent of male participants and 65 percent of female participants reported that they had sexual intercourse during the past year (the year before completing the survey). Of these sexually active people, 28 percent of the men and 39 percent of the women experienced at least one sexual dysfunction or problem.

Among sexually active men, the most common sexual dysfunctions were early ejaculation (14% of respondents) and erectile difficulties (10%). Among the women, the most common sexual problems were lack of sexual interest (21%), inability to experience orgasm (16%), and lubrication difficulties (16%).

Among the sexually active respondents, 18 percent of the men and 18.8 percent of the women had sought medical help for their problems, and almost 40 percent had spoken about their sexual problem(s) with their partners. According to the survey results, physicians asked only 9 percent of respondents about their sexual health during routine office visits in the previous three years.

Among GSSAB participants, men generally had higher sexual well-being scores than women. In the United States, Canada, Europe, and other Western nations, 71 percent of men were extremely or very satisfied emotionally with their relationships, compared with 63 percent of women. In Mediterranean nations (such as Algeria, Egypt, Israel, and Turkey), the corresponding percentages for relationship satisfaction were 52 percent for men and 41 percent for women, and in China, Japan, Indonesia, and other East Asian nations, they were 30 percent for men and 23 percent for women.

In general, the survey found that feelings of sexual satisfaction and well-being correlated with levels of physical activity. People, especially men, who were more physically active tended to have higher levels of sexual well-being.

Almost 50 percent of men and 32 percent of women in Western nations indicated that sex was extremely or very important in their lives. Both men and women in Mediterranean and Asian nations gave less importance to sex than in Western nations.

Men who had multiple partners were more likely than monogamous men to believe that sex was important, but they were less likely to be satisfied in their relationships. Women generally placed greater importance on emotional satisfaction than physical satisfaction in their relationships compared with men.

Among the conclusions reached by the GSSAB researchers were that sexual desire and sexual activity are widespread in the forty-to-eighty age group and that desire and activity persist into old age. Also, sexual dysfunctions tend to occur at a relatively high rate in this age group, and the dysfunctions become more prevalent with increasing age, especially in men.

A. J. Smuskiewicz

See also: Sexual Disorders, Female; Sexual Disorders, Male; Sexual Dysfunction, Treatment of; Sexuality among Older Adults.

Further Reading

Laumann, E. O., Paik, A., Glasser, D. B., Kang, J. H., Wang, T., Levinson, B., … & Gingell, C. (2006). A cross-national study of subjective sexual well-being among older women and men: Findings from the Global Study of Sexual Attitudes and Behaviors. *Archives of Sexual Behavior, 35*(2), 145–161.

Nicolosi, A., Buvat, J., Glasser, D. B., Harmann, U., Laumann, E. O., & Gingell, C. (2006). Sexual behaviour, sexual dysfunctions and related help seeking patterns in middle-aged and elderly Europeans: The global study of sexual attitudes and behaviors. *World Journal of Urology, 24*(4), 423–428.

Nicolosi, A., Laumann, E. O., Glasser, D. B., Moreira, E. D., Paik, A., & Gingell, C. (2004). Sexual behavior and sexual dysfunctions after age 40: The global study of sexual attitudes and behaviors. *Urology, 64*(5), 991–997.

PFLAG

PFLAG purports to be the largest nonprofit organization in the United States working to unite families and allies with individuals from the lesbian, gay, bisexual, transgender, and queer (LGBTQ) community. Prior to 2014, PFLAG as an acronym stood for "Parents and Friends of Lesbians and Gays." PFLAG's strategic vision is "PFLAG envisions a world where diversity is celebrated and all people are respected, valued, and affirmed inclusive of their sexual orientation, gender identity, and gender expression." The mission of the organization is concentrated on three major domains: support, education, and advocacy for the LGBTQ community.

The founding of PFLAG is credited to Jeanne Manford and tied to her 1972 participation in New York City's Christopher Street Liberation Day March (an early precursor to modern-day LGBTQ Pride celebrations). During this time of rampant cultural homophobia, Manford marched in the parade alongside her gay son, Morty, while holding a protest sign that read "Parents of gays unite in support of our children." During the parade, Manford is said to have been approached by a number of gay and lesbian crowd members who begged her to speak with their non-LGBTQ-affirming parents. Following this experience, Manford decided to begin a support group linking LGBTQ-identified individuals with heterosexual family members and allies of the community.

The first official PFLAG meeting took place on March 26, 1973, at the Metropolitan–Duane Methodist Church in Greenwich Village, New York City. The group was initially referred to as Parents FLAG (Parents and Friends of Lesbians and Gays) and had about twenty people in attendance at the first meeting. As word about Parents FLAG began to spread, additional support groups came into existence across the country. After the 1979 National March for Gay and Lesbian Rights in Washington, D.C., representatives from these various groups met together for the first time. The following year, Parents FLAG began to establish itself as a national resource for education on the gay and lesbian community by distributing information to educational institutions and leaders of various faith communities. Soon thereafter, a major moment for PFLAG occurred when "Dear

Abby" mentioned the support groups in her advice column. The ,publicity reportedly generated over 7,000 letters requesting more information about PFLAG.

In 1981, spurred by the "Dear Abby" publicity, members decided to form a national organization, and the first PFLAG National office was created in Los Angeles under founding president Adele Starr. The 1980s and 1990s represented a period of significant growth for the organization, during which time it was granted nonprofit tax-exempt status, relocated its national office several times, began to organize itself into a chapter-based structure, and became increasingly involved in local and national advocacy work on behalf of the LGBTQ community.

In 1993, PFLAG added the word "Families" to the name. For the first time, the organization also specifically included bisexual people in its mission and advocacy work. In 1998, PFLAG also added transgender people. In 2014, the organization officially changed its name from "Parents, Families, and Friends of Lesbians and Gays" to the abbreviated "PFLAG" in order to reflect growing inclusivity related to the diverse LGBTQ community served by the organization.

PFLAG National is currently headquartered in Washington, D.C., and overseen by both elected leadership and paid staff members. At its highest level, PFLAG is governed by a twenty-one-member board of directors, consisting of elected volunteers serving three-year terms. A major responsibility of the board of directors is to elect the PFLAG national president and executive director.

PFLAG is separated into fourteen regions throughout the United States, with each region electing a regional director who serves a two-year term. Six regional directors are elected to serve on the PFLAG board of directors, and these positions act as a link between PFLAG members and the national office. On a local level, PFLAG is organized into chapters. It currently boasts over 400 chapters and 200,000 members across all fifty states. Chapters officially consist of three or more individuals or families working to further the vision and mission of PFLAG and have significant autonomy with regard to planned member activities and events.

PFLAG's first foray into national advocacy occurred in the 1980s when the organization became involved in opposing Anita Bryant's crusade against gay rights. In the 1990s, local Massachusetts PFLAG chapters helped pass the first Safe Schools legislation in the country. Also during this time, a PFLAG-affiliated family was involved in the Department of Education's ruling that Title IX protects gay and lesbian students from harassment based on sexual orientation. More recently, PFLAG's advocacy work has included significant involvement in the U.S. marriage equality rulings, support for the Equality Act, legislative bans on conversion therapy for LGBTQ youth, federal employment protections for transgender people, and working with Congress to promote LGBTQ rights as a global foreign policy priority.

Jennifer A. Vencill

See also: Gay-Straight Alliance (GSA); LGBTQ+.

Further Reading

PFLAG. (2019). About PFLAG. Retrieved from https://pflag.org/about

Pheromones

Pheromones are chemical substances that are released into the environment by many species of animals as communication signals that influence the behavior of other members of their species. These signals are usually in the form of chemicals that can be smelled, tasted, or detected by a special structure called the vomeronasal organ (VNO). Animals known to communicate with pheromones include insects, mollusks, reptiles, rodents, dogs, cats, hogs, and monkeys. A few plants are known to release pheromone-like chemicals when grazed upon (prompting the production of other chemicals in surrounding plants of the same species that make them less tasty to animals). The existence of pheromone communication among human beings has long been suspected, but it has been difficult to prove scientifically that such chemicals influence human behavior.

Pheromones play a number of important social roles in animal species, including territory marking, threat warnings, and the attraction of mates and other reproduction-related purposes. Many kinds of male mammals, such as wolves, tigers, monkeys, and deer, mark the boundaries of their territories with oily liquid secretions containing pheromones. These chemicals serve as signals to attract females and repel other males. The chemicals also serve to protect food resources within the animal's territory.

Warning-type pheromones are released by certain kinds of ants, snails, and mice when they are injured or threatened by enemies. When the airborne chemical signals are detected by other members of the species, they have the effect of driving those individuals out of the area.

Animal pheromones serve various purposes related to mating and reproduction. Queen bees (the females that reproduce in bee colonies) secrete pheromones that block the sexual development of other females in a colony, causing them to become worker bees instead. Female silk moths secrete a powerful pheromone that can attract male moths from several miles away. Female tree snakes emit pheromones that prompt both the start and end of male courtship behaviors. Some male mice secrete pheromones that speed the development of puberty in young female mice. Pheromones released by some female mice, hamsters, and other rodents attract and sexually arouse males of their species. In hogs, the smell of a boar's saliva can prompt a sow to stand in a mating position.

Many researchers suspect that the sweaty secretions of armpits, the groin area, and other body regions contain pheromones that influence human sexual and reproductive behaviors as well as other emotions and behaviors.

Some research suggests that pheromones released into the air by ovulating women cause testosterone levels to increase in nearby men. Many observations indicate that women who spend a lot of time together—such as women who live together in college dormitories—tend to develop menstrual cycles that become increasingly in synch over time. Some unusual research has demonstrated that the smell of the sweat of people who have just jumped out of airplanes with parachutes makes other people more attentive to details—suggesting a type of chemical alarm signal might be contained in the sweat.

In other perspiration research, the smell of men's sweat has been shown to make some women feel more relaxed. In addition, women were found to prefer the smell of sweaty T-shirts that had been worn by men who had versions of a gene called MHC that were different than their own MHC genes. That finding implied that a pheromone in men's sweat might guide women to select mates who would enhance the genetic diversity, and thus the health, of their future offspring.

Research published in 2011 indicated that pheromone odors released by glands in a mother's nipples help guide newborns to the breasts to suckle for milk. Other research suggests that pheromones released by breastfeeding women can alter the moods of nearby women who do not have children, increasing their sexual desire.

Despite the many observations that suggest important social and behavioral roles for human pheromones, none of these observations have been confirmed by large-scale, placebo-controlled scientific studies. The complexity of human behavior, compared to the relatively simple behaviors of most animals, further complicates the scientific evaluation of pheromone influences on people. In addition, although some people have tiny VNO ducts behind their nostrils—similar to the pheromone-detecting VNOs of animals—not all people have such structures, and the structures, when present, have not been shown to actually function.

Moreover, unlike the specific chemical compounds that have been identified as pheromones in animals—such as bombykol in female silk moths and androstenone in boar saliva—no particular chemical substances have been confirmed as human pheromones. The best candidate for a human pheromone is androstadienone, a compound in sweat that the body makes from testosterone—the scent of which has been shown to alter brain activity in people. However, more research is needed before androstadienone can be proven to consistently function as a behavior-modifying pheromone.

A. J. Smuskiewicz

See also: Arousal; Menstruation; Ovulation; Sex Hormones.

Further Reading

Hadhazy, A. (2012, February). Do pheromones play a role in our sex lives? *Scientific American.* Retrieved from https://www.scientificamerican.com/article/pheromones-sex-lives/

Wyatt, T. D. (2003). *Pheromones and animal behaviour: Communication by smell and taste.* Cambridge: Cambridge University Press.

Yuhas, D. (2014). Are human pheromones real? *Scientific American.* Retrieve from https://www.scientificamerican.com/article/are-human-pheromones-real/

Phimosis

Phimosis is a condition in which the foreskin (prepuce) cannot retract over the glans (head) of the penis. It is normal among male children before adolescence. Attempting to retract the foreskin before the foreskin releases from the glans can cause pain and scarring. Medical personnel advise treatment only when phimosis affects sexual relations. A variety of treatments are available, ranging from conservative, noninvasive actions to radical circumcision.

At birth, the foreskin is adhered to the glans of the penis. This developmental phimosis is normal and in most cases will disappear as the child matures. "Pathological phimosis" is the term used when an uncircumcised adult male's foreskin will not retract. The most common cause is that the tip of the foreskin is too narrow to pass over the glans. The condition is relatively rare and occurs in only 1–5 percent of uncircumcised males. The most common and conservative treatment is the application of topical steroidal medications to the tip of the foreskin. This medication will accelerate growth of the tip of the foreskin, making it larger and allowing it to pass over the glans. This treatment is often accompanied by dilation and stretching. This can be done through manual stretching or the use of medical devices. Constant tension will cause the skin to grow new cells, making the foreskin larger. Steroids and stretching are both painless and have a rate of success of around 85 percent. They also preserve the foreskin tissue, which protects nerves that gives heightened pleasure during intercourse.

More extreme treatments include several types of surgery, known as preputioplasty. One version involves a slit in the foreskin parallel to the length of the penis. The opening is then closed in a transverse manner, making the foreskin looser. This operation is less painful and requires less recovery time than a circumcision. Traditional surgical treatment for phimosis was total circumcision, which was more painful and ran the risk of greater infection than modern preputioplasty. In addition, the loss of the foreskin may result in decreased sensitivity during intercourse.

Tim J. Watts

See also: Circumcision; Foreskin; Penis.

Further Reading

Better Health Channel. (2014). Foreskin care. Retrieved from https://www.betterhealth.vic.gov.au/health/conditionsandtreatments/foreskin-care

National Health Service. (2018). Tight foreskin (phimosis and paraphimosis). Retrieved from https://www.nhs.uk/conditions/phimosis/

UCSF Department of Urology. (2019). Phimosis. Retrieved from https://urology.ucsf.edu/patient-care/children/phimosis

Physical Attractiveness

There are many things that can make people seem attractive. Some people are attracted to others' intelligence, or to their kindness, or to their sense of humor. Oftentimes, people are attracted to others who share similar attitudes and values. Being attracted to a person has been reported as the number one reason why people have sex, and physical attractiveness plays a major role.

Physical attractiveness is important to overall attractiveness when selecting a partner, and it tends to be most important during a first meeting or when making a first impression of a potential partner. In addition, physical attractiveness may be especially important when considering a short-term sexual partner as compared to a long-term relationship. Physical attractiveness is important to both males and females, although some gender differences have been noted. In general, among heterosexual individuals, men tend to place more importance on physical attractiveness than women.

What is considered physically attractive varies by culture and changes over time. And, while physical attractiveness is ultimately subjective to the individual—what one person finds physically attractive is often different from what another person finds attractive—there are some general consistencies.

In terms of facial attractiveness, people tend to rate faces that are symmetrical and those that are "averaged" as most attractive. It is important to note that "averaged" in this context means that all facial features are proportionate to each other. The eyes are neither too close together nor too far apart, and the ears and nose are neither too big nor too small. All features are balanced and "averaged." This preference for symmetry and "averaged" faces has been shown to be present among men and women and across a variety of cultures. Female faces that are considered to have more feminine traits, such as large eyes, are also generally considered to be more attractive.

In terms of bodily attractiveness, body mass index (BMI) and waist-to-hip ratios have been the most studied. BMI is a value that considers the individual's height and mass. Someone who is tall and has a lower body mass has a lower BMI than someone who is short and has a higher body mass. Waist-to-hip ratios consider the diameter of someone's waist in relation to the diameter of their hips. Someone with a waist smaller than their hips has a waist-to-hip ratio less than 1.0, whereas someone whose waist is larger than their hips has a waist-to-hip ratio greater than 1.0. In current Western culture, female bodies that are lower than average with respect to BMI and waist-to-hip ratios tend to be rated as more attractive; however, those that are much lower or much greater than average are generally rated as less attractive than those that are closer to the average. Among male bodies, lower levels of body fat and higher rates of muscle are generally considered more attractive, as are waist-to-hip ratios that are less than but nearer to 1.0. Cultural differences in preferred BMI and waist-to-hip ratios have been noted.

Ultimately, physical attractiveness is subjective, and different people are attracted to different physical characteristics in their partners. Some people find height attractive, while other people prefer a short partner. Some people find blonde hair attractive, while others prefer those with brown hair. And while physical attractiveness is important, especially when considering a casual sex partner, it is not the only characteristic that is considered, and it generally becomes less important when considering a long-term romantic relationship partner.

Heather L. Armstrong

See also: Desire; Evolutionary Perspectives on Gender and Sexual Behavior; Romantic Attraction and Orientation; Same-Sex Attraction and Behavior.

Further Reading

Apicella, C. L., Little, A. C., & Marlowe, F. W. (2007). Facial averageness and attractiveness in an isolated population of hunter-gatherers. *Perception, 36*, 1813–1820.

Little, A. C., Jones, B. C., & DeBruine, L. M. (2011). Facial attractiveness: Evolutionary based research. *Philosophical Transactions B, 366*, 1638–1659.

Luo, S., & Zhang, G. (2009). What leads to romantic attraction: Similarity, reciprocity, security, or beauty? Evidence from a speed-dating study. *Journal of Personality, 77*(4), 933–963.

Marlowe, F., & Wetsman, A. (2001). Preferred waist-to-hip ratio and ecology. *Personality and Individual Differences, 30*(3), 481–489.

Meston, C. M., & Buss, D. M. (2007). Why human have sex. *Archives of Sexual Behavior, 36*, 477–507.

Smith, K. B. (2017). Attraction, intimacy, and love. In C. F. Pukall (Ed.), *Human sexuality: A contemporary introduction* (2nd ed.). Don Mills, ON: Oxford University Press.

Planned Parenthood

Planned Parenthood Federation of America (PPFA), usually shortened to Planned Parenthood, is a nonprofit organization that offers reproductive and other health services, sexuality education, and advocacy for reproductive justice. It is the largest U.S. provider of reproductive health care. PPFA's services include screening for cancer; testing, counseling, and treatment for sexually transmitted infections; contraception; and abortion. Contraception accounts for about one-third of PPFA's services, and testing and treatment for sexually transmitted infections accounts for 42 percent. PPFA provides nearly 300,000 abortions each year among the 2.7 million people it serves with health care annually.

According to their mission statement, "Planned Parenthood believes in the fundamental right of each individual, throughout the world, to manage his or her fertility, regardless of the individual's income, marital status, race, ethnicity, sexual orientation, age, national origin, or residence."

The organization began in Brooklyn, New York, when Margaret Sanger opened the first birth-control clinic in 1916. She founded the American Birth Control League in 1921, which became part of Planned Parenthood Federation of America in 1942. Since then, PPFA has expanded and contracted in size. As of 2015, it had sixty-one locally governed affiliates nationwide. The affiliates operate approximately 700 health centers. In addition, Planned Parenthood affiliates provide educational programs to 1.5 million young people and adults. PPFA is an affiliate of the International Planned Parenthood Federation.

When Margaret Sanger opened the first clinic in Brooklyn, poor women often suffered serious health problems from multiple pregnancies and having more children than they were able to support. Information about birth control was judged "obscene," and Sanger was arrested eight times as she advocated for its use.

Planned Parenthood has been attacked for Margaret Sanger's early support of negative eugenics, in which she said that there were irresponsible and reckless people whose religious scruples "prevent their exercising control over their numbers." She said, "There is no doubt in the minds of all thinking people that the procreation of this group should be stopped." Her strategy was that they should be offered birth control.

Others have opposed the work of Planned Parenthood by suggesting that the organization targets African American communities in an attempt at genocide.

They point to the percentages of African American women who get abortions as compared to white women. A major factor for all women seeking abortion is economics, and according to the Pew Research Center, "the median wealth of white households is 18 times that of Hispanic households and 20 times that of black households" (Kochhar, Fry, & Taylor, 2011).

Again, some of these attacks on PPFA stem from the belief that Margaret Sanger wanted to employ eugenics on the African American population. In 1930, she opened a birth control clinic in Harlem at the request of black leaders and staffed it with African American doctors and nurses. Martin Luther King Jr. commended Sanger in his acceptance speech for an award named in her honor.

In 1948, PPFA provided a small grant to Dr. Gregory Pincus to explore the possibility of a hormonal contraceptive. In 1953, based on Dr. Pincus's encouraging research, Sanger persuaded philanthropist Katherine Dexter McCormick to underwrite the development of a birth control pill, which resulted in Enovid, the first oral contraceptive. It was approved by the U.S. Food and Drug Administration in 1960 and had a profound effect on society. Within five years, one out of every four married women in the United States under the age of forty-five had used the pill.

In 1970, President Richard Nixon signed into law Title X of the Public Health Service Act. This made contraceptives available to low-income women and provided funding for educational programs to reduce teenage pregnancy. Planned Parenthood affiliates were recipients of these funds, enabling them to provide birth control to poor women and young people. In 1973, the Supreme Court decision in *Roe v. Wade* overturned state laws that outlawed abortion. Planned Parenthood began offering abortion services at several of their affiliates and increasingly advocated for reproductive justice.

The Planned Parenthood Action Fund, the nonpartisan advocacy and political arm of PPFA, publicizes issues and organizes people to support "women's full equality in health care access." This includes the right to abortion, and opponents of abortion have long criticized PPFA for offering this service. In the 1980s and 1990s, Planned Parenthood affiliates were subject to murders of staff, clinic bombings, arson attacks, and anthrax scares. Abortion rights continue to be a significant part of PPFA's advocacy agenda. Lawmakers regularly propose laws to restrict access to abortion, and Planned Parenthood and other organizations work to ensure that women are able to get an abortion when they need one. In addition, PPFA works "for commonsense policies that foster the sexual and reproductive health and rights of individuals, families, and communities" (Planned Parenthood, 2014).

Michael J. McGee

See also: Abortion Legislation; Contraception; Family Planning Clinics; *Planned Parenthood v. Casey*; *Roe v. Wade*; Sanger, Margaret; Sexual Health; Sexual Rights.

Further Reading

Chesler, E. (1992). *Woman of valor: Margaret Sanger and the birth control movement in America.* New York: Simon & Schuster.

Kochhar, R., Fry, R., & Taylor, P. (2011, July 26). Wealth gaps rise to record highs between Whites, Blacks, Hispanics. *Pew Social Trends*. Retrieved from http://www.pewsocialtrends.org/2011/07/26/wealth-gaps-rise-to-record-highs-between-whites-blacks-hispanics/

Planned Parenthood Federation of America. (2014). *2013–2014 Annual Report*. New York: Author.

Planned Parenthood Federation of America. (2019). Planned Parenthood. Retrieved from http://www.plannedparenthood.org/

Sanger, M. (1921, November 18). The morality of birth control. Retrieved from https://www.nyu.edu/projects/sanger/webedition/app/documents/show.php?sangerDoc=238254.xml

Planned Parenthood v. Casey

Planned Parenthood v. Casey was a 1992 Supreme Court decision about abortion rights. An earlier landmark Supreme Court case, *Roe v. Wade*, had made abortion legal in the United States in 1973. However, in the 1980s, a group of Pennsylvania laws were passed that required a woman to notify her spouse before obtaining an abortion. In addition, her doctor had to provide her with specific information that might change her mind, and she had to wait at least twenty-four hours before the procedure could take place. If she was a minor, she needed to get the consent of at least one of her parents or permission from a judge to have the abortion. Further, the Pennsylvania law said that a woman could only get an abortion if it was a medical emergency. Finally, the law imposed certain reporting requirements on facilities providing abortion services. Before any of these laws could take effect, Planned Parenthood of Southeast Pennsylvania, five abortion clinics, and a physician representing himself and other doctors who provided abortions brought the case against the state, led by governor Robert Casey. The plaintiffs said these laws were unconstitutional. The district court agreed that the provisions of the law were unconstitutional and stopped their enforcement. The court of appeals later affirmed some of the provisions but struck down the husband notification provision. In some ways, these laws were a challenge to the findings in *Roe v. Wade*. Since the *Roe* decision, many states have tried to overturn it or to limit women's access to abortion by putting restrictions on the procedure.

When the *Planned Parenthood v. Casey* case came to the Supreme Court, the court reaffirmed *Roe* but upheld most of the Pennsylvania provisions. For the first time, the justices imposed a new standard to determine the validity of laws restricting abortions. It asked if a state regulation imposes an "undue burden," which is defined as a "substantial obstacle in the path of a woman seeking an abortion before the fetus attains viability" (Wharton, Frietsche, & Kolbert, 2006). Under this standard, the only part of the law to fail the undue burden test was the husband notification requirement. The court said that the rest of the provisions were constitutional and were not an "undue burden."

Casey ruled that states may regulate abortions so as to protect the health of the mother and the life of the fetus and may outlaw abortions of "viable" fetuses. This means that the state could enact laws prohibiting abortions if the fetus was developed enough to live outside the woman's body. Casey held that states could now pass regulations about the first trimester (before the fetus is viable) but only to protect a woman's health, not to limit a woman's access to abortion. The court also said that, with newer life-preserving medicines and technology, the point at which a fetus might become "viable" (the point at which states may constitutionally outlaw abortions) could now be earlier than six months into the pregnancy.

The court ruled that the mandatory twenty-four-hour waiting period was not an undue burden and was thus constitutional. They said the provision's purpose, to promote well-considered abortions, was legitimate and only slightly limited access to abortions. They also ruled that the spousal consent provision was an undue burden because husbands could resort to abuse and obstruction when they learned of the woman's abortion plans. The court upheld the remaining portion of the law, including a parental consent provision for minors.

Casey v. Planned Parenthood, though less famous than *Roe v. Wade*, is actually a more important case. *Casey* not only affirmed *Roe*'s abortion right but also broadened the states' authority to regulate it. The *Casey* decision crafted a new undue burden analysis and, for the first time, made it the controlling standard for evaluating all abortion restrictions. The decision remains as controversial as *Roe*. Many legal scholars think the "undue burden" test is more ambiguous and difficult to apply. The justices' decision was intended to provide a level of protection for the abortion right that was consistent with *Roe*'s main objective of "ensur[ing] that the woman's right to choose not become so subordinate to the State's interest in promoting fetal life that her choice exists in theory but not in fact" (Nossiff, 2007). As Supreme Court justices change over time, this standard may mean that future legal challenges to abortion rights may succeed and that access to safe and legal abortion may be diminished.

Michael J. McGee

See also: Abortion, Elective; Abortion Legislation; Planned Parenthood; *Roe v. Wade.*

Further Reading

CQ Almanac. (1992). Supreme Court's decision on Pennsylvania case. In *CQ Almanac 1992* (48th ed., 30-E-34-E.). Washington, DC: Congressional Quarterly. Retrieved from http://library.cqpress.com/cqalmanac/cqal92-845-25185-1106699

Nossiff, R. (2007). Gendered citizenship: Women, equality, and abortion policy. *New Political Science, 29*(1), 61–76.

Wharton, L. J., Frietsche, S., & Kolbert, K. (2006). Preserving the core of Roe: Reflections on Planned Parenthood v. Casey. *Yale JL & Feminism, 18*, 317.

PLISSIT Model of Sex Therapy

The PLISSIT model of sex therapy represents points of intervention created to assist health care providers in providing a sex-positive space for patients while simultaneously aiding in the shaping of more positive health behaviors. Adults and adolescents alike frequently possess concerns related to their sexual health and sexual trajectory and the ways in which physical and mental factors can influence their sex lives. Various physical and psychological conditions (such as diabetes, cancer, neurological disease, depression, anxiety, and grief) can negatively affect sexual health and sexual satisfaction. In addition, factors such as lack of training to address sexual health issues, biases related to sexual and sexuality-related concerns, or discomfort around discussing sexuality-related topics with patients act as barriers to individuals receiving information that will aid in increasing their sexual autonomy and chances of engaging in sexual health–promoting behaviors.

The first stage of the PLISSIT model is "permissions." The act of gaining permission from a patient to administer assistance regarding sexual concerns is a crucial step used to reinforce the basic autonomy a patient should feel in making their sexual decisions. Seeking permission from a patient is used as a way to avoid offending the patient at any point of assessment. Furthermore, granting the patient permission works to normalize the patient's sexual fantasies, desires, behaviors, and boundaries while screening for engagement in any behaviors that may be harmful to self or others. Ways clinicians can foster permission in the treatment setting are to engage in routine questioning, generalizing and normalizing patients' experiences, and asking open-ended questions to further assess patients' symptoms.

The second stage of the PLISSIT model is "limited information." The sharing of limited information emphasizes the caring professional as a point of informational resource for the patient. Information that caregivers can provide includes, but is not limited to, male, female, and nonbinary anatomy and physiology; the impact of various diseases on sex drive and sexual function; information on gender, gender expression, sexual orientation, and modes of sexual expression; and avenues of sexual exploration that may be open to patients. While the health professional wants to provide a wealth of information, it is important to note that this information should be centered around the patient's primary concern(s) so as not to overburden the patient with information that may not address their needs.

The third stage of the PLISSIT model is "specific suggestions." If patients respond positively to the permission and limited information phases of the model, caregivers may want to provide the patient with specific suggestions on how to address their concerns. These suggestions may involve reading printed materials related to the concern, engaging in a behavior that exposes the patient to the concern, or working with the patient to consider medicinal options that may address the concern. Specific suggestions are not rules for the patient to follow but are instead tools the patient may or may not choose to use.

The final stage of the PLISSIT model is "intensive therapy." The level of intensive therapy in the PLISSIT model usually involves an expert or highly trained therapist, counselor, social worker, or psychiatrist. This level of the PLISSIT model is reserved for more complex concerns the patient may be experiencing. Some of the interventions that could be involved in this step could potentially include trauma-informed therapies, aggressive medication management, or other therapeutic treatment that may intervene in more crisis-related health concerns.

Many investigations of the PLISSIT model highlight it as a tool to assist patients in navigating their sexualities when they have experienced some sort of physical or mental health trauma. This model has been used to assist health care providers in administering competent care when patients have encountered sexual difficulties related to interactions with cancers, diabetes, emotional trauma, grief, and other health issues. The PLISSIT model can also be used with adolescents to assist in clarifying their concerns around sexual identities and sexual decision making.

Shadeen Francis and Patrick R. Grant

See also: Disabilities, Sexual Function and; Psychosexual Therapy; Sexual Dysfunction, Treatment of; Sexual Health.

Further Reading

McInnes, R. (2003). Chronic illness and sexuality. *The Medical Journal of Australia, 179*(5), 263–266.

Nusbaum, M. R. H., & Hamilton, C. D. (2002). The proactive sexual health history. *American Family Physician, 66*(9), 1705.

Polyamory

"Polyamory," also known as "poly," comes from the Greek and Latin languages and means "many loves." Polyamory is a relationship style that reflects shared intimacy, emotion, friendship, or sexual connectedness between two or more people. Though the dynamic most often seen is couples having other relationships outside of the duo, within polyamory, the person does not have to be partnered with another person but can give and receive love, care, intimacy, and emotional support as a single person with multiple people. Other examples of relationship styles within polyamory include polyfidelity ("in which two people, possibly two or more couples, form a sexually exclusive group") and open marriages (Easton & Hardy, 2009, p. 275). Polyamory gives people an alternative relationship configuration to monogamy, where two people are committed to each other in their relationship (hence polyamory sometimes being called nonmonogamy). People who choose to be involved in a polyamorous relationship vary in sex, gender, gender expression, and sexual orientation.

Though there is no one significant incident that sparked polyamory as it is seen and negotiated today, there have been many reasons for this idea to grow: whether through the attempts to personalize expressions of love for more than one person, dismantle larger systems of patriarchy and capitalism, or to rearrange these same systems to benefit the needs of women. Though making sexual and emotional connections with people outside of primary relationships has been happening since relationships existed, the organized and structured idea of nonmonogamy began to take shape in the 1960s in the United States. From the mentality of the 1950s, where sex outside of monogamous relationships was cheating but more acceptable for men who were "sowing wild oats" as opposed to women being "loose," the blossoming idea in the 1960s of open marriages, polyamory, and free love became an alternative. Sexual and social revolutions (including feminism and anarchy), particularly in the United States and Europe (where much of the research and information has been focused), were movements that not only changed attitudes toward social justice, equality, and the self but also expanded the search for authenticity, claiming autonomy, and resisting authority.

"Swinging" was one of the first organized forms of nonmonogamy for people who identified as heterosexual and bisexual. Swinging, the practice of couples exchanging partners, usually for sexual pleasure, can be seen within the Hollywood scene in the 1930s and 1940s. Researchers also note swinging among Air Force pilots and their wives during World War II at military installments. Their research shows that swinging was used as a way for wives to be supported by the surviving pilots due to the fatality rate during the war. This practice of nonmonogamy still exists today among couples trying to explore different sexual orientations as well as kink and BDSM (bondage/domination, sadism/masochism) practices with others.

Due to there being at least two or more people involved within this relationship dynamic, it is important to have a foundation of, or skills to build a foundation of, communication, honesty, trust, and boundaries. Good communication prevents assumptions around the needs of each person in the relationship. Exploration around what the individual person or multiple people want may include discussions of how many people are going to be involved in the relationship(s), how time will be managed and valued among those involved, what intimacy looks like with each person, and so on. From these conversations, boundaries may be generated to protect and respect the wants, desires, needs, and sensitivities of the individuals and to prevent unwanted hurt or emotional pain as best as possible. This is to say that communication and boundaries do not always avoid emotional pain, as words, gestures, and nuances can be misunderstood, but these qualities are a start in building a solid foundation in polyamorous relationships for all to be heard.

Two concepts that are a part of conversations in polyamory but constantly misconceived are jealousy and compersion. Jealousy is an emotion usually brought up by "expression of insecurity, fear of rejection, fear of abandonment, feeling left out, feeling not good enough, feeling inadequate, [and/or] feeling awful" (Easton & Hardy, 2009). Even though jealousy is usually an emotion people try to avoid feeling, it is a feeling that may come up for some people if they are involved with another person or multiple people. For example, if Billy is in a polyamorous relationship with Steve and Jamie, Jamie may get jealous of the time Steve is spending with Billy, vice versa, or it can be experienced by all. Again, with communication, honesty, trust, and boundaries, partners can further discuss where those feelings are coming from to help alleviate or redirect the emotion. Compersion, on the other hand, is the positive expression a person feels toward their partner about their partner's romantic or intimate interest in another. Steve, for example, may be excited that Jamie and Billy are going to the movies together since Steve is not interested in participating in that activity.

A concern that comes with being physically intimate with multiple partners is the fear of spreading sexually transmitted infections (STIs) among partners. There are several ways this can be resolved, mostly using the foundation of communication. Some, or all, of the partners within the relationship may choose to use barriers such as condoms, dental dams, or rubber gloves. Partners may also use some form of birth control to prevent unintended pregnancies.

Some, or all, partners who are sexually active may also practice a method called "fluid bonding" or "fluid monogamy," where the partners will engage in sexual activity without barriers. Before this method of intimacy is practiced, all individuals are tested for STIs and HIV so the health status of all participants is known. Continued conversations among the partners involved help them to decide what boundaries are placed around sexual activities for the safety of all.

Though polyamory is usually seen as a way for two or more people to coordinate their love and commitment to one another, polyamory can also be seen as a way to build and support families while distributing resources such as money, energy, and time among the group, even without sex being involved. For example, in the Nandi communities in Kenya (and also South Africa), the females took on "female husbands" (defined as women who are "promoted" to the status of "man" through their marriages to other women). This had not only the benefits of negating gender roles but also the wife of a female husband "is free to engage in sexual liaisons with men of her own choosing"; as such, she has the advantage of sexual freedom (Murray & Roscoe, 1998). Though these relationships are still within the structure of marriage, they also show the freedom negotiated in relationships in order to meet sexual and economic needs to sustain the community. The practice has now grown throughout communities as a way to sustain partnerships, raise children, and create individual freedoms of loving for people of all genders and sexual orientations.

Currently, nonmonogamy in all forms is expanding and being given more visibility, even within the media, to challenge the traditional idea of monogamy. Literature by authors such as Tristan Taormino (*Opening Up—A Guide to Creating and Sustaining Open Relationships*, 2008), Wendy-O Matik (*Redefining Our Relationships*, 2002), and the well-known resource *The Ethical Slut* by Dossie Easton and Janet Hardy (1997), give people who identify as nonmonogamous a guide related to their lifestyle. These books contain a wide variety of information to help answer questions and ease anxiety around topics such as how to deal with jealousy, STIs and safer sex, coming out to family members and friends, family planning, and speaking to one's children about nonmonogamy and family structure.

The internet is also a source for general information about nonmonogamy and is often used to find "meet-ups," such as LovingMore.com and Polyamory.org. Spokespeople such as Anita Wagner Illig for practicalpolyamory.com, and organizations such as the Woodhull Freedom Foundation, have committed their mission to educating and supporting people within various types of nonmonogamous relationships and advocating for their rights (Woodhull Freedom Foundation, 2019). These resources, as well as TV shows such as *Polyamory: Married and Dating*, help the experienced and curious person alike to offset the negative views and stigma attached to relationships outside of the traditional two-person dynamic.

Shane'a Thomas

See also: Communication, Sexual; Monogamy; Open Marriage; Polygamy; Sexual Revolution; Swinging.

Further Reading

Easton, D., & Hardy, J. W. (2009). *The ethical slut: A practical guide to polyamory, open relationships & other adventures* (2nd ed.). New York: Celestial Arts.

Munson, M., & Stelboum, J. P. (1999). Introduction: The lesbian polyamory reader: Open relationships, non-monogamy, and casual sex. In M. Munson & J. P. Stelboum (Eds.), *The lesbian polyamory reader: Open relationships, non-monogamy, and casual sex* (1–7). New York: Harrington Park Press.

Murray, S. O., & Roscoe, W. (1998). *Boy-wives and female husbands: Studies in African homosexualities.* New York: St. Martin's Press.

Taormino, T. (2008). *Opening up: A guide to creating and sustaining open relationships.* San Francisco: Cleis Press.

Woodhull Freedom Foundation. (2019). Home page. Retrieved from https://www.woodhull foundation.org

Polyandry

"Polyandry" is a broad term used to refer to the cultural practice in which one woman is simultaneously married to two or more men. Polyandry is a relatively rare custom in contemporary societies but is thought to have been somewhat more common in the past. At any rate, polyandry has been found around the world, most often in egalitarian societies.

Polyandry is a variety of polygamy, where an individual may have more than one spouse at a time. Polygamy is often confused with polygyny, where it is customary for a man to have more than one wife at a time. Polyandry is sometimes practiced alongside polygyny in a society, which forges a system referred to as polygynandry. These cultural practices can result in less partitioning of family land holdings and other assets, restricted population growth, and expanded opportunities with respect to domestic economic activities.

Polyandry is generally understood to have an economic basis rather than a status or sexual basis. It is most often associated with extreme conditions, such as severe poverty, which might frequently be correlated with the practice of female infanticide. That sort of situation produces a surplus supply of males for whom mates can be rather difficult to find. A similar result can be produced in polyandrous societies that do not commit adequate resources to caring for female children, apparently in response to poor probabilities of their being able to marry. Endemic warfare, such as that reported among the Yanomama Shirishana of Brazil, can also create an unbalanced sex ratio, which might lead to the practice of intermittent polyandry. Male absenteeism, such as that associated with prolonged military service or priestly duties, is another factor commonly associated with the cultural practice of polyandry. In a polyandrous marriage, the woman does not acquire extra husbands for sexual satisfaction, nor does she gain any additional status for the number of husbands she has. The woman usually has little to no say over whether or not to take on additional husbands in a polyandrous marriage.

Fraternal polyandry is the most common variant of polyandry that has been documented ethnographically and historically. For instance, the Nyinba of northwestern Nepal, who are culturally similar to many Tibetan ethnic groups, practice fraternal polyandry, as do many of their Tibetan neighbors. In these cultures, most men who have brothers marry polyandrously, and all the brothers tend to remain in these marriages for the rest of their lives to maintain coresidence patterns associated with their system of property inheritance and succession to positions of household authority. A sociobiological explanation for fraternal polyandry that has been suggested is that since brothers demonstrably have more genetic material in common with each other than with others they are not related to, raising the children of one's brother is a way to ensure that your gene pool is more likely to survive. Fraternal polyandry is frequently associated with the belief in partible paternity, which holds that a child can possibly have more than one biological father. At any rate, brothers who can keep all their family resources together by being in a polyandrous marriage are clearly able to maintain greater collective wealth than those who divide resources and establish separate family units.

An alternative variant of polyandry involves a woman who has two or more husbands who are not related. This type of polyandry has been reported, for example, among the Nayar of Kerala, India. The Nayars are a caste among whom a man's property is inherited by the children of his sisters, not by his own biological children. Under this polyandrous system, only the women know who are their biological children. It is thought that polyandry among the Nayar arose in response to men being employed in the military; this could have created a shortage of laborers to work on family farms, with polyandry developing as a cultural adaptation. Other castes in Kerala who practiced this form of polyandry include the Kammalans and the Thiyyas.

Victor B. Stolberg

See also: Marriage; Marriage, Cross-Cultural Comparison of; Polygamy; Polygyny.

Further Reading

Beall, C. M., & Goldstein, M. L. (1981). Tibetan fraternal polyandry: A test of sociobiological theory. *American Anthropologist, 83*, 5–12.

Levine, N. E. (1988). *The dynamics of polyandry: Kinship, domesticity, and population on the Tibetan border.* Chicago: University of Chicago Press.

Peters, J. F., & Hunt, C. H. (1975). Polyandry among the Yanomama Shirishana. *Journal of Comparative Family Studies, 6*, 197–207.

Raha, M. K., & Coomar, P. C. (1987). *Polyandry in India.* Delhi: Gian Publishing House.

Polycystic Ovary Syndrome (PCOS)

Polycystic ovary syndrome (PCOS) is a condition in which multiple fluid-filled follicles, called cysts, develop within the ovaries, resulting from an imbalance in hormones. People with PCOS generally have higher levels of androgen hormones (otherwise known as male hormones) such as testosterone. Every person with PCOS is affected differently and demonstrates an array of different symptoms. Those diagnosed with PCOS are often prescribed oral birth control pills to aid with the symptoms.

The causes of PCOS are unknown. There is a debate as to whether PCOS may be a product of environmental factors, such as hormone-containing preservatives within foods, or genetic factors, such as the hereditary passage from mother to daughter. Other factors that seem to be related to the development of PCOS are obesity and insulin resistance. Insulin is secreted by the pancreas and is used to help absorb glucose (sugar) into cells from the blood stream. When a person has insulin resistance, the level of glucose increases in the bloodstream. High insulin production may also affect the endocrine system by promoting the production of androgens that lead to hormone imbalance and thus relate to PCOS.

There are a variety of symptoms associated with PCOS. One of the most common symptoms is irregularities in the menstrual cycle. People with PCOS may have fewer than nine menstruations within a year, absent menstruations, or heavy bleeding. Other symptoms of PCOS include adult acne, excessive body hair growth (hirsutism), and weight gain that often leads to obesity. In addition, PCOS is related to high blood pressure, sleep apnea, depression, uterine bleeding, endometrial cancer, and infertility. PCOS may contribute to the development of type II diabetes or heart disease. It is important to know that people with PCOS are affected differently and may each demonstrate a different combination of symptoms.

There is no single test for PCOS. Doctors often diagnose PCOS through a list of criteria that includes hyperandrogenism, ovulatory dysfunction, and polycystic ovaries. Patients must exhibit two out of the three criteria to be diagnosed. Tests that will aid in diagnosis include physical exams, pelvic exams, various blood tests, and ultrasounds. The quickest way to identify PCOS is through an ultrasound, which will show the cysts within the ovaries on the screen of the machine. However, it is important that doctors first rule out hyperthyroidism and hypothyroidism, both of which can cause similar symptoms and conditions to PCOS. Doctors use the physical and pelvic exams to look for symptoms such as excessive hair growth and adult acne. Doctors may also inquire as to the patient's medical history as well as the medical history of the patient's mother and grandmother due to the potential hereditary aspects of the syndrome.

There is no treatment for PCOS that will rid the ovaries of their follicles and correct the hormone imbalance. However, there are treatments to aid with the symptoms of PCOS. The most common treatment prescribed by doctors is birth control. Oral birth control pills with estrogen and progestin aid with regulating menstrual cycles and help to lower the androgen. Lower androgen levels help eliminate acne and excessive hair growth. Other forms of birth control, such as the vaginal ring, can also be used.

Metformin may be prescribed to help lower insulin levels and to aid in regulation of the menstrual cycle and weight loss. People who want to become pregnant but are experiencing issues related to PCOS may be prescribed clomiphene, follicle-stimulating hormone and luteinizing hormone, spironolactone, or steroids.

There are no techniques to prevent PCOS. However, for people with a family history of PCOS, living a healthy lifestyle that encompasses a low-carbohydrate diet and daily moderate to vigorous activity levels may help with related symptoms.

Camilla Loggins

See also: Androgens; Birth Control Pills, Estrogen-Progestin; Estrogen; Infertility; Menstruation; Ovaries; Testosterone.

Further Reading

American College of Obstetricians and Gynecologists. (2017). *Polycystic ovary syndrome (PCOS).* Retrieved from http://www.acog.org/-/media/For-Patients/faq121.pdf?dmc=1&ts=20150930T0048253696

Mayo Clinic. (2019). Polycystic ovary syndrome (PCOS). Retrieved from http://www.mayoclinic.org/diseases-conditions/pcos/basics/definition/con-20028841

Sheehan, M. T. (2004). Polycystic ovarian syndrome: Diagnosis and management. *Clinical Medicine & Research, 2*, 13–27.

Polygamy

Polygamy is the cultural practice of having more than one spouse at a time. Essentially polygamy is the form of marriage that permits an individual to have more than one husband or wife at the same time. There are two basic forms of polygamy: polygyny, in which a man can have more than one wife, and polyandry, in which a woman can have more than one husband at a time. Polygyny is far more common than polyandry, but collectively polygamy is more prevalent than monogamy. Monogamy, the practice of having one spouse at a time, is the predominant pattern in modern Western societies, but across cultures and over time, polygamy is the most widely preferred marriage form.

The term "polygamy" comes from two Greek words: "polloi" meaning "many" and "gamos" meaning "marriage." Thus, the literal meaning of polygamy is marriage to several mates at once.

Certain religions permit the practice of polygamy, generally polygyny. According to the Quran and sanctioned under Sharia law, Islam allows a man to take as many as four wives. Hinduism has no limit on the number of wives a man can have. Buddhism does not prohibit polygamy. Ancient Judaism, as described in the Old Testament, allowed kings, princes, and other male members of the upper classes to have multiple wives (Deuteronomy 21:15; Judges 8:30; II Samuel 3:2–5; I Kings 11:1–3). Up until it was banned in 1890, the Church of Jesus Christ of Latter-Day Saints, or the Mormons, openly practiced polygyny, which they erroneously referred to as polygamy, resulting in confusion to this day; splinter Mormon sects and other Christian fundamentalist groups still practice polygynous marriages, although the U.S. Congress passed a law prohibiting polygyny in 1862.

The custom of taking multiple wives was practiced in pre-Communist China and continues today in many countries, primarily in Africa, the Middle East, and Asia. For example, Thailand legally accepted polygyny up until 2010, and it is still legal in neighboring Myanmar (Burma). In fact, polygyny was practiced in many places up until modern times, including Ireland, Japan, Oceania, and Turkey. Polygamy remains legal in over 150 countries around the world. Polyandry, the custom of a single wife with two or more husbands at a time, was practiced by peoples like the Inuit, many Native Americans, the Todas of India, and some groups in Nepal and Tibet.

There is generally an economic rationale behind polygamy. Multiple spouses can clearly expand the resources available. For example, when the Blackfoot of North America switched from beaver to buffalo fur trading, cowives made more sense as buffalo skin tanning was a labor-intensive task exclusive to women, and more wives dramatically increased a man's financial potential. Similarly, Sinuai women in the Solomon Islands take on the primary responsibilities for raising pigs, a major signifier of wealth; thus, more wives help generate more wealth. There can be strong political and economic factors supporting polygamy, including the establishment of alliances and supporting descent ties between groups. Other factors are also involved; in some societies, if there was a shortage of men, such as resulting from warfare, then polygyny might be more likely, such as is the case among the Yanomamo of southern Venezuela and northern Brazil; conversely, if there was a shortage of women, such as associated with female infanticide, then polyandry might be a cultural response.

Victor B. Stolberg

See also: Marriage; Marriage, Cross-Cultural Comparison of; Monogamy; Polyamory; Polyandry; Polygyny.

Further Reading

Chagnon, N. A. (1977). *Yanomano: The fierce people.* New York: Holt, Rinehart and Winston.

Conaty, G. T. (1995). Economic models and Blackfoot ideology. *American Ethnologist, 22*(2), 403–409.

Gordon, S. B. (2003). The Mormon question: Polygamy and constitutional conflict in nineteenth-century America. *Journal of the Supreme Court History, 28*(1), 14–29.

Hayase, Y., & Liaw, K.-L. (1997). Factors on polygamy in sub-Saharan Africa: Findings based on the demographic and health surveys. *The Developing Economies, 35*(3), 293–327.

Rehman, J. (2007). The Sharia, Islamic family laws and international human rights law: Examining the theory and practice of polygamy and talaq. *International Journal of Law, Policy and the Family, 21*(1), 108–127.

Polygyny

Polygyny is a marital pattern in which a man has more than one wife at a time. Polygyny and polyandry are different forms of polygamy. Polygyny is practiced by the majority of societies around the world, particularly in non-Western countries.

Polygyny was a dominant practice across many ancient societies. In this regard, polygyny featured prominently among peoples discussed in the Old Testament. The patriarchs, such as Abraham (Genesis 16:1–16) and Jacob (Genesis 29:20–29) were polygynous; Abraham had three wives, and Jacob had four. In ancient Israel, kings and other male members of the upper social classes in particular were permitted more than one wife (Deuteronomy 21:15; Judges 8:30). The most famous kings of ancient Israel, David (I Samuel 25:39–44; I Samuel 27:3; II Samuel 3:2–5) and Solomon (I Kings 11:12), were polygynous in the extreme. The harem of

Solomon surpassed that of even his father (I Kings 11:1–8); Solomon is said to have had seven hundred wives and three hundred concubines (I Kings 11:3). Rehoboam, Solomon's son, continued the family tradition, as he had eighteen wives and sixty concubines, who collectively bore him twenty-eight sons and sixty daughters (II Chronicles 11:21). Polygyny was practiced by kings of other ancient Near Eastern kingdoms as well, including the Sumerians, Babylonians, Assyrians, Hittites, and Egyptians. Many reasons were given to explain polygyny in ancient times, including love, procreation, trade alliances, and political diplomacy.

It is estimated that about 70 percent of the world's cultures permit polygyny. This, of course, does not mean that 70 percent of the world's population practice polygyny. In fact, even in societies that allow polygyny, most men only have one wife at a time. There are many reasons polygyny is not the most common form of marriage, even where it is permitted. Only a small proportion of men in societies that say they prefer polygyny actually are able to practice it due, in no small measure, to the economic burden of acquiring and maintaining more than one wife. In addition, in societies that permit polygyny, there is inequality in the ability of a man to sexually reproduce.

Polygyny is more common in societies with marked age stratification, as older males with more status and wealth acquire wives as a way to demonstrate this. On the other hand, polygyny is also more common in societies where women exert more control over resources and thus are less dependent on male parental investments.

Polygynous marriages often require financial support and approval from a large group of kin. Substantial bridewealth, the compensation expected by the family of the bride from the groom and his family, is often necessary to acquire a bride. In many pastoral societies, for example, several head of livestock are commonly expected for the "purchase" of a bride. Most potential grooms must draw on the resources of extended kin groups to accumulate sufficient bridewealth. Kin in polygynous societies are less likely to contribute to paying bridewealth for additional wives. Unless a man is very successful financially and has considerable status, it may be considered culturally inappropriate for him to seek an additional wife. In some polygynous societies, a man must be able to provide and maintain separate households for each wife, which can present considerable financial demands. It has also been found that in some societies where women are seen as an economic liability, where men do the majority of the work, that polygyny is less common. For instance, among the Sinuai of the Solomon Islands, women do much of the work of raising pigs, a highly valued resource, and also contribute to labor in the gardens; consequently polygynous households tend to have more pigs and thus greater economic resources, granting more status to polygynous husbands.

Another factor contributing to the difficulties of polygynous marriages is the interpersonal dynamics of balancing the demands of multiple wives. Considerable administrative skills may be needed to manage two or more wives and their children and households. If the relationships between cowives are not congenial, this can add to the stressors upon a polygynous husband. There may need to be complex calculations made as to things like which wife a man sleeps with, whom to eat food from, and whose children to allocate resources to.

There are other social pressures restricting polygyny, even where it is possible. For example, a study of retired Zulu migrant workers in South Africa found that although polygyny is considered to be the culturally preferred practice, the majority of Zulu men are monogamous. White South Africans and largely white Christian churches promote socially dominant values in opposition to polygyny, to which many Zulu decide to conform.

In addition to the disadvantages of polygyny, there are also several advantages cited. As mentioned, a polygynous husband typically acquires higher status and more social prestige by having more wives. Having multiple wives is often a signifier of wealth and power. A wife's status also often increases as her husband acquires more wives. Contrary to what might be assumed, polygyny can naturally contribute to population control. For example, among the Shipibo of the Amazon in Peru, polygyny allows women to have longer intervals between birthing children when paired with postpartum sexual abstinence; this practice also lowers infant mortality as mothers can breastfeed longer with the net result of suppressed birthrates. Some cultures practice sororal polygyny where a man marries sisters or other closely related females, which may help lessen jealousy between cowives and also maintains closer kinship relationships for offspring. In some cultures, the senior wife wields relative authority over junior wives, which can aid in maintaining smoother dynamics as she can often help mediate conflicts and disputes between cowives. Many ethnographic studies report on the degree of cooperation and harmony between cowives who can assist each other in the performance of labor-intensive activities.

Victor B. Stolberg

See also: Marriage; Marriage, Cross-Cultural Comparison of; Monogamy; Polyamory; Polyandry; Polygamy.

Further Reading

Hern, W. M. (1992). Family planning, Amazon style. *Natural History, 101*(12), 30–37.

Moller, V., & Welch, G. J. (1990). Polygamy, economic security, and well-being of retired Zulu migrant workers. *Journal of Cross-Cultural Gerontology, 5*(3), 205–216.

Oliver, D. (1955). *A Solomon Island society*. Cambridge, MA: Harvard University Press.

Tonkinson, R. (1978). *The Mardudjara aborigines: Living the dream in Australia's desert*. New York: Holt, Rinehart and Winston.

Pornography

The earliest use of the word "pornography" in the United States was in 1843 in a book that described pictures of naked women in ancient Rome. Today, pornography is defined as the depiction of sexual material that is intended to be sexually arousing. The word "pornography" is often used to describe sexual content in a negative way. Erotica, on the other hand, is a more positively evaluated form of sexual content and comes from a Greek word meaning "love poem."

Sometimes people equate pornography and erotica with obscenity. "Obscenity" is a legal term, and while there is subjectivity in its application, it describes material that, applying contemporary community standards, appeals to the prurient interest; depicts or describes, in a patently offensive way, sexual conduct specifically defined by the applicable state law; and lacks serious literary, artistic, political, or scientific value. Sexually explicit material that meets those conditions is illegal. Many pornographic materials that were once deemed in court to be obscene were later appealed and found to be acceptable under the First Amendment, freedom of speech.

The first pornographic book printed on a printing press, *I Modi*, was published in Rome in 1527 and included sixteen sonnets about various sexual positions that were accompanied by engraved illustrations. The first pornographic novel, *Memoirs of a Woman of Pleasure, or Fanny Hill*, was written in England in 1758 and is one of the most banned books in history. When it was published in the United States in the 1960s, it was banned, but when the case was appealed to the Supreme Court, it was found that it did not meet the standard of obscenity.

Pornography in the United States became a big business in the 1840s. Prior to then, erotic books and pictures were imported from France and England. Beginning in 1846, a New York publisher, William Haines, who had previously imported sexual materials began to produce them. By the time he died in 1872, he had published 320 pornographic books. Haines was the most successful publisher of pornography of the time, but he was hardly alone. Thousands of books, magazines, pamphlets, and photographs of explicit sexual content were produced in New York City throughout the nineteenth century and distributed nationally through the mail.

The proliferation of these materials and their delivery through the mail prompted the first federal obscenity law, the Comstock Act of 1873. The law made it illegal to send through the mail erotica, contraceptives, abortifacients, sex toys, or any information about these items. The Comstock Act was named for Anthony Comstock, an antivice reformer from New York whose job became to monitor the mail and confiscate and destroy obscene materials. He was very effective in his work, and due to his efforts, the flourishing pornography trade in New York City declined, only to be taken up in Philadelphia, St. Louis, Chicago, and San Francisco.

Shortly after the motion picture was developed, French producers made short films of women taking off their clothes. With profits to be made, producers in many countries began to make pornographic films. Men who could afford the projector bought the "stag films" discreetly and showed them at private parties. Eventually, pornographic movies would be distributed to adult theaters, and then, in the 1970s, made available on videotape, which consumers could view in the privacy of their homes.

Nowadays, sexually explicit material is available in magazines on newsstands, in bookstores, on television and DVDs, and, most pervasively, on the internet. It is estimated that, in the United States, pornography revenues equal $13 billion annually. A book series known for its erotic storyline, *50 Shades of Grey*, has sold over

125 million copies, and a follow-up book sold another million copies within days of its release.

With so much consumption of pornography, many people are concerned about its effects. Among mental health professionals, there is debate about whether or not pornography use is harmful to healthy sexual development and intimate relationships. Many professionals view its use as problematic because some people use it compulsively, others experience relationship difficulties when one partner feels left out or inadequate because of their partner's porn use, or an individual feels a lack of satisfactory sexual performance when comparing real life with the fantasies portrayed in pornography.

There has been a long-standing argument that exposure to pornography increases violence against women. However, Milton Diamond's analysis of data from around the world shows that as pornography becomes more available, sex crimes either decrease or remain constant. Sexually explicit material has wide acceptance and use and is tolerated for adults. Among the studies on attitudes about pornography, the only constant finding is that adults want to prevent its exposure to children. One researcher suggests that sexually explicit material functions in a variety of ways, such as increasing the consumer's knowledge, illustrating a range of intimate behaviors, helping to develop a sexual identity, and offering a context for expressing gender and sexuality.

As with all representations of sexuality in the media, explicit content expresses a set of values and a point of view. In most pornography, the people portrayed are highly sexual and available for sexual behavior at any time. The focus is typically on pleasure (most often the male's) rather than on the relationship between the characters. The bodies of the people in the story, picture, or video are most often idealized, and models with attractive attributes are used as the talent. In the case of professionally produced films, lighting, music, camera angles, and editing are skillfully combined to create the most arousing effects. Critics of pornographic films point out that the fantasy aspect of the content leads viewers, especially younger viewers, to expect that this is how shared sexual behavior is or should be.

Research also suggests that unhappy adults who use sexually explicit media are most likely to be negatively influenced by it. Because so much pornography presents an extremely casual view of sex, consumers without a steady partner may view sexual behavior without being in a relationship as desirable. The risk for these people is that they are more likely to engage in casual sex with people not known to them, and there is an increased potential for sexual aggression, contracting sexually transmitted infections, and being part of an unintended pregnancy.

The casual view of sex in pornography is also a factor in young people's expectations of what they might anticipate as they begin dating. Among early adolescents, exposure to sexually explicit media is an important factor in sexual socialization and leads to more permissive, earlier sexual behavior. Among teen boys who consume pornography, three-quarters report committing some form of sexual harassment. A strategy that parents and youth serving professionals can take to diminish the impact of exposure to porn is to provide comprehensive sexuality education in conjunction with media literacy education. Adults can help young people to view all media with a critical eye and to understand that it is created in particular ways for profit and influence.

Research suggests that as consumers of sexually explicit material get used to a particular type of porn, they seek novelty by viewing more intense or unusual behaviors that can lead to "porn addiction." The next step in the process suggests that users get habituated to the new, more intense content and wind up back where they started, seeking yet another, more intense behavior. At this point, they begin acting out sexually, as they no longer get satisfaction from viewing porn. Whether or not this theory is accurate is a matter of debate.

Much of the concern about porn is that it will cause someone to behave in unhealthy, addictive, or relationship-damaging ways. In a review of the research, analysts found that more porn use is related to higher levels of libido or sexual arousal. Individuals who report being more aroused by porn also use it more and report higher levels of sexual desire. Thus, a higher need or desire for sensation predicts more frequent use of porn in both adolescents and adults. It is valuable for all users of sexually explicit material to consider their motivation to use it and to work to understand its role in their life. Developing a healthy relationship to fantasy and pornography is an indicator of sexual maturity.

The first peer-reviewed journal about the study of pornography, *Porn Studies*, began publication in 2014.

Michael J. McGee

See also: Advertising, Sex in; Arousal; Commission on Obscenity and Pornography; Media and Sexuality; *Miller v. California*; Pornography Addiction; Sex Education.

Further Reading

Attwood, F. (2005). What do people do with porn? Qualitative research into the consumption, use and experience of pornography and other sexually explicit media. *Sexuality and Culture, 9*(2), 65–86.

Attwood, F., & Smith, C. (2014). Porn studies: An introduction. *Porn Studies, 1*(1–2), 1–6.

Brown, J. D., & L'Engle, K. L. (2009). X-rated: Sexual attitudes and behaviors associated with U.S. early adolescents' exposure to sexually explicit media. *Communication Research, 36*(1), 129–151.

Dennis, D. (2009). *Licentious Gotham: Erotic publishing and its prosecution in nineteenth-century New York.* Cambridge, MA: Harvard University Press.

Diamond, M. (2009). Pornography, public acceptance and sex related crime: A review. *International Journal of Law and Psychiatry, 32*(5), 304–314.

D'Orlando, F. (2011). The demand for pornography. *Journal of Happiness Studies, 12*(1), 51–75.

Hardingham-Gill, T. (2015, June 23). *The new Fifty Shades of Grey novel has already smashed UK book sales records.* Retrieved from http://metro.co.uk/2015/06/23/the-new-fifty-shades-of-grey-novel-has-already-smashed-uk-book-sales-records-5261225/

Ley, D., Prause, N., & Finn, P. (2014). The emperor has no clothes: A review of the "pornography addiction" model. *Current Sexual Health Reports, 6*(2), 94–105.

Library of Congress. (1873). American memory from the Library of Congress. *Statutes at Large: U.S. Congressional Documents.* Retrieved from http://memory.loc.gov/ammem/amlaw/lwsl.html

Maltz, W., & Maltz, L. (2008). *The porn trap: The essential guide to overcoming problems caused by pornography*. London: HarperCollins.

Slade, J. W. (2006). Eroticism and technological regression: The stag film. *History & Technology, 22*(1), 27–52.

Smith, W., & Anthon, C. (Eds.). (1843). *A dictionary of Greek and Roman antiquities*. New York: American Book Company.

Wright, P. J. (2015). A longitudinal analysis of US adults' pornography exposure. *Journal of Media Psychology, 24*(2), 67–76.

Wright, P. J., Tokunaga, R. S., & Bae, S. (2014). More than a dalliance? Pornography consumption and extramarital sex attitudes among married US adults. *Psychology of Popular Media Culture, 3*(2), 97.

Pornography Addiction

Pornography involves the depiction of sexual behaviors in ways intended to cause sexual arousal or satisfaction. Common forms of pornography include pictures, videos, and written accounts of sexual features or behaviors. At present, pornography is primarily accessed by users in North America through the internet, though print magazines and sexually explicit films remain available. Problematic pornography use is sometimes referred to as "pornography addiction" or "pornography compulsion," though the use of these terms varies among professionals. Problematic pornography use may cause relational, occupational, legal, financial, spiritual, and mental health distress.

The American Society of Addiction Medicine defines addiction as "a primary, chronic disease of brain reward, motivation, memory and related circuitry. Dysfunction in these circuits leads to characteristic biological, psychological, social and spiritual manifestations. This is reflected in an individual pathologically pursuing reward or relief by substance use and other behaviors." According to this model, an individual with pornography addiction will find it very difficult or impossible to avoid pornography use, will crave the activity, and will often have difficulty acknowledging the damage done to personal relationships (such as those with a romantic or sexual partner, children, extended family, or friends) or other areas of functioning. Addiction models employ a medical model and view the behavior as chronic, involving cycles of relapse and remission. Addiction is often seen as progressive, worsening over time if the individual does not participate in recovery and treatment activities.

While an addiction model may be an appropriate one to apply to some individuals' use of pornography, the bulk of the research on pornography use indicates that most users of pornography do not experience clinically significant distress and impairment in biological, psychological, or social domains of functioning as a result of pornography use. There is also some disagreement among mental health professionals about whether problematic pornography use is better understood in terms of an addiction model or a compulsion model. In a compulsion model, an individual repeatedly engages in behaviors that they feel driven to perform in response to another stressor, such as anxious thoughts. Some clinicians prefer to use a compulsion model to describe problematic pornography use because it better fits the symptoms reported by their clients. Finally, an individual may experience problems related to pornography use that do not fit either an addiction or compulsion model, such as relationship strain due to pornography use, even if the use is infrequent or time-limited.

Research suggests that there is no single cause for problematic pornography use. It is often more helpful to look at several biological, psychological, social, and spiritual contributors to this and other problematic behaviors. Some sex researchers have focused on the important role of an individual's arousal template in pornography use. The template is the individual's pattern of sexual arousal in response to internal stimuli (such as thoughts and images) and external stimuli (the sights, sounds, smells, tastes, and touches that the individual finds arousing). It is likely the product of biological predispositions and both classical and operant conditioning during adolescence and early adulthood. Early exposure to pornography may significantly shape an individual's arousal template in terms of what they find arousing later in life; also, an individual may specifically seek out pornography to find the features of a sexual scenario that they find arousing, particularly if it is difficult to find those features in a face-to-face relationship or encounter.

Assessment of pornography use can be difficult for many reasons. Individuals are often reluctant to disclose the frequency and duration of pornography use as well as the specific content of what is used. Individuals often underreport pornography use due to embarrassment, concerns about judgment from the assessor, or a lack of awareness of the scope of the pornography use. Further, the individual may see it as a more or less problematic behavior than the assessor. For example, men often report that pornography use is less problematic compared to women's descriptions of the same behaviors. Some individuals see any pornography use as inherently problematic, while a sex therapist or educator may view the individual's behavior as normal. The *DSM-5* does not include a diagnosis for a pornography-related disorder among its descriptions of substance-related and addictive disorders, though some individuals may display symptoms consistent with an unspecified paraphilic disorder.

Several brief assessments of pornography problems are available, such as the Internet Sex Screening Test. A consultation with a mental health professional that specializes in sexual concerns is recommended before determining if an individual has a pornography problem. Treatment often focuses on anxiety management, depression treatment, conflict resolution, and identifying face-to-face means of meeting sexual needs and interests. Treatment may be offered in inpatient hospital settings, outpatient counseling, twelve-step groups, and online programs.

Elizabeth A. Maynard

See also: Compulsivity, Sexual; Online Sexual Activity; Out-of-Control Sexual Behavior; Pornography.

Further Reading

American Psychiatric Association. (2011). *Diagnostic and statistical manual of mental disorders* (5th ed.). Arlington, VA: American Psychiatric Association.

American Society of Addiction Medicine. (2019). Retrieved from www.asam.org

Cooper, A. (Ed.). (2013). Cybersex: The dark side of the force (special issue). *Journal of Sexual Addiction and Compulsivity, 19*(1–2), 1–160.

Grant, J. E., Potenza, M. N., Weinstein, A., & Gorelick, D. A. (2010). Introduction to behavioral addictions. *The American Journal of Drug and Alcohol Abuse, 36*(5), 233–241.

Twohig, M. P., & Crosby, J. M. (2010). Acceptance and Commitment Therapy as a treatment for problematic Internet pornography viewing. *Behavior Therapy, 41*(3), 285–295.

Preejaculate Fluid

Preejaculate fluid (preseminal fluid, precum) is a fluid created mainly by the bulbourethral glands (Cowper's glands). The Cowper's glands are two small glands along the urethra. This fluid is necessary to reduce the acidity of the urethra and provides lubrication for the ejaculate. Discharged from the urethra during foreplay, masturbation, and sexual arousal, most men are unable to control the release of preejaculate fluid and do not feel it happening. This fluid is known as preejaculate because it occurs before orgasm and ejaculation.

For sperm to survive, it must be in a neutral or alkaline environment. Preejaculatory fluid neutralizes the urethra, which can be an acidic environment due to the presence of urine, increasing the viability of sperm. Like the urethra, the vagina is also an acidic environment and is hostile toward sperm. Preejaculatory fluid may neutralize the vagina, increasing sperm's survival and motility. Along with neutralizing the urethra and vagina, preejaculatory fluid may be a lubricant for the glans (head of the penis) and aid in penetration.

Preejaculate fluid is clear, colorless, and chemically different from semen. The amount of fluid an individual produces varies widely, with some individuals not producing any. Some individuals are uncomfortable or embarrassed by the amount of preejaculate they produce. This overproduction of preejaculate is rare and might be treatable with an alpha-5-reductase inhibitor. Preejaculate, like semen, can contain sexually transmitted infections (STIs), including HIV, that can be transmitted to uninfected people if barrier methods, such as condoms or dental dams, are not used.

A widely debated topic regarding preejaculate is whether or not this fluid contains sperm. The quick answer is it is unlikely that preejaculatory fluid contains viable sperm; however, it is possible, so precautions should be taken. Research into whether preejaculatory fluid contains sperm has produced mixed results with some studies showing that no viable sperm are present in preejaculate and other studies showing many viable sperm in preejaculate samples. If there is semen present in the urethra from a prior ejaculation, it is possible for sperm to enter the preejaculatory fluid and be released from the urethra before climax and ejaculation. Some sexuality and health educators advise people to urinate after ejaculation to remove semen from the urethra, reducing the possibility of the preejaculate fluid containing sperm.

Some individuals use the knowledge that it is unlikely that preejaculate fluid contains sperm as reason to use the withdrawal method (coitus interruptus, pull-out method) as a form of pregnancy prevention. In the event that preejaculatory fluid does not contain sperm, the withdrawal method may still not be the most reliable birth control option because not everyone can determine when they will ejaculate, and therefore they may not pull out in time. This method also leaves people susceptible to STI and HIV infection as these diseases can be transmitted via preejaculatory fluid. It is advised that individuals use barrier methods to protect themselves against disease transmission and to reduce the risk of pregnancy.

Damiene Denner

See also: Bulbourethral Glands; Ejaculation; Semen; Sexually Transmitted Infections (STIs); Withdrawal Method.

Further Reading

American Pregnancy Association. (n.d.). Can you get pregnant with pre-cum? Retrieved from http://americanpregnancy.org/getting-pregnant/can-you-get-pregnant-with-precum/

Herbenick, D. (2005). Q&A: Can you get pregnant from pre-cum? *Kinsey Confidential.* Retrieved from http://kinseyconfidential.org/can-you-get-pregnant-from-pre-cum/

Killick, S. R., Leary, C., Trussell, J., & Guthrie, K. A. (2011). Sperm content of pre-ejaculatory fluid. *Human Fertility, 14*(1), 48–52.

Pregnancy

The thought of having a baby might excite some people, scare some people, or do both for some people. Some people may decide not to continue a pregnancy, and sometimes a pregnancy ends in an unexpected miscarriage. If the pregnancy continues for a full forty weeks, though sometimes sooner, a baby is born through a process called birth. Birth happens via vaginal delivery or through cesarean section. Not everyone who is pregnant becomes the parent of a baby after they give birth to the baby, as some people may place the baby for adoption or may be acting as surrogates for other people. However, most people who give birth to a baby become the parent of that child.

Only people with uteruses can become pregnant. An egg from an ovary and a sperm from a testicle need to combine to begin a pregnancy. The egg is fertilized by the sperm, and this creates something called a zygote. A zygote has all the genetic information about the person the sperm came from and the person the egg came from in addition to the blueprints for continuing to grow. This zygote then grows enough to be called a blastocyst. When the blastocyst attaches to the uterus, it can then be called an embryo. The embryo is called a fetus when it grows for a few more weeks. This fetus then continues to grow for about another six months before it is born. Full gestation is considered forty weeks or roughly nine months.

People often become pregnant while in a relationship with another person. The most common way a pregnancy occurs is through penis-in-vagina sex, though this is not the only method. Some people become pregnant through other methods of bringing sperm and eggs together, often called assisted reproductive technology, so that the zygote can implant into a uterus and grow.

People often learn that they are pregnant from a pregnancy test. Many people take a home pregnancy test where they place urine on a device that tests for something called human chorionic gonadotropin (hCG). A pregnant person's body starts to produce hCG about two to three weeks after conception (or about four weeks since the beginning of the last menstrual period). When taking a pregnancy test, it can be useful to take the test first thing after waking up in the morning because hCG concentrations will be highest after not urinating for a while. If a test comes back positive, meaning the person is pregnant, that is almost always the case as there are very few false positives. However, false negatives are more common, so if a home pregnancy test is negative, the person can try again in a week to be sure. Some people also do urine tests at doctors' offices instead of on their own at home. Blood tests by a doctor are not more accurate and cannot be done any earlier than a home pregnancy test using urine. If an at-home test is positive, the person should schedule an appointment with a doctor. If they expect to continue the pregnancy, all alcohol, substance, tobacco, and hormonal birth control use should be stopped.

It is not always easy for someone to become pregnant, and sometimes repeatedly trying to conceive changes the way someone feels about their body and sexuality. When people are trying to conceive, doctors often prescribe medications to increase the chances of an egg and a sperm combining and for a blastocyst to attach to the uterus. These medications often cause other changes to the way a person's body feels and whether they are in the mood to sexually connect with a partner. Trying to conceive might also include one or more miscarriages for the people trying to become parents. Almost always, a miscarriage is completely unavoidable and is not anyone's fault. Sometimes people do not tell others they are pregnant for the first twelve weeks, or the first trimester, as the first trimester has the highest chances of a miscarriage occurring. Trying to conceive is a great time for couples to talk about what they most enjoy during sex and ways to continue having sex that is fun for everyone involved.

There are many changes that occur to the pregnant person's body as the fetus grows. Some of these changes affect the way a person experiences and expresses their sexuality. For example, breasts feel fuller, clothing no longer fits the same way, some people get upset stomachs almost daily, most pregnant people are very tired, and the pregnant person usually notices they can feel movement from the fetus inside their uterus. Many people talk about feeling uncomfortable being sexual while a fetus is developing inside their uterus. Sometimes people are afraid penetrative sex might be dangerous to the fetus or painful. Vaginal sex will not contact the fetus. Very early on in a pregnancy, a barrier develops to block off the uterus from the vagina. In general, sex should not cause undesired pain, so if a pregnant person notices pain, they should contact their doctor.

During the first trimester, or the first twelve weeks of the pregnancy, many changes occur. Often, people will be unaware that they are pregnant until after they miss a period and take a pregnancy test, which usually happens around weeks four or five. Some people will have no pregnancy symptoms at all. Others may experience early pregnancy symptoms, which may include sore breasts, nausea or morning sickness, mood swings, tiredness, headaches, food cravings, a heightened sense of smell, vaginal discharge, a need to urinate more frequently, cramping, changes to hair and skin, and feeling boated. During this stage, the zygote grows from being just a few cells to being a fetus about two inches long. In addition, the fetus's nervous system and brain develop, the heart forms and starts to beat, other internal organs form, and facial features and limbs start to develop.

During the second trimester, weeks thirteen to twenty-seven, the pregnant person forms a small bump in their midsection that continues to grow for the duration of the pregnancy. Breasts also start to enlarge, and the placenta forms around week fourteen. Usually the symptoms of pregnancy are less severe in the second trimester. In addition to the symptoms noted above, some people may also experience trouble with their gums; aches and pains, especially around the belly; nosebleeds; gastric complaints; trouble sleeping; and bladder or vaginal infections, among others. The fetus is continuing to grow and develop during this phase and will grow from about 2.5 inches long to about 14.4 inches long. It also becomes possible for the pregnant person to feel the fetus moving inside them.

During the third and final trimester, the fetus continues to grow, and the pregnant person's body readies itself for birth. Commonly, people in the third trimester of pregnancy may experience heartburn and indigestion, aches and pains, and tiredness. Other symptoms mentioned above may still be present. Toward the end of the trimester, people may begin to feel Braxton-Hicks contractions, or a tightening of the muscles of the uterus. The fetus continues to grow and gain weight until birth. It continues to be active and can respond to sound and light. At week thirty-seven, the fetus is considered to be full term, meaning it's likely big enough and developed enough to survive in the outside world without medical intervention should it be born. Most births occur during weeks thirty-nine to forty-one. Typically babies are about twenty inches long when they are born and often weigh around seven to eight pounds, although some can be much lighter or much heavier.

Being a parent also affects how individuals might be able to sexually connect with each other. It is often very difficult to find time and energy to have sex when caring for an infant who wakes up every two hours and needs regular feeding and diaper changes. Most parents work full-time jobs and worry about how to financially afford this new addition to their family. Some new parents also suffer from postpartum depression, which causes feelings of deep sadness and hopelessness. Doctors and therapists can help people with postpartum depression. Very little alone time, not enough sleep, and lots of stress do not help people have sex. It is very important for new parents to set aside time to go on regular dates once the baby is old enough to be cared for by someone other than a parent.

Rosara Torrisi

See also: Assisted Reproductive Technology; Fertility; Infertility.

Further Reading

Boggs, B. (2016). *The art of waiting: On fertility, medicine, and motherhood.* Minneapolis: Graywolf Press.

Cavallucci, D., & Fulbright, Y. K. (2008). *Your orgasmic pregnancy: Little sex secrets every hot mama should know.* Alameda, CA: Hunter House Publishers.

Kerner, I., & Raykeil, H. (2009). *Love in the time of colic: The new parents' guide to getting it on again.* New York: William Morrow Paperbacks.

National Health Service. (2020). Week-by-week guide to pregnancy. Retrieved from www.nhs.uk/start4life/pregnancy/week-by-week/

Tsiaras, A. (2010). Conception to birth. Presented at INK Conference TED Talk. Retrieved from https://www.ted.com/talks/alexander_tsiaras_conception_to_birth_visualized?language=en

Premarital Sex

Premarital sex is sex that takes place before marriage. Survey results from the early 2010s indicate that around 90 percent of ever-married Americans under the age of forty-five years had sex before they married. Nearly half of American high school students admit to having engaged in sexual intercourse. Discussions of youthful premarital sex, in particular, often focus on topics such as immorality and emotional immaturity. There are negative consequences to society in terms of unwanted pregnancies and the spread of sexually transmitted infections (STIs).

Premarital sex most often takes place after puberty when hormonal changes greatly escalate the sex drive, the desire for sexual activity. The age at which puberty occurs varies by individual but is typically before or during the early teen years. Menarche is the onset of menstrual periods. Scientists have found that the average age at which girls experience menarche declined from around sixteen years old during the early 1900s to less than thirteen years old in the early 2000s. Research suggests that boys are also beginning puberty at earlier ages than in decades past. The reasons for this trend are not yet clear.

The U.S. Census Bureau collects detailed data about the marital status of Americans. One statistic of particular interest is the age at first marriage. Between 1970 and 2009, the median age at first marriage for women increased from twenty-one to twenty-seven years; the median age for men increased from twenty-three to twenty-eight years. In 1970, nearly half (42%) of women marrying for the first time were teenagers; by 2009, that number had dropped to only 7 percent. Overall, the data indicate that Americans are marrying for the first time at older ages than in the past.

The combination of younger puberty ages and older ages at first marriage translates to a longer time period during which premarital sex can occur. This wide window of opportunity is a modern phenomenon. In ancient times, girls first married around or even before the onset of puberty. This greatly reduced the chances of premarital sex taking place. There are still societies in the twenty-first century in which child brides or young teen brides are common, primarily parts of Africa and Asia.

The U.S. Centers for Disease Control and Prevention (CDC) conducts surveys in which it asks Americans about their marital status and sexual history. During surveys conducted from 2011 to 2013, the CDC found that 89 percent of ever-married women aged fifteen to forty-four years and 92 percent of ever-married men aged twenty to forty-four years said they had engaged in premarital sexual intercourse.

Every two years, the CDC conducts a national Youth Risk Behavior Survey (YRBS) in which it surveys students in ninth through twelfth grades in U.S. public and private schools. Results indicate that in 2017, 39.5 percent of the students said they had engaged in sexual intercourse. This percentage is down from 54 percent in 1991.

The YRBS data specifies premarital sex rates by race and ethnicity. In 2017, black or African American teens had the highest rate of premarital sex at 45.8 percent. They were followed by Hispanic or Latino teens (41.1%) and white teens (38.6%). According to the YRBS, a small fraction (3.4%) of all the ninth to twelfth graders asked in 2017 said they had sexual intercourse for the first time before they were thirteen years old. This compares with 10 percent in 1991. Another subject addressed in the YRBS is number of sexual partners. Some 9.7 percent of the ninth to twelfth graders surveyed in 2017 said they had engaged in sexual intercourse with at least four people. This percentage is down from 19 percent in 1991. Having multiple sexual partners is considered risky because it raises the chances of unwanted pregnancies and STIs.

Attitudes about premarital sex are often driven by religious beliefs or cultural sensibilities. Sex outside of marriage (and hence premarital sex) is deemed immoral in religions such as Christianity, Islam, and Judaism. In some cultures, premarital sex is considered inappropriate not because of religious restrictions but because it violates long-standing cultural traditions regarding marriage. In addition, there is widespread belief that youths lack the maturity needed to make rational decisions about engaging in sex and the possible consequences of doing so. Physical intimacy often adds psychological complexity to a relationship. This may be difficult for teenagers to process emotionally; for example, they may confuse sexual passion with love.

Premarital sex can result in pregnancy. According to the CDC, unmarried teenage girls accounted for nearly 195,000 U.S. births during 2017. This equated to a rate of around 18.8 births per 1,000 unmarried girls in this age range. However, the teen birth rate has declined dramatically since the early 1990s. YRBS survey data indicate that more than half (53.8%) of the sexually active ninth to twelfth graders surveyed in 2017 said they used a condom during their most recent sexual intercourse, and 20.7 percent said they used birth control pills. However, 13.8 percent of the sexually active teens reported using no method of birth control.

The spread of STIs is a major public health problem. People who have sex with multiple partners have the greatest risk of contracting these diseases. Preteens and teens who engage in premarital sex are high-risk groups because they begin having sex at such a young age. This increases the likelihood that they will have multiple partners during their sex lives. According to the CDC, during the early 2010s, there were 10 million new STIs among persons aged fifteen to twenty-four years in the United States. These youths accounted for 50 percent of all new infections, even though they comprised just over a quarter of the sexually active population.

Kim Masters Evans

See also: Casual Sex; Dating, Cross-Cultural Comparison of; Hookup Culture; Marriage; Religion, Diversity of Human Sexuality and; Teen Pregnancy.

Further Reading

Copen, C. E., Daniels, K., Vespa, J., & Mosher, W. D. (2012). First marriages in the United States: Data from the 2006–2010 National Survey of Family Growth. *National Health Statistics Reports, 49*, 1–21.

Kann, L., McManus, T., Harris, W. A., Shanklin, S. L., Flint, K. H., Queen, B., ... Ethier, K. A. (2018). Youth risk behavior surveillance—United States, 2017. *MMWR Surveillance Summaries, 67*(8), 1–114.

Martin, J. A., Hamilton, B. E., Osterman, M. J., Curtin, S. C., & Matthews, T. J. (2015). Births: Final data for 2013. *National Vital Statistics Reports, 64*(1), 1–65.

U.S. Centers for Disease Control and Prevention. (2016). Trends in the prevalence of sexual behaviors and HIV testing: National YRBS: 1991–2013. Retrieved from http://www.cdc.gov/healthyyouth/data/yrbs/pdf/trends/us_sexual_trend_yrbs.pdf

U.S. Centers for Disease Control and Prevention. (2017). Key statistics from the National Survey of Family Growth: Premarital sex. Retrieved from http://www.cdc.gov/nchs/nsfg/key_statistics/p.htm#premarital

U.S. Centers for Disease Control and Prevention. (2017). Sexually transmitted diseases: Adolescents and young adults. Retrieved from http://www.cdc.gov/std/life-stages-populations/adolescents-youngadults.htm

U.S. Centers for Disease Control and Prevention. (2019). Reproductive health: Teen pregnancy. Retrieved from https://www.cdc.gov/teenpregnancy/index.htm

U.S. Centers for Disease Control and Prevention. (2019). Teen births. Retrieved from http://www.cdc.gov/nchs/fastats/teen-births.htm

Premature Ejaculation

Premature ejaculation (PE, also known as rapid ejaculation, premature climax, or early ejaculation) occurs when someone uncontrollably ejaculates before or immediately upon sexual penetration, often with minimal sexual stimulation. While this primarily affects males, some females also experience PE. PE is fairly common and is more likely to occur in younger males. It is estimated that PE affects most men at some point in their life.

Diagnostic criteria for PE include ejaculation within one minute of penetration, the inability to delay ejaculation all or nearly all the time, and the feeling of distress and frustration that may lead to the avoidance of sexual intimacy. PE can be primary or secondary. Primary PE is lifelong, beginning with the individual's first sexual encounter, and occurs nearly all the time. Secondary PE is acquired and develops after the individual has had sexual experiences without ejaculatory issues. Symptoms of PE do not always meet diagnostic criteria and may be categorized as natural variable PE instead. Natural variable PE occurs when an individual has periods of premature ejaculation and normal ejaculation.

Premature ejaculation often has no clear cause. Certain situations, such as a new partner or a long time since last ejaculation, may increase the potential for PE. For some individuals, PE may only occur in specific sexual situations.

Early sexual experiences are thought to establish sexual patterns that often persist into adult life and can be difficult to change. When individuals are hurried to reach climax or associate feelings of guilt that lead to a tendency to rush to orgasm and end sexual activities, PE can result. Relationship problems may also contribute to PE. Anxiety, especially anxiety regarding sexuality or sexual performance, can affect ejaculation. If an individual is anxious about prematurely ejaculating, this anxiety can increase the chances of future PE. Anxiety regarding erectile dysfunction (having or maintaining an erection) may create a pattern of rushed ejaculation because the individual tries to climax before losing their erection. Rushing to ejaculation is not always something the individual knows they are doing, making it difficult to identify.

PE can have biological causes, including abnormal hormone and neurotransmitter levels. The ejaculatory system is a reflex, and this reflex can become damaged, causing PE. Inflammation and infection of the prostate or urethra and nerve damage may also affect ejaculation.

Embarrassment concerning PE is common and can impede individuals from seeking medical and therapeutic assistance. Sexual experience and age can help individuals learn how to delay ejaculation and, in many instances, PE will resolve itself over time. Some individuals may be relieved to know that PE is common and treatable.

Gaining more control over an individual's orgasm can decrease the instances of PE. Masturbating to climax an hour or two before partnered sexual activities may allow an individual to better control their orgasm during sex. Reducing or eliminating the use of alcohol, tobacco, and recreational drugs may also improve an individual's control. Communicating with a partner to slow or stop stimulation when ejaculation is approaching, using different positions during sexual activities, and using condoms and medications that reduce sensation may allow an individual to better control ejaculation. Certain creams, gels, and sprays (topical anesthetics) that are applied before sexual activities to reduce sensation can be used to delay ejaculation, although these should be discussed with a medical professional before use. Some of these medications may also transfer to the individual's partner(s) during sexual activity and reduce the partner's sensation. Methods that reduce sensation may also reduce sexual pleasure.

Use of the pause-squeeze technique may be an effective therapy to delay ejaculation. To do this technique, sexual activity should begin as usual up until the point where the individual is about to ejaculate. At this point the penis should be compressed between the shaft and head for several seconds until the urge to ejaculate subsides. After the squeeze is released, the individuals should wait roughly thirty seconds before continuing sexual activity. Repeat the squeeze technique again when the individual feels like they are about to ejaculate. This technique can be repeated as many times as necessary until the individual is able to enter their partner without ejaculating.

Reducing anxiety associated with ejaculation is another possible treatment, especially because these thought patterns can lead to more episodes of PE. Thinking of nonsexual matters and using relaxation techniques may delay ejaculation. Focusing on other types of sexual activity, apart from penetrative sex, may reduce pressure and anxiety associated with sexual activity. Counseling and behavioral therapy may also be useful in reducing anxiety that is related to PE.

Damiene Denner

See also: Ejaculation; Performance Anxiety; Retrograde Ejaculation; Sexual Disorders, Male; Start-Stop Technique.

Further Reading

Harvard Health Publishing. (2017). Premature ejaculation. Retrieved from https://www.health.harvard.edu/a-to-z/premature-ejaculation-a-to-z

Mayo Clinic. (2018). Premature ejaculation. Retrieved from https://www.mayoclinic.org/diseases-conditions/premature-ejaculation/symptoms-causes/syc-20354900

NHS. (2019). Ejaculation problems. Retrieved from https://www.nhs.uk/conditions/ejaculation-problems/

Premenstrual Dysphoric Disorder (PMDD)

Premenstrual dysphoric disorder (PMDD) is a depressive disorder characterized by a severe form of premenstrual syndrome (PMS) in which mood swings, depression, irritability, or anxiety significantly impair everyday functioning. Both PMS and PMDD have physical and emotional symptoms. However, PMDD causes extreme mood shifts that can disrupt the individual's work and relationships. In both PMS and PMDD, symptoms typically begin seven to ten days before the menstrual period starts and continue for the first few days of the period. Both PMS and PMDD can cause fatigue, bloating, breast tenderness, and changes in sleep and eating patterns. However, in PMDD, at least one of the following emotional or behavioral symptoms stands out: extreme moodiness, marked irritability or anger, overwhelming sadness or hopelessness, and extreme anxiety or tension.

According to the fifth edition of the *Diagnostic and Statistical Manual of Mental Disorders* (*DSM-V*), women can be diagnosed with PMDD if they exhibit a pattern of symptoms during the final week before the onset of their menstrual cycle. The symptoms should start to improve within a few days after the onset of the menstrual cycle and be minimal or absent in the following week. These symptoms include marked mood swings, irritability, anger, and increased interpersonal conflicts. They also include depressed mood, feelings of hopelessness, anxiety, feelings of being "on edge," and decreased interest in usual activities. Other symptoms may include difficulty concentrating, a lack of energy, a change in appetite or sleep pattern, breast tenderness, food cravings, weight gain, and a sense of being overwhelmed. These symptoms must be significantly distressing and impair the individual's ability to function in important areas of life. Finally, this condition cannot have been caused by substance use, medical conditions, or other mental disorders.

Just as with PMS, the cause of PMDD is not well understood. As with other mental disorders, several factors appear to be involved. First among these are hormones. Hormonal changes during the menstrual cycle can trigger some of the symptoms of this disorder. In addition, changes in levels of serotonin, a neurotransmitter thought to regulate mood, can trigger these symptoms. For instance, low levels of serotonin can cause premenstrual depression, fatigue, and sleep problems. Other factors include stress, which can increase symptom intensity, and poor nutrition. Eating highly salty foods can cause fluid retention, while consuming alcohol and caffeine can cause moodiness and fatigue. Low levels of vitamins and minerals and a previous history of depression may also increase the likelihood of having PMDD.

Medications, counseling, or psychotherapy have a place in treating PMDD. Commonly prescribed medications include selective serotonin reuptake inhibitors, which can help with the symptoms of depression, fatigue, sleep problems, and food cravings. Over-the-counter pain medications can ease cramping and breast tenderness. Diuretics can reduce swelling and bloating. Oral contraceptives can stabilize hormonal swings, and hormone injections or contraceptive injectables can temporarily stop menstruation and the accompanying pain. Psychotherapy can also help those with this disorder to develop more effective coping strategies. The use of stress management and mindfulness practices can increase relaxation, acceptance, and living in the present.

Len Sperry

See also: Diagnostic and Statistical Manual of Mental Disorders (*DSM*); Menstruation; Premenstrual Syndrome (PMS); Sex Hormones.

Further Reading

Huston, J. E., & Fujitsubo, L. C. (2002). *PMDD: A guide to coping with premenstrual dysphoric disorder*. Oakland, CA: New Harbinger Publications.

Sperry, L. (Ed.). (2015). *Mental health and mental disorders: An encyclopedia from androgyny to zolpidem*. Santa Barbara, CA: Greenwood.

Premenstrual Syndrome (PMS)

Premenstrual syndrome, often referred to as PMS, is a combination of psychological and physiological symptoms that occur in relation to a person's menstrual cycle. PMS symptoms can begin up to two weeks prior to the menstrual cycle. Once the person's period starts, the symptoms typically end within four days or less. These premenstrual symptoms can be so severe that they interfere with how the person is able to interact with their daily activities. There is a wide range of experiences with PMS. Some individuals barely notice symptoms, while others suffer debilitating symptoms. PMS is most common among individuals between twenty and forty years old. Premenstrual syndrome has a wide range of psychological and physical symptoms, and each person's experience is different. PMS is typically diagnosed when an individual has psychological and physical symptoms five days before their period for three consecutive menstrual cycles.

Physiological symptoms of PMS include, but are not limited to, fatigue, bloating and/or weight gain, skin issues (i.e., acne), abdominal pain (i.e., cramping), breast tenderness, headaches and migraines, general aches and pains throughout the body, constipation or diarrhea, and vomiting.

PMS can also affect one's cognitive processes and emotional state. Often these psychological shifts are negative and cause distress. These symptoms of psychological distress could be incorrectly attributed to other external stimuli outside of

PMS. Psychological symptoms of PMS include, but are not limited to, hostility or irritability, exhaustion, food cravings, depression, mood swings, change in libido, anxiety, insomnia, and social withdrawal.

Currently, there is no research that has proven the cause of PMS; however, it is thought to be due to changes in hormone levels that occur throughout menstruation and ovulation. Stress may be an additional contributor to the intensity of the symptoms of PMS.

If an individual experiences PMS, it is best for them to consult with their health care provider to find a treatment that works best for their body. Hormone and symptom levels are different for each individual; therefore, there is no one-size-fits-all solution. That said, there are some home remedies that can reduce the symptoms from PMS. Medication used to treat symptoms of PMS include hormonal contraceptives, nonsteroidal anti-inflammatory drugs (e.g., ibuprofen), antidepressants, and diuretics (i.e., water pills). There are also lifestyle adjustments that may help alleviate the uncomfortable symptoms presented with PMS, including eating a well-balanced diet; decreasing sugar, salt, and caffeine consumption; getting seven to eight hours of sleep every night; and participating in regular exercise, as exercise helps to release endorphins, which can help psychological symptoms such as depression and anxiety. Individuals may also benefit from activities that help to reduce stress, such as meditation, yoga, massage therapy, and other forms of relaxation therapy.

Overall, living a well-balanced and healthy lifestyle can help treat many unwanted physical and psychological symptoms caused by PMS. If changes in lifestyle do not help with painful and distressing PMS symptoms, then further medication and medical advice from a health care provider may be required.

Nicole Williams

See also: Menstruation; Premenstrual Dysphoric Disorder (PMDD); Sex Hormones.

Further Reading

American College of Obstetricians and Gynecologists. (2015). Premenstrual syndrome (PMS). Retrieved from https://www.acog.org/Patients/FAQs/Premenstrual-Syndrome-PMS

Freeborn, D., Revino, H., & Burd, I. (2019). Premenstrual syndrome (PMS). Retrieved from https://www.urmc.rochester.edu/encyclopedia/content.aspx?contenttypeid=85&contentid=p00581

Mayo Clinic. (2018). Premenstrual syndrome (PMS). Retrieved from https://www.mayoclinic.org/diseases-conditions/premenstrual-syndrome/symptoms-causes/syc-20376780

National Institutes of Health. (2019). Premenstrual syndrome. Retrieved from https://medlineplus.gov/premenstrualsyndrome.html

Office on Women's Health. (2018). Premenstrual syndrome (PMS). Retrieved from https://www.womenshealth.gov/menstrual-cycle/premenstrual-syndrome

Priapism

A priapism is a persistent, painful, and unwanted erection of the penis. Priapism causes erections that are not the result of sexual desire or arousal. Typically, the engorged portions of the penis become tender and painful during a priapism, and the symptoms can last a few hours, days, or weeks. Priapism is rare and most often occurs in children between five and ten years old and adults between twenty and fifty years of age. Clitoral priapism can occur in females when the clitoris becomes engorged with blood for prolonged periods of time, resulting in a tender, painful, and unwanted erection of the clitoris.

There are two kinds of priapism: ischemic (low flow) and nonischemic (high flow). Ischemic priapism is characterized by blood not being able to leave the penis and is the most common kind of priapism. Nonischemic priapism occurs when there is too much blood flowing into the penis. This kind of priapism is often less painful than ischemic priapism. Prognosis for priapism is often good; however, the longer medical attention is delayed, the greater the risk for permanent injury.

There are several causes of priapism, including nervous system disorders, mechanical disorders, alcohol and other drug use, prescription medication, blood disorders, and injury. Nervous disorders that can lead to priapism include disorders of the spinal nerves or peripheral nerves that lead to the reproductive tract. Syphilitic involvement of the nervous system can also cause priapism in children and adults. Mechanical causes of priapism include obstructions in the penis, such as blood clots or tumors, and occasionally prolonged and rough sexual activity in the case of chronic priapism. Causes of priapism in children may include local irritation, prolonged masturbation, and a full bladder. Congenital syphilis, leukemia, sickle cell anemia, and infections of the reproductive tract can also lead to priapism in children.

Priapism that lasts longer than four hours requires immediate treatment. If left untreated, priapism can lead to urine retention in the bladder, kidney disease, penile disfigurement, and permanent impotence (inability to achieve or maintain an erection). Priapism that lasts less than four hours does not require immediate medical assistance but should be brought to the attention of a doctor so future episodes can be prevented and the cause can be determined.

Ischemic and nonischemic priapism are treated differently. Nonischemic priapism is often treated with a watch-and-wait approach because this kind of priapism can be resolved with no treatment and poses little risk to the penis. In the event that treatment is needed, surgery to put material in the body that blocks the flow of blood to the penis may be recommended. The application of pressure and ice to the perineum and penis to reduce swelling may also be an effective treatment for nonischemic priapism.

There are several ways to treat ischemic priapism. Aspiration, the draining of blood from the penis via syringe, may relieve pain and stop the erection. Medication that constricts blood vessels, such as phenylephrine, can be injected into the spongy tissue of the penis (corpus cavernosum) to increase the flow of blood out of the penis. Surgery that reroutes blood using a device (shunt) implanted in the penis may also be helpful in treating priapism. Treatment of sickle cell anemia, leukemia, and damaged arteries and tissue may also be necessary for successful treatment of priapism.

Damiene Denner

See also: Erection; Penis.

Further Reading

American Urological Association. (2010). Priapism. Retrieved from https://www.auanet.org/guidelines/priapism-guideline

Mayo Clinic. (2019). Priapism. Retrieved from https://www.mayoclinic.org/diseases-conditions/priapism/symptoms-causes/syc-20352005

National Health Service. (2017). Priapism (painful erections). Retrieved from https://www.nhs.uk/conditions/priapism-painful-erections/

Progesterone

Progesterone is a hormone produced primarily in female bodies by the ovaries and, during pregnancy, by the placenta. Small amounts of progesterone are also produced by the adrenal glands and by male testicles. Progesterone is classified as belonging to a group of steroid hormones called progestogens.

The main role of progesterone is to prepare the uterus for pregnancy. During the middle of the menstrual cycle, one of the two ovaries releases an egg. Immediately after this ovulation, the corpus luteum (the structure left in the ovary after the egg is released) begins secreting large amounts of progesterone into the bloodstream. These secretions continue for approximately ten to twelve days, causing the endometrium (the lining of the interior walls of the uterus) to develop a thickened layer of blood vessels, cells, and glands.

Should the released egg be fertilized by a sperm cell, the fertilized egg implants itself into this thickened uterine lining. As the endometrium is penetrated, tissues from the embryo become intertwined with tissues from the uterus, forming the placenta, which carries food and oxygen to, and waste away from, the embryo (and, later, the fetus). The large amount of progesterone secreted by the placenta keeps the uterine muscle relaxed during pregnancy, preventing the baby from being born prematurely. The progesterone from the placenta works with other hormones to induce development of cells in the breasts that secrete milk and to strengthen the pelvic wall in preparation for birth. Immediately after birth, progesterone levels begin to decline.

If the egg is not fertilized and pregnancy does not occur, the extra lining of the uterus and the corpus luteum are discharged through the vagina in menstrual bleeding (commonly called a period). Whether or not pregnancy occurs, the monthly increase in progesterone levels may cause body temperature to increase and breasts to enlarge and become more sensitive.

Progesterone plays important roles in the nervous system for all people. It helps to protect nerve cells, including the neurons of the brain, and to regulate the transmission of nerve impulses by interacting with proteins at sites on nerve cells called receptors. Progesterone aids the normal development of brain neurons, and it may help to protect the brain against traumatic injury by reducing inflammation.

Additional functions of progesterone are associated with regulation of blood clotting, cellular oxygen levels, conversion of fat into energy, and insulin secretion by the pancreas. It also plays a role in keeping the bronchial tubes of the lungs open and clear.

Progesterone, or synthetic versions of it known as progestin, is used as medication to treat certain conditions involving the female reproductive system, including menstrual bloating, irregular menstruation, and premenstrual syndrome (characterized by a variety of physical and psychological symptoms that may occur up to two weeks before menstruation). Some people take progestin as part of hormone replacement therapy (HRT) to manage the symptoms of menopause; estrogen is usually also part of HRT. Progesterone-based medications are sometimes prescribed as part of treatment for breast, uterine, or kidney cancer, and for weight loss related to cancer or AIDS. The hormone is typically taken in pill form.

Progestin is also used in birth control pills, either by itself or combined with estrogen. Progestin-only pills are commonly called the minipill because they contain a lower dose of the hormone than the progestin-and-estrogen combination pill. The pills work mainly by thickening the mucus of the cervix (the neck of the uterus) to block sperm from entering and by suppressing ovulation. The progestin-only pill generally carries less risk of adverse effects, such as stroke and uterine cancer, than the combination pill, though it is somewhat less effective at preventing pregnancy. Progestin is the active ingredient in the injectable contraceptive (medroxyprogesterone acetate) and in many intrauterine devices.

Topical cream or gel products containing progesterone are sold for a variety of purposes, including as treatments for menopausal symptoms, osteoporosis, allergies, headaches, and irritability. However, there is conflicting scientific evidence regarding the effectiveness of such products.

Because of its role in neuron protection, researchers are investigating the use of progesterone in treating patients with nervous system disorders, such as multiple sclerosis.

A. J. Smuskiewicz

See also: Birth Control Pills, Estrogen-Progestin; Birth Control Pills, Progestin-Only; Contraceptive Implants; Contraceptive Injectables; Contraceptive Patch; Estrogen; Hormone Replacement Therapy; Intrauterine Device (IUD); Ovulation; Pregnancy; Sex Hormones.

Further Reading

Goldstein, S. R. (2019). Progesterone. Retrieved from http://www.healthywomen.org/condition/progesterone

ScienceDirect. (2019). Progesterone. Retrieved from https://www.sciencedirect.com/topics/neuroscience/progesterone

Pronoun Usage

A pronoun is a word used in place of a noun to refer to a specific subject. When pronouns are used to refer to people, they create linguistic and mental shortcuts related to the perception of a person's gender identity, which then informs how others refer to them. In the English language and using societal conventions, a person's gender and pronouns are often assumed from a person's looks and behaviors, and these assumptions are often based on a binary understanding of gender (exclusively male or masculine and female or feminine). For example, one may use the masculine pronoun "he" for someone assumed to be a male or man, whereas the feminine pronoun "she" may be used for someone assumed to be a female or woman. Gendered assumptions and expectations may be imposed onto others (whether intentionally or not) by assuming a person's pronouns and using the assumed pronouns to reference the person. It is important to ask people what their personal pronouns are instead of using pronouns based on gendered assumptions. Pronouns are important to some individuals and may be one way a person may assert their own gender identity.

Of note, labels for gender identity (e.g., transgender, genderqueer, agender) are growing and changing quickly. "Cisgender" is a term describing individuals whose gender identity is congruent with their birth-assigned sex. Individuals who identify as cisgender may feel comfortable with pronouns that are associated with societal expectations (i.e., a person assigned male at birth feeling comfortable being referenced with pronouns "he, him, or his"). For individuals who identify within the transgender and gender-nonconforming community, as well as for some cisgender individuals (such as cisgender individuals whose gender expression does not align with societal expectations), using pronouns associated with their birth-assigned sex may cause discomfort or even distress. When a person is called by a pronoun with which they do not identify, the person may feel invisible, frustrated, sad, upset, annoyed, and so on. Also, a person who repeatedly asks others to use the pronouns they identify with or who frequently educates others about pronoun usage may experience tiredness and exhaustion.

Similar to gender identity labels, pronouns are changing and frequently being created, meaning some people may be unfamiliar with the use of these words. Some individuals are comfortable using binary pronouns to indicate feminine (e.g., she, her, hers, herself) and masculine (e.g., he, him, his, himself) identities. In the English language, some individuals use pronouns that neutralize gendered language (e.g., they, them, their, theirs, themself). For example, instead of saying, "She went by herself to the store," one would say, "They went by themself to the store." Some individuals who do not identify with binary or they, them, their, theirs, and themself pronouns may use other gender neutral pronouns like ze, hir, hirs, hirself or xe, xem, xyr, xyrs, and xemself. Moreover, some individuals may prefer to not use any pronouns and would rather just have others use their name when referring to them.

G. Nic Rider and Leonardo Candelario-Pérez

See also: Binary Gender System; Gender; Gender Expression; Gender Identity; Gender Transition; Nonbinary Gender Identities; Transgender.

Further Reading

Bongiovanni, A., & Jimerson, T. (2018). *A quick and easy guide to they/them pronouns.* Portland, OR: Limerence Press.

Gender Neutral Pronoun Blog. (n.d.). The need for a gender-neutral pronoun. Retrieved from https://genderneutralpronoun.wordpress.com/

Prostate

The prostate, also called the prostate gland, is a walnut-sized organ that is part of the male reproductive system. It is located below the bladder, just in front of the rectum.

A whitish fluid that makes up much of semen is produced in the prostate. This fluid contains proteins, fats, minerals, and other substances that provide nourishment to the sperm cells. Other parts of the seminal fluid—which provides a medium in which the sperm can be transported out of the body—are produced in glands called seminal vesicles and bulbourethral glands (also called Cowper's glands).

After sperm cells are produced in the testicles, they travel to the prostate through the vas deferens tubes. The sperm then becomes mixed with the fluid from the prostate and the other glands. In ejaculation, the semen passes out of the body via the urethra, a tube that runs from the bladder and prostate through the penis. The urethra is the same tube that carries urine out of the body.

Physical stimulation of the prostate can play a role in sexual arousal, leading to orgasm and ejaculation. The prostate is most effectively stimulated by massaging the skin around the anus or the skin between the anus and testicles. This stimulation can be performed with fingers, a penis, or a sex toy, such as a vibrator or "p-spot" massager.

The prostate commonly becomes enlarged in men who are older than fifty. In some cases, the enlarged gland puts so much pressure on the urethra that the individual feels a frequent urge to urinate, though it may be difficult to urinate when they try to do so. Treatment for an enlarged prostate depends on the severity of the symptoms and whether the enlargement is benign (noncancerous) or the result of cancer. In cases of benign enlargement, called benign prostatic hyperplasia, many patients can be treated successfully with medications, such as alpha-blockers. If symptoms persist, all or part of the gland may be removed in surgery.

Treatment of prostate cancer typically consists of surgical removal of the entire gland and radiation therapy. Medications that reduce levels of testosterone may also be used because prostate cancer cells use this hormone to grow. Prostate cancer usually grows slowly before it reaches a fatal stage. Thus, many physicians recommend that older men avoid surgery and radiation, which each carries certain risks, while continuing to have the growth of the cancer monitored.

Prostate cancer is the most common cancer among men, and more men die of prostate cancer than any other form of cancer except lung cancer. There is a genetic basis to prostate cancer, with greater risk among those who have a family history of the disease. African American men are at the greatest risk. Treatment has a high success rate if it is started before the cancer spreads beyond the prostate, with almost all patients alive five years after diagnosis. However, after the cancer has spread to lymph nodes, bones, or other tissues, five-year survival rates drop to less than 30 percent.

Many physicians recommend that middle-aged and older men get annual tests to detect early signs of prostate cancer. One such test is a digital rectal examination, in which the doctor feels the gland with a finger inserted into the anus, checking for a lump or hard spot that may be indicative of cancer. In another test, called the prostate-specific antigen (PSA) test, levels of the PSA protein are measured in a blood sample. Higher-than-normal levels may indicate cancer.

Prostatitis is an inflammation of the prostate that may be caused by an infection. Treatment for this condition often involves the use of antibiotics.

A. J. Smuskiewicz

See also: Benign Prostatic Hyperplasia; Prostate Cancer; Prostatectomy; Prostatitis; Semen.

Further Reading

Carter, H. B., & Couzens, G. S. (2013). *The whole life prostate book: Everything that every man—At every age—Needs to know about maintaining optimal prostate health.* New York: Free Press/Simon & Schuster.

Cohen, J. S. (2014). *Prostate cancer breakthroughs 2014: New tests, new treatments, better options: A step-by-step guide to cutting-edge diagnostic tests and 12 medically proven treatments.* Del Mar, CA: Oceansong Publishing.

Walsh, P. C. (1995). *The prostate: A guide for men and the women who love them.* Baltimore: The Johns Hopkins University Press.

Prostate Cancer

Prostate cancer is the abnormal, uncontrolled multiplication of cells within the prostate. This cancer is the most common cancer among men, and it kills many men every year. However, if diagnosed and treated early, it is one of the more curable forms of cancer.

In 2020, it has been estimated that there will be 191,930 new cases of prostate cancer diagnosed in the United States, representing 10.6 percent of all new cancer cases. It is also expected that more than 33,000 Americans will die of the disease in 2020, representing 5.5 percent of all cancer deaths. Prostate cancer is responsible for more deaths among American men than any other form of cancer except lung cancer.

All ethnic groups can get prostate cancer, but African American men are at the highest risk. This cancer is rarely diagnosed before age forty-five, though African Americans are at risk around age forty. Prostate cancer is most commonly diagnosed between the ages of sixty-five and seventy-four.

Prostate cancer has a lower mortality rate than most cancers. If diagnosed and treated early, people with prostate cancer have a good chance of long-term survival. The average five-year survival rate for patients with prostate cancer is 99 percent. If treatment is begun very early, this rate rises to 100 percent. However, if the cancer is not diagnosed and treated until after it has spread to other parts of the body, the five-year survival rate drops to 28 percent.

The risk of prostate cancer steadily increases with age, especially after age forty-five. By age eighty, about 80 percent of men have some cancer cells in their prostate.

Prostate cancer runs in families. Men who have relatives who have had prostate cancer are at elevated risk for the disease themselves. This risk more than doubles for men who have fathers or brothers diagnosed with prostate cancer.

Heredity factors alone cannot explain most cases of prostate cancer. There are other factors that increase risk, though these factors are little understood. A high-fat diet, smoking, and exposure to certain environmental toxins (such as heavy metals) are suspected of increasing risk.

Early stages of prostate cancer produce few if any symptoms. Those with more advanced prostate cancer may experience pain or discomfort in the pelvic area, lower back, ribs, or upper thighs, as well as an abnormally frequent urge to urinate. However, passing urine may be difficult. These symptoms are caused by the abnormal enlargement of the prostate gland, which puts pressure on the bladder and the urethra.

Physicians can perform tests to check for prostate enlargement and to determine if this enlargement is the result of cancer or some other, less serious condition. In a digital rectal examination, the patient's prostate is felt by the physician's finger, which is inserted into the rectum. Abnormal hardness or lumps suggest the presence of cancer. In a test known as prostate-specific antigen (PSA) test, the blood is analyzed for levels of the PSA protein. Elevated levels of this protein are indicative of cancer.

If cancer is suspected based on these tests, an ultrasound examination is usually conducted to produce a detailed image of the prostate. Using this image, the physician inserts needles through the rectum wall to obtain tissue samples from the prostate. Microscopic examination of these biopsy samples will reveal if the tissue is malignant or benign. If malignant, further tests are performed to determine the stage of cancer development—whether the cancer is confined to the prostate or if it has metastasized to other parts of the body.

If the cancer is confined to the prostate, surgical removal of the gland and/or radiation therapy can often cure the patient. These procedures may lead to urinary incontinence and/or sexual impotence in patients. Some advanced surgical procedures may be able to remove the cancerous tissue while preserving nerves necessary for sexual functioning.

If the cancer has spread to tissues and organs beyond the prostate, additional treatments beyond prostate surgery and radiation therapy are necessary. These treatments may include orchiectomy (removal of the testes) and administration of certain hormones or other medications. These treatments lower the levels of the male hormones that "feed" the growth of prostate cancer cells.

The earlier treatment for prostate cancer is initiated, the more successful the treatment is likely to be. To catch this cancer in an early, curable stage of development, many doctors recommend that men over age forty get annual digital rectal examinations and PSA tests. PSA tests are able to detect smaller, earlier growths of cancer than rectal exams. Some doctors recommend routine rectal exams but not routine PSA tests, because PSA tests may reveal small cancers that grow so slowly that they will never become life-threatening. Treatment for such small cancers could lead to unnecessary potential complications for patients. Thus, when small cancers are detected in the prostate, some doctors recommend waiting to see if the cancer spreads before beginning treatment.

A. J. Smuskiewicz

See also: Penile Cancer; Prostate; Prostatectomy; Testicular Cancer.

Further Reading

National Cancer Institute. (2020). Cancer stat facts: Prostate cancer. Retrieved from http://seer.cancer.gov/statfacts/html/prost.html

Walsh, P. C., & Worthington, J. F. (2012). *Dr. Patrick Walsh's guide to surviving prostate cancer*. New York: Grand Central Life & Style.

Prostatectomy

Prostatectomy is the partial or total removal of the prostate gland. The prostate gland is part of the reproductive system, and it secretes prostate fluid found in semen. The muscles of the prostate gland also help to project the seminal fluid into the urethra during ejaculation. Not all of the functions of the prostate are known. The prostate is located directly below the bladder, and the urethra, the tube-like structure that carries urine from the bladder during urination, passes through the center of the prostate gland.

Prostatectomies are typically performed as part of the treatment plan for prostate cancer and can be performed along with several other treatments, including chemotherapy, hormone therapy, and radiation. The procedure of a prostatectomy involves removing the prostate, or part of the prostate, any cancerous tissue, nearby lymph nodes, and the seminal vesicles. A radical prostatectomy is the removal of the entire prostate and more related tissues, while a simple prostatectomy is used more to treat obstructive lower urinary tract symptoms produced by benign prostatic hyperplasia.

A radical prostatectomy can be performed by three different methods: robot-assisted radical prostatectomy, open radical prostatectomy, and laparoscopic radical prostatectomy. The robot-assisted radical prostatectomy uses a robotic device guided precisely by a surgeon at a remote console that displays a 3-D view of the prostate and surgical field by feeding specialized instruments through the small incisions in the lower abdomen. The open radical prostatectomy is retropubic surgery, where a surgeon makes one incision in the lower abdomen and accesses the prostate manually through that incision site. The laparoscopic radical prostatectomy is where the surgeon again makes small incisions in the lower abdomen and uses highly specialized tools to move through those incisions and remove the prostate. The risks of any of the radical prostatectomy methods include bleeding, urinary tract infection, urinary incontinence, impotence, narrowing of the urethra or bladder, lymphoceles, possible change in the length of the penis, and sterility. Each method has its own benefits and disadvantages and requires thoughtful discussion and consideration with a physician and social support system to decide the method best suited to the individual.

Prostatectomies are done under general anesthesia, and antibiotics are typically given immediately prior to surgery in order to prevent infection. A urinary catheter, a flexible tube placed within the urethra to allow urine flow to avoid obstruction while in recovery, is typically placed after a prostatectomy and kept in place for five to ten days postoperation. After the procedure, pain medications are administered intravenously, and patients are encouraged to walk the day of the surgery. It is common for patients to be discharged from the hospital the day after the procedure with outpatient postoperative visits as needed. It may take several months to a year for sexual function to return to normal after a prostatectomy. Though semen will continue to be produced, it is simply reabsorbed harmlessly by the body and will not be able to be projected through the urethra without the prostate gland's assistance. Prostatectomies are useful and effective interventions to remove and treat prostate cancer but are invasive and carry lifelong changes that must be considered before proceeding with this intervention.

Cassia Araujo-Lane

See also: Benign Prostatic Hyperplasia; Prostate; Prostate Cancer; Prostatitis; Seminal Vesicles.

Further Reading

Johns Hopkins Medicine. (2019). Radical prostatectomy. Retrieved from https://www.hopkinsmedicine.org/health/treatment-tests-and-therapies/radical-prostatectomy

Kim, E. H., Larson, J. A., & Anriole, G. L. (2016). Management of benign prostatic hyperplasia. *Annual Review of Medicine, 67*(1), 137–151.

Mayo Clinic. (2019). Prostatectomy. Retrieved from https://www.mayoclinic.org/tests-procedures/prostatectomy/about/pac-20385198

Rincones, O., Sidhom, M., Mancuso, P., Wong, K., Berry, M., Forstner, D., … Girgis, A. (2019). Robot or radiation? A qualitative study of the decision support needs of men with localised prostate cancer choosing between robotic prostatectomy and radiotherapy treatment. *Patient Education and Counselling, 102*(7), 1364–1372.

Prostatitis

Prostatitis is an infection involving the prostate. The disease can be subdivided into two types: acute bacterial prostatitis and chronic bacterial prostatitis. Most infections are bacterial in origin and are caused by the movement of bacteria into the prostate via the urethra; however, bacteria may also be introduced via surgery or manipulation of the surrounding structures. The most common agents involved in prostatitis are gram-negative bacteria, including *Escherichia coli, Enterococcus*, and *Proteus* species. Prostatitis may also be caused by *Chlamydia trachomatis* and *Trichomonas vaginalis.*

Acute bacterial prostatitis (ABP) may present with lower abdominal pain, pain with urination, frequent urination, urinary urgency, painful erections, fever, blood in the ejaculate fluid, and chills. Characteristics that increase the risk for infection include diabetes, having a chronic indwelling catheter, and performing self-catheterization. On examination, the prostate may be tender and swollen. Special care needs to be taken with prostate exams, as excessive massage of the prostate may lead to spread of the bacteria, resulting in sepsis (when an infection spreads to the bloodstream). Evaluation may be performed with a gram stain or urine culture to uncover the causative organism. While a blood culture is not often called for, it may be used if someone presents with systemic symptoms such as low blood pressure, as this may be a sign of sepsis. Blood cultures can also be performed for people with a high risk of developing sepsis or severe infections, such as heart lesions. ABP is treated with antibiotics. A potential complication of this infection is urinary retention.

Chronic bacterial prostatitis (CBP) may develop from ABP that is not treated appropriately or if bacteria is spread to other areas through the blood into the prostate, if it is refluxed into the prostate with urine during recurrent urinary tract infections, or if an ascending infection occurs through the urethra. On rare occasions, infections may be caused by fungi or *Mycobacterium tuberculosis*. Smokers and individuals with diabetes may have a higher risk. Otherwise, the risk factors mostly mirror those associated with ABP. Often, individuals with CBP may be asymptomatic or have symptoms similar to a mild urinary tract infection (pain with urination, urinary urgency, increased frequency, or abdominal pain). Laboratory evaluation is performed by testing the urine or prostatic fluid, and treatment requires an extended course of antibiotics (more than six weeks). Chronic pelvic pain may also occur as a result.

Rachel Snedecor

See also: Benign Prostatic Hyperplasia; Prostate; Prostate Cancer; Prostatectomy; Sexually Transmitted Infections (STIs).

Further Reading

Chuang, A. Y., Tsou, M. H., Chang, S. J., Yang, L. Y., Shih, C. C., Tsai, M. P., ... Hsueh, P. R. (2012). Mycobacterium abscessus granulomatous prostatitis. *The American Journal of Surgical Pathology, 36*(3), 418–422.

Dickson, G. (2013). Prostatitis: Diagnosis and treatment. *Australian Family Physician, 42*(4), 216–219.

Meyrier, A., & Fekete, T. (2019). Acute bacterial prostatitis. Retrieved from https://www.uptodate.com/contents/acute-bacterial-prostatitis

Schaeffer, A. J. (2006). Clinical practice: Chronic prostatitis and the chronic pelvic pain syndrome. *New England Journal of Medicine, 355*, 1690–1698.

Yoon, B. I., Kim, S., Han, D. S., Ha, U. S., Lee, S. J., Kim, H. W., ... Cho, Y. H. (2012). Acute bacterial prostatitis: How to prevent and manage chronic infection. *Journal of Infection and Chemotherapy, 18*(4), 444–450.

Prostitution

Prostitution is generally recognized as the practice of performing sexual acts in exchange for monetary payment, be it sexual intercourse or other forms of noncoital sex. Prostitutes are sex workers and are pejoratively referred to as "hookers"; customers are typically called "Johns," referring to the term "John Doe." The legal status of prostitution varies within and across countries around the world. In the United States, prostitution is predominantly considered a crime, except for some counties in Nevada, but exists in other places of the world as a regulated profession or a permissible but unregulated offense. Like many other types of sex work, this profession is typically degraded and considered obscene or immoral. This may be due to religious convictions surrounding sexual deviance and monogamy, individual or collective erotophobia, an association with premarital and extramarital sex, or even more practical concerns regarding the spread of sexually transmitted infections. There are many reasons people solicit the services of prostitutes and other sex workers, as commercial sex is often easily accessible, sexually gratifying, and customizable (i.e., physical characteristics or interest in a particular act).

Informally referred to as "the oldest profession in the world," the exchange of sex for resources is present throughout human history, and the practice has even been reported in various animal species. Currently measured as a worldwide billion-dollar industry, prostitution continues to thrive. That is not to say this perceivably natural phenomenon has existed without challenge. Christian traditions and sexuality beliefs during the Middle Ages in Europe were challenging for prostitution. Interestingly, prostitution was openly condemned but frequently valued in juxtaposition by the church as a "necessary evil" to preserve the proper sanctity of marriage. The persistent advertisement of a clear division between dishonorable sexuality and wholesome reproduction within the household inspired Sigmund Freud's theory of the Madonna/whore dichotomy and many of Michel Foucault's philosophical ponderings. The proposed discrepancy was so pervasive that medieval medical models of the prostitute began to emerge describing sex workers as infertile. This concept was meant to explain a lack of recurring gestation based on the notion that a womb was inhospitable to pregnancy when it became too "slippery" to allow for conception (as per indiscriminate and transient sexual encounters). These presumptions were inaccurate and failed to account for the regular use of contraception or the enlistment of abortion procedures.

Such dehumanizing constructs vastly differ from the respected high-class traditions of the Eastern world and earlier periods of antiquity when prostitution was more welcome as a form of commerce or even prestigiously anointed. Sacred prostitution among temple priestesses of ancient Mesopotamia, the "living artwork" of the Japanese geisha, and the hetaerae of ancient Greece are all examples of coveted sexual exchange. Inanna, the Sumerian goddess of love, was seen as patron of ritual sexuality, brothels, and male prostitution. The craft of the Japanese geisha is still practiced today, adored as an artisan of beauty and desire, although their services are not always associated with sexual interactions. Reportedly more autonomous than their Eastern counterparts were the renowned courtesans of ancient Greece. Not to be confused with common "pornai," hetaerae were economically independent and regularly took part in the city symposia. Unable to marry, the hetaerae maintained lower social status but were the most educated and influential women in all of Greece.

Today, prostitution is typically viewed as demeaning regardless of professional ranking. Modern prostitution in the United States is generally composed of streetwalkers, those who work in massage parlors or brothels, and call girls or escorts. Streetwalking is the most stigmatized form of prostitution and often the most dangerous. Visible to the public, streetwalkers are more likely to be arrested and to experience physical violence and sexual abuse. Little control over their working conditions leaves streetwalkers faced with dangerous hazards such as kidnapping, robbery, and rape. Brothel and massage parlor workers are safer in their reliable working spaces. Working in these establishments reduces the likelihood of arrests, as sensuous massage parlors may limit or disguise services advertised to avoid legal difficulties, and brothels are legal where permitted by law. Brothels are also usually equipped with safety features like panic buttons, surveillance devices, support staff, and prophylactics, and they require regular employee medical exams. While many customers enjoy frequenting these businesses, some prefer the privacy of arranging appointments with professional escorts. Call girls may be independently managed or have appointments arranged by employers who advertise their services. High-end call girls are considered the highest-ranking form of prostitution because they serve wealthier clientele and can charge higher fees than the average sex worker.

The "fast cash" appeal of the sex industry is not the only reason people become sex workers and is definitely not exclusive to women. While most prostitutes are female, both men—sometimes referred to as gigolos—and trans individuals are also drawn to sex work. Not all who are involved in prostitution are motivated by socioeconomic issues, drugs, or homelessness, although these are common incentives. Some also genuinely enjoy being paid for sex. However, not everyone who engages in sex work actively chooses to do so. In the United States, coercive parties have been known to "groom" vulnerable adolescents by providing gifts and attention only to eventually exploit them sexually. In many countries, people, many of whom are minors, may be deceived with seemingly harmless work opportunities in order to be trafficked or may be blatantly kidnapped and sold into sex slavery. While voluntary participation (of those meeting the lawful age of consent) in sex tourism markets is often legal, the forced labor of commercial sex exploitation is explicitly illegal worldwide. Although nonconsensual sex work will most likely always remain illegal, advocacy efforts to legalize consensual prostitution continue in many places where it is currently not permitted.

Due to advancing research, modern debate surrounding the legalization of prostitution is evolving. Regardless of moral conviction, greater attention to the benefits of prostitution is being objectively explored. Commercial regulation of prostitution has the potential to provide safer conditions for both clients and sex workers, legal access for sexually marginalized communities such as the disabled when professional sexual surrogacy is inaccessible, and a general normalization of human sexual needs. Historically, the assistance of sex workers has also played a significant role in a wide range of scientific research, particularly in the field of sexology. When members of the general population may be apprehensive to participate in investigative physiological reports or sexual history surveys for research projects, adequate compensation of sex workers allows for readily available participant samples. Clearly, the relationship between modern society and prostitution is complex and multifaceted.

Ilyssa Boseski

See also: Age of Consent; Madonna/Whore Dichotomy; Religion, Diversity of Human Sexuality and; Sex Tourism; Sex Work; Sex Workers, Male; Sexual Slavery; Sugar Daddies and Sugar Babies.

Further Reading

Bullough, V. L. (1994). *Science in the bedroom: A history of sex research.* New York: Basic Books.

Charnov, E. L. (1982). *The theory of sex allocation. Monographs in Population Biology* (MPB-18). Princeton, NJ: Princeton University Press.

International Labour Organization, International Labour Office. (2009). *Executive summary of 2009 Global Report on Forced Labour "The cost of coercion."* Retrieved from http://www.ilo.org/global/docs/WCMS_106387/lang--en/index.htm

Lacquer, T. (1990). *Making sex: Body and gender from the Greeks to Freud.* Cambridge, MA: Harvard University Press.

Lovelock, B. (2013). *The ethics of tourism: Critical and applied perspectives.* New York: Routledge Taylor & Francis Group.

National Center for Victims of Crime. (2012). Grooming dynamic. Retrieved from https://www.victimsofcrime.org/media/reporting-on-child-sexual-abuse/grooming-dynamic-of-csa

Pomeroy, S. (1995). *Goddess, whores, wives, and slaves: Women in classical antiquity.* New York: Schocken Books.

Ringdal, N. J. (2005). *Love for sale: A world history of prostitution.* New York: Gross Press.

Yarber, W. L, Sayad, B. A., & Strong, B. (2010). *Human sexuality: Diversity in contemporary America* (7th ed.). New York: McGraw-Hill.

Psychosexual Therapy

Psychosexual therapy assists with sexual difficulties and dysfunctions, including erectile concerns, loss of sexual desire, sexual avoidance, and fear of sex. Sexual difficulties and dysfunctions vary in complexity and severity and can be the result of physical or psychological illness as well as emotional and relational distress. Psychosexual therapy focuses on psychoeducation, bolstering communication skills, intimacy development, implementing behavioral techniques, and utilizing self-monitoring techniques to systematically desensitize anxious responses that may occur during sexual situations. Traditional psychosexual therapy focuses primarily on sensitization and desensitization techniques to lower anxiety related to sexual experiences. In particular, the focus is on verbal and nonverbal communication with the intent of improving intimacy, dispelling negative thoughts, and potentially temporarily abstaining from sexual intercourse in order to reduce anxiety.

The effective implementation of psychosexual therapy is strongly based on the initial evaluation and assessment of an individual or couple. Due to the intimate nature of psychosexual therapy, it is essential that a strong therapeutic alliance is formed, focused on promoting unconditional positive regard and genuineness. As the therapist begins the assessment process, special attention is paid to collecting a detailed sexual history. The alliance built in the beginning of therapy will be utilized during the evaluation and assessment process to develop a comfortable environment where sexual issues can be explored. Rao and colleagues (2018) speak to the importance of confidentiality during this stage of therapy, as a lack of privacy regarding sexual concerns may impede accurate history taking. Psychosexual history should include assessment of current complaints, duration of the issue, associated symptoms, onset, frequency, and severity of the issue or issues. In addition, sexual practices, intimacy and relationship problems, and current sexual functioning must be addressed. After thorough assessment and evaluation, tenets of psychosexual therapy may be implemented.

Numerous models of psychosexual therapy exist to best serve clients as specific needs arise, including treatment modalities focused on systemic therapy and sexology. One modality, the Sexual Wellness Enhancement and Enrichment Training model, proposes a mind-body skills interaction aiming to improve sexual wellness through adequate and educational self-care. The PLISSIT model of psychosexual therapy addresses permission, limited information, specific suggestion, and intensive sexual therapy to improve communication and arousal behaviors between the client couple. Other forms of psychosexual therapy incorporate aspects of cognitive behavioral therapy, mindfulness, and psychoeducation.

Clinical results of psychosexual therapy allege differences in treatment efficacy outcomes. Frühauf, Gerger, Schmidt, Munder, and Barth (2013) propose that psychological interventions may especially improve female hypoactive sexual desire disorder and female orgasmic disorder. However, further updated outcome studies are needed to assess efficacy in treating other sexual dysfunctions and the long-term effects of psychosexual therapy. O'Donoghue (1996) suggests various obstacles to treatment when practicing psychosexual therapy. While the process can improve sexual performance, efficacious outcomes rely heavily on couple dynamics and involvement. Obstacles to treatment may include, but are not limited to, sexual dysfunction in extramarital affairs, lack of partner involvement, ethical concerns, past sexual history (rape, sexual abuse, etc.), religious beliefs, and reproduction conflicts. Another concern is the efficacy of therapy when used with diverse populations, such as LGBTQ+ persons or young adults. Binik and Meana (2009) assert that psychosexual therapy falls short of standards for evidence-based practice.

Further considerations for the future include changing the vehicle through which therapy is delivered. Hall (2004) conducted a pilot study exploring the efficacy of online psychosexual therapy. Feedback provided by participants included increased self-awareness, greater sexual knowledge, and an improvement in sexual dysfunction. While challenges remain in conducting psychosexual therapy online, Hall provides a framework from which to work. In the age of technology, this may be a strong option for accessing psychosexual therapy.

Kyndel L. Tarziers and Franco Dispenza

See also: Performance Anxiety; PLISSIT Model of Sex Therapy; Sensate Focus; Sexual Disorders, Female; Sexual Disorders, Male; Sexual Dysfunction, Treatment of.

Further Reading

Baker, A. C., & Absenger, W. (2013). Sexual Wellness Enhancement and Enrichment Training (SWEET): A hypothetical group model for addressing sexual health and wellbeing. *Sexual & Relationship Therapy, 28*(1–2), 48–62.

Binik, Y. M., & Meana, M. (2009). The future of sex therapy: Specialization or marginalization? *Archives of Sexual Behavior, 38*(6), 1016–1027.

Frühauf, S., Gerger, H., Schmidt, H., Munder, T., & Barth, J. (2013). Efficacy of psychological interventions for sexual dysfunction: A systematic review and meta-analysis. *Archives of Sexual Behavior, 42*(6), 915–933.

Hall, P. (2004). Online psychosexual therapy: A summary of pilot study findings. *Sexual & Relationship Therapy, 19*(2), 167–178.

Markovic, D. (2012). Psychosexual therapy in sexualised culture: A systemic perspective. *Sexual & Relationship Therapy, 27*(2), 103–109.

Masters, W. H., Johnson, V. E., & Kolodny, R. C. (1988). *Masters and Johnson on sex and human loving.* Boston: Little, Brown and Company.

O'Donoghue, F. (1996). Psychological management of erectile dysfunction and related disorders. *International Journal of STD & AIDS, 7*(Suppl. 3), 9–12.

Rao, T. S. S., Maheshwari, S., George, M., Chandran, S., Manohar, S., & Rao, S. S. (2018). Psychosocial interventions for sexual dysfunction in addictive disorders. *Indian Journal of Psychiatry, 60*, S506–S509.

Ridley, J. (2006). The subjectivity of the clinician in psychosexual therapy training. *Sexual & Relationship Therapy, 21*(3), 319–331.

Puberty

Puberty is the beginning of the process of a child growing into an adult. There are many physical, mental, and social changes that occur during this time.

Puberty begins when the maturing pituitary gland sends a signal to the body to start producing sex hormones; for people assigned male at birth this includes testosterone and some estrogen, and for people assigned female at birth this includes estrogen, progesterone, and some testosterone. These hormones affect the adolescent body in many ways, both physically and mentally.

For all genders, puberty is a process that takes place over several years. For folks assigned female at birth, puberty often begins between the ages of nine and fifteen but can sometimes occur earlier or later. For folks assigned male at birth, puberty usually begins a little later, most often between the ages of eleven and sixteen. The age of the onset of puberty may depend on a number of factors, including heredity (the age at which one's parent or other family members began puberty), body weight, racial background, environment, and other influences. Historically, all genders are reaching puberty at younger ages than in previous decades, which some experts believe may be due to changing environmental influences.

Some of the physical changes that occur during puberty happen for all genders. Everyone will grow taller, although some folks may have a more significant height increase than others. An increase in natural oil production also takes place, which can cause the hair and scalp to become more oily and lead to acne (pimples) on the face and upper body. Changes in the tone of voice also happen during this time. This is most noticeable for adolescents who were assigned male at birth, as their voices may deepen significantly, and they may experience several stages of embarrassing voice-cracking and squeaking in the process. Though less noticeable, the voices of folks who were assigned female at birth change slightly as well.

Another change that affects all genders is the development of body hair. For people with more testosterone, this includes a thickening of the hair on the legs and arms, hair around the genitals, underarm hair, and sometimes new hair growth on the chest, stomach, back, and face (though this may occur much later). For people who have more estrogen, hair growth includes the legs, underarms, around the genitals, and sometimes on the face as well.

In addition to the many physical changes that puberty brings, there are also mental changes. The onset of puberty jump-starts additional brain development, which allows adolescents to understand and engage in much more abstract, complex, and new ways of thinking. The hormonal surges and fluctuations can also bring about sudden shifts in moods and emotional reactions. The sex hormones that are instrumental in puberty may also contribute to adolescents becoming naturally more curious about sex and sexuality, thinking sexual thoughts, and becoming sexually excited.

Puberty often brings about some social changes as well. In addition to becoming more curious about sexuality, some adolescents may begin experimenting sexually with each other. Youth at various stages of puberty also tend to become much more self-conscious than previously and sometimes feel quite awkward and clumsy as they adjust to all the changes happening inside and outside their bodies. Close, intimate friendships also become very important and common during this time. Along with this, some young adults may become even more concerned with fitting in with their peers than previously, and bullying may also become more of a concern during these years.

The bodily changes that occur during puberty for people who have a uterus usually begin with the development of breast buds that will later become breasts. The growth of body hair (legs, underarms) and pubic hair (hair around the genitals) often follows. Vaginal discharge is also common during the year leading up to a person's first menstrual period, which often occurs within around a year or two of developing breast buds. During this time, many people will also begin to gain some extra "padding" of fat around the hips, buttocks, and thighs, and the bones of their hips and pelvis may also begin to widen in order to allow a baby to safely pass through the pelvis during childbirth in the future. Usually, the most notable stage of puberty for people who have a uterus is the first menstrual period (menarche). A period comes in the form of blood and tissue from the uterus that pass out of the body through the vaginal opening. Although someone with ovaries is born with all their eggs (ova) already in the ovaries, they do not start releasing these eggs until puberty, when sex hormones trigger the first ovulation (release of an egg). This begins the menstrual cycle that marks a person's new capability to become pregnant. A person's first period can be both frightening and exciting, depending largely on how well prepared and informed they are before experiencing their first period. Many young folks' periods will be irregular and sporadic at first, usually becoming more regular (occurring about every twenty-eight days or so) over the next several years.

For people who have a penis, puberty often begins with an increase in height, developing body hair and pubic hair, and possibly growing some facial hair, though this often develops a few years later. Around this time, their voices may also begin to deepen. In addition to growing taller, they also gain an increase in muscle mass. The sex hormones involved in puberty begin the production of sperm cells in a person's testicles, which will allow them to begin ejaculating and therefore also makes them capable of contributing to beginning a pregnancy. About half of all adolescents with penises will experience nocturnal emissions during puberty as the body releases an overproduction of semen during sleep in the form of an ejaculation. Like a first period, nocturnal emission may also be a frightening experience if a person is not prepared or if they are unaware that this is a normal occurrence. Once masturbation or sexual activity is initiated, nocturnal emissions tend to cease. Nearly all young people who have a penis will also experience spontaneous erections during puberty. This is where the spongy tissue of the penis fills with blood and becomes firm (erect). During puberty, some adolescents may be thinking sexual thoughts or become sexually excited more easily, which can contribute to frequent erections, but often this happens for no apparent reason at all. This can be an embarrassing situation but is extremely common and completely normal. This may also happen to adult males, though significantly less often.

Puberty is often celebrated in many different cultures as the beginning of a young person's journey into maturity, new responsibilities, and adulthood. Other cultures simply consider it to be a private event and prefer to keep it hidden and not spoken of, while some societies view the onset of puberty with much stigma and superstition, particularly for girls experiencing menarche. In U.S. society, many schools include puberty education as part of health class, though often well after many young people have already begun experiencing the changes of puberty. There are still many schools that do not include lessons on puberty at all, or leave out important information. Many adolescents in the United States receive a majority of their reproductive health information from peers or from the internet, which are not always reliable sources.

Lyndsay Mercier

See also: Adolescent Sexuality; Adrenarche; Breast, Female; Menarche; Menstruation; Nocturnal Emissions; Ovulation; Pubic Hair; Semen; Sex Hormones.

Further Reading

Boston Women's Health Book Collective. (2005). *Our bodies, ourselves.* New York: Scribner.

Harris, R. H. (2018). *It's perfectly normal: Changing bodies, growing up, sex, and sexual health.* Somerville, MA: Candlewick Press.

Puberty, Delayed

Delayed, or late, puberty refers to the lack of sexual maturation (evidenced by bodily changes occurring during the transition from childhood to adulthood) in a young adolescent. In most cases, the delay is not caused by illness or disease and is simply a late start in the onset of adolescence. Sometimes, however, delayed puberty is caused by medical conditions, medicines, or malnutrition. Treatment options vary based on the cause of the delay.

An increase in the production of sex hormones (testosterone in males and estrogen in females) is responsible for the onset of puberty, or sexual maturation. In female adolescents, these hormonal changes result in a growth spurt, the development of breasts and pubic hair, and the onset of menstruation. Male adolescents begin to grow pubic and facial hair, have a growth spurt, their testicles and penis get larger, and the body becomes more muscular. These changes take place over a number of years, and the age at which it starts and ends varies widely. Puberty generally begins between the ages of seven and thirteen for girls and between the ages of nine and fifteen for boys. Delayed puberty occurs when the signs of sexual maturation exceed this age range.

Roughly estimated to occur in about 3 percent of children, delayed puberty can have several causes. In over 90 percent of cases, delayed puberty is due to what is known as a constitutional delay in growth and puberty (being a late bloomer), a condition ten times more common in boys than in girls. This type of delay tends to run in families, and affected children are usually shorter in stature than their peers. Sometimes delayed puberty and growth can be secondary to a chronic illness, such as diabetes (high blood sugar), cystic fibrosis (an illness affecting the lungs and digestive system), and celiac disease, a digestive intolerance to a protein found in wheat, barley, and rye. Also, some young girls who undergo intense physical training for a sport start puberty later than usual. Another culprit is malnutrition, which may be due to an eating disorder such as anorexia. In other cases, the delay in puberty occurs because of a long-term medical condition known as hypogonadism, in which the sex glands (the testes and ovaries) produce few or no hormones or the parts of the brain involved in sending hormones to the sex glands—the hypothalamus and pituitary—fail to function properly.

Treatment is usually a matter of watching and waiting with regular checks on height, weight, and levels of relevant hormones. In some instances, medication such as testosterone injections, skin patches, or gels, or estrogen in skin patch or pill form, can jump-start puberty. Growth hormones may also be prescribed if the pituitary is not working well enough. Whatever the cause, if the delay causes psychological or emotional stress, medical professionals can offer children ways to cope and manage the delay more effectively.

Linda Tancs

See also: Adrenarche; Hypogonadism; Puberty; Sex Hormones.

Further Reading

Ann & Robert H. Lurie, Children's Hospital of Chicago. (2019). Late puberty. Retrieved from https://www.luriechildrens.org/en/specialties-conditions/delayed-puberty/

Mayle, P. (1975). *What's happening to me? A guide to puberty.* New York: Kensington Publishing.

Pubic Hair

Pubic hair develops for people of all genders during puberty. In addition to protecting the skin from friction during sex, it may also help trap bacteria and other pathogens before they reach the reproductive organs.

Social trends and preferences for pubic hair styling vary greatly across time and by culture. In contemporary Western societies, it has been noted that females with visible body hair, including hair in the pubic region, can incur social castigation and be positioned as aggressive, less sociable, less happy, and less sexually attractive. The regime of removing part or all of the pubic hair (particularly for females) has differing historical roots. Some researchers claim that pubic hair shaving had all but ceased in the latter part of the nineteenth century in Westernized societies, with natural pubic hair being the norm in terms of genital appearance. Nevertheless, this practice reemerged in the 1980s and ranges from removal of hair from the bikini line (outer pubic hair) to the Brazilian (a small strip of central pubic hair remains) to the complete removal of all pubic hair. This cultural change has largely been influenced by pornography and the prevalence of social norms around the removal of all pubic hair, which are often seen in the media. This regime is mirrored within online pornography, where films of females who have not shaved are considered a sexual preference "specialty" in terms of appearance and appeal.

Reflecting this trend is the rising amount of research into why females choose to remove all or most of their pubic hair, with research participants citing hygiene, aesthetics, and sexual attraction as primary driving forces, particularly within heterosexual relationships. It has been noted that alternative identities such as older females, feminists, and lesbians may actively abstain from pubic hair removal. Nevertheless, the cultural dominance of hair removal has led some to claim that "it is now unusual for a clinician . . . to examine any woman under the age of 30 who still has all her pubic hair" (Riddell, Varto, & Hodgson, 2010).

With respect to males, pubic hair removal and grooming appear to have less importance, but research by Hildebrandt (2003) claims the display of natural pubic hair between males and females may be narrowing. Male body hair has been socially constructed as a visible sign suggesting virility and masculinity, but some recent research suggests that it is becoming more of a social norm for males to trim and tidy up around the genital region, but it is still not the social norm for complete pubic hair removal (although pornographic imagery can display men with no visible pubic hair).

Lesley-Ann Smith

See also: Femininity; Masculinity; Media and Sexuality; Pornography; Puberty.

Further Reading

Boroughs, M., Cafri, G., & Thompson, K. J. (2005). Male body depilation: Prevalence and associated features of body hair removal. *Sex Roles, 52*(9–10), 637–644.

Braun, V., Tricklebank, G., & Clarke, V. (2013). It shouldn't stick out from your bikini at the beach: Meaning, gender and the hairy/hairless body. *Psychology of Women Quarterly, 37*(4), 478–493.

Caselli, D. (2006). "The wives of geniuses I have sat with": Body hair, genius and modernity. In K. Lesnik-Oberstein (Ed.), *The last taboo: Women and body hair* (18–47). Manchester, UK: Manchester University Press.

Fahs, B. (2014). Genital panics: Constructing the vagina in women's qualitative narratives about pubic hair, menstrual sex and vaginal self-image. *Body Image, 11*, 210–218.

Fahs, B. (2014). Perilous patches and pitstaches: Imagined versus lived experiences of women's body hair growth. *Psychology of Women Quarterly, 38*(2), 167–180.

Fahs, B., & Delgado, D. (2011). The specter of excess: Constructing race, class, and gender in women's body hair narratives. In C. Bobel & S. Kwan (Eds.), *Embodied resistance: Breaking the rules, challenging the norms* (13–25). Nashville, TN: Vanderbilt University Press.

Hildebrandt, S. (2003). The last frontier: Body norms and hair removal practices in contemporary American culture. In H. Tschachler, M. Devine, & M. Draxlbauer (Eds.), *The embodiment of American culture* (59–73). Munster, Germany: Litverlag.

Ramsey, S., Sweeney, C., Fraser, M., & Oades, G. (2009). Pubic hair and sexuality: A review. *The Journal of Sexual Medicine, 6*, 2102–2110.

Riddell, L., Varto, H., & Hodgson, Z. G. (2010). Smooth talking: The phenomenon of pubic hair removal in women. *The Canadian Journal of Human Sexuality, 19*(3), 121–130.

Toerien, M., Wilkinson, S., & Choi, P. Y. L. (2005). Body hair removal: The "mundane" production of normative femininity. *Sex Roles, 52*(5), 399–406.

Pubic Lice

A common name for pubic lice is crabs, because under magnification, they look very much like crabs. Pubic lice are organisms that are similar to those organisms that cause scabies, body lice, and head lice, and they all live on the human body and consume human blood.

Pubic lice are tannish to grayish-white, six-legged ectoparasitic organisms (parasites that live on the host surface) that are approximately two millimeters by two millimeters in size. Their scientific name is *Pediculosis phthirus pubis*. Lice are found worldwide and are not racially discriminatory. They are known to infest the hair of the pubic area primarily, which includes the groin, genitalia, and anogenital region (space between anus and genitalia). However, pubic lice can infest facial hair if there is intimate contact, such as during oral sex. If pubic lice are found in the eyebrows or eyelashes in children, it is important to realize that this may be a sign of sexual abuse.

Pubic lice have three forms: the egg (also called a nit), the nymph, and the adult. The nits are lice eggs, often challenging to see but found firmly attached to the hair shaft. Adult female lice typically lay about thirty eggs in their nearly month-long life span. The nits are oval and usually yellow to white in color. Pubic lice nits take approximately six to ten days to hatch. When the nits hatch, they become nymphs, which are immature lice. A nymph looks like an adult pubic louse but smaller. After hatching, the pubic lice nymphs take about two to three weeks to mature into adult lice. The pubic lice are capable of reproducing only in their adult form, not as nymphs. In order for a nymph to survive, it must feed on the blood of the human host via burying its head in the skin, similar to the action of a tick.

When the nymph matures into an adult, the adult female is larger than the male louse. Pubic lice have a broader body than head lice. The pubic louse has two front legs that are very large and look like the pincher claws of a crab, which is how they received their nickname "crabs." Within twenty-four hours of mating, the mature female louse begins laying seven to ten eggs (nits) daily, and repeated fertilization is not required. If the louse falls off a person and does not land on another human host, it will die within one to two days.

The biggest differences between scabies, pubic lice, and body and head lice are how they are acquired and their locations on the body. Scabies are known to reside in the webs between the fingers and under the fingernails, but if someone scratches their groin on a regular basis, they can be transmitted to the groin and genital regions. Body lice usually reside in hairy regions, like armpits, the chest if hair is present, and in areas of tight-fitting clothes. Body lice are typically passed by sharing unwashed clothes from person to person.

Pubic lice are the only organisms in this family that are known to be transmitted by sexual contact. And if a person has acquired pubic lice, though lice are not specific carriers for disease, the individual should be evaluated for other sexually transmitted infections (STIs). It is important to realize that STIs frequently occur simultaneously, as they have the same mode of transmission, and the majority of STIs can be asymptomatic. Therefore, any time a person is diagnosed with one STI, they should be tested for all of them.

Risk factors for acquiring pubic lice include poor hygiene, having intercourse with a person infected with pubic lice, having multiple sexual partners, and sharing bedding, towels, or clothing with an infected person. Despite much concern about the spread of STIs through public restrooms, public spread of pubic lice rarely occurs.

Once this parasite takes hold, it is easily transmitted from person to person. The infection can be extremely uncomfortable, with intense itching that is oftentimes worse at night. This itching sensation may start soon after being infected, or it may start as late as two to four weeks after contact. In addition to the itch, there is often a reaction to the parasite consuming the blood, which causes the skin to turn bluish-gray in color. Vigorous scratching often leads to sores and secondary bacterial skin infections.

The treatment for pubic lice is not intense, but it can be laborious, and it must be performed and completed to fully treat the infection. All partners should be treated at the same time to avoid passing the infection back and forth. All the individuals' clothing and bedding, as well as any cloth or fabric items they may have come in contact with within their homes, should be treated.

Topical treatments are the mainstay of treatment. Shampoos with 1 percent permethrin are the favorite treatments used for the elimination of pubic lice and can be purchased over the counter (OTC). Other products include OTC therapies like antilice shampoo or a mousse substance containing pyrethrins and piperonyl butoxide. Another option, if the OTC medications do not help, is to contact a doctor for a prescription of 0.5 percent malathion lotion, or lindane shampoo, which is an option for therapy. This treatment is usually reserved for later use because of the potential neurotoxic side effects on the brain, especially in infants and pregnant people. The final medication option known at this time is oral ivermectin (a broad-spectrum antiparasitic medication used all over the world for parasitic infections), which can kill the adults and nymphs but cannot kill the nits. In addition to medications, those with pubic lice must use a fine-toothed comb to comb through pubic hair and remove nits.

People may believe that if they have a cleanly shaven pubic region, this eliminates either the risk of acquiring pubic lice or serves as a treatment to eliminate the lice after infestation has occurred, but these are myths. After acquiring pubic lice, trimming pubic hair can help treatment but is not necessary. The trimming aids in eliminating the nits but does not eliminate the adults or nymphs. Trimming allows for ease in the application of medication and better visualization of the louse. If a person shaves after infestation, they run the risk of leaving the head of the louse in the skin, which can end up causing a superficial skin infection.

Usually a single course of treatment is all that is needed. But if another treatment is necessary or recommended, then one should contact their doctor, and the subsequent treatment should be done four days to one week after the previous.

Howard W. MacLennan Jr.

See also: Pubic Hair; Scabies; Sexually Transmitted Infections (STIs).

Further Reading

Grimes, J. A., Smith, L. A., & Fagerberg, K. (2013). *Sexually transmitted disease: An encyclopedia of diseases, prevention, treatment, and issues.* Santa Barbara, CA: Greenwood.

McAnulty, R. D., & Burnette, M. M. (Eds.). (2006). *Sex and sexuality.* Santa Barbara, CA: Praeger.

Newton, D. E. (2009). *Sexual health: A reference handbook.* Santa Barbara, CA: ABC-CLIO.

Public Displays of Affection

Public displays of affection (PDA) are characterized by physical acts of intimacy in a public setting. Although PDAs are often associated with conventional social settings such as schools and parks, PDA can also take place in cyber social spaces. Social media provides a communication platform in which individuals often develop and maintain their relationships, including romantic ones.

PDA can take place in both romantic and nonromantic relationships and ranges from platonic displays such as holding hands, hugging, and putting one's arm around someone else's shoulder, to more intimate acts such as kissing and posting pictures on social media demonstrating physical intimacy or closeness with a romantic partner. Although intimate acts of affection take place in both the public and private spheres, researchers argue that in the public sphere these acts have the intentional effect of demonstrating the intimate status of the individuals' relationship to others.

There are significant cultural differences that inform how PDA is displayed and interpreted. As explained by social scientists, these differences are better understood by how cultures express communication in their relationships, or high-context versus low-context communication. In high-context cultures, verbal communication is less explicit, and greater emphasis is placed on physical contact such as closeness and touch. In lower-context cultures, verbal communication is more explicitly expressed, and individuals derive meaning from the words found in messages. It is important to note that the context of cultures is not static. For instance, Finland has traditionally been considered a high-context culture, but researchers have recently observed that this trend is changing.

Cultural attitudes about race and PDA can intersect. For example, interracial couples in the United States are less likely to engage in PDA due to the stigma surrounding interracial relationships. Compared to intraracial couples, studies have found that adolescents in interracial romantic relationships engage in less PDA, suggesting that individuals learn at a young age what kinds of PDA are culturally acceptable and valued.

Gender and gender expression play an integral part in PDA. In many societies, same-sex and same-gender PDA is stigmatized, prohibited, and even punishable by law. Therefore, due to stigma and the fear of violence, some scholars have found that PDA is less common among same-sex and same-gender couples. Those who decide to engage in PDA have to be very strategic about simple acts such as holding hands in order to protect themselves from retaliation and hate crimes. It should be noted, however, that same-sex and same-gender PDA is perceived differently in various cultures. For example, although in many Arab countries same-sex romantic relationships are prohibited, two men holding hands is not perceived to be romantic.

The stigmatization of same-sex and same-gender PDA is learned at an early age. For example, schools in the United States disproportionately punish lesbian, gay, bisexual, transgender, and queer (LGBTQ) youth for engaging in PDA. This form of discrimination toward LGBTQ youth leads to consequences such as expulsion from school and contributes to increased mental health concerns in LGBTQ youth. More broadly, this double standard is indicative of negative cultural beliefs and attitudes toward the LGBTQ community in the United States.

To sum, PDA is a phenomenon that is observed across diverse groups of individuals worldwide. However, there are differences in terms of culture, gender, gender expression, and sexual identity, among others, that must be considered in how PDA is interpreted.

Roberto L. Abreu and Jacob Huff

See also: Dating, Cross-Cultural Comparison of; Gender Expression; Heterosexism; Kissing; Media and Sexuality; Touching, Sexual Arousal and.

Further Reading

Charton, L., & Boudreau, J. A. (2017). "We or them," "you and I," and "I": Spaces of intimacy and (not so) public displays of affection in Hanoi. *Gender, Place & Culture, 24,* 1303–1322.

de Oliveira, J. M., Costa, C. G., & Nogueira, C. (2013). The workings of homonormativity: Lesbian, gay, bisexual, and queer discourses on discrimination and public displays of affections in Portugal. *Journal of Homosexuality, 60,* 1475–1493.

Seidman, G., Langlais, M., & Havens, A. (2019). Romantic relationship-oriented Facebook activities and the satisfaction of belonging needs. *Psychology of Popular Media Culture, 8*(1), 52.

Vaquera, E., & Kao, G. (2005). Private and public displays of affection among interracial and intra-racial adolescent couples. *Social Science Quarterly, 86,* 484–508.

Purity Pledges

Purity pledges, also known as virginity pledges or abstinence pledges, are commitments made by people—usually young women—not to have sex until married. Most purity pledges are religious in nature, even if they are not directly involved with a particular church. Although many cultures have similar expectations about remaining sexually chaste until married, purity pledges are unique in that they involve an explicit vow and often mark those vows with a ring. The pledges are most common in the United States, although they can also be found in some South American countries as well.

In addition to purity rings, other artifacts or events can mark purity pledges. In the United States, greeting cards and religious pamphlets are often produced for parents to use as part of the purity pledge process. Prewritten contracts can also be downloaded online or purchased from vendors that outline the details of the pledge. Some families or groups of families hold purity balls, sometimes-elaborate ceremonies where daughters take the vow in front of friends and families. In some purity balls, daughters bring their fathers as dates and pledge that until they have another man in their life—specifically, a husband—they will avoid sex and sexual activity. As such, many people—especially those outside of Evangelical Christian communities—have critiqued purity pledges as a sexist practice that is especially focused on girls and young women.

Many families and individuals point to religious convictions as the reason for having their children make purity pledges. Particularly, they argue that cultural sexual mores and rituals are out of line with traditional Christian practices. To that end, most pledges involve religious language in the purity contract and the use of prayer to ask for the pledge to be successful. Even though some critique purity pledges as old-fashioned and counterculture, advocates of purity pledges point to how many U.S. celebrities—most notably, the Jonas Brothers and Jessica Simpson—have publicly worn purity rings. Fathers often espouse that they see it as their duty to protect the sexuality of their daughters, as do mothers; and, thus, the pledges are encouraged. Children, especially daughters, often report that they are happy to make the pledges because they mean so much to their parents and, to a lesser degree, because they also believe in the principles that the pledge represents.

Research has revealed that, despite their popularity, purity pledges do not tend to have any impact on whether or not someone will have sex before marriage. If a child introduces the idea of the pledge to the family, then it is more likely that the pledge will be successful. Overall, however, there is no compelling scientific evidence that purity pledges have any effect on choices to not be involved in sexual relationships. A relationship has been established, however, between taking purity pledges and not being prepared for safer sexual activity. Links between being bullied and wearing purity rings have also been established. Still, many families contend that even if pledges are not efficacious, they represent shared values and meaning between family members.

Jimmie Manning

See also: Adolescent Sexuality; Abstinence; Religion, Diversity of Human Sexuality and; Virginity.

Further Reading

Bruckner H., & Bearman P. S. (2005). After the promise: The STD consequences of adolescent virginity pledges. *Journal of Adolescent Health, 36*, 271–278.

Gardner, C. J. (2011). *Making chastity sexy: The rhetoric of evangelical abstinence campaigns*. Berkeley: University of California.

Manning, J. (2014). Exploring family discourses about purity pledges: Connecting relationships and popular culture. *Qualitative Research Reports in Communication, 15*(1), 92–99.

Rosenbaum, J. E. (2009). Patient teenagers? A comparison of the sexual behavior of virginity pledgers and matched nonpledgers. *Pediatrics, 123*, 110–120.

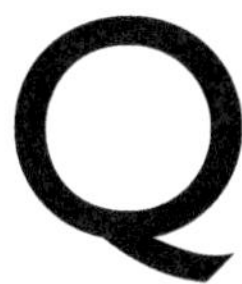

Queer

"Queer" is a word that broadly refers to sexual and gender minorities. A queer person, then, is someone who is not heterosexual (attracted to people of a different sex) or is not cisgender, meaning a typically masculine male or a typically feminine female. Queer is often considered to be an identity, one that can be claimed by a person or that is placed on another person. Queer is highly contextual, meaning that the way it is interpreted often depends on context cues such as surrounding words and sentences as well as nonverbal cues such as tone of voice. Although frequently used to identify lesbian, gay, bisexual, or transgender (LGBT) people, queer can indicate any gender or sexuality that is not the norm.

The word "queer" originally had nothing to do with sex or gender but instead was a word that meant peculiar, weird, or strange until the late 1800s. Then the word started being used to identify and antagonize people who were attracted to the same sex. As that suggests, even though "queer" can be a positive word that empowers people, some use it in a negative way as a put-down even today. That is why the word is often contested, or debated, among LGBT people. Some feel that because it is rooted in a negative use, it is not a good way to refer to those who are LGBT. That sentiment is becoming less common, especially among younger people who grew up with the word being used in a positive context.

One way that the word "queer" became transformed into a positive identity marker was its use by political activists. This use was especially evident in the United States in the late 1980s and early 1990s when the AIDS crisis had many people frustrated that the government was not helping sick gay men. One group named itself Queer Nation, noting that the word "queer" in their title made their name more noticeable and directly confronted the stigma and prejudice aimed at sexual minorities. Members of Queer Nation would rally and chant, "We're here! We're queer! Get used to it!" as a way of making people take notice that queer people and their rights were being ignored. This activist use of "queer," as well as others, became a radical way of asserting rights. Many continued to use the word "queer" in this sense; in the present day, it is less radical but still noticeable by people.

Around the time activists started to use "queer," a similar movement developed in colleges and universities as many professors, especially those in women's studies, began to use the word. Queer theory developed as an intellectual movement that theorized about heteronormativity, the idea that societies construct the ways that gender and sexuality are supposed to be and that people who do not follow those norms should not be oppressed or shamed. Queer theory continues to be developed by scholars, often involving research that examines how heteronormativity is unrealistic, problems related to sexuality or gender and privacy, and cultural pressures for people to assimilate into cisgender or heterosexual roles and behaviors.

Jimmie Manning

See also: Gay Rights Movement; Gender; Genderqueer; LGBTQ+; Pronoun Usage; Sexual Identity; Sexual Rights.

Further Reading

Lovaas, K. E., Elia, J. P., & Yep, G. A. (2006). Shifting ground(s): Surveying the contested terrain of LGBT studies and queer theory. *Journal of Homosexuality, 52*, 1–18.

Manning, J. (2009). Because the personal *is* the political: Politics and unpacking the rhetoric of (queer) relationships. In K. German & B. Dreshel (Eds.), *Queer identities/political realities* (1–12). Newcastle: Cambridge.

Rand, E. J. (2014). *Reclaiming queer: Activist and academic rhetorics of resistance.* Tuscaloosa: University of Alabama.

Sedgwick, E. K. (1990). *Epistemology of the closet.* Berkeley: University of California.

Questioning

"Questioning" is a term used to discuss how individuals explore and wonder about their sexual orientation, sexual identity, or gender identity. "Questioning" can be used to refer to the process of such exploration and potential change in orientation or identity. "Questioning" can also be used by an individual as an identity during this process, or at times to express rejection of trying to fit one's individual experience into existing identity labels.

The process of questioning, and identifying as questioning, is often discussed in the context of teens and adolescents, for whom navigating emerging roles and identities is particularly salient. Physiological changes associated with pubertal development, emerging and crystallizing sexual interests, changes in peer interactions (e.g., start of dating and partnered sexual activity), and changes in gendered social expectations and roles are all potentially relevant factors during this entry into adulthood. However, questioning of sexuality or gender may be relevant for individuals of any age. For some, this can reflect a lifelong process of flexibility and change in their orientation and identity.

Questioning represents an important part of development of gay, lesbian, bisexual, and other sexual minority orientations and identities. Adoption of a gender minority identity, such as a transgender identity, or transitioning from one gender to another, often starts with a process of questioning. Our society has a baseline presumption that people are heterosexual and cisgender, and questioning often involves the individual realizing that society's expectations are not consistent with their own experience. They often must actively seek out information and navigate the challenges associated with differing from the heteronormative and cisnormative mainstream. This can include coping with distress as the result of discrimination directed toward LGBT individuals. Questioning can also involve navigating self-acceptance and integration of a nonheterosexual and noncisgender identity, where internalized homophobia or transphobia can be a significant source of difficulty for some individuals.

Questioning can be especially complex among individuals whose experiences do not fit easily into existing categories of the gender binary (male versus female) or gendered attractions (heterosexual versus homosexual). They can face pressure from both outside and inside the LGBT community to decide on a category or label. For example, an individual may be expected to decide if they are definitively male or female, when their actual gender identity involves both masculine and feminine features. Some individuals may find less common but more applicable identities for themselves (e.g., pansexual, agender), while others may decide against labeling themselves at all.

Questioning can overlap with sexual orientation and identity formation in sexual and gender minority individuals, but it is not synonymous with having an "unformed" or "developing" identity. Indeed, heterosexual cisgender individuals may also engage in questioning their gender and sexual identities. In some cisgender heterosexual university samples, about half of the men and two-thirds of the women reported having questioned their sexual orientation in the past. However, after a process of questioning and exploration, these individuals returned to a heterosexual orientation as the best descriptor of their own sexuality.

Recently, there has been an increase in adolescents who are less interested in maintaining a specific gender or sexual identity. This may be associated with increasing societal acceptance of gender fluidity and sexual minorities. Questioning youth include those who see that there are a large number of ways people can label and understand their sexual and gender identities, and they are consequently not interested in foreclosing on a specific identity (without more experience and information). For some individuals, questioning becomes a lifelong process in recognition of how gender and sexual identities can change in response to changing stages, circumstances, and relationships across the life span.

The process of questioning can take on many forms and involve different behaviors. Introspection and reflection on one's motivations, feelings, thoughts, and sense of self are common. For example, individuals consider which people and groups they have (or do not have) romantic and sexual attractions to. They may also compare their relative levels of attraction toward one gender or sex versus another. Individuals may also notice experiences such as an intrinsic sense of "maleness" or "femaleness" or other sexual/gender identities. A person may become aware of a sense of difference from societal norms or expectations, such as difference from heteronormative romantic or sexual attractions, or a lack of fit with expectations and roles prescribed to their assigned gender. For some, this may be accompanied by significant distress and dysphoria; for others, it may be a sense of "lack of fit" with a heterosexual or cisgender identity.

New sexual behaviors or gender presentation may also be explored. For example, individuals questioning sexual orientation may reflect on whether past sexual and romantic activities with different genders or sexes were enjoyable, repulsive, or neutral. Individuals questioning gender identity may experiment with different aspects of gender presentation (e.g., hairstyle, clothes, names, pronouns) in private or public and whether these behaviors feel more or less congruent with their internal sense of self. Prospective behaviors may also be explored through hypothetical thinking and perspective taking. This can include imagining engaging in sexual activities with different genders and sexes or imagining living or presenting as a different gender (or gender fluid) and noting positive, negative, or ambivalent or neutral reactions within oneself.

Exposure to information related to other identities and orientations, and interactions with individuals with those identities and orientations, can have a significant impact on questioning individuals. Learning about other orientations and identities in sex education class, through the media, from family and peers, and from other sources can be crucial for helping questioning individuals identify and contextualize their own experiences. For youth, opportunities to meet and engage with diversity in sexuality and gender, such as through gay-straight alliance organizations in school, is often reported to be important for supporting questioning individuals. Having a trusted mentor who has similar experiences with sexual or gender identity can also be valuable for questioning youth as a source of support and information. With the proliferation of the internet, questioning individuals also have more opportunities to seek out information and supportive communities online.

Questioning identity can map onto several existing models of identity development. Some models are based on developmental stages, and questioning often represents the early stages of these models. For example, Cass's (1979) model of homosexual identity development states that sexual identity is acquired and progresses linearly through six distinct stages: identity confusion, identity comparison, identity tolerance, identity acceptance, identity pride, and identity synthesis. For emerging gay or lesbian individuals, questioning can map onto the stages of identity confusion (where the individual realizes that their experiences are incongruent with heteronormative expectations) and identity comparison (where the individual examines whether a gay or lesbian identity may be suitable for them).

Other models are based on developmental processes rather than stages. For example, Cox and Gallois's (1996) social identity model highlights two major processes involved in identity development: self-categorization (which involves self-labeling with a group and adoption of norms and values of a group) and social comparisons (which involves varying levels of dependence on having a group membership and contrasts between values and norms of different groups). Both appear important in the questioning process; questioning involves exploration of which social groups the individual fits into and the social impacts of adopting certain identities. For example, questioning involves widening the range of self-labels and groups that are available to the individual. The questioning process may also become more complicated or protracted if adoption of a new gender or sexual identity or orientation will precipitate conflict with other important group memberships (e.g., family, existing peer groups).

Some authors have used an intersectionality approach to examine questioning. This paradigm emphasizes how sexuality and gender exist within a broader sociocultural and individual interpersonal context, which include factors such as cultural values and norms, socioeconomic status, education, age, and personal relationships and life experience. Questioning is then a reflection of the dynamic interaction between an individual's self-identity within this broader context. This approach also emphasizes that sexuality and gender, although conceptually different, are often interactive and interrelated. Questioning of one may lead to new experiences and subsequent further questioning of the other. Questioning can become a lifelong process that allows greater flexibility and fluidity in response to changing individual circumstances and often involves rejection of clear labels and categories in favor of a more personally relevant and integrated sense of self-identity.

Silvain S. Dang

See also: Adolescent Sexuality; Binary Gender System; Coming Out; Fluidity, Gender; Fluidity, Sexual; Gender Dysphoria; Gender Identity; Gender Identity Development; Gender Roles, Socialization and; Gender Transition; Genderqueer; Homophobia, Internalized; LGBTQ+; Queer; Sexual Identity; Sexual Orientation.

Further Reading

Cass, V. C. (1979). Homosexual identity formation: A theoretical model. *Journal of Homosexuality, 4*(3), 219–235.

Cox, S., & Gallois, C. (1996). Gay and lesbian identity development: A social identity perspective. *Journal of Homosexuality, 30*(4), 1–30.

Diamond, L. M., & Butterworth, M. (2008). Questioning gender and sexual identity: Dynamic links over time. *Sex Roles, 59*, 365–376.

Hollander, G. (2000). Questioning youth: Challenges to working with youths forming identities. *School Psychology Review, 29*, 173–179.

Morgan, E. M., Steiner, M. G., & Thompson, E. M. (2010). Processes of sexual orientation questioning among heterosexual men. *Men and Masculinities, 12*(4), 425–433.

Morgan, E. M., & Thompson, E. M. (2011). Processes of sexual orientation questioning among heterosexual women. *Journal of Sex Research, 48*(1), 16–28.

Steinmetz, K. (2017, May). Beyond "he" or "she": The changing meaning of gender and sexuality. *Time.* Retrieved from http://time.com/4703309/gender-sexuality-changing/

R

Rape

Rape involves the penetration of a person's bodily orifice, which includes the oral cavity, vagina, or anus. It can involve any object, but the typical instrument of insertion is a penis. Rape exists when consent is not present. People traditionally viewed rape as only involving women as victims. However, modern legal statutes in many countries acknowledge that men experience rape. This changing conception of victimization relates to shifts in cultural beliefs and values of gender and sexuality.

The concept of rape has existed since the beginning of recorded history. Greek mythology notes several instances of rape. Interestingly, several stories have themes related to bestiality, with gods taking the form of animals to engage in forced copulation with women. This includes the story of Europa. Zeus took the form of a bull, embedded himself in a herd belonging to her father, and raped her. Other ancient accounts of rape exist in the Code of Hammurabi and the Bible. Throughout time, rape has been a part of cultures in various ways. This includes bridal arrangements between families, carnal rewards associated with war victories, and slavery. A commonality with these examples involves patriarchal standards of male aggression and ideas that women are the property of males. Gender equality has changed much of this. Consider that in the United States it used to be legal for husbands to rape their wives, sometimes referred to as marital rape. All states had removed laws involving marital rape exemptions by 1993. Recent movements within the United States have even advocated the existence of "rape culture." This involves social settings where rape is prevalent, partly because popular culture and the media excuse themes associated with it. The argument is that rape culture thrives when the use of misogynistic language and the objectification of women's bodies is acceptable. For example, consider the debate around Robin Thicke's song "Blurred Lines."

There are several different forms of rape. Molestation concerns an adult using a child for sexual stimulation. It is not just family related and can occur in a variety of settings, including educational and religious contexts. Dynamics involving people in positions of power over children and the inability for children to provide legal consent are key. Statutory rape involves the prohibition of intercourse between people of a specified legal age regardless of consent. The age of consent in most areas of the United States is between fourteen and eighteen. Acquaintance rape involves someone the victim knows. Research shows that one-quarter of women report at least one rape experience. Up to 95 percent of those women indicate the assailant was an acquaintance. Rape by an acquaintance is more likely with adolescents. Scholars are skeptical of statistics in this area, and with rape in general, since surveys indicate only 4 percent of rape victims report the crime to law enforcement. Date rape is a type of acquaintance rape involving situations where the victim agreed to accompany the perpetrator to an entertainment-based event, social gathering, or dining encounter. The perpetrator may establish sex as a necessary exchange for paying for the date. Other themes involve the encouragement of intoxication, the use of drugs to limit the victim's mental capacity, and social isolation to reduce detection. Group rape involves fraternities, athletic teams, and gangs. These are all-male groups that promote masculine, physical aggression in their behaviors and have an elevated sense of group identity. Dynamics involve advanced planning by a group leader, victim selection, victim humiliation, and systematic coverup if the event becomes public knowledge. Some theories argue that homoerotic tendencies are involved in group rape. Western culture has traditionally frowned on homosexual contact between groups of males with close emotional ties. Therefore, a group rape involving a female victim provides males with an indirect outlet for sexual contact with other males. Criminal convictions for group rape are uncommon.

In the United States, there is legal variation with the term "rape." In some states, statutes refer to sexual assault instead of rape. Sexual assault involves actions against a victim's will or without consent, using force or threats related to force, and/or manipulation. Other acts involving sexual motivation not falling under the traditional definition of rape can apply. This includes consensual sex between two people of legal age where one is an authority figure working in an official capacity for the government. Consider a teacher or juvenile detention officer having a sexual relationship with someone eighteen years or older. Some states simply use the words "rape" and "sexual assault" interchangeably. Once under prosecution, research shows that rapists will defend themselves in ways that refocus responsibility to the victim. This includes claiming that the victim's seduction was irresistible, the victim wanted it despite saying "no," the victim enjoyed it, or the victim has a history of promiscuity, making the likelihood of rape impossible. These motives often emerge after the assault to justify the crime and are not necessarily rationalizations that provide good legal standing during court proceedings. However, literature implies that in cases involving female victims, whether or not the person was engaging in what culture defines as wholesome activities before an assault can make a difference with some judges and juries. Sexual assault penalties vary in the United States, with most having one- to two-year minimum sentences. Mitigating and aggravating circumstances, such as the number of previous offenses, influence punishment. Castration is an option for some offenders. This is more likely to involve a chemical component that lowers testosterone levels, but some offenders have volunteered for physical castration. Critics argue that rape can be more about power and control and less about sexual gratification. In turn, physical castration might limit the ability of a rapist to use his penis for penetration, but the possibility of using other objects still exists. Upon release from prison, over 50 percent of convicted rapists commit some criminal offense within five years.

Due in part to the influence of the feminist movement in the early 1970s, the public, and more importantly the legal system, started paying attention to the aftermath of rape. Rape crisis centers emerged, and the idea of addressing psychological reactions to rape became relevant. Associated with posttraumatic stress disorder, "rape trauma syndrome" entered the lexicon of clinical fields associated with sexual assault responses. It involves symptoms including, but not limited to, shock, nausea, headaches, stomach pains, sleep irregularity, trouble eating, crying, being startled easily, radical lifestyle changes, substance abuse, and suicidal tendencies.

Jason S. Ulsperger

See also: Date Rape; Rape, Abuse and Incest National Network (RAINN); Rape Shield Laws; Rape Trauma Syndrome; Sexual Abuse; Sexual Assault; Statutory Rape.

Further Reading

Cocca, C. (2004). *Jailbait: The politics of statutory rape laws in the United States*. Albany: State University of New York Press.

Denton, M. (2018). *Rape culture: How can we end it?* New York: Lucent Press.

Horeck, T. (2014). #AskThicke: Blurred lines, rape culture, and the feminist hashtag takeover. *Feminist Media Studies, 14*(6), 1105–1107.

Reddington, F., & Kreisel, B. (2017). *Sexual assault: The victims, the perpetrators, and the criminal justice system*. Durham, NC: Carolina Academic Press.

Smith, M. (2018). *Encyclopedia of rape and sexual violence*. Santa Barbara, CA: ABC-CLIO.

Rape, Abuse and Incest National Network (RAINN)

The Rape, Abuse and Incest National Network, also known as RAINN, is one of the United States' largest anti-sexual-violence agencies. It created and runs the National Sexual Assault Telephone Hotline and National Sexual Assault Online Hotline, which are composed of independent RAINN affiliates answering a twenty-four-hour hotline that can be reached via phone or the internet (800-656-HOPE and online.rainn.org). RAINN also provides education about sexual violence, leads efforts to prevent sexual violence, and helps to improve services to victims throughout the United States.

Scott Berkowitz cofounded RAINN in 1994, along with Tori Amos, who was the organization's first national spokesperson. RAINN was founded through monetary help from Atlantic Records and Warner Music Group. At the time of its founding, RAINN was composed of 347 centers across the United States that helped provide victim support. RAINN has continually grown and now has more than 1,100 affiliated centers. Scott Berkowitz is still the president of RAINN, and Christina Ricci is currently RAINN's national spokesperson.

RAINN manages two different hotlines, the National Sexual Assault Hotline and the National Sexual Assault Online Hotline, and since opening in 1994, the organization has helped more than two million people. RAINN is able to provide this support by partnering with more than 1,100 local sexual assault agencies across the nation to bring free and confidential services twenty-four hours a day, seven days a week. Individuals who contact the national hotline phone number will be routed to sexual assault service providers in their area.

RAINN expanded its services in 2007 by starting the first confidential online instant messaging program that enabled individuals to talk with trained staff members through a secure and confidential web-based interface. The plan to go digital was due to the fact that half of sexual assault victims are younger than eighteen, and this age group is more likely to embrace online technology than to make a phone call. Both hotlines provide confidential support, referrals for medical help, resources, and legal information. The hotline can be contacted by victims or loved ones looking for information about sexual violence.

The U.S. Department of Defense (DoD) has also contracted RAINN to operate the DoD Safe Helpline. This helpline is solely for members of the Department of Defense community and can be reached via phone or the internet. Individuals trained specifically on topics of military sexual assault operate these hotlines and provide appropriate help and services based on the caller's request. The DoD Safe Helpline is also confidential, and identifying information will not be shared with the DoD.

RAINN also works closely with the entertainment industry to help educate people and prevent sexual violence. RAINN provides information and educational statistics to news junkets across the United States and also runs television ads with the help of celebrities. These celebrities offer monetary support to RAINN to help keep their services going. Above all is their informative and educational website, RAINN.org, that provides not only statistics on sexual violence but also information on the effects of sexual assault along with other important educational information. RAINN's website also provides lists of local services and tips on how to be safer in public and on the internet. RAINN's mission is to help decrease the number of sexual violence incidents across the nation, and it continually provides new information and support to make this happen.

Amanda Baker

See also: Date Rape; Incest; Rape; Sexual Abuse; Sexual Assault.

Further Reading

DoD Safe Helpline. (n.d.). About Safe Helpline. Retrieved from https://www.safehelpline.org/about

Finn, J., & Hughes, P. (2008). Evaluation of the RAINN National Sexual Assault Online Hotline. *Journal of Technology in Human Services, 26*(2–4), 203–222.

RAINN. (2019). About RAINN. Retrieved from https://rainn.org/about-rainn

RAINN. (2019). About the national sexual assault telephone hotline. Retrieved from https://rainn.org/get-help/national-sexual-assault-hotline

Rape Shield Laws

The term "rape shield law" refers to a set of conventions guiding the disclosure of information about the background of a person who is alleging a sexual assault. Colloquially, "rape shield law" can be used to describe two different things:

disclosure of a victim's background in the press or exposure of a victim's background during the prosecution of the assailant.

While there is no set law prohibiting the press from disclosing personal information about someone alleging a sexual assault, popular convention has deterred the publication of a victim's name or likeness. Many media outlets avoid publishing any type of information that could potentially identify an alleged rape victim. The widespread expansion of news and social media facilitated by the explosion of wireless and internet technology can affect the trend of protecting rape victims' identities, and this becomes amplified if it is a high-profile case, such as if a celebrity is being accused.

There are laws governing the use of the victim's background in the prosecution of a sexual assault case, and these laws can vary jurisdictionally (Galvin, 1986). The name of a complaining witness is usually a part of the accusatory instrument, and thus a part of the case, but there are different guidelines regarding the use of information about a victim's past sexual history. The prejudicial nature of this evidence can outweigh its evidentiary value.

While many jurisdictions prohibit the introduction of evidence of a victim's past, there are circumstances under which information about a victim's sexual past may be introduced as evidence. One is if the victim and the defendant have been intimate prior to the alleged incident, such as if they were in a sexual relationship or married. Another is if the victim has had a past conviction of a sex crime, notably a prostitution offense. A sex work conviction may be introduced as evidence, regardless of its connection to the current case or the time since the conviction. Another exception to rape shield laws is if there is evidence that may be used to impeach a witness or prove perjury. This can occur in a rape prosecution if the complainant asserts they have never had sex before and the prosecution has a credible witness who testifies that they had sex with the complainant. Here, the testimony is used to challenge credibility, but it also has the effect of introducing information about the complainant's sexual past. Evidence may also be introduced if it can show that forensic evidence found on the victim originated from someone other than the defendant.

Rachel Kalish

See also: Date Rape; Rape; Sexual Assault.

Further Reading

Anderson, M. J. (2002). From chastity requirement to sexuality license: Sexual consent and a new rape shield law. *George Washington Law Review, 70*, 51.

Galvin, H. R. (1986). Shielding rape victims in the state and federal courts: An approach for the second decade. *Minnesota Law Review, 70*, 763.

Haddad, R. I. (2005). Shield or sieve? *People v. Bryant* and the rape shield law in high profile cases. *Columbia Journal of Law and Social Problems, 39*, 185.

Rape Trauma Syndrome

"Rape trauma syndrome" was coined by two therapists, Ann Burgess and Lynda Holmstrom, to refer to a series of symptoms that are commonly experienced by rape victims. Since this syndrome has been named, it has been used in countless trials to help survivors have a voice. Rape trauma syndrome is a collection of emotional, physical, and behavioral reactions that are experienced by victims of attempted or completed rape. Burgess and Holmstrom identified two stages: the first, known as the acute phase, is the immediate phase of disruption and disorganization; the second phase is the long-term process of reorganization. A third phase, known as the underground phase, has since been recognized. Phase length varies, and individuals may go back and forth between the phases. The names of the stages have also changed over time and may differ depending on the source of information. This article uses the language used by the creators.

The acute stage occurs immediately after the assault. The physical and emotional reactions in this stage are intense, and sometimes victims are in disbelief or shock because of what has happened to them. Other emotions that may be experienced include fear, humiliation, shame, guilt, self-blame, anger, and revenge. Due to the range of emotions, the victims may demonstrate this stage in a variety of ways, from crying to a composed calmness. Physically, the victim may feel soreness all over the body, generalized pain, and bleeding. They may react with fear and confusion and have difficulty completing daily tasks. This phase usually lasts from a few days to a few weeks.

The underground phase follows the acute stage. During this phase, the victim tries to return to what their life was prior to the rape, and often they may try to act as if nothing has happened. Throughout this phase, they may not want to discuss what has happened or to have reminders of the incident. Individuals can remain in this stage for years and may give off the appearance that they are over what happened to them.

The final stage is the reorganization stage. This stage is often started off by a trigger and returns the victim to a phase of emotional turmoil. This process is often long term and may require outside help and therapy. Through this phase, the individual can become very frightened of returning to the stage of emotional pain. Fears and phobias can develop; fantasies of revenge may also come up, and the individual may experience eating and sleeping disturbances. As this stage develops, the individual will hopefully be able to work through these difficult emotions and behaviors and toward returning to a life where the rape is not at the forefront. The context of the assault, such as the individual's developmental stage in life, who committed the assault, cultural background, and the nature of the assault, can have a significant effect on the process through the reorganization stage.

Amanda Baker

See also: Child Sexual Abuse; Date Rape; Rape; Rape, Abuse and Incest National Network (RAINN); Sexual Abuse; Sexual Assault.

Further Reading

Burgess, A. W. (1983). Rape trauma syndrome. *Behavioral Sciences & the Law, 1*(3), 97–113.

Burgess, A. W., & Holmstrom, L. L. (1974). Rape trauma syndrome. *American Journal of Psychiatry, 131*(9), 981–986.

Rape Crisis Cape Town Trust. (2019). Rape trauma syndrome (RTS). Retrieved from http://rapecrisis.org.za/information-for-survivors/rape-trauma-syndrome/

Reimer, David

David Reimer was the child at the center of the controversial "John/Joan" gender experiment conducted by Dr. John Money, a celebrated psychologist in practice at Johns Hopkins Gender Identity Clinic in Baltimore, Maryland.

Reimer was an identical twin. The infants were born August 22, 1965, in Winnipeg, Manitoba, Canada, and named Bruce Peter Reimer and Brian Henry Reimer. At eight months old, Bruce's penis was completely severed during a botched circumcision. After the accident, the twins' parents, Ron and Janet Reimer, were referred to Dr. Money for advice on how to care for their son after his accident.

A well-known sexologist and researcher, Dr. Money believed that human gender identity is malleable and can be instructed or influenced by outside factors. He is, in fact, credited with coining the term "gender role," meaning the behavior "learned by a person as appropriate to their gender, determined by the prevailing cultural norms."

Meeting the Reimer family inspired Money to devise an experiment to prove his theory. With an identical twin to serve as the control, the circumstances seemed nearly perfect. Money encouraged Reimer's parents to authorize sex reassignment surgery on the baby, raise him as a girl, and never tell either of the twins (or anyone else) what had happened.

Reimer was the first documented case of sex reassignment of a child born developmentally normal. Over the course of more than a decade, Money subjected the Reimer twins to a number of sexually explicit exercises and activities, some of which were photographed and/or witnessed by half a dozen colleagues or more. Throughout the experiment, Money continued to report that Brenda (formerly Bruce) had transitioned successfully and was doing just fine as a girl. He gained more and more power and fame for his work, and his findings were discussed in medical textbooks and psychology lectures worldwide.

In reality, however, nothing was further from the truth. Both twins struggled with depression and anxiety. Brenda, consistently sullen and angry, experienced severe gender dysphoria and was bullied in school for being too masculine. At age thirteen, Brenda threatened to commit suicide if made to see Money again.

The twins were fifteen when Ron Reimer finally told his sons what had happened. Immediately, Brenda assumed the name David and began living as male. David attempted to put the past behind him, but he remained tortured by the trauma. He attempted to end his life on more than one occasion, and he so longed for revenge that he went so far as to buy an unregistered handgun with the intention of killing the doctors involved. By age twenty-two, he had begun testosterone therapy and had undergone chest reconstruction surgery to remove the breasts that had resulted from the estrogen pills he had been subjected to since he was eleven years old. David later went on to have additional surgical procedures to construct a penis. In 1997, he married Jane Fontane, who had three young children.

The truth about David's experience was uncovered by another sex researcher, Dr. Milton Diamond of the University of Hawaii, who wanted to know what had become of the twins who had likely entered adulthood. He also wondered why

Money had not published or spoken of the twins' case for more than a decade. Intrigued, Dr. Diamond hunted down the Reimers and soon learned the real story and published an article refuting Money's claims.

The media eventually caught wind of the study gone awry, and David's life became front-page headlines. After they hit it off during an interview, David agreed to let *Rolling Stone* reporter John Colapinto write his life story. Published in 2000, the resulting book *As Nature Made Him: The Boy Who Was Raised as a Girl,* shined a very unflattering light on the now-infamous story of Dr. Money's experiment.

In 2002, David's brother Brian died after overdosing on antidepressant medication. David was struggling financially, and he had grown quite weary of the invasion to his privacy. In May 2004, his wife, Jane, told him she wanted a divorce. Two days later, David shot himself.

Money's lies had ramifications far beyond just the Reimer family. His reports were used by the medical community as justification for sex reassignment surgeries for thousands of children born with ambiguous genitals or other intersex conditions; this is a nonconsensual practice that has only recently begun to wane after significant work by intersex community advocates.

C. Michael Woodward

See also: Circumcision; Diamond, Milton; Gender Dysphoria; Gender Identity; Gender Roles, Socialization and; Money, John; Sex Reassignment Surgery.

Further Reading

Colapinto, J. (2000). *As nature made him: The boy who was raised as a girl.* New York: HarperCollins Publishers.

Gaetano, P. (2017, November 15). *David Reimer and John Money gender reassignment controversy: The John/Joan case.* Retrieved from https://embryo.asu.edu/pages/david-reimer-and-john-money-gender-reassignment-controversy-johnjoan-case

Religion, Diversity of Human Sexuality and

There are many philosophical perspectives from which to examine the intersection of religion and sexuality. A French philosopher, Michel Foucault (1978), discusses sexuality as socially constructed and suggests that its meaning is derived from the language that is used to discuss it. When institutions dialogue about sex and sexuality, John Gagnon (1990) describes this reality as having an instructional system around sexuality. Religion is one such institution or system.

Religion can be defined as an organized system of beliefs based on a worldview about the relational interconnectedness between humans, nature, the universe, creation, or a divine presence. Some key components of religion include community, group worship, a set of dogma or doctrine, a set of moral values, rituals, and a creation story about how the world came to be to help explain the universe and humanity's relationship to it. Religions also have what is called a metanarrative, or a story from which the religious system stems that differentiates it from other religious systems. In Christianity, this is the story of the passion, death, and resurrection of Jesus from the Christian Bible; for Islam, it is the story of Muhammad told in the Qur'an; in Buddhism, the metanarrative is the story and life of Siddhartha Gautama, or the first Buddha. All these aspects are crucial in the interpretation of the religion. These interpretations then affect the institution's view of the human condition, part of which is sexuality.

Because of the various worldviews and experiences that led to the creation of multiple religions, it follows that each religion has a different way of viewing human sexuality. How a religion views the purpose of our existence will affect how it is believed we should operate around sexuality. The view of how humans relate to the Divine or the universe is called a theological or cosmological anthropology.

As religion attempts to make sense of various human experiences, it has inevitably been met with the reality of sexuality. Many ancient religions understood that fertility was a natural human process that exhibited great power. The creation and perpetuation of humanity quite literally depended on fertility. Fertility of humans, fertility of land and soil after the dawn of agriculture, and fertility of livestock were all seen as powers of nature so great that many religions have specific fertility deities. Prayers, sacrifice, and service were all paid to these deities to appease them so that nature would work in their favor. Many ancient rituals involved retelling or reenacting stories of fertility to bring about good fortune or luck to situations in which fertility was unsure or not guaranteed. Differences in fertility practices or sexual behaviors were often a point of pride for a new religion as it emerged and distinguished itself and its doctrines from the surrounding religious systems.

One of the ways religion attempts to make sense of sexuality is by having codes or rules and regulations around sexual behavior. Because religion is concerned with how humans relate to the world, it often has proscriptions on how to live in it as well. Most societies throughout history have had some rules on what was considered acceptable and unacceptable sexual behavior. While the overall view can range from seemingly negative views of human sexuality to viewing sexuality as an ultimate form of divine love, sexuality has been present in much of the dialogue around morality.

Within religions, the purpose of humanity is often closely tied to what is sexually right and wrong. For example, in some religious belief systems, the body is viewed as bad or weak compared to the soul. This sense of dualism affects how the religion views sexual pleasure or the effects of procreation. In Christianity, St. Augustine of Hippo, influenced by Manicheism (a dualistic religion that stresses a dichotomy between light and dark), felt that sexual intercourse even for procreation is still sinful. The Christian view that sexuality is for procreation stems from the metanarrative in which God tells Abraham to be fruitful and multiply. The official Christian church did not accept Augustine's teaching that all sexual activity was sinful, but his sentiments of sexuality being innately harmful have persisted throughout history.

In other religions, sexuality can be more readily seen as a holistic part of the human experience. In these religions, rules of sexual morality may focus more on appropriate times in life to be sexual or understand a multiplicity of ways to be sexual. In Hinduism, the understanding of sexual orientation and gender identities guides what is or is not moral based on the fact that there is a place in society for those with differing sexual experiences and identities.

The word "pornography" is an excellent example of how sexual morality works in society. The Greek word "porneia" means "illicit" or "illegal sex." This refers to any sexual behavior that is deemed wrong or inappropriate for society. In a religious context, primarily the Christian Bible, this word is translated to mean fornication, adultery, or otherwise sexually immoral behavior.

Rituals are extremely important to religious systems. Many religions today have rituals around sexuality, just as they might have rituals around initiation or death. Sexual rituals involve a symbolic act or recognition of power. Some religions, like Judaism, have rituals around circumcision or menstruation. Other religions have specific prayers for sexual intercourse between spouses or special rituals for accessing various sexual energies. For example, religions that focus on psychic energy and the role of sexuality in that view of humanity may engage in sex magic—a harnessing of sexual energy to transcend the average human experience.

People may ascribe to a religion for many reasons: because it resonates most with their worldview, answers questions, gives them security, supplies them with a space that feels sacred, gives them a community, has been what their family practiced, or provides a feeling of closeness to a Divine presence and more connection than another system of belief. Whatever the reason, one's religious and sexual identities will likely intersect. For some individuals, navigating this intersection is simple and aligns with their experience of sexuality. For others, however, this intersection can be a point of contention, pain, or sexual discomfort or dysfunction. A Christian raised with the understanding that sex before marriage is bad may have internalized this message so much that sex after marriage may be difficult or impossible because of sexual aversion. A Jewish rabbi who feels pressured to get married may feel so overwhelmed by the implicit sexual obligations of marriage that they avoid the topic all together. Topics of sexual orientation, gender identity, differences in sexual development, marital structures and lifestyles (monogamy, nonmonogamy, polyamory, etc.), and sexual development or behaviors are all places that this dissonance can occur.

The cognitive dissonance that can come with having a sexual identity contrary to what one's religion may identify as morally good can be difficult to reconcile. Some people may seek the help of their religious leaders or religiously sensitive counselors and therapists. When this identity discord arises, learning about one's own religious system and cosmological or theological anthropology can help identify and resolve the internal and external issues present in the situation.

The concept of sexuality being socially constructed is only one paradigm or philosophical disposition about the nature of sexuality. Many religions view sexuality as essential—an integral part of the human experience, whether or not it is discussed on a societal level. The true nature of sexuality is seen to be discoverable or able to be uncovered by society. In such a view, it is often seen as the responsibility of the religious leader, theologian, or philosopher to describe that nature and help others in society strive toward what is morally good. The rituals, prayers, rules, and regulations are all in existence because somewhere throughout history it was thought to be a good idea to institute such practices. When examining other codes of sexual morality, it is helpful to know the cosmological or theological anthropology from which a system works in order to identify why it is held to be the morally good option. The diversity of the ways religions deal with human sexuality is vast. A common theme, however, has been that sex and sexuality have been important enough to make rules about and even honor in certain ways. In our present society, the intersection of how various cultures and religions deal with sexuality can be seen in the hotly debated topics of abortion, premarital sex, sexual pleasure, masturbation, and sexuality education. Each voice in these discourses comes from a position that is possibly connected to a religious identity trying to resolve dissonance.

Mark A. Levand

See also: Antigay Prejudice; Circumcision; Fertility; Menstruation; Reparative Therapy; Roman Catholic Church Sexual Abuse Scandal; Tantric Intercourse.

Further Reading

Foucault, M. (1978). *The history of sexuality: Volume 1, an introduction* (R. Hurley, Trans.). New York: Pantheon.

Gagnon, J. H. (1990). The explicit and implict use of the scripting perspective in sex research. *Annual Review of Sex Research, 1*, 1–43.

Reparative Therapy

Reparative therapy (also known as gay conversion therapy or sexual reorientation therapy) is intended to convert individuals having a homosexual orientation to a heterosexual one. Targeted primarily toward white male homosexuals, these programs are based on the assumptions that same-sex attraction is a pathological or deviant condition and that this orientation can be changed. Beginning in the 1990s, reparative therapies underwent extensive scrutiny as to their theoretical validity, effectiveness, and potential to inflict harm. These practices are currently opposed by all major mental health and medical organizations and are banned in some states, with increasing support for national prohibition. In the face of this, many organizations that had offered these therapies have closed. Nonetheless, some reparative therapy programs continue to operate with primary support from conservative religious organizations.

Discussion of reparative therapies has existed since the 1920s, and over time, treatments utilized to "cure" homosexuality have included brain surgery, medical hormonal castration, and behavioral aversion therapy pairing homoerotic images with sensations of pain or nausea. More recently, less intrusive and more traditional talk therapy approaches including visualization and skills training have been emphasized in conversion programs, as have spiritually based interventions.

Historically, proponents of reparative therapy based their theoretical foundation for this treatment on psychoanalytic theory. Reasoning that abnormal development patterns resulted in male homosexuality, early indications of homosexual orientation were thought to be evidenced through an abnormally large amount of time spent with one's mother and a lack of interest in sports, physical confrontations with other males, and flirtation and sexual harassment of females. Ironically, this interpretation's use of psychoanalytic theory is at odds with the opinion voiced by Sigmund Freud that homosexuality was not a feature that could be, or perhaps should be, changed. It is also inconsistent with other psychoanalytic interpretations of male homosexual identity development.

Theoretically, reparative therapy conflicts with mainstream beliefs in two ways. First, it views homosexuality as pathological and in some cases even criminal or immoral. In contrast, homosexual orientation has not been considered a disorder by professional mental health organizations since 1973 and has also received increasing social and political acceptance. Second, there is no theoretical or empirical support for viewing homosexual orientation as changeable rather than innate to the individual. There are no empirical studies indicating these programs are successful in changing sexual orientation. Results reported by programs are also questionable in that they often measure success based on reported homosexual activity rather than sexual orientation so that a lack of homosexual activity would be considered a success. Further, many programs believe that a homosexual cannot have sex with an other-sex partner, so engaging in heterosexual sex indicates a successful conversion. Finally, participant reports indicate coercive factors may influence reported results as participants may indicate changes to please program therapists or to avoid alienation or exclusion from group affiliations, such as expulsion from schools.

Beyond failing to change sexual orientation, reparative therapy programs can cause harm to participants. Programs may not ethically inform participants that this therapy is deemed ineffective and banned by mental health organizations and that their assumptions are at odds with majority views on the nature of homosexuality as reflecting normal versus pathological development. They may provide misinformation as to the connection of homosexual orientation to other pathologies, fail to allow for informed consent, and create false impressions of program effectiveness. As a result of the misinformation and intervention approaches used in reparative therapy, participants may suffer from depression and suicidal ideation, anxiety, reduced self-esteem, relational disruption, feelings of alienation and isolation, and identity confusion.

Given that the professional literature is rich with information that is critical of reparative therapy, the lack of theoretical or research foundation for these programs supports criticism that they are based on personal opinion and social bias rather than scientific evidence. The content of websites promoting reparative therapy offer two main justifications for the treatment. The first is that of professional therapists who feel those who want this type of treatment have a right to have it, regardless of the negative evaluation of this therapy in the professional community. The second is that of religious counselors who believe homosexuality is sinful and should be changed on moral grounds. Those reparative therapy programs that continue to operate tend to have religious themes and emphasize the belief that homosexuality can be changed yet stress the responsibility of the participant for results and make no promises for change.

Mary McClure

See also: Antigay Prejudice; Gay Affirmative Therapy; Homophobia; Homosexuality; Religion, Diversity of Human Sexuality and; Sexual Identity; Sexual Orientation.

Further Reading

Arthur, E., McGill, D., & Essary, E. H. (2014). Playing it straight: Framing strategies among reparative therapists. *Sociological Inquiry, 84*(1), 16–41.

Bright, C. (2004). Deconstructing reparative therapy: An examination of the processes involved when attempting to change sexual orientation. *Clinical Social Work Journal, 32*(4), 471–481.

Haldeman, D. C. (1994). The practice and ethics of sexual orientation conversion therapy. *Journal of Consulting and Clinical Psychology, 62*(2), 221–227.

Shidlo, A., & Schroeder, M. (2002). Changing sexual orientation: A consumers' report. *Professional Psychology: Research and Practice, 33*(3), 249–259.

Reproductive Coercion

Reproductive coercion, also called coerced reproduction, is a form of domestic violence that occurs when a sexual partner destroys, or fails to use, a form of contraception without telling their partner; threatens a partner who does not want to become pregnant; forces a partner to carry a pregnancy against their wishes; or forces a partner to terminate a pregnancy. Essentially, one partner is preventing the other from making their own reproductive decisions. While reproductive coercion can happen in relationships of all genders, sexes, and sexual orientations, it is most frequently seen in mixed-sex couples in which the male partner inflicts reproductive coercion on their female partner. During reproductive coercion, certain reproductive health behaviors are used to maintain power and control over another person in the relationship in an attempt to keep them in an abusive relationship. The behaviors can include intimidation, verbal threats, or acts of violence that are used to influence a person's reproductive decision making with the intent to pressure or coerce a partner into becoming a parent or ending a pregnancy.

These behaviors generally take three forms: pregnancy pressure, pregnancy coercion, and birth control sabotage. Pregnancy pressure and coercion occur when one partner is pressured or coerced by the other partner to have unprotected sex to get pregnant, to continue an unwanted pregnancy, or to terminate a pregnancy.

Birth control sabotage can be verbal or behavioral and is defined as pressure to become pregnant or not to use birth control. Verbal sabotage includes statements such as "You would have my baby if you loved me," or "I'll leave you if you don't get pregnant." Behavioral sabotage includes acts such as poking holes in or breaking a condom, throwing away birth control pills and replacing them with placebos, hiding or destroying birth control, removing a condom during intercourse without the other partner knowing, or the forceful removal of contraceptive devices such as vaginal rings or intrauterine devices. It may also include the use of force to have unprotected sex.

The direct relationship between physical violence and reproductive coercion is not entirely known, and birth control sabotage does not occur solely in violent relationships, but several studies have demonstrated a strong link between domestic violence and birth control sabotage. The risk of unintended pregnancy increases dramatically for women in physically abusive relationships. If a woman has a physically abusive partner, that partner is likely to engage in reproductive coercion as well. And this coercion affects women across the socioeconomic and educational spectrum. An important strategy to help reduce reproductive coercion is to focus on the training of health care providers, and in particular OB/GYNs, to recognize victims of reproductive coercion and direct these patients to agencies and hotlines, such as the National Domestic Violence Hotline, that help women who are abused.

Currently in the United States, it is not a crime to destroy birth control pills or a condom. However, it is a crime to force a woman to ingest a substance or a pill that induces an abortion without her knowledge.

Amy Reynolds

See also: Contraception; Pregnancy; Rape, Abuse and Incest National Network (RAINN); Sexual Abuse; Sexual Rights.

Further Reading

Murray, R. (2013, June). More men are sabotaging women's birth control to get them pregnant: ACOG. *NY Daily News*. Retrieved from http://www.nydailynews.com/life-style/health/men-sabotaging-women-birth-control-article-1.1361932

Trawick, S. M. (2012). Birth control sabotage as domestic violence: A legal response. *California Law Review, 100*(3), 721–760.

Retrograde Ejaculation

"Retrograde ejaculation" (RE) refers to the backward movement of semen into the bladder as opposed to the typical movement expulsion pattern via the urethra during ejaculation. This results in what is referred to as a "dry orgasm" or "dry ejaculation," where little to no semen is externally released. RE is not a physically harmful or painful condition but may be permanent depending on its cause and other contributing factors. Infertility is common among those with RE, and additional treatment may be required in order to conceive. Although RE may feel as pleasurable as a typical orgasm, psychological issues may arise if the individual experiences feelings of inadequacy derived from social expectations placed on masculinity and sexual performance.

Antegrade or forward-moving ejaculation (AE) occurs when sperm is transported from the testes to the prostate via the muscular vessel referred to as the vas deferens. Once in the prostate, the sperm mixes with prostatic secretions and seminal fluid to produce the male ejaculate known as semen. This ejaculate is then propelled through the urethra before exiting the penis externally. For this function to be performed, the muscle located at the opening of the bladder, otherwise known as the bladder neck, closes to prevent the entry of semen into the bladder. During RE, these muscles fail to contract, allowing for semen to enter the bladder instead of traveling through the urethra. This dysfunction can be attributed to anatomical, surgical, neurological, or drug-induced causes and will vary according to each case. Signs indicative of RE include urine that appears to be cloudy after orgasm, expelling little or no semen from the penis during ejaculation, and infertility among different-sex couples trying to conceive.

The most common causes of RE include medications and surgical procedures that relax the bladder neck. If a person believes they are experiencing RE due to medication, they may consult with a physician regarding the discontinuation or alteration of their medication. Neurological issues related to RE include, but are not limited to, spinal cord injury, diabetes, and multiple sclerosis. Certain surgeries surrounding the prostate, urethra, and bladder may also lead to RE by causing damage to the prostatic muscles responsible for contracting and the bladder neck. Retroperitoneal lymph node dissection (RLND), for example, is common among people with RE. RLND is a surgical procedure that is used to identify and treat testicular cancer. During this surgery, the nerves that control the bladder neck may be injured, leading to ejaculatory dysfunction. Of the several notable causes mentioned, RE induced by medication tends to be the easiest to treat and shows the most successful reversal rate.

RE is not physically harmful, nor does it cause physical pain or discomfort in most cases. While the ejaculatory fluid does not physically exit from the penis, having an orgasm is entirely possible, and the sensation typically resembles that of an orgasm with AE. Although a person may be physically healthy, it is important to consider the emotional and psychological implications that may result from feelings of inadequacy or emasculation. These feelings are likely to be derived from issues pertaining to infertility and concerns about sexual performance.

Cognitive awareness and subjective perception of self are highly influential while evaluating RE and how it affects quality of life. A man's relationship with his sexuality is often heavily influenced by societal standards and expectations surrounding masculinity. The often strong correlation between masculinity and the ability to reproduce may leave one feeling as though they are evolutionarily inferior and incomplete in their masculinity. This unfortunate misconception may then lead to issues such as performance anxiety or distress, leading to a decrease in sexual satisfaction. Inaccurate associations surrounding personal and partnered relationships with sex and intimacy is another possible result.

If infertility is a concern, there are viable options that allow for the successful retrieval of sperm. Postejaculation sperm retrieval followed by a postejaculate urine analysis is a noninvasive and promising option for many experiencing RE. Since the seminal fluid is redirected to the bladder during orgasm, a urine sample containing the semen can be collected post ejaculation. This method can be completed in a few easy steps with the guidance of a physician and is the most favorable option due to its noninvasive nature. Artificial stimulation of emission and ejaculation is a less favorable option as it is more invasive and requires anesthetic. Artificial stimulation is typically recommended for individuals with RE stemming from a spinal cord injury.

Although RE is noted as a common form of ejaculatory dysfunction in males, the topic is rarely discussed or researched from an evidence-based standpoint. It is, however, known that RE poses no physical threat and does not have to deter an individual from having a fulfilling sexual, intimate, and social life. Infertility resulting from RE is a prominent concern, and modern methods used to retrieve sperm for artificial insemination purposes have proven to be hopeful and viable options. Overall, people experiencing RE may suffer from both medical and psychological concerns. The extent of distress experienced by the individual is dependent on both the cause of the dysfunction as well as social and emotional stressors associated with male sexuality and performance.

Cheyenne Taylor

See also: Ejaculation; Infertility; Male Sexuality; Masculinity; Performance Anxiety; Premature Ejaculation; Semen; Testicular Cancer.

Further Reading

Harvard Health Publishing. (2018). Retrograde ejaculation. Retrieved from https://www.health.harvard.edu/a_to_z/retrograde-ejaculation-a-to-z

Kamischke, A., & Nieschlag, E. (2002). Update on medical treatment of ejaculatory disorders. *International Journal of Andrology, 25*(6), 333–344.

Mayo Clinic. (2019). Retrograde ejaculation. Retrieved from https://www.mayoclinic.org/diseases-conditions/retrograde-ejaculation/symptoms-causes/syc-20354890

Mehta, A., & Sigman, M. (2015). Management of the dry ejaculate: A systematic review of aspermia and retrograde ejaculation. *Fertility and Sterility, 104*(5), 1074–1081.

Memorial Sloan Kettering Cancer Center. (2018). Retrograde ejaculation. Retrieved from https://www.mskcc.org/cancer-care/patient-education/retrograde-ejaculation

Metro Vancouver Urology. (2013). Retrograde ejaculation and anejaculation. Retrieved from http://www.metrovanurology.com/content/retrograde-ejaculation-and-anejaculation

Yavetz, H., Yogev, L., Hauser, R. Lessing, J. B., Paz, G., & Homonnai, Z. T. (1994). Retrograde ejaculation. *Human Reproduction, 9*(3), 381–386.

Roe v. Wade

Roe v. Wade is a landmark legal decision issued on January 22, 1973, in which the U.S. Supreme Court struck down Texas laws banning abortion. This decision in effect legalized the procedure for all of the United States.

In the early nineteenth century, a woman could get a legal abortion. It was legal if it was done before "quickening," when the woman felt the fetus move, usually about the fourth month of pregnancy. Over time, states made it illegal in response to women dying from abortions that were done by untrained people or under unsafe conditions. In the late 1850s, the new American Medical Association began calling for laws against abortion. This was partly to eliminate doctors' competition from midwives and homeopaths who performed the procedure. In 1873, Congress passed the Comstock Law, which made it illegal to distribute birth control and abortion-inducing drugs through the U.S. mail. Eventually abortion was illegal in all the states.

In the 1960s, the sexual revolution and women's rights movement resulted in public pressure to make abortion laws less restrictive. Some women resorted to illegal, dangerous, "back-alley" abortions or aborted the fetus themselves. In the 1950s and 1960s, the estimated number of illegal abortions in the United States ranged from 200,000 to 1.2 million per year. When a few states began to relax abortion restrictions, some women found it relatively easy to travel to a state where the laws were less stringent. Some women could find a doctor who was willing to certify that there was a medical necessity for an abortion. Poor women, however, often could not afford to travel outside their state for the procedure. The state laws that were in place were often unclear, so doctors did not really know whether they were committing a serious crime by providing an abortion. In this time of social change, government interference in sexual matters was beginning to be questioned by people who were shifting their conception of privacy.

The *Roe v. Wade* case began in 1970 when "Jane Roe," a fictional name used to protect the identity of the plaintiff, Norma McCorvey, filed suit against Henry Wade, the district attorney of Dallas County, Texas. The case challenged the state law banning abortion. McCorvey was young, unmarried, poor, and pregnant for the third time. Two recent law school graduates, Sarah Weddington and Linda Coffee, took her case and won it. After the district court found the Texas law unconstitutional, Wade appealed to the Supreme Court.

Sarah Weddington argued the case in the higher court as well. In the *Roe* decision, Justice Blackmun's majority opinion explicitly rejected a fetal "right to life" argument. He wrote that these Texas laws in most cases violated a woman's constitutional right of privacy. He found it to be implicit in the liberty guarantee of the due process clause of the Fourteenth Amendment ("nor shall any state deprive any person of life, liberty, or property, without due process of law"). The court also said that this right must be balanced against the state's interests in regulating abortions, protecting women's health, and protecting the potential for human life.

There is no right to privacy explicitly guaranteed in the Constitution, but the Supreme Court has long recognized some right to privacy. Starting in the 1960s, the court's position on privacy came to be seen as a right connected to a person rather than to a location. The change in conceptions of privacy can be seen in the landmark decision of *Griswold v. Connecticut* (1965). The Supreme Court ruled that a Connecticut statute outlawing access to contraception violated the U.S. Constitution because it invaded the privacy of married couples to make decisions about their families. Since 1973, many court cases in the states have narrowed the scope of *Roe v. Wade* but have not overturned it. In *Planned Parenthood v. Casey* (1992), the Supreme Court established that restrictions on abortion are unconstitutional if they place an "undue burden" on a woman seeking an abortion before the fetus is viable (able to live outside the woman's body). Advocates both for and against abortion rights continue to debate the issue, and many people are concerned about changes in the makeup of the Supreme Court that could alter the law in one direction or the other.

Michael J. McGee

See also: Abortion Legislation; *Planned Parenthood v. Casey.*

Further Reading

Gold, R. B. (2003). Lessons from before Roe: Will past be prologue? *Guttmacher Report on Public Policy, 6*(1), 8–11.

Reagan, L. J. (1997). *When abortion was a crime: Women, medicine, and law in the United States, 1867–1973.* Berkeley: University of California Press.

Torr, J. D. (2006). *Abortion: Opposing viewpoints.* Farmington Hills, MI: Greenhaven Press/Thomson Gale.

Roman Catholic Church Sexual Abuse Scandal

The Roman Catholic Church sexual abuse scandal was named a scandal for the way that American Catholic bishops handled sexually offending priests. In 2002, a series of stories surfaced of people being sexually abused as minors by Catholic priests. Many bishops had a common practice of removing offending priests from one parish and placing them in another parish, with further opportunity to offend. The legality of these cases could often be overlooked because many of the victims never formally brought charges against offending priests. The stories of abuse originated in the archdiocese of Boston and created a space for other victims to tell their stories.

Awareness of sexual abuse in the Catholic Church had been growing steadily over the years leading up to the scandal. In 1992, the archbishop of Chicago, Cardinal Joseph Bernardin, commissioned a board of primarily nonclerical (lay) Catholics to review charges brought against bishops and priests. Another recognition of the sexual misconduct of priests was the creation of the VIRTUS program by the National Catholic Risk Retention Group in 1998. This program was designed to inform people of what the organization calls human relationship, including relationships between adults and children as well as other vulnerable populations. Ultimately, in January 2002, the *Boston Globe* began publishing stories of people who were sexually abused by priests. Thousands of other articles began arising all over the country. People who had been abused as minors finally had a space and a community to go to with their stories that they had not had before. Later that year, in Dallas, the U.S. bishops had a general meeting at which they approved the Charter for the Protection of Children and Young People. This charter created a board that commissioned the John Jay College of Criminal Justice to conduct a study to help understand the causes and context of the scandal. This report became known as *The Causes and Context of Sexual Abuse of Minors by Catholic Priests in the United States, 1950–2010*, or *The John Jay Study*.

As a result of the scandal, many other Catholic organizations around the world began examining their own policy around priests that have sexually abused minors. After a similar scandal took place in Ireland in the spring of 2010, Pope Benedict XVI wrote a pastoral letter to the Catholics of Ireland expressing feelings of true sorrow and apologizing for the sinful and criminal mistakes made by members of the church.

The *John Jay Study* came under attack from both Catholic and non-Catholic sources for having authority limitations. In addition, an unusually high number of sexual abuse incidences in the report (about 40%) seemed to take place within a six-year time span, from 1975 to 1980. The report did, however, make a point to dispel the myth that if a priest is gay, he has a higher likelihood of sexually abusing a minor.

Pope Francis I approved a specific tribunal (a church committee) to hear the cases of bishops accused of failing to protect minors in which high-ranking church members will be held accountable for their cover-ups. The scope of this tribunal will be to address the specific cases of high-ranking clerics who had been virtually immune to repercussions for their actions.

Mark A. Levand

See also: Child Sexual Abuse; Religion, Diversity of Human Sexuality and; Sexual Abuse.

Further Reading

Dempsey, J. Q., Gorman, J. R., Madden, J. P., & Spilly, A. P. (1992). *The cardinal's commission on clerical sexual misconduct with minors.* Chicago: Archdiocese of Chicago.

National Catholic Risk Retention Group. (1999). Taking bigger and bigger steps. *Communicare, 1*(1), 1–4.

Pope Benedict XVI. (2010). Pastoral letter of the Holy Father Pope Benedict XVI to the Catholics of Ireland. Retrieved from http://w2.vatican.va/content/benedict-xvi/en/letters/2010/documents/hf_ben-xvi_let_20100319_church-ireland.html

Roberts, T. (2011). Critics point to John Jay study's limitations. *National Catholic Reporter.* Retrieved from http://ncronline.org/news/accountability/critics-point-john-jay-studys-limitations

Terry, K. J., Smith, M. L., Schuth, K., Kelly, J. R., Vollman, B., & Massey, C. (2011). *The causes and context of sexual abuse of minors by Catholic priests in the United States, 1950–2010: A report presented to the United States Conference of Catholic Bishops by the John Jay college research team.* Washington, DC: United States Conference of Catholic Bishops.

Romantic Attraction and Orientation

Romantic attraction and orientation are concepts similar to sexual attraction and orientation. Just as people can be sexually attracted to others of the same sex/gender, another sex/gender, both same and other sexes/genders, or not at all, people can be romantically attracted to others of the same sex/gender, another sex/gender, both same and other sexes/genders, or not at all.

Many people, including scientific researchers, use the term "sexual orientation" to account for all types of attraction (e.g., romantic, sexual) to other people. However, some biological and psychological research has indicated that sexual attraction (who people want to have sex with) and romantic attraction (who people want to love or be in a romantic relationship with) are two different constructs with different brain systems.

For most people, it is expected that their romantic attraction and orientation matches with their sexual attraction and orientation. In other words, individuals who are sexually attracted to other-sex/gender individuals (e.g., people who are heterosexual or straight) are also romantically attracted to other-sex/gender individuals or that people who are sexually attracted to same-sex/gender individuals (e.g., people who are gay or lesbian) are also romantically attracted to same-sex/gender individuals. However, this is not always the case.

Some bisexual individuals report being sexually attracted to both men and women but only romantically attracted to one sex/gender or the other. Alternatively, some may be romantically attracted to both sexes/genders but may only experience sexual desire for either the same or other sex/gender.

The construct of romantic attraction and orientation may be especially relevant to people with an asexual sexual orientation. People with an asexual sexual orientation report a lack of sexual attraction to other people, regardless of sex or gender. However, not all people with an asexual sexual orientation report a lack of romantic attraction. Some asexual individuals desire and want to be in intimate and romantic relationships with other people. Further, these people could be romantically interested in the same sex/gender (homoromantic), other sex/gender (heteroromantic), or any sex/gender (biromantic, panromantic). If a person experiences neither sexual attraction nor romantic attraction, they may identify as asexual and aromantic.

Interestingly though, given that sexual attraction and romantic attraction are two distinct constructs, this means that people who experience sexual attraction (i.e., those with a sexual orientation other than asexuality) can potentially also be aromantic. For these people, they may desire to have a sexual relationship with a single person or with multiple people, but they do not desire to, or are unable to, experience a romantic connection with their partner(s).

Given that most research on attraction and sexual orientation assumes that romantic attraction is a component of sexual orientation, more research on the distinction between sexual attraction and romantic attraction, and the outcomes when these two concepts do not align, is needed.

Heather L. Armstrong

See also: Asexuality; Bisexuality; Kinsey's Continuum of Sexual Orientation; Sexual Identity; Sexual Orientation.

Further Reading

Bogaert, A. F. (2015). *Understanding asexuality.* Lanham, MD: Rowman & Littlefield.

Diamond, L. M. (2003). What does sexual orientation orient? A biobehavioral model distinguishing romantic love and sexual desire. *Psychological Review, 110*(1), 173–192.

Fisher, H. E., Aron, A., Mashek, D., Li, H., & Brown, L. L. (2002). Defining the brain systems of lust, romantic attraction, and attachment. *Archives of Sexual Behavior, 31*(5), 413–419.

S

Safer Sex

"Safer sex" is an umbrella term for a range of practices that people can employ to reduce the risk of contracting or transmitting a sexually transmitted infection (STI) during consensual sexual encounters. STIs are infections that can be passed on through genital contact, body fluids, or, sometimes, skin-to-skin contact. Sex has, of course, risks that are not just physical, such as emotional and relational risks. However, "safer sex" is a term commonly used to refer to the management of physical risks associated with sexual practices, mainly the transmission of STIs, including HIV.

One of the main practices under the safer sex umbrella is the use of condoms for insertive and receptive sexual activities. To be effective, condoms need to be used from the beginning of sexual contact—for example, before inserting a penis into a vagina or anus. Condoms can be insertive—that is, placed on the penis or toys that are then inserted into an orifice, such as the mouth, vagina, or anus. This is the most common type of condom, which is usually distributed in safer sex kits and can be easily found in a range of stores, from pharmacies to gas stations. Receptive condoms are less popular, as they have only been in use since the early 1990s. They are placed in the vagina or anus and are commonly known as female condoms. Condoms are available in both latex and nonlatex materials, and using lube at the same time reduces friction and thus the risk of breaking the condom during sexual intercourse. Condoms are for single use only, which means that multiple condoms can be used in a single sexual encounter, if there are multiple insertions. Condoms can also be used on toys to decrease exposure to other people's bodily fluids when switching toys between partners or in sexual encounters with multiple people. The use of condoms reduces the risk of pregnancy and STI transmission, even though those risks can never be completely eliminated during a sexual encounter with another person.

The choice and use of sex toys also need to be considered for safer sex. Some sex toys are made from porous materials, which might encourage the pooling of harmful bacteria, and some are made from toxic materials, which should not come into contact with genitals. Generally, silicone, glass, and metal sex toys are the safest and easier to clean, including the ability to sterilize them through boiling. It is important to not insert a toy in the anus first and then into the vagina, even when masturbating or when inserting it in the same person, given that the bacteria in the anus can cause infection in the vaginal area.

Safer sex practices can include the use of contraceptives, such as oral hormonal pills, intrauterine devices, diaphragms, spermicides, contraceptive sponges, vaginal rings, implants, and so on. However, those methods only reduce the risk of pregnancy and do not stop the transmission of STIs, including HIV. Regular HIV and STI testing is also part of safer sex practices, especially when a higher number of sexual partner is involved or when new sexual partners are introduced.

Alex Iantaffi

See also: Barrier Contraceptive Methods; Condoms, Female (Receptive); Condoms, Male (Insertive); Contraception; Intercourse; Sex Toys; Sexual Health; Sexually Transmitted Infections (STIs); Testing, STI.

Further Reading

Farr, G., Gabelnick, H., Sturgen, K., & Dorflinger, L. (1994). Contraceptive efficacy and acceptability of the female condom. *American Journal of Public Health, 84*(12), 1960–1964.

Stabile, E. (2013). Getting the government in bed: Regulating the sex toy industry. *Berkeley Journal of Gender, Law & Justice, 28*, 161–184.

Steiner, M., Piedrahita, C., Glover, L., Joanis, C., Spruyt, A., & Foldesy, R. (1994). The impact of lubricants on latex condoms during vaginal intercourse. *International Journal of STD & AIDS, 5*(1), 29–36.

World Health Organization. (2007). *Global strategy for the prevention and control of sexually transmitted infections: 2006–2015: Breaking the chain of transmission.* Geneva: World Health Organization.

Same-Sex Attraction and Behavior

Same-sex attraction and same-sex behavior are two components of what is commonly referred to as "sexual orientation." "Sexual orientation" refers to an individual's pattern of sexual desire for others, their sexual behavior in relation to others, and their sexual identity or label; it is a predominantly Western way to understand sexual diversity. For most people, their sexual behavior, attraction, and identity label all align; however, this is not always the case. For example, some people may self-identify as "straight" but may have same-sex attraction or behavior. Many bisexual people who are in committed, monogamous relationships experience bisexual attraction and may self-identity as "bisexual," but they may only have sex with one person and therefore one sex or gender.

Alfred Kinsey (1948) conceptualized sexual orientation as a single behavioral continuum ranging from "exclusively heterosexual" to "exclusively homosexual." Subsequent models of sexual orientation have considered additional dimensions, such as sexual attraction, sexual fantasies, emotional preference, social preference, and self-identity. Various scales have been developed to measure these components—for example, the Klein Sexual Orientation Grid. Quite recently, sexuality theorists have posited new models for understanding sexual orientation that consider partnered sexualities (gender or sex and partner number).

Most of the scales developed to measure sexual orientation were and continue to be based on a binary gender/sex system. This binary gender or sex system has been problematized by queer theorists in the West. Historical and modern studies of non-Western cultures document different frameworks and conceptualizations of gender or sex and sexual orientation that have been devalued and erased via European colonization. For most of human history, the concept of sexual orientation as it is understood today did not exist, and the acceptability of same-sex sexual behavior and attraction has varied with time and place. In what is now North America, many indigenous peoples recognized two-spirit individuals, a term that encompasses a diversity of gender/sex identities and roles. Prior to colonization, similar attitudes were found among many indigenous peoples; for example, same-sex relationships were accepted and relatively common among the Maori, the indigenous people of New Zealand.

In Europe, a strong Christian tradition resulted in any sexual activity other than procreative sex within marriage being seen as sinful. Sodomy in particular, regardless of the gender/sex of the individuals involved, was considered to be against the "natural law" that governed human behavior and was therefore illegal as well as immoral. With the development of modern Western medical practices—including psychiatry—in the nineteenth century, however, these views shifted, and sexual orientation was framed first as a matter of health or illness and then as an inherent and fixed characteristic and a key feature of an individual's sexual self. Previous understandings of same-sex attraction and behavior were replaced by this new conceptualization.

Within this current Western framework, a number of theories have been proposed to explain the development of sexual orientation. Masters and Johnson (1979) suggested a behavioral explanation, that sexual orientation is determined by the reinforcement or punishment of same-sex or different-sex sexual behavior via pleasurable sexual experiences or unpleasant ones. Subsequent behavioral research conducted within this theoretical framework has provided mixed results; it seems that experience may have some influence on sexual orientation, but it is likely not the only factor.

Biological theories focus on genetics, hormones, and physiology as the potential causes of nonheterosexual sexual orientations. Studies with identical and fraternal twins indicate a possible genetic component: individuals whose identical twin is gay or lesbian are more likely to be gay or lesbian themselves, although this has been examined far more in gay men than in women, and the limited evidence regarding this phenomenon in women is not as strong. In addition, the fact that not all identical twins have the same sexual orientation suggests that other factors may play a role. Exposure to differing levels of hormones during prenatal development as well as the anatomy of specific brain structures have been suggested as additional influences, although the mechanism of these influences is not yet clear. The connection between orientation and brain anatomy in particular has not been satisfactorily determined; it is not known whether these anatomical differences determine sexual orientation or whether sexual orientation may result in these differences developing later in life.

In contrast to biological theories, social constructionist theories emphasize that the categories and frameworks used to understand sexual orientation are socially constructed while recognizing the significant impact that categories such as gay, lesbian, bisexual, and heterosexual have on individuals' lives. In his key work *The History of Sexuality,* Michel Foucault outlined the substantial shifts in how sexuality has been viewed across time and place, arguing that sexuality is not an inherent characteristic of individuals but rather is defined by cultures through the delineation of certain kinds of relationships and behaviors as sexual, specifically as "heterosexual" or "homosexual."

Regardless of the underlying cause(s) of sexual orientation, the social categories and valuing of alignment between attraction, behavior, and identity further marginalize, pathologize, and cause distress for people and communities with diverse experiences and social locations. In her sexual configurations theory, van Anders (2015) summarized a number of shortcomings in existing theories and research related to sexual orientation, such as the implication that sexual orientation is about attraction to biological sex rather than gender; the privileging of heterosexuality as a desired, natural default; and the failure to account for the fact that attraction and behavior are not always fixed and may shift over the course of an individual's lifetime. In addition, she provides a framework that includes sexual attraction, behavior, and identity as well as a diversity of partnered sexualities with regard to sex/gender and relationship structure. The variations in alignment between sexual identity label, sexual attraction, and sexual behavior as well as the fluid nature of these constructs have been noted by Diamond (2016) and others and may be more common than previously thought.

Nathan Lachowsky and Karyn Fulcher

See also: Binary Gender System; Biological Theories of Sexual Orientation; Kinsey's Continuum of Sexual Orientation; Sexual Orientation.

Further Reading

Aspin, C., & Hutchings, J. (2007). Reclaiming the past to inform the future: Contemporary views of Maori sexuality. *Culture, Health & Sexuality, 9*(4), 415–427.

DeLamater, J. D., & Hyde, J. S. (1998). Essentialism vs. social constructionism in the study of human sexuality. *Journal of Sex Research, 35*(1), 10–18.

Diamond, L. M. (2016). Sexual fluidity in males and females. *Current Sexual Health Reports, 8*, 249–256.

Epstein, R., & Robertson, R. E. (2014). How to measure sexual orientation range and why it's worth measuring. *Journal of Bisexuality, 14*(3–4), 391–403

Fausto-Sterling, A. (2000). *Sexing the body: Gender politics and the construction of sexuality.* New York: Basic Books.

Foucault, M. (1980). *The history of sexuality. Volume one: An introduction.* (R. Hurley, Trans.) New York: Vintage Books.

Galupo, M. P., Lomash, E., & Mitchell, R. C. (2017). "All of my lovers fit into this scale": Sexual minority individuals' responses to two novel measures of sexual orientation. *Journal of Homosexuality, 64*(2), 145–165.

Kinsey, A. C., Pomeroy, W. B., & Martin, C. E. (1948). *Sexual behavior in the human male.* Oxford: Saunders.

Masters, W. H., & Johnson, V. E. (1979). *Homosexuality in perspective.* Boston: Little, Brown.

Van Anders, S. (2015). Beyond sexual orientation: Integrating gender/sex and diverse sexualities via sexual configurations theory. *Archives of Sexual Behaviour, 44*, 1177–1213.

Same-Sex Marriage

"Same-sex marriage" refers to the legal union of two individuals of the same sex—in other words, the marriage of two men or two women. These marriages can occur in civil (i.e., nonreligious) or religious ceremonies. Same-sex marriage has long been a topic of political, social, and religious debate, with opponents contrasting it to a "traditional" or heterosexual marriage between one man and one woman.

Same-sex unions are not new, and records dating from ancient Greece, Rome, and China show loving relationships, sometimes formalized through ritual proceedings, between two men and two women. However, while same-sex unions have been recorded across varying times and cultures, legal recognition of these unions is relatively new. In 2001, The Netherlands became the first country to legalize same-sex marriages, followed by Belgium (2003) and Spain (2005) in Europe, and Canada (2005) in North America. As of summer 2020, twenty-nine countries now perform same-sex marriages, including much of Europe, all of North America, several in Central and South America, Australia, New Zealand, and South Africa. The United States extended the right to marry to all citizens with a historic Supreme Court ruling on June 26, 2015. Several additional countries recognize marriages performed internationally and/or allow for civil unions between same-sex couples.

Marriage offers numerous benefits to committed couples, both mixed-sex and same-sex. Married couples are immediately entitled to practical, legal benefits such as family law, adoption, pension and health benefits, tax benefits, immigration, and inheritance and power of attorney. Without these rights, same-sex couples have been denied the ability to start families and to care for their loved ones during sickness and death. Same-sex marriage also provides social support for couples, with recently married couples reporting greater acceptance of relationships by family and friends. Legalization of same-sex marriage also increases social support on a greater scale, with public support of same-sex marriage significantly increasing after laws are passed. This greater social acceptance may also contribute to decreases in internalized homophobia, which in turn is associated with better mental and physical health outcomes for gay, lesbian, and bisexual individuals. In addition, gay and bisexual men living in Massachusetts reported significantly fewer medical and mental health care visits and decreased health care costs following the legalization of same-sex marriage in that state, regardless of their own marital status, suggesting that same-sex marriage may benefit all sexual minority individuals. Finally, marriage also contributes to greater relationship satisfaction. After being married, same-sex couples tend to report increased commitment and connection as well as greater feelings of love and closer emotional bonds toward their partners.

Given the recent legalization of same-sex marriage in the United States, it is likely that research into the effects of marriage on individuals, couples, families, and society at large will expand over the next few years. Studies on same-sex divorce may also be forthcoming.

Heather L. Armstrong

See also: Antigay Prejudice; Civil Union; Gay Rights Movement; Marriage; Marriage, Cross-Cultural Comparison of.

Further Reading

Alderson, K. (2004). A phenomenological investigation of same-sex marriage. *The Canadian Journal of Human Sexuality, 13*, 107–122.

Hatzenbuehler, M. L., O'Cleirigh, C., Grasso, C., Mayer, K., Safren, S., & Bradford, J. (2012). Effect of same-sex marriage laws on health care use and expenditures in sexual minority men: A quasi-natural experiment. *American Journal of Public Health, 102*, 285–291.

Lannuti, P. J. (2008). "This is not a lesbian wedding": Examining same-sex marriage and bisexual-lesbian couples. *Journal of Bisexuality, 7*, 237–260.

MacIntosh, H., Reissing, E. D., & Andruff (Armstrong), H. (2010). Same-sex marriage in Canada: The impact of legal marriage on the first cohort of gay and lesbian Canadians to wed. *The Canadian Journal of Human Sexuality, 19*, 79–90.

Newcomb, M. E., & Mustanski, B. (2010). Internalized homophobia and internalizing mental health problems: A meta-analytic review. *Clinical Psychology Review, 30*, 1019–1029.

Ramos, C., Goldberg, N. G., & Badgett, M. V. L. (2009). *The effects of marriage equality in Massachusetts: A survey of the experiences and impact of marriage on same-sex couples.* Los Angeles: The Williams Institute, UCLA.

Sanger, Margaret

Margaret Higgins Sanger (1879–1966) was a nurse, activist, sexuality educator, and advocate for birth control. She was born in Corning, New York, to Michael Higgins, an Irish immigrant stonemason, and his wife, Anne. The sixth of their eleven children, she always believed her mother's death at fifty was due to having had eighteen pregnancies and caring for so many children. Margaret learned self-reliance early when she had to leave school at sixteen to take care of her dying mother.

After her mother's death, Margaret studied nursing at White Plains Hospital. In 1902, she married William Sanger, an architect. They had three children. Sanger worked as a visiting nurse and midwife on the Lower East Side, where she saw the struggles of immigrant women in poor health who had too many children to provide for.

At this time, there were few options for preventing pregnancy, and it was illegal to even give information about "any drug or medicine, or any article whatever, for the prevention of conception." This was the Comstock Law, enacted by Congress in 1873. Anthony Comstock, a crusader "for the suppression of vice" in New York City, drafted the law. In his role as special agent in the U.S. Post Office, he was able to confiscate "immoral" materials sent through the mail and arrest those who sent them.

Despite the law, Margaret Sanger published a monthly newsletter, *The Woman Rebel*, which advocated for women's right to control their own bodies. She promoted the term "birth control," which spoke directly to preventing pregnancy. At the same time, she wrote "Family Limitation," a sixteen-page pamphlet that described specific methods of contraception.

Under the Comstock Law, Sanger was arrested in 1914 for publishing *The Woman Rebel*. While awaiting trial, she fled to Europe and remained there until October 1915. She learned more from experts in Holland and England about contraceptives and human sexuality. During her ten months in Europe, William Sanger was tricked into selling a copy of "Family Limitation" to a Comstock cohort. He was arrested and spent thirty days in jail. His arrest prompted influential newspapers to print more stories about Margaret and contraception. Public opinion was turning. In February 1916, the charges against her were dropped.

The following October, Margaret Sanger opened the first birth control clinic in the United States, staffed by herself; Ethel Byrne, her sister who was a registered nurse; Fania Mindell, a volunteer who spoke three languages; and Elizabeth Stuyvesant, a social worker. Ten days after the clinic opened, the vice squad arrested Sanger and Mindell. After paying a fine, they were released and promptly reopened the clinic, only to be arrested again with Ethel. While the clinic was open, they saw 464 women.

Several weeks later, Ethel Byrne was tried, convicted, and sentenced to a month in the Blackwell's Island workhouse. She went on a hunger strike, and four days later the police began to force-feed her through a tube, a historical first. Publicity about Ethel's imprisonment further influenced public opinion about women's rights. The trials of Margaret Sanger and Fania Mindell began in January 1917. Sanger was convicted but offered a more lenient sentence if she promised to not break the law again. She said, "I cannot respect the law as it exists today" and spent thirty days in jail.

She appealed the conviction, and in 1918, the court ruled partly in her favor, that doctors could prescribe contraception for medical purposes. This victory enabled Margaret Sanger to found the American Birth Control League in 1921 and the Clinical Research Bureau in 1923. Both organizations gained support from middle-class and wealthy donors and advocates. She worked successfully to convince physicians to endorse family planning.

To change the laws regarding access to contraceptives, she ordered diaphragms from Japan, knowing the authorities would confiscate them. In 1936, the government's case against her resulted in a decision to overturn the Comstock Law. The following year, the American Medical Association accepted contraception as a normal part of clinical practice.

In 1942, the organizations that Margaret Sanger founded were renamed Planned Parenthood Federation of America. Four years later, she helped found the International Planned Parenthood Federation. Sanger was the organization's first president and continued in that role until she was eighty years old.

In the 1920s, Sanger had begun to propose that mentally disabled women not be allowed to have children, and she became involved in the eugenics movement, whose goal was to improve the genetic quality of the human race. She was also accused of trying to limit births in the African American population, though she maintained that her goal was to provide better birth control to better the lives of African American women and their families.

She died in 1966 in Tucson, Arizona. People opposed to abortion, as well as those who are in favor of abortion rights, have criticized her views on race and eugenics. Nonetheless, Margaret Sanger is regarded as a leader of the American reproductive and woman's rights movements.

Michael J. McGee

See also: Contraception; Planned Parenthood; Sexual Rights.

Further Reading

Chesler, E. (1992). *Woman of valor: Margaret Sanger and the birth control movement in America.* New York: Simon & Schuster.

Coates, P. W. (2008). *Margaret Sanger and the origin of the birth control movement, 1910–1930: The concept of women's sexual autonomy.* Lewiston, NY: Edwin Mellen Press.

Dennis, D. (2009). *Licentious Gotham: Erotic publishing and its prosecution in nineteenth-century New York.* Cambridge, MA: Harvard University Press.

Satcher, David

Dr. David Satcher, MD, PhD (1941–) was the U.S. surgeon general from 1998 to 2002. He was the sixteenth surgeon general and is the only person in history to be surgeon general and assistant secretary for health simultaneously. In 2001, he issued a report titled "The Call to Action to Promote Sexual Health and Responsible Sexual Behavior." The purpose of the report was to address the public health challenges surrounding Americans' sexual health and to promote responsible sexual behavior. At the time the report was published, there were approximately 12 million new cases of sexually transmitted infections (STIs) each year in the United States (Office of the Surgeon General, 2001) and approximately 800,000 persons living with HIV. In addition, 22 percent of women and 2 percent of men were victims of a forced sexual act.

The mission of the report was to start an open and honest discussion about sexuality and sexual health within the nation. The report explained that sexual health is intimately tied to a person's mental and physical health. In the same manner that mental and physical illnesses can affect sexual health, sexual issues often affect mental and physical health. The report discussed the benefits of healthy sexual interactions, which include bonding, intimacy, pleasure, and reproduction.

In the report, several terms were defined. "Sexual health" was defined as being broader than just the absence of disease and dysfunction. It is defined as the ability to make informed sexual decisions in a responsible manner without the presence of sexual abuse or discrimination. Sexual responsibility requires that individuals be aware of their level of sexual development and their personal sexuality. In addition, individuals should have the information and skill set needed to estimate the risk of a situation and the possible outcomes. Respect for self and partner is essential, and there should be tolerance for different sexual orientations. The importance of ensuring that pregnancies occur in a welcoming environment was also addressed.

The report came forth at a time where it took courage to talk about sexuality in American culture. The previous surgeon general, M. Joycelyn Elders, had taken the risk to discuss masturbation and suffered political backlash. Elders was the fifteenth surgeon general and was the first African American surgeon general. In December 1994, at a United Nations conference on AIDS, she was asked whether it would be appropriate to teach schoolchildren about masturbation, to which she replied that masturbation was a part of human sexuality. President Bill Clinton's administration requested that Elders step down from her post on December 9. Despite being fully aware of what had occurred to the surgeon general just before him, Satcher let his mission of greater health for all Americans guide him to publishing his report on sexual health.

A native of Anniston, Alabama, Satcher has extensive experience with health. At two years old, he contracted whooping cough and became severely ill. His family was unable to take him to the local hospital because it did not admit African Americans. However, they were able to reach an African American physician, Dr. Fred Jackson, who traveled to tend to the toddler's illness. At age six, Satcher decided he wanted to follow in Jackson's footsteps and become a physician. He attended Morehouse College, where he was class president. At Morehouse, he often attended lectures by Dr. Martin Luther King Jr. that inspired him to play an active role in the civil rights movement. He attended Case Western Reserve University, where he earned a MD and PhD.

In 1993, Satcher became director of the Centers for Disease Control and Prevention (CDC) and administrator of the Agency for Toxic Substances and Disease Registry. He was in that position for five years. During his time at the CDC, he focused on continuing the public health gains in HIV/AIDS, cervical and breast cancer screening, and childhood vaccinations. In addition, he addressed the emerging epidemic of obesity that was overtaking the nation. At the same time he was addressing these issues, he was strengthening the infrastructure of the CDC.

Satcher and his wife, Nola Satcher, are parents to four children. Satcher is currently founding director and senior adviser of the Satcher Health Leadership Institute at Morehouse School of Medicine in Atlanta, Georgia. He was previously president of Morehouse School of Medicine from 2004 to 2006 and president of Meharry Medical College in Nashville, Tennessee, from 1982 to 1993.

Renée M. Haynes

See also: Sexual Health.

Further Reading

Creelan, M. (2013). David Satcher (b. 1941). *New Georgia Encyclopedia.* Retrieved from https://www.georgiaencyclopedia.org/articles/science-medicine/david-satcher-b-1941

Jehl, D. (1994, December). Surgeon general forced to resign by White House. *New York Times.* Retrieved from http://www.nytimes.com/1994/12/10/us/surgeon-general-forced-to-resign-by-white-house.html

Office of the Surgeon General (US). (2001). The Surgeon General's call to action to promote sexual health and responsible sexual behavior. Rockville, MD: Office of Population Affairs (US).

Satcher, D. (2007). CDC's 60th anniversary: Director's perspective: David Satcher, M.D., Ph.D., 1993–1998. *MMWR, 56*(23), 579–582. Retrieved from http://www.cdc.gov/mmwr/preview/mmwrhtml/mm5623a3.htm

Schemo, D. J. (2001, June). Surgeon General's report calls for sex education beyond abstinence. *New York Times.*

U.S. Department of Health and Human Services. (2007). David Satcher (1998–2002). Retrieved from https://www.hhs.gov/surgeongeneral/not-found/about/previous/biosatcher.html

Savage, Dan

Dan Savage is a gender and sexuality advocate, a writer, a father, a husband, and an outspoken gay man who has used his words to change history. Whether it is sexual or political, Dan Savage has exercised his ability to write and seek clarity for the masses.

He is a modern-day Dear Abby or Ann Landers, advising for almost thirty years with *Savage Love*, an internationally syndicated weekly sex advice column with a focus on relationships, sex toys, and sexual freedom. Writing this column began as a joke and was only supposed to last six months. The joke was that Dan Savage wanted to use the same gay rhetoric imposed on gay communities on straight communities. He is continuously surprised and humbled to receive the gravity of questions he has over the past three decades. He has been quoted as saying that he will never stop writing his column and that "it will be pried out of his dying hands." He uses humor, reality, and snark heavily in his column. Ironically, he writes his column on the desk of Anne Landers, as he had purchased it from her estate.

Dan Savage was born in Chicago, Illinois, in 1964 and attended the University of Illinois at Urbana-Champaign, where he received a bachelor of fine arts in acting. His parents had encouraged him to enter religious life, as they had both been very active within their Roman Catholic community; his father was a deacon and his mother a lay minister.

He adopted his son DJ in 1999 with his boyfriend, Terry Miller, through open adoption, and they were married in 2015 immediately as the legalities allowed. He has been electrically vocal on how these moments have shaped his life.

In an infamous quote exemplifying his stance on cultural religiousness versus indoctrinated religious behavior, Dan said, "We can learn to ignore the bullshit in the Bible about gay people. The same way we have learned to ignore the bullshit in the Bible about shellfish, about slavery, about dinner, about farming, about menstruation, about virginity, about masturbation."

In 2010, Dan and Terry created a notable reflection of honesty, empathy, and mental health awareness entitled "It Gets Better" in reaction to the suicide of a young queer person. This reflection is a collection of user-submitted YouTube videos to document how life can get better, help to erase any pain, manage loneliness, eliminate bullying, and expose gender and sexuality stigmas. This social media platform has given Savage the opportunity to reach an audience of fearful and impressionable LGBTQ+ youth and provides optimistic examples, mentors, and mental health resources to help curb the epidemic of suicides and self-harming behaviors.

Savage has written and collaborated on several books, notably *Savage Love*, *The Kid*, *Skipping Towards Gomorrah*, *The Commitment*, *It Gets Better*, and *American Savage*. He continues to open and have conversations related to religious intolerance, sexual stigma, heteronormative ideologies, and political injustice.

Michele Montecalvo

See also: LGBTQ+; Media and Sexuality.

Further Reading

Savage, D. (2019). Savage love. Retrieved from https://www.thestranger.com/savage-love

Savage, D. (2019). Savage lovecast [podcast]. Retrieved from https://www.savagelovecast.com

Savage, D., & Miller, T. (2019). It gets better project. Retrieved from https://itgetsbetter.org/

Scabies

Scabies is a very itchy, highly contagious skin infection caused by the mite (parasite) *Sarcoptes scabiei.* This mite exclusively lives and grows in humans and is spread from person to person (through any type of direct skin-to-skin contact). However, it can live without a human host for up to thirty-six hours, or even longer when in a cold environment. As such, more infections are seen in the winter than in the summer. Scabies are very small and usually cannot be seen by the human eye. They cause a skin reaction by burrowing underneath the surface of the skin and laying their eggs in a tunnel. The itching that is characteristic of this infection is thought to be due to an allergic reaction against the mite, its feces, and eggs.

Scabies causes an intensely itchy skin reaction consisting of small red bumps located in specific parts of the body. The symptoms are worst at nighttime. The most common locations are between and on the sides of fingers, the buttocks, waist, armpits, bottom of feet, upper thighs, along the skin folds of the elbows, knees, and wrists; on the penis and scrotum, and around the nipples.

Scabies is usually not seen on the face or head. Occasionally, people can see the tunnels that the mites made as they travel under the skin. The tunnels appear as brown-gray lines that can be up to 0.6 inches (1.5 centimeters) long. Less commonly, people can get large, itchy, red, round, dome-shaped bumps, known as nodules, in the groin or armpits.

People who have weak immune systems, such as those with human immunodeficiency virus (HIV), can develop a very contagious form of scabies called crusted scabies. A person with crusted scabies typically has large, red, itchy, and crusty-looking skin patches or bumps that are usually on the hands, feet, or head.

Scabies is passed from person to person through direct contact, including genital-genital or genital-skin contact. This infection is a commonly known sexually transmitted infection (STI), especially among young adults across the world. However, it is not exclusively sexually transmitted, as any skin-to-skin contact, regardless of the body part infected, can lead to infection in another person. Infections are commonly spread throughout entire families once one family member is infected. The infection is very contagious, and close contact for just fifteen to twenty minutes is enough time for it to move from one person to another. Scabies is different from many other STIs because (although less common) a person can also get the infection from touching clothing, bedding, furniture, or other objects that have the mites on them (e.g., by wearing the same shirt that someone with an active scabies infection just wore). There is a higher risk of getting scabies from direct skin-to-skin contact than from object-skin contact because there are usually more mites on a person's skin than on clothes. Symptoms usually start developing about three to six weeks after a person has been infected. A person who gets reinfected with scabies can develop symptoms much sooner—within three to five days after infestation.

A doctor can diagnose scabies based on someone's symptoms (including information about any close contacts with scabies) and exam, and if a burrow or tunnel is seen on exam, this makes the diagnosis more certain. Sometimes a doctor can perform a skin scraping or an adhesive tape test to look for mites or eggs. Although these tests can confirm a diagnosis, they are not necessary for diagnosis. In fact, a result that is negative for mites does not prove against scabies as the cause of infection.

Scabies can be treated and potentially cured with proper use of medication and cleaning techniques at home. Standard treatment is with permethrin cream. The steps for applying the cream must be strictly followed. The cream must be applied to every inch of skin from the neck down and kept on overnight, or between eight and fourteen hours, and then washed off. The treatment must be repeated one week later. Any close contacts (family members, dorm roommates, sexual partners), even those who do not have symptoms, also must receive the same medical treatment. There is also a pill—ivermectin—that is just as effective as the cream. One pill is taken to initiate treatment, and a second dose is taken fourteen days later. Ivermectin is used to treat crusted scabies. The pill may be harder to find, and more costly, and so this option should be discussed with a doctor.

Even after treatment, itching may still continue for two weeks. This lingering symptom can be treated with allergy medications, also known as antihistamines, such as over-the-counter diphenhydramine or loratadine.

To prevent reinfecting oneself or infecting close contacts, all clothing, bedding, and cloth products or toys that were used in the week prior to starting treatment should be washed in hot water and then dried in a hot dryer. If something cannot be washed, it should be placed in a airtight sealed plastic bag for three days. Floors should be vacuumed. Even if only one partner is infected, sex should be postponed until both partners complete treatment; otherwise the infection will just continue to be passed back and forth between partners.

Condoms do not prevent against transmission of scabies but should still be used to prevent the transmission of other STIs.

There is no vaccine to prevent scabies. One way to decrease the risk of getting it is by limiting the number of sexual partners.

Mona Dalal

See also: Pubic Lice; Sexually Transmitted Infections (STIs).

Further Reading

Grimes, J. A., Smith, L. A., & Fagerberg, K. (2013). *Sexually transmitted disease: An encyclopedia of diseases, prevention, treatment, and issues.* Santa Barbara, CA: Greenwood.

McAnulty, R. D., & Burnette, M. M. (Eds.). (2006). *Sex and sexuality.* Santa Barbara, CA: Praeger.

Newton, D. E. (2009). *Sexual health: A reference handbook.* Santa Barbara, CA: ABC-CLIO.

Scrotum

The scrotum is an external sac of skin that holds the testes in some male mammals, including humans. Its placement is apparently an evolutionary development intended to keep the sperm produced by the testes cooler than the normal body temperature. For humans, sperm develops and matures best at a temperature several degrees below normal body temperature. An external location for the testes may also prevent inadvertent emptying of the testes before sperm is mature due to normal contraction and relaxing of the abdominal muscles. Common medical problems associated with the scrotum include the development of masses, which may impair reproductive function.

The scrotum is located in human males between the penis and the anus. It is composed of a thin layer of skin over smooth muscle and includes a large number of oil-producing and sweat glands. The scrotum is divided into two compartments by a ridge known as the raphe, which connects to a muscular internal partition that separates the compartments. Within each compartment are the testes, the epididymis, and a large number of nerves and blood vessels. The muscles in the scrotum help to regulate the temperature of the testes. In cold conditions, the muscles contract, drawing the scrotum closer to the abdomen to increase its temperature. Under warmer conditions, the muscles relax, allowing the scrotum to lengthen and more air to circulate around it. Higher temperatures around the scrotum cause the male's fertility to decrease.

The scrotum is vulnerable to blisters caused by chafing and scratching, especially when damp. Skin irritation may also occur because of exposure to soaps, detergents, and other irritants. Scrotal masses may also develop. Symptoms include unusual lumps, sudden pain, dull aching pain, tender or swollen testicles, and nausea or vomiting. Fever, frequent urination, and pus or blood in the urine may also be indications of problems with the scrotum. Regular self-examinations are important to identify problems at an early stage. Common causes of scrotal masses include testicular cancer, spermatocele, and epididymitis. Inguinal hernias may also occur when part of the small intestine pushes through the abdominal wall into the groin.

Tim J. Watts

See also: Epididymis; Testicles; Testicular Cancer.

Further Reading

Harvard Health Publishing. (2016). Lumps or pain within the scrotum. Retrieved from https://www.health.harvard.edu/decision_guide/lumps-or-pain-within-the-scrotum

Jewell, T. (2018). Scrotum overview. Retrieved from https://www.healthline.com/human-body-maps/scrotum

Mayo Clinic. (2019). Scrotal masses. Retrieved from https://www.mayoclinic.org/diseases-conditions/scrotal-masses/symptoms-causes/syc-20352604

Semen

Semen (seminal fluid) is produced by the male reproductive system and is a fluid that may contain spermatozoa (sperm). Composed of several kinds of fluid and components, semen provides a protective and nutritive environment for sperm and aids in the fertilization of an ovum, or female egg. In order for fertilization to occur, sperm (with pH 7.2 to 8.0) must survive in the acidic environment of the female reproductive organs and reach an ovum in the fallopian tubes. Semen increases the viability of sperm and is comprised of fructose, prostaglandins, enzymes, and other substances that create a more alkaline environment for the sperm. These fluids also enhance sperm's motility, increasing the possibility that a sperm will reach an egg. The seminal vesicles, prostate gland, and bulbourethral glands (Cowper's glands) contribute the various fluids that comprise semen. Sperm, produced in the testes, makes up less than 5 percent of semen, and there are roughly 200 million to 500 million sperm in a single ejaculate. The average ejaculate is roughly one teaspoon (approximately three to five milliliters) in volume; however, this volume is affected by several factors, such as hydration, age, and the length of time since last ejaculation. After a vasectomy, ejaculate will be roughly the same volume because sperm is only a small part of the composition of semen.

Typically, semen is translucent and tinted a white, gray, or yellowish color. Semen also has a distinct smell and flavor. A very strong odor or unusual color could signal a medical problem, such as a prostate infection, and may require a doctor. Upon ejaculation, semen is a gel-like consistency because it begins to coagulate. After a period of fifteen to thirty minutes, the semen becomes a liquid again due to prostate-specific antigen, which causes decoagulation. Researchers believe semen coagulates upon ejaculation so it is less susceptible to gravity and can remain in the vagina for longer, increasing the possibility of fertilization.

Semen is safe to ingest; however, it can transmit sexually transmitted infections (STIs) such as herpes, human papillomavirus, chlamydia, gonorrhea, and HIV. Transmission of STIs is a risk if individuals are engaging in unprotected oral sex. Infection of the genitals (vagina, penis, anus) is also possible when contact with semen occurs. It is recommended that individuals use a barrier method for protection, such as a condom or dental dam, during any sexual act that might put them at risk for disease transmission.

Although rare, some individuals are allergic to semen. Known as human seminal plasma sensitivity, this allergy is characterized by a localized allergic response when the individual comes in contact with seminal fluid. Desensitization treatment has been found to be successful for human seminal plasma sensitivity.

Semen cryopreservation is a process that stores semen for several years and allows sperm to retain its fertility. The fertility of semen is assessed by a sperm count that determines how many viable sperm are in the semen sample. With this technology, sperm can be kept viable outside of the human body for a long period of time and used for fertilization of an ovum.

Damiene Denner

See also: Bulbourethral Glands; Ejaculation; Prostate; Seminal Vesicles; Sexually Transmitted Infections (STIs); Sperm.

Further Reading

Human Fertilization & Embryology Authority. (n.d.). Sperm freezing. Retrieved from https://www.hfea.gov.uk/treatments/fertility-preservation/sperm-freezing/

Joannides, P. (2013). *Guide to getting it on* (7th ed.). Waldport, OR: Goofy Foot Press.

Mandal, A. (2019). What is semen? Retrieved from http://www.news-medical.net/health/What-is-Semen.aspx

Seminal Vesicles

The seminal vesicles are two glands in the human male as well as many other mammals. They help produce semen used in reproduction. Fluid from the seminal vesicles provides nutrients for sperm as well as helping make conception possible. Seminal vesicles sometimes are affected by congenital deformities as well as certain diseases, including tuberculosis.

Seminal vesicles are associated with the vas deferens. They are elongated, saclike glands that are about two to three inches long. They sit below the urinary bladder and above the prostate gland, and their ducts, along with those of the vas deferens, form the ejaculatory ducts that place semen in the urethra. A muscular lining of smooth muscle contracts during ejaculation to force the contents of the seminal vesicles into the urethra. Inside the seminal vesicles, a lining of convoluted, folded tissue is found. This lining secretes a fluid that joins the sperm and other fluids from the vas deferens to form semen that is ejaculated by the male. The fluid from the seminal vesicles constitutes up to 60 percent of the volume of the semen that is ejaculated. This yellowish fluid is composed partially of fructose, which provides energy for the sperm. It also includes proteins, citric acid, phosphorus, potassium, and prostaglandins. The semen is slightly alkaline, which helps counteract the acidity of the vagina and improves the survival rate of the sperm. The semen also includes clotting factors, which makes it thicker and sticky. This factor allows the semen to cling to the walls of the female reproductive tract and increases the ability of the sperm to make their way to the ovum (egg).

Few abnormalities are associated with the seminal vesicles. Congenital cysts sometimes develop in the seminal vesicles and the prostate, but they are normally small and do not cause problems. A more serious problem is associated with cystic fibrosis. The seminal vesicles in this case are usually malformed or completely absent. As a result, the male is sterile. In other cases, the ducts may become blocked, either from trauma or from calcification. Infection from tuberculosis may spread to the seminal vesicles as well, causing scarring or alterations in shape that prevents the glands from working.

Tim J. Watts

See also: Ejaculation; Semen; Vas Deferens.

Further Reading

ScienceDirect. (2019). Seminal vesicles. Retrieved from https://www.sciencedirect.com/topics/neuroscience/seminal-vesicle

Seladi-Schulman, J. (2018). What are the seminal vesicles and what is their purpose? Retrieved from https://www.healthline.com/human-body-maps/seminal-vesicles/male

Seminiferous Tubules

The seminiferous tubules are located in the male testes and are coiled, long, thin, ramen noodle–like tubules. They are made up of a variety of cells and are the site of germination, maturation, and transportation of sperm cells. The outside of the tubules is made of stem cells that will divide into two separate cells through mitosis. As the stem cells divide, they move inward and create the inside walls of the tubules. Within the tubules are Sertoli cells, which are column-like cells that line the wall of the tubules. The tubules also contain spermatogenic cells, which will later turn into sperm cells. These cells allow for spermatogenesis, the process that creates mature sperm.

To create sperm cells, the spermatogenic cells divide twice into four separate cells within the tubules. The early-stage spermatozoa, otherwise known as the spermatogonia, will flow throughout the tubules for around sixty days, passing through the central tubule as they head to the rete testis. The rete testis is a network of delicate tubules located on the upper back portion of each testicle. The sperm then flow through the efferent ducts to the epididymis to be stored until they are passed to the vas deferens. During the sperm's travel through the seminiferous tubules, the spermatogonia mature and receive nutrients from the Sertoli cells. By the end of their trip, the spermatogonia transition into spermatozoa, or mature sperm cells; however, they will still need to develop their tails.

Seminiferous tubules go through many changes as the individual grows from birth to adulthood. In newborns, the seminiferous tubules only contain spermatogonia and Sertoli cells. Around the time of puberty, the seminiferous tubules begin to produce sperm. After this point, the testes begin to enlarge due to the size increase of the seminiferous tubules. The seminiferous tubules also contain over 200 compartments that are divided by walls that belong to the corpora cavernosa of the penis.

There are two different kinds of tubules. Convoluted tubules are located on the lateral side of the testes, while straight tubules occur when the tubule begins to connect and form the duct that leads to the outside of the testis. The tubules are formed from the testis cord that is developed from the gonadal cords. This gonadal cord is formed from the gonadal ridge during embryonic development.

Sperm are very fickle, and they must have regulated temperature. Spermatogenesis works best at a temperature slightly less than core body temperature. Due to this fact, the scrotum will move toward or away from the body to maintain a temperature of about 95 degrees Fahrenheit. The movement of the scrotum is administered by the cremaster muscle. When the testicles need to be closer to the body, the cremaster muscle contracts. When the testicles need to be farther from the body, the cremaster muscle relaxes. The cremaster muscle also responds to stress. For example, if an individual is in a threatening situation, the testicles may move closer to the body so that they are protected.

Casey T. Tobin

See also: Epididymis; Sperm; Testicles.

Further Reading

Barclay, T. (2015). Seminiferous tubules. Retrieved from http://www.innerbody.com/anatomy/male-reproductive/seminiferous-tubules

Jones, R. E., & Lopez, K. H. (2014). *Human Reproductive Biology.* San Diego, CA: Academic Press.

Marieb, E. N., & Hoehn, K. (2016). The reproductive system. In *Human anatomy and physiology* (10th ed., 1029–1030). London: Pearson Education.

Sensate Focus

Many couples seek couples therapy and sex therapy to improve their relationships. Sensate focus is a specific technique utilized by sex therapists to aid in improving the sexual relationship between two people.

Sex researchers William Masters and Virginia Johnson first described sensate focus in 1970. Helen Singer Kaplan, a sex therapist, developed it further in 1974. Sensate focus involves a series of exercises that systematically desensitize participants' sexual anxiety and negative associations to sex.

Sensate focus exercises span several weeks and are done in specific steps. These exercises require one partner to be the "giver" and one partner to be the "receiver." Both partners will experience being the "giver" and "receiver" as they switch roles halfway through each sensate focus experience they have together. Each exercise should be done about three times a week until the exercise does not elicit anxiety (usually one to two weeks). Each partner should take a turn as the "giver" and as the "receiver," spending about twenty minutes in each role. Typically, intercourse is prohibited until the completion of the exercises.

The first phase of sensate focus exercises involves the giver touching their partner's body without touching the breasts or genitals. This involves different types of touch using the hands and mouth. The goal of this phase of sensate focus is to explore different types of touch and sensation, not to sexually arouse one's partner. Though sexual arousal often occurs, it is not the purpose of the exercise, and one should not try to have an orgasm or give their partner an orgasm.

In the second phase of the exercises, touching that occurred in phase one is still encouraged. In addition, breast and genital exploration is permitted. However, as in phase one, orgasm is not the goal and should not be attempted. Intercourse is not allowed during this phase, and touching that would lead to an orgasm is not permitted. In the third phase, mutual touching will occur simultaneously as opposed to taking turns as the giver and receiver. Stage four begins with incorporating elements from all the prior phases. In addition, the couple may begin to rub their genitals together and eventually have intercourse. Orgasm is permitted during this phase.

If an erection is achieved during phases one to three, stimulation should be halted until the penis returns to a flaccid state. The purpose of this is to aid in reducing anxiety about losing an erection and not being able to obtain one again. During all phases of the exercises, communication is important. Focusing on one's own pleasure is of utmost importance.

Sensate focus exercises are often employed during sex therapy when one or both partners experience sexual anxiety. The exercises may help treat erectile dysfunction that is often a result of psychological stress or anxiety. Sensate focus works by helping to alleviate anxiety and obsessive thoughts that may prevent someone from obtaining or maintaining an erection. By introducing the individual slowly and without pressure to different forms of stimulation, anxiety may lessen and sexual functioning may be restored.

In addition, sensate focus exercises may help improve sexual communication as they encourage couples to feel more comfortable discussing their sexual likes and dislikes. Couples may experience different sensations and have a forum to explore their sensuality. Sensate focus allows both partners to understand their body and their partner's body better, which can improve overall sexual satisfaction. Couples learn to give and receive pleasure in a relaxed environment without any pressure to perform sexually. The increased communication and sensual experiences a couple experience together may lead to an increase in emotional and sexual intimacy.

There are nine primary functions of engaging in sensate focus exercises:

1. It helps individuals understand their body more thoroughly and the sensations that are desired.
2. It has each partner focus on their own pleasure as opposed to worrying about the pleasure of their partner, which may cause anxiety.
3. It enhances sexual communication.
4. It helps partners understand their partner's sexual needs more.
5. It expands sexual exploration.
6. It allows each partner to appreciate sensual and sexual touch without the need for orgasm.
7. It helps create a positive relationship and relational expression.
8. It aids in building sexual desire.
9. It enhances feelings of closeness, intimacy, caring, and love in a relationship.

Amanda Manuel

See also: Communication, Sexual; Johnson, Virginia; Kaplan, Helen Singer; Masters, William H.; Masters and Johnson Four-Stage Model of Sexual Response; Performance Anxiety; Psychosexual Therapy; Sexual Dysfunction, Treatment of.

Further Reading

Hertlein, K. M., Weeks, G. R., & Gambescia, N. (2009). *Systemic sex therapy.* New York: Routledge.

Long, L. L., Burnett, J. A., & Thomas, R. V. (2006). *Sexuality counseling: An integrative approach.* Upper Saddle River, NJ: Pearson/Merrill Prentice Hall.

Serial Monogamy

"Serial monogamy" refers to the practice of having a succession of romantic or sexual relationships with one individual at a time. Each relationship lasts for a relatively long period compared with a "hookup" or a brief, casual dating relationship. For example, a woman may have a pattern of dating one man exclusively for several weeks or months before breaking up with him to date another. Or a man may be married to a series of women, remaining faithful to each woman for years before the marriage ends in divorce.

Precise definitions of serial monogamy, as well as estimates of its prevalence, vary. However, many people practice serial monogamy, and, according to some definitions and estimates, it is actually the most prevailing style of romantic and sexual relationship in the United States and other Western countries today.

A key aspect of serial monogamy is that the individual tends to spend as little time as possible being alone or single; they typically move into a new relationship as soon as the previous relationship is over. Psychologists note that this tendency may suggest a form of personal insecurity in which the individual fears to spend much time alone. Perhaps constantly being in one relationship or another serves as a distraction from having to think about or deal with unpleasant aspects of the individual's personal life. Or perhaps the relationships give the individuals a temporary sense of self-confidence that they lack on their own.

Serial monogamy might also imply a genuine desire to be faithful to a loved one but a simultaneous fear of remaining seriously committed to that person for very long. Some psychologists note that the relationships in serial monogamy could offer certain individuals a good compromise—the relationships provide a sense of stability, love, and limited commitment while at the same time avoiding permanent commitment.

The chances of pregnancy and sexually transmitted infections are generally easier to control in a serial monogamous relationship than in relationships in which multiple partners are involved. Both partners in a serial monogamous relationship typically are aware of each other's birth control and safer sex practices.

A. J. Smuskiewicz

See also: Dating; Dating, Cross-Cultural Comparison of; Hookup Culture; Monogamy; Polyamory.

Further Reading

Andersson, C. (2015). A genealogy of serial monogamy: Shifting regulations of intimacy in twentieth-century Sweden. *Journal of Family History, 40*(2), 195–207.

Ben-Zeév, A. (2008, October). Is serial monogamy worth pursuing? *Psychology Today.* Retrieved from https://www.psychologytoday.com/blog/in-the-name-love/200810/is-serial-monogamy-worth-pursuing

Sex Chromosomes

A sex chromosome is a type of chromosome (a thread-like structure made up of DNA that maps the human body) that participates in one's determination as either biologically male or female. Generally occurring in a pair, they carry not only the genes that determine male and female traits but also those for some other characteristics. An abnormal number of sex chromosomes results in disorders that can interfere with normal growth.

Humans and most other mammals have two sex chromosomes, known as the X and Y chromosomes. Females have two X chromosomes, and males have an X chromosome and a Y chromosome. A female's egg cells always have one X chromosome, while a male's sperm cells may carry either an X or a Y chromosome. This arrangement means that it is the male cell that determines the sex of the offspring when fertilization occurs. The joining of a female X chromosome with a male X chromosome will result in a female child, and the joining of a female X chromosome with a male Y chromosome will result in a male child.

Both X and Y chromosomes determine characteristics other than sex. The X chromosome is large, containing about 1,098 genes. Most of these genes code for something other than female anatomical traits. In fact, many of the non-sex-determining X-linked genes are responsible for a variety of conditions. Some of the most common human genetic disorders are red-green color blindness (a color vision deficiency in which an individual cannot perceive red and green in the same way as people with normal vision) and male pattern baldness. Another condition linked to X genes is hemophilia, a blood-clotting disorder resulting in prolonged bleeding from even minor cuts and injuries. Duchenne muscular dystrophy, a gradual and irreversible wasting of skeletal muscle, is also linked to the X chromosome. Contrary to the X chromosome, the much smaller Y chromosome has only twenty-six genes, and one is responsible for male anatomical traits. Most of the remaining Y chromosome genes are involved either with cellular health or sperm production. When any of the genes involved in sperm production are missing or defective, the result is usually very low sperm counts and subsequent fertility challenges or infertility.

Other disorders are linked to the quantity or quality of the chromosomes. Two of the most common conditions are Turner syndrome and Klinefelter syndrome. Turner syndrome occurs when one of a female's two X chromosomes is abnormal or missing, causing short stature and developmental problems with the ovaries and production of sex hormones. Although there is no cure, treatment includes human growth hormone and estrogen hormone replacement therapy. Another condition affecting about one in one thousand females is triple X syndrome, a condition in which a female has three X chromosomes instead of two. This condition usually results from an error in the formation of an egg cell, a sperm cell, or an embryo. Symptoms vary in severity and may include developmental delays. Males with Klinefelter syndrome are born with an extra X chromosome (XXY instead of XY), which can slow sexual development because of lowered testosterone and can cause increased breast growth. Depending on its severity, the condition is treatable with testoterone replacement therapy, breast reduction, and counseling.

Linda Tancs

See also: Biological Sex; Chromosomal Sex; Gender; Klinefelter Syndrome; Turner Syndrome; X Chromosome; Y Chromosome.

Further Reading

Easter, C. (n.d.). Sex chromosomes. Retrieved from https://www.genome.gov/genetics-glossary/Sex-Chromosome

ScienceDirect. (2019). Sex chromosome. Retrieved from https://www.sciencedirect.com/topics/biochemistry-genetics-and-molecular-biology/sex-chromosome

Weingarten, C. N., & Jefferson, S. E. (2009). *Sex chromosomes: Genetics, abnormalities, and disorders.* Hauppauge, NY: Nova Science Publishers.

Sex Differentiation of the Brain and Sexual Orientation

Sex differentiation, the process of developing as male, female, or somewhere on the intersex spectrum, begins in the sixth week of pregnancy. Embryos that contain a Y chromosome typically develop testes, while embryos with two X chromosomes typically develop ovaries. After fetal gonads (testes or ovaries) are developed, other organs in the body also start to develop male or female characteristics, including the brain. While the mechanisms for many sex-linked characteristics continue to be studied, it is now widely accepted that the complex interactions between brains, genes, hormones, and the intrauterine environment (the womb) underlie the development of not only sex but also sexual orientation.

To understand the development of sexual orientation, it is necessary to understand that the development of sex is a complex biological process that affects the development of not only the body but also the brain. Indeed, sex arises from a complex interaction between a mother's womb, a baby's genes, hormones (such as estrogen and testosterone), and the immune systems of both mother and child. Interactions between these factors cause the brains of males and females to change. This is despite conflicting results in studies examining specific sex differences in the brain. Indeed, given (1) the many ways that male and female brains could be compared (e.g., volume, mass, connectivity), (2) the large number of comparable brain structures, and (3) the wide variation in these structures within each sex, it is difficult to fully characterize the differences between male and female brains. Furthermore, differences in the brains of adult men and women do not necessarily arise from biological sex alone. It is also possible that environmental influences, such as gendered roles for boys and girls, also influence how the brain develops.

Nevertheless, despite the difficulties associated with this research, sex differences in how the brain works and how people behave are widely recognized. Likewise, there is now lots of evidence that shows brains also differ by sexual orientation and not just biological sex. These studies mirror those that compare physical differences between homosexual and heterosexual subjects by demonstrating differences in the brain structure and function between homosexual and heterosexual individuals. For example, on average, the part of the brain in gay men that is associated with male-typical sexual behavior (the anterior hypothalamus) has more similarities with the female brain relative to heterosexual men. It has been suggested that the "feminization" of this structure may lead homosexual men to, among other things, respond similarly to women when exposed to male body odors. Aside from the hypothalamus, other differences in the brain have also been identified, and the existing evidence from this body of literature strongly supports other findings that suggest sexual orientation, like sex, is related to changes that fetuses undergo while in their mother's womb.

Kiffer G. Card

See also: Biological Theories of Sexual Orientation; Gender; Sex Hormones; Sexual Dimorphism; Sexual Orientation.

Further Reading

Balthazart, J. (2011). *The biology of homosexuality.* New York: Oxford University Press.

Fisher, A. D., Ristori, J., Morelli, G., & Maggi, M. (2018). The molecular mechanisms of sexual orientation and gender identity. *Molecular and Cellular Endocrinology, 467,* 3–13.

Garcia-Falgueras, A., & Swaab, D. F. (2010). Sexual hormones and the brain: An essential alliance for sexual identity and sexual orientation. *Pediatric Neuroendocrinology, 17,* 22–35.

LeVay, S. (2016). *Gay, straight, and the reason why: The science of sexual orientation* (2nd ed.). New York: Oxford University Press.

McCarthy, M. M., Nugent, B. M., & Lenz, K. M. (2017). Neuroimmunology and neuroepigenetics in the establishment of sex differences in the brain. *Nature Reviews Neuroscience, 18*(8), 471–484.

Ngun, T. C., Ghahramani, N., Sánchez, F. J., Bocklandt, S., & Vilain, E. (2011). The genetics of sex differences in brain and behavior. *Frontiers in Neuroendocrinology, 32*(2), 227–246.

O'Hanlan, K. A., Gordon, J. C., & Sullivan, M. W. (2018). Biological origins of sexual orientation and gender identity: Impact on health. *Gynecologic Oncology, 149*(1), 33–42.

Roselli, C. E. (2018). Neurobiology of gender identity and sexual orientation. *Journal of Neuroendocrinology, 30*(7), e12562.

Ruigrok, A. N. V., Salimi-Khorshidi, G., Lai, M.-C., Baron-Cohen, S., Lombardo, M. V., Tait, R. J., & Suckling, J. (2014). A meta-analysis of sex differences in human brain structure. *Neuroscience and Biobehavioral Reviews, 39*(100), 34–50.

Savic, I. (2014). Pheromone processing in relation to sex and sexual orientation. In C. Mucignat-Caretta (Ed.), *Neurobiology of chemical communication.* Boca Raton, FL: CRC Press/Taylor & Francis. Retrieved from http://www.ncbi.nlm.nih.gov/books/NBK200984/

Sex Education

The history of sex education in the United States is quite short, beginning in 1913 when schools began to teach sex education. By the 1930s, most secondary schools provided some sort of sex education, but it was not mandatory nor regulated by the federal or state governments. Whether or not students were taught about sex was not an issue for state governments until the emergence of HIV/AIDS in the early 1980s. At this time, states mandated that schools teach about HIV/AIDS and how to stop it from spreading in order to curb the sudden outbreak. It was required that schools help stop the rapid spread of HIV, but the government did not provide a specific way to do so. Groups pushing for abstinence-based programs had existed since the 1960s as a way to counteract the Supreme Court cases *Griswold v. Connecticut*, which made contraception legal in 1965, and *Roe v. Wade*, which made abortion legal in 1973. These groups believed that the Supreme Court rulings signified an end to sexual purity in the United States, and they sought to protect students' innocence. The existence of these groups prior to states requiring some form of sex education in the 1980s influenced how students were taught about sex.

In the late 1980s, another enthusiastic push for abstinence-only education came as more teenagers became pregnant, resulting in high numbers of single mothers and abortions. This perpetuated the belief that the United States' moral fabric was unraveling. Pro-abstinence-only groups dominated the emerging political conversation about sex education at this time and lobbied for more control. This resulted in the federal and state governments giving schools across the country about $1.5 billion from 1996 to 2007 under Title V of the Social Security Act to support and develop abstinence-only curriculum.

During this time, many countries around the world, and especially in Europe, were implementing a different kind of sex education, one that was comprehensive and included information about anatomy, sexual development, sexually transmitted infections (STIs), contraception, pregnancy, childbirth, abortion, and healthy relationships. This type of fact-based education teaches students from elementary school through high school about different aspects of sex and sexuality from different perspectives and gradually builds in content as the students get older. Not surprisingly, countries with this approach have lower rates of unplanned pregnancies, abortions, and STIs, and rates continue to decrease. Meanwhile, the U.S. rates are significantly higher.

In 2010, as part of the Affordable Care Act, the U.S. government passed the Personal Responsibility Education Program in an effort to expand sex education curriculum past abstinence-only curriculum to include teaching students about the various forms of contraceptives available and how to use them. This is the first federally funded sex education curriculum that combines abstinence-only teachings with fact-based curriculum. This is one step that the United States has taken to try to improve the nation's ineffective sex education. Unfortunately, even though this legislation was passed by both political parties, schools across the country have consistently rejected the funds from the program in order to keep teaching students the abstinence-only curriculum.

Not only is the sex education curriculum in the United States outdated in the ideals about sex, but the programs do not effectively prevent teenage pregnancies or STIs. The teenage birth rate in the United States is three times higher than in France, four times higher than in Germany, and five times higher than in the Netherlands. Similarly, the United States does not have the best statistics regarding STIs. According to the Centers for Disease Control and Prevention, young adults, ages fifteen to twenty-four, are at a higher risk of acquiring STIs than older generations. As of 2015, all the nationally reported STIs (chlamydia, gonorrhea, and syphilis) have seen increases between 6 percent and 19 percent in the number of infections reported. The U.S. youth population is about six times more likely to be diagnosed with HIV/AIDS than in Europe, and U.S. youth are far less likely to use any contraception. The lack contraception use in the United States is not surprising seeing that abstinence-only education wrongly teaches that condoms do not work. We even see differences in these statistics within in different U.S. states. In states where sex education is more comprehensive, as opposed to the abstinence-only approach, there are lower rates of unplanned pregnancies and STIs.

A positive consequence of teaching children about sexuality is that it builds a foundation for future learning and growth. As students age, their sex education needs change. For example, teaching about the physical, mental, and emotional changes that happen during puberty helps students understand that what is happening is supposed to happen. When young people do not properly understand what is to be expected during puberty, it can lead to eating disorders, excessive use of anabolic steroids, depression, and increased use of legal and illegal substances. Understanding the changes in their bodies helps build confidence in talking about these changes, which promotes communication between students and trusted adults if something is wrong or if they have questions.

Research shows that the majority of people in the United States prefer that schoolchildren receive a complete and comprehensive sex education similar to programs found in Europe. Many teachers, parents, doctors, and politicians are trying to replace abstinence-only programs based on the research showing it is ineffective, looking to Europe's more comprehensive sexuality education approach. However, there are still many deep-seated religious ideals and misconceptions about the science of adolescent development that are held by many Americans and continue to perpetuate outdated curriculum.

Former president Barack Obama proposed eliminating a $10 million-a-year grant that funds abstinence-only sex education. However, the Republican-led Senate and House of Representatives extended federal funding through the beginning of the next presidency, giving control of the budget to the Donald Trump administration. President Trump proposes to increase support for abstinence-only sex education by nearly $300 million.

Carson Clark and Karen S. Beale

See also: Abstinence; Contraception; Puberty; Religion, Diversity of Human Sexuality and; Sexual Health; Sexual Learning; Teen Pregnancy.

Further Reading

Guttmacher Institute. (2019). Sex and HIV education. Retrieved from https://www.guttmacher.org/state-policy/explore/sex-and-hiv-education

Ponzetti, J. J., Jr. (2016). *Evidence-based approaches to sexuality education: A global perspective.* New York: Routledge/Taylor & Francis Group.

Sex Guilt

Sex guilt is the feeling of regret or remorse after engaging in a sexual activity. It can occur after engaging in any sexual activity, including masturbation, but it is typically discussed in regard to sexual intercourse. It is often confused with sex anxiety or sexual shame. Sex anxiety is the feeling of apprehension or worry that may occur before a sexual encounter or about anything sex related. Sexual shame comes from the fear of disgrace or humiliation from others about sex or a sex-related behavior. Simply put, sex guilt is privately experienced based on a specific behavior, sexual shame is more publicly oriented, and sex anxiety is a more generalized emotion.

The feelings of regret and remorse following a sexual encounter are experienced by an individual if they believe that they have acted contrary to their beliefs or values. For example, sex guilt may be experienced by a person raised in a strict religious environment who engaged in sex before marriage. However, sex guilt can also be experienced for other reasons, such as because they cheated on their significant other, because they had sex with someone they didn't love, because they were intoxicated during the sexual encounter, or because they engaged in a sex behavior that they did not want to. Sex guilt is reported more often by women, likely due to the sexual double standard.

Scientific research on sex guilt really began in the 1960s and 1970s, likely due to researchers trying to understand the phenomenon of "free love" and the sexual revolution. In the 1980s and 1990s, there was very little research published on this topic, but recently, more researchers are beginning to study it again to try to better understand why it occurs and the effects it can have on an individual and their relationships.

Sex guilt can cause cognitive dissonance (an unpleasant feeling when one's beliefs or values do not match their behaviors). Because cognitive dissonance is so emotionally painful, people experiencing it must make a choice: they must either change their behavior, by no longer engaging in the sexual activity, or they must change their beliefs or values about sex. Sex guilt can also lead to decreased self-esteem, increased sex anxiety, and decreased sexual satisfaction in relationships. Extreme cases can lead to sexual dysfunction and depression.

Because sex guilt stems from the mismatch between a person's behaviors and their beliefs or values, it can be particularly difficult to overcome and avoid negative results. Many people seek help from a counselor, a minister, a sex educator, or a trusted friend. Working through these feelings is very important in order to maintain sexual health.

Rachael Zaffiro and Karen S. Beale

See also: Cheating and Infidelity; Double Standards, Sexual; Performance Anxiety; Premarital Sex; Religion, Diversity of Human Sexuality and.

Further Reading

Hackathorn, J., Ashdown, B., & Rife, S. (2016). The sacred bed: Sex guilt mediates religiosity and satisfaction for unmarried people. *Sexuality & Culture, 20*(1), 153–172.

Janda, L. H., & Bazemore, S. D. (2011). The Revised Mosher Sex-Guilt Scale: Its psychometric properties and a proposed ten-item version. *Journal of Sex Research, 48*(4), 392–396.

Sex Hormones

Sex hormones are any of several chemical substances secreted by various glands that are responsible for human sexual and reproductive characteristics and behaviors. While typically classified as male and female, all people have varying levels of each of the sex hormones. The main male sex hormones are testosterone, androsterone, and other androgens. The main female sex hormones are estrogen and progesterone. Sex hormones are steroids, fat molecules that have a core structure made of three rings of six carbon atoms and one ring of five carbon atoms. Besides their natural functions, sex hormones and synthetic versions of them have a number of medical uses.

Testosterone is the most active and powerful male sex hormone. Most testosterone is produced by the connective tissue cells surrounding the sperm-producing tubules in the testes, or testicles. Small amounts of testosterone are also secreted by the adrenal glands, on top of the kidneys, and by the ovaries.

Androsterone plays a supportive role for the functions of testosterone, and it also plays roles in other physiological processes. Androsterone and certain other androgens—including androstenedione, dehydroepiandrosterone (DHEA), and dehydroepiandrosterone sulfate (DHEA sulfate)—are produced mainly in the adrenal cortex, the outer portion of the adrenal glands. The testes and ovaries also produce some of these hormones, and DHEA and DHEA sulfate can be converted into testosterone or androstenedione in adipose (fat) tissues and other body tissues.

Testosterone and androgen levels increase in males during puberty, typically starting between the ages of twelve and fourteen. As the testes release testosterone into the bloodstream, it flows throughout the body, prompting the development of physical and behavioral characteristics that mark male sexual maturity. These characteristics include the growth of hair on the face and body, the buildup of muscle mass, the growth of the penis and testes, and the deepening of the voice.

Testosterone and other androgens promote male sexual arousal and general aggressiveness, peaking during sexual interest and arousal. Healthy forms of aggressiveness, such as a competitive drive and high motivation and energy, are associated with high testosterone levels. Some research has found associations between high testosterone levels and criminal sexual aggression, including rape, in certain men. Other functions of testosterone, for all people, include the promotion of cognitive functions—such as thinking ability, memory, concentration, and focus—and spatial awareness. Testosterone also helps the ovaries produce estrogen.

In cases in which boys or men do not produce sufficient amounts of androgens, testosterone or androgen replacement therapy can promote the development and functioning of male reproductive organs and normal sperm cells. Trans men opting for gender transition may also take testosterone or androgen therapy in order to promote masculinization of their physical features. Synthetic versions of these hormones may be administered as injections, pills, creams, gels, patches, or implants. Androgen replacement is also used as treatment for men who have low sex drives.

Androgens can be used to treat people who have other disorders, including breast cancer, anemia, skin problems, and abnormally delayed growth. Androgen drugs known as "anabolic steroids" are used by some athletes to build muscle strength. However, such use can result in serious physical and psychological side effects, including cardiovascular problems, liver damage, testicular shrinkage, and excessive aggression.

Estrogen begins to be secreted in large amounts by the ovaries at the start of puberty, usually between the ages of ten and twelve. Among the various forms of estrogen, the strongest and most important is estradiol. As these hormones flow through the bloodstream, they produce physical changes that mark female sexual maturity. These changes include the development of breasts, rounded hips, and mature vaginal and clitoral tissues.

Estrogen also stimulates the beginning of the menstrual cycle, in which, once a month, an ovary releases a mature egg. During the menstrual cycle, estrogen works in conjunction with progesterone to thicken the lining of the uterus in preparation for pregnancy. If pregnancy occurs, the hormones continue to be produced in large amounts, maintaining the uterine lining and prompting the various developments of pregnancy. If pregnancy does not occur, the hormone levels decrease, leading to the shedding of the thickened uterine lining in menstruation.

During middle age, usually between the ages of about forty-five and fifty-five, the secretion of estrogen by the ovaries gradually decreases. When estrogen levels in the blood become suitably low, ovulation and menstrual periods stop, and menopause beings. Postmenopausal women can no longer become pregnant.

In addition to the estrogen secreted by the ovaries, smaller amounts of estrogen are secreted by the adrenal glands and the testes. Small amounts are also produced in adipose tissue and other tissues, through the metabolic conversion of other hormones. The functions of estrogen in men are not clearly understood, though it likely plays a role in promoting blood clotting and strengthening bones.

Progesterone is secreted primarily by the ovaries and, during pregnancy, by the placenta. Like estrogen, small amounts of progesterone are also produced by the adrenal glands and the testes.

As previously indicated, during the menstrual cycle, one of the ovaries releases an egg and begins secreting large amounts of progesterone. These secretions cause the endometrium (the lining of the interior walls of the uterus) to develop a thickened layer of blood vessels, cells, and glands. Should the released egg be fertilized by a sperm cell, the fertilized egg develops into an embryo, which implants in the uterine lining. Tissues from the embryo become intertwined with tissues from the uterus, forming the placenta. Large amounts of progesterone secreted by the placenta keep the uterine muscle relaxed during pregnancy, preventing the fetus from being born prematurely. The placenta's progesterone works with other hormones to induce development of milk-secreting cells in the breasts and to strengthen the pelvic wall in preparation for birth. Immediately after birth, progesterone levels begin to decrease.

If the egg is not fertilized and pregnancy does not occur, menstruation occurs and progesterone levels immediately decline. Whether or not pregnancy occurs, the monthly increase in progesterone levels may increase body temperature and cause the breasts to enlarge and become more sensitive.

In addition to its sexual and reproductive functions, progesterone, in all people, helps to regulate the transmission of nerve impulses; aids in the development and protection of brain neurons; and plays roles in the regulation of blood clotting, cellular oxygen levels, conversion of fat into energy, and insulin secretion by the pancreas.

Drugs made with synthetic estrogen, sometimes mixed with synthetic progesterone (progestin), are used in oral contraceptives (birth control pills). Estrogen-progestin pills are known as "the combination pill," while progestin-only pills are commonly called "the minipill." The combination pill contains a higher dose of progestin than the minipill. These pills prevent pregnancy by blocking ovulation, thinning the uterine lining, and thickening the mucus of the cervix.

Estrogen and progestin pills, creams, patches, implants, and injections are also used in hormone replacement therapy (HRT) to reduce some of the unpleasant symptoms of menopause (such as hot flashes, skin itchiness and dryness, and brittle bones). Progesterone-based medications are sometimes prescribed as treatments for irregular menstruation; premenstrual syndrome; breast, uterine, or kidney cancer; and weight loss related to cancer or AIDS. HRT may also be used by trans women during the gender transition process.

A. J. Smuskiewicz

See also: Androgens; Estrogen; Hormone Replacement Therapy; Oxytocin; Progesterone; Synthetic Hormones; Testosterone.

Further Reading

Baker, S. (2007). The sex hormone secrets. *Psychology Today*. Retrieved from https://www.psychologytoday.com/gb/articles/200701/the-sex-hormone-secrets

Our Bodies Ourselves. (2019). Hormones that affect sexual desire. Retrieved from https://www.ourbodiesourselves.org/book-excerpts/health-article/hormones-affecting-sexual-desire/

ScienceDirect. (2019). Sex hormones. Retrieved from https://www.sciencedirect.com/topics/neuroscience/sex-hormones

Sex Reassignment Surgery

"Sex reassignment surgery" (SRS), also called "genital reconstruction surgery" or "gender affirmation surgery," refers to surgical procedures in which the body is either masculinized or feminized as desired or required. Some, but not all, transgender people seek this type of surgical intervention as part of their gender transition process. Surgeries may include chest, genital, or facial reconstruction.

Most transgender people who choose to undergo SRS will have also used hormone therapy and may have had other procedures, such as electrolysis to remove facial hair. The types of interventions and procedures chosen will depend on the individual, their identity and expression, as well as additional factors such as financial access and access to appropriate medical care. SRS first became publicly available in the United States in the 1950s.

SRS procedures will vary across people. During construction of a neovagina (vaginoplasty), the testicles are removed, as is the interior muscle tissue of the penis. The neovagina is then created from the inverted skin of the penis or from skin grafts. A nerve-sensitive portion of the penis head is shaped into a clitoris to preserve sexual stimulation—though some nerve tissue may be lost in the operation. Following the surgery, the neovagina must be regularly cleaned and lubricated because sufficient natural lubrication is not produced. In addition, the vaginal opening must be frequently dilated with a special device to maintain an adequate width and depth to the vagina as the body has a natural tendency to try to close the opening. For some, it may be possible to orgasm during sexual stimulation of the neovagina, although this will vary among people.

Construction of a neophallus is more complicated than construction of a neovagina and the results more varied. The first step is to remove the uterus, fallopian tubes, ovaries, and vaginal tissues. Testicular implants are then inserted into the vulvar tissue to create a scrotum. Next, in a procedure called phalloplasty, the surgeon attempts to create a functioning, sufficiently sized penis from the nerve-containing clitoral tissue, together with vascularized (blood vessel–containing) tissue taken from other body areas, such as the abdomen, thigh, or forearm. To enable the person to have an erection, the surgeon usually implants a penile prosthesis within the newly formed penile tissue. The prosthesis is either semirigid or inflatable. In addition, the urethra must be lengthened using any available vascularized genital skin. Given the difficulty of these procedures, there may be complications and nerve damage resulting in loss of sexual pleasure and function. As such, the benefits and risks of these procedures need to be carefully considered by the individual in consultation with their health care providers.

Reliable statistics regarding SRS procedures and their outcomes are difficult to obtain. Various sources place the approximate number of SRS procedures performed in the United States each year at anywhere from one hundred to one thousand or more—with feminization surgeries far more common than masculinization surgeries. Hundreds to thousands more SRS procedures are performed every year in other countries throughout the world, especially in Thailand, which has been dubbed the "SRS capital" of the world. Although the precise number of these surgeries is uncertain, it is clear that the number of these operations has increased in recent decades. While many people are satisfied with the results of their surgeries, others are not and later report regret at having completed the procedures.

A. J. Smuskiewicz

See also: Gender Diversity; Gender Transition; Transgender.

Further Reading

Coleman, E., Bockting, W., Botzer, M., Cohen-Kettenis, P., DeCuypere, G., Feldman, J., . . . Monstrey, S. (2012). Standards of care for the health of transsexual, transgender, and gender-nonconforming people, version 7. *International Journal of Transgenderism, 13*(4), 165–232.

The Gender Centre Inc. (2019). Female to male information kit. Retrieved from https://gendercentre.org.au/resources/kits-fact-sheets/female-to-male

The Gender Centre Inc. (2019). Male to female information kit. Retrieved from https://gendercentre.org.au/resources/kits-fact-sheets/male-to-female

Guss, C., Shumer, D., & Katz-Wise, S. L. (2015). Transgender and gender nonconforming adolescent care: Psychosocial and medical considerations. *Current Opinion in Pediatrics, 26*(4), 421–426.

Iantaffi, A., & Barker, M. J. (2017). *How to understand your gender: A practical guide for exploring who you are.* London: Jessica Kingsley Publishers.

Sex Tourism

"Sex tourism" refers to traveling for the specific purpose of procuring sex, intimacy, exoticism, or unconstrained sexual experiences. Although sex tourism can be found almost anywhere in the world, it tends to be most popular in regions where the cost of sex is lower (e.g., the Caribbean, Cambodia, Thailand, Philippines, Bangladesh, Jamaica, and Dominican Republic). The high demand for sex tourism in these areas is a significant source of income that many of these countries rely on for economic performance or contribution for gross domestic product. From a tourist perspective, Eastern cultures are popular sex tourist destinations because of the desire to have sexual experiences with others that are exotic or non-Western. Traditionally, sex tourists were thought to be predominately heterosexual men traveling to have sex with women. In recent decades, however, it has been discovered that the dynamics and demographics of the sex tourism industry are much more complex; women, men who have sex with men, and locals are now known to also engage in the industry.

Though prostitution is legal in many popular sex tourism destinations, the sex tourism industry contributes to one of the largest criminal industries in the world—human trafficking. Given the demand for child sex tourism, children are especially vulnerable to human trafficking; child sex tourism is currently a multibillion-dollar industry that affects over 2 million children each year. Despite most countries having laws to protect children against sex tourism, unenforced laws make it feasible to avoid charges of sex crimes. The advancement of internet and mobile technology, as well as an upsurge in global users, has provided an increase in anonymity and hidden avenues to access child sex tourism. Such advancements have also contributed to decreased risk of arrest and an increase of sexual exploitation of children in the travel and tourism industry.

Nicole C. Doria and Matthew Numer

See also: Prostitution; Sex Work; Sex Workers, Male; Sexual Slavery.

Further Reading

Centers for Disease Control and Prevention (CDC). (2013). Sex tourism. Retrieved from https://wwwnc.cdc.gov/travel/page/sex-tourism

Hawke, A., & Raphael, A. (2016). Offenders on the move: Global study on sexual exploitation of children in travel and tourism. Retrieved from https://www.ecpat.org.uk/offenders-on-the-move-global-study-on-sexual-exploitation-of-children-in-travel-and-tourism-2016

Kosuri, M., & Jeglic, E. (2017). Child sex tourism: American perceptions of foreign victims. *Journal of Sexual Aggression, 23*(2), 207–221.

Richards, T., & Reid, J. (2015). Gender stereotyping and sex trafficking: Comparative review of research on male and female sex tourism. *Journal of Crime and Justice, 38*(3), 1–20.

SexInfo. (2018). Sex tourism. Retrieved from http://www.soc.ucsb.edu/sexinfo/article/sex-tourism

Sex Toys

The term "sex toy" can be used to describe a number of objects and accessories that are used to increase sexual pleasure or support sexual activity, either solo or partnered. Sex toys refer to items that are used by people of all gender identities, sexual orientations, and types of relationships and can be used all over the body, including on, around, and in genitalia. In the United States, items designated as sex toys can only be purchased by individuals eighteen years of age and older. However, it is not illegal for young people to own sex toys, and other countries have different laws, some more lenient and others more restrictive.

Archaeologists have discovered stone carvings from over 8,000 years ago (between 4000 BCE and 6000 BCE) that resemble phalluses, indicating that objects have been used to facilitate sexual pleasure throughout the history of humanity and is not limited to current usages and technologies. Historically, modern sex accessories were only available in sex stores or porn shops, which later expanded to include sex toy stores (designed specifically for the purpose of peddling these items), and now, many sex toys are available in drugstores and on major online retail sites. This demonstrates how sex toys have become more accepted in the mainstream, and this is mirrored by the centering of sex toys in certain TV shows like *Sex and the City*, movies, and in popular books, such as *50 Shades of Grey* and the *Marketplace Series*.

A vibrator is any object used sexually that vibrates in some way. These items can be used externally for clitoral, vulvar, penile, scrotal, or nipple stimulation, or internally for vaginal or anal stimulation (items should only be used anally if they have a base wider than the rest of the toy). One of the most frequently recognized sex toys is the rabbit-style or dual stimulator vibrator, made popular on *Sex and the City*, although vibrators come in all shapes, sizes, colors, and styles. Many use batteries from AAA to D, some are rechargeable, and a few types still plug into the wall for their power source.

Following vibrators, another popular sex toy are dildos, insertable toys for the mouth, vagina, or anus. Some dildos may vibrate, while many do not; the names can be interchangeable for vibrating dildos, often based on the primary function of the toy. Dildos can be held in the hand or strapped onto the body via a harness. Just as vibrators offer diverse options, dildos are offered in a plethora of lengths, widths, colors, levels of realism, and styles. The most commonly used type of harness for a dildo is worn around the waist, but harnesses are also manufactured that can be worn on the forehead, chin, chest, palm, thigh, or foot, depending on the preference of the wearer. People of all genders can penetrate others or be penetrated themselves by dildos, and people of all sexual orientations may engage in strap-on sexual activity, using one or more dildos and harnesses.

There are a variety of different sex toys designed for use in the anus. These include, but are not limited to, anal dildos, butt plugs, anal beads, and anal probes. Dildos are meant to be used in motion, while butt plugs, anal beads, and anal probes are meant to be used in a stationary manner inside the anus to provide a feeling of fullness and anal stimulation. It is important to note that any toy used in the anus should have a flared based (wider than the rest of the toy) to keep it from slipping inside the body and getting stuck in the anal canal, or eventually, in the intestines. Also, toys used anally should be designated for that purpose, used with a condom, or made of a sterilizable material because anal bacteria can cause oral and vaginal infections during cross-contamination even in the same body. People of all genders and sexual orientations may enjoy using anal toys, and the enjoyment of anal stimulation is not limited to any sexual orientation.

Penis rings, sometimes referred to as "cock rings," are usually worn around the testicles and penis in order to permit blood to flow into the penis but not back out again. This can somewhat increase the length, width, and time of erection temporarily as well as provide a more intense orgasm for the wearer. It should be noted that these objects should not be worn longer than fifteen to twenty minutes at a time in order to prevent discomfort and potential medical problems. Some rings also have a vibrating function. These may also be worn on nonvibrating dildos to add a vibrating effect. Penis rings are frequently suggested as a first step to treat erectile dysfunction, sometimes partnered with a penis pump in order to have an erection.

Another group of sex toys can be considered more sexual health toys. These are items that help to strengthen vaginal and pelvic floor muscles. Because having strong pelvic floor muscles can help with bladder control (including during pregnancy and aging), easier recovery after vaginal birth, and stronger orgasms, toned muscles can be supportive for a number of positive health outcomes. While Kegel exercises can be done independently of toys, once inserted, these items can help the body to do these exercises subconsciously when the wearer is moving. Typically, these are round balls specifically designed to be worn for hours at a time, allowing the wearer to build stronger Kegel muscles by triggering the muscles to subconsciously contract and then release during any movement.

Any sex toy that is made from a jelly material (some called sil-a-gel, gelee, Jel-ee, etc.) is not guaranteed to be safe for use inside the body. These materials contain something called phthalates, which are rubber softeners (like what they use on shower curtains), and not only do they often smell bad, but they can leach into the body during use, causing irritation, pain, and even potentially cancer, based on research studies commissioned by Smitten Kitten and Tantus (The Coalition Against Toxic Toys). As sex toys are not regulated by the FDA in the United States, manufacturers are not restricted to body-safe materials. Sex toy materials that are phthalate free and more safe for use on and in bodies include hard plastic, elastomer, TPR, medical-grade silicone, glass or Pyrex, metal (aluminum or stainless steel), ceramic, Corian, granite, polyurethane-coated wood, and marble. If a material is unknown, using a condom over a toy is an effective method for barring transfer of phthalates to the body. When a sex toy will be used by multiple partners, it is considered best practice to either use a condom on the toy in order to prevent the potential spread of bacteria and sexually transmitted infections or to choose a sex toy material that can be sterilized, such as medical-grade silicone, metal, ceramic, Corian, or glass. These materials can be sterilized by being wiped down with 10 percent bleach solution or toy-specific sterilizer, being boiled for three to five minutes, or being put through the dishwasher on the top shelf (the latter two options should only be used for nonvibrating toys).

There are a variety of other toys not specifically discussed here. Many of these toys are specific to kink or BDSM play, such as floggers, paddles, nipple clamps, wrist and ankle restraints, spreader bars, ball gags, whips, ropes, and others. In addition, new sex toys are placed on the market on a regular basis, and while they may fall into one of the categories discussed above, they often have unique qualities, like a vibrator that can be worn as a glove, a dildo that can simulate ejaculatory fluid, or a vibrating toy that can be controlled via the internet (referred to as "teledildonics").

Shanna K. Kattari

See also: Afterplay; Anal Intercourse; Arousal; Clitoris; Foreplay; Grafenberg Spot (G-spot); Kegel Exercises; Masturbation; Oral Sex; Orgasm; Pelvic Floor Muscles; Sex Education; Sexual Satisfaction.

Further Reading

BadVibes. (n.d.). Smitten Kitten. Retrieved from http://badvibes.org/the-smitten-kitten

Health Services Brown University. (2015). Sex toys. Retrieved from https://www.brown.edu/campus-life/health/services/promotion/sexual-health-sex-101/sex-toys

Moskowitz, C. (2010, July). Stone age carving: Ancient dildo? *Live Science*. Retrieved from http://www.livescience.com/9971-stone-age-carving-ancient-dildo.html

Scarleteen. (2019). Sex toys. Retrieved from http://www.scarleteen.com/tags/sex_toys

Teen Health Source. (n.d.). Sex toys. Retrieved from http://teenhealthsource.com/sex/sex-toys/

Venning, R., & Cavanah, C. (2003). *Sex toys 101: A playfully uninhibited guide*. New York: Simon & Schuster.

Sex Work

"Sex work" refers to sexual services or erotic entertainment provided for material or monetary compensation. The use of the term "sex work" underscores the employment and labor aspect of commercial sex while at the same time encompassing a variety of erotic services that do not involve direct sexual contact. A sex worker includes any individual working in the adult entertainment or sex industry, such as an exotic dancer or stripper, burlesque dancer, phone sex operator, dominatrix, fetish or role-play artist, erotic model, erotic masseur, peepshow performer, porn actor or actress (including internet webcam performer and print model), and prostitute (including brothel worker, street-based worker, bar prostitute, call girl, gigolo or hustler, and escort).

The term "sex work," coined by Carol Leigh circa 1979, was created to decrease stigma and to raise awareness of the safety and rights of those who trade sexual services as their work. The development of this perspective can be traced back to the beginning of the prostitutes' rights movement, which evolved into the sex workers' rights movement, as prostitutes began to reference their work as legitimate labor. In the beginning, use of the term "sex work" had generally applied to prostitutes. Rather than using the term "prostitution," "sex work" was created as a more inclusive term that identifies sex work as an occupation with multiple positions, including prostitution.

Many sex workers have faced challenges to have their work identified and accepted as legitimate work from which one can maintain a sustainable living and have employment protections. During the 1970s and 1980s, feminists frequently debated about pornography and prostitution. While the dominant discourse was on the negative effects and consequences, some feminists presented a more liberated view of female sexuality and work options. Such feminists birthed a wave of sex work activists who began to challenge the dominant discourse on prostitution and pornography in defense of women's sexual freedom, expression, and labor choices.

Call Off Your Old Tired Ethics (COYOTE), the first prostitutes' rights organization in the United States, spurred by Margo St. James and others, was formed in 1973. COYOTE, also later referred to as the North American Task Force on Prostitution, formed to address issues from the sex worker perspective via self-made pamphlets, posters, and conference papers. Throughout the following decades, more sex worker organizations developed, created publications, established platforms for sex worker voices and concerns to be heard, and began raising awareness about sex work and the conditions that some sex workers face, especially in the wake of the HIV/AIDS epidemic.

Since some sex work requires sexual contact, sexual health is a primary concern. In the early stages of the HIV/AIDS epidemic, prostitutes were accused of being a conduit for the spread of the virus. Early information about HIV was written in gay publications as well as sex-worker publications in order to debunk myths and provide factual information. For example, in an article from the 1980s publication *Tucson Whores and Tricks*, a writer provided research statistics and current information, for that time, about the documented risks of HIV/AIDS to prostitutes rather than the assumed risks that came from prostitutes: "There has been an overemphasis on the danger of contracting AIDS from prostitutes, and an underemphasis of the dangers to prostitutes. . . . Of the approximately 14,000 cases of AIDS, 1% have contracted through heterosexual sex. That amounts to 140 people. The media has not made it clear that 90% of these cases represent women who have caught AIDS from men" (Unknown, 1985).

Considering the risk of sexually transmitted infections, including HIV, condoms are crucial for sex workers who have sexual contact with clients. However, it is common practice to use carrying condoms as evidence against people who are accused of prostitution, and this has been a practice in several countries for decades. In recent years, some sex worker organizations and human rights organizations have taken up this issue as an infringement of people's rights to protect themselves and as a public health issue.

Sex workers face particular scrutiny in society and in mainstream media. Using sex work concepts to sell products, activities, and clothing has become increasingly popular. More recent examples of sex work portrayed in the media depict varied portrayals of sex work and the sex industry. Examples include pole dancing classes (of which many are offered by former and current exotic dancers); stiletto-style shoes that are marketed to the average working woman (similar to those worn by many sex workers); exotic dancers appearing in music videos; phone sex operators in movies such as Spike Lee's *Girl 6* and music videos like *Hotline Bling* by Drake; TV shows depicting sex workers, such as the HBO series *Cathouse*, featuring a legal brothel in Nevada; the Showtime series *Secret Life of a Call Girl*, which focuses on the fictitious account of the life of a call girl in London; and the realty TV show *Kendra on Top*, featuring a former *Playboy* model's life after leaving the sex industry.

Although prostitution is said to be the "world's oldest profession," it has yet to be recognized as a profession. One researcher wrote, "Sex work, like other expressions of sexuality that deviate from the norm, will be oppressed, and sex workers discriminated against" (Hunter, 1991). This refers to policies and laws that continue to make sex work a crime, stigmatize sex workers, and tolerate violence against sex workers. Though sex work in its various forms has increasingly become part of the discourse in academia and mainstream media, issues of legalization and decriminalization continue to be at the forefront of the current debates for sex worker rights organizations.

Kevicha Echols

See also: Pornography; Prostitution; Sex Workers, Male; Sexual Rights; Sexually Transmitted Infections (STIs); Sugar Daddies and Sugar Babies.

Further Reading

Centers for Disease Control and Prevention. (2019). HIV among women. Retrieved from http://www.cdc.gov/hiv/group/gender/women/index.html

Francoeur, R., & Koch, P. B. (1998). Prostitution—sex workers. In R. Francoeur, P. B. Koch, & D. Weis (Eds.), *Sexuality in America* (196–201). New York: Continuum.

Gall, G. (2007). Sex worker unionization: An exploratory study of emerging collective organization. *Industrial Relations Journal, 38*(1), 70–88.

Hunter, A. (1991). The development of theoretical approaches to sex work in Australian sex worker rights groups. In S. A. Gerull & B. Halstead (Eds.), *Sex industry and public policy conference* (110). Canberra, Australia: Australian Institute of Criminology.

Koken, J. A. (2010). The meaning of the "whore": How feminist theories on prostitution help research on female sex workers. In M. Ditmore, A. Levy, & A. Willman (Eds.), *Sex work matters: Power and intimacy in the global sex industry.* London: Zed Books.

McElroy, W. (1996). *Sexual correctness: The gender-feminist attack on women.* Jefferson, NC: McFarland.

Unknown. (1985). Sex in the age of AIDS: Information for women in the sex industry. *Tucson Whores and Tricks: A Journal of Health and Politics for Sex Professionals,* 6–9.

Sex Workers, Male

Male sex workers include men who exchange, barter, or trade sex and sex-related services for money, goods, or other forms of capital. Male sex work can include, but is not limited to, prostitution, escorting, modeling, pornographic acting, webcam sex performances, live sex shows, and other entertainment and commercial endeavors. In some instances, male sex workers engage in "survival sex," which is an attempt to make money to support basic human needs such as food and housing. Clients or consumers of male sex workers can include women, men, transgender persons, persons living with disabilities, as well as couples. Furthermore, male sex workers may identify as gay, bisexual, queer, heterosexual, or "gay-for-pay." Male sex workers who sell sex to men may not necessarily be attracted to men;

and vice versa, male sex workers who sell sex to women may not necessarily be attracted to women.

Male sex workers exist in many of today's societies despite the fact that male sex workers are less prevalent than female sex workers. Male sex workers are diverse in terms of social demographics and motivations to work in the commercial sex industry. Although many male sex workers engage in commercial sex trade at massage parlors, brothels, and bars, male sex workers also utilize the internet at high frequencies. Internet and mobile phone technology platforms (e.g., geosocial mobile applications, social media applications) have increased the global visibility of male sex workers. For instance, there are over sixty countries worldwide that advertise male escorts through websites, and some of these websites advertise sexual services. Legality of male sex work, in general, varies by country and region.

Documented cases of male sex work date as far back as ancient Greece and Rome, but scholars have taken more concerted efforts in recent years to research male sex workers. Scholarship produced between the 1940s and 1970s focused on sociopathy and social deviance of male sex workers, whereas scholarship from the 1980s and 1990s examined implications of male sex work on public health. When compared to female sex workers and men in the general population across many different countries, researchers have reported that HIV and sexually transmitted infections were higher among men who engaged in sex work. Researchers are continuing to track the social and public health implications of male sex work.

Franco Dispenza

See also: Pornography; Prostitution; Sex Work.

Further Reading

Baral, S. D., Friedman, M. R., Geibel, S., Rebe, K., Bozhinov, B., Diouf, D., … Caceres, C. (2015). Male sex workers: Practices, contexts, and vulnerabilities for HIV acquisition and transmission. *Lancet (London, England), 385*(9964), 260–273.

Kumar, N., Minichiello, V., Scott, J., & Harrington, T. (2017). A global overview of male escort websites. *Journal of Homosexuality, 64*(12), 1731–1744.

Minichiello, V., & Scott, J. (Eds.). (2014). *Male sex work and society.* New York: Harrington Park Press.

Minichiello, V., Scott, J., & Callander, D. (2013). New pleasures and old dangers: Reinventing male sex work. *Journal of Sex Research, 50*(3–4), 263–275.

Sexaholics Anonymous

Sexaholics Anonymous (SA) is an organization designed to help people recover from sexual "addictions" or out-of-control sexual behavior, with the only membership requirement being "a desire to stop lusting and become sexually sober." The recovery program used by SA is based on the twelve steps developed by Alcoholics Anonymous (AA). Members meet in local groups in which they share their experiences to help one another solve their common problems. The organization is financially supported through nonmandatory contributions from its members. SA is headquartered in Brentwood, Tennessee.

Unlike some other organizations designed to help sex addicts, SA does not believe it is possible to control or limit, and still enjoy, sexual obsessions or compulsions. Rather, it advocates completely stopping the problematic sexual behaviors.

SA was founded in the 1970s by an individual known as "Roy K." (Members prefer to maintain their anonymity by using only the first letter of their last name.) In 1979, Roy K obtained permission from AA to use its twelve steps as the core of SA's own recovery program. Roy K's strict, conservative, evangelical religious ideas are reflected not only in the adaptation of AA's twelve steps but also in the main guidebook used by SA, officially titled *Sexaholics Anonymous* but often referred to as *The White Book*. The text of this book and of SA's official website elaborate on the group's conservative ideas. The website, for example, describes how people become "sexaholics" by becoming disconnected from family and friends and tuning out "with fantasy and masturbation."

As described by SA, the way to stop sexual compulsions lies in a combination of physical, emotional, and spiritual healing. The "sexaholic" can achieve such healing only by turning away from the "isolating obsession" and by turning to the fellowship of SA group meetings, by turning to God, and by improving relations with other people.

The uncompromisingly conservative messages of SA—which include opposition to same-sex couples, to sex with anyone other than a spouse, to masturbation, and to other behaviors that are generally accepted, or at least tolerated, elsewhere in society—are a source of much criticism among the group's detractors. Furthermore, many psychologists argue that the group's strict definition of sexual sobriety is not useful or helpful for many people struggling with sexual compulsions. Despite such criticism, many members of SA have testified to the ways in which the organization has helped them conquer serious problems that had previously been destroying their lives.

A. J. Smuskiewicz

See also: Compulsivity, Sexual; Hypersexuality; Out-of-Control Sexual Behavior; Pornography Addiction.

Further Reading

Sexaholics Anonymous. (2001). *Sexaholics anonymous*. Brentwood, TN: Sexaholics Anonymous.

Sexaholics Anonymous. (2019). Home page. Retrieved from http://www.sa.org

Sexism

Sexism is discrimination and bias that devalues a person or group of people—namely women and that which is considered feminine based on sex or gender. The term "sexism" was introduced during the 1960s, but the beliefs and practices associated with it pervade human history and have persistently lowered the quality of women's lives and devalued all things feminine.

The terms "sex" and "gender" are often seen as interchangeable, but scholars make a clear distinction in that "sex" refers to one's physical reality (secondary sex characteristics, genitalia, reproductive system), whereas "gender" is either the socially constructed expectations (gender stereotypes, feminine, masculine), sex-based social roles, or an aspect of one's identity (a person with an assigned sex of male may have a gender identity of female). Sexism is oppressive to both women (sex) and feminine (gender) stereotypes, roles, and identity. It is important to note that as much as these distinctions are useful in advancing scholarship, common usage must be respected. These concepts are complex, amorphous, and often overlapping. For example, a transgender person with an assigned sex of female may indeed consider themselves to be a man, regardless of whether there have been alterations to secondary sex characteristics or genitalia.

Can a woman be sexist toward men? No. A woman, or any person, may indeed have prejudices and negative views of men and masculinity (misandry). But sexism, like racism, must be understood within the larger edifice of hegemony that results in structurally reinforced oppression of certain types of humans. The history of world cultures clearly shows that the vast majority have been and are today patriarchal, both formally and implicitly. Sexism—biases and discrimination against women and the feminine—is embedded in patriarchy. Men have not experienced systematic oppression and so are not the object of sexism. The fact that this distinction has only recently been established is itself evidence of the capacity of patriarchy. It is further support for the adage that "privilege is invisible to those who have it." It was once presumed that women (feminine) *or* men (masculine) could be the object of sexism. Those in power, men, who benefited from patriarchy, were blind to the reality that social structures, language, and tacit norms systematically oppress women.

Peter Glick and Susan Fiske developed a model of *ambivalent* sexism that distinguishes between *hostile* and *benevolent* sexism. The former refers to explicit, negative, and harmful biases that contend women and femininity are inferior to men and masculinity. It is explicit and, like racism, it is based on a general antipathy toward a type of person. Benevolent sexism has a veneer of positivity, for it is based on a perceived affection instead of antipathy. Further, it is often associated with helping behaviors, such as offering to carry a woman's package or picking up a dinner bill. Despite this, it is constructed on damaging stereotypes of women (incompetent, weak) and the superiority of men. It perpetuates the patronizing attitude that women require men's protection and help.

Others have compared *old-fashioned* and *modern* sexism. Old-fashioned sexism is the essentialist belief that biological forces result in universal and clear sex differences. This view is seen in many Western faith traditions and is often used to justify societal gender roles that place men in positions of power (provider, public or professional leader, head of house). Modern sexism is the false belief that the unequal treatment of the sexes is a historical reality that no longer exists. Such a view denies that women are still discriminated against and is hostile toward current policies (workplace, governmental) designed to create equity between the sexes.

Finally, *internalized* sexism occurs when a girl or woman incorporates the sexist images, assumptions, and beliefs of society into her view of herself and of other women. This results in a perception that women, including oneself, are mere objects of desire, are incompetent, and are powerless. Internalized sexism leads to an invalidation and derogation of the feminine.

Sexism oppresses women and girls in that it provides the ideological underpinnings of patriarchy. Sexist discrimination of women and femininity is woven throughout the entire fabric of a patriarchy. This includes, but is not limited to, institutional structures, language, workplace practices, division of household labor, placement into leadership positions, public policy, interpersonal relations, sexual conduct, judicial procedures, and individual attitudes.

The history of world cultures demonstrates sex disparities in a number of life quality markers. Women have disproportionally been the victims of sexual objectification, intimate partner violence, employment discrimination, pay inequity, and stress-related physical ailments (e.g., chronic pain, irritable bowel syndrome, asthma). It is sexism that perpetuates these disparities.

Ed de St. Aubin and Alexandria Colburn

See also: Feminist Theory; Gender; Stereotypes, Gender; Stereotypes, Sexual.

Further Reading

Glick, P., & Fiske, S. T. (2012). An ambivalent alliance: Hostile and benevolent sexism as complementary justifications for gender inequity. In J. Dixon & M. Levine (Eds.), *Beyond prejudice: Extending the social psychology of conflict, inequity and social change* (70–88). New York: Cambridge University Press.

Swim, J. K., & Hyers, L. L. (2009). Sexism. In T. D. Nelson (Ed.), *Handbook of prejudice, stereotyping, and discrimination* (407–430). New York: Psychology Press.

Sexology

Rich in its history, sexology is the scientific study of human sexuality. Over recent centuries, the area of expertise has legitimized itself as a scholarly discipline composed of various branches from the field of biology (e.g., anatomy, physiology, evolutionary theory) and the social sciences (e.g., psychology, anthropology, history, philosophy). Periodically trivialized or regarded as obscene, this serious field of study examines sexual diversity of the human condition by means of rigorous scientific research. In search of how "natural" and "healthy" sexuality manifests, sexologists have historically challenged the assumptions and cultural boundaries surrounding sexual behavior and desire. In an attempt to discover the scientific laws of sexuality, early sex research was primarily focused on the construction of a medical model for professional reference regarding what was deemed sexual dysfunction (according to the time period) (McGann, 2011; Roberts, 2011). Since that time, sexological ventures have expanded on both physiological and behavioral research and have provided an array of normalizing evidence used to advocate for the social justice of sexual minorities and, in more recent decades, encourage informative pleasure-based models of instruction.

Although many have sought to analyze the internal and external factors influencing one's sexual health as far back as Hippocrates and Aristotle, modern sexology is an innovation of approximately the past 200 years. Fluctuating motives and parties involved have left a complex legacy across the development of sexology as a professional field. Originally introduced by Elizabeth Osgood Goodrich Willard in 1867, the term "sexology" is often attributed to the early German pioneer Iwan Bloch and his innovative exploration of sexuality as a scientific study. Bloch illustrated the concept of *Sexualwissenschaft* (sexology) in his work *Das Sexualleben unserer Zeit in seinen Beziehungen zur modernen Kultur* (The Sexual Life of Our Time in Its Relations to Modern Civilization, 1908); although the earlier work *Psychopathia Sexualis with Especial Reference to Contrary Sexual Instinct: A Medical Study* (1886) by German psychiatrist Richard Freiherr von Krafft-Ebing is often considered the founding text substantiating sexology as a scientific discipline. Krafft-Ebing's examination of sexual behavior among criminals founded his assertion of four major types of sexual abnormality: lack of sex drive, excessive sex drive, poorly regulated sex drive, and perversions "contrary to sexual instinct." In addition, he coined the terms "sadism," "masochism," and "fetishism" in order to better describe the various activities he deemed perverse.

The groundbreaking work in Europe of the late nineteenth and early twentieth century was also heavily influenced by English physician Henry Havelock Ellis and German physician Magnus Hirschfeld. Ellis's book entitled *Studies in the Psychology of Sex* (1896) popularized the significance of individual and cultural relativity in relation to sexual behaviors and their assumed connotations. This was revolutionary in an era where concepts such as masturbation and homosexuality were severely pathologized. As for Hirschfeld, some of his significant contributions to the field of sexology include the inception of transgender advocacy; publishing the first journal dedicated to sexology, *Sexualwissenschaft* (1908); founding the first society for sexology, *Ärztliche Gesellschaft für Sexualwissenschaft und Eugenik* (Medical Society for Sexual Science and Eugenics, 1913), alongside Bloch; and founding the first institute dedicated to sexual research in Berlin, *Institut für Sexualwissenschaft* (Institute for Sexual Research) (1919).

After the tyrannical Nazi pillaging of medical collections and scientific contributions of Jewish scholars, Europe relinquished the lead in sexological developments of the early twentieth century to American scholars such as Alfred Kinsey. While Hirschfeld's notoriously extensive data collections supported many of Kinsey's subsequent findings, it was Kinsey's meticulously unprecedented research that would ultimately set the standards for modern sexology. His books *Sexual Behavior of the Human Male* (1948) and *Sexual Behavior of the Human Female* (1953), known as "The Kinsey Reports," took the world by storm as he exposed myths regarding the frequency of premarital and extramarital sex, the presence of same-sex behavior, and the publicly muted capacity of female arousal (Kinsey et al., 1948, 1953). In addition, the introduction of Kinsey's Continuum of Sexual Orientation, aptly known as "The Kinsey Scale," familiarized the public with a more fluid space between homosexuality and heterosexuality, which was later expanded on by Fritz Klein. Klein's expansion measured seven separate components of sexuality (attraction, behavior, fantasies, lifestyle, emotional preference, social preference, and self-identification) as they relate to a person's past, present, and ideal future for a more comprehensive representation of experiential variation. Klein also published *The Bisexual Option: A Concept of One Hundred Percent Intimacy* (1978), based on his original research, and founded the *Journal of Bisexuality* (1999).

Also similar to Kinsey's studies was the work of Dr. William Masters and Virginia Johnson, who began conducting laboratory research in the late 1950s. With the evolution of technology, Masters and Johnson were able to thoroughly explore physiological response during sexual arousal and sexual intercourse. Their book *Human Sexual Response* (1966) continued to dispel colloquial assumptions, much like the work of Alfred Kinsey. Innovative equipment developed by Masters and Johnson allowed the pair to measure a variety of physiological responses, the most peculiar of which included a transparent phallic mechanism equipped with a small camera in order to record vaginal contractions.

Decades after the work of Masters and Johnson, the scientific research of Helen Singer Kaplan further explored sexual functioning with particular focus surrounding dysfunction and desire. Kaplan's three-phase model of sexual response addressed desire as a significant component of the human sexual response cycle and sexual functioning. Her books *The New Sex Therapy* (1974) and *Disorders of Sexual Desire* (1979) afforded countless therapists scientific explanation and treatment interventions for practical application. This movement toward pleasure-based functioning, and away from behavioral pathology, continued with the hands-on body work of Betty Dodson. Dodson's work during and after the sexual revolution included the formation of BodySex Workshops for guided exploration and masturbation instruction for women (Hooper & Holford, 2004); subsequently, male body workshops to address performance anxiety were later adapted (Hooper & Holford, 2004). Some more well-known pleasure-based contributions to the field include the work of John Perry and Beverly Whipple in their exploration of Grafenberg spot (G-spot) functions; Dr. Ruth Westheimer's promotion of sexual literacy and better interpersonal communication within sexual relationships; and Sue Johanson's candid sex education and popularized endorsement of sexual health aids such as sex toys.

The complexity of contemporary sexuality has far surpassed the limited notions of conception, coital positions, and sexual orientation many might assume. Although often faced with censorship, the greater purpose of sexology has not been short-lived. Comprehensive biopsychosocial considerations have expanded the field further than any intentions of early contributors, far beyond what many of them may have even been able to anticipate. At this point, sexology has grown from an attempt to adequately quantify and categorize the operations of reproductive body parts and human behavior into a theoretical exploration of sexuality as its own social phenomena.

Ilyssa Boseski

See also: Desire, Models of; Dodson, Betty; Ellis, Henry Havelock; Hirschfeld, Magnus; Johnson, Virginia; Kaplan, Helen Singer; Kaplan's Triphasic Model; Kinsey, Alfred; Kinsey's Continuum of Sexual Orientation; Krafft-Ebing, Richard von; Masters and Johnson Four-Stage Model of Sexual Response; *Sexual Behavior in the Human Male* and *Sexual Behavior in the Human Female*; Society for the Scientific Study of Sexuality (SSSS).

Further Reading

Bullough, V. L. (1994). *Science in the bedroom: A history of sex research.* New York: Basic Books.

Haeberle, E. J. (1983). *The birth of sexology: A brief history in documents.* (n.p.)

Hoenig, J. (1977). Dramatic personae: Selected biographical sketches of 19th century pioneers in sexology. In J. Money and H. Musaph (Eds.), *Handbook of sexology* (21–43). Holland: Elsevier/North Holland Biomedical Press.

Hooper, A., & Holford, J. (2004). *Anne Hooper's Sexology 101: From Victorian transvestites to '70's swingers and internet Viagra.* Berkeley, CA: Ulysses Press.

Kinsey, A. C., Pomeroy, W. R., & Martin, C. E. (1948). *Sexual behavior in the human male.* Bloomington: Indiana University Press.

Kinsey, A. C., Pomeroy, W. R., Martin, C. E., & Gebhard, P. H. (1953). *Sexual behavior in the human female.* Bloomington: Indiana University Press.

Kuefler, M. (2007). *The history of sexuality sourcebook.* Orchard Park, NY: Broadview Press.

McGann, P. J. (2011). Healing (disorderly) desire: Medical-therapeutic regulation of sexuality. In S. Siedman, N. Fischer, & C. Meeks (Eds.), *Introducing the new sexuality studies* (427–437). New York: Routledge Taylor & Francis Group.

Oosterhuis, H. (2000). *Stepchildren of nature: Krafft-Ebing, psychiatry, and the making of sexual identity.* Chicago: Chicago University Press.

Roberts, C. (2011). Medicine and the making of a sexual body. In S. Siedman, N. Fischer, & C. Meeks (Eds.), *Introducing the new sexuality studies* (67–74). New York: Routledge Taylor & Francis Group.

Siedman, S. (2011). Theoretical perspectives. In S. Siedman, N. Fischer, & C. Meeks (Eds.), *Introducing the new sexuality studies* (3–12). New York: Routledge Taylor & Francis Group.

Siedman, S., Fischer, N., & Meeks, C. (2011). *Introducing the new sexuality studies* (2nd ed.). New York: Routledge Taylor & Francis Group.

Szuchman, L. T., & Muscarella, F. (Eds.). (2000). *Psychological perspectives on human sexuality.* New York: John Wiley & Sons.

Yarber, W. L., Sayad, B. A., & Strong, B. (2010). *Human sexuality: Diversity in contemporary America* (7th ed.). New York: McGraw-Hill.

Sexting

Sexting is the "willing interactive exchange of sexual-oriented messages using a digital mobile communications device" (Manning, 2013). As that definition suggests, several elements must come together for sexting to occur. It must be consensual, meaning that both the sender and receivers of sext messages want to participate. A person sending a sext message to another person who does not want it would not be considered sexting. Sexting must also be interactive. If a person were simply making sexual messages for himself or herself to read, that would not be sexting. The messages involved with sexting are sexually oriented, whether that is explicitly sexual statements or images or even subtle hints about sex. Finally, sexting involves mobile communications devices such as cell phones. Sexual interaction on a home computer or laptop would be cybersex, as the device is not as portable.

Although most studies now demonstrate that a majority of adults sext, initial studies about sexting were inconsistent in showing how many people were sexting. The accepted explanation for this is that many of these studies did not offer a clear definition of sexting. Sexting is also considered to be a cultural practice, meaning that people in different areas and communities might be more likely to sext than people from others.

Research reveals that people sext for many reasons. These include exploring possibilities of what their partners enjoy sexually, using the sext messages for self-pleasure, or simply to pass time.

Early studies about sexting mostly focused on adolescent sexting practices. These studies examined the harms of sexting, such as the possibility for nude photos shared during sexting to be shared with others, causing hurt or humiliation. These studies found that many young people were practicing sexting, and, as one might expect, people tend to sext more as they approach adulthood. Some scholars have critiqued these studies as alarmist because they only focused on the negative aspects of sexting and might overstate the harms.

Legal scholars have also researched sexting, placing a focus on how sexting would be interpreted under laws that were created before sexting existed. This includes questions about age of consent, or when, legally, people are old enough to sext. Legal scholars have also pointed out how sharing sext images of underage adults could be considered as the illegal distribution of child pornography.

Because sexting is a relatively new practice, sexting research about both adults and adolescents is still in its early stages. Although researchers have some good ideas about how many people sext and why, they still have much to learn about sexting. Given that adolescents do run into problems with sexting, most of the research will probably investigate their sexting habits. Other researchers have started examining how sexting can be beneficial for adults, especially when it comes to exploring sexual needs and desires.

Jimmie Manning

See also: Adolescent Sexuality; Age of Consent; Online Dating; Online Sexual Activity.

Further Reading

Döring, N. (2014). Consensual sexting among adolescents: Risk prevention through abstinence education or safer sexting? *Cyberpsychology: Journal of Psychosocial Research on Cyberspace, 8*(1), article 9.

Humbach, J. A. (2010). Sexting and the First Amendment. *Hastings Constitutional Law Quarterly, 37*, 433–486.

Lounsbury, K., Mitchell, K. J., & Finkelhor, D. (2011). The true prevalence of "sexting." Retrieved from http://www.unh.edu/ccrc/pdf/Sexting%20Fact%20Sheet%204_29_11.pdf

Manning, J. (2013). Interpretive theorizing in the seductive world of sexuality and interpersonal communication: Getting guerilla with studies of sexting and purity rings. *International Journal of Communication, 7*, 2507–2520.

Sexual Abuse

Sexual abuse is defined as any sexual act or game where the aggressor is at a more advanced psychosexual stage in life than the intended victim or is in a position of power over the intended victim. It is also sometimes referred to as molestation, sexual violence, or sexual victimization. Sexual abuse can include acts where physical contact does not take place, such as harassment, taking photographs, or showing unwanted sexual material. Research on sexual abuse has increased over the past few decades. Often, "sexual abuse" is used as an umbrella term for all types of sexual violence. However, sexual abuse can be looked at as a sexual encounter that lacks consent, equality, respect, trust, and safety. Sexual abuse in research is mainly studied as sexual violence that occurs between an adult and a child (eighteen years old and below). Sexual assault can also be sexual violence that takes place between adults. It is also important to know that not all sexual abuse is traumatic or all reactions severe; each experience is different for the individual and should be understood and treated as such.

The majority of sexual abuse victims do not report the assault, so it can be difficult to know or even estimate the prevalence. Some research has shown that sexual abuse is reported by 28–30 percent of women. Research has also shown that 12 percent of men and 17 percent of women were sexually abused before adolescence.

Survivors of sexual abuse may show a number of negative symptoms throughout their life, such as mental health problems, substance abuse, suicidal thoughts/attempts, and sexual dysfunctions. One area that seems to be strongly affected by sexual abuse is intimate partner relationships. Research shows that in a relationship where one partner has suffered from childhood sexual abuse, victims may have poor attachment boundaries, decreased levels of communication within the relationship, less understanding of each other, and a loss of connection and cohesion over the trauma. Also, trauma transmission may is likely to appear within these same relationships. Due to a lack of relationship and sexual satisfaction among sexual abuse victims, they become more likely to be in high-conflict relationships or to avoid sexual and intimate relationships all together.

Sexual harassment includes unwelcomed sexual advances, sexual requests, and other sexual conduct and is considered a type of sexual abuse when the abuser is in a position of power over the victim. Sexual harassment can happen in the workplace, between teachers and students, between doctors and patients, and in any other setting where the abuser holds power over the victim prior to the onset of the abuse. Studies have shown that 41 percent of women and 32 percent of men have experienced sexual harassment in the workplace at least once.

Childhood sexual abuse is any form of sexual activity that takes place with a minor and is a form of child abuse. This abuse can occur in a variety of ways and does not have to involve physical contact. A child cannot give consent to engage in sexual acts because of their age. Types of childhood sexual abuse can include but are not limited to digital interactions (sexting or phone calls that are sexual in nature); fondling or touching the child; exposing oneself to the child; masturbating in front of or forcing the child to masturbate; intercourse of any kind (oral, vaginal, or anal); having, seeing, or sharing any type of images or videos of children with sexual content; sex trafficking; or any other sexual misconduct that can be harmful to a child. Any of these actions can lead to legal consequences, and each state in the United States has its own varying legal definition of child sexual abuse.

Starting in 2002, development of a sexual abuse scandal in the Catholic Church was detailed in the media. Many individuals came forward, stating that they had been abused by their priests and clergymen when they were children. This type of sexual abuse not only dealt with the abuser being in a position of power over their victim but was also a form of childhood sexual abuse due to the victims being below the age of consent.

Individuals who have developmental disabilities are more likely to be sexually abused. The perpetrators are usually known to the victims and may be family members, friends, service providers, psychiatrists, personal care staff, or residential care staff. It is important to note that oftentimes this abuse goes undiscovered due to the lack of oversight of care and lack of sexual education and consent taught to the victims.

Help from individual therapy and counseling has been shown to lessen the symptoms of the trauma and can help victims become survivors. There have been numerous studies on how individual therapy works with sexual abuse survivors. Research has showed that using eye movement desensitization and reprocessing individual therapy with survivors had long-lasting gains and improved the symptoms of sexual abuse trauma. Little research has been done on how couples therapy could help relationship satisfaction for a couple where one partner is a survivor of sexual abuse. One theoretical foundation that has been helpful for survivors of sexual abuse, as well as couples, is narrative therapy.

Amanda Baker

See also: Child Sexual Abuse; Date Rape; Incest; Psychosexual Therapy; Rape; Rape Trauma Syndrome; Roman Catholic Church Sexual Abuse Scandal; Sexual Assault; Sexual Consent; Sexual Harassment.

Further Reading

Cobia, D., Sobansky, R., & Ingram, M. (2004). Female survivors of childhood sexual abuse: Implications for couples' therapists. *The Family Journal, 12*(3), 312–318.

Crooks, R., & Baur, K. (2005). *Our sexuality.* Belmont, CA: Thomson/Wadsworth.

Edmond, T., & Rubin, A. (2004). Assessing the long-term effects of EMDR: Results from an 18-month follow-up study with adult female survivors of CSA. *Journal of Child Sexual Abuse, 13*(1), 69–86.

Habigzang, L. F., & Koller, S. H. (2013). Evaluation of the therapeutic process in cases of sexual abuse. *Revista Latinoamericana de Psicologia, 45*(2), 201–210.

Jeary, K. (2005). Sexual abuse and sexual offending against elderly people: A focus on perpetrators and victims. *Journal of Forensic Psychiatry & Psychology, 16*(2), 328–343.

Kane, M. N. (2008). Investigating attitudes of Catholic priests toward the media and the US Conference of Catholic Bishops response to the sexual abuse scandals of 2002. *Mental Health, Religion & Culture, 11*(6), 579–595.

King, B. M. (2012). *Human sexuality today* (7th ed.). Upper Saddle River, NJ: Prentice Hall.

Mahoney, A., & Poling, A. (2011). Sexual abuse prevention for people with severe developmental disabilities. *Journal of Developmental & Physical Disabilities, 23*(4), 369–376.

RAINN. (2019). Child sexual abuse. Retrieved from https://www.rainn.org/get-information/types-of-sexual-assault/child-sexual-abuse

Sexual Assault

Sexual assault is a coerced or forced sexual act between two people where one is engaged in the activity against their will. This is a form of sexual violence and sexual victimization and can happen in a number of ways. Sexual assault includes rape (forced oral, vaginal, or anal penetration or by use of a date rape drug), sexual activities with a minor, fondling, unwanted kissing, or any form of unwanted sexual torture. Sexual assault is a crime, and each U.S. state has its own varying legal definition. "Sexual assault" can also be used as an umbrella term for sexual abuse, sexual violence, and sexual victimization. "Sexual assault" is the usual wording for legal definitions. Research often differentiates between sexual assault and sexual abuse by stating that sexual assault refers to sexual violence that takes place between adults while sexual abuse is sexual victimization that takes place between a victim and someone with power.

Rape is a form of sexual assault that can include oral, anal, or vaginal penetration through actual or threat of physical, emotional, or psychological harm and coercion without consent from the victim. Rape can happen to anyone of any gender, age, or sexual orientation. "Rape" is often used interchangeably with "sexual assault." Definitions of rape differ from state to state and between federal agencies. The common theme of rape is the offender's willingness to disrespect the victim's right to consent and to take advantage of a nonconsenting individual.

Date rape drugs are drugs or alcohol used to hinder a person's ability to consent to sexual activity. This is called drug-facilitated sexual assault. Any drug that can affect a person's judgment and behavior can be a date rape drug. There are many different types of drugs that can be used, and drug-facilitated sexual assault takes place not only on dates but also while out with friends at a bar and in many other scenarios. Alcohol is the most common drug used. Other date rape drugs are gamma hydroxybutyrate (GHB), Rohypnol (roofies), and ketamine (Special K). It is important to know that regardless of the drug used or a person's behavior, a victim is not to be blamed for what happened.

Sexual assault is one of the biggest public health concerns on college campuses. Anywhere from 20–25 percent of females are sexually assaulted in some way during their undergraduate years. Sexual assault on college campuses has gained national attention within the last few years and has gained a lot of research attention as well. Sexual assault on college campuses includes harassment, rape, date rape, and other forms. Many universities have started to look at the use of violence prevention education and modalities to help decrease the frequency of sexual assaults on campuses.

Amanda Baker

See also: Child Sexual Abuse; Date Rape; Rape; Rape Trauma Syndrome; Sexual Abuse; Sexual Consent; Sexual Harassment.

Further Reading

Crooks, R., & Baur, K. (2005). *Our sexuality.* Belmont, CA: Thomson/Wadsworth.

Exner, D., & Cummings, N. (2011). Implications for sexual assault prevention: College students as prosocial bystanders. *Journal of American College Health, 59*(7), 655–657.

King, B. M. (2012). *Human sexuality today* (7th ed.). Upper Saddle River, NJ: Prentice Hall.

RAINN. (2019). Drug-facilitated sexual assault. Retrieved from https://rainn.org/get-information/types-of-sexual-assault/drug-facilitated-assault

Sexual Avoidance

"Sexual avoidance" refers to actively avoiding all sexual activity. Unlike a motivation to abstain from sexual activity for religious reasons or due to particular circumstances (e.g., to focus on other aspects of life or because the individual is not in a relationship), the term "sexual avoidance" is typically used to describe the avoidance of sexual activity motivated by feelings of anxiety, fear, or shame.

In some cases, sexual avoidance is a result of hypoactive sexual desire (desire that is persistently deficient or absent); sexual activity is avoided because the person has no interest in engaging in it. Men and women with other sexual dysfunctions may engage in sexual avoidance in order to avoid an unsatisfactory sexual encounter. For example, men with erectile disorder may take steps to ensure they do not have sex with their partner, such as going to bed after the partner has gone to sleep and not initiating sex or even nonsexual contact for fear that it may lead to sex. At times, the partner of the person with the sexual dysfunction may also avoid sexual activity as a means of avoiding rejection or a disappointing sexual encounter.

Sexual aversion disorder is another possible cause of sexual avoidance. With sexual aversion disorder, the avoidance of sexual activity goes beyond a lack of interest or a desire to avoid an unsatisfactory sexual encounter. People with sexual aversion disorder may be mistaken for having low desire, but aversion includes an intense fear or revulsion of some or all sexual activities, a type of phobic response.

Some people use the term "sexual anorexia" as a synonym for sexual avoidance. Used in this manner, sexual avoidance is seen as similar to sex addiction. With sex addiction, individuals are seen as acting out sexually to avoid negative feelings and intimacy. With sexual anorexia, individuals are seen as acting in by cutting themselves off from sex and intimacy. Rather than a lack of desire or phobic response preventing sexual activity, the individual avoids sex out of compulsion.

Sexual avoidance is diagnosed through the use of a thorough sexual history. Treatment for the condition typically consists of sex therapy, a specialized form of psychotherapy or talk therapy. Therapy includes the attempt to determine the cause of the avoidant behavior, and treatment is determined based on this cause. In the case of sexual aversion, antianxiety medication combined with systematic desensitization may be used. Systematic desensitization involves gradual exposure to the situations that cause the phobic response while using relaxation techniques to reduce anxiety.

Treatment for sexual dysfunctions such as low desire, erectile disorder, premature ejaculation, and pain disorders may include medical intervention and sex therapy. Sexual avoidance may cause significant distress for the individual and for their partner if they are in a relationship. A component of the sex therapy treatment may include couple therapy to address the impact of the avoidant behavior and to improve any relational factors that may be contributing to or maintaining the problem.

Adrienne M. Bairstow

See also: Abstinence; Desire Disorders; Erotophilia and Erotophobia; Psychosexual Therapy; Sex Guilt; Sexual Dysfunction, Treatment of.

Further Reading

Encyclopedia of Mental Disorders. (2019). Sexual aversion disorder. Retrieved fromhttp://www.minddisorders.com/Py-Z/Sexual-aversion-disorder.html

Hartney, E. (2018). What you should know about sexual anorexia. Retrieved from http://addictions.about.com/od/sexaddiction/a/what_is_sexual_anorexia.htm

Katehakis, A. (2014). The devasting pain of "sexual anorexics." Retrieved from https://www.psychologytoday.com/blog/sex-lies-trauma/201408/sexual-anorexia-the-shadow-addiction

Sexual Behavior in the Human Male and *Sexual Behavior in the Human Female*

Published in 1948, *Sexual Behavior in the Human Male*, and its companion published in 1953, *Sexual Behavior in the Human Female*, are collectively known as "The Kinsey Reports." They were written by Alfred Kinsey and colleagues based on his studies of human sexual behavior. The books were the first to bring the study of human sexuality to the public and mainstream media and were associated with a shift in public attitudes toward sex and sexuality.

In 1938, Alfred Kinsey was teaching a marriage course at Indiana University. His students wanted to learn a wide range of topics surrounding marriage, and they wanted the course to include both male and female students. To learn more about his students, Kinsey required them to fill out a survey about their sexual histories. Members of the Indiana University faculty disliked what Kinsey was teaching, and the research he was doing along with it, so they petitioned the president of the university to remove him from the course. The president gave Kinsey a choice to keep his class or do research but not both. Kinsey chose the research.

Kinsey's research team included Clyde Martin, who handled the statistical analysis; Wardell Pomeroy, a psychologist; and Paul Gebhard, a trained anthropologist. Providing almost all the data were 5,994 females and 5,300 males, with the majority of participants being younger white adults with some college education. Kinsey used in-depth, face-to-face interviews by highly trained interviewers. In each interview, a subject would be questioned about their history on up to 521 items, depending on their specific experience. Histories covered social and economic data, physical and physiologic data, marital histories, sexual outlets, heterosexual histories, and homosexual histories.

Sexual Behavior in the Human Male became a best seller, making Kinsey a household name. Included in the male Kinsey Report was Kinsey's heterosexual-homosexual rating scale, better known simply as the Kinsey Scale. Kinsey reported that people did not fit into neat and exclusive heterosexual and homosexual categories but that sexual behavior, thoughts, and feeling are inconsistent across time.

Other topics of the book included anal sex, bisexuality, coitus, erogenous zones, extramarital sex, fantasy, foreplay, homosexuality, masturbation, nudity, oral sex, orgasm, peak performance or maximum sexual activity, premarital sex, sadomasochism, and sex with prostitutes. The controversial and shocking findings challenged conventional beliefs about sexuality and other taboo topics. While some criticized Kinsey's research as an unsuitable public topic, others criticized his research methods. One critique was on his sampling method. Some believed his sample was not a true representation of the U.S. population since he mostly interviewed college students, prostitutes, and prison inmates.

The most important contribution of the female edition was the exploration of basic male-female similarities and differences. Kinsey broke the myth that women merely engaged in sex for procreation or to please their male partners. While the female sexual behavior findings advocated for female sexuality, outrage again broke out over the findings, as it had over the male version. Critiques again questioned his research methods, arguing that the statistics could not be accurate because good women would not engage in the activities that are discussed in the book or, if they had, they would not have revealed their experiences to Dr. Kinsey.

Lauren Ewaniuk

See also: Kinsey, Alfred; Kinsey's Continuum of Sexual Orientation.

Further Reading

Kinsey, A. C., Pomeroy, W. R., & Martin, C. E. (1948). *Sexual behavior in the human male.* Bloomington: Indiana University Press.

Kinsey, A. C., Pomeroy, W. R., Martin, C. E., & Gebhard, P. H. (1953). *Sexual behavior in the human female.* Bloomington: Indiana University Press.

Sexual Consent

Consent, the ability to make fully informed decisions, is a human right, essential to our sexual rights of sexual autonomy and bodily integrity. According to the World Association of Sexual Health, "Everyone has the right to control and decide freely on matters related to their sexuality and their body. This includes the choice of sexual behaviors, practices, partners and relationships with due regard to the rights of others. Free and informed decision making requires free and informed consent prior to any sexually-related testing, interventions, therapies, surgeries, or research." Informed consent and sexual consent describe the process of ensuring our sexual right to freely choose to participate in sex-related interventions or research and to pursue sexual activity, respectively.

Informed consent precedes participation in sexuality-related research or sexuality-related testing and interventions. Informed consent has three dimensions: ensuring individuals have the competence to provide consent, understand the activities to which they consent, and are participating entirely voluntarily. In research, for example, researchers inform the participant about the purpose of the research project, the activities expected of participants, and the potential benefits and risks. Researchers carry the responsibility to ensure that participants have understood the procedures and are competent to make a qualified choice about their participation. Participation is completely voluntary; participants have the right to decline or withdraw from the study at any time. This informed consent process mirrors sexual consent.

Sexual consent is a conscious, clear, voluntary agreement to pursue sexual activity and other sex-related matters. Like informed consent, a person must have a thorough understanding of the sexual activities that will be pursued as well as the risks and benefits of engaging in such activities. At the time of consent, individuals must have the capacity to fully comprehend the meaning of the sexual activity and its social, emotional, and physical consequences. Sexual consent requires that individuals must be willing and freely agree to participate at the outset and throughout the duration of the activity. Crucially, individuals have the right to decline or withdraw from sexual activities at any time, for any reason, and without any aversive consequences.

This definition indicates that pursuing sexual activity with a person who lacks the ability to provide consent is nonconsensual. Legally, individuals are unable to provide consent when they are mentally incapacitated (e.g., severe cognitive disabilities, intoxicated from substances or alcohol), physically helpless (e.g., unconscious, sleeping), lack independence (e.g., children), or otherwise lack comprehension of the significance of sexual activity. The requirement of clear, voluntary agreement means that sexual consent can never be assumed based on subtle cues or context. Legally, consent cannot be supposed from a person's silence or failure to resist sexual activity. When a partner says "stop," "I'm not sure," or "maybe later," or is silent, pulls away, or acts ambivalent in any way, they are declining consent. Moreover, flirtation, sexy clothing, sexual settings (e.g., strip club, sex party, sex work), and prior or existing sexual or romantic relationships do *not* imply consent. Finally, if a person initially consents to sexual activity and withdraws consent for any reason, at any point during sexual activity, continued sexual activity is nonconsensual. Essentially, pursuing sexual activity without clear consent is nonconsensual and constitutes sexual coercion and violence, which violates both the sexual health principles and the law.

Importantly, sexual consent, which describes willingness and agreement to engage in sexual activity, differs from sexual desire or "wanting" to engage in the activity. Individuals may want to engage in sexual activity or experience physiological arousal (e.g., erection, lubrication, increase in heart rate) without being willing to participate in sexual activity. Ensuring a person's willingness, in addition to pleasure, safeguards pleasurable, safe, consensual sexual experiences.

Most people effortlessly obtain sexual consent, although some believe sexual consent is complicated. Researchers argue that gendered expectations and sexual double standards contribute to this belief. In the United States, individuals receive vastly different sociocultural messages about sexuality based on gender. Feminine individuals receive messages around risk and immorality, while, paradoxically, equating their worth with sexual prowess (e.g., look "hot" but not "slutty"; be popular but not prudish). Feminine ideals to be "nice" and passive conflict with pressure to firmly resist sexual activity. In contrast, masculine individuals face pressure to be constantly interested in and ready for sexual activity, are taught to persistently seek sexual activity, and gain social status through acquiring sexual experiences. These gendered messages are associated with traditional sexual scripts (heterosexual norms for negotiating sexual activity), which portray that the person who initiates sexual activity (usually a masculine individual) assumes that their partner (usually a feminine individual) consents, until the partner refuses the initiator's advances. Research has demonstrated that sexual consent occurs less often when individuals more strongly adhere to gendered expectations and traditional sexual scripts. In addition, same-gender partners who lack social norms to guide their sexual behavior are more likely to obtain sexual consent than those in heterosexual relationships.

Sexual consent can become complicated when individuals feel uncertain or lack effective communication to express their unwillingness (due to intoxication or confusion, the behavior happening too quickly to refuse, etc.). Moreover, individuals may be concerned about the social consequences of refusing (e.g., hurting the other's feelings). Research has shown that while people believe a direct verbal "no" is the most effective way to refuse, saying no can feel awkward and embarrassing. As a result, many people soften their refusals ("I'm not ready yet," "I like you, but . . . ," or give excuses rather than state their unwillingness), which leads to confusion. As such, individuals should assume nonconsent until clear, unambiguous sexual consent is granted.

A popular myth about consent is the erroneous belief that obtaining verbal consent will "kill the mood." Yet, the "mood" of sexual activity depends on the ability to actively attend and respond to one's partner's verbal and nonverbal expressions of sexual willingness and enjoyment. Sexual pleasure diminishes when individuals do not attend to or ignore the verbal and nonverbal expressions of their partner. Moreover, research has demonstrated that the vast majority of people report consenting to their last sexual encounter *both* nonverbally *and* verbally. Nonverbal indicators of consent include a *combination* of direct (undressing themselves or their partner, touching their partner) and indirect nonverbal behaviors (not resisting their partner's attempts while *also* reciprocating their partner's advances, caressing, getting closer). When combined with verbal indicators of consent (e.g., expressing desire and willingness), the sexual consent process can enhance the "mood."

The sexual consent process begins with obtaining a clear agreement to initiate a specific sexual activity, agreeing to progress to more intimate activities, and stopping sexual activity when consent becomes unclear or is withdrawn. As a preliminary step, individuals need to understand their feelings, boundaries, and degree of willingness to engage in specific sexual behaviors with their partner. To initiate sexual activity, these feelings are expressed to the partner(s), verbally and nonverbally. Consent is an ongoing process, involving continuously observing one's partner's enjoyment and willingness and seeking additional agreement to progress to more intimate behaviors. Suppose an individual obtained consent to unbutton their partner's shirt. As an ongoing process, they would observe their partner's facial expressions and bodily movements as they move from one button to the next, looking for evidence of pleasure versus discomfort, using nonverbal and verbal cues. Sexual behavior proceeds when individuals and partners exhibit clear willingness and pleasure, and it stops when the individual's *or* their partner's pleasure and willingness become unclear or withdrawn (silence, pulling away, looking away, saying no, slowing down, not actively participating, etc.). Inquiring about the other's feelings after stopping sexual activity facilitates clarity while easing social awkwardness. This process affirms everyone's right to freely choose or withdraw from sexual activity, at any time, without negative consequences. The key to mutually positive sexual interactions is to be sensitive to your partner's desires, needs, and willingness.

Sexual consent is a fundamental right. Each person has the responsibility to ensure that they have the consent of others. Sexual consent safeguards everyone's bodily integrity and the right to have safe, consensual sexual interactions. Wanted, pleasurable, consensual sex is abundantly more satisfying that nonconsensual sex. By ensuring that all parties involved are willing and freely enjoying themselves, sexual consent maximizes the capacity for sexual pleasure.

Janna A. Dickenson and Itor Finotelli Jr.

See also: Age of Consent; Communication, Sexual; Rape; Sexual Assault; Sexual Rights; Sexual Script; Statutory Rape.

Further Reading

Archard, D. (1998). *Sexual consent.* Boulder, CO: Westview Press.

Kismödi, E., Corona, E., Maticka-Tyndale, E., Rubio-Aurioles, E., & Coleman, E. (2017). Sexual rights as human rights: A guide for the WAS declaration of sexual rights. *International Journal of Sexual Health, 29*(Supl), 1–92. doi: 10.1080/19317611.2017.1353865

Muehlenhard, C. L., Humphreys, T. P., Jozkowski, K. N., & Peterson, Z. D. (2016). The complexities of sexual consent among college students: A conceptual and empirical review. *The Journal of Sex Research, 53*(4–5), 457–487.

Sexual Dimorphism

"Sexual dimorphism" refers to the anatomical differences between males and females of the same species, excluding their sexual organs. Multitudes of animal species are sexually dimorphic, including humans. The opposite of sexual dimorphism is sexual monomorphism, which is when males and females of the same species appear identical except for their sexual organs. Sexual dimorphism is manifested in a variety of different ways, including size, coloration, and secondary sex characteristics. Sexual dimorphism stems from evolution and is often a result of sexual selection. While there are apparent physical differences between human males and females, they are more physically similar to one another when compared to the level of differentiation in many other species.

Sexual dimorphism is a result of evolution. In a sexually dimorphic species, each sex has evolved to further traits that are advantageous and reduce traits that are not. It is thought that sexual selection is an evolutionary mode of driving sexual dimorphism. Sexual selection is a form of natural selection; members of one sex look for certain characteristics in the other sex when choosing mates. This interaction results in differences between the sexes, because the favorable characteristics in each sex are increasingly passed on genetically over time. For example, the females of a species may prefer larger males because this is a visual sign of their capability to fight and survive. Over time, larger males will have more offspring, and so the genes for larger size are passed on to future generations, and, eventually, the males of the species evolve to be larger to compete for female attraction. It is hypothesized that sexual selection may be the reason human females have larger breasts filled with fatty tissue. Humans are the only mammals in which females always have breasts—not only during lactation. Therefore, it is thought that female humans evolved to have breasts as a signal of fertility to attract mates.

Sexual dimorphism can be expressed in visually extreme ways or in subtle ways. For example, male and female peafowl look dramatically different: the males display ornate tail feathers, while the females have subdued feathers. As another example, mandrills have different coloration on their faces and are extremely different in size. In humans, the sexes are more similar to one another when compared to many species with extremely different appearances. For example, human males are typically larger than females, but the difference is not as pronounced as it is in many primates, like the mandrills.

Nevertheless, there are apparent differences between human males and females. As previously mentioned, males are generally larger than females. According to the National Health Statistic Reports, males in the United States are 9 percent taller than females on average. In development, females go through puberty at an earlier age, and they are typically taller than males in early adolescence. In addition, males have a higher percentage of muscle mass than females. Females store more fat on their bodies, partially due to having a lower average basal metabolic rate than males.

Secondary sex characteristics are also examples of sexual dimorphism in humans. These are characteristics that typically appear during puberty but are not part of the reproductive system. For example, females have larger breasts, wider hips, and a distribution of fat deposits around the buttocks, hips, and thighs. These differences are due to females having a higher level of estrogen than males. Females also tend to have rounder features, such as face shape, and softer, plumper skin. In turn, males have broader shoulders and a lower body fat percentage than females. Males grow facial hair, and they often have thicker body hair present on areas such as the chest and back. Also, males have a larger larynx, commonly known as an Adam's apple. Males also have more testosterone, which aids in increasing muscle mass and the length of vocal cords and growing facial and body hair.

Sexual dimorphism in the brains of human males and females is a controversial subject. Overall, scientists have found greater similarities between male and female brains than they have found differences. However, researchers have found some significant differences as well. Male brains tend to be slightly larger in volume than female brains on average. Researchers have attempted to determine which structures of either sex's brain have more or less volume and tissue density, but it has proven to be difficult research. A study of 2,750 females and 2,466 males found differences in the thickness of cortices—the researchers found that women have thicker cortices on average than males. The same study found that volumes of subcortical regions were higher in males than females; these subcortical regions included the hippocampus and amygdala. Scientists have long attempted to determine if anatomical brain differences may be attributed to behavioral or intelligence differences between males and females, but no conclusions can be drawn with certainty.

Sexual dimorphism is widely variable among human males and females. The different characteristics between males and females do not occur in the same proportion for each individual. In addition, an estimated 1.7 percent of the population is intersex—people born with sexual anatomy and characteristics that do not fit the typical presentation for male or female. Furthermore, gender identity is a complicated topic and is increasingly discussed in today's society. Sex is assigned at birth, but someone's personal gender identity does not always correspond with the gender typically assigned to one's sex. Essentially, an individual's anatomical presentation is not always an indicator of their gender identity. Some transgender people may choose to undergo a transition process. This sometimes includes hormone replacement therapy and/or sex reassignment surgery. Both can result in an individual's sex characteristics and anatomy being altered to fit the desired presentation of their gender identity. Therefore, characteristics differentiating male and female humans are not always as clearly determined as they may be in nonhuman animals.

Sexual dimorphism is found across the spectrum of animal species and can include extreme differences as well as less obvious ones. The range of differentiation also varies widely among individuals, and there are people whose characteristics do not align with the sexual binary. Ultimately, human males and females are more similar than dissimilar.

Casey T. Tobin

See also: Biological Theories of Sexual Orientation; Breast, Female; Evolutionary Perspectives on Gender and Sexual Behavior; Female Sexuality; Gender Identity; Intersexuality; Male Sexuality; Puberty; Sex Differentiation of the Brain and Sexual Orientation.

Further Reading

Leary, C. (2016). Nine of the most dramatic examples of sexual dimorphism. Retrieved from https://www.mnn.com/earth-matters/animals/blogs/9-most-dramatic-examples-sexual-dimorphism

McDowell, M. A., Fryar, C. D., Ogden, C. L., & Flegal, K. M. (2008). Anthropometric reference data for children and adults: United Sates, 2003–2006. *National Health Statistics Reports, 10.* Retrieved from https://cdc.gov/nchs/data/nhsr/nhsr010.pdf

Ritchie, S. J., Cox, S. R., Shen, X., Lombardo, M. V., Reus, L. M., Alloza, C., … Deary, I. J. (2018). Sex differences in the adult human brain: Evidence from 5216 UK Biobank participants. *Cerebral Cortex, 28*(8), 2959–2975.

Viloria, H. (2015). How common is intersex? An explanation of the stats. Retrieved from https://intersexequality.com/how-common-is-intersex-in-humans/

Wolchover, N. (2011). Men vs. women: Our key physical differences explained. Retrieved from https://livescience.com/33513-men-vs-women-our-physical-differences-explained.html

Sexual Disorders, Female

Female sexual disorders are broadly referred to as female sexual dysfunctions. A sexual dysfunction is any physical or psychological problem that affects sexual health and well-being. Female sexual dysfunctions affect one or more aspects of a woman's sexual function and can be related to arousal, desire, orgasm, or pain. In order for a sexual problem to be considered a disorder, it must be persistent, consistent, and cause "clinically significant" distress to the individual. Sexual disorders are defined slightly differently based on the professional setting (medical or psychological, for instance). In the medical field, sexual disorders are classified based on the *International Classification of Diseases, Eleventh Revision* (*ICD-11*). Here, sexual dysfunctions are defined as syndromes that comprise the various ways in which adult people may have difficulty experiencing personally satisfying, noncoercive sexual activities. Sexual response is a complex interaction of psychological, interpersonal, social, cultural and physiological processes and one or more of these factors may affect any stage of the sexual response. In order to be considered a sexual dysfunction, the dysfunction must: 1) occur frequently, although it may be absent on some occasions; 2) have been present for at least several months; and 3) be associated with clinically significant distress (World Health Organization, 2018).

In *ICD-11*, sexual dysfunction is broken down into hypoactive sexual desire dysfunction, sexual arousal dysfunctions, orgasmic dysfunctions, and dysfunctions related to pelvic organ prolapse.

In comparison, for mental health professionals, sexual dysfunctions are defined in the *Diagnostic and Statistical Manual of Mental Disorders, Fifth Edition* (*DSM-5*). Similarly, in the *DSM*, sexual disorders are defined as a "clinically significant disturbance in a person's ability to respond sexually or to experience sexual pleasure. An individual may have several sexual dysfunctions at the same time" (American Psychiatric Association, 2013). Female sexual dysfunctions in the *DSM-5* include female orgasmic disorder, female sexual interest/arousal disorder, and genito-pelvic pain/penetration disorder. If a woman meets criteria for one of these disorders, and her symptoms are not better explained by a psychological or medical condition, her doctor may diagnose her with a sexual disorder and will consider the time of onset (lifelong versus acquired; generalized versus situational) and the severity of the dysfunction (mild, moderate, severe). For instance, if a woman experiences pain with intercourse, a provider would want to understand when this began—whether it has always been an issue (lifelong) or if it has occurred more recently (acquired). The health care provider would also want to better understand if the pain occurs during all kinds of penetration, both sexual and nonsexual (e.g., using tampons or wearing tight clothing) (generalized) or if it is specific to a particular partner or activity such as penetrative intercourse (situational).

There is no single cause of female sexual dysfunctions. When considering treatment, many factors must be considered, including (1) partner factors (e.g., does the partner have any sexual problems or health concerns); (2) relationship factors (e.g., conflict, communication); (3) individual factors (e.g., poor body image, history of abuse, lack of education about sexuality), psychiatric concerns (e.g., anxiety, depression), or current stressors (e.g., job loss, pregnancy); (4) cultural or religious factors (e.g., shame around sexual activity, negative attitudes toward sexuality); and (5) medical factors relevant to prognosis, course, or treatment.

Treatment of female sexual dysfunctions varies depending on the specific dysfunction but can include a thorough medical evaluation and medical interventions such as medications, individual or couple's sex therapy, and pelvic floor physical therapy.

Abby Girard

See also: Anorgasmia; Arousal; Desire Disorders; *Diagnostic and Statistical Manual of Mental Disorders* (*DSM*); Dyspareunia; Female Sexuality; *International Classification of Diseases, Eleventh Revision* (*ICD-11*); Sexual Disorders, Male; Sexual Dysfunction, Treatment of.

Further Reading

American Psychiatric Association. (2013). Diagnostic and statistical manual of mental disorders (5th ed.). Arlington, VA: American Psychiatric Publishing.

Mayo Clinic. (2016). Female sexual dysfunction. Retrieved from https://www.mayoclinic.org/diseases-conditions/female-sexual-dysfunction/symptoms-causes/syc-20372549

World Health Organization. (2018). *International statistical classification of diseases and related health problems* (11th rev.). Retrieved from https://icd.who.int/browse11/l-m/en

Sexual Disorders, Male

Male sexual disorders are broadly referred to as male sexual dysfunctions. A sexual dysfunction is any physical or psychological problem that affects sexual health and well-being. Male sexual dysfunctions can affect all men, but most are more common in men as they age. Male sexual dysfunctions affect one or more aspects of a man's sexual function and can be related to desire, erection, or orgasm. In order for a sexual issue to be considered a disorder, it must be persistent, consistent, and cause "clinically significant" distress to the individual. Sexual disorders are defined slightly differently based on the professional setting (medical or psychological, for instance). In the medical field, sexual disorders are classified based on the *International Classification of Diseases, Eleventh Revision* (*ICD-11*). Here, sexual dysfunctions are defined as syndromes that comprise the various ways in which adult people may have difficulty experiencing personally satisfying, noncoercive sexual activities. Sexual response is a complex interaction of psychological, interpersonal, social, cultural and physiological processes and one or more of these factors may affect any stage of the sexual response. In order to be considered a sexual dysfunction, the dysfunction must: 1) occur frequently, although it may be absent on some occasions; 2) have been present for at least several months; and 3) be associated with clinically significant distress (World Health Organization, 2018).

In *ICD-11*, sexual dysfunction is broken down into hypoactive sexual desire dysfunction, sexual arousal dysfunctions, orgasmic dysfunctions, and dysfunctions related to pelvic organ prolapse.

In comparison, for mental health professionals, sexual dysfunctions are defined in the *Diagnostic and Statistical Manual of Mental Disorders, Fifth Edition* (*DSM-5*). Similarly, in the *DSM* sexual disorders are defined as a "clinically significant disturbance in a person's ability to respond sexually or to experience sexual pleasure. An individual may have several sexual dysfunctions at the same time" (American Psychiatric Association, 2013). Male sexual dysfunctions as classified in *DSM-5* include erectile disorder, delayed ejaculation, male hypoactive sexual desire disorder, and premature (early) ejaculation. If a man meets criteria for one of these disorders, and his symptoms are not better explained by a psychological or medical condition, his doctor may diagnose him with a sexual disorder and will consider the time of onset (lifelong versus acquired; generalized versus situational) and the severity of the dysfunction (mild, moderate, severe). For instance, if a man experiences difficulty with erection, a provider would want to understand when this began—whether it has always been an issue (lifelong) or whether it occurred more recently (acquired). The health care provider would also want to know if the difficulty with erections occurs all the time (e.g., during masturbation and partnered sexual acts, regardless of the partner or situation; generalized) or if the difficulty is specific to a particular partner or activity such as penetrative intercourse only (situational).

There is no single cause of male sexual dysfunctions. When considering treatment, many factors must be considered, including (1) partner factors (e.g., does the partner have any sexual problems or health concerns); (2) relationship factors (e.g., conflict, communication); (3) individual factors (e.g., poor body image, performance anxiety, lack of education about sexuality), psychiatric concerns (e.g., anxiety, depression), or current stressors (e.g., job loss, work stress); (4) cultural or religious factors (e.g., shame around sexual activity, negative attitudes toward sexuality); and (5) medical factors relevant to prognosis, course, or treatment.

Treatment of male sexual dysfunctions varies depending on the specific dysfunction but can include a thorough medical evaluation and treatment with medication, individual or couple's sex therapy, and pelvic floor physical therapy.

Abby Girard

See also: Arousal; Desire Disorders; *Diagnostic and Statistical Manual of Mental Disorders* (*DSM*); Erectile Dysfunction; *International Classification of Diseases, Eleventh Revision* (*ICD-11*); Male Sexuality; Orgasm; Performance Anxiety; Premature Ejaculation; Sexual Disorders, Female; Sexual Dysfunction, Treatment of.

Further Reading

American Psychiatric Association. (2013). *Diagnostic and statistical manual of mental disorders* (5th ed.). Arlington, VA: American Psychiatric Publishing.

Cleveland Clinic. (2019). Sexual dysfunction in males. Retrieved from https://my.clevelandclinic.org/health/diseases/9122-sexual-dysfunction-in-males

Mayo Clinic. (2018). Female sexual dysfunction. Retrieved from https://www.mayoclinic.org/diseases-conditions/female-sexual-dysfunction/symptoms-causes/syc-20372549

World Health Organization. (2018). *International statistical classification of diseases and related health problems* (11th rev.). Geneva: World Health Organization. Retrieved from https://icd.who.int/browse11/l-m/en

Sexual Dysfunction, Treatment of

"Sexual dysfunction" refers to any of a number of problems that may impair a person's sexual ability or sexual satisfaction. Sexual dysfunctions are one category included in the *Diagnostic and Statistical Manual of Mental Disorders* (*DSM*), which includes the following diagnoses for men: delayed ejaculation (ejaculation that takes an extended period of time), erectile disorder (the inability to obtain or maintain an erection sufficient for penetration), male hypoactive sexual desire disorder (lack of or reduced sexual interest), premature (early) ejaculation disorder (ejaculation occurring soon after the start of sexual activity or within one minute of penetration), substance or medication-induced sexual dysfunction, and unspecified sexual dysfunction.

The *DSM* includes the following sexual dysfunction diagnoses for women: female orgasmic disorder (the delay or absence of orgasm, or a reduction in intensity of orgasmic sensations), female sexual interest/arousal disorder (lack of or reduction in sexual interest or arousal), gentio-pelvic pain/penetration disorder (difficulty with vaginal penetration, or pain or fear of pain with penetration), substance/medication-induced sexual dysfunction, and unspecified sexual dysfunction.

Although sexual dysfunctions are included in the *DSM*, the term is more commonly used to refer to conditions that negatively affect an individual's sexual function, regardless of whether they are due to physical, psychological, or combined factors. Even in the case of conditions with biological causes, there are often psychological factors that contribute to or maintain the problem. For example, heart disease may have the physical side effect of erectile disorder. However, once a man experiences erectile disorder on one occasion, he may become anxious about sex. This anxiety can itself lead to erectile disorder even once the physical condition has been resolved. For this reason, sexual dysfunction should be assessed for biological, psychological, and social factors, all of which should be treated for optimal outcome.

Sexual dysfunction often includes impairment of function in one of the phases of the sexual response cycle: excitement, plateau, orgasm, and resolution. It should be noted, however, that sexual pain, while commonly considered a sexual dysfunction, may not impair any of the phases of the sexual response cycle. Sexual dysfunction may also be categorized as lifelong (present from the first sexual experience) or acquired (a condition that developed after a period of problem free sexual activity) and as generalized (occurring with various situations, sexual activities, and partners) or situational (occurring with only some types of situations, activities, and partners).

Treatment for sexual dysfunction begins with a thorough medical history and exam to determine if there are any physical causes for the dysfunction. The prescribed treatment is dependent on the specific sexual impairment. Treatment may include medication (for example, for conditions including premature ejaculation or sexual pain), pelvic physical therapy (for conditions such as sexual pain), and sex therapy (a specialized form of psychotherapy or talk therapy). As mentioned above, even in the cases of biology-based sexual dysfunction, psychological factors may be involved in contributing to or maintaining the problem. As a result, sex therapy can be useful in conjunction with other treatments.

Sex therapy includes a thorough sexual history of both partners. This is important as in some cases both partners have a sexual dysfunction. Assessment will also determine if there are any social factors that contribute to the problem (such as a lack of sexual knowledge or negative views about sex) or relational factors (such as conflict or communication difficulties). It is common for couples affected by sexual dysfunction to engage in sexual avoidance, wherein one or both partners avoids sexual activity in order to avoid being rejected or to avoid a disappointing sexual experience. In some cases, couples begin to avoid even nonsexual touch for fear that it will lead to sex.

A common component of sex therapy treatment for sexual dysfunction includes the use of sensate focus exercises. Sensate focus exercises are a series of nondemand pleasuring activities. Couples are given instructions for each activity and make a commitment to complete the exercises in the privacy of their home at a time when they will not be interrupted. The exercises start with touching activities that do not include the breasts or genitals so that the couple can become accustomed again to intimate touch without the pressure of expectations around erections or orgasms. The goal is merely to experience pleasurable touch. The exercises progress to genital touch and eventually to penetrative sex if possible and desired by the couple.

Adrienne M. Bairstow

See also: Desire Disorders; *Diagnostic and Statistical Manual of Mental Disorders* (*DSM*); Psychosexual Therapy; Sensate Focus; Sexual Satisfaction.

Further Reading

American Psychiatric Association. (2013). *Diagnostic and statistical manual of mental disorders* (5th ed.). Washington, DC: Author.

Cleveland Clinic. (2019). Sexual dysfunction. Retrieved from http://my.clevelandclinic.org/health/diseases/9121-sexual-dysfunction

Pietrangelo, A. (2016). What is sexual dysfunction? Retrieved from http://www.healthline.com/health-slideshow/what-sexual-dysfunction#1

U.S. National Library of Medicine. (2016). Sexual problems in men. Retrieved from http://www.nlm.nih.gov/medlineplus/sexualproblemsinmen.html

U.S. National Library of Medicine. (2016). Sexual problems in women. Retrieved from http://www.nlm.nih.gov/medlineplus/sexualproblemsinwomen.html

Sexual Expression

Sexual expression is the way individuals convey their sense of their sexual self, which can include their gender, their sexual orientation, and their sensuality.

Gender expression is a form of sexual expression, as it affects someone's maleness, femaleness, or other combination. How does the individual convey male or female styles? In traditional sex-role stereotyped ways, with women in dresses, primarily wearing pink, or men in suits or blazers with pants? Or with more flexibility, with women wearing more androgynous clothing, pants, T-shirts, jeans, and with men wearing more typically feminine clothing, including dresses, makeup, and even high-heeled shoes? Women seem to have more flexibility wearing men's clothing than men do wearing women's clothing. For example, women who dress as men, in suits and even ties, are given a pass, whereas men who wear women's clothing are often ridiculed, mocked, and worse, beaten up or murdered. They are seen as unmanly, feminine, or gay, which is seen as threatening to some men.

Sexual orientation, different from gender, is about how individuals resonate with a partner or partners. Perhaps they are heterosexual or straight. Perhaps they are gay or lesbian. Maybe they are bisexual, relating to both men and women. They might be asexual, with no sexual feelings toward another person. Or pansexual, where they are attracted to all genders, basing their choice on the individual rather than the gender. Sexual orientation is part of a person's sexual self and is not a choice.

Sexual expression also includes how individuals manage or convey their sexuality. Are they monogamous or polyamorous? Are they sexual with intercourse or without? Are they sexual with themselves and with others? Are they sensual? Do they walk or carry themselves with an awareness of themselves as sexual beings? Do they sparkle with personality? Do they make others feel good about themselves? Are their clothes sensual, with styles and soft fabrics such as velvet or silk? Sexual expression also includes how often a person has sex by themselves or with others. It can include what kind of sex they are having, whether oral, anal, or vaginal sex, sex without intercourse, using toys such as vibrators, or if they have sex with others, or in a group, or if they are into kink, which could include sadism and masochism, S&M, which some refer to as sexuality and mutuality. Even the way someone kisses, or does not like to kiss, is part of their sexual expression. Are they physically affectionate? Are they huggers or not? Even arousal to paraphilic objects is part of sexual expression, which can include certain pieces of clothing, high heels, rubber, costumes, leather, or tools, such as boots and whips.

The important idea is to make sure all partners are consenting and that no one is being forced to do something they do not want to do. Consent is essential in sexual relationships. Otherwise the sexual acts or expressions of sexuality are called sexual assault, sexual abuse, sexual coercion, sexual violence, sexual battery, molestation, or rape, with often traumatic consequences for the victim (or survivor) and possible consequences for the perpetrator.

Sexual expression is a combination of gender, gender expression, sexual orientation, and the ways someone has sex, including frequency, number of partners, and sexual acts. Each person's sexual expression is unique. The challenges and opportunities are to learn more about the sexual expression of others as well as to learn more about one's own sexual expression and then to share that information with a partner. This is what helps create true intimacy.

Judith Steinhart

See also: Gender Expression; Gender Identity; Paraphilias; Sexual Identity; Sexual Orientation; Stereotypes, Gender; Stereotypes, Sexual.

Further Reading

DeLamater, J. (2012). Sexual expression in later life: A review and synthesis. *Journal of Sex Research, 49*(2–3), 125–141.

Sprecher, S., & Cate, R. M. (2005). Sexual satisfaction and sexual expression as predictors of relationship satisfaction and stability. In J. H. Harvey, A. Wenzel, & S. Sprecher (Eds.), *The handbook of sexuality in close relationships* (235–256), New York: Routledge.

Sexual Harassment

Sexual harassment includes any sort of unwanted physical contact, such as hugging, touching clothing, and patting or stroking hair or body parts; verbal and written communications including suggestive comments, requests for sexual favors, comments about someone's body or clothing, rumor spreading, or threats of sexual contact or assault; and nonverbal actions such as staring and making suggestive gestures or expressions. Not all forms of sexual harassment are sexual in nature in that sexual harassment can also occur based on a person's sex, gender, or sexual orientation. For example, if someone continually makes derogatory comments about a particular sexual orientation, this could be considered sexual harassment. When these actions or a combination of several of these actions create an uncomfortable or hostile environment, particularly if it occurs in a work or school setting, it is considered sexual harassment.

There are two general types of sexual harassment that may be experienced. The first type, hostile environment, is the more common, but it is also difficult to define. Typically, a hostile environment will involve another person making inappropriate and unwanted sexual comments or suggestively touching or acting sexually inappropriate with another person. The second type of sexual harassment is the quid pro quo. This type of harassment involves someone, often an employer or another person in a position of power, suggesting that someone perform a sexual favor in return for a benefit, such as a job position, promotion, or better grade.

Sexual harassment offenders can be of any sex and any gender identity, although significantly more females report being sexually harassed. This could either be due to actual higher rates of perpetration against females or a lack of reporting from male victims. In either case, it is important for victims of sexual harassment to know their rights and what steps they should take to make sure that the harassment ends. First, and foremost, victims need to voice their concerns and document the events that are making them uncomfortable. This may include confronting the perpetrator about their behavior. Sometimes that person does not realize their actions could be deemed sexual in nature and that they are making someone feel uncomfortable. If the victim is uncomfortable approaching the perpetrator, support may be available from a supervisor, a human resources representative, or any other coworker or peer with whom they feel comfortable disclosing their story. Although not all environments and companies have sexual harassment policies, it is still strongly encouraged to take steps to prevent sexual harassment. Many companies and organizations have preestablished policies and procedures in place so that anyone that learns of sexual harassment, particularly in the workplace or at school, is able to contact the appropriate person or department to file a formal complaint.

If policies are in place, once a formal complaint has been filed, an internal investigation about the incident(s) will commence. This procedure varies from environment to environment but often includes interviewing the victim and the accused perpetrator. Victims should be aware that the person who has made them feel uncomfortable will most likely continue to work or study alongside them throughout the investigation and possibly after as well, depending on the outcome. In a work setting, employers are required to remain impartial during the investigation and therefore are not able to terminate or demote the accused employee unless the investigation determines that the accusations were valid. Incidents of sexual harassment, isolated or continued, can cause poor workplace, educational, or other environmental conditions for not only the victim of the harassment but also the surrounding people.

If the sexual harassment occurred in a work or school environment, in the event the internal investigation determines there was either insufficient evidence to prove an incident of sexual harassment or that the event(s) that occurred were not sexual in nature, the accused person may maintain their employment or position with the organization. An investigation that ends in this manner can be very distressing for victims because they will continue to be in a situation that may be uncomfortable. Since sexual harassment is considered a form of workplace discrimination, employees are protected under Title VII of the Civil Rights Act of 1964; if it occurs in an educational environment, people are protected under Title IX. With respect to sexual harassment in the workplace, Title VII is a U.S. federal law that states that it is illegal for a company or employer to discriminate against an individual based on their sex. Therefore, victims can contact the Equal Employment Opportunity Commission directly and file a formal complaint, and they will then conduct their own investigation.

Whether the victim can get justice or not, sexual harassment can have lasting effects on their physical and social well-being. These symptoms can include headaches, nausea, weight fluctuations, lowered self-esteem, sexual dysfunction, and sleeping troubles. Experiencing these symptoms could also lead to more serious disorders, such as depression, anxiety, or posttraumatic stress disorder. These symptoms or disorders could eventually lead to the victim being unable to perform in their daily life activities, including at their job, and could result in job loss or demotion, lack of educational opportunity, or lack of or impaired other daily life activities.

Casey T. Tobin

See also: Rape; Sexual Abuse; Sexual Assault; Sexual Harassment in College; Sexual Harassment in Education; Sexual Harassment in the Workplace.

Further Reading

Crouch, M. (2001). *Thinking about sexual harassment: A guide for the perplexed.* New York: Oxford.

Grossman, J. (2016). *Nine to five: How gender, sex, and sexuality continue to define the American workplace.* Cambridge: Cambridge University Press.

Sexual Harassment in College

Fueled by a newfound independence, freedom, and possible substance experimentation, sexual harassment on college campuses is quite prevalent, so prevalent that it seems as if experiencing sexual harassment sometime over the course of a college education is inevitable. Sexual harassment encompasses a wide variety of behaviors. From a physical standpoint, sexual harassment includes any unwanted physical contact including, but not limited to, hugging, touching of clothes or hair, touching body parts, sexual assault, and rape. It also includes any form of unwanted verbal, written, or nonverbal communication, such as heckling, requesting sexual favors, sending pictures of naked body parts or sex-related content, making suggestive gestures or expressions, and threats of sexual contact or assault. Any nonsexual discrimination or aggression based on gender identity or sexual orientation is also considered sexual harassment. For example, if an administrator, professor, staff member, or student were to make comments about a particular sexual orientation being less successful than the rest of the population, it would be considered sexual discrimination and, therefore, also sexual harassment. Any of these actions, singularly or in conjunction, that creates an uncomfortable, hostile, or fear-inducing environment is considered sexual harassment.

People of all gender identities can be the victims and the perpetrators of sexual harassment on college campuses. Sexual harassment is not limited to faculty-to-student cases. Students, instructors, interns, professors, residence life staff, administrators, and supporting staff can be victims or perpetrators of sexual harassment. Females report the highest rates of experiencing harassment, with males reported as the most frequent perpetrators. This could be an actual representation of the incidence of sexual harassment; however, it is important to consider that males may underreport being the victims of harassment. Many male victims are reluctant to report sexual harassment for fear of the stigma of being weak or vulnerable. In general, it is known that sexual harassment is underreported across all demographics.

At federally funded educational institutions, students and faculty are protected against sexual harassment and discrimination under Title IX of the Education Amendments of 1972. This federal law requires all schools to make it publicly known and posted that sexual harassment and discrimination is prohibited and will not be tolerated under any circumstances. The college must provide a clear grievance procedure for victims to make a formal complaint or start an investigation regarding sexual harassment. It is required that institutions investigate every allegation and remedy the situation in a timely manner. Title IX also ensures both the victim and the accused perpetrator are given the same rights during the investigation and hearings. If any institution fails to adhere to the regulations of Title IX, it could possibly lose federal funding. However, since the law was established in 1972, this has yet to occur. If the victim is unsatisfied with the outcome of the school's investigation and hearing, that individual may choose to file a lawsuit against the institution for sexual discrimination.

Sexual harassment can lead to significant and potentially long-lasting psychological effects. Victims of all gender identities have reportedly experienced loss of self-esteem, guilt, shame, inability to concentrate, sexual dysfunction, and self-harm. As a student, these effects have a significant academic and social impact that may result in a student missing many of the typical college experiences. Students' academic success may be impeded by the urge to drop classes, switch schools, or withdraw from the university to avoid contact with the person harassing them. The psychological effects paired with a decline in academic performance could lead to more serious mental health disorders, including depression, anxiety, eating disorder, posttraumatic stress disorder, and suicidal thoughts or attempts.

If the accused perpetrator is found guilty of sexual harassment, they may face a number of consequences depending on the severity of the harassment. These repercussions can include a referral for counseling, probation, suspension, or expulsion from the institution. If legal action was taken outside of the college, perpetrators could face significant fines and possible incarceration.

Sexual harassment can have an impact on people beyond the harasser and the harassed. The institution may suffer because students may lose their sense of a safe learning environment. If sexual harassment is an issue on a campus, this could have a significant impact on the reputation of the college, which in turn could affect the likelihood of top-rated professors coming to their campus, number of applicants, and fund-raising efforts. In order to prevent sexual harassment on college campuses, many institutions have adopted prevention programs that include sexual harassment, discrimination, and sexual assault awareness. These programs aim to educate students, faculty, staff, and administrators about the topics of harassment and consent, knowing when to intervene, and when to report suspected sexual harassment.

Casey T. Tobin

See also: Rape; Sexual Assault; Sexual Harassment; Sexual Harassment in Education; Sexual Harassment in the Workplace.

Further Reading

Crouch, M. (2001). *Thinking about sexual harassment: A guide for the perplexed.* New York: Oxford.

Kipnis, L. (2017). *Unwanted advances: Sexual paranoia comes to campus.* New York: Harper.

Watts, M. (2015). *Sexual violence on campus: Overview, issues and actions.* Hauppauge, NY: Nova Science Publishers.

Sexual Harassment in Education

In the United States, under Title IX of the Education Amendments of 1972, sexual harassment in school is defined as any unwelcome conduct that is sexual in nature and interferes with a student's ability to participate in or benefit from educational programs. Specifically, Title IX states that sexual harassment is a form of sex discrimination and requires all public and private educational institutions that receive federal funds to decrease and eliminate sexual harassment in schools.

Nevertheless, according to recent reports, sexual harassment remains pervasive in American schools.

Title IX is designed to protect students from sexual harassment perpetrated not only by teachers and other school employees but also by fellow students and anyone else involved with school activities (e.g., visiting speakers). Conduct that is considered sexual harassment can be both verbal and physical and includes sexual propositions, touching of a sexual nature, displaying or distributing sexually explicit drawings and pictures, performing sexual gestures, telling dirty jokes, and circulating or showing emails or websites of a sexual nature.

Unlawful sexual harassment is divided into two categories: quid pro quo harassment and hostile environment harassment. Quid pro quo harassment occurs when teachers or other school employees explicitly or implicitly ask students to submit to unwelcome sexual advances as a condition for better grades, better assignments on sport teams, or other rewards. All other types of sexual harassment are considered hostile environment harassment and can be perpetrated by school employees, students, or others associated with school programs and activities. To be recognized as unlawful, the hostile environment harassment claim must show the actual impact on the victimized student in an academic setting.

National surveys conducted among high school students in the United States indicate that 40–50 percent experience at least one sexual harassment incident in a given year, and the percentage increases to 80 percent at some point over their high school career. Peer harassment (i.e., a student or a group of students harassing another student) is the most common form of sexual harassment in school, and female students are more likely to become the targets. Although students are sexually harassed more frequently in person, online forms of sexual harassment such as through texting, email, and social media are on the rise. Cases of harassment by teachers and other authority figures are far less frequent, but they do occur, often with serious consequences.

Recently, the rising incidences of bullying in schools have received considerable attention. It is important to note that many of these bullying incidents involve sexual harassment, targeting vulnerable populations such as gay, lesbian, and transgender students. As a first step toward eliminating these incidences, schools should establish clear policies against sexual harassment and bullying and spell out how they intend to implement these policies.

Yoko Crume

See also: Sexual Harassment; Sexual Harassment in College; Sexual Harassment in the Workplace.

Further Reading

Hill, C. A, & Kearl, H. (2011). *Crossing the line: Sexual harassment at school.* Washington, DC: AAUW.

Hornor, G. (2012). Emotional maltreatment. *Journal of Pediatric Health Care, 26*(6), 436–442.

The U.S. Department of Education. (2008). *Sexual harassment: It's not academic.* Washington, DC: U.S. Department of Education.

Sexual Harassment in the Workplace

Sexual harassment is a form of sex discrimination that encompasses unwelcome sexual advances, requests for sexual favors, and other verbal or physical harassment of a sexual nature. Although many victims are reluctant to report their experiences, surveys show that it affects more women than men. Prompt reporting helps resolve issues quickly, and workplace training aids in preventing further occurrences.

A federal law known as Title VII of the Civil Rights Act of 1964 prohibits many forms of discrimination, such as sexual harassment. Title VII applies to private employers with fifteen or more employees, including state and local governments. It also applies to employment agencies, labor organizations, and the federal government regardless of the number of employees. To be unlawful, conduct must explicitly or implicitly affect an individual's employment; unreasonably interfere with an individual's work performance; or create an intimidating, hostile, or offensive work environment. In the workplace, actions such as touching colleagues, repeatedly requesting dates, making sexual comments, and using vulgar language are all potentially problematic.

Because of low reporting rates, it is difficult to quantify the experience of sexual harassment in the workplace. Low reporting rates are due to a variety of factors, such as fear of retaliation from employers, concern for the harasser, shame, belief in the futility of the grievance process, or fear of being blamed for the harassment. Reporting is also complicated by varying perceptions of what constitutes sexual harassment. For example, the offensive conduct can take place between members of the same sex. In addition, the harasser can be the victim's supervisor, an agent of the employer, a supervisor in another area, a colleague, or an outside party. The victim does not have to be the person harassed but could be anyone affected by the offensive conduct. Unlawful sexual harassment may also occur without economic injury to or discharge of the victim. Despite the challenges in determining the prevalence of sexual harassment, studies show that it affects women more than men, with at least one-third of women in the United States experiencing some form of sexual harassment. One in ten men report experiencing it as well, and a quarter of men say they worry about being falsely accused of sexual harassment.

It is important to file a complaint with a supervisor or human resources department promptly to increase the chance of a quick resolution. Once a harassment complaint is filed, it cannot be retracted. An employer is obligated to investigate all complaints, and supervisors are obligated to report any suspected or known harassment. Employees who have filed complaints should continue to perform their normal work duties and report any retaliation. The retaliation laws are broad and may protect coworkers of the victim as well as witnesses in the investigation.

Prevention is the best tool to eliminate sexual harassment in the workplace. Many employers take steps to prevent sexual harassment from occurring by communicating to employees that sexual harassment will not be tolerated. One common method for doing so is by providing a written antiharassment policy to employees, outlining what harassment is, telling all employees that harassment will not be tolerated, and setting out how employees should respond to incidents of harassment. Other methods of dealing with harassment include sexual harassment training and establishing an effective complaint or grievance process offering immediate and appropriate action when an employee complains.

Linda Tancs

See also: Sexual Harassment; Sexual Harassment in College; Sexual Harassment in Education.

Further Reading

Saguy, A. C. (2003). *What is sexual harassment? From Capitol Hill to the Sorbonne* (3rd ed.) Oakland: University of California Press.

U.S. Equal Employment Opportunity Commission. (n.d.) *Facts about sexual harassment.* Retrieved from http://www.eeoc.gov/eeoc/publications/fs-sex.cfm

Sexual Health

The World Health Organization defines sexual health as "a state of physical, emotional, mental, and social well-being in relation to sexuality; it is not merely the absence of disease, dysfunction, or infirmity. Sexual health requires a positive and respectful approach to sexuality and sexual relationships, as well as the possibility of having pleasurable and safe sexual experiences, free of coercion, discrimination, and violence. For sexual health to be attained and maintained, the sexual rights of all persons must be respected, protected, and fulfilled" (WHO, 2006).

Based on this definition, the World Association for Sexual Health has developed a Declaration of Sexual Rights, which outlines the sexual rights that are "essential for the achievement of the highest attainable sexual health" (WAS, 2014).

Based on these, someone who could be considered a sexually healthy person would

- have accurate sexual knowledge so they can have happy relationships and enjoyable sex
- know how to avoid infections and seek safe and effective treatment if they have symptoms of a sexually transmitted infection
- know how to plan for a baby when they (and their partner[s]) want one, know how to avoid unintended pregnancies, and know that safe methods of abortion are available in the event of an unexpected pregnancy
- manage their sexual relationships so that their intimacy and pleasure needs are satisfied without harming other people

Looking at this in another way, a sexually healthy person can be described as having an ethical approach to their sex life. The fundamentals of human ethics are the concepts of autonomy, nonmaleficence, and beneficence. Put simply, a sexually healthy person has sex when there is consent (agreement) and an expected positive outcome (enjoyment, pleasure, satisfaction) without harm for all participants. Of course, sexual events are rarely perfect; sometimes orgasm does not happen, sometimes there is pain, sometimes a vagina stays dry or a penis stays flaccid or an anus does not relax, or sometimes a throat gag reflex is overreactive. All these things come and go, and there are ways, both through knowledge and actions, to deal with these sexual challenges as they arise—the important thing is to practice sexual loving kindness.

While some people choose to only have sex with someone they love, and others find anonymous sex more to their preference, everyone can have sex in a loving way, whether they are "in love" with the person or otherwise. This is not to say that casual, or quick, or mutually consensual "rough" play is not healthy. On the contrary, loving means respect for the other person(s) and a commitment to mutual satisfaction and pleasure, however that is found.

Sexual knowledge, and access to this knowledge, is a sexual right that many in the world are unable to exercise due to legal, religious, economic, and other structural barriers. While the fundamentals and mechanics of reproductive sex may well be "instinctual," there is much a person needs to learn about themselves and their potential sexual partner(s) before they meet the criteria of a sexually healthy person. Sexual knowledge is more than techniques or positions; a sexually healthy person can develop an attitude that is open to pleasure, intimacy, connection, excitement, consideration, and compassion for themselves and their partners.

Sexually transmitted infections (STIs) are only one component of the definition of sexual health. Many people may consider "the absence of an STI" as a good definition of sexual health; however, many people have chronic, sometimes lifelong, viral infections that are sexually transmitted (e.g., herpes, HPV, hepatitis, HIV) and can still be sexually healthy. Everyone can respect and be honest with their sexual partners by using condoms for intercourse and enjoying outercourse or nonpenetrative sex. Sexually healthy people can have regular tests for STIs and can take medications to manage any viral or bacterial STIs. A sexually healthy person is also able to be honest and communicate with the people they have had sex with and let them know if an STI appears or is found following an STI test.

Sexually healthy people who have sex with members of the other sex use effective contraception when they do not wish to reproduce, and if an unintended pregnancy occurs, they can seek out a safe termination of the pregnancy using medications or a small operation. Unsafe abortions are a major cause of death and disability in women in many parts of the world. Sexually healthy people think about contraception as well as STI prevention, pleasure, and orgasm when having sex with members of the other sex.

Sexually health people manage their sexual relationships so that their intimacy and pleasure needs are satisfied without harming other people. It is self-evident how someone who forces their needs for pleasure onto another, without regard for the other's desires or wishes, is sexually unhealthy. A sexually healthy individual is able to listen and read their partner's verbal and nonverbal body language and respond to what their partner's body or voice is saying. A sexually healthy person can negotiate and communicate their needs for hugs, orgasm, and sex while respecting the response of their partner. A sexually healthy person can also masturbate to meet their immediate needs if they are aroused and their partner is not in the mood for sex or there is currently no partner available.

In summary, a sexually healthy person is a good lover, both in and out of the bedroom, and, as a consequence, a sexually healthy person creates happier and healthier communities.

Kelwyn Browne

See also: Communication, Sexual; Intimacy, Sexual and Relational; Sex Education; Sexual Rights; Sexually Transmitted Infections (STIs).

Further Reading

World Association for Sexual Health. (2014). Declaration of sexual rights. Retrieved from http://www.worldsexology.org/wp-content/uploads/2013/08/declaration_of_sexual_rights_sep03_2014.pdf

World Health Organization. (2006). Defining sexual health. Retrieved from https://www.who.int/reproductivehealth/topics/sexual_health/sh_definitions/en/

Wylie, K. R. (Ed.). (2015). *ABC of sexual health* (3rd ed.). Chichester: Wiley-Blackwell.

Sexual Identity

"Sexual identity" refers to how individuals view and understand themselves as sexual beings. "Sexual identity" is often incorrectly seen as synonymous with "sexual orientation identity," but the two are very different concepts. Individuals' sexual orientation identity refers to their understanding of their sexual orientation, or to whom they are emotionally, romantically, or sexually attracted, whereas sexual identity is a much broader concept. Sexual identity encompasses all personal and social aspects of individuals' lives related to their sexual orientation identity, sexual or romantic thoughts and desires, sexual or romantic beliefs, and sexual or romantic activities.

The first well-known exploration of individuals' sexual development was written by Sigmund Freud in the early 1900s. Freud suggested that individuals are sexual from birth and go through a series of stages during which they come to understand, manipulate, and exercise their sexual impulses in socially appropriate ways. In the mid-twentieth century, Erik Erikson (1950/1985) expanded on Freud's work by developing a theory of ego identity development that detailed the process through which individuals come to understand themselves and establish how they interact with others throughout their lives.

Building on Erikson's work, researchers and theorists began to explore how individuals incorporate aspects of their identities, such as their race or ethnicity, culture, and sexuality into their global identity, or their sense of themselves as a whole person. The term "sexual identity" began being used in social science literature extensively in the late 1970s. Two of the first researchers to focus on individuals' understandings of themselves as sexual individuals were Vivienne Cass and Richard Troiden, both of whom did research with gay men. Their models came to be known as models of sexual identity development even though they were actually models that sought to explain how individuals came to understand themselves as a sexual minority, accept themselves as a sexual minority, reveal their sexual minority identity to others, and then integrate their sexual minority identity into their global identity. Cass's (1984) and Troiden's (1988) models were later expanded on by other researchers and theorists, but the work generally continued to focus on sexual minorities.

The late 1990s and early 2000s saw a shift toward recognizing that all people have sexual identities, not just those who identify as sexual minorities. This required a reevaluation of how the term "sexual identity" was being used, as it needed to be expanded to include aspects of sexuality in the lives of those who identify as heterosexual as well. Within the academic literature, Eliason (1995) was among the first to explore sexual identity development among individuals who identified as heterosexual. Rather than exploring sexual identity as a temporal process, his work sought to classify individuals' level of exploration or commitment to their sexual identity. Eliason's findings indicated that most individuals who identify as heterosexual had not given much thought to their sexual identity and had committed themselves to identifying as heterosexual without much thought as to what being heterosexual meant or exploring any other possibilities.

Around this time, the term "sexual orientation identity" began to be used to differentiate between individuals' sexual orientation and their overall sexual identities, even though academic, professional, and popular literature often continues to use "sexual identity" to refer to sexual orientation identity. Worthington and his colleagues developed a theory of how individuals who identify as heterosexual develop their sexual identity. This work sought to identify where individuals were on four aspects of sexual identity development: commitment, which indicates an individual has committed to a sexual identity without exploring the various components of sexual identity; exploration, which represents the degree to which individuals are actively exploring aspects of their sexual identity; synthesis and integration, which indicates an individual has gone through the process of exploring their sexual identity, has come to a more advanced understanding of it, and has integrated it into their global identity; and sexual orientation identity uncertainty, which represents the degree of uncertainty individuals feel about their sexual orientation identity.

Worthington and his colleagues found individuals who identify as sexual minorities generally spend more time considering their overall sexual identity as they are already required to examine their sexual orientation identity, and this introspection spreads to other areas of sexual identity exploration. More advanced sexual identity development has been linked with positive sexual health outcomes, indicating it is an important process in individuals' lives. Worthington's model is generally considered to represent the most comprehensive way of understanding sexual identity among all individuals as it considers not just individuals' sexual orientation identities but all aspects of their lives that make up their sexual identity.

Richard A. Brandon-Friedman

See also: Gender Identity; Gender Identity Development; Romantic Attraction and Orientation; Sexual Orientation.

Further Reading

Argüello, T. M. (2018). Identity development. In M. P. Dentato (Ed.), *Social work practice with the LGBTQ community* (71–96). New York: Oxford University Press.

Brandon-Friedman, R. A. (2018). *The impact of sexual identity development on the sexual health of youth formerly in the foster care system.* Manuscript submitted for publication.

Brandon-Friedman, R. A. (2018). *Youth sexual identity development theories: A guide for social workers.* Manuscript submitted for publication.

Cass, V. C. (1984). Homosexual identity formation: Testing a theoretical model. *Journal of Sex Research, 20*, 143–167.

Eliason, M. J. (1995). Accounts of sexual identity formation in heterosexual students. *Sex Roles, 32*, 821–834.

Erikson, E. H. (1985). *Childhood and society: 35th anniversary edition.* New York: W. W. Norton & Company. (Original work published 1950)

Freud, S. (2000). *Three essays on the theory of sexuality* (J. Strachey, Trans.). New York: Basic Books. (Original work published 1915)

Troiden, R. R. (1988). *Gay and lesbian identity: A sociological analysis.* Dix Hills, NY: General Hall.

Worthington, R. L., Navarro, R. L., Savoy, H. B., & Hampton, D. (2008). Development, reliability, and validity of the Measure of Sexual Identity Exploration and Commitment (MoSIEC). *Developmental Psychology, 44*(1), 22–33. doi: 10.1037/0012-1649.44.1.22

Sexual Learning

Sexual learning is a lifelong normative experience socializing people into appropriate sexual behaviors and beliefs, including expectations of the appropriate gender partner and an implied progression of intimate behaviors. Sexual learning happens both through formal sex education and informally through peers, family, and media.

Sex is taboo yet drenched in intrigue. Many parents feel schools should provide sex education, so they do not have to. Formal sex education is affected by social and political forces and can be abstinence or contraception based, yet it often involves clinical reproductive biology disconnected from pleasure or relationships. Dissatisfied with formal sex education, young people learn about sex from peers and older siblings. This education is often reliant on stereotypes, myths, and misinformation.

Many theories in sociology and psychology assert how people learn to be sexual, such as social scripts and social learning theory, which posit a link between behaviors and environmental cues.

Scripting theory is based on the assertion that behavior is shaped by the social environment, so actors will engage in acts they believe to be socially preferable. As social forces shift over time, so do attitudes about sex. Due to these changes regarding sexuality, scripts instructing what is acceptable to do sexually, when, and with whom are affected by age, cultural context, and social location (Gagnon & Simon, 2005). The shared nature of these beliefs facilitates sexual learning.

Scripts operate on three interconnected levels: the cultural, the interpersonal, and the intrapsychic. The cultural level encompasses media, political forces, and large-scale ideologies. Put simply, cultural messages tell people what they are supposed to do, interpersonal scripts provide feedback from partners, and intrapsychic scripts inform how people are supposed to feel. The best example of an instructive sexual script is the baseball analogy, which instructs actors to start with kissing ("first base"), as they progress through steps of intimacy. Regardless of personal experience, actors know this appropriate progression.

Similar to sexual scripts, social learning theory asserts that people learn behavioral cues from exposure in their social environment, yet this is mediated by perceiving rewards and consequences so that rewarded actions are encouraged and punished actions discouraged. Social learning theory recognizes reciprocal determinism—or the effects of the combination of cognition, environment, and behavior—and notes that behavioral reinforcement can be both direct or vicarious.

Media expand the possibility for sexual learning, formal and informal. Internet technology makes people aware of new research and ideological debates. Technology expands informal knowledge by increasing exposure to different practices, creating new narratives upon which people can draw in sexual decision making. Due to this, media can supersede peers as a socialization agent and create endless possibilities for sexual learning.

Rachel Kalish

See also: Media and Sexuality; Sex Education; Sexual Script; Social Learning Theory, Gender and; Stereotypes, Gender; Stereotypes, Sexual.

Further Reading

Bandura, A. (1971). *Social learning theory.* New York: General Learning Press.

Gagnon, J. H., & Simon, W. (2005). *Sexual conduct: The social sources of human sexuality* (2nd ed.). New Brunswick, NJ: Aldine Transaction.

Levine, J. (2003). *Harmful to minors: The perils of protecting children from sex.* New York: Thunders Mouth Press.

Simon, W., & J. H. Gagnon. (1984). Sexual scripts. *Society, 22*, 53–60.

Sexual Orientation

Sexual orientation is the interaction between thoughts and feelings that produces attraction, sexual desire, and feelings of love for other people. Some individuals experience these thoughts and feelings toward members of the other sex—referred to as a heterosexual (straight) orientation. Others' thoughts and feelings are directed to members of the same sex—referred to as a same-sex, or gay or lesbian, orientation. Still others experience attraction and desire toward both sexes (bisexual orientation) or toward neither sex (asexual orientation). As our understanding of sexual orientation and gender grows, people are beginning to use new language to describe their sexual orientation to a variety of genders, including pansexual and skoliosexual.

Sexual orientation is sometimes, but not always, reflected in people's behaviors and choice of relationship partner or partners. Many people will engage in sexual activity and have relationships with those to whom they are attracted. For example, many heterosexual people will engage in sex with members of the other sex and will typically have other-sex partners. Likewise, many gay and lesbian people will engage in sex with members of the same sex and often have relationships with same-sex partners. However, this is not always the case, and some people, both heterosexual and gay or lesbian, report having had sexual encounters with members of both sexes. Similarly, if a person is not sexually active (e.g., they are a virgin and/or they practice celibacy for personal, religious, or medical reasons), this does not mean that they stop having a sexual orientation, only that they are not currently engaging in some or all types of sexual behavior. This is especially important to remember for individuals who identify as bisexual but are in a committed, monogamous relationship with one partner.

Sexual orientation is also distinct from sexual identity. Across all times and cultures, some individuals experience heterosexual, gay or lesbian, bisexual, or asexual orientations. However, how we label and understand these orientations and subsequent behavior varies by culture and across time. For example, before 1869 there were no "homosexuals" because the word had not even been invented yet; "heterosexuals" were not "invented" until 1892, more than twenty years later. In the present time, culture influences how we understand same- and other-sex orientations. Within each culture, different labels and words will be used to describe this same basic phenomenon. For example, in Western culture, people may use the words "straight," "gay," "bisexual," "asexual," "pansexual," "queer," "kinky," and so on. These terms reflect subjective sexual identities and are often related to, but not necessarily the same as, one's sexual orientation.

Sexual orientation is often considered to be binary—gay or lesbian versus straight or heterosexual. The problem with this distinction is that it ignores the great amount of variability that is seen among people. Another way of conceptualizing sexual orientation is as a spectrum. Most characteristics within the human population fall somewhere on a spectrum. For example, think of height—some people are very short, some people are very tall, and most people fall somewhere in between. This idea has also been suggested as a way of describing sexual orientation. Some people are exclusively gay or lesbian, some people are exclusively heterosexual, and some fall somewhere in between. A third way of considering sexual orientation was proposed by Michael Storms in 1980. Storms suggested that instead of considering gay and straight as "opposites," it might make more sense to consider desire for men as distinct from desire for women. What this means is that an individual can have high desire for men and low desire for women (e.g., a gay male or a straight female), high desire for women and low desire for men (e.g., a lesbian woman or a straight man), or high desire for both men and women (e.g., bisexual men and women). The benefit of this model of sexual orientation is that it can also be used to explain asexual orientation as a low (or no) desire for both men and women, something that a gay or straight binary or gay or straight spectrum is unable to do.

One of the most frequently asked questions about sexual orientation is about prevalence. How many people are straight? How many are gay or bisexual? How many asexual individuals are there? While this may seem like a straightforward question, it is actually quite hard to measure, and what specifically is measured can lead to different answers. In a recent U.S. national probability sample of almost 6,000 men and women ages fourteen to ninety-four, 92.2 percent of adult men and 93.1 percent of adult women self-identified as heterosexual; 4.2 percent of adult men and 0.9 percent of adult women identified as gay or lesbian; 2.6 percent of men and 3.6 percent of women identified as bisexual; and 1.0 percent of men and 2.3 percent of women identified as "other." When considering same-sex behavior in this same sample, 9.3 percent of men aged twenty to twenty-four had received oral sex from a male partner, while 9.3 percent had given oral sex to a male partner, and 10.8 percent had received anal sex; the numbers were higher for women: 16.8 percent had received oral sex and 14 percent had given it to a female partner. Some studies suggest that when asked about same-sex attraction, rates are much higher with as many as two to three times more people reporting attraction as compared to behavior or identity. Finally, while asexuality is a relatively new area of scientific research, national probability samples from both the United States and the United Kingdom indicate that roughly 1.0 percent of the population identifies as asexual.

Another commonly asked question about sexual orientation is whether it is something people are born with or whether it is a choice someone makes. The vast majority of scientists and researchers believe there is sufficient evidence to indicate that sexual orientation is something that people are born with and not something that is chosen or that can be changed. There is growing evidence that genetics, birth order and handedness, and anatomical brain structures all contribute to one's sexual orientation, suggesting that there is not one specific "cause" of sexual orientation but rather many possible causes with biological origins. That said, while nurture doesn't "cause" one's sexual orientation, the culture in which someone is raised influences many aspects of their life, including how they express themselves sexually and define their identities, roles, and behaviors. Consequently, both nature and nurture need to be considered when discussing and understanding sexual orientation.

Heather L. Armstrong

See also: Asexuality; Biological Theories of Sexual Orientation; Bisexuality; Demisexuality; Heterosexuality; Homosexuality; Kinsey's Continuum of Sexual Orientation; Pansexuality; Romantic Attraction and Orientation; Sex Differentiation of the Brain and Sexual Orientation; Sexual Identity; Storms's Model of Sexual Orientation.

Further Reading

Alderson, K. (2014). Sexual/affectional orientations and diversity. In C. F. Pukall (Ed.), *Human sexuality: A contemporary introduction.* Don Mills, ON: Oxford University Press.

Blanchard, R., Cantor, J. M., Bogaert, A. F., Breedlove, S. M., & Ellis, L. (2006). Interaction of fraternal birth order and handedness in the development of male homosexuality. *Hormones and Behavior, 49*, 405–414.

Bogaert, A. F. (2004). Asexuality: Its prevalence and associated factors in a national probability sample. *The Journal of Sex Research, 41*, 279–287.

Bullough, B. L., & Bullough, B. (1997). The history of the science of sexual orientation 1880–1980. *Journal of Psychology & Human Sexuality, 9*, 1–16.

Chandra, A., Mosher, W. D., & Copen, C. (2011, March). *Sexual behavior, sexual attraction, and sexual identity in the United States: Data from the 2006–2008 National*

Survey of Family Growth. National Health Statistics Reports, No. 36. Washington, DC: U.S. Department of Health and Human Services.

Herbenick, D., Reece, M., Schick, V., Sanders, S. A., Dodge, B., & Fortenberry, J. D. (2010). Sexual behavior in the United States: Results from a national probability sample of men and women ages 14–94. *Journal of Sexual Medicine, 7*(Supp 5), 255–265.

Jannini, E. A., Blanchard, R., Camperio-Ciani, A., & Bancroft, J. (2010). Male homosexuality: Nature or culture? *Journal of Sexual Medicine, 7*, 3245–3253.

Kinsey, A. C., Pomeroy, W. B., & Martin, C. E. (1948). *Sexual behavior in the human male.* Philadelphia: W. B. Saunders Company.

Kirk, K. M., Bailey, J. M., & Martin, N. G. (2000). Etiology of male sexual orientation in an Australian twin sample. *Psychology, Evolution & Gender, 2*, 301–311.

Poston, D. L., & Baumle, A. K. (2010). Patterns of asexuality in the United States. *Demographic Research, 23*(18), 509–530.

Savic, I., & Lindstrom, P. (2008). PET and MRI show differences in cerebral asymmetry and functional connectivity between homo- and heterosexual subjects. *Proceedings of the National Academy of Sciences, 105*, 9403–9408.

Savin-Williams, R. C. (2006). Who's gay? Does it matter? *Current Directions in Psychological Science, 15*(1), 40–44.

Storms, M. D. (1980). Theories of sexual orientation. *Journal of Personality and Social Psychology, 38*, 783–792.

Sexual Revolution

The sexual revolution was a period during the 1960s and 1970s when social attitudes toward human sexuality became substantially more tolerant, liberal, and broad-minded, especially in the United States and western Europe. As a result of these liberalized attitudes, many women felt freer to engage in certain behaviors that were previously socially frowned upon. These behaviors included having casual sex outside of marriage, wearing sexually provocative clothing, and pursuing careers that had been mostly restricted to men. Thus, the sexual revolution was inextricably linked with the women's liberation movement of the same period. However, the sexual behaviors and social attitudes of men also became more liberal and free during this period.

Many social scientists attribute the events of the sexual revolution primarily to two developments in the United States: the development and legalization of birth control pills and the legalization of abortion.

In 1960, the U.S. Food and Drug Administration approved the first oral contraceptive (birth control pill) for general use by women. Within three years, more than two million American women were using the Pill to prevent pregnancy. The Pill allowed women the freedom to have sexual intercourse anytime and with anyone they pleased without the risk of pregnancy. In addition to birth control pills, other new forms of contraception became widely available for women during the 1960s, including intrauterine devices.

In 1973, the U.S. Supreme Court ruled in the *Roe v. Wade* case that abortion was legal during the first trimester of pregnancy. Previous to this ruling, women who wanted an abortion had to resort to illegal procedures that were often dangerous. If caught getting an abortion, a woman could be charged with murder or manslaughter. The legalization of abortion meant that women who did not intend to become pregnant and did not wish to keep the pregnancy could get a professional and safe abortion.

Some social scientists argue that the sexual revolution should not be attributed to these court rulings. Rather, they view the sexual revolution as part of the overall civil rights movement of the era, in which various socially marginalized groups—such as African Americans, hippies and other young people, and antiwar demonstrators—fought for greater influence, freedom of expression, or social equality. Whatever the causes, following the contraceptive and abortion rulings, there was a fairly rapid change in sexual behaviors. Studies revealed that between 1965 and 1975, the number of American women having sexual intercourse before marriage dramatically increased.

Coinciding with the new ability of women to have sex without the fear of pregnancy, women began to assert their rights in other areas. These developments were referred to as women's liberation (women's lib). Fashion trends throughout the 1960s and early 1970s were dominated by the liberation of female sexuality in the form of overtly sexual and revealing styles, including tight miniskirts, colorful low-cut tops, and dancer-type go-go boots. Women began wearing their hair longer and started to use more provocative makeup styles.

In addition to the superficial trends of fashion, there were more substantially positive results of the sexual revolution for women. One of these developments was an increase in the number of women attending colleges and universities in the United States—a number that by the 2000s exceeded the number of male students. As a result, more women entered white-collar professional careers in business, medicine, science, and other areas that were previously dominated by men.

Areas of popular culture that both reflected and promoted aspects of the sexual revolution included magazines, television, movies, and music, which all increased their sexual content during the 1960s and 1970s. Hardcore pornographic magazines, such as *Hustler* (first published in 1974), became available on magazine stands alongside the softcore *Playboy* (first published in 1953). *Love American Style*, a TV comedy that aired from 1969 to 1974, was one of many television programs that showed people in risqué sexual situations that were new to that entertainment medium. *Carnal Knowledge* (1971) and *Last Tango in Paris* (1972) were among the popular movies of the time that pushed the boundaries of depicting sexual situations. Pop songs that did the same included "Let's Spend the Night Together" by the Rolling Stones (1967) and "Lola" by the Kinks (1970).

As the social transformations of the sexual revolution were taking place, many conservative, traditional people in the United States strongly objected to these trends as immoral and socially harmful. They claimed that the liberalized sexual attitudes were corrupting traditional values and leading to excessive promiscuity, including among teenagers. The clashes that pitted social conservatives against feminists and other social liberals marked the beginning of the United States' "culture wars," which continue to divide the population today.

The results of the sexual revolution have been mixed in terms of positive and negative effects. Whether one views these results as good or bad often depends on one's political and cultural perspective. Conservative critics argue that the "free love" attitudes of the 1960s and 1970s led to a culture in which casual sex and hookups became common for both men and women. These critics link an increase in the prevalence of sexually transmitted infections, as well as the emergence of HIV/AIDS in the 1980s, to the sexual promiscuity of the sexual revolution. Other social trends often associated with the sexual revolution are increases in the numbers of divorces, out-of-wedlock births, and single mothers.

Liberal defenders of the sexual revolution counter that such unfortunate trends are outweighed in importance by the fact that women have made enormous strides in many measures of freedom and success, including economic independence, career achievement, and sexual liberation. Furthermore, the sexual liberation of women that began in the 1960s and 1970s has continued to spread to other segments of the population, such as the LGBT (lesbian, gay, bisexual, transgender) community.

A. J. Smuskiewicz

See also: Abortion Legislation; Estrogen-Progestin Birth Control Pills; Female Sexuality; Gay Rights Movement; Male Sexuality; *Roe v. Wade*; Sexual Rights.

Further Reading

Allyn, D. (2000). *Make love, not war: The sexual revolution: An unfettered history*. Boston: Little, Brown and Company.

PBS. (n.d.). The pill and the sexual revolution. Retrieved from http://www.pbs.org/wgbh/amex/pill/peopleevents/e_revolution.html

Thompson, K. M. J. (2013). A brief history of birth control in the U.S. Retrieved from https://www.ourbodiesourselves.org/book-excerpts/health-article/a-brief-history-of-birth-control/

Sexual Rights

Sexual rights, often referred to more inclusively as sexual and reproductive rights, is the concept of human rights as they apply to sexuality and reproduction. Sexual rights include a wide range of issues that often overlap and intersect in important ways. For example, sexual rights issues may include sexuality education, improving access to health care services focused on sexuality and reproduction (e.g., screenings for sexually transmitted infections, prenatal care), sexual pleasure, violence against women, sex work, and protection for those with diverse sexual orientations and gender identities. Such sexual rights are embedded in a larger concept of human rights, which typically includes the right to privacy, freedom from violence, freedom of thought, equality and freedom from discrimination, and the right to health and well-being.

Sexual and reproductive rights are most typically championed by nonprofit and/or nongovernmental organizations (NGOs) working toward equality and social justice at both regional levels and across the globe. Some of the most notable NGOs that fight for sexual rights include Amnesty International, the

International HIV/AIDS Alliance, the International Planned Parenthood Federation (IPPF), the World Association for Sexual Health (WAS), and the World Health Organization (WHO).

Depending on the organization and its major areas of focus, the term "sexual rights" has been defined in a number of ways. For example, some definitions include reproductive justice, whereas others are more distinctly focused on goals such as freedom of sexual expression and pleasure. Sexual rights have been increasingly included in definitions of sexual health as well as overarching conceptualizations of health and well-being. In a historic 2002 report, part of an effort to create a clear description for use in policy development, aid work, and health care, the WHO defined sexual rights in the following manner:

> Sexual rights embrace human rights that are already recognized in national laws, international human rights documents and other consensus statements. They include the right of all persons, free of coercion, discrimination and violence, to:
>
> - the highest attainable standard of sexual health, including access to sexual and reproductive health care services;
> - seek, receive and impart information related to sexuality;
> - sexuality education;
> - respect for bodily integrity;
> - choose their partner;
> - decide to be sexually active or not;
> - consensual sexual relations;
> - consensual marriage;
> - decide whether or not, and when, to have children; and
> - pursue a satisfying, safe and pleasurable sexual life.

The WHO further identified sexual rights as a fundamental component of sexual health, and the organization has embraced the position that sexual health cannot be maintained unless individuals' sexual rights are protected and upheld (WHO, 2002).

Members of WAS, a worldwide, multidisciplinary umbrella organization for scientific societies, professionals, and NGOs working in the field of human sexuality, penned what is believed to be the first official documentation of sexual rights. The Declaration of Sexual Rights was first proclaimed in 1997 at the Thirteenth World Congress of Sexology in Valencia, Spain. In 1999, at the Fourteenth World Congress of Sexology in Hong Kong, the document was revised and formally adopted by the WAS General Assembly. This revised version included eleven sexual rights, though it has subsequently been expanded. The 2014 WAS Declaration of Sexual Rights outlines and discusses the following sixteen sexual rights:

- the right to equality and nondiscrimination
- the right to life, liberty, and security of the person
- the right to autonomy and bodily integrity
- the right to be free from torture and cruel, inhuman, or degrading treatment or punishment
- the right to be free from all forms of violence and coercion

- the right to privacy
- the right to the highest attainable standard of health, including sexual health, with the possibility of pleasurable, satisfying, and safe sexual experiences
- the right to enjoy the benefits of scientific progress and its application
- the right to information
- the right to education and the right to comprehensive sexuality education
- the right to enter, form, and dissolve marriage or other similar types of relationships based on equality and full and free consent
- the right to decide whether to have children, the number and spacing of children, and to have the information and the means to do so
- the right to the freedom of thought, opinion, and expression
- the right to freedom of association and peaceful assembly
- the right to participation in public and political life
- the right to access justice, remedies, and redress

The WAS Declaration of Sexual Rights further outlines the importance of attending to the interaction of "biological, psychological, social, economic, political, cultural, legal, historical, religious, and spiritual factors" in considering sexual rights and health (World Association for Sexual Health, 2013).

The IPPF, a global NGO committed to promoting sexual and reproductive health, has also published a declaration of sexual rights. Sexual Rights: An IPPF Declaration, published in 2008, has three main parts. First, a preamble introduces the declaration as it is relevant to the mission and vision of the IPPF. The document then addresses seven "guiding principles," which introduce key concepts related to human rights and explain how such universal human rights apply to sexuality. The final section of the IPPF Declaration is titled "Sexual Rights Are Human Rights Related to Sexuality" and outlines the following sexual rights:

- Article 1: Right to equality, equal protection of the law and freedom from all forms of discrimination based on sex, sexuality or gender
- Article 2: The right to participation for all persons, regardless of sex, sexuality or gender
- Article 3: The rights to life, liberty, security of the person and bodily integrity;
- Article 4: Right to privacy
- Article 5: Right to personal autonomy and recognition before the law
- Article 6: Right to freedom of thought, opinion and expression; right to association
- Article 7: Right to health and to the benefits of scientific progress
- Article 8: Right to education and information
- Article 9: Right to choose whether or not to marry and to found and plan a family, and to decide whether or not, how and when, to have children
- Article 10: Right to accountability and redress

Sexual Rights: An IPPF Declaration (International Planned Parenthood Federation, 2013) overlaps in many ways with other declarations of sexual rights;

however, it is notable for including significantly greater detail about rights surrounding family planning (Article 9), a major emphasis of the organization.

Jennifer A. Vencill

See also: Consent; Planned Parenthood; Reproductive Coercion; Safer Sex; Sex Education; Sex Work; Sexual Assault; Sexual Health; Sexual Slavery; Sexually Transmitted Infections (STIs).

Further Reading

Herdt, G. (Ed.). (2009). *Moral panics, sex panics: Fear and the fight over sexual rights.* New York: NYU Press.

International Planned Parenthood Federation. (2013). *Sexual rights: An IPPF declaration.* Retrieved http://www.ippf.org/resource/Sexual-Rights-IPPF-declaration

Lind, A. (2010). *Development, sexual rights, and global governance.* New York: Routledge.

Sexual Rights Initiative. (2016). *Intro to sexual rights.* Retrieved from https://www.sexualrightsinitiative.com/sexual-rights

World Association for Sexual Health. (2013). *Declaration of sexual rights.* Retrieved from https://worldsexualhealth.net/resources/declaration-of-sexual-rights/

World Health Organization. (2002). *Defining sexual health. Report of a technical consultation on sexual health 28–31 January 2002, Geneva.* Retrieved from http://www.who.int/reproductivehealth/topics/gender_rights/defining_sexual_health/en/

Sexual Satisfaction

Sexual satisfaction is complicated and very subjective. What one person enjoys will not necessarily be the same thing that someone else, maybe even their partner, also likes. For the purposes of research, sexual satisfaction has been defined as “an affective response arising from one’s subjective evaluation of the positive and negative dimensions associated with one’s sexual relationship” (Lawrance & Byers, 1995). In other words, sexual satisfaction (or dissatisfaction) is the way an individual feels about their sexual relationship based on all the good and bad elements of that relationship.

E. S. Byers and colleagues have studied what leads to sexual satisfaction in a relationship in depth over the last twenty years and have developed the interpersonal exchange model of sexual satisfaction (IEMSS) as a conceptual framework to explain and predict sexual satisfaction. The IEMSS posits that within a sexual relationship, there are costs and rewards. Sexual costs are things that require effort, either mental or physical, or things that produce pain, embarrassment, or anxiety. A general example could be engaging in a sexual activity that your partner really enjoys but that is not particularly exciting for you. Conversely, sexual rewards are things that are pleasurable and gratifying; this could be the feeling of connection you have with your partner after sex or the physical pleasure of a really good orgasm. Within a relationship and over time, if an individual’s sexual rewards are greater than their sexual costs, the individual will feel sexually satisfied. If the costs become higher than the rewards, and this continues for a prolonged period of time, then the individual will likely feel dissatisfied.

The IEMSS also accounts for an individual's expectations about their relationship (called their comparison level). If the costs and rewards of the relationship are greater than or in line with the expectations of the individual, then satisfaction occurs. If an individual feels as though their expectations are not being met, even if the rewards outweigh the costs, they will likely feel dissatisfied. There is one additional component to the model. Satisfaction will be greatest in a relationship when rewards and costs are seen as equal between partners. If one partner is getting many rewards and one partner is experiencing many costs, then the satisfaction of both partners will decrease. The IEMSS has been used to study satisfaction in long-term and short-term relationships as well as in varying cultures.

Sexual satisfaction has been studied extensively, and there are several things that, in addition to the components of the IEMSS, are consistently linked with sexual satisfaction. First, relationship satisfaction is highly intertwined with sexual satisfaction; those who are happy in their relationships are generally sexually satisfied and vice versa. Sexual function is also closely linked with sexual satisfaction; when people experience sexual dysfunction, their satisfaction tends to drops. Finally, many studies have examined gender differences in sexual satisfaction, and, in general, both men and women report comparable levels of satisfaction.

Heather L. Armstrong

See also: Communication, Sexual; Desire; Psychosexual Therapy; Sensate Focus; Sexual Disorders, Female; Sexual Disorders, Male.

Further Reading

Armstrong, H. L., & Reissing, E. D. (2013). Women who have sex with women: A comprehensive review of the literature and conceptual model of sexual function. *Sexual and Relationship Therapy, 28*, 364–399.

Byers, E. S., Demmons, S., & Lawrance, K.-A. (1998). Sexual satisfaction within dating relationships: A test of the interpersonal exchange model of sexual satisfaction. *Journal of Social and Personal Relationships, 15*, 257–267.

Byers, E. S., & MacNeil, S. (2006). Further validation of the interpersonal exchange model of sexual satisfaction. *Sex & Marital Therapy, 32*, 53–69.

Lawrance, K.-A., & Byers, E. S. (1995). Sexual satisfaction in long-term heterosexual relationships: The interpersonal exchange model of sexual satisfaction. *Personal Relationships, 2*, 267–285.

Raisi, F., Yekta, Z. P., Ebadi, A., & Shahvari, Z. (2015). What are Iranian married women's rewards? Using interpersonal exchange model of sexual satisfaction: A qualitative study. *Sexual and Relationship Therapy, 30*(4), 475–489.

Sánchez-Fuentes, M. D. M., & Santos-Iglesias, P. (2015). Sexual satisfaction in Spanish heterosexual couples: Testing the interpersonal exchange model of sexual satisfaction. *Journal of Sex & Marital Therapy, 42*(3), 223–242.

Sánchez-Fuentes, M. D. M., Santos-Iglesias, P., & Sierra, J. C. (2014). A systematic review of sexual satisfaction. *International Journal of Clinical and Health Psychology, 14*, 67–75.

Stephenson, K. R., & Meston, C. M. (2011). The association between sexual costs and sexual satisfaction in women: An exploration of the interpersonal exchange model of sexual satisfaction. *The Canadian Journal of Human Sexuality, 20*, 31–40.

Sexual Script

Gagnon and Simon (1973) developed sexual script theory in their influential book *Sexual Conduct*. Their theory shifted the view in sexological studies from largely biological and psychoanalytic to include cultural and social aspects as well. Since its development, sexual script theory has been one of the most cited modern theories of understanding sexual behavior and has gone on to incorporate views of learning, sociobiology, postmodern, and feminist perspectives.

A sexual script is a cognitive schema or a mental template that serves to signal how one should understand or behave in a sexual situation. A script is typically signaled by one event that sets in action the anticipation of the following sequence that might unfold. Some of these events can be seen to increase the probability that the next step in the chain will occur; others may be seen to decrease that probability.

Sexual scripts have been broken down into three different levels: the cultural, interpersonal, and intrapersonal. Cultural scripts are those that individuals learn from media and different social institutions, such as law, religion, and school. Cultural scripts shape our understanding of what are appropriate and inappropriate sexual choices within society or culture. Some sexual behavior is considered taboo, illegal, or admonished, while others are encouraged, lauded, and envied. Interpersonal scripts involve specific actors engaging within the framework of cultural scripts and concretely enacting these abstract ideas. Interpersonal scripts have two levels. On one level, they are the reinforcement of cultural scripts in a more social or interactional manner. On another level, interpersonal scripts are also a way of direct learning from others through the response to the immediate cues and actions of others. In other words, they are a way of acting out cultural scripts. When all the actors involved share similar scripts, there is relative harmony. However, when there are differences, conflict, improvisation, and learning through assimilation and accommodation may happen. Intrapsychic scripts are the unique ways in which a person internalizes the cultural and interpersonal scripts with their sexual interest, desires, and preferences. Intrapsychic scripts develop an internal mental eroticism containing fantasies, memories, and mental rehearsals. It also includes the process of negotiating interpersonal scripts with others within the cultural script context.

Sexual script theory has been applied to a broad array of research, including gender roles in sexual initiation, casual sex, HIV/AIDS epidemic, rape, and use of pornography, to name a few. Researchers using sexual script theory tend to use two broad approaches to analysis: critical review and self-report. Critical review methods explore cultural-level scripts through the analysis of cultural artifacts, such as mass media, or an already accrued body of research. Self-report methods instead use participants who are asked to describe sexual scripts or validate the existence of hypothetical scripts. In this paradigm, participants may be asked to describe what happened in a specific sexual scenario or to respond to a hypothetical scenario.

Alexander Kovic

See also: Gender Roles, Socialization and; Sex Education; Stereotypes, Gender; Stereotypes, Sexual.

Further Reading

Gagnon, J., & Simon, W. (1973). *Sexual conduct: The social sources of human sexuality.* Piscataway, NJ: Aldine Transaction.

Krahé, B., & Tomaszewska-Jedrysiak, P. (2011). Sexual scripts and the acceptance of sexual aggression in Polish adolescents. *European Journal of Developmental Psychology, 8*(6), 697–712.

Masters, N. T., Casey, E., Wells, E. A., & Morrison, D. M. (2013). Sexual scripts among young heterosexually active men and women: Continuity and change. *Journal of Sex Research, 50*(5), 409–420.

McCormick, N. B. (2010). Preface to sexual scripts: Social and therapeutic implications. *Sexual and Relationship Therapy, 25*(1), 91–95.

Morrison, D. M., Masters, N. T., Wells, E. A., Casey, E., Beadnell, B., & Hoppe, M. J. (2015). "He enjoys giving her pleasure": Diversity and complexity in young men's sexual scripts. *Archives of Sexual Behavior, 44*(3), 655–668.

Simon, W., & Gagnon, J. H. (2003). Sexual scripts: Origins, influences and changes. *Qualitative Sociology, 26*(4), 491–497.

Wiederman, M. W. (2015). Sexual script theory: Past, present, and future. In J. DeLamater & R. F. Plante (Eds.), *Handbook of the sociology of sexualities* (7–22). Cham, Switzerland: Springer Press.

Sexual Slavery

Sexual slavery is a form of oppressive dominance over an individual or group of people through the overt and comprehensive control of sex or sexuality. The term "slavery" is generally used to differentiate individuals who are coerced into sexual behavior from individuals who engage voluntarily in prostitution. Other relevant terms often used by scholars include "forced sexual labor," "trafficking in the sex industry," and "commercial sexual exploitation."

Humanity unfortunately has witnessed several potent examples of sexual slavery throughout history. For example, "comfort women" were kept by the Japanese military during World War II, raped multiple times per day, endured immense physical and psychological pain from sexually transmitted infections and forced abortions, and were often threatened with death. Indeed, an estimated 75 percent of them died during their capture. More recently, an estimated 20,000 women in Yugoslavia were methodically raped as a strategy for "ethnic cleansing" during conflict there in the 1990s, and many Yazidi women were sexually enslaved at the hands of ISIS during the civil war in Syria and surrounding areas.

Although we often only consider egregious examples, sexual slavery is undoubtedly present in day-to-day society and throughout the world. A 2017 report by the International Labour Organization estimates that approximately 4.8 million individuals are exposed to forced sexual exploitation (i.e., "persons in forced labor and services imposed by private actors for sexual exploitation") every year. Moreover, because of the hidden nature of sexual exploitation and the victims who are involved, the few estimates that exist likely underestimate the magnitude of the problem. The vast majority of victims are women and children (usually girls), and in contrast to assumptions often made by policy makers and the general public, they often remain within a single country as opposed to being trafficked across international borders.

Sexual slavery is a multibillion-dollar industry and the third-largest profit earner for international organized crime after drugs and weapons. The potential for financial gain is a clear motivator for traffickers to engage in this behavior, with the industry reaping approximately $44.3 billion. Some scholars suggest that the glamorization of pimping in modern culture (i.e., through film and music) may also play a role in motivating traffickers to engage in this behavior.

Perpetrators use many notable techniques to lure individuals into sexual slavery to maximize their own personal gain and minimize their risk of being caught. In particular, they often prey on vulnerable young women or others (e.g., those facing homelessness or living in group homes; lesbian, gay, bisexual, or transgender youth), sometimes targeting them at bus stations or shopping centers. Many contextual and situational factors make an individual vulnerable to being forced into sexual labor, such as experiences of poverty, childhood violence, family dysfunction, inadequate education, illicit substance dependency, and the presence of prostitution markets. As highlighted by a few researchers, risk factors can be broken down into four categories: individual characteristics (e.g., history of substance abuse, runaway, being a sexual minority), family dynamics (e.g., parental dysfunction, family violence), community (e.g., gang membership, transient male population), and sociocultural and economic (e.g., high crime rates, poverty or unemployment. Perpetrators may provide initial financial or emotional support and may even engage in intimate relations with their victims before increasingly using and abusing them. Others pose online as supportive peers or place job advertisements on the internet promising a purportedly legitimate employment opportunity within a country or across international borders. As victims become ensnared in sexual slavery, victims who cross international borders can be classified as illegal immigrants by the country they have traveled to, leaving them with little or no legal recourse against their attackers. Furthermore, because a victim may form a complex attachment with the perpetrator, they may be unaware of being exploited and remain resistant to outside intervention.

Most survivors of sexual slavery who manage to escape the horrific conditions imposed on them experience severe posttraumatic stress. A meta-analysis evaluating negative outcomes of sex trafficking highlights depression, anxiety, and posttraumatic stress disorder as the most common mental health symptoms experienced by victims. A study evaluating the psychosocial outcomes of the "comfort women" described above found that many of these women experienced learned helplessness throughout their capture, which kept them from actively seeking shelter. Some reported experiencing extreme bouts of anger throughout their capture and suffered from sexually transmitted infections. Long-term symptoms of the abuse included anxiety disorders and substance abuse, and almost all the survivors who were interviewed recounted that their social functioning had been severely impaired by their experiences.

To deal with the problems of sexual slavery, U.S. governmental policies have been implemented, albeit often with very limited scope or impact. For example, the Mann Act of 1910 (aka the White Slave Traffic Act) prohibited the transportation of any girl or woman for immoral purposes across borders. As an expansion, the International Convention for the Suppression of the Traffic in Women and Children notably changed the term "white slavery" to "trafficking." In 2000, the U.S. government enacted the Trafficking Victims Protection Act, which only aids undocumented immigrants exposed to *severe* trafficking unless they are under the age of eighteen years old. To support survivors of sexual slavery and reduce the overall prevalence, engaged governments recognize the necessity of ensuring the availability of appropriate housing, food and clothing, mental health counseling, legal services, and other necessities to vulnerable populations. Some notable programs in the United States to mitigate the harm caused by sex trafficking include the Early Intervention Prostitution Program and the Commercial Sexual Exploitation of Children Community Intervention Project Training Institute. A 2018 qualitative study by Bruhns and colleagues noted that victims under eighteen years old were typically forcefully prevented from leaving the sex trade by their exploiters, emphasizing the need for intense and comprehensive resources including safe houses and witness protection programs for these victims. In contrast, the study suggests that older victims require logistical information to help them exit.

Overall, the most effective worldwide legal policies on sexual exploitation are based on empirical evidence rather than on theoretical ideologies. A more widespread understanding of forced sexual labor, and improved policy to combat it, may help ease feelings of negative judgment and bias often experienced by survivors.

Laura Kabbash and Scott T. Ronis

See also: Child Sexual Abuse; Prostitution; Rape; Rape Trauma Syndrome; Sex Tourism; Sexual Abuse.

Further Reading

Bruhns, M. E., del Prado, A., Slezakova, J., Lapinski, A. J., Li, T., & Pizer, B. (2018). Survivors' perspectives on recovery from commercial sexual exploitation beginning in childhood. *Counseling Psychologist, 46*(4), 413–455.

Felner, J. K., & DuBois, D. L. (2017). Addressing the commercial sexual exploitation of children and youth: A systematic review of program and policy evaluations. *Journal of Child & Adolescent Trauma, 10*(2), 187–201.

Hepburn, S., & Simon, R. J. (2010). Hidden in plain sight: Human trafficking in the United States. *Gender Issues, 27*(1–2), 1–26.

Hoffman, Y., Grossman, E., Shrira, A., Kedar, M., Ben-Ezra, M., Dinnayi, M., ... Zivotofsky, A. (2018). Complex PTSD and its correlates amongst female Yazidi victims of sexual slavery living in post-ISIS camps. *World Psychiatry, 17*(1), 110–112.

International Labor Organization. (2017). *Global estimates of modern slavery: Forced labour and forced marriage.* Geneva, Switzerland. Retrieved from https://www.ilo.org

Kotrla, K. (2010). Domestic minor sex trafficking in the United States. *Social Work, 55*(2), 181–187.

Lee, J., Kwak, Y.-S., Kim, Y.-J., Kim, E.-J., Park, E. J., Shin, Y., … Lee, S. I. (2018). Psychiatric sequelae of former "comfort women," survivors of the Japanese military sexual slavery during World War II. *Psychiatry Investigation, 15*(4), 336.

Lerum, K., & Brents, B. G. (2016). Sociological perspectives on sex work and human trafficking. *Sociological Perspectives, 59*(1), 17–26.

Miller-Perrin, C., & Wurtele, S. K. (2017). Sex trafficking and the commercial sexual exploitation of children. *Women & Therapy, 40*(1–2), 123–151.

O'Brien, J. E., White, K., & Rizo, C. F. (2017). Domestic minor sex trafficking among child welfare–involved youth: An exploratory study of correlates. *Child Maltreatment, 22*(3), 265–274.

Oram, S., Stöckl, H., Busza, J., Howard, L. M., & Zimmerman, C. (2012). Prevalence and risk of violence and the physical, mental, and sexual health problems associated with human trafficking: Systematic review. *PLoS Medicine, 9*(5), 1–13.

Woolman, S., & Bishop, M. (2006). State as pimp: Sexual slavery in South Africa. *Development Southern Africa, 23*(3), 385–400.

Sexuality across the Life Span

Sexuality develops and changes throughout a person's life. While there are times, like puberty, when changes are pronounced, sexuality continues to influence people's lives in many ways from birth (and even before) until death. Further, sexual development is influenced by many things, including biological, social, and psychological experiences. Knowing what to expect and how sexuality can affect someone can help people have realistic expectations, manage changes successfully, and lead healthy sexual lives.

Sexual development begins before birth as the fetus grows and develops sexual characteristics and organs. Infants and young children can experience pleasure from physical contact, and it is common for them to self-stimulate, either manually or by rubbing their genitals on something such as a blanket or toy. It is important to note that behaviors that may seem sexual to observing adults are motivated by curiosity, pleasure, and self-soothing rather than by sexual desire as young children do not yet have an understanding of sexuality. Likewise, as children age, they become aware of their bodies and the bodies of others, and they begin to recognize physical differences between males and females. Curious children may play games like "doctor" in which they compare their bodies with other children. Again, this play is not sexually motivated and is done as a way for children to learn and understand theirs and others' bodies. Knowing these behaviors are normal and to be expected can help parents manage this behavior if they observe it among their own children. Parents' reactions to their children's sexual behavior can have an important effect on later sexual development. If parents react negatively and punish their children, the child may learn to feel ashamed and guilty about their sexuality. As such, it is preferable for parents to teach their children appropriate ways in which to express their sexuality. Sex education is a lifelong process, and parents play a key role in teaching their children to feel good about their bodies, to be respectful of themselves and others, and to feel comfortable asking their parents questions about sexuality.

In preadolescence and adolescence, children's interest in sex increases, and masturbation is common. While many activities and friendships occur primarily with same-sex peers, interest in dating also increases. Social norms tend to be strictly enforced, and many adolescents face peer pressure to behave in socially accepted ways. Importantly, adolescents go through puberty and so experience many physical, cognitive, and emotional changes that affect their sexual development. During later adolescence, many people begin to form romantic relationships and may begin to experiment with partnered sexual behaviors. Typical sexual exploration follows the sexual script that begins with kissing and progresses to genital touching, oral sex, and finally sexual intercourse. Generally speaking, the average age of first sexual intercourse is seventeen for both males and females, and a positive first experience has been shown to be related to better sexual adjustment later in life. As adolescents become sexually active, they need to be aware of safer sex practices to protect themselves and their partners from sexually transmitted infections and, if having sex with other-sex partners, unintended pregnancy.

As adults, people are likely to have a variety of sexual experiences and relationships. Most people will be single at some point, either intentionally or because they have not yet found a long-term partner. During this time, some may be abstinent, while others may have casual sex with one or multiple partners. Most people will also experience dating and getting to know a partner in a more intimate way. Some people will live with partners, and most people marry at least once in their lives. Some of these will experience divorce and infidelity. All these experiences teach people about their own sexuality and the sexuality of their partners. Communication is key between partners in order to have positive and healthy sexual experiences.

As people age, their bodies change, and some aspects of sexual function, like having an erection or experiencing vaginal lubrication, may become more challenging. However, there is much diversity among people. Some older adults experience less sexual activity, while others continue to have sex on a regular basis; one study found that more than half of adults over seventy-five were engaging in sexual activity three or more times per month. As the body changes, as in puberty, it is important for people to know what to expect so that they can be prepared and make adjustments as needed. Sexual expression in older adults may place more of an emphasis on the emotional and intimate connection between partners and may focus more on kissing and sexual touching rather than penetrative sex.

All life stages and relationship experiences provide the opportunity for people to grow and develop sexually. Being aware of sexuality at all stages of life is important for the sexual health of individuals and their partners. Once people know what to expect, they can prepare, respond, and make informed decisions about their sexual lives.

Heather L. Armstrong

See also: Adolescent Sexuality; Childhood Sexuality; Puberty; Sexual Health; Sexuality among Older Adults; Sexuality among Younger Adults.

Further Reading

Haffner, D. (2008). *From diapers to dating.* New York: Newmarket Press.

O'Sullivan, L. F., Cheng, M. M., Harris, K. M., & Brooks-Gunn, J. (2007). I wanna hold your hand: The progression of social, romantic and sexual events in adolescent relationships. *Perspectives on Sexual and Reproductive Health, 39*(2), 100–107.

Reissing, E. D., Andruff (Armstrong), H. L., & Wentland, J. J. (2012). Looking back: The experience of first sexual intercourse and current sexual adjustment in young heterosexual adults. *The Journal of Sex Research, 49*(1), 27–35.

Reissing, E. D., & Armstrong, H. L. (2020). Sexuality over the lifespan. In C. F. Pukall (Ed.), *Human sexuality* (3rd ed.) (203–221). Don Mills, ON: Oxford University Press.

Waite, L. J., Laumann, E. O., Das, A., & Schumm, L. P. (2009). Sexuality: Measures of partnerships, practices, attitudes, and problems in the National Social Life, Healthy, and Aging Study. *The Journals of Gerontology. Series B, Psychological Sciences and Social Sciences, 64B*(Supp 1), i56–i66.

Sexuality among Older Adults

Sexuality involves a focus on sexual matters and involvement in sexual activity. Sexual activity declines as people age, but interest and ability to engage in sex remain in later life. Sexual satisfaction is a significant contributor to quality of life with older adults, ranking close to religious commitments. Differences in sexuality between older adult men and women exist.

Sexuality is a blend of biological, psychological, and cultural aspects of life. In other words, it has physiological origins, but it also represents socially constructed realities that shift. For example, biological constraints limit sexual behavior at certain ages. This leads people to believe older adults do not have as much sex because it is not physically possible. However, research shows higher levels of sexual activity among older adults now compared to previous decades. Though physical limitations exist, cultural acceptance of sexuality in old age is increasing and leading to more sex. Keep in mind, medical advances related to erectile dysfunction, facilitating the production of vaginal lubrication, and certain hormone therapies have contributed to this as well.

Statistics on populations up to the age of eighty-five years show over 50 percent of older adults engage in sexual activity regularly. Numbers are as high as 73 percent around the age of sixty but as low as 25 percent around the age of eighty. The most common reason for giving up sex involves physical limitations. This includes perceived health concerns related to heart disease and strokes, exhaustion and pain related to respiratory disease and arthritis, and lowered self-confidence after surgeries affecting appearance, such as mastectomies. Regardless, sexual activity has the ability to increase health and well-being. Sex leads to a lower risk of heart attack, less cancer, and more restful sleep. Another reason for reduced sexual activity in old age is lack of an available partner. This is specifically problematic for women. The likelihood of having a sexual partner decreases for women as they age due to higher mortality rates for men. There is also a higher level of cultural acceptance related to older men marrying younger women, which reduces the dating pool for females who lose significant others or go through divorces late in life. Data show less than 1 percent of older women have multiple partners in any given year, but even in situations involving lifelong partners, sexual activity decreases due to an increase in familiarity and sexual boredom. Management of aging parents and care provided for grandchildren also contribute.

Current estimates indicate that by 2030 up to six million people in the United States will identify as lesbian, gay, or bisexual. People in older diverse populations such as these report higher levels of life satisfaction than earlier in life. This is primarily due to having already managed problems associated with a culturally stigmatized identity. Stereotypes involving people with alternative sexual orientations have diminished significantly, such as the dissolving perception of older gay men as lonely or predatory. However, problems related to sexuality persist with institutional discrimination, victimization, and specific issues connected to health care and human services access. Consider limitations for life partners related to access to pensions and visitation barriers related to medical contexts. Over 60 percent of older people in the LGBTQ community have younger sexual partners. This creates unique challenges due to generational variation. Older men who have sex with other men are at higher risk of HIV and other sexually transmitted infections. Compared to heterosexual populations, older lesbian and bisexual women have more chronic health problems and alcohol abuse issues, which adversely affects behavior patterns related to sex.

Sexual urges do not cease when older adults move into elder care facilities. However, health care providers often have problems viewing older adults as sexual beings. Sexual activity, especially masturbation, is viewed as problematic, not enriching. With sexually active adults in elder care environments, including older adult housing, males are more likely to seek out multiple partners. Females may insulate themselves from risk by building a personal relationship first and engaging in sex later. Both rarely use protection, including condoms. In some facilities, such as nursing homes, policies restrict older adults from going to private places to engage in intimacy. Facilities also place multiple residents in one room, which lowers the availability of locations for those wanting privacy for sexual activities. Furthermore, over half of nursing homes have policies requiring family approval for sexual activity if a resident has any sign of cognitive impairment, with around 12 percent requiring approval regardless of mental state. Some even require written physician orders allowing a resident to have sex.

Jason S. Ulsperger

See also: Sexual Health; Sexuality across the Life Span; Sexuality among Younger Adults.

Further Reading

Baumle A. (2013). *International handbook on the demography of sexuality.* Dordrecht, Netherlands: Springer.

Fredriksen-Goldsen, K., Kim, H., Shui, C., & Bryan, A. (2017). Chronic health conditions and key health indicators among lesbian, gay, and bisexual older US adults, 2013–2014. *American Journal of Public Health, 107*(8), 1332–1338.

Jen, S. (2017). Older women and sexuality: Narratives of gender, age, and living environment. *Journal of Women & Aging, 29*(1), 87–97.

Lester, P., Kohen, I., Stefanacci, R., & Feuerman, M. (2016). Sex in nursing homes: A survey of nursing home policies governing resident sexual activity. *Journal of the American Medical Directors Association, 17*(1), 71–74.

Ulsperger, J. S., & Knottnerus, J. D. (2015). *Elder care catastrophe: Rituals of abuse in nursing homes and what you can do about it.* London: Routledge.

Sexuality among Younger Adults

Puberty ends at between eighteen and twenty-four years of age, and by the time early adulthood is reached, physical and sexual development have reached maturation for males and females. Height and weight may increase slightly around this time, and physical abilities will peak in early adulthood. Adult females have developed breasts, underarm and pubic hair, and widened hips. For most females, menstruation is a monthly occurrence, and having children may be considered. Males have reached their maximum height, gained a deeper voice, attained broader shoulders, increased in muscle mass, and have underarm and pubic hair.

Around middle adulthood, many changes begin to occur in adults. Changes include an increased sensitivity to sound, having skin that is not as elastic and results in wrinkles and dryness, vision variations, graying and thinning hair, being more prone to illnesses than before, and a possible decrease in reproduction capabilities. Many common illnesses and diseases have an impact on an adult's sexuality. These illnesses or complications include heart disease, diabetes, hypertension, digestive problems, glaucoma, arthritis, and prostate issues.

Once males reach the age of twenty-five, testosterone levels begin to slowly decline, which may influence sexual desire and activity. Over time, males may not be able to have an erection as easily as they once had, or may not be able to sustain an erection once they have one. The quantity of semen released decreases as a man ages, as does the strength of his ejaculation. However, healthy males continue producing sperm until death, and so they are capable of fathering a child later in life.

Of the many eggs a female begins with, only 400–500 will go through ovulation. The number of eggs declines over time, and those that remain during adulthood may decline in quality. As adulthood progresses, females' fertility gradually declines as the individual begins to move into perimenopause (forty to forty-five years old). During this time, individuals experience irregular periods and a decline in estrogen levels, which may result in decreased vaginal lubrication, lack of sexual desire, and possible mood changes.

Psychological and social development have different implications in adulthood because the process is no longer defined by significant physical and cognitive changes. Much of a person's life span is in adulthood, significant psychosocial gains are evident, and often adults report higher levels of satisfaction with their sex life if they are in a committed relationship compared to their single peers. In part, the emotional bond that forms between partners over time often leads to sexual intimacy. Sexual schemas, the perspective one has about their own sexual aspects, are further developed in adulthood. As one moves through adulthood, often they will have a wide variety of sexual techniques and experiences, allowing for a more positive perspective of their own sexuality. As adults age, the process and purpose of sexual experiences tend to move toward emotional connections and intimacy rather than sexual orgasm.

Typically, pregnancies occur between ages twenty and forty, and childbirth can influence an individual and their partner(s)' sex life immensely. The frequency of sexual activity may drop after pregnancy because of hormonal changes, stress, self-esteem, changes in responsibilities, and involvement with children. Pregnancy within a relationship has an impact on all parties involved. Whether it is a same-sex partnership, a mixed-sex partnership, or a polyamorous partnership, pregnancy and the birth of a child will have an impact on intimacy, private time, sexual encounters, financial responsibilities, and emotional reactions to one another and to the child.

Sexual social development continues in adulthood with factors that include sexual satisfaction, reproductive decisions, sexually transmitted infection prevention, intimate relationships, relationship status, and lifestyle choices. Many people reach adulthood with previous sexual experiences in adolescence. Younger adults tend to have more sexual freedom and experiment more than middle-aged or older adults, possibly because they are not in a committed relationship. As young adults navigate the dating scene, many of them form a series of relatively short-term, monogamous relationships. However, in Western cultures, the social expectation is for adults to eventually settle down and commit to a partner for a long-term relationship.

During early adulthood, sexual capabilities peak. It is not uncommon for people to have multiple partners during this time, but this tendency does make this age group more prone to acquiring sexually transmitted infections and unplanned pregnancies than adults who are in monogamous relationships. Although long-term, monogamous relationships are still valued by young adults, they tend to occur later in life. In young adults, people tend to focus more on obtaining a college education, developing their career, and gaining financial stability before they settle down with a lifelong partner. Many opt for cohabitation before getting married for financial reasons and to learn more about each other before making the commitment of marriage.

Casey T. Tobin

See also: Adolescent Sexuality; Marriage; Pregnancy; Sexuality across the Life Span; Sexuality among Older Adults.

Further Reading

Cavanaugh, J., & Blanchard-Fields, F. (2015). *Adult development and aging* (7th ed.). Stamford, CT: Cengage.

Darling, C., Cassidy, D., & Powell, L. (2014). *Family life education: Working with families across the lifespan* (3rd ed.). Long Grove, IL: Waveland Press.

Edelman, C. L., Mandle, C. L., & Kudzma, E. C. (2013). *Health promotion throughout the life span.* St. Louis, MO: Elsevier Health Sciences Mosby.

Sexualization

The American Psychological Association defines sexualization as "the inappropriate imposition of sexuality upon a person, whether through objectification, overvaluing or emphasizing the person's appearance or sexual behavior, or some other means" (Grinnell, 2018). To sexualize something or someone can mean to make them sexual when they are not being or feeling sexual. It can mean to think about them in a sexual way when they are not thinking of themselves that way.

Many people are critical of the tactics that advertisers and the media use to sexualize young people. That is, they are concerned about how ads, TV shows, and movies attach adult sexual meanings to the way children and teenagers look, feel, and behave. For a long time, women have objected to the ways in which they have been sexualized as well. The concern is that sexualization suggests that the worth of a woman is based on her sexual desirability rather than her abilities or intelligence.

Dr. Dennis Dailey describes sexualization as the use of sexuality to influence, manipulate, or control another person. His holistic model of sexuality has been used in many textbooks and educational settings. His view is that sexualization involves how we use our sexuality and may include manipulating or controlling others. In this interpretation, the behaviors are personal between two people. These can range from mild behaviors, like flirting, to more serious activities, like seduction, withholding sex from an intimate partner to punish them or to get something, sexual harassment, sexual abuse, incest, and rape.

Sexualization is sometimes considered the "darker" side of sexuality, as it describes a range of behaviors from the relatively harmless to the violent, cruel, or criminal. The reality is that no one has the right to exploit someone sexually. Some of the behaviors, particularly "flirting" and "seduction," can have a positive or negative impact. It depends on the intent of the person engaging in such behavior as well as the way in which it is interpreted by the person on the receiving end.

Flirting is a relatively harmless behavior, but it can be an attempt to manipulate someone else, and it can cause the person who is manipulated to feel hurt or shame. Flirting with a police officer to get out of a speeding ticket may not be harmful, but flirting with the new girl in school on a dare may be hurtful and embarrassing.

Seduction is the act of enticing someone to engage in sexual activity. This may be mutually pleasurable for both parties, but it can be a negative experience if someone is manipulated into doing something to which they have not fully consented.

Sexual harassment is illegal. It means bothering someone with unwanted sexual words or behaviors. It can be making the space where someone works, studies, or lives feel sexually unsafe. It could mean unwanted touching, such as hugging an underling or patting someone's buttocks. It could mean a teacher, supervisor, or other person in authority asking for sexual activity in exchange for grades, hiring, raises, and so on. The laws provide protection against sexual harassment.

Rape is a crime in which someone forces genital contact with another. Force can include using physical strength, threats, weapons, or implied threats that cause fear in the person who is raped. It can also involve drugs or alcohol that reduces the ability for someone to consent to have sex.

Incest is forced sexual contact of a minor who is related to the perpetrator by birth or marriage. Incest is always illegal and betrays the trust that children and youth give to their families. Like sexual harassment, rape, and sexual assault, incest should be reported to the authorities.

On a social level, researchers have studied the impact of the media's widespread use of sexualization. They found that people who consume sexualized media are more likely to consider themselves as sex objects. Current media puts an emphasis on sexual appearance, physical beauty, and sexual appeal to others. Most people do not have the idealized physical attributes of models or performers on television, in movies, video games, and advertisements. Those who view themselves as sex objects tend to pay chronic attention to their physical appearance and feel less valuable or authentic than others. When a person's value comes only from their sexual appeal or behavior to the exclusion of other characteristics, they can have low self-esteem, anxiety, and shame. In research on the effects of sexualization by the media, the objectification effect was more pronounced for participants using video games or online media. The effect of media use on self-objectification equally affected men and women, older and younger participants, and participants of several ethnic backgrounds.

Michael J. McGee

See also: Advertising, Sex in; Media and Sexuality; Sexual Consent; Sexual Harassment; Sexual Health.

Further Reading

Advocates for Youth. (2007). *Life planning education: A comprehensive sex education curriculum.* Washington, DC: Advocates for Youth.

Dailey, D. M. (1981). Sexual expression and aging. In F. J. Berghorn & D. E. Schafer (Eds.), *The dynamics of aging: Original essays on the process and experiences of growing old* (311–330). Boulder, CO: Westview Press.

Grinnell, R. (2018). Sexualization. *Psych Central.* Retrieved from https://psychcentral.com/encyclopedia/sexualization/

Karsay, K., Knoll, J., & Matthes, J. (2018). Sexualizing media use and self-objectification: A meta-analysis. *Psychology of Women Quarterly, 42*(1), 9–28.

Sexually Transmitted Infections (STIs)

Sexually transmitted infections (STIs) are infections that are passed from person to person through intimate sexual contact, including oral, vaginal, and anal sex. STIs affect people of all genders, sexual orientations, backgrounds, economic levels, and cultures. In the United States, approximately 20 million new infections occur each year, and half of these are among those ages fifteen to twenty-four. The most common STIs generally fall into one of three categories: bacterial STIs consisting of bacterial vaginosis (BV), gonorrhea, syphilis, and chlamydia; viral STIs consisting of genital herpes, viral hepatitis, HIV, and human papillomavirus (HPV); and parasitic STIs consisting of pubic lice (crabs) and trichomoniasis. STIs such as those listed above can be transferred in a variety of ways during both sexual and, in some cases, nonsexual contact. While some people experience symptoms when they contract an STI, many do not. Therefore, regularly STI screening is recommended for most sexually active people.

Bacterial STIs include bacterial vaginosis (BV), gonorrhea, syphilis, and chlamydia. BV is an imbalance of the bacteria present in the vagina and can sometimes occur after a sexual encounter with a new sex partner or with multiple sex partners. BV can also occur due to nonsexual things such as antibiotic use; vaginal douching; or using perfumed soaps, shower gel, or bubble bath. Semen may also trigger BV, so using a condom during sexual intercourse with a male partner may be preventative. Gonorrhea infection can occur in the vagina, uterus, cervix, urethra, anus, mouth, eyes, and throat. Gonorrhea can be passed through oral, anal, and vaginal sex with a partner who has gonorrhea. In addition, it can also be spread through contact by touching an infected area and then touching another place on the body where the infection can enter, such as the eyes or genitals. Syphilis is usually spread through direct contact with a syphilis sore during vaginal, oral, and anal sex. As such, syphilis usually appears on the penis, or around the vagina or anus, but it can occur elsewhere, such as the mouth. Chlamydia is passed through condomless oral, anal, or vaginal intercourse with a partner who has chlamydia. It is the most commonly reported STI in the United States, and in 2017, 1,708,569 infections were reported. Rates of chlamydia are increasing in the United States, especially among women. This is worrisome as many women do not experience symptoms, and, left untreated, chlamydia can cause infertility, ectopic pregnancy, and chronic pelvic pain.

Viral STIs include herpes, hepatitis, HIV, and HPV. In humans, two types of herpes virus, HSV1 and HSV2, can be spread through genital-to-genital, oral-to-genital, or oral-to-oral contact. Transmission is most likely to occur when herpes blisters (also known as cold sores if located on the mouth or lips) are present; however, transmission can occur when symptoms are not present. Hepatitis A is typically transmitted by consuming food or drinking water that has been contaminated with human fecal matter containing the virus, although it can also be transmitted through sexual contact with a person who has the virus. Hepatitis B is spread from person to person through direct contact with blood, sexual fluids such as semen, and needles from drug use. Hepatitis C is also spread through contact with blood containing the virus, commonly through sharing needles or other equipment used to inject drugs. HIV is spread through contact with blood, semen, vaginal fluids, and other bodily fluids such as spinal fluid, breast milk, and amniotic fluid. Advances in HIV treatment now mean that people living with HIV who are virally suppressed through treatment are not able to transmit the virus. HIV can enter the body through the mucous membranes, damaged tissues, or through the bloodstream. It then proceeds to attack and destroy the immune system's infection-fighting cells, making copies of itself, and then killing the healthy cells. HPV is a group of common viruses that includes more than one hundred different types, some of which can be spread through oral, anal, or vaginal sexual contact. HPV can cause genital warts but, importantly, also causes cervical, vaginal, vulvar, penile, anal, and oral cancers, depending on the site of infection.

STIs can also be caused by parasites. Pubic lice are usually spread through sexual contact or by contact with clothing, bed linens, or towels that have been used by a person with pubic lice. Also known as crabs, pubic lice are parasitic insects that prefer to invade the pubic or genital region of human beings, though it is not unusual to find them in other areas with coarse hair, such as armpits or beards. Trichomoniasis (also known as trich) is caused by a tiny parasite called *Trichomonas vaginalis*. This parasite typically infects the vagina and urethra, although the head of the penis or prostate gland can also be infected. It is spread through condomless vaginal or anal sex.

Symptoms may vary with each individual STI and with each individual person. Often, people experience no symptoms at all. In general, symptoms may include pelvic pain, smelly discharge, itching and burning, abdominal pain, fever, pain during sex, pain with urination, and/or changes in menstrual cycle. If any of these symptoms are experienced, it is important to speak with a health care professional for testing and treatment.

Diagnosis of STIs may be through examination of the genitals or pelvic area by a physician, or, in some cases, through fluid sampling, blood tests, or even biopsies of the area. Attempted self-diagnosis, home treatments, or ignoring symptoms can lead to more severe problems. Yearly check-ups with a physician that include honest dialogue about sexual activities and genital checks are highly recommended for most sexually active people, and more frequent testing is recommended for individuals who have new or multiple partners. Early diagnosis and treatment is important for the individual's health and to prevent the onward spread of STIs.

Most STIs can usually be successfully treated and cured. Treatments vary depending on the type and how long the infection has been present. HIV and herpes infection presently have no cure, although treatment is available for symptoms and to reduce the presence of the viruses in the body. People living with HIV who are virally suppressed through treatment are not able to transmit the virus to others.

In order to reduce the likelihood of acquiring an STI, prevention strategies such as using condoms and avoiding sexual contact during an active infection are recommended. Vaccines are also available for hepatitis and HPV. Clear and honest communication between partners about past sexual history and previous STI infection is important. Yearly exams by a qualified physician or sexual health professional, as well as testing for STIs before having condomless sex or after a potential exposure event, will help reduce the rate of STIs.

When engaging in any type of sexual contact, correctly used condoms provide the best protection against STIs. There are two types of condoms. The most common is placed over a penis (insertive), while the other is placed within a vagina or rectum (receptive). If a person has a latex allergy, polyurethane condoms should be used instead. Dental dams also offer protection from STIs during oral sex when used correctly. Importantly, other forms of birth control (e.g., the Pill, an IUD) do not offer protection from STIs, so condoms or dental dams should still be used.

Linda D. Hinkle

See also: Bacterial Vaginosis; Chancroid; Chlamydia; Condoms, Female (Receptive); Condoms, Male (Insertive); Dental Dam; Gonorrhea; Hepatitis, Herpes; Human Immunodeficiency Virus (HIV); Human Papillomavirus (HPV); Molluscum Contagiosum; Pubic Lice; Safer Sex; Scabies; Syphilis; Testing, STI; Trichomoniasis.

Further Reading

Brianti, P., De Flammineis, E., & Mercuri, S. R. (2017). Review of HPV-related diseases and cancers. *New Microbiology, 40*(2), 80–85.

Centers for Disease Control and Prevention. (2017). Sexually transmitted diseases: Adolescents and young adults. Retrieved from https://www.cdc.gov/std/life-stages-populations/adolescents-youngadults.htm

Centers for Disease Control and Prevention. (2018). Sexually transmitted disease surveillance, 2017: Chlamydia. Retrieved from https://www.cdc.gov/std/stats17/chlamydia.htm

Drumright, L. N., Gorbach, P. M., & Holmes, K. K. (2004). Do people really know their sex partners?: Concurrency, knowledge of partner behavior, and sexually transmitted infections within partnerships. *Sexually Transmitted Diseases, 31*(7), 437–442.

Holmes, K. K., Levine, R., & Weaver, M. (2004). Effectiveness of condoms in preventing sexually transmitted infections. *Bulletin of the World Health Organization, 82*(6), 454–461.

National Health Service. (2018). Trichomoniasis. Retrieved from https://www.nhs.uk/conditions/trichomoniasis/#

Rodger, A. J., Cambiano, V., Bruun, T., Vernazza, P., Collins, S., van Lunzen, J., … Lundgren, J. (2016). Sexual activity without condoms and risk of HIV transmission in serodifferent couples when the HIV-positive partner is using suppressive antiretroviral therapy. *JAMA, 316*(1), 171–181.

Shepard, Matthew

Matthew Shepard (1976–1998) became a symbol for the LGBTQ+ rights movement after he was the victim of a vicious hate crime in October 1998. Shepard was a gay college student in Laramie, Wyoming, who was attacked after meeting two men, Aaron McKinney and Russell Henderson, at a bar. Five days later, he died in the hospital. His death provoked discussions about the violence and discrimination experienced by individuals of the LGBTQ+ community. Shepard's story has been documented in many books, movies, and plays, including *The Laramie Project* and *Matthew Shepard Is a Friend of Mine*.

Matthew Shepard was born on December 1, 1976, to Judy and Dennis Shepard in Casper, Wyoming. He had one younger brother. Shepard attended school in Casper until his junior year, when his family moved to Saudi Arabia. He graduated high school from The American School in Switzerland. While living abroad, he learned how to speak German and Italian. He was also very involved in community theater.

At age twenty-one, Shepard became a freshman at the University of Wyoming, studying political science, foreign relations, and languages. He was chosen to be the student representative for the Wyoming Environmental Council, and he also became a member of a gay alliance club on campus. On the night of October 6,

1998, Shepard went to the Fireside Bar in Laramie alone after seeing some friends at a local restaurant. He met McKinney and Henderson, who allegedly led Shepard to believe they were gay.

Shepard left the bar with McKinney and Henderson, and they took him to a remote location several miles east of Laramie. There, they robbed, beat, and pistol whipped Shepard, and they tied him to a fence and left him to die in freezing temperatures. Nearly eighteen hours later, Shepard was discovered by a cyclist, who initially thought he was a scarecrow. He was taken to Ivinson Memorial Hospital in Laramie, but due to his severe injuries, he needed to be transferred to a hospital outside of Fort Collins, Colorado.

Shepard died from his injuries early on October 12, surrounded by his family. McKinney and Henderson were convicted of felony murder and sentenced to two consecutive life sentences. Despite the nature of the attack, the men could not be charged with a hate crime because no such laws existed in Wyoming at the time.

Shepard's murder elicited protests and an increased advocacy for federal legislation for LGBTQ+ victims of violence. Shepard's parents founded the Matthew Shepard Foundation to honor their son's memory and to advocate for acceptance for LGBTQ+ individuals. His mother became a vocal activist for the LGBTQ+ community.

Over a decade after Shepard's murder, President Barack Obama signed the Matthew Shepard and James Byrd Jr. Hate Crimes Prevention Act (HCPA) in 2009. The HCPA is a federal law that added sexual orientation and gender identity to the list of protected classes against biased crimes. This means that the U.S. Department of Justice is able to investigate and prosecute bias-motivated crimes of violence against individuals for either their gender identity or sexual orientation.

Sarah Gannon

See also: Antigay Prejudice; Gay Rights Movement; LGBTQ+.

Further Reading

Anti-Defamation League. (n.d.). Matthew Shepard and James Byrd Jr. Hate Crimes Prevention Act (HCPA): What you need to know. Retrieved from https://www.adl.org/sites/default/files/documents/assets/pdf/combating-hate/What-you-need-to-know-about-HCPA.pdf

Hassanein, R. (2019). Remembering and honoring Matthew Shepard. Retrieved from https://www.hrc.org/blog/remembering-and-honoring-matthew-shepard

Hurst, J. C. (1999). The Matthew Shepard tragedy. *About Campus, 4*(3), 5.

Matthew Shepard Foundation. (2019). Frequently asked questions. Retrieved from http://www.matthewshepard.org/faq/

Medium. (n.d.). Matthew's Place. Retrieved from https://medium.com/matthews-place

Slut Shaming

Slut shaming, also known as slut bashing, is a form of stigma and bullying directed at people (most often women and girls) who are perceived or believed to have violated some form of traditional expectations for sexual behaviors. It involves attacking a person and making them feel guilty and ashamed for their sexual behaviors—real or perceived—that deviate from societal norms. Such norms are often gendered and stereotypical in nature—for example, the myth that "good girls" do not or should not want sexual activity. Viewed through this lens, slut shaming is often considered a method of sociocultural regulation of patriarchal sexual values (e.g., that sex is the acquisition of pleasure from a woman, something one "takes" from a woman) as well as a major component of rape culture. Slut shaming has garnered national attention in recent years due to its increasing presence online as a form of cyberbullying and harassment, particularly of women and girls.

Typical practices of slut shaming involve attacking a woman or girl for being sexual (in any capacity), having one or more sexual partners, or expressing or acting on their sexual feelings. Other circumstances in which women and girls have been "slut shamed" include violating accepted dress codes by wearing attire that is judged to be too sexually provocative, using or fighting for access to birth control, and after being sexually assaulted. In this latter example, slut shaming is akin to victim blaming by contending that the crime of sexual violence was caused, fully or in part, by the woman's sexually provocative behaviors or clothing, thereby absolving the perpetrator of any wrongdoing.

Though its exact definition varies by historical era, the term "slut" is typically used in a derogatory fashion to describe a woman who is sexually promiscuous, unclean, or disgusting. Slut shaming may, though does not necessarily, involve use of the term "slut" or related insults (whore, tramp, etc.). At its core, the act of slut shaming is less about the word "slut" and more significantly involves the implication that if a woman is sexual in a way that traditional society disapproves of, she is and should feel inferior. Thus, slut shaming might involve anything from direct verbal abuse or spreading rumors and gossip about a person's sexual behaviors to online harassment, sharing sexual photos or videos of a person without their consent, or physical intimidation or assault.

Slut shaming appears to be increasing in the age of social media and technology and has far-reaching negative consequences, again particularly for women and young girls. Data reveal that two out of five girls in the United States have had sexual rumors spread about them, three out of four have received unwanted sexual comments or looks, and one in five has had negative sexual messages written about her in a public area. Being publicly shamed and denigrated in this manner—often for ongoing and lengthy periods of time—can be highly traumatic, resulting in subsequent mental health concerns such as anxiety, depression, and, in some cases, suicide. In addition, it has been noted that once a person has been slut shamed and labeled a "slut" or "whore," they are more likely to become a target of sexual violence as they are now viewed as inferior or even deserving of the violence. As noted above, if the person actually is sexually assaulted or harassed, the label of "slut" is often used to rationalize the behavior and protect the perpetrator.

A major cultural response to slut shaming was the growth of the SlutWalk protest march. SlutWalk, which has become a global movement, started in 2011 in response to an incident in which a Toronto law enforcement officer told a group of students that "women should avoid dressing like sluts" in order to prevent sexual assault. The protest most often takes the form of a march where some participants dress in "slutty" attire, such as short skirts and high heels. Other SlutWalks have encouraged participants to wear any form of clothing in which they have been slut shamed or sexually assaulted as a way of highlighting that sexual violence can and does occur regardless of attire that is deemed sexually provocative.

Jennifer A. Vencill

See also: Double Standards, Sexual; Female Sexuality; Madonna/Whore Dichotomy; Sexual Assault; Sexual Harassment; Stereotypes, Sexual.

Further Reading

Friedman, J. (2011). *What you really really want: The smart girl's shame-free guide to sex and safety.* New York: Seal Press.

Tanenbaum, L. (2000). *Slut! Growing up female with a bad reputation.* New York: HarperCollins Publishers.

Tanenbaum, L. (2015). *I am not a slut: Slut-shaming in the age of the Internet.* New York: HarperCollins Publishers.

Smegma

Smegma is a combination of fats and oils, exfoliated skin cells, and moisture produced by human genitals. In males, it is produced by the foreskin of the penis and can accumulate between the foreskin and the glans of the penis. In females, it is produced generally by glands around the clitoris and accumulates around the clitoris and in the folds of the labia minora. It is believed that smegma evolved as a natural lubricant for sexual intercourse. Problems with smegma are relatively minor and can be solved with good hygiene.

Most discussion of smegma concentrates on what is produced by males. Researchers have argued about the value of smegma and why it is produced by the body. Tests show that it is composed of more than 25 percent fats and 13 percent proteins. Much of this comes from skin cells that are shed by the penis and the foreskin. When newly produced, smegma has a smooth, moist texture. It acts as a lubricant to help the foreskin slide back to expose the glans during intercourse. During childhood, little if any is produced. However, during adolescence, the male begins to produce more and more, reaching peak production about the time of sexual maturity. During middle age, production declines. By old age, men produce almost no smegma. Individual experiences may differ somewhat. The opponents and supporters of male circumcision often include a discussion of the benefits and drawbacks of smegma, because a circumcised penis does not produce smegma.

As smegma ages, it becomes greasy or hardens onto the penis. Because it contains dead skin cells and bacteria, an unpleasant odor may also result. Dirt, sand, and other particles may accumulate under the foreskin with the smegma. This can result in irritation to the penis and even an infection. Early researchers believed smegma could also increase the chances of cancer, but this has now been discounted. Smegma can easily be removed with gentle daily washing with soap and water. Excessive washing with soap can lead to dermatitis and should be avoided.

Tim J. Watts

See also: Circumcision; Foreskin; Labia; Penis.

Further Reading

The Circumcision Decision. (2013). Smegma. Retrieved from http://thecircumcisiondecision.com/smegma/

Lentz, M. (2017). Smegma removal: How to clean smegma in males and females. Healthline. Retrieved from https://www.healthline.com/health/how-to-get-rid-of-smegma

Social Learning Theory, Gender and

Social learning theory was developed by Albert Bandura through his laboratory experiments focusing on modeling and behavior. A famous experiment of his, conducted in 1965, involved three groups of four-year-old children and Bobo dolls. All the children were shown a film where a model exhibited aggressive behavior toward an inflated Bobo doll, but the three groups were shown three different consequences for this behavior: the actor was punished for his actions, the actor was ignored for his actions, or the actor was rewarded with treats for his actions. Based on the consequences shown to the groups, the children's behaviors, including their actions and speech, imitated the observed model, showing that learning involves a cognitive process whereas behaviors are modeled on the observed behavior of others and the consequences of that behavior. From this experiment, Bandura used social learning theory as a way to explain how behavioral responses of people are a function of a cognitive process through attention, retention, motor reproduction, and incentive and motivational processes. These four concepts can also be used to explain how gender identity and expression is shaped by the various influences within society.

Gender identity, as conceptualized by behavioral psychologist John Money in his book *Man and Women, Boy and Girl* (1972) and challenged later by the biophysical work of Milton Diamond and philosopher Judith Butler, is a person's own psychological awareness of their gender, whether it be male, female, transgender, or another diverse identity. Gender identity can be the same or different from one's biological sex, how a person is labeled as male, female, or intersex based on the specific combinations of their chromosomes, gonads, and hormone levels. While biological sex is based on a person's physical body, gender identity and expression are shaped by society's expectations of how the biological sex should act, appear, and behave on a personal (hairstyle, clothing, voice), interpersonal (how one performs their gender gives signals to another person on how to act or treat someone), and institutional basis (masculinity characteristics are more valued than feminine characteristics).

Being able to perform these attributes in a socially favorable manner produces rewards or incentives. Through social learning theory's concept of attention, the person must pay attention to the social cues around them to learn and then imitate the behavior. For example, if a young girl sees her mother always crossing her legs while sitting in a chair (but never her father), she will believe that crossing her legs is something that girls do. With the concept of retention, if the young girl watches TV and further sees that women mostly cross their legs while sitting in order to be "ladylike," these constant examples will help her retain this information so that she is more likely to perform this activity again. Having the ability to remember the motor reproductive process of the expected activity (sit in chair, cross one leg over the other, place hands on knees to keep legs closed), along with the observation (all women cross their legs when sitting), is also a sign of cognition influencing behavior. Finally, the incentive and motivational process for the young girl is when she receives affirmative messages about crossing her legs when sitting ("She is sitting like such a lady!"), but her behavior and thinking is also shaped by any negative messaging that she receives ("Real women keep their legs closed!"). Social learning theory recognizes that both positive and negative messages and the increase or lack of incentives or punishments can shape how one expresses their gender.

For people who identify as gender diverse, transgender, genderqueer, or who are outside of the gender dichotomy of male and female, some of the social understanding of how to perform as a certain gender can be challenging, confusing, and frustrating. The further away one is from the dichotomy of gender (masculine to feminine), the more negative the consequences and the fewer incentives one may receive. This dynamic between gender-diverse people and society does not always provide a safe space for one to create, dress, live, or behave, which increases the chance of discrimination when one does not express their gender in socially accepted ways.

Shane'a Thomas

See also: Binary Gender System; Gender; Gender Diversity; Gender Expression; Gender Identity; Gender Identity Development; Gender Roles, Socialization and; Genderqueer; Intersexuality; Stereotypes, Gender; Transgender.

Further Reading

Fausto-Sterling, A. (2012). *Sex/gender: Biology in the social world.* New York: Routledge.

Lehmiller, J. J. (2014). *The psychology of human sexuality.* Hoboken, NJ: Wiley-Blackwell.

Longres, J. (2000). *Human behavior in the social environment* (3rd ed.). Belmont, CA: Wadsworth/Thomson Learning.

Mazur, J. (1998). *Learning and behavior* (4th ed.). Upper Saddle River, NJ: Prentice-Hall.

Seidman, S. (2012). Theoretical perspectives. In S. Seidman, N. Fisher, & C. Meeks (Eds.), *Introducing the new sexuality studies* (2nd ed., 3–12). New York: Routledge.

Tauches, K. (2012). Transgendering: Challenging the "normal." In S. Seidman, N. Fisher, & C. Meeks (Eds.), *Introducing the new sexuality studies* (2nd ed., 135–139). New York: Routledge.

Society for the Scientific Study of Sexuality (SSSS)

The Society for the Scientific Study of Sexuality (SSSS, pronounced "quad S") is an international nonprofit organization committed to sexuality research. Founded in 1957, SSSS is the oldest professional organization for the study of sexuality in the United States. Through various academic and professional endeavors, SSSS maintains an interdisciplinary network of professionals who believe in the importance of the rigorous study of sexuality at the clinical, educational, and social levels. Within this network lives a diverse grouping of professionals, including therapists, anthropologists, medical practitioners, theologians, lawyers, sexologists, psychologists, educators, researchers, therapists, activists, and policy makers. The range of perspectives held by SSSS members has supported the growth of sexual science as an academic and professional field of study.

Albert Ellis (1973–2007) was an American psychologist who was passionate about human sexuality. Considered a key player in the American sexual revolution, Ellis worked alongside well-known sexologists, including Alfred Kinsey. Amid publishing books and papers on sexual liberation, guilt-free sexuality, and love, Ellis rallied support from other academics to create an organization where sexuality could be the primary focus of research. This gathering of minds in the realm of sexual science came to be known as the Society for the Scientific Study of Sexuality.

There are more than 700 members in SSSS among seven categories of membership: general members, fellows, chartered members, students, developing professionals, lifetime members, and honorary members. Membership benefits include discounted attendance to society events, regional and national members meetings, awards for professional excellence and public service, and connections to the organization's directory of professional resources. Both members and nonmembers have access to the public events offered by the SSSS, such as conferences, scholarly publications, and newsletters.

SSSS is committed to the future of sexual science. The SSSS student mentorship program was instituted to connect people that would otherwise be stratified by geographical location and work experience. All SSSS members are eligible to be mentors or mentees. In this way, students and developing professionals can learn from researchers and fellows, and those established in their careers can contribute to the field of sexology in a new way.

Members of SSSS are strongly encouraged to be involved in the organization. Members are seen as community leaders, and through an ambassador program, young and old SSSS members are equally supported to plan futures in professional, community, or academic leadership.

SSSS has three primary publications in circulation. The most well-known publication is the *Journal of Sex Research*, which is a scientific quarterly reputed to contain the latest in sexual science research. The *Annual Review of Sex Research* is the yearly equivalent to the *Journal of Sex Research*. Its purpose is to synthesize recent advances in theory and research. The least academic of the three publications is *Sexual Science*, an online newsletter sharing information on upcoming trainings, conferences, job opportunities, and more.

Shadeen Francis

See also: Ellis, Albert; Kinsey, Alfred; Sexology.

Further Reading

Society for the Scientific Study of Sexuality. (2019). Home page. Retrieved from http://www.sexscience.org

Taylor and Francis Group. (2010). Annual review of sex research. Retrieved from http://www.tandfonline.com/loi/hzsr20#.VxlvhIrJE4

Sodomy Laws

"Sodomy laws" refer to any laws against certain sexual acts deemed by society to be immoral, unnatural, and harmful. The term "sodomy" is used for such acts. Throughout history, the laws of many different societies and cultures have recognized different definitions for sodomy. In a general historical sense, sodomy laws were targeted against the typical sexual acts engaged in by men with other men, especially anal and oral sex. However, depending on the culture, such laws might also encompass certain other sexual acts, including anal and oral sex between mixed-sex partners as well as sexual relations with animals (bestiality), dead bodies (necrophilia), and children (pedophilia).

The word "sodomy" is derived from the biblical tale of Sodom and Gomorrah, two cities used as examples of extreme sexual immorality. Despite the biblical condemnation, sodomy—in the sense of relations between men and relations between men and boys—was fairly common and acceptable in many societies during ancient times.

During the late 1900s, sodomy laws began to be modified or eliminated in many states within the United States as societal attitudes toward same-sex behavior became more liberal and tolerant. Still, as of 2019, sixteen states maintain some version of sodomy laws. Furthermore, such laws remain important aspects of social order in numerous other nations, such as those controlled by strict Islamic governments.

Until the 1960s, sodomy—including mutually consensual sex between same-sex partners—was classified as a serious felony crime throughout the United States, with standard punishments consisting of fines and imprisonment. In 1961, Illinois became the first state to eliminate criminal punishment for mutually consensual sodomy between adults. This move followed recommendations made in 1955 by a group of liberal lawyers and law professors called the American Law Institute.

Many—but not all—other states either eliminated or reduced their criminal penalties for sodomy or same-sex sexual behavior during the 1970s. Some states kept their sodomy laws but did not enforce them. Penalties described in remaining sodomy laws—whether or not they were enforced—ranged up to life in prison.

A 1986 ruling by the U.S. Supreme Court, in the case of *Bowers v. Hardwick*, upheld a Georgia law criminalizing oral and anal sex in both mixed-sex and same-sex sexual activity. That ruling was used by some lawyers as justification for sodomy laws in several states, though other lawyers believed that the issue remained unsettled.

In 2003, the Supreme Court, in the case of *Lawrence v. Texas*, ruled that an existing sodomy law in Texas was unconstitutional because it violated the Fourteenth-Amendment right of adults to engage in private, mutually consensual sexual conduct. That ruling had the legal effect of constitutionally invalidating most remaining sodomy laws in other states as well—seemingly resolving the issue in the United States. Nevertheless, of the fourteen states that had sodomy laws at the time of the ruling, only two—Montana and Virginia—moved to repeal their laws. Not even Texas formally repealed its sodomy law, though the state added a disclaimer to the law noting that the high court ruled it to be unconstitutional.

Despite the 2003 Supreme Court decision, sixteen states maintain sodomy laws within their criminal statutes as of 2019: Alabama, Florida, Georgia, Idaho, Louisiana, Maryland, Massachusetts, Michigan, Minnesota, Mississippi, North Carolina, Oklahoma, and South Carolina; laws in Kansas, Kentucky, and Texas target only same-sex behavior. Most of these laws are vaguely worded as to what constitutes criminal behavior, using such phrases as "any unnatural and lascivious act" or "abominable and detestable crime against nature." Political pressure from socially conservative communities within these states tends to prevent legislators from repealing such sodomy laws. However, these laws are usually not actively enforced. Although a small number of people, mainly gay men, continue to be arrested by local police under these laws, prosecutors do not pursue these cases, so the arrested individuals are soon released. If adults engaging in consensual sex were to be prosecuted under sodomy laws, the criminal prosecutions would likely be struck down by state courts, using the 2003 high court decision as a basis.

As of 2019, mutually consensual sexual activities between same-sex adults—constituting acts of "sodomy"—are illegal in seventy countries. Most of these countries are in Africa and the Middle East. In some of these nations—including Afghanistan, Brunei, Iran, Mauritania, Pakistan, Nigeria, Qatar, Saudi Arabia, Somalia, Sudan, the United Arab Emirates, and Yemen—sexual acts between men could be punishable by death. In several other nations in these regions, sodomy is punishable with life in prison.

A. J. Smuskiewicz

See also: Anal Sex; Dating, Cross-Cultural Comparison of; Gay Rights Movement; Homosexuality; Oral Sex; Same-Sex Attraction and Behavior.

Further Reading

American Civil Liberties Union. (2019). Getting rid of sodomy laws: History and strategy that led to the Lawrence decision. Retrieved from https://www.aclu.org/getting-rid-sodomy-laws-history-and-strategy-led-lawrence-decision

Duncan, P. (2017, July). Gay relationships are still criminalised in 72 countries, report finds. *The Guardian.* Retrieved from https://www.theguardian.com/world/2017/jul/27/gay-relationships-still-criminalised-countries-report

Human Dignity Trust. (2019). Map of countries that criminalise LGBT people. Retrieved from https://www.humandignitytrust.org/lgbt-the-law/map-of-criminalisation/

Somnus Orgasm

Somnus orgasm is the uniquely female (assigned female at birth) phenomenon of experiencing orgasm during sleep. Most often, people born with a vulva/vagina who have an orgasm during sleep will wake during the orgasm, but this is not always the case. Some may sleep through the experience and recall it later upon waking or might not remember it occurring at all. As many as 42.7 percent of women will likely experience an orgasm during sleep by the age of seventy-eight, and the number of women could potentially be higher as this is a vastly understudied area of sexuality research.

Some research suggests that somnus orgasm prevalence and frequency may be more common during certain periods or life events. For example, some women report experiencing orgasm during sleep when going through long periods of sexual abstinence, during pregnancy, or at certain times of their menstrual cycle. Some experts suggest that there may also be a relationship between somnus orgasm and lucid dreaming, level of education (or future level of education), sexual liberalism, likelihood of experiencing other types of orgasm, and previous knowledge of somnus orgasm, though more research needs to be conducted before these possible relationships can be better supported. Many women also report that their sleep orgasm experiences occur most often during sexual dreams, but this is not always the case.

While somnus orgasms have some similarities with the male experience of nocturnal emission, there are several significant differences. The most notable distinction is that somnus orgasms do not only occur during puberty such as male nocturnal emissions do. Girls and women who experience orgasm during sleep may experience their first occurrence before the age of five years old or at any other point in their lives. In addition, many girls and women who experience somnus orgasms continue to do so regularly throughout their entire life. In fact, Alfred Kinsey's monumental sexuality studies suggested that somnus orgasms may potentially be more prevalent and frequent among older women, which is the opposite of male nocturnal emission frequency, which diminishes or ceases altogether following adolescence. Another major difference is that, as far as current research has found, women who experience orgasm during sleep do not appear to ejaculate during these events like males during nocturnal emissions. Though female ejaculation itself is well documented, it has not yet been formally studied in regard to somnus orgasms. This is why some women may not be aware of an orgasm happening at all, as there is no obvious physical evidence.

Women and girls who have experienced orgasm during sleep have often been pathologized, thought to be suffering from various diseases or ailments, believed to be promiscuous, or even persecuted for witchcraft. The earliest records suggest that girls and women who reported having an orgasm while asleep were assumed to be having an affair with the devil and therefore practicing witchcraft. Later, it was commonly believed that virginal girls could not experience orgasm during sleep, so it was thought to be a sign of promiscuity or sexual deviancy. One supernatural explanation that has been common throughout history, and still very much believed today by some, is that an orgasm during sleep is the result of a demonic sexual assault from an incubus (a sex demon who is thought to attack women in their sleep). Even today, as many people are still unaware that somnus orgasms are a normal event, some women seeking information from their doctors or therapists are misdiagnosed with epilepsy or schizophrenia. Research has also demonstrated that while most women and girls view their sleep orgasm experiences as enjoyable and pleasurable, many (especially those who were young during their first or early somnus orgasm events) felt embarrassed, ashamed, guilty, or frightened. This serves to illustrate the importance of accurate sexual health education both in schools and at home.

Lyndsay Mercier

See also: Female Sexuality; Nocturnal Emissions; Orgasm.

Further Reading

King, F. (2012). *Waking into "the big O."* North Charleston, SC: Createspace.

Kinsey, A., Pomeroy, W., Martin C., & Gebhard, P. (1953). *Sexual behavior in the human female.* Philadelphia: W. B. Saunders Company.

Mercier, L. (2020). *Things that go bump in the night: Prevalence, predictors, and experiences of women who orgasm during sleep.* Dissertation. Widener University.

Sperm

Sperm are the male sex cells produced by the testicles, or testes. As a result of penile-vaginal intercourse or other enhanced fertility treatments, a sperm cell may fertilize an egg cell to form a zygote (fertilized egg), which develops into an embryo. The embryo, in turn, develops into a fetus. Sperm carry the male deoxyribonucleic acid (DNA), making up half of the genetic material inherited by the baby. The other half comes from the female egg. At the time of fertilization, the twenty-three chromosomes (structures that carry genes) in the sperm join with the twenty-three chromosomes in the egg to produce the baby's complete genetic makeup of forty-six chromosomes.

Sperm are produced in the seminiferous tubules that fill the interior of the testes. They then travel to a coiled tube at the rear of the testes called the epididymis, where they complete their development. During sexual arousal, the sperm are released outside the testes into long tubes called vas deferens. The sperm next become mixed with nourishing fluids from the prostate, seminal vesicles, and bulbourethral glands before passing out of the body through the penis during ejaculation in a sticky mixture called semen. An average, healthy ejaculation of semen contains approximately one hundred million sperm cells.

To fertilize an egg—a process that usually occurs within one of the fallopian tubes just outside the uterus—a sperm cell has to penetrate the surface of the egg. Enzymes released by the head of the sperm break down the egg's coating to allow entry into the egg. Before that, however, the long tail, or flagellum, behind the head of the sperm whips from side to side to propel the sperm cell forward as it makes its journey through the female reproductive tract. Sperm may remain viable inside the female body for approximately five days after sexual intercourse.

The health and viability of sperm decline with age, especially after age fifty. To be successful in fertilization, sperm must meet three main qualifications: (1) they must exist in large numbers in the ejaculate—typically more than 15 million to 20 million sperm cells per milliliter; (2) they must have normal shapes—with an oval head and a long whip-like tail; and (3) they must be able to move through the vagina, cervix, and uterus to reach the egg in the fallopian tube. It is common for a certain percentage of sperm to have abnormal shapes or abnormal movements. In a man who is fertile, at least 40 percent of his sperm typically have normal structure and movement.

Some research suggests that the sperm of older men carry an increased risk of producing offspring with certain conditions, including autism and schizophrenia. In addition, the risk of miscarriage may increase in pregnancies caused by older men.

Several things can be done in order to maintain fertility and the health of sperm. Practicing safer sex—that is, using condoms or other protections against sexually transmitted infections—can help prevent problems with fertility and sperm. Eating a healthy, well-balanced diet; maintaining an appropriate weight; and limiting cigarette smoking and drug and alcohol intake can also help preserve sperm health. Regular physical exercise and the reduction of stress are two additional factors that have been shown to be important in maintaining fertility.

A. J. Smuskiewicz

See also: Conception; Contraception; Ejaculation; Fertility; Ova; Semen; Seminiferous Tubules; Sex Chromosomes; Testicles.

Further Reading

Cleveland Critics. (2017). 7 things you can do to keep your sperm healthy. Retrieved from https://health.clevelandclinic.org/7-things-you-can-do-to-keep-your-sperm-healthy/

Mayo Clinic. (2018). Healthy sperm: Improving your fertility. Retrieved from http://www.mayoclinic.org/healthy-living/getting-pregnant/in-depth/fertility/art-20047584

NHS. (2019). Low sperm count. Retrieved from https://www.nhs.uk/conditions/low-sperm-count/

Spermicides

Spermicides are a contraceptive method that can be used alone or with another contraceptive method in order to increase effectiveness. They are composed of a spermicidal agent in a carrier (cream, gel, foam, film, pessary, or suppository) that allows dispersion and retention in the vagina. In order to prevent pregnancy, the spermicide must be inserted into the vagina next to the cervix at least fifteen minutes (and not more than three hours) before intercourse. The active agent, nonoxynol-9, forms a chemical barrier that destroys the membrane of sperm cells, either killing them or slowing them down so that they fail to pass through the cervix and reach the ovum. This method is not widely used, being one of the least effective of all birth control methods, with effectiveness rates ranging from 71–82 percent.

Spermicides are more effective when combined with another barrier method such as a condom, diaphragm, or cervical cap. Contrary to popular belief, nonoxynol-9 does not protect against sexually transmitted infections. In fact, research shows that spermicides actually increase the risk of contracting HIV. This is because the chemicals they contain can damage the vaginal mucus, causing vaginal irritation and small lesions on the vaginal walls, which raises the risk of HIV transmission. Consequently, spermicides are not recommended for individuals who are allergic to nonoxynol-9, are at greater risk for contracting HIV, are living with HIV, are using antiretroviral therapy, or have a history of toxic shock syndrome.

Before each instance of vaginal intercourse takes place, the spermicide must be placed deep into the vagina using an applicator or else placed directly on a condom. Generally, it should be applied within one hour before intercourse, although some gels have longer effectiveness. Some spermicides are effective immediately after insertion, while others, such as suppositories and films, take ten to fifteen minutes to become effective. It is important to read the instructions carefully so that the spermicide is used correctly and inserted at the optimal time.

Spermicides have certain advantages and disadvantages. Conveniently, a consultation with a health care provider is not required. Spermicides have no hormonal side effects, and there is immediate return to fertility after use. They also help lubricate the vagina. Furthermore, because they can be inserted ahead of time, they do not interrupt the sexual activity. An added benefit is that they can be inserted into the vagina without a partner's collaboration, which gives the person with a vagina control over the contraception strategy. On the downside, spermicides are one of the least effective birth control methods, especially when used alone. They can cause irritation or burning of the vagina or penis, and some individuals are allergic to the chemical content. They also have an unpleasant odor and taste. Finally, spermicides provide no protection against sexually transmitted infection and may actually increase susceptibility.

Sylvie Lévesque

See also: Barrier Contraceptive Methods; Contraception; Pregnancy; Sexually Transmitted Infections (STIs); Sperm; Vaginitis.

Further Reading

Black, A., Guilbert, E., Costescu, D., Dunn, S., Fisher, W., Kives, S., ... Todd, N. (2015). Canadian contraception consensus (Part 2 of 4). *Journal of Obstetrics and Gynaecology Canada, 37*(11), 1036–1039.

Glasier, A., & Gebbie, A. E. (2008). *Handbook of family planning and reproductive healthcare.* (5th ed.). London: Churchill Livingstone.

McVeigh, E., Guillebaud, J., & Homburg, R. (2013). *Oxford handbook of reproductive medicine and family planning.* Oxford: Oxford University Press.

Society of Obstetricians and Gynaecologists of Canada. (2019). Retrieved from www.sexandu.ca

World Health Organization. (2018). Family planning: A global handbook for providers. Retrieved from https://www.who.int/reproductivehealth/publications/fp-global-handbook/en/

Sponge, Contraceptive

The sponge—more precisely called the vaginal sponge or the contraceptive sponge—is a device inserted deep into the vagina to prevent pregnancy. It is disc-shaped, soft, about two inches (five centimeters) in diameter, and made of polyurethane foam.

The device works both by physically blocking the entry of sperm into the cervix (neck of the uterus) and by releasing spermicide, a chemical compound (nonoxynol-9) that kills sperm. Only one brand of sponge is approved for use in the United States by the Food and Drug Administration; it became available in 1983. Additional brands are available in other countries.

The sponge is generally easy and convenient to use, inexpensive, and requires no prescription. Before inserting the sponge, it must be moistened with water to activate the spermicide. The device can be left in place for as long as thirty hours. It remains effective for twenty-four hours, during which time the woman can have sexual intercourse as often as she likes. It should be kept in place at least six hours after intercourse to prevent pregnancy. Many people prefer the sponge as a contraceptive because, unlike birth control pills, it does not disrupt their hormone balance and, thus, does not have the side effects associated with hormonal changes.

However, the sponge is less effective than birth control pills and many other methods of contraception. It is most effective for people who have never given birth, with about nine to twelve out of every hundred becoming pregnant when using the sponge as directed. For those who have previously given birth and who use the sponge as directed, about twenty to twenty-four out of every hundred will become pregnant. The sponge's effectiveness at preventing pregnancy is enhanced if the partner uses a condom or if the penis is withdrawn before ejaculation. A condom will also help protect against sexually transmitted infections (STIs), for which the sponge offers no protection.

The sponge is safe to use for most people. However, those who have hypersensitivities (allergies) to polyurethane or sulfa drugs should not use the device as it may cause skin irritation and dryness, resulting in small open wounds that raise the risk of STIs. The device may also be inappropriate for people who have had a history of toxic shock syndrome (TSS) as the sponge raises the risk of TSS—which is characterized by fever, rash, dizziness, confusion, and, in the worst cases, multiple organ failure—if it is left in place longer than thirty hours; if it is used during vaginal bleeding; or if it is used soon after childbirth, miscarriage, or abortion. The sponge may also lead to problems for those who have had frequent yeast or urinary tract infections, particularly by raising the risk of such infections if it is left in place for too long.

Some people experience difficulties inserting or removing the sponge, but most, with practice, can easily learn to use it. The device is most easily inserted while in a squatting position, using one or two fingers to slide it up the vagina as far as it will go. The device has a strap, which is pulled to remove it.

A. J. Smuskiewicz

See also: Barrier Contraceptive Methods; Cervix; Contraception; Spermicides.

Further Reading

Health Link BC. (2017). Contraceptive sponge for birth control. Retrieved from https://www.healthlinkbc.ca/health-topics/tw9510

Mayo Clinic. (2019). Contraceptive sponge. Retrieved from https://www.mayoclinic.org/tests-procedures/contraceptive-sponge/about/pac-20384547

Planned Parenthood. (2019). Birth control sponge. Retrieved from https://www.plannedparenthood.org/learn/birth-control/birth-control-sponge

Start-Stop Technique

The start-stop technique is used to aid in the treatment of early (premature) ejaculation. A urologist, Dr. James Semans, first described the start-stop technique in 1955. However, the technique was not popular at the time and did not become popularized until years later when Dr. Helen Kaplan wrote about it as a successful technique to delay ejaculation. The start-stop technique is now a common intervention that sex therapists teach their clients who are seeking treatment for premature or early ejaculation.

The start-stop technique works by allowing the person to learn how to better control when they ejaculate. By stopping stimulation to the penis periodically, the person is able to learn their body's signals for when they are close to ejaculating. When the person is able to take note of these signs, they may withhold stimulation prior to the point of no return, or the point at which ejaculation is inevitable regardless of continued stimulation or not. Practicing stopping prior to the point of no return allows the person to gain control over their ejaculation and reduce the occurrence of early ejaculation.

It is best to begin practicing the start-stop technique independently during masturbation. The person can stimulate their penis and increase arousal. When they become highly excited, stimulation of the penis is stopped completely for several seconds (or potentially a bit longer) with the intention of decreasing arousal. An erection should still be maintained during this break. After this short break, stimulation may begin again. This process should be repeated several times before ejaculation is permitted. The start-stop technique takes practice. Sex therapists recommend that practice during masturbation occur several times per week for thirty to sixty minutes per session for several weeks. Improved ejaculatory control should be noticed after several weeks of this practice. As control improves, stimulation may be decreased during practice instead of stopping it completely.

When the individual has become comfortable using this technique by themselves, they may try using this with their partner. During sex, the individual may stop moving, pull out, or take a short break by switching positions in order to decrease excitement and delay ejaculation. As control improves with the partner, they may also choose to change the intensity of the stimulation instead of stopping completely. Sexual communication with a partner is important while trying the start-stop technique. An individual may ask their partner to change the type of stimulation or the intensity of it during this practice.

The aim of the start-stop technique is to allow the person to hold themselves in the plateau phase of the sexual response cycle for their desired amount of time. This phase of the sexual response cycle comes after arousal, when the penis is erect, but prior to orgasm or ejaculation. Mastering the start-stop technique allows the person to stay in this phase for as long as desired.

Amanda Manuel

See also: Arousal; Communication, Sexual; Ejaculation; Masturbation; Orgasm; Premature Ejaculation.

Further Reading

Herbenick, D. (2012). *Sex made easy.* Philadelphia: Running Press.

Yarber, W., Sayad, B., & Strong, B. (2010). *Human sexuality: Diversity in contemporary America* (7th Ed.). New York: McGraw-Hill.

Statutory Rape

Statutory rape (SR) is consensual sex between two people, one of whom is under the "age of consent," the minimum age at which someone is legally capable of understanding the consequences of sex. The federal age of consent is sixteen. It is a crime in all states for anyone thirty years or older to have sex with someone fifteen years or younger. However, individual states vary with regard to sexual relations between persons close in age; some states might prosecute an eighteen-year-old who had sex with a fifteen-year-old, but others would not. This highlights the tension between SR laws' original impetus—protecting minors from predatory adults—and allowing for sexual relations among peers. Around half of high school students have had sex, one in three within the past three months.

Up until the mid-1990s, SR laws were sporadically enforced relative to how frequently they occurred. For example, in California, between 1975 and 1978, around 400 cases were prosecuted annually while over 50,000 underage teens gave birth outside marriage, a trend that continued for decades. Finally, in 1996, Congress instituted welfare reform laws that called for aggressive prosecution of SR in an effort to reduce adolescent pregnancy rates. Subsequent analysis of over 7,500 SR cases reported between 1996 and 2000 across twenty-one states revealed that 60 percent of victims were fourteen- or fifteen-year-old females, 55 percent of perpetrators were males age twenty or younger, and 29 percent said they were "boyfriend and girlfriend."

The criminal characterization of SR depends on the state and ages of victim and offender. It may be called "statutory rape," "sexual abuse," or "encouraging delinquency," with a range of punishments from one to twenty years in jail and lifetime registration as a sex offender. In general, the older the age of the perpetrator, the more severe the penalty. A victim's willingness to engage in sex is not a defense against SR charges, nor is an offender being mistaken about the minor's age.

Enforcement of SR law has been undermined by race and sexual politics throughout America's history. White men accused of sexual involvement with black girls were typically never prosecuted, whereas black men were almost always arrested, convicted, and severely punished up until the 1950s. Similarly, women involved with young boys were rarely arrested until relatively recently as these relations were considered "appropriate initiation." But male-on-male SR cases typically ended in conviction due to concerns for "inculcating a homosexual lifestyle."

Today, arrest and conviction rates for SR still depend on the age, race, and gender of victim and offender as well as whether they report being in a romantic versus casual relationship. For example, among romantic SR pairings, there are sixteen arrests of female-on-female cases for every one arrest of a male-on-female case. And, compared to arrest rates for more common white-on-white SR cases, black-on-black pairings have a 17 percent less likelihood of arrest.

In some states, SR is governed by mandatory reporting. Health care providers, teachers, and others who work with adolescents must report known or suspected SR cases to police or face criminal charges themselves. The concern is that this may cause young people to cover up their relationship, and, if pregnant, avoid essential prenatal care for fear of getting themselves or their partners in trouble.

Ultimately, adolescents are likely to be confused about SR laws because in some states they are legally allowed to consent to sex-related medical care, such as obtaining treatment for sexually transmitted infections, before they can legally consent to sex.

David J. Reynolds

See also: Adolescent Sexuality; Age of Consent; Sexual Consent; Sugar Daddies and Sugar Babies.

Further Reading

Chaffin, M., Chenoweth, S., & Letourneau, E. J. (2016). Same-sex and race-based disparities in statutory rape arrests. *Journal of Interpersonal Violence, 31*, 26–48.

Eaton, D. K., Kann, L., Kinchen, S., Shanklin, S., Flint, K. H., Hawkins, J., … Wechsler, H. (2012). Youth risk behavior surveillance—United States, 2011. *Morbidity and Mortality Weekly Report*, *61*, 1–162.

Troup-Leasure, K., & Snyder, H. N. (2005). Statutory rape known to law enforcement. *Juvenile Justice Bulletin* No. NCJ 208803. Washington, DC: Office of Juvenile Justice & Delinquency Prevention.

Stereotypes, Gender

Gender stereotypes are socially constructed expectations that boys and men ought to be masculine and that girls and women should be feminine. They are two related clusters of beliefs, images, and assumptions about what male and female should be. These stereotypes may be positive or negative, but they are ultimately oppressive, especially for women. Gender stereotypes influence nearly all spheres of one's psychosocial existence during every phase of the life span.

Feminine stereotypes submit that girls and women are fragile, overly emotional, and passive (negative) as well as nurturing, empathic, pure, and gentle (positive). Masculinity is defined as aggressive, crude, emotionally constrained, entitled (negative) and independent, assertive, competent, and courageous (positive). Note that whether certain adjectives are positive or negative varies by context. There are cultures, for example, in which aggressiveness is highly valued. This is true for passivity as well.

Whether or not aspects of these stereotypes are viewed as positive or negative, they are all repressive: they limit one's ability to freely express the full range of human sentiments and modes. Research has consistently shown that those who do not conform to gender stereotypes in U.S. society experience social rejection and more negative mental and physical health outcomes. Transgender women, for example, are at a high risk for being targets of violence. Further, the research on gender stereotypes during childhood demonstrates that current norms are more condemning of boys who exhibit feminine qualities when compared to the acceptance, in general, of girls who show masculine tendencies. A girl labeled a "tom boy" in her first decade of life is applauded for her vigor and adventurousness, whereas a boy with feminine interests is devalued. While this results in a more constricted developmental path for boys, it further highlights the notion that gender stereotypes present that which is feminine as inferior to the masculine. The social scripts associated with childhood gender valuations are slowly shifting.

As stereotypes, these differences between masculine and feminine are not aligned with actual differences between the sexes (male, female, intersex), biological or otherwise. There are indeed distinctions between women and men: genitalia, secondary sex characteristics, hormone levels, reproductive functions, and so on, However, even assumed biological differences—that were thought to be based on divergent survival modes during our species's evolutionary past—have been challenged as recent research finds that survival demands were quite similar for men and women. Further, the latest science demonstrates that the brains of men and women do not differ in volume or neuro-connectivity. Turning to more widely held stereotypes about sex differences in behaviors and abilities (e.g., math, leadership), a literature review highlights that there is more variation *within* groups of women or of men than there are *between* men and women. That is to say, men and women, as groups, are more similar than they are different.

While gender stereotypes are potentially damaging to the lives of men, women, and genderqueer or nonconforming individuals, this damage is far from equal. Globally pervasive structural dynamics, those perpetuated by tacit and explicit rules of society and its institutions (laws, health care, employment) favor men and masculinity while devaluing women and femininity. Such hegemony within gender stereotypes is associated with a host of beliefs and practices that severely reduce the quality of life for women. For example, the stereotype that women are only competent at household tasks and overly emotional directly aligns with policies of several societies that bar women from higher education or driving. The stereotype of male entitlement maintains ideas held in many parts of the world that women are the property of men, and therefore, a husband can rape and abuse his wife without legal consequence. These stereotypes are also at work in U.S. society in both more obvious (e.g., division of household labor, pay disparities, sexual assault policy) and subtle ways (e.g., expected dating behaviors, assessment of a political candidate, "acceptable" extracurricular activities).

The impact of gender stereotypes must be understood from an intersectional lens. This highlights the way that overlapping structures of oppression (e.g., sexism, racism, heterosexism, ageism, classism) intersect to shape lives and experiences. For example, the gender stereotypes that are connected to being a black man are different in important ways than those associated with being a white man. Two men representing these different demographics will experience quite distinct encounters with socially constructed expectations of their race and gender together, which is also likely influenced by their sexual orientation, age, social class, and so on.

Another dangerous consequence of gender stereotypes is that they reinforce false binaries (female *or* male; feminine *or* masculine) and fail to account for widely accepted variations in both sex and gender. There are not just two sexes, nor are ways of being a human simplistically organized into two discrete categories.

In sum, gender stereotypes impose limiting expectations on individuals that stifle the full expression of human experiences. These clusters of beliefs, images, and assumptions regarding how people of different genders are *supposed* to think, behave, and relate are based on a false essentialism that wrongly posits biological underpinnings. Further, gender stereotypes reinforce an incorrect binary perspective on sex and gender that carries important implications for the well-being and safety of those who live outside these false binaries.

Ed de St. Aubin and Lauren B. Yadlosky

See also: Binary Gender System; Childhood Gender Nonconformity; Evolutionary Perspectives on Gender and Sexual Behavior; Female Sexuality; Femininity; Gender; Gender Roles, Socialization and; Male Sexuality; Masculinity; Sexism; Stereotypes, Sexual.

Further Reading

Dyble, M., Salali, G. D., Chaudhary, N., Page, A., Smith, D., Thompson, J., … Migliano, A. B. (2015). Sex equality can explain the unique social structure of hunter-gatherer bands. *Science, 348*, 796–798.

Ellemers, N. (2018). Gender stereotypes. *Annual Review of Psychology, 69*, 275–298.

Hyde, J. (2014). Gender similarities and differences. *Annual Review of Psychology, 85*, 616–626.

Joel, D., Berman, Z., Tavor, I., Wexler, N., Gaber, O., Stein, Y., … Liem, F. (2015). Sex beyond the genitalia: The human brain mosaic. *Proceedings of the National Academy of Science, 112*, 15468–15473.

Stereotypes, Sexual

Sexual stereotypes are culturally ingrained ideas about biological sex, gender, and sexuality that shape a person's understanding of their own identity as it relates to their interpersonal and intimate relationships. Because people use stereotypes to inform how they see the world, stereotypes can have a powerful influence on how people behave, how they present to others, and what they believe to be attractive. Oftentimes, people accept stereotypes as truths without realizing the effect they have. Individuals might accept that men are more "aggressive, powerful, and adventurous," while women are "mild-mannered, emotionally expressive, and passive." Although most people understand that these generalizations cannot possibly be true for everyone, socialization may make them difficult to refute. Without a critical lens, stereotypes can promote systemic gender and sexual imbalances. Cognitively, the main function of stereotyping is to allow people to quickly and efficiently make judgments about someone's behavior. However, by saying, for instance, that "men don't cry" or women "cry too often," a dangerous dichotomy is created so that neither sex can express their feelings without being perceived negatively. These sorts of stereotypes also negate the experiences of transgender, nonbinary, and queer individuals, who may not be recognized or included within a sexual or gender binary.

Sexual stereotypes are informed by a number of factors beyond gender, including race, sexuality, and class. Many stereotypes are deeply rooted in colonialism and harken back to the time when two cultures initially collided. For instance, the Jezebel stereotype, which refers to an overtly sexual woman with "uncontrollable urges," is a contemporary stereotype about black women from the Book of Kings that has been perpetuated through EuroAmerican literature and society since the nineteenth century. This attribution was originally formed after Europeans colonized, assaulted, and enslaved African woman, sometimes showcasing them due to their "extraordinary" bodies, which were seen as "objectively" more sexual than white bodies. In more recent research on the effects of sexual stereotypes for gay men, participants reported feeling that black gay men were most likely to be "dominant" sexually, while Latinx gay men were thought to be more "passionate and hot" overall. The study found that these assumptions affected the way participants chose their partners, the way they performed during sexual encounters, and their level of sexual risk. These sorts of studies make it clear that sexual stereotypes are formed by more than sexuality alone.

There are a number of potential explanations for why these stereotypes exist, ranging from sociocultural influences to evolutionary biology. Sociocultural factors like television, music, and internet use have a large potential to affect the development of sexual stereotypes. Television continues to play a large role in the content and exposure children receive while they are developing their perceptions of gender and sex. Certain genres of music, pornographic material, and internet content can also contribute to higher endorsement of stereotypes about gender and sex. Peers and communities also influence how individuals see sex, gender, and stereotypes; people are more likely to adopt the perspectives of those around them and ascribe to the sexual stereotypes of their peer group, despite actual sexual behavior.

Sexual stereotypes may also be based on hardwired behavior adapted through evolution. Stereotypes act as mental shortcuts in order to make decisions, assess others' intent, and perceive possible threats. When it comes to sexual stereotypes, women's intent is often seen as "warm and trustworthy," while they are perceived as nonthreatening and low in competence. For men, it is the opposite. From propaganda to neurological imaging, certain groups are repeatedly dehumanized and vilified through stereotypes that reinforce an "us" versus "them" or in-group or out-group mentality. Interestingly, evolutionary psychology also suggests that stereotypes help connect people with potential mates. There are reasons that women are assumed to prioritize partnership and monogamy, while men are assumed to prioritize many sexual partners and are more sexually assertive. Those reasons are based on the ways in which human ancestors were able to procreate and ensure family survival. Since female ancestors were anchored by child care, it was important to be discerning about which mate would come back with food. Hence, sexual stereotypes are not just social constructs; they are part of the human biological legacy.

While biological perspectives have empirical support, people, thankfully, are not doomed to behave according to patterns dictated hundreds or thousands of years ago by cave-dwellers or colonial invaders. Newer research has begun to challenge the evolutionary rationale for sexual stereotypes. For example, the sense of power, not gender, could be responsible for the typically male stereotyped experience of sexual assertiveness and satisfaction, challenging the previously believed evolutionary view of male sexual behavior. In addition, when women gain more occupational and financial power, "passive" stereotypical behavior decreases. Some social movements also show that stereotyping can be neutralized. For example, the different waves of the feminist movement have been able to fight sexual stereotypes such that women now outnumber men in all levels of higher education, despite stereotypes of women having less intellect. Younger generations endorse traditional sexual stereotypes and roles less over time, thanks to feminist movements, same-sex rights, and social justice, telling people that stereotypes can change as culture does too.

The impact of sexual stereotypes is pervasive and can affect several areas related to personal well-being. Research shows that "stereotype threat," the idea that an individual conforms to stereotypes about them when they are made aware of the stereotype, can increase someone's potential for mental and physical health problems. Sexual stereotypes can also increase sexual risk taking. For instance, studies have shown that race-related sexual stereotypes (e.g., believing that some groups of people are more likely to be living with HIV than others) can greatly affect contraceptive use and sexual risk taking. And while some people may like the stereotypes associated with their race or ethnicity, research suggests that, overall, many people of color, and especially queer people of color, feel sexually objectified and are more likely to experience adverse health consequences. This becomes amplified when things like discrimination and prejudice factor into how someone sees their sexual and gender identities.

Fortunately, there are proven strategies for fighting the stereotypes many people unconsciously believe. For one, people can watch media that encourages a range of behaviors, roles, and appearances for different genders. While completely eliminating stereotypical content might not be realistic, challenging the images and themes within this content can help people balance their potential impact. For instance, the more aware someone is of stereotype threat, the more the harm of that stereotype might be neutralized. Simply understanding and purposefully negating stereotypes helps to lessen their influence.

Providing information and education can also help to decrease the influence of stereotypes. Since stereotypes are mental shortcuts to help fill voids of information, if people are provided with factual information, they are more likely to hold accurate opinions and make more accurate judgments. When people know specific personal information about friends, coworkers, or colleagues, they are less apt to use stereotypes to fill in the blanks. Allowing people to get to know each other as individuals, and not from a distance, might decrease the use of stereotypes. Social psychological research has also shown that when people reject prejudice as a community, stereotypes can change. When given tasks that require teamwork, people are able to look beyond the stereotypes they know and connect as individuals.

Alex M. Rivera and Marissa C. Floro

See also: Evolutionary Perspectives on Gender and Sexual Behavior; Female Sexuality; Gender; Male Sexuality; Sexual Identity; Sexual Script; Stereotypes, Gender.

Further Reading

Calabrese, S. K., Earnshaw, V. A., Magnus, M., Hansen, N. B., Krakower, D. S., Underhill, K., & Dovidio, J. F. (2018). Sexual stereotypes ascribed to black men who have sex with men: An intersectional analysis. *Archives of Sexual Behavior, 47*(1), 143–156.

Davis, S., & Tucker-Brown, A. (2013). Effects of black sexual stereotypes on sexual decision making among African American women. *Journal of Pan African Studies, 5*(9), 111–128.

Lammers, J., & Stoker, J. I. (2019). Power affects sexual assertiveness and sexual esteem equally in women and men. *Archives of Sexual Behavior, 48*(2), 645–652.

Newcomb, M. E., Ryan, D. T., Garofalo, R., & Mustanski, B. (2015). Race-based sexual stereotypes and their effects on sexual risk behavior in racially diverse young men who have sex with men. *Archives of Sexual Behavior, 44*(7), 1959–1968.

Siegel, K., & Meunier, É. (2019). Traditional sex and gender stereotypes in the relationships of non-disclosing behaviorally bisexual men. *Archives of Sexual Behavior, 48*(1), 333–345.

Ward, L. M., Merriwether, A., & Caruthers, A. (2006). Breasts are for men: Media, masculinity ideologies, and men's beliefs about women's bodies. *Sex Roles, 55*, 703–714.

Wesche, R., Espinosa-Hernández, G., & Lefkowitz, E. (2016). Gender's role in misperceptions of peers' sexual motives. *Sexuality & Culture, 20*(4), 1003–1019.

Sterilization

"Sterilization" refers to any procedure that permanently ends an individual's physical capacity to reproduce. It is used as a method of voluntary birth control by persons who either wish to never reproduce or feel they have already produced the maximum number of children they wish to have. Sterilization has also been used as an involuntary control on the fertility of persons deemed "undesirable" by various governments. Forced sterilization policies have touched most of the world over the past two centuries, have their roots in racism and eugenics, and are closely associated with genocide and "ethnic cleansing."

Sterilization techniques involve permanently blocking the tubes that transport gametes. A vasectomy refers to cutting and closing the vas deferens, which transport sperm from the testicles, where it is produced, to the prostate, where it is mixed with other fluids before leaving the body through the urethra. In most cases, a vasectomy is performed through a small surgical incision in the scrotum as an outpatient procedure. Tubal ligation refers to a number of techniques that cut or block the fallopian tubes. The fallopian tubes allow sperm to travel to mature ova and fertilized eggs to travel into the uterus. Transluminal tubal ligation uses an intravaginal catheter to place expanding fiber inserts, springs, or coils that occlude, or block, the tubes. Tablets of the pharmaceutical quinacrine are also sometimes used off-label for tubal occlusion. Surgical tubal ligation is performed through either a small incision (laparoscopy) or large incision (laparotomy) in the abdominal wall. It may be performed under local or general anesthesia and is sometimes performed during cesarean birth or other abdominal surgery. Other surgical procedures such as ovariectomy (removal of the ovaries), hysterectomy (removal of the uterus), and castration (removal of the testicles), also result in permanent sterility but are no longer primarily used for this purpose.

There is currently no such thing as pharmaceutical sterilization, though public outcry has followed reports of fictitious drugs circulated in internet hoaxes and conspiracy theory campaigns. One urban legend involving a fictitious, sterility-inducing "date rape drug" called Progestrex periodically surfaces. More troubling, public health campaigns in developing nations—including Kenya, Nicaragua, Tanzania, Mexico, and the Philippines—have been targeted with the claim that their vaccines contain sterility drugs. The vaccine most frequently targeted is a tetanus shot given to women aged fifteen to forty-five to prevent newborn tetanus—a fatal condition spread through unsanitary birthing conditions and unhygienic umbilical cord care, which kills around 60,000 newborn babies annually. The conspiracy theory states that the tetanus vaccine contains an antibody to the pregnancy hormone human chorionic gonadotropin and will cause a woman's immune system to attack all future fertilized eggs. It is important to note that while such an antibody has featured in research involving contraceptive vaccines, such vaccinations have to be repeated at least every twelve weeks to be effective and cannot render women permanently sterile.

However, history provides justification for fears of forced sterilization. Forced sterilization is performed either without a person's consent or knowledge, under coercion, or as a requirement for receiving lifesaving benefits or health care. Between 1907 and 1979, over thirty U.S. states and territories passed laws requiring or allowing the forced sterilization of certain people. Enforcement was overseen by state eugenics boards, which employed physicians and social workers to target individuals for forced sterilization. Physicians who performed such sterilizations were granted immunity from malpractice suits. Targeted persons were overwhelmingly female, and most were black, Latina, or Native American. Sterilization was by hysterectomy or tubal ligation and was frequently performed without parental or patient consent on children undergoing other medical procedures ranging from appendectomy to routine vaccination. Criteria for legal forced sterilization included "feeblemindedness," "idiocy," "imbecility," institutionalization, incarceration, epilepsy, mental illness, alcoholism, suspected hereditary illness, blindness, deafness, "deformity," homosexuality, and transgender expression (including women who wore "male clothing"); "moral delinquency," including unwed motherhood, prostitution, being a victim of rape or incest, and showing evidence of "unbridled sexual desire," such as by having many children; and "dependency," including receiving public welfare funds or public health services, homelessness, poverty, and being an orphan or foster child. Over 60,000 people were forcibly sterilized in the continental United States, outside of Indian reservations, through 1979. In Puerto Rico, over one-third of women of childbearing age had been forcibly sterilized by 1968. On reservations, half of Native American women had been forcibly sterilized by 1976. Though most U.S. forced sterilization laws were overturned by 1980, reports continue to surface, such as a 2013 case revealing the forced sterilization of at least 148 female inmates in California prisons between 2006 and 2010.

Angela Libal

See also: Essure Coil; Fertility; Tubal Ligation; Vasectomy.

Further Reading

Carmon, I. (2014, June). For eugenic sterilization victims, belated justice. Retrieved from http://www.msnbc.com/all/eugenic-sterilization-victims-belated-justice

Krase, K. (2014). History of forced sterilization and current U.S. abuses. Retrieved from https://www.ourbodiesourselves.org/book-excerpts/health-article/forced-sterilization/

Lombardo, P. (n.d.). Eugenic sterilization laws. Retrieved from http://www.eugenicsarchive.org/html/eugenics/essay8text.html

Planned Parenthood. (2019). Sterilization. Retrieved from https://www.plannedparenthood.org/learn/birth-control/sterilization

Rutecki, G. W. (2010). Forced sterilization of Native Americans: Late twentieth century physician cooperation with national eugenic policies. Retrieved from https://cbhd.org/content/forced-sterilization-native-americans-late-twentieth-century-physician-cooperation-national-

Walden, R. (2013). CIR prison investigation opens another chapter on sterilization of women in U.S. Retrieved from http://www.ourbodiesourselves.org/2013/07/cir-prison-investigation-opens-another-chapter-on-sterilization-of-women-in-u-s/

Sternberg's Triangular Theory of Love

Psychologist and educator Robert Sternberg developed Sternberg's triangular theory of love in 1986. This theory outlines different types of love relationships and the dynamics of these types of love. Sternberg argues that love is comprised of three elements, marking the points of the triangle. These three elements are intimacy, passion, and commitment. These three elements may be combined into seven different types of love. Over the course of a relationship, each quality may be present in different amounts, and these amounts can fluctuate and change over time. The fluctuation of these elements may affect the quality of the relationship.

The three elements are components that are present in relationships. The variety in the intensity and presence of these elements reflects how one feels toward the other in a relationship. Intimacy involves mutual feelings of trust; there is a sense of connectedness and openness where people share feelings and experiences. Passion refers to physical attraction and sexual desire toward a person. Commitment is linked to a decision to make a relationship long term.

Isolating or combining these three elements may create seven love styles. "Liking" is a love style that occurs when only intimacy is present. This may be experienced as a friendship. "Infatuation" occurs when passion is the only present element. Some may think of this love style as lust. "Empty love" is connected only to commitment. An example of this love style is when a couple remains married even though their sexual and emotional connection has dissolved.

"Romantic love" is characterized by the combination of passion and intimacy. This may occur in a new dating relationship. When passion and commitment are shared, "fatuous love" results. This may be best described as a sudden marriage after love at first sight. "Companionate love" is the result of blending intimacy and commitment. Many long-term relationships may experience this type of love as sexual attraction may wane at times during the course of a relationship.

The joining of all three elements—intimacy, passion, and commitment—produces "consummate love." According to the theory, this is the most desirable love type for a romantic relationship. The marked absence of all three elements results in an eighth love style called "nonlove." This may occur after a relationship has ended.

This theory utilizes language laced with strong connotations. For example, "empty love" has a negative connotation that some may view as ethnocentric as this type of love has been used to describe arranged marriages. This theory also assumes people want relationships that include elements of intimacy, passion, and commitment, as "consummate love" is celebrated as the highest form of love, which may be invalidating to some with other relationship styles with which they are very satisfied.

Research has shown that the three components of love become more pronounced as individuals age from adolescence to young adulthood. Commitment becomes most prominent in adult relationships and is highly regarded in adults' understanding of love. Research has noted that there are only very modest differences between genders in regard to the three elements of love.

Amanda Manuel

See also: Attachment Theory of Love; Companionate Love; Consummate Love; Desire; Intimacy, Sexual and Relational; Lee's Theory of Love Styles; Love.

Further Reading

Sternberg, R. J. (1986). A triangular theory of love. *Psychological Review, 93*, 119–135.

Sumter, S. R., Valkenburg, P. M., & Peter, J. (2013). Perceptions of love across the lifespan: Differences in passion, intimacy, and commitment. *International Journal of Behavioral Development, 37*(5), 417–427.

Yarber, W., Sayad, B., & Strong, B. (2010). *Human sexuality diversity in contemporary America* (7th Ed.). New York: McGraw-Hill.

Stonewall Riots

The Stonewall Inn, located in the Greenwich Village neighborhood of New York City, is the birthplace of the modern LGBTQ+ movement. On June 28, 1969, the patrons of the Stonewall Inn fought back against a police raid. For the first time, gay people refused to accept the status quo of oppression and stood up for themselves against regular city-sanctioned harassment. The Stonewall riots paved the way for future LGBTQ+ people to be treated fairly and as equal to other members of society.

In 1969, police raids on gay bars occurred regularly as it was illegal to serve gay people alcohol or for gay people to dance with one another. During a typical raid, the customers would be lined up to have their identification checked. Those without identification or those dressed in drag were arrested. Women were required to wear feminine clothing and would be arrested if their clothing was deemed too masculine. Employees and management of the bars were also typically arrested.

On June 28, 1969, at 1:20 a.m., eight police officers arrived at the Stonewall Inn for a planned raid, but the 200 patrons refused to cooperate. Standard procedure was to line up the patrons, check identification, and have female officers take customers dressed as women to the bathroom to verify their sex, upon which any men dressed as women would be arrested. Those dressed as women that night refused to go with the officers. Men in line began to refuse to produce their identification. The police decided to take everyone present to the station, but the patrol wagons had not arrived, leaving the arrested patrons to wait. Those not arrested were allowed to leave, but instead of leaving, they stayed outside of the bar to see what was unfolding. Within minutes over a hundred people congregated outside.

While waiting for the patrol wagons, a scuffle broke out when a woman in handcuffs complained that her handcuffs were too tight. She was hit in the head with a baton for complaining. She tried to escape repeatedly, but eventually an officer was able to pick her up and heave her into the back of the wagon, which was the last straw for the angry crowd.

The crowd continued to grow, and the police were greatly outnumbered. Some police officers barricaded themselves inside the Stonewall Inn for their own safety. The crowd had overturned a police wagon, and bottles, rocks, and bricks were being thrown at the wagon and at the police inside the inn. The tactical police force arrived to free the trapped police and arrest anyone they could. By 4:00 a.m., the streets had been cleared of the crowd. Thirteen people were arrested, four police officers were injured, and much of the crowd was hospitalized.

News of the riot spread, and the next night thousands of people gathered in front of the Stonewall Inn. Rioting, fires, and violence broke out again. More than a hundred police officers arrived, but the riot continued until 4:00 a.m. On the third night, around 1000 protestors gathered again. Another riot took place, with injuries to both demonstrators and police, looting in local shops, and arrests of five people.

The riots produced from a bar raid became a literal example of gays and lesbians fighting back and a symbol for many people. Many were moved by the rebellion and sensed an opportunity to act. As a result of the Stonewall riots, gay rights groups were established in every major American city. Before the riots at the Stonewall Inn, homosexuals were harassed, oppressed, and despised. The events of June 28, 1968, were one of the first instances of LGBTQ+ people fighting back and demanding equal rights.

Lauren Ewaniuk

See also: Drag; Gay Rights Movement; LGBTQ+.

Further Reading

Carter, D. (2004). *Stonewall: The riots that sparked the gay revolution.* New York: St. Martin's Press.

Duberman, M. (1994). *Stonewall.* New York: Plume.

Editors, C. R. (2015). *The Stonewall riots: The history and legacy of the protests that helped spark the modern gay rights movement.* Scotts Valley, CA: CreateSpace.

Storms's Model of Sexual Orientation

Storms's model of sexual orientation was proposed by Michael Storms in 1980. Storms expanded on the model of sexual orientation described by Alfred Kinsey and suggested that rather than one spectrum of sexual orientation from exclusively gay to exclusively straight, there were two spectrums of sexual attraction or fantasy, one indicating level of attraction or fantasy to same-sex/gender people and the other indicating level of attraction or fantasy to other-sex/gender people.

There are many ways to conceptualize sexual orientation, some of which are more accurate than others. Some people think of sexual orientation as being made up of discreet categories: people are either gay, straight, or bisexual. Because the categories are discreet, people have to be in one category or another. This model of sexual orientation was predominant until Alfred Kinsey began studying sexuality in a more scientific manner. Based on his interviews with people about their sexual behaviors, Kinsey proposed that there is a spectrum or a continuum of sexual orientation. Kinsey believed that while some people were exclusively gay or lesbian and some people were exclusively heterosexual, most people fell somewhere in between. As such, he developed a scale in order to measure sexual orientation, which ranges from zero (exclusively straight or heterosexual) to six (exclusively gay or homosexual); people with scores of one to five on this scale fall somewhere in between exclusively straight and exclusively gay and may be considered as some degree of bisexual.

Expanding on Kinsey's model, Storms proposed a new model of sexual orientation based on people's fantasies and attractions to members of the same sex/gender and members of the other sex/gender. He proposed that rather than one continuum (gay to straight), there were actually two continuums. Storms's continuums or dimensions of sexual orientation were attraction/fantasy to people of the same sex/gender (homoeroticism) and attraction or fantasy to people of the other sex/gender (heteroeroticism). If someone indicated that they were high in heteroeroticism and had no homoeroticism, then they would have a straight or heterosexual sexual orientation. Similarly, if someone indicated that they were high in homoeroticism and had no heteroeroticism, then they would have a gay or lesbian sexual orientation. If someone indicated that they experienced both high heteroeroticism and high homoeroticism, meaning that they experienced sexual attraction and fantasy to both people of the same and other sex/gender, then they would have a bisexual sexual orientation.

Storms's model is conceptually important because it allows for a range of attractions to same- and other-sex/gender people. For example, the model allows for someone to report high heteroeroticism and moderate homoeroticism. It is also important because it allows for and can theoretically explain asexuality. According to Storms's model, if someone reports no heteroeroticism and no homoeroticism, they would then have an asexual sexual orientation. This is a significant development and improvement over the original Kinsey scale, which could not account for an asexual sexual orientation.

Heather L. Armstrong

See also: Asexuality; Bisexuality; Kinsey's Continuum of Sexual Orientation; Sexual Identity; Sexual Orientation.

Further Reading

Storms, M. D. (1980). Theories of sexual orientation. *Journal of Personality and Social Psychology, 38*(5), 783.

Swan, D. J. (2018). Models and measures of sexual orientation. In D. J. Swan & S. Habibi (Eds.), *Bisexuality: Theories, research, and recommendations for the invisible sexuality* (19–36). Cham, Switzerland: Springer.

Sugar Daddies and Sugar Babies

Sugar daddies are usually older, wealthier men who have emotional or sexual relationships with younger women or men (sugar babies) in exchange for money, material goods, housing, or other luxury items. This mutually beneficial relationship is known as sugar dating and has become more prevalent in dating culture since the launch of the website Seeking Arrangement in 2006 (the largest sugar dating site). Today, Seeking Arrangement has an active community of ten million members across more than 139 countries with translations in ten languages. The community includes eight million sugar babies and two million sugar daddies and mommies. This is one of many platforms that are now available to facilitate sugar dating. The increase in sugar dating can be attributed to the increased desire for a superficial and affluent lifestyle and the internet's ability to accommodate these desires through sugar dating websites. Sugar dating, however, as a means of income (specifically to finance a higher education), is also a recent trend in North America.

Sugar dating has been criticized for being a new form of prostitution, and it has been argued that it should be illegal. Others believe that this claim is inaccurate because it does not take into consideration the different types of arrangements that occur within sugar dating: exchange of sex for money without companionship, exchange of sex for money with little companionship, or high level of companionship where sex and money accompany the relationship as they do in traditional dating. Given that prostitution excludes engagement in sexual activity as a result of social companionship, sugar dating often does not fall within the realm of prostitution. Further, prostitution charges are rarely made as a result of sugar dating or engagement with sugar dating websites.

Nicole C. Doria and Matthew Numer

See also: Online Dating; Prostitution; Sex Work.

Further Reading

Brouard, P., & Crewe, M. (2012). Sweetening the deal? Sugar daddies, sugar mummies, sugar babies and HIV in contemporary South Africa. *Agenda, 26*(4), 48–56.

Miller, A. (2012). Sugar dating: A new take on an old issue. *Buffalo Journal of Gender, Law and Social Policy, 20*, 33.

Motyl, J. (2013). Trading sex for college tuition: How sugar daddy "dating" sites may be sugar coating prostitution. *Penn State Law Review, 117*(3), 927–957.

Reed, L., Sharpe, C., Coker, K., & Harrington, E. (2015). *Sugar babies, sugar daddies, and the perceptions of sugar dating.* ProQuest Dissertations and Theses.

Seeking Arrangement. (2019). About us. Retrieved from https://www.seeking.com/about-us

Surrogate, Sexual

A sexual surrogate (also known as a "surrogate partner") is a specially trained intimacy skill professional. Surrogates work alongside supervising sex therapists to better cultivate client sexual and relational intimacy skills by guiding sensuality, sexual arousal and touching, relaxation techniques, and effective forms of communication. This triangulated intervention helps clients develop the social skills necessary to engage in satisfying sexual relationships as sexually healthy persons when dating in their own lives. Surrogate services support a variety of client challenges, including severe anxieties, trauma recovery, specific sexual dysfunction, physical disability, and the sexual rehabilitation of those sustaining various injuries. As sexual difficulties can often be psychological rather than (or in addition to) physical, these challenges can cause relationship problems, negative body image issues, sexual avoidance, and an array of other significant life obstacles.

According to the International Professional Surrogate Association (IPSA), the leading authority on sexual surrogacy, gradual progress through diagnostic, skill-building, and healing exercises offer the shared physical intimacies that "facilitate development of healthy self-concepts and improve sexual functioning" (IPSA, n.d.). It is important to note that surrogate relationships do not always include sexual intercourse or any particular form of sexual contact. Surrogate partner relationships are initiated under the premise of a finite and structured treatment plan. While clients may voluntarily terminate support at any time, the sex therapy team (client, surrogate partner, and therapist) is normally expected to collaborate on the point of closure. Typically, clients attend weekly one- to two-hour sessions with surrogate partners in addition to meetings held with supervising therapists, for a total of at least thirty hours; more intensive therapy treatments are structured over shorter periods of time to best serve clients with limited access to local surrogate partner therapy.

Due to the sensitive nature of this type of therapy, comprehensive training programs and strict ethical codes are put in place for certified surrogate partners. In addition to various bodywork techniques, surrogate interns are educated in psychological, physical, and emotional human needs. Such training allows these professionals to provide qualified referrals for operating therapists and appropriate client-focused services. By initiating a therapeutic client relationship, sexual surrogates agree to, above all else, recognize the client's welfare as "the chief focus and primary ethical responsibility" (IPSA, 1973). Surrogate partners are also expected to uphold confidentiality; conduct themselves as professionals representative of all surrogate partners and their respective organizations; ensure they themselves, as well as their clients, are properly safeguarded against sexually transmitted infections and conception; respect the boundaries of expertise as applied strictly from the position of a surrogate (if other topical degrees or certifications are present); and recognize and address any personal limitations of competency. These regulations maintain the integrity of the practice by reducing the potential for client exploitation or services otherwise inadequate or harmful to client development.

Ilyssa Boseski

See also: Communication, Sexual; Disabilities, Sexual Function and; Intimacy, Sexual and Relational; Sex Education; Sexual Avoidance; Sexual Health.

Further Reading

International Professional Surrogates Association. (1973). *Code of Ethics of the International Professional Surrogates Association.* Retrieved from https://www.surrogatetherapy.org/ipsa-mission/code-of-ethics/

International Professional Surrogates Association. (n.d.). Surrogate partner therapy. Retrieved from http://www.surrogatetherapy.org/what-is-surrogate-partner-therapy/

Surrogate Mothers

Surrogate mothers are women who carry and bear children for other women, typically women who are infertile or who are otherwise unable to bear children. In some countries, surrogates may receive payment for their childbearing services, though they may also offer their services out of a desire to help people. In other countries, this type of payment is illegal, although health care costs and other costs related to the pregnancy may be covered by the adoptive parents. There are two types of surrogate mothers: traditional and gestational surrogates.

A traditional, or partial, surrogate is inseminated with the male's sperm through the process of artificial insemination. Because the sperm fertilizes an egg of the surrogate, the surrogate is technically the fetus's biological mother. After carrying the fetus to term and delivering it, the surrogate gives the baby up to the parents. Typically, the surrogate will never see the baby again. However, some people using surrogate services agree to let the surrogate mother visit the child from time to time. In a mixed-sex couple or same-sex male couple, the male partner, or one of the male partners, may donate his own sperm. However, if he is unable to produce viable sperm, of in the case of a same-sex female couple, the surrogate could be inseminated with sperm from an anonymous donor.

Traditional surrogacy is the original form of surrogacy, and it has been used for thousands of years, if one considers surrogate sexual intercourse. Modern-type surrogacy involving artificial insemination, paid surrogates, and legal contracts dates to about 1980. Reliable statistics on the numbers of traditional surrogate births are unavailable because many cases go unreported.

A gestational, or full, surrogate is implanted with an embryo that was produced in the laboratory through in vitro fertilization (IVF), usually using the egg of the intended mother and the sperm of the intended father, if carrying for a mixed-sex couple. Thus, the gestational surrogate—unlike the traditional surrogate—is not the fetus's biological mother. She simply carries the fetus in her womb until birth, which makes her the child's "birth mother." She then gives the child over to the parents who will raise it. In some cases, such as for same-sex couples, or if a mixed-sex couple is experiencing infertility, eggs or sperm from donors will be used in the IVF process.

Gestational surrogacy was first used in 1985. The number of gestational surrogate births in the United States has been increasing steadily throughout the 2000s, from at least 740 in 2004 to at least 1,600 in 2011, according to the Society for Assisted Reproductive Technology (SART). SART notes that the actual numbers of these births are probably higher than suggested by these statistics because many clinics do not report their surrogate procedures.

There are many reasons that people may choose to use a surrogate. Mixed-sex couples may wish to have a child but may experience infertility problems. Often these couples will have previously tried other assisted-reproduction techniques such as IVF. Also, some women may choose to use a surrogate because of their own health concerns, such as problems with their uterus (uterine cancer, fibroids, polyps) that would make pregnancy risky or impossible. In addition, conditions in other parts of the body, such as severe cardiovascular disease, could also raise the health risks of pregnancy and childbirth and as such doctors may recommend considering surrogacy. Older women may also choose to use a surrogate to avoid age-related complications with pregnancy. Same-sex couples, especially same-sex male couples, may also wish to use surrogate mothers to have children, as might single men who wish to become fathers. Although such individuals could choose to adopt children, they might prefer using surrogacy because it produces a genetic connection to the child or because they feel it offers some other personal connection that adoption may not provide.

Some surrogates are friends or relatives of the people for whom they perform the service. Using such surrogates is generally less expensive than paying a surrogate agency, which is the option used by most people in the United States. In some countries, including the United States, an agency, for a substantial charge, helps an individual or couple find a suitable surrogate and handles arrangements involving legal documentation and fees paid by the individual or couple to the surrogate.

Most surrogate agencies follow certain guidelines for the women they select as surrogates. Agencies generally prefer to use women who are between the ages of twenty-one and forty, who have previously given birth to at least one healthy baby without complications, who have passed a professional psychological screening, and who can provide personal references. The surrogate must also sign a legal contract detailing her responsibilities, including providing proper prenatal care for the fetus and giving the baby to the parents after birth. Finally, surrogates must pass thorough medical examinations, including tests for infectious diseases and for the health of the uterus.

In the United States, the cost of using agency-based surrogacy services is often at least $100,000 (and much more in some cases). The surrogate herself typically receives anywhere from about $15,000 to $35,000 for a single pregnancy—in addition to medical, legal, and travel costs.

The growing practice of surrogacy has raised a number of complicated legal issues, mostly in regard to the parental legal rights of the child's biological mother or the woman who delivers the child versus the woman who raises the child. In some cases, the surrogate mother may refuse to give the child to the partners or may later desire to see the child she gave birth to. She may also seek to take possession of the child away from the couple that has been raising it. When such cases arise, they must go through court procedures according to the relevant state laws. There are no federal laws that specifically address or restrict surrogacy.

Because gestational surrogates are not biologically related to the children they give birth to, they rarely have firm legal grounding for later wanting to see the child. Since this fact makes legal matters less potentially complicated for couples wishing to use the services of surrogate mothers, gestational surrogacy is believed to be more common than traditional surrogacy.

Laws in some states require individuals using surrogacy services to formally adopt the child after birth or to obtain a formal "declaration of parentage" for the child. In other states, a legal contract between the surrogacy users and the surrogate mother is all that is needed. In any case, an experienced attorney should be used by anyone involved in this process to ensure that the responsibilities of all parties are properly carried out.

A. J. Smuskiewicz

See also: Artificial Insemination; Assisted Reproductive Technology; Infertility; Ova Donation; Pregnancy.

Further Reading

Cohen, D. L. (2013, March). Surrogate pregnancies on rise despite cost hurdles. Retrieved from http://www.reuters.com/article/2013/03/18/us-parent-surrogate-idUSBRE92H11Q20130318#8JgIWZ7wPEpE5sLo.97

Fenton-Glynn, C. (2019, April). Surrogacy: Why the world needs rules for "selling" babies. *The Guardian.* Retrieved from https://www.bbc.co.uk/news/health-47826356

Propst, A. (2017). Gestational carriers (surrogacy). Retrieved from http://www.babycenter.com/surrogacy

Swinging

The act of swinging, often referred to as "the lifestyle," is the engagement of sexual relationships with people outside of the traditional couple arrangement. Swinging can involve two or more couples or a couple and a single person. Swinging can be done in public at places like sex clubs, or it can be practiced in private. Motivations for swinging vary and can range from a couple wanting to diversify their sexual routine to being a way to allow a bisexual partner to fulfill their same-sex attraction and sexual needs. Swinging is an activity that requires healthy and competent sexual communication between all parties involved.

Monogamy, or being in a sexually exclusive two-person relationship, is a cultural norm within Western societies. Laws, civil partnerships, and religious ceremonies reinforce this arrangement of relationships via legal rights and religious vows said during the processes of marriage. Monogamy is so dominant in Western society that people or couples who deviate away from the norm and who choose to engage sexually and consensually with other people or other couples are often considered to be deviant or immoral and may be seen as threatening to society and the traditional family structure.

The terms "swinging" and "swingers" emerged in the 1970s to replace the label of wife-swapping, a term used by the media in the 1950s. Shortly after World War II on air force bases, Gay Talese (1980) noted that couples engaged in the swapping of spouses as a random exercise whereby car keys were placed in a hat and husbands would pick a key by chance to determine who they would have sexual engagements with that evening. It would be reasonable to suggest that swinging is generally more organized now with some areas having formalized swinging clubs that offer a wide array of sexual activities.

Research on swinging is limited. However, one study found that married couples who identified as swingers had higher rates of happiness within their marriages than nonswinging married couples. This research suggests that "emotional monogamy" was seen as integral to maintaining a successful coupling rather than focusing on sexual monogamy within a relationship.

Lesley-Ann Smith

See also: Communication, Sexual; Extramarital Sex; Marriage; Monogamy; Open Marriage; Polyamory.

Further Reading

Barker, M. (2013). *Rewriting the rules: An integrative guide to love, sex and relationships.* East Sussex: Routledge.

Bergstrand, C., & Williams, J. B. (2000). Today's alternative marriage styles: The case of swingers. *Electronic Journal of Human Sexuality, 3*(10). Retrieved from http://www.ejhs.org/volume3/swing/body.htm

Fernandes, E. M. (2009). The swinging paradigm: An evaluation of the marital and sexual satisfaction of swingers. *Electronic Journal of Human Sexuality, 12.* Retrieved from http://www.ejhs.org/Volume12/Swinging2.htm

Gould, T. (1999). *The lifestyle: A look at the erotic rites of swingers.* Buffalo, NY: Firefly.

Talese, G. (1980). *Thy neighbour's wife.* New York: Dell Publishing.

Synthetic Hormones

Synthetic hormones are compounds synthesized in a laboratory to mimic molecules made by organs in the human body. Also known as hormone replacements, they are best known to the general public for their use in hormonal birth control options and in hormone replacement therapy (HRT) for women going through menopause. However, synthetic hormones are widely used to replace or supplement many of the human body's naturally occurring hormone molecules in the treatment of thyroid disorders, diabetes, joint pain, and a number of other conditions.

Scientists first began to isolate and study hormones produced by the human body in the 1930s. Among the first hormones to be widely studied—and later synthesized—were estrogen and progesterone. After the discovery of these hormones' roles in pregnancy and fertility, early family planning activists such as Margaret Sanger began to advocate for the production of an oral contraceptive pill. As a result of Sanger's activism and research conducted by American biologist Gregory Pincus, the world's first oral contraceptive, Enovid, was approved by the Food and Drug Administration in 1960. Estrogen and progesterone have come to be the world's most widely used artificial hormones.

A good deal of controversy exists over the differences among synthetic hormones and so-called natural or bioidentical hormones. While hormone sources and production methods vary widely, any hormone introduced into the human body that is not made by the human body has gone through some process of artificial manufacture or synthesis in a laboratory.

In general, synthetic hormones are created chemically, without the aid of living organisms. So-called natural hormones are derived at least in part from living organisms and are typically produced by converting plant or animal compounds into molecules that either resemble or are identical to hormone molecules made in the human body.

Examples of "natural" hormones include estrogen and progesterone replacements whose initial building blocks come from soybeans and wild yams (although many of these hormones now are made chemically as well). Another example is insulin hormone replacement for diabetics. In the past, artificial human insulin was made by purifying insulin taken from cattle and pig pancreases; today insulin is more commonly produced through the use of genetically modified yeasts and bacteria. Both of these processes would fall under the broad umbrella of "natural" hormone production.

Greater confusion exists around the term "bioidentical." The Endocrine Society, a scientific organization dedicated to endocrinology and hormone research, defines bioidentical hormones as "compounds that have exactly the same chemical and molecular structure as hormones that are produced in the human body." In comparison, nonbioidentical hormones have structures that imitate hormones produced in the human body and can act as a substitute, but they are not identical to human hormones.

There is no standard agreement on approved sources or manufacturing methods for bioidentical hormones. As a result, bioidentical hormones may be purely synthetic (manufactured chemically in a lab), or they may be derived from plants or other organisms and then altered to have the exact structure of the human hormones they replace. The lack of clarity on definitions of "synthetic," "natural," and "bioidentical" has led some doctors to argue that, in the end, any hormone introduced to a human body is in fact a synthetic hormone.

Whatever their sources or production methods, synthetic hormones are used to treat a large and growing array of human health issues that are caused by either a complete absence or a shortage of specific human-produced hormones. As mentioned above, the most common uses of synthetic hormones are hormonal birth control methods and HRT. Synthetic estrogen, progesterone, or testosterone may also be used as part of fertility treatments and by transgender individuals to change their bodies to better reflect their gender identity.

Synthetic thyroid hormones are given to replace those that the thyroid is no longer producing (as in the case of hypothyroidism) or to suppress the growth of thyroid tissue in patients with thyroid cancer. The most common thyroid replacement hormone is thyroxine, which is chemically produced. Dried animal thyroid tissue, taken mainly from pigs, also is available and in the past was the standard treatment for hypothyroidism. However, the American Thyroid Association cautions that human and pig thyroids do not produce the same proportions of individual active thyroid hormones.

Beginning in the 1960s, human growth hormone (HGH) was given to children whose pituitary glands were not producing enough of the substance. Originally, the only source of HGH was the pituitaries of human cadavers. However, it was discovered that some of this "natural" HGH had come from a cadaver infected with Creutzfeldt-Jakob disease, leading to a public health crisis and a ban on HGH by 1985. Six months later, a synthetic version of HGH, known as recombinant HGH, was created and marketed as Protropin and later as Kigtropin. Today the illegal use of synthetic HGH by professional athletes and bodybuilders has raised concerns about dangerous side effects.

Other synthetic hormone–related controversies include the use of certain artificial growth hormones to increase growth or milk production in livestock. The best known of these is recombinant bovine growth hormone. Among ecologists and environmental advocates, there is growing concern over the increasing presence of a number of synthetic hormones—most notably those used in birth control pills—in water supplies worldwide. Because not all synthetic hormones are absorbed by the body, many are excreted through urine and end up in septic systems and sewage treatment plants. There is currently no effective method for removing these artificially created molecules from the water, and many are beginning to accumulate in watersheds, creating problems for fish and other wildlife and, potentially, humans.

Terri Nichols

See also: Estrogen; Estrogen-Progestin Birth Control Pills; Gender Transition; Hormone Replacement Therapy; Intrauterine Device (IUD); Menopause; Progesterone; Progestin-Only Birth Control Pills; Sex Hormones.

Further Reading

Files, J. A., Ko, M. G., & Pruthi, S. (2011). Bioidentical hormone therapy. *Mayo Clinic Proceedings, 86*(7), 673–680.

Holtorf, K. (2009). The bioidentical hormone debate: Are bioidentical hormones (estradiol, estriol, and progesterone) safer or more efficacious than commonly used synthetic versions in hormone replacement therapy? *Postgraduate Medicine, 121*(1), 73–85.

PBS. (2019). The development of synthetic hormones. Retrieved from http://www.pbs.org/wgbh/amex/pill/peopleevents/e_hormones.html

Syphilis

Syphilis is one of the sexually transmitted infections (STIs) that can cause genital ulcer disease (GUD) as well as other bodily complications, depending on how long an individual has the infection before being treated. Included in the GUD group are granuloma inguinale, lymphogranuloma venereum, and the herpes simplex virus. And, just like other STIs, syphilis can be present in a person without causing signs or symptoms of disease. Similar to the other bacterial causes of GUD, there are tests available to diagnose, antibiotics that currently work to treat, and, happily, syphilis can be effectively prevented by the use of condoms for sexual intercourse.

Syphilis seems to have been around in humans for a long time, and it may have evolved to infect humans after "jumping" from other species, such as llamas or primates. The first recorded cases of syphilis in the Western world were during the epidemic in 1495, during a war in France, and following the return of Christopher Columbus and his sailors from their travels to America. Mobile populations have long been known to transmit new pathogens from one population to another. Soldiers and sailors were early travelers who engaged in population mixing (sexual and casual contact) with new groups of people, and subsequently infections were transmitted both to and from host and visitor. Some infections were not a big problem; others became epidemics. This new STI (syphilis) quickly spread across Europe and had a devastating impact, including death. Just as now, different groups blamed each other for transmission instead of talking practically about prevention.

The World Health Organization estimates there are close to 1 million new cases of treatable STIs every day in the world, with 5.6 million new cases of syphilis every year, or 15,342 cases every day. Globally, syphilis is on the increase again. While anyone who has sex without a condom can theoretically catch syphilis, it is more common in populations who have more sexual activity with more people, compared to the general population. For example, sex workers and men who have sex with men usually have more sexual events with more numbers of people than other populations and so are at increased risk of exposure to and acquisition of syphilis. These populations are also stigmatized, socially marginalized, and are illegal in many countries of the world, making it more difficult to test and treat them to prevent further transmission as well as prevent complications.

Syphilis is a bacteria known as *Treponema pallidum*, subspecies *pallidum*, which under the microscope is shaped like a spiral (spirochete) and uses a corkscrew-like mechanism to gain entry into the body. Despite syphilis being around since before antibiotics were discovered, unlike most other STIs, *Treponema pallidum* remains sensitive to penicillin, so the infection is easily treated with an injection of benzathine penicillin.

Transmission can happen when having sexual activity with someone who has the bacteria and a lesion. The bacteria often causes a lesion (sore) at the site of entry into the body, for example on the lip, tongue, anus, vulva, or penis. The lesion may be hidden inside the anus, mouth, vagina, or under the foreskin in the penis, and if it is painless, which it often is, the person may not know they have it. If a condom is used, then the risk of transmission is much reduced. However, a condom may not protect if the lesion is on a part of the anatomy not covered by the condom, for example, on the scrotum or labia. Fortunately, this is not as common. If an individual is having sex with someone and notices a lesion on their genitals or mouth, it is best to politely encourage the partner to see a doctor for testing and treatment and to put sex on hold until the lesion has healed.

Syphilis has four recognized disease phases. Primary syphilis is described above, as a lesion occurring approximately three to six weeks after having sex with a person who has syphilis. The lesion may be painful but most often is painless. Without treatment, the lesion goes away by itself, but the bacteria remain in the person's body and then cause secondary syphilis a few months after primary. In secondary syphilis, a skin rash occurs most commonly, and then the lesions come back and there may be more than one. The lesions may also be present in other parts of the body, including under the arms, on the anus, and on the face. The person may also experience body aches and fever. Without treatment, syphilis then goes into a latent stage where signs of infection are not visible but a blood test can still detect the infection.

Primary, secondary, and early latent syphilis are also known as early syphilis because these symptoms of infection happen in the first two years and are still easily treatable with benzathine penicillin. Tertiary syphilis is much more dangerous and can happen twenty years or more after the initial exposure if the person did not receive effective treatment in the early stages. Tertiary syphilis can cause damage in several body organ systems, including the brain and heart. While it is harder to treat, it is still treatable, but any damage done may be permanent and can even be fatal. Thankfully, tertiary syphilis is rare now due to the wide availability of early testing and effective treatment.

If a pregnant person has untreated syphilis, the fetus can be become infected while in the uterus. Luckily, effective treatment of the pregnant person in the early stages of pregnancy ensures the fetus is also effectively treated. Without treatment, many pregnancies end in stillbirth or the baby is born with congenital syphilis and may have developmental problems. As such, all pregnant people in many countries are encouraged to have a syphilis test during pregnancy.

A simple blood test can determine if syphilis is present and if treatment is needed. Having regular sexual health checkups is one way to maintain sexual health. Some people have a yearly check, while others who have more sexual activity with more people may need a checkup every three months or more often. Using condoms for intercourse and having a good look for lesions before oral sex is also a good idea to reduce risk. Syphilis remains a problem STI globally but is easily tested and easily, cheaply, and effectively treated with a penicillin injection.

Kelwyn Browne

See also: Condoms, Female (Receptive); Condoms, Male (Insertive); Sexually Transmitted Infections (STIs); Testing, STI; Tuskegee Syphilis Study.

Further Reading

Australian Sexual Health Alliance. (2018). Australian STI management guidelines for use in primary health care: Syphilis. Retrieved from http://www.sti.guidelines.org.au/sexually-transmissible-infections/syphilis

Centres for Disease Control and Prevention. (2019). STD surveillance report, 2018. Retrieved from http://www.cdc.gov/std/

STD Prevention Online. (2019). Home page. Retrieved from http://www.stdpreventiononline.org

World Health Organization. (2016). Global health sector strategy on sexually transmitted infections, 2016–2021. Retrieved from http://www.who.int/reproductivehealth/publications/rtis/ghss-stis/en/

Wylie, K. R. (Ed.). (2015). *ABCs of sexual health* (3rd ed.). Chichester: Wiley Blackwell UK.

T

Tantric Intercourse

Tantric intercourse is a sexual practice that originated in India and has roots in East Asian religions such as Hinduism, Buddhism, and Taoism; it is based on spiritual practices and philosophies, including yoga and meditation. Tantric sex emphasizes the importance of consciousness and enlightenment, which can be achieved through sexual experience. Energy also plays an important role in Tantric sex. Sexual energy within the body is believed to flow through the individual and to connect the individual with their partner and with the larger natural and spiritual world. This energetic connection is often described as being cosmic and transcendental.

Although Tantra has been practiced for thousands of years, it is a relative newcomer to Western society, and while interest is increasing, it is still seen as falling into the category of "new age" practices. In general, Western cultures tend to emphasize orgasm as the objective of sexual encounters, and orgasm is generally considered as a biological and functional experience. While some foreplay may occur, sexual intercourse is seen as the "main event," and the sexual experience typically ends when one or both partners experiences an orgasm—a process that lasts on average about six minutes. Tantric sex, on the other hand, is generally a prolonged experience between partners. Rather than a focus on orgasm, the focus becomes a spiritual and energetic connection, which can lead to increased sexual pleasure. Key components include extended foreplay, deep breathing, slow sexual intercourse, and delayed ejaculation. Male practitioners of Tantric sex may learn to control their orgasm so that it occurs without ejaculation, thus allowing them to have multiple orgasms without a refractory period. Orgasms themselves are seen as energetically charged, expansive events that enhance physical, cognitive, affective, and psychic experiences. Further, orgasms are considered to have individual, partnered, and spiritual or transcendental qualities.

Some of the basic practices of Tantric sex may be useful in the treatment of physical and sexual difficulties. For instance, the emphasis on extended foreplay may help to promote orgasm in individuals (often women) who are unable to orgasm during a typical sexual experience. Similarly, focusing on pleasure and connection with the partner as well as extended breath work and slow sexual intercourse may help prolong the length of time it takes for a man to orgasm, one of the most common male sexual concerns. The emphasis on energy and connection with the partner may also help to improve and develop intimacy within the relationship. Finally, because Tantric orgasm focuses on an energetic and spiritual experience, individuals with severe physical difficulties that affect their sexual functioning (e.g., severe neck or back injuries, paralysis) report being able to experience orgasms that are described as being sexual, physical, and mental. Thus, Tantra may be a hopeful option for individuals who wish to remain sexual after a physically limiting injury or other disability that affects or prevents typical sexual activity. Although scientific research in this field is presently limited, future research may help expand our understanding of Tantra and its use in treating sexual dysfunction.

Heather L. Armstrong

See also: Anorgasmia; Foreplay; *Kama Sutra*; Orgasm; Religion, Diversity of Human Sexuality and; Sexual Dysfunction, Treatment of.

Further Reading

Lousada, M., & Angel, E. (2011). Tantric orgasm: Beyond Masters and Johnson. *Sexual and Relationship Therapy, 26*, 389–402. doi: 10.1080/14681994.2011.647903

Rei, K. (2008). *Tantric sex: The path to sexual bliss.* New York: Dorling Kindersley.

Richardson, D. (2003). *The heart of Tantric sex.* Alresford: O Books.

Voigt, H. (1991). Enriching the sexual experience of couples: The Asian traditions and sexual counseling. *Journal of Sex & Marital Therapy, 17*, 214–219.

Waldinger, M. D., McIntosh, J., & Schweitzer, D. H. (2009). A five-nation survey to assess the distribution of the intravaginal ejaculatory latency time among the general population. *The Journal of Sexual Medicine, 6*, 2888–2895. doi: 10.1111/j.1743-6109.2009.01392.x

Teen Pregnancy

"Teen pregnancy" refers to any pregnancy that occurs to any female under twenty years old, regardless of intention or relationship status. Teen pregnancy is both a highly personal issue and an important societal concern. The young pregnant person may or may not have intended to become pregnant, and they may or may not be in a position to take care of and support a baby. They also may or may not have a willing partner, husband, or parents to help. If not, and the individual chooses to have and keep the baby, taxpayer-funded social services may be required to support the baby. Alternatively, abortion or adoption may be considered. Whatever the case may be, there are likely to be many considerations for the individual, their family, and society at large.

According to statistics compiled by the Centers for Disease Control and Prevention (CDC), a total of 194,377 babies were born to women between the ages of fifteen and nineteen in 2017—making for a birth rate of 18.8 per 1,000 teen women. This birth rate represented a decrease of 7 percent compared with 2016. The birth rates from 2016 to 2017 decreased for all ethnic groups—though birth rates for African American, Hispanic, and indigenous teens remained more than twice as high as rates for white teens. In addition, teen birth rates were significantly higher in southern states and rural areas than in northern states and urban areas.

While reasons for the declining birth rate are not entirely clear, the CDC suggests that more teens may be abstaining from sex, and those who are sexually active may be more likely to use some form of birth control. The CDC also notes that with respect to the ethnic and regional disparities in birth rate, higher birth rates are associated with lower education and income, fewer community opportunities for youth activities or employment, and participation in child welfare, foster care, or juvenile justice systems.

The CDC further notes that addressing these issues of disparity could lead to additional drops in teen pregnancy and birth rates—which, despite the decreases, continue to be substantially higher in the United States than in most other Western industrialized nations. To try to meet this objective, the CDC and other government health institutions fund and participate in programs involving training, education, counseling, community outreach, clinical care, and research focusing on teen pregnancy.

Surveys of teen mothers conducted by the CDC from 2006 through 2010 revealed that 23 percent of the moms had intended for the pregnancy to occur, while 77 percent had not intended it to happen. About 58 percent of the mothers said that although they would have liked to eventually become pregnant, their pregnancy happened too soon. Teen births accounted for 5 percent of all births in the United States in 2017.

The CDC notes that teen pregnancy is a leading reason that girls drop out of high school. Only about 50 percent of teenage mothers receive a high school diploma by the time they are twenty-two, compared to about 90 percent of girls who do not give birth as teenagers. Teen pregnancy is associated with poverty and with receiving public benefits in order to support the family. Some reports indicate that relatively few teen mothers receive child support payments from the father.

Children born to teen mothers are more likely than other children to drop out of high school themselves, more likely to have health problems, more likely to commit criminal acts and be incarcerated, more likely to be unemployed as adults, and, if female, more likely to also give birth while still a teen.

Considering these factors, the CDC reported that teen pregnancy and childbirth accounted for an estimated $9.5 billion in costs to U.S. taxpayers in 2010. Those costs included health care, foster care, eventual incarceration of the children of teen mothers, and lost tax revenue resulting from lower education and income among teen mothers. While this number has declined in recent years, teenage pregnancy continues to have a massive social and economic impact in the United States.

The prevention of teen pregnancy is considered a major public health priority because of the potentially adverse consequences of pregnancy at a young age. In this regard, the CDC recommends that young women be educated about the following points:

- knowledge of sexual issues, including sexually transmitted infections and methods of preventing pregnancy
- the benefits of abstinence and limiting the number of partners
- the usefulness of condoms and remembering to use condoms
- dealing with perceptions of peer norms regarding sexual behavior
- understanding an individual's ability and right to refuse sex
- avoiding places and situations that might lead to sex

- communication with parents or other adults about sex, pregnancy, and contraception
- access to youth-friendly clinical services
- understanding the role of public health agencies in reducing teen pregnancy

Open and honest communication between parents and their teenaged children about these and other points can be very helpful in preventing unintended pregnancies. Parents have a responsibility to discuss these matters with their sons as well as their daughters. Research suggests that conversations between parents and their children about sex, relationships, birth control, and pregnancy tend to have several positive effects on teen behavior, such as delaying sexual intercourse to a later age. If teens do have sex, they tend to have it less often than other teens, and they are more likely to use condoms and other birth control methods.

Family planning clinics play an important role in teen pregnancy prevention by providing teens with counseling and information about sex, contraception, pregnancy, and sexually transmitted infections, as well as basic care. Clinics can also offer guidance to parents about these issues. A reproductive health clinic is legally obligated to ensure the confidentiality of the care they provide to teens—meaning that the clinics generally cannot share teens' health information with parents or anyone else without the written permission of the teens. There are certain exceptions to this confidentiality rule, such as when the clinic is concerned that the teen might harm themselves. The CDC reported in 2014 that almost 60 percent of sexually active teens aged seventeen or younger visited a family planning clinic for contraception services during the previous year.

According to the CDC, an estimated 90 percent of teens aged fifteen to seventeen used some form of contraception the last time they had sex, most commonly condoms or birth control pills. Only about 1 percent of teens in that age group use long-acting reversible contraception (LARC) methods, such as intrauterine devices or hormonal implants. If more teens used LARC methods, unintended pregnancies would likely decrease because those methods are highly effective and easy to use as they do not require taking a pill every day or being prepared in advance of a sexual encounter.

A. J. Smuskiewicz

See also: Abortion, Elective; Adolescent Sexuality; Contraception; Family Planning Clinics; Pregnancy; Premarital Sex.

Further Reading

U.S. Centers for Disease Control and Prevention. (2019). Reproductive health: Teen pregnancy. Retrieved from https://www.cdc.gov/teenpregnancy/index.htm

U.S. Centers for Disease Control and Prevention. (2019). Teen births. Retrieved from http://www.cdc.gov/nchs/fastats/teen-births.htm

Teena, Brandon

Brandon Teena (1972–1993) was a transgender man murdered on New Year's Eve in 1993 in Nebraska. Approximately one week prior, Jon Lotter and Marvin

Nissen attacked and raped Teena, reportedly because they discovered Teena's biological sex was different from his gender identity. At this time, few images of transgender individuals were portrayed in the media. This crime was recounted in the documentary *The Brandon Teena Story* and the major motion picture *Boys Don't Cry*.

Brandon Teena was born as Teena Marie Brandon on December 12, 1972, in Lincoln, Nebraska. Teena was assigned as a female at birth. His mother was a sixteen-year-old widow who had another daughter three years older than Teena. Teena's father was killed in a car accident before Teena's birth.

Teena attended Catholic school until his expulsion senior year. When he attended counseling, he disclosed that he was sexually abused by his uncle for four years as a child. It is reported that around the time Teena experienced puberty, he began dressing and presenting as male and started dating women.

Throughout Teena's life, he had a handful of arrests and criminal charges, many related to forgery. In 1993, a warrant was issued for Teena's arrest after he violated probation. It was around this time he began fully living as Brandon Teena. He developed a friendship and moved in with a young mother, Lisa Lambert, who resided in a farmhouse in Humboldt, Nebraska. Through Lambert, Brandon met Lotter and Nissen. He also developed a close friendship speculated to be romantic with Lana Tisdel.

Teena seemed to be accepted by Lotter and Nissen, until his arrest in December 1993. He was placed in jail when he could not make bail, and staff discovered Teena was a biological female. He was placed in the women's section of the jail until Tisdel posted bail. Teena's arrest and biological sex were printed in the local newspaper.

On Christmas Eve, Teena attended a party where Lotter and Nissen pulled his pants down, wanting to see his genitals. Once they discovered Teena's biological sex, they spent the day assaulting and raping him, later locking him in Nissen's bathroom. Teena escaped to Tisdel's house, where they notified authorities. Teena was taken to a hospital, where a rape kit was conducted and later lost.

Despite Teena reporting the attack, having a rape kit conducted, and having witnesses to corroborate his account of the events, Sheriff Charles Laux did not make an arrest. It was reported that Teena was mistreated by Sheriff Laux, even referring to him as "it." Laux brought Lotter and Nissen in for questioning, and even with a partial confession, he made no arrests.

On December 31, 1993, Lotter and Nissen drove to Lambert's farmhouse, where Teena was staying. They shot and stabbed Teena, Lambert, and a third person to death. After being charged, Lotter was sentenced to death, while Nissen received life imprisonment in exchange for testifying against Lotter.

Teena's treatment by law enforcement and tragic murder helped bring awareness to the transgender community. It also showcased the violence and discrimination experienced by transgender individuals. This and other instances of violence experienced by the LGBTQ+ community prompted individuals to begin lobbying for more hate crime laws regarding gender identity and sexual orientation in the United States.

Sarah Gannon

See also: Rape; Transgender; Transphobia.

Further Reading

Bass, A. (2011). *Telling Brandon Teena's story accurately.* GLAAD. Retrieved from http://www.glaad.org/2011/05/05/telling-brandon-teenas-story-accurately

Buist, C., & Stone, C. (2014). Transgender victims and offenders: Failures of the United States criminal justice system and the necessity of queer criminology. *Critical Criminology, 22*(1), 35–47.

Friedman, H. J. (2006). *Brandon: An American tragedy.* Retrieved from web.archive.org/web/20071010043900/http://www.friedmanlaw.com/news-teena-brandon.php

Sloop, J. M. (2000). Disciplining the transgendered: Brandon Teena, public representation, and normativity. *Western Journal of Communication, 64*(2), 165.

Woods, C. S., Ewalt, J. P., & Baker, S. J. (2013). A matter of regionalism: Remembering Brandon Teena and Willa Cather at the Nebraska History Museum. *Quarterly Journal of Speech, 99*(3), 341–363.

Testicles

Testes, also called testicles, are two oval glands of the male reproductive system. They are located in a fleshy sac called the scrotum, which is located behind the penis. Testes produce the male sex cells, known as sperm, as well as the male sex hormones, mainly testosterone.

Each testicle is the size of a large olive, measuring about 1.5 inches (4 centimeters) by 1.25 inches (3 centimeters). They are filled with dense masses of fibrous tissue and small twisting tubes between the tissue. These tubes, known as seminiferous tubules, are the sites of sperm production and development. All the seminiferous tubules join to form twelve to fifteen larger tubes called efferent ducts, which carry the sperm to a coiled tube at the rear of the testicle called the epididymis. There, the sperm complete their development.

During sexual arousal, the sperm are released outside the testes into long tubes called the vas deferens. The sperm then become mixed with nourishing fluids from the prostate, seminal vesicles, and bulbourethral glands before passing out of the body during ejaculation in a sticky mixture known as semen. The semen passes through the penis via the urethra.

Testosterone is produced by cells in the testes called Leydig cells. The production of this hormone reaches high levels at puberty, which typically starts between the ages of twelve and fourteen. High levels of testosterone lead to the development of male secondary sex characteristics, such as beard growth, a deeper voice, increased muscle mass, and an enlarged penis and scrotum.

Disorders of the testes include cancer, infections, hormone abnormalities, and injuries. Testicular cancer, the most common type of cancer in men younger than age thirty-five, is characterized by a painless lump or hard area in one testicle. Individuals may also feel aches in the groin or lower abdomen. Physicians recommend that young men routinely examine their testicles for abnormalities so that this type of cancer can be detected early, before it spreads to other tissues or lymph glands. A diagnosis of testicular cancer can be confirmed with a blood test measuring levels of certain chemicals and a biopsy. Treatment usually consists of removal of the affected testicle. Even if an individual has only one testicle, they may still retain their fertility.

The removal of one or both testicles is known as an orchiectomy. Besides testicular cancer, orchiectomies may also be performed for other reasons, including treatment for prostate cancer and during gender transition for trans women.

In hypogonadism, the testes produce abnormally low levels of testosterone. In some cases, this condition is congenital (present at birth) and may be associated with other congenital conditions, such as undescended testicles (in which the testes fail to move down into the scrotum) or Klinefelter syndrome (in which the individual has an extra X chromosome). In other cases, hypogonadism may occur later in life as a result of trauma, adverse effects of certain medications, disorders of the pituitary gland, or aging. Hormone-based therapies are often used to treat patients with hypogonadism.

Testicles can be injured in sports activities by being hit, kicked, or crushed. The wearing of an athletic cup helps to prevent such traumatic injuries. Another sports-related injury happens when the vas deferens and surrounding tissue become twisted, cutting off the blood supply to a testicle. Such testicular torsion requires emergency surgery.

A. J. Smuskiewicz

See also: Hypogonadism; Orchiectomy; Scrotum; Seminiferous Tubules; Sperm; Testicular Cancer; Testosterone; Vas Deferens.

Further Reading

National Cancer Institute. (2011). *21st century adult cancer sourcebook: Testicular cancer*. Los Gatos, CA: Progressive Management/Smashwords.

National Institutes of Health. (2015). Male reproductive system. Retrieved from http://www.nlm.nih.gov/medlineplus/malereproductivesystem.html

Testicular Cancer

Testicular cancer is cancer of the testicles (also called testes), the two oval glands of the male reproductive system, located in the scrotum. Testicular cancer is the most common type of cancer in men younger than age thirty-five, though it can occur at any age. The average age at diagnosis is thirty-three. Each year, according to the American Cancer Society, approximately 8,800 new cases of testicular cancer are diagnosed, and about 380 men die of the disease, in the United States.

More than 90 percent of testicular cancers begin in cells known as germ cells, where sperm is produced. The cancer gradually spreads to adjoining tissues and, if left untreated, to other parts of the body. Cancerous cells called seminomas, which are more common in older men, spread more slowly than nonseminomas, which are more common in teenagers and younger men. Some types of testicular cancers begin in stroma, the tissue where testosterone is produced.

The precise causes of testicular cancer are unknown. Unlike breast cancer, no specific genes have been identified that increase an individual's risk of testicular cancer. Scientists have found, however, that many individuals with testicular cancer have extra copies of a section of chromosome 12 called isochromosome 12p.

The role of genetics in testicular cancer is further suggested by the fact that white men are four to five times more likely to be diagnosed with testicular cancer than black men. Scientists have also found that individuals with certain other conditions, including an undescended testicle or HIV infection, are also more likely to develop testicular cancer.

The most common early symptom of testicular cancer is a painless lump, swelling, or hard area in one testicle, though both testicles are sometimes affected. Individuals may also feel aches in the groin or lower abdomen. Additional symptoms, in rare cases, may include soreness or growth of the breasts. This breast growth is caused by a hormone that is secreted by some testicular tumors.

Advanced cases of testicular cancer often include pain in the lower back—an indication that the cancer has spread to the abdominal lymph nodes or to the liver. Cancer that has spread to the lungs typically causes coughing and breathing difficulties.

Physicians recommend that people with testicles—especially young individuals—routinely examine their testicles for abnormalities so that cancer can be detected early, before it spreads to other tissues or lymph glands. To properly examine the testicles, the individual should move the penis out of the way, gently roll each testicle between the thumbs and fingers with both hands, and feel and look for any lumps or changes in size or shape. Any suspicious findings should prompt a visit to a physician.

A physician makes a diagnosis of testicular cancer with a physical examination and certain tests. The first test is usually an ultrasound examination to create images that aid in distinguishing cancerous tumors from benign (noncancerous) growths. Next, a blood test may be performed to evaluate the levels of certain protein markers that are indicative of cancer, such as alpha-fetoprotein, human chorionic gonadotropin, and lactate dehydrogenase. Finally, the cancer diagnosis may be confirmed with a biopsy, in which a small piece of the tumor is surgically removed and examined under a microscope. However, the physician may choose not to conduct a biopsy to avoid the risk of spreading the cancerous cells during the procedure.

If cancer if diagnosed, additional imaging techniques may be used to determine the stage of the cancerous growth. Such techniques usually include computed tomography or magnetic resonance imaging.

Treatment for patients with testicular cancer depends on the stage of cancer and other aspects of the patient's case. A team of doctors collaborates to determine the wisest course of treatment, typically including a urologist (who specializes in the urinary and reproductive systems), a radiation oncologist (who specializes in radiation therapy), and a medical oncologist (who specializes in chemotherapy).

Most cases of testicular cancer will require a combination of treatments. In many cases, the affected testicle (or testicles) will need to be removed in a procedure called an orchiectomy. If the cancer has spread beyond the testicles, further surgical interventions will likely be required. After surgery, the patient will probably require follow-up treatment with radiation therapy or chemotherapy (drug therapy).

Treatment success is directly related to the patient's stage of cancer—whether it was localized in only the testicle(s), whether it had spread regionally (to nearby lymph nodes or other tissues), or whether it had spread to distant locations (such as the lungs or brain). The five-year survival rate for treated patients with localized testicular cancer is 99 percent; for treated patients with regional testicular cancer, 96 percent; and for treated patients with testicular cancer that has spread to distant parts of the body, 74 percent.

Many famous people have had testicular cancer and have survived to be diagnosed as cancer-free. These people include cyclist Lance Armstrong, figure skater Scott Hamilton, hockey player Brandon Davidson, and jockey Bob Champion.

A. J. Smuskiewicz

See also: Orchiectomy; Penile Cancer; Prostate Cancer; Testicles.

Further Reading

American Cancer Society. (2019). Testicular cancer. Retrieved from http://www.cancer.org/cancer/testicularcancer/index

National Cancer Institute. (n.d.). Testicular cancer. Retrieved from http://www.cancer.gov/cancertopics/types/testicular

Testing, STI

In terms of screening guidelines for sexually transmitted infections (STIs), most health care providers in the United States follow the recommendations of the United States Centers for Disease Control and Prevention (CDC) and the United States Preventative Services Task Force. The purpose of screening is to target at-risk populations, limit the spread of disease, and provide treatment to responsive diseases. Complications associated with STIs include infertility, chronic pelvic pain, infections of the upper genital tract, cervical cancer, and chronic hepatitis.

For chlamydia and gonorrhea, infections may be asymptomatic or present with mild symptoms. However, if they go without treatment, serious complications can occur in women, such as pelvic inflammatory disease, infertility, chronic pelvic pain, and issues with pregnancy. For men who have sex with men (MSM), there is a higher risk of exposure to STIs. As a result, they may benefit more from frequent screening. Additional guidelines exist for transgender individuals, pregnant people, and MSM for specific STIs. The CDC 2015 guidelines recommend screening both men and women under twenty-four years of age annually for gonorrhea and chlamydia. For MSM, screening every six to twelve months is recommended. For all screening efforts, it is recommended that all of the sites of sexual contact be sampled (vaginal, penile, oral, and rectal). Sampling can be performed by swabbing the sites or collecting a urine sample to perform a nucleic acid amplification test, which will detect the organism. For those who complete recommended treatments, a test of cure is not recommended.

All individuals who seek screening and treatment for STIs should also be offered testing for HIV (recommended for ages thirteen to sixty-four by the CDC). MSM should be screened at least annually if their status is negative, unknown, if they have new partners, or if their partners have had at least one new partner.

For syphilis, screening is recommended for those who are at high risk, such as MSM, people who are living with HIV, and pregnant people. This is performed by using a screening assay such as rapid plasma reagin or a treponemal test such as enzyme-linked immunosorbent assay on a blood sample. Further evaluation can be performed with additional tests.

Screening for oncogenic forms of human papilloma virus (HPV) takes place through cervical cancer screening via Pap smears in women over twenty-one years old. Otherwise, it is not recommended in younger women or male partners of women with HPV. While it is recommended that Pap smears start at age twenty-one, specific HPV testing is not performed until age thirty. Hepatitis B screening is recommended for MSM and others at high risk, and hepatitis C screening is recommended for men and women who are at high risk or were born between 1945 and 1965. MSM at high risk, born between 1945 and 1965, or who are living with HIV should also be screened for hepatitis C. Of note, vaccines are available for HPV, hepatitis A, and hepatitis B. Screening is currently not recommended for bacterial vaginosis, trichomoniasis, *Mycoplasma genitalium*, vulvovaginal candidiasis, or diseases that cause genital, anal, or perianal ulcers (herpes simplex virus or chancroid) in asymptomatic individuals who have not been in contact with an infected partner.

Rachel Snedecor

See also: Chlamydia; Gonorrhea; Hepatitis; Herpes; Human Immunodeficiency Virus (HIV); Human Papillomavirus (HPV); Sexually Transmitted Infections (STIs); Syphilis; Trichomoniasis.

Further Reading

Ghanem, K. G., & Tuddenham, S. (2019). Screening for sexually transmitted infections. Retrieved from https://www.uptodate.com/contents/screening-for-sexually-transmitted-infections

Kohl, K. S., Markowitz, L. E., & Koumans, E. H. (2003). Developments in the screening for Chlamydia trachomatis: A review. *Obstetrics and Gynecology Clinics of North America, 30*(4), 637–658.

LeFevre, M. L. (2014). Screening for chlamydia and gonorrhea: U.S. Preventive Services Task Force recommendation statement. *Annals of Internal Medicine, 161*(12), 902–910.

U.S. Preventive Services Task Force. (2016). Final recommendation statement: Syphilis infection in nonpregnant adults and adolescents: Screening. Retrieved from http://www.uspreventiveservicestaskforce.org/Page/Document/RecommendationStatementFinal/syphilis-infection-in-nonpregnant-adults-and-adolescents

Workowski, K. A., & Bolan, G. A. (2015). Sexually transmitted diseases treatment guidelines, 2015. *MMWR, 64*(3), 2–110.

Testosterone

Testosterone is the main male sex hormone. It and other male sex hormones, collectively known as androgens, are secreted primarily by the testes, or testicles. Small amounts of these hormones are also secreted by the adrenal glands and by the ovaries.

Testosterone levels increase when a male reaches puberty, typically starting between the ages of twelve and fourteen. At puberty, the pituitary gland releases a hormone that stimulates the testes to boost their testosterone production. The testosterone is released into the bloodstream and flows throughout the body, prompting the development of male secondary sex characteristics. These characteristics include the growth of hair on the face and body, the buildup of muscle mass, the growth and maturing of the penis and testicles, and the deepening of the voice. The changes of puberty occur over a period ranging from two to five years.

The small amount of testosterone produced in the female body is necessary for normal female sexual development. The chemical activity of this "male" hormone helps the ovaries produce estrogens, which are the main hormones responsible for the development and maintenance of female secondary sex characteristics.

Besides its role in physical development, testosterone also influences behaviors, including sexual arousal and general aggressiveness. Levels of testosterone spike during sexual arousal and interest. Links have been found between testosterone and sexual aggression, including rape, in some men. In some criminals who repeatedly engage in such behaviors, orchiectomy (surgical removal of the testes, also called castration) has successfully reduced their aggressive tendencies. Healthy forms of aggressiveness, such as a competitive drive to succeed and high levels of motivation and energy, have also been linked to testosterone. Furthermore, studies suggest that testosterone helps promote cognitive functions, such as thinking ability, memory, concentration and focus, and spatial awareness.

Testosterone levels peak during early adulthood, at approximately age twenty. Levels begin to decline at roughly age thirty at a normal rate of about 1 percent per year. As their testosterone levels decline, some middle-aged men may experience reduced sexual desire, difficulty with erection, insomnia, lack of energy, and depression. Having such symptoms is commonly referred to as "low T." Testosterone-based medications in the form of injections, pills, patches, gels, or implantable pellets are available to relieve these symptoms. However, these drugs carry a number of health risks, including heart attack, blood clots, an enlarged prostate, testicle shrinkage, and enlarged breasts, as well as drastic mood swings. Careful, medically supervised use of testosterone drugs can minimize their risks. Testosterone levels can be boosted in alternative ways not involving the use of drugs. These ways include high-intensity exercise, such as weight lifting, combined with a diet low in fructose (fruit sugar) and high in saturated fats.

People concerned about their testosterone levels can have them measured in blood, urine, or saliva tests. Blood tests are the most common way to evaluate testosterone levels. One or two repeat measurements are usually made, preferably in the morning, because testosterone levels fluctuate throughout the day. Normal male testosterone levels range from about 300–1000 nanograms per deciliter (ng/dL). Normal female levels range from about 15–17 ng/dL.

It is normal for testosterone levels to decline with age. However, one abnormal cause for testosterone decline is a condition called hypogonadism, in which the testes do not secrete enough of the hormone because of various congenital (present at birth) problems, a malfunctioning pituitary gland, traumatic injury, or other factors. Testosterone-containing drugs are used to treat hypogonadism.

Abnormally low levels of testosterone may also be caused by excessive amounts of iron in the blood, kidney or liver disease, inflammation of the lungs, obesity, and adverse reactions to radiation treatment or chemotherapy for cancer. In addition, people under a great deal of stress and those who drink alcohol excessively tend to have reduced levels of testosterone.

Anabolic steroids are synthetic versions of testosterone that can be used to treat some of the previously mentioned low-testosterone conditions. However, these drugs are best known for being used by athletes in attempts to increase their strength and enhance their performance. Such uses are neither legal nor safe. The risks carried by all testosterone-based drugs are magnified when they are used in unapproved, unsupervised ways. Because anabolic steroids disrupt the normal hormonal balance in the body, they can lead to development of female sex characteristics in males and male sex characteristics in females.

Abnormally high levels of testosterone are much less common than abnormally low levels. Limited evidence suggests that excessive amounts of testosterone—that is, levels outside the normal range—may be associated with increased likelihood to become an alcoholic, to smoke cigarettes, and to engage in high-risk sports and sexual activities. Such outcomes would logically lead, in turn, to greater likelihood for cirrhosis of the liver, lung cancer, sexually transmitted infections, and injuries. However, most physicians doubt these associations and do not consider high testosterone to be a clinically meaningful condition. Rare cases of excess testosterone could be related to hyperthyroidism (an overactive thyroid gland) or tumors in the testicles or adrenal glands. The most common causes of abnormally high testosterone levels are hormone therapy for low testosterone levels and abuse of anabolic steroids.

Finally, testosterone therapy may also be used by trans men as part of their gender transition process.

A. J. Smuskiewicz

See also: Androgen Insensitivity Syndrome; Androgens; Andropause; Gender Transition; Hypogonadism; Male Sexuality; Puberty; Sex Hormones; Testicles; Testosterone Replacement Therapy.

Further Reading

Brizendine, L. (2011). *The male brain.* New York: Harmony Books/Crown Publishing Group.

Mayo Clinic. (2018). Testosterone therapy: Potential benefits and risks as you age. Retrieved from https://www.mayoclinic.org/healthy-lifestyle/sexual-health/in-depth/art-20045728

Testosterone Replacement Therapy

Testosterone replacement therapy (TRT), also known as androgen replacement therapy, is a common prescription treatment for cisgender men whose testosterone levels are abnormally low. Testosterone is also typically prescribed to treat intersex conditions as well as masculine-identified transgender and nonbinary individuals suffering from gender dysphoria.

In cisgender men, testosterone naturally declines with age but can become low any time for a variety of reasons. This condition is known as hypogonadism. Treatment is generally only prescribed when symptoms are present. Symptoms of low testosterone may include low libido, erectile dysfunction, fatigue and poor energy level, decreased muscle mass, body and facial hair loss, difficulty concentrating, depression, irritability, or low sense of well-being.

Testosterone is highly effective in the treatment of gender dysphoria for individuals who were assigned female at birth but who identify as male or nonbinary, or for intersex individuals who want to masculinize their appearance. In ovary-based bodies, TRT causes changes to secondary sex characteristics such as redistribution of body fat, increased muscular mass, growth of facial hair, deepening of the voice by thickening of vocal cords, increased libido, clitoral enlargement, cessation of menses, increased risk of male pattern baldness, and thickening of skin. Heredity limits response to hormones. Cross-sex hormone treatment appears acceptably safe over the short to medium term, though long-term data is lacking. The goal is to improve the patient's quality of life by facilitating their transition to a physical state that more closely represents their sense of themselves. Weekly or biweekly injection is the traditional treatment method and tends to bring on changes most rapidly. Changes are reported to have a more rapid onset after hysterectomy or menopause. Once started, treatment is usually lifelong, unless fully masculinized effects are not desired. Though it has been prescribed off-label for this purpose since the mid-twentieth century, use of the cross-hormone replacement therapy for transgender people has not been approved by the Food and Drug Administration.

The World Professional Association for Transgender Health (2011) recommends the following guidelines for prescribing hormone therapy for a transgender individual:

- persistent, well-documented gender dysphoria
- capacity to make an informed decision and consent
- legal age of majority (eighteen years or older in the United States)
- other medical and mental health issues under control
- one recommendation letter by mental health provider

Small doses of testosterone are occasionally considered as an option for treating cisgender women with low libido. A number of studies have shown, however, that the unwanted masculinizing side effects and other health risks usually outweigh the marginal effectiveness.

Risks of TRT include acne, elevated cholesterol and decreased high-density lipoprotein, increased triglycerides, potential liver toxicity, potential polycythemia, and potential insulin resistance. Total mortality was not higher than in the general population.

Testosterone may be administered as an injection, via a gel or cream application, skin or oral patch, buccal lozenges, or slow-release implant. Pills are not recommended due to the extra strain placed on the liver by oral testosterone. Dosage may change with age or surgery.

Testosterone is considered a controlled substance; as such, patients may have trouble using mail-order pharmacy services or getting prescriptions filled for more than a thirty-day supply.

C. Michael Woodward

See also: Androgen Insensitivity Syndrome; Androgens; Andropause; 5-Alpha-Reductase Deficiency; Gender Dysphoria; Gender Transition; Hormone Replacement Therapy; Hypogonadism; Sex Hormones; Testosterone.

Further Reading

Gooren, L. J., Giltay, E. J., & Bunck, M. C. (2008). Long term treatment of transsexuals with cross-sex hormones: Extensive personal experience. *The Journal of Clinical Endocrinology & Metabolism, 93*, 19–25.

Khatri, M. (2016, October 20). Is testosterone replacement therapy right for you? Retrieved from https://www.webmd.com/men/guide/testosterone-replacement-therapy-is-it-right-for-you#1

Maxey, K., & Woodward, C. M. (2014). *Caring for transgender people.* Tucson: University of Arizona College of Medicine.

Urology Times. (2016, November 17). Testosterone therapy in women: Is there a benefit? Retrieved from http://www.urologytimes.com/modern-medicine-feature-articles/testosterone-therapy-women-there-benefit

World Professional Association for Transgender Health. (2011). *Standards of care for the health of transsexual, transgender, and gender nonconforming people, 7th Version.* Retrieved from http://www.wpath.org

Touching, Sexual Arousal and

Touch is a necessary and natural human experience. Scholars of touch discuss how important it is for infants to be touched as well as for people throughout their life span. Often called the "Freud of touch," Ashley Montagu (1971) discussed the utmost importance of touch during human development in his book *Touching: The Human Significance of the Skin.* Touching can release important hormones in the body that enhance the immune system as well as promote bonding between people.

People have differing levels of desire for touch. Dennis Dailey, a sexuality educator, calls this need for touch skin hunger. He uses this term to discuss how people differ in their need to give and receive touch. Some people like to be touched, hugged, or cuddled a lot. Others feel comfortable not touching much at all—a high five may be enough physical contact for them. People with varying degrees of skin hunger can enjoy touch in both sexual and nonsexual ways.

Sexual arousal from touch is a common experience. A person can become sexually aroused from touch (called responsive desire—responding to a touch stimuli). When a person is in a sexually aroused state, touch can increase this arousal. Touching erogenous zones (or sexually sensitive areas) may bring so much pleasure to a person they may achieve orgasm. Sexual arousal can make touches that would otherwise be uncomfortable (such as tickling or scratching) very pleasurable.

In addition to feeling pleasurable, touch also has many other physical and emotional benefits. Moderate massage can lead to decreased depression and enhanced immune functioning. Frequent hugging between romantic partners has been shown to lower blood pressure and increase oxytocin, or "the love hormone," which enhances emotional bonding between partners. Skin-to-skin contact also helps people to maintain a sense of normalcy as things are changing due to aging or illness. With all its many benefits, touch and sexual arousal can come from many different sources.

A person may want to touch themselves in a sexual way. Masturbation or self-stimulation of the genitals is the most obvious form of sexually arousing self-touch. Touching oneself in various places in a sensual manner may heighten sexual arousal when engaged in sexual behaviors with another person. Self-touch can also be healing in nonsexual ways and can help people calm down when they are stressed.

Consensually giving and receiving touch can enhance intimacy with others in both sexual and nonsexual ways. Holding hands, hugging, and cuddling with friends and family can enhance closeness and feelings of safety and trust, thereby strengthening the relationship. Engaging in more sensual touch with a romantic or sexual partner can enhance feelings of both physical and emotional intimacy, thereby enhancing the romantic or sexual bond.

There are also instances in which individuals engage in nonconsensual touching. Sometimes, bodies respond to touch in a sexual way even when an individual is not consenting. Emily Nagoski (2015) discussed this in her book *Come as You Are*. The things that bodies do during sexual arousal—erections, vaginal lubrication, and so on—can often feel good when experienced in a situation where that touch is wanted. During times of unwanted touch, like rape or sexual molestation, bodies may also respond sexually whether the victim is sexually aroused or not. It is important to know that touch is a way to express and explore sexuality, but on its own, when a body responds sexually, it does not mean that it was a wanted or consensual experience.

Consensual touch can have many physical and emotional benefits. Touch can promote physical health in the short and long term and can also help people to feel better about themselves. Mutually consensual touch also helps people to feel more connected to friends, family, and romantic and sexual partners. The need for touch or skin hunger varies widely, and we must engage in ongoing conversations with those we touch to make sure that we are meeting their skin hunger needs in consensual and pleasurable ways.

Mark A. Levand and Stephanie C. Chando

See also: Arousal; Erogenous Zones; Intimacy, Sexual and Relational; Masturbation; Oxytocin; Public Displays of Affection.

Further Reading

Advocates for Youth. (2007). *Life planning education: A comprehensive sex education curriculum*. Washington, DC: Author.

Field, T. (2014). *Touch* (2nd ed.). Cambridge, MA: A Bradford Book.

Leonard, K. E., & Kalman, M. A. (2015). The meaning of touch to patients undergoing chemotherapy. *Oncology Nursing Forum*, *42*(5), 517–526.

Montagu, A. (1971). *Touching: The human significance of the skin*. New York: Columbia University Press.

Nagoski, E. (2015). *Come as you are: The surprising new science that will transform your sex life*. Delran, NJ: Simon & Schuster.

Redelman, M. J. (2008). Is there a place for sexuality in the holistic care of patients in the palliative care phase of life? *American Journal of Hospice & Palliative Medicine*, *25*(5), 366–371.

Transexual Menace

Transexual Menace was an advocacy organization founded in 1994 in New York City by Riki Wilchins and Denise Norris. "The Menace" was the first known direct-action political group specifically focused on transgender inclusion. Like the HIV/AIDS advocacy group ACT UP! of the same era, they took their advocacy to the streets in the form of protests and awareness activities.

The Menace organizers were trailblazers in the early days of the visible transgender civil rights movement, defining themselves, demanding their legal rights, and fighting for medical care and against job discrimination (Wilchins, 2017). The group's first gathering was held in response to the exclusion of transgender people from gay pride events, a regular occurrence before the more-inclusive LGBTQ+ movement took hold. The name Transexual Menace was inspired by feminist activist Betty Friedan, founder of the National Organization for Women, who referred to lesbians involved in the feminist movement as the "lavender menace" because she felt they detracted from the "real" women's movement. Cofounder Wilchins preferred the British spelling of "transexual" with one S rather than the more common American spelling, "transsexual."

At a time when transgender people were generally expected to blend in with mainstream society in order to avoid harassment, Transexual Menace sought to be visible. The Menace may, in fact, be best known for its logo, which featured a pair of large red lips and the name "Transexual Menace" in blood-dripping letters against a stark black background, closely resembling the instantly recognizable logo of the cult classic *The Rocky Horror Show* film and stage production.

Hoping to bring more media attention to antitransgender hate crimes, Menace members showed up en masse in public in their dramatic black and red T-shirts. Among other activities, The Menace organized vigils during the trials of those accused of crimes against transgender people, such as Tom Nissen and John Lotter, two of the alleged killers of Nebraska trans man Brandon Teena.

Although Transexual Menace was never a legally established organization, it grew to as many as forty loosely affiliated chapters, both across the United States and abroad. Wilchins once mused that one simply needed to express interest in starting a chapter to consider it done. A surprisingly high number of chapters were in conservative areas of the United States, such as Indiana, Texas, and Arizona.

Transexual Menace's story caught the attention of filmmaker Rosa von Praunheim, who developed a feature-length documentary about the group in 1996. The film, *Transexual Menace*, was originally developed for television but was also screened at a number of film festivals around the country in subsequent years.

Among the Menace's most impactful work was on behalf of transgender athletes competing in the 1994 Gay Games. The Menace descended on a board meeting of the games' organizers to protest the overly vigorous and invasive process transgender women were forced to endure in order to compete. The Menace convinced board members to change the regulations to be more equitable for the 1994 games; unfortunately, those regulations were reinstated for the 1998 games, and transgender athletes were not fully embraced until the 2002 games in Sydney, Australia.

Wilchins later went on to form GenderPAC (GPAC) in 1995, a national coalition of trans rights groups specifically dedicated to transgender rights and public policy, again in response to the lack of trans inclusion in the work being done by national gay and lesbian organizations; GPAC later evolved into TrueChild, which works to bring a "gender transformative" approach to policies and programs that affect the healthy development of children and youth.

C. Michael Woodward

See also: GenderPAC; Teena, Brandon; Transgender; Transsexual.

Further Reading

TrueChild. (2017). Home page. Retrieved from https://www.truechild.org

Wilchins, R. (2017). *TRANS/gressive: How transgender activists took on gay rights, feminism, the media & congress...and won!* New York: Riverdale Avenue Books.

Transgender

The term "transgender," which gained popularity in Western societies in the 1990s, refers to individuals who do not identify as their gender or sex assigned at birth. "Trans," as a prefix, means "across"; thus, in relation to gender, "transgender" refers to someone who does not identify with their sex or gender label assigned as birth or who has moved across gender categories. Furthermore, "trans," as a shorthand, is often used as an umbrella term when discussing transgender and gender-diverse people contemporarily. Transgender is a gender identity, not a sexual orientation. Gender identity refers to one's inner sense of gender, regardless of gender or sex assignment at birth. Being transgender is also not the same as being a drag performer, though some drag performers do identify as transgender.

To date, there are few studies with good estimates on the prevalence of transgender identities in society. Estimates include numbers from the *Diagnostic Statistical Manual*, Dutch studies, and estimates collected by transgender people themselves. Currently, the best prevalence numbers come from data analyzed and summarized by the Williams Institute at UCLA, which estimates that approximately 0.3 percent of individuals living in the United States identify as transgender, or about 700,000 individuals. Worldwide, the estimate is that there are around 15 million transgender people.

There are two known early sources for the word "transgender," though debate on the origin continues. The most frequently cited source of the term is an early trans activist and trans person named Virginia Prince (1912–2009). Prince, in 1969, identified herself as a "transgenderal," or, according to her definition, someone who wanted to change their gender but not necessarily their sex. The second, and less widely known, source of the term originated in a 1965 medical text written by psychiatrist John F. Olivan. The specific term used by Olivan was "transgenderism," indicating an individual who wished to change their gender or sex (both "gender" and "sex" were used in this definition, highlighting the historical confusion over the separation of these two distinct concepts).

The category of transgender, due to its wide definition and cultural or historical shifts, has taken many different connotations. Caution should be taken when applying this term to other time periods and other cultures. There are also cultural variations of transgender terminology in specific communities, notably racial and ethnic differences.

When discussing transgender people, there are many subcategories of identity. Common identities under the trans umbrella include, but are not limited to, trans woman (or male-to female transgender), trans man (or female-to-male transgender), genderqueer, bigender, gender nonconforming, nonbinary, agender, and so on. Trans women are individuals assigned male at birth but who identify and live as women, commonly using the pronouns she, her, or hers, and who may employ medical intervention to feminize their bodies. Trans men are individuals assigned female at birth but who identify and live as men, commonly using the pronouns he, him, or his, and who may employ medical intervention to masculinize their bodies. Genderqueer, gender nonconforming, and nonbinary individuals embody gender in many different ways, often blurring the boundaries between masculine and feminine in specific and purposeful ways.

There is no one way to be transgender. Trans people often undergo a series of steps to transition from their gender or sex assignment at birth to a different gender identity and gender expression (that is, the outward signs of gender such as clothing, hair, etc.). Transition for a trans person is a highly individualized process, and no blueprint exists. Common steps include coming out to one's self, friends, family, coworkers, and employers; seeking mental health care to discuss the desired outcome of transition and referral letters for medical care; hormone transition including the administration of various hormone treatments from a medical provider; and gender-affirming surgeries. There are many different hormonal and surgical options available, and, notably, not all trans people want hormone intervention or surgical interventions.

Jay A. Irwin

See also: Agender; Bigender; Biological Sex; Cisgender; Drag; Gender Diversity; Gender Identity; Gender Transition; Genderqueer; Nonbinary Gender Identities; Pronoun Usage; Transexual Menace; Transphobia; Transsexual.

Further Reading

Erickson-Schroth, L. (Ed.). (2014). *Trans bodies, trans selves: A resource for the transgender community.* New York: Oxford University Press.

Gates, G. J. (2011). How many people are lesbian, gay, bisexual, and transgender? Los Angeles: The Williams Institute, UCLA School of Law. Retrieved from http://williamsinstitute.law.ucla.edu/wp-content/uploads/Gates-How-Many-People-LGBT-Apr-2011.pdf

Stryker, S. (2008). *Transgender history.* Berkeley, CA: Seal Press.

Transphobia

"Transphobia" refers to attitudes and beliefs about transgender people that stigmatize and antagonize people within the transgender community. The word "transgender" (or "trans") is often used as an umbrella term to refer to any gender-nonconforming person, behavior, expression, or identity, including people who cross-dress, are transsexual, are genderqueer, are drag queens and kings, as well as a host of other terms that people use to categorize their gender.

Transphobia, like other forms of stigma and discrimination, is manifested across three main levels: structural, interpersonal, and internalized transphobia. Structural forms of transphobia include laws and policies that discriminate against trans individuals and include health care access barriers. The fact that transgender individuals can be currently fired in thirty-two states because of their nonconforming gender identity is an example of structural transphobia. Interpersonal forms of transphobia include sexual violence, hate crimes, workplace discrimination, and family rejection of trans people. For example, at least 50 percent of trans people experience sexual assault or rape at least once in their life due to their gender identity or expression. Lastly, internalized transphobia is a set of negative beliefs and attitudes toward trans or gender nonconforming features in oneself and in others.

Transphobia across its three levels negatively affects the mental and physical well-being of transgender individuals. According to the transgender minority stress model, trans people experience chronic stress due to the stigma attached to their gender identities or expressions, which in turn leads to poor mental and physical health. For example, transgender individuals often experience depression, substance abuse, high blood pressure, HIV infection, and low self-esteem due to stigma and discrimination. Furthermore, many doctors refuse to provide service to trans patients because of transphobic views, and as a result, trans people often do not receive adequate health care and are therefore unable to develop positive well-being. High incidence of suicide due to experiencing stigma also affects trans people; in one study, 41 percent of transgender people reported having attempted suicide.

Members of the trans community who possess multiple stigmatized identities may experience more severe and chronic forms of transphobia. Due to societal pressures that favor masculinity over femininity, trans women often experience more frequent and severe sexual harassment and violence. Furthermore, trans women of color experience disproportionate levels of harassment and violence, which leads to many deleterious health outcomes.

Research provides evidence on reducing transphobia. Both family acceptance and social support, for example, help mitigate the negative consequences of interpersonal transphobia experienced by trans individuals. Useful interventions to counteract one's internalized transphobia include reducing shame around one's transgender identity. Similarly, acceptance and sensing pride of one's transgender identity also protect against the negative effects of experiencing transphobia among trans people.

Caitlin Monahan and Nadav Antebi-Gruszka

See also: Antigay Prejudice; Homophobia; Transgender.

Further Reading

Bockting, W. O., Miner, M. H., Swinburne Romine, R. E., Hamilton, A., & Coleman, E. (2013). Stigma, mental health, and resilience in an online sample of the US transgender population. *American Journal of Public Health, 103*(5), 943–951.

Bradford, J., Reisner, S. L., Honnold, J. A., & Xavier, J. (2013). Experiences of transgender-related discrimination and implications for health: Results from The Virginia Transgender Health Initiative Study. *American Journal of Public Health, 103*(10), 1820–1829.

Clements-Nolle, K., Marx, R., Guzman, R., & Katz, M. (2001). HIV prevalence, risk behaviors, health care use, and mental health status of transgender persons: Implications for public health intervention. *American Journal of Public Health, 91*(6), 915–921.

Coleman, E., Bockting, W., Botzer, M., Cohen-Kettenis, P., Decuypere, G., Feldman, J., ... Zucker, K. (2012). Standards of care for the health of transsexual, transgender, and gender-nonconforming people, version 7. *International Journal of Transgenderism, 13*(4), 165–232.

Grant, J. M., Mottet, L. A., Tanis, J., Herman, J. L., Harrison, J., & Keisling, M. (2010). *National transgender discrimination survey report on health and health care.* Washington, DC: National Center for Transgender Equality and the National Gay and Lesbian Task Force.

Hill, D. B., & Willoughby, B. L. (2005). The development and validation of the genderism and transphobia scale. *Sex Roles, 53*(7–8), 531–544.

Hughto, J. M., Reisner, S. L., & Pachankis, J. E. (2015). Transgender stigma and health: A critical review of stigma determinants, mechanisms, and interventions. *Social Science & Medicine, 147,* 222–231.

Macnish, M., & Gold-Peifer, M. (2014). Families in transition: Supporting families of transgender youth. In T. Nelson & H. Winawer (Eds.), *Critical topics in family therapy* (119–129). New York: Springer International Publishing.

Sevelius, J. M. (2012). Gender affirmation: A framework for conceptualizing risk behavior among transgender women of color. *Sex Roles, 68*(11–12), 675–689.

Stotzer, R. L. (2009). Violence against transgender people: A review of United States data. *Aggression and Violent Behavior, 14*(3), 170–179.

Transsexual

The term "transsexual" has meant different things in different time periods. The contemporary usage of the term typically refers to a person who desires to or who has modified their body to transition from one gender or sex to another through the use of medical technologies such as hormones or surgeries. Previous definitions operated as a catch-all term for people with different genders than their sex assigned at birth. Occasionally, an alternate spelling of the word is used—"transexual" instead of "transsexual." It is important to note that, currently, there is debate over the term "transsexual" within the transgender community. Some individuals find the term antiquated or pejorative, while others use the term to self-describe themselves. Currently, "transgender" or "trans" is the larger umbrella term to refer to individuals who do not identify as the sex they were assigned at birth. Transsexual, while still used by some individuals, should be used with caution as it is not adopted uniformly.

The term "transsexual" is often traced back to Magnus Hirschfeld, the German sexologist and physician who advocated for the acceptance of sexual minorities during the late 1800s and early 1900s. The term gained popularity in medical communities largely due to the work of Harry Benjamin in the 1950s and 1960s (e.g., the popular work *The Transsexual Phenomenon* of 1966). The term "transsexual" became more known in a widespread audience when Christine Jorgensen's transition from male to female became a worldwide headline in 1952. The term was designed to show a difference between individuals wishing to physically alter their bodies (transsexuals) and individuals who only wished to wear differently gendered clothing (transvestite).

Social movement groups associated with transgender rights have also adopted the term "transsexual" in various time periods. The most well-known group using the term is The Transexual Menace, an early direct-action group that advocated for transgender acceptance and rights that was formed by advocate Riki Wilchins in the 1990s.

The most widespread usage of the term "transsexual" is currently in the medical community to refer to individuals utilizing various medical transition steps. Transition can look many different ways depending on the individual's goals and the steps needed to maximize a person's comfort within their own body and sense of self. Within the medical community, many guidelines exist to assist physicians working with transsexual patients through their transition process. The most holistic guideline is produced by the World Professional Association for Transgender Health and is called the Standards of Care.

A chief complaint against the term "transsexual" within the trans community is the overly medicalized and pathologized nature of the term. Historically, individuals who identified as transsexual were often diagnosed as having gender identity disorder, the psychological category that is now referred to as gender dysphoria or gender dysphoric disorder. Diagnosis with one of these clinical terms was historically required before a trans person could begin their medical transition. Requiring individuals to be diagnosed with a mental illness before medical transition has been loosened in the most recent Standards of Care, but the inclusion of such a category in the *Diagnostic Statistical Manual of Mental Disorders* can be seen as stigmatizing.

Two major transsexual categories exist—trans women and trans men. Trans women, or male-to-female transsexual people, are assigned male at birth and undergo various medical interventions to alter their bodies to achieve a more typical female look. Trans men, or female-to-male transsexual people, are assigned female at birth and undergo various medical interventions to alter their bodies to achieve a more typical male look. Increasingly diverse ways of identifying, modifying, and presenting gendered characteristics are acknowledged within trans communities. Typically for transsexual-identified individuals, a more binary expression of gender is endorsed. In other words, individuals who adopt a transsexual self-identity often prefer more gender-typical gender expression. Trans women who identify as transsexual may endorse more stereotypically female gender expressions and attitudes, and trans men who identify as transsexual may endorse more stereotypically male gender expression and attitudes.

Jay A. Irwin

See also: Benjamin, Harry; Gender Dysphoria; Gender Transition; Genderqueer; Hirschfeld, Magnus; Jorgenson, Christine; Transexual Menace; Transgender; Transphobia; World Professional Association for Transgender Health (WPATH).

Further Reading

Coleman, E., Bockting, W., Botzer, M., Cohen-Kettenis, P., DeCuypere, G., Feldman, J., … Zucker, K. (2012). Standards of care for the health of transsexual, transgender, and gender-nonconforming people, version 7. *International Journal of Transgenderism, 13*(4), 165–232.

Erickson-Schroth, L. (Ed.). (2104). *Trans bodies, trans selves: A resource for the transgender community.* New York: Oxford University Press.

World Professional Association Transgender Health. (2019). Home page. Retrieved from https://www.wpath.org

Transvestite

A transvestite is an individual who dresses in clothes characteristic of another gender. The term typically refers to a man who dresses in women's clothing such as a dress, pantyhose, and high heels. Society generally considers this behavior to be unusual. By contrast, it is generally more socially acceptable for a woman to wear men's clothing, such as a suit or tuxedo. Whatever the views of society, most psychologists view transvestism as a healthy form of self-expression for most of the individuals who engage in the behavior.

The term "transvestite" is commonly used interchangeably with "cross-dresser." Some people distinguish one term from the other based on the motivations of the dresser or other criteria, and some people find one term or the other offensive. However, there is a range of views regarding this terminology within the LGBT (lesbian, gay, bisexual, transgender) community, and the use of "transvestite" or "cross-dresser" comes down to a matter of personal preference.

There is a fairly clear distinction between a transvestite and someone who is transgender or transsexual. For example, a male transvestite enjoys dressing in women's clothing, but he generally self-identifies as male most of the time. By contrast, a genetic male who is transgender always self-identifies as female, with many such individuals eventually transforming their bodies through female hormones and sex reassignment surgery. In some cases, some people who identify as a transvestite may experience change in their gender identity over time and later identify as transgender. Transvestism is not a reflection of sexual orientation, and a transvestite may be straight, gay, bisexual, or another sexual orientation.

The reasons that a transvestite dresses in other-gender clothes vary among individuals—and may even vary from one time to another in the same individual. Some male transvestites find a sense of peace and a relief from stress while wearing soft, feminine clothes. While they pretend to be a woman, they may also find escape from the demands and expectations that society places on them as a man. Many transvestites become sexually aroused by the way they feel and look in women's clothes. Some transvestites dress to entertain others. If male, these individuals are often called female impersonators, gender illusionists, or drag queens. Some women dress as men to "pass" as male in order to get certain jobs.

Some transvestites dress only in the privacy of their homes, but others enjoy going out in public while dressed as the other gender. Going out in public is a huge step that many transvestites are afraid to take, but those who do often discover a sense of personal liberation that they do not otherwise know. They may find that they enjoy living in public as a woman, even if only for a few hours at a time. Some transvestites can successfully "pass" as a woman in public. Others cannot pass but find that they are still accepted by others in social situations. Unfortunately, some transvestites experience intolerance and violence from certain people.

The prevalence of transvestism is unknown, as are the causes. It is known, however, that most transvestites appear to be born with a tendency for the behavior, which is often first manifested in childhood, and the behavior appears to last a lifetime for most. Some transvestites feel guilty about their dressing and repeatedly try to stop the behavior with "purges" of their female wardrobe, but they typically eventually restock the wardrobe. Many transvestites are happy and well adjusted with their behavior. But for those who feel confused or disturbed by their behavior, professional therapy can help them to accept themselves.

Transvestism has been known throughout history in all cultures, with varying degrees of social acceptance. Some famous female transvestites have been Joan of Arc, a French soldier in the 1400s; Isabelle Eberhardt, a Swiss explorer in the late 1800s and early 1900s; and Dorothy Lawrence, an English writer and soldier in the 1900s. Some famous male transvestites have been Elagabus, a Roman emperor in the third century; Francois Timoleon de Choisy, a French writer from the mid-1600s to early 1700s; Ed Wood, an American movie director in the mid-1900s; and the modern-day performers Eddie Izzard and RuPaul.

A. J. Smuskiewicz

See also: Drag; Gender Expression; Gender Roles, Socialization and; Transgender.

Further Reading

Coleman, V. (2014). *Men in bras, panties, and dresses: The secret truths about transvestites.* Seattle, WA: Amazon Digital Services.

Novic, R. (2005). *Alice in Genderland: A crossdresser comes of age.* Bloomington, IN: iUniverse.

Tri Ess: The Society for the Second Self. (2019). Home page. Retrieved from http://www.tri-ess.org

Trichomoniasis

Trichomoniasis is the most common nonviral sexually transmitted infection (STI). The single-celled parasite causes more than 7 million infections per year in the United States, which is almost twice the number of gonorrhea and chlamydia cases combined. Worldwide, there are more than 180 million cases annually. Given the impressive number of people infected, it is surprising that most people have never heard of this infection. The good news is that trichomoniasis is easily treated with antibiotics, so perhaps part of the reason that it is not well known is the fact that this infection can be completely cured. The bad news is that trichomoniasis is often difficult to diagnose.

Trichomoniasis is the infection caused by a single-celled parasite, *Trichomonas vaginalis.* Viewed under the microscope, trichomonas (called "trich" for short) is roughly the same size and shape as a white blood cell, appearing somewhat pear shaped. Trich has five tails, called flagella, that whip around to propel the organism. If a clinician looks at a freshly prepared slide under the microscope, the trich parasites will be easy to identify as they tumble and move across the viewing field. However, if the slide sits out on the microscope for more than a minute, the slide dries out and the trichomonas quickly stop moving, making them much more difficult to identify as they sit side by side with the numerous white blood cells that typically accompany trichomonal infections.

Trichomonal infections can be passed from partner to partner by direct genital contact. Trich infections are the only STI that is passed through neither oral nor anal sex. Transmission is, therefore, most often from genital intercourse between a male and female or through sharing sex toys between two or more females. Latex condoms greatly decrease the transmission of trichomonas, though not when there is failure of the condom via breakage or improper use. Trichomonas cannot be passed by kissing, hugging, or other casual contact, nor is it transmitted in public restrooms, hot tubs, swimming pools, or bed linens. While trichomonas can remain viable in moist areas such as damp towels or underwear, transmission resulting in infection has never been documented.

Trich can infect any person, but 90 percent of male infections are completely asymptomatic; the men are totally unaware of any symptoms. For the 10 percent of men who do notice a problem, the most common complaints are a discharge from their urethra and pain with urination or ejaculation. In females, the symptoms often come and go over weeks, months, or even years. Burning or discomfort while urinating, a light yellow or green frothy vaginal discharge, or a bad odor (from the discharge) can signal the presence of trich. Another common female symptom may be simply the new onset of pain or discomfort during sex, with or without any of the other complaints.

Because the symptoms can wax and wane, or even disappear without treatment, trichomonal infections can and often do persist for a long time. Women with trich infections that show up as a vaginal discharge may assume they have a vaginal yeast infection. After using an over-the-counter product for several days, the discharge and irritation seem to resolve, which further confirms to that individual that they did, indeed, have a yeast infection, which is now treated and gone. However, all that has really happened is that, following the natural history of trich infections, a discharge, discomfort, and odor may be noticed for several days to a week, and then the symptoms fade, but the infection persists. Weeks later, the symptoms recur, but people may not connect the dots to realize it is the same infection.

Trichomoniasis can also present with burning and irritation with urination, and in this case, the same scenario often replays via a presumed bladder infection. This time, the individual may call or go in to see a clinician and may be prescribed an antibiotic for a urinary tract infection. When the medical provider performs the routine dipstick test on the urine, they will detect white blood cells, which are a sign of inflammation and infection. The same will be seen with a quick glance under the microscope (as mentioned earlier). These white blood cells are exactly what the clinician is expecting, and many will base their treatment on the patient's symptoms—burning and discomfort with peeing—and these simple tests. This diagnosis does not routinely call for a pelvic exam in this setting, so the physical exam is likely to be normal. The doctor may then write a prescription for an antibiotic to treat the bladder infection, but the common medications that are used to treat bladder infections will not affect the trichomonas. So, the symptoms go away because of the natural course of the infection, but the infection remains and can cause problems again down the road.

However, if the doctor sends the urine off for a culture (to confirm suspicion of a bladder infection as well as to see which bacteria is causing it), but the real cause of the symptoms is a trichomonal infection, the culture will come back as negative, which means no bacteria were present. In this situation, the patient is typically notified that they can stop their antibiotic and to follow up if the symptoms recur. The take-home message here is not that every presumed bladder infection should have a confirmatory culture but that if a patient has recurrent infections or a single classic infection with a negative culture, then further exams and tests are indicated to look for other masquerading infections such as trichomoniasis.

Fortunately, trichomonas does not cause permanent damage to the reproductive or genitourinary tracts in the manner that other infections such as gonorrhea and chlamydia do. However, there are some serious concerns with trichomonal infections. Perhaps the most important issue with trich is that the presence of a trich infection, along with the irritation and inflammation that it causes, greatly increases that person's risk of contracting another STI—particularly the viral infections. Trich infection at least triples the risk of contracting HIV from a partner with HIV, with studies showing between three to five times increased risk. Trichomonas is also linked with an increased risk of pelvic inflammatory disease and infertility.

Another very significant issue with trichomonal infections is the increased incidence of low-birthweight and even premature infants when a pregnant person contracts trichomoniasis.

Trichomonal infections can be diagnosed by urine or vaginal or urethral discharge samples. Clinicians can immediately examine these specimens under microscopy, and as mentioned earlier, if the parasites are still swimming around, it is a very obvious diagnosis. However, current studies show the sensitivity (the ability to detect the organism if it is present) of these wet preps as roughly 60–70 percent. The accuracy of this test, though, known as the specificity (if the test is positive, it really is trichomonas), is 98 percent. When these unicellular organisms are bouncing along in their characteristic manner, it is very obvious. Culturing the sample yields fairly accurate information, with 95 percent sensitivity, but can take up to a week to get results. Newer tests include ELISAs and direct fluorescent antibody tests. Their 80–90 percent sensitivity rate is much better than the wet preps, with results typically available in a couple of days. Newly developed rapid diagnostic tests use polymerase chain reaction DNA probes and boast excellent sensitivity (97%) and specificity (98%). This new technology comes at a price, of course—up to $200 per test for patients choosing to test directly from an outpatient lab.

Pap smears are another source of detection for trichomonal infections, though they should not be thought of as a good screening tool for this purpose. Pap smears are designed to detect precancerous or cancerous changes of the cervix. However, because of the high volume of Pap tests, even though they have a low sensitivity of detecting trichomonas, many people are indeed diagnosed with trichomonal infections from their Pap test. (Note that a normal Pap test does not mean that the individual definitely does not have trichomonas, nor any other STI.) Pap tests have been shown to have anywhere from 25 percent to 60 percent sensitivity in detecting trichomonas. This low number should come as no surprise for two reasons: (1) obviously the trich are immobile by the time a pathologist receives the slide, so they appear very similar to white blood cells, and (2) remember the pathologist is focused on looking for precancerous changes in the cervical cells, not necessarily zooming in on the neighboring ever-present white blood cells (which may, in fact, be a trichomonas parasite).

There are also some clues on the physical exam that could lead the clinician to look for trichomonas. People with vaginal infections may have a characteristic frothy, light green discharge, along with a foul odor. This discharge may be noticed only on speculum exam, although often the patient will be aware of it on their underwear. In addition, the cervix or vaginal wall may have several small bright red spots, called petechiae. Roughly one in ten vaginal trichomonal infections will produce a classic strawberry cervix that is covered with these red spots, and this presentation is virtually diagnostic of trichomonas.

There are only two antibiotics that can cure trichomoniasis: metronidazole and tinidazole. The preferred choice is metronidazole. Unfortunately, this antibiotic has a relatively high rate of side effects. Nausea (10 %), gastrointestinal discomfort or cramps (7%), metallic taste (9%), and headaches (18%) are the most common complaints. Also, the patient must abstain from all alcohol while taking metronidazole and for at least twenty-four hours after completing the course of antibiotic. Metronidazole can be given in a single dose of two grams or in twice-a-day dosing of five hundred milligrams for a week. To minimize side effects and maximize patient compliance, the single dose is typically recommended. However, if that single dose fails to clear the infection, then a full week of metronidazole is used. This drug should not be used in the first trimester of pregnancy.

A second-line antibiotic is tinidazole. This medication is given as a single two-gram dose, and alcohol should be avoided for at least three days after the treatment dose. Tinidazole, too, has side effects of bitter taste (6%) and nausea (5%), though slightly less than metronidazole. It should not be given during the first trimester of pregnancy or when breastfeeding.

Both the person diagnosed with the trichomonal infection and their current partner need to be treated with antibiotics at the same time (while abstaining from intercourse during treatment) to avoid being reinfected. Due to the difficulty of detecting trichomonas, physicians typically treat any potentially exposed partners without actually testing them to confirm that they are infected as well. Depending on where the patient lives, their physician may or may not be allowed to write prescriptions for the appropriate antibiotic for the person to give to their partner(s). This is called expedited partner therapy, and legal restrictions vary from state to state in the United States.

Alternative therapies such as herbs, vinegar, or douching do not cure trichomonal infections. In fact, douching is associated with adverse side effects and could potentially push infections upward in the genital tract or create microtrauma in the vaginal mucosa, which breaks down the lining enough to increase susceptibility to other STIs.

Trichomonas is passed from person to person only during vaginal intercourse or through shared sex toys, so abstaining from sex will certainly prevent trichomoniasis, and consistent use of condoms will also greatly reduce risk. Risk factors for contracting trichomoniasis are similar to those for most STIs, and the more partners and individual has, the higher the risk.

The question of developing a preventative trichomonas vaccine has been raised. A vaccine could potentially reduce societal costs from trich-related pregnancy complications, increased incidence of HIV disease, and other medical costs due to this difficult to detect, yet very common, disease.

Jill A. Grimes

See also: Sexually Transmitted Infections (STIs); Testing, STI; Vaginal Secretions; Vaginitis; Yeast Infection (Candidiasis).

Further Reading

Grimes, J. A., Smith, L. A., & Fagerberg, K. (2013). *Sexually transmitted disease: An encyclopedia of diseases, prevention, treatment, and issues.* Santa Barbara, CA: Greenwood.

McAnulty, R. D., & Burnette, M. M. (Eds.). (2006). *Sex and sexuality.* Santa Barbara, CA: Praeger.

Newton, D. E. (2009). *Sexual health: A reference handbook.* Santa Barbara, CA: ABC-CLIO.

Tubal Ligation

A tubal ligation—commonly called "getting your tubes tied"—is a surgical procedure for permanent contraception. In this relatively simple procedure, the surgeon cuts, ties, or blocks the fallopian tubes, the tubes that carry eggs from the ovaries to the uterus. Sperm normally fertilizes the egg in one of the two fallopian tubes prior to the fertilized egg implanting itself in the uterine wall. Thus, a tubal ligation is designed to prevent the sperm and egg from meeting, making fertilization (and, by extension, pregnancy) impossible.

Tubal ligation is a common surgical sterilization procedure. After a tubal ligation, there is no need to use birth control pills or other forms of contraception. The procedure has the added possible benefit of decreasing the risk of ovarian cancer.

A tubal ligation can be performed with various techniques. The fallopian tubes can be cut and sealed with a cauterization (burning) tool. The tubes can be closed by tying, clipping, or banding them, such as with plastic rings or clips. Another option is to insert small metal coiled devices, called tubal implants, into the tubes. These implants seal off the tubes and require no cutting or tying.

In most cases, tubal ligation is a minimally invasive surgical procedure performed through one or two small abdominal incisions with laparoscopes—thin, tubelike devices with surgical tools or cameras at the ends. Tubal ligation may be performed as either an outpatient or inpatient surgical procedure with the use of either regional anesthesia (known as an epidural) or short-acting general anesthesia. The insertion of tubal implants is typically a ten-minute nonsurgical procedure in which the physician inserts the implants up through the vagina and uterus and into the fallopian tubes.

Many people choose to have a tubal ligation while they are having other abdominal operations, such as a cesarean section (C-section). Many others choose to get "postpartum" tubal ligations within twenty-four to thirty-six hours after vaginal childbirth, when the fallopian tubes are higher in the abdomen and easier for the surgeon to access.

Most people can go home several hours after an outpatient tubal ligation. When performed in conjunction with childbirth, a tubal ligation does not usually add to the hospital stay. Following the procedure, it is normal to experience minor discomfort and pain at the site of the laparoscopic incision for a few days as well as slight vaginal bleeding and bloating (caused by the gas used to lift the skin and muscles away from the abdominal organs during the ligation procedure). The individual may also feel some fatigue and dizziness.

Tubal ligation carries some risks and may not be suitable for everyone. For example, the procedure is associated with complications in people who have histories of previous pelvic or abdominal surgery, pelvic inflammatory disease, type 2 diabetes, or obesity. Those conditions may cause complications because they sometimes leave scarring or adhesions (sticking together) of tissues in the abdomen—creating difficulties for the surgeon performing the tubal ligation. In other cases, tubal ligation can result in complications by causing damage to the bowel, bladder, or blood vessels; by producing a wound that does not heal or that becomes infected; or by causing prolonged pelvic or abdominal pain. A medical appointment one or two weeks after a tubal ligation is typically recommended to check the status of the patient's healing and to look for any signs of complications.

In approximately one out of every hundred women, tubal ligation is ineffective, and the woman may become pregnant. Ineffective tubal ligations are most common in young women. Pregnancy can occur if a new open passage forms within blocked tubes or if cut tubes grow back together. A pregnancy that occurs after a tubal ligation has a relatively high chance of being ectopic—that is, the fertilized egg becomes implanted in a location outside the uterus, usually in a fallopian tube. Ectopic pregnancies can occur several years after a tubal ligation. These are emergency, life-threatening situations that require immediate medical attention.

Some tubal ligations can be reversed, should pregnancy be desired at a later date. However, a reversal is a complex type of operation—and it is often not successful.

A. J. Smuskiewicz

See also: Contraception; Essure Coil; Fallopian Tubes; Sterilization; Vasectomy.

Further Reading

Johns Hopkins Medicine. (2019). Tubal ligation. Retrieved from https://www.hopkinsmedicine.org/health/treatment-tests-and-therapies/tubal-ligation

Mayo Clinic. (2018). Tubal ligation. Retrieved from https://www.mayoclinic.org/tests-procedures/tubal-ligation/about/pac-20388360

National Health Service. (2018). Female sterilization. Retrieved from https://www.nhs.uk/conditions/contraception/female-sterilisation/

Turner Syndrome

Turner syndrome is a chromosomal atypicality associated with the X chromosome. Individuals with Turner syndrome have one normal X chromosome and either a partially missing or completely missing second X chromosome. If an individual is completely missing their second X chromosome, they have the chromosome structure XO. Most pregnancies with Turner syndrome fail to progress, and so it is relatively rare; it occurs in about 1 in every 2,500 newborn females worldwide. The missing or absent structure of the second X chromosome affects development before and after birth. Most people with Turner syndrome identify as female or intersex.

Among humans, the typical sex chromosomal structure is either two XX chromosomes in females or one X and one Y chromosome in males. Because individuals with Turner syndrome do not have a Y chromosome, they develop in utero as female and have female reproductive organs, including a uterus and ovaries, although ovarian function is usually significantly reduced or they may completely stop functioning in early life.

Signs and symptoms of Turner syndrome vary among people. The most common characteristic is short stature, which can be noticeable during infancy or childhood. Other characteristics of Turner syndrome include a broad chest, low-set ears, variations with arm and leg structure, variations with hand and foot structure, and underdeveloped female sex characteristics, such as breasts. About a third of people with Turner syndrome have extra folds of skin on the neck, a low hairline, skeletal abnormalities, swelling of the hands and feet, or kidney problems. Up to half of individuals may also experience heart abnormalities that can be life-threatening.

Some individuals may be diagnosed before birth during prenatal screening or via ultrasound, which may show heart or kidney abnormalities. Some individuals with Turner syndrome may be diagnosed at birth or as children if physical symptoms are present. If no symptoms are noticed, diagnosis may not occur until the individual is a teenager or young adult, and this may be as the result of slowed growth and an absence of puberty, which does not begin as expected.

Many people with Turner syndrome require growth hormone therapy during childhood, and many also require hormone replacement therapy to begin puberty. Some individuals may also require hormone replacement therapy throughout their life. Because of problems with ovarian development and function, and subsequent hormonal effects, many people with Turner syndrome are infertile.

Turner syndrome is considered to be a random chromosome abnormality. There does not appear to be a genetic or family history influence.

Heather L. Armstrong

See also: Chromosomal Sex; Intersexuality; Sex Chromosomes; X Chromosome.

Further Reading

Bondy, C. A. (2007). Care of girls and women with Turner syndrome: A guideline of the Turner Syndrome Study Group. *The Journal of Clinical Endocrinology & Metabolism, 92*(1), 10–25.

Chivers, M. (2017). Gender. In C. F. Pukall (Ed.), *Human sexuality: A contemporary introduction* (2nd ed.). Don Mills, ON: Oxford University Press.

Hjerrild, B. E., Mortensen, K. H., & Gravholt, C. H. (2008). Turner syndrome and clinical treatment. *British Medical Bulletin, 86*, 77–93.

Mayo Clinic. (2019). Turner syndrome. Retrieved from https://www.mayoclinic.org/diseases-conditions/turner-syndrome/symptoms-causes/syc-20360782

National Institutes of Health. (2019). Turner syndrome. Retrieved from https://ghr.nlm.nih.gov/condition/turner-syndrome#sourcesforpage

Tuskegee Syphilis Study

The Tuskegee Syphilis Study of Untreated Syphilis in the Negro Male was an unethical study conducted by the United States Public Health Service (USPHS) between 1932 and October 1972. This study was the longest nontherapeutic study in medical history. The USPHS began the study, working with the Tuskegee Institution, to gain access to the African American community and nearby medical facilities. The USPHS also invited other African American doctors and nurses to be part of the experiment. The study enrolled 600 predominately poor and uneducated African American men; 399 of the men had previously contracted syphilis, while 201 men did not have syphilis and acted as controls. The men with syphilis were not told they had this infection; rather they were told they had "bad blood." The purpose of the study was to see exactly what the disease would do to a human being if left untreated. By 1947, it was known that penicillin could cure syphilis; however, doctors in the study knowingly failed to treat participants in the study. They also failed to tell the participants about penicillin, and they prevented them from accessing available treatment from other sources. By the end of the study in 1972, twenty-eight men had died of syphilis, one hundred died from complications of syphilis, forty of their wives were infected, and nineteen of their children were born with congenital syphilis.

Syphilis is a sexually transmitted infection that can cause long-term complications if not treated correctly. According to the Centers for Disease Control and Prevention (CDC), syphilis is divided into four stages: the primary stage, secondary stage, latent stage, and the late or tertiary syphilis stage. Syphilis is spread through direct contact with syphilis sores and is transmitted vaginally, anally, orally, or through birth if the mother has syphilis infection.

During the first stage of syphilis, a person may notice a single, painless sore, or chancre, in the infected area that will go away on its own in three to six weeks. If the sore is not noticed, possibly because it is located inside the anus, vagina, or cervix, or if the person ignores it and does not seek treatment, the syphilis infection will progress into stage two. During the second stage of syphilis, approximately one to three months after the primary infection, a person will develop a skin rash most commonly on their abdomen, back, arms, and legs, including the palms and soles of the feet. The rash can look red, rough, and reddish-pink and may be formed of many flat, whitish lesions. Other possible symptoms are fever, sore throat, headache, weight loss, fatigue, muscle ache, patchy hair loss, and swollen lymph glands.

Even if the rash of secondary syphilis is not treated, it will eventually clear on its own. If continually left untreated, the latent stage of syphilis occurs. During this stage, which can last for years, the body does not experience any signs or symptoms. The final stage, or tertiary syphilis, can occur approximately three to fifteen years or longer after primary infection, although some people with syphilis infection will never develop tertiary syphilis. However, when it does happen the symptoms are very serious. During the last stage of syphilis, the bacteria attack the neurological and cardiovascular systems of the body, ultimately damaging the heart, brain, spinal cord, skin, bones, and other organs.

Prior to the Tuskegee Syphilis Study, in 1929, the USPHS conducted the "Wasserman Survey." The survey was held in six counties, including Macon County, Alabama, which had the highest rate of untreated syphilis, to determine the prevalence of syphilis among African Americans in the South. In 1932, the Rosenwald Fund withdrew their support of the Wassermen Survey and decided to focus the study on African Americans exclusively in Macon County, Alabama.

Residents of Macon County were under the impression that doctors were coming to begin a new health program. During recruitment for the Tuskegee Syphilis Study, individuals were screened by doctors who were determined to find a good study group of African American males, twenty-five years of age or older, who had been living with syphilis for more than five years.

The subjects of the experiment were under the impression that they were patients of a joint federal and local medical and nursing program at the Tuskegee Institute. As a way to encourage the men to participate in the study, they received free medical exams, free meals, and free burial insurance. The study was originally projected to be a six-month experiment but subsequently lasted forty years. The men were under the impression that they would be examined and treated but were misled because they were not given all the facts required to give consent. Subsequently the men never received adequate treatment for the disease, were never offered treatment, and were even prevented from accessing treatment from other sources. In 1972, the Tuskegee Syphilis Study ended. The experiment was the cover story of the *New York Times*, condemning the unethical, unjustified forty-year experiment.

In 1972, Charlie Pollard, a Macon farmer, went into the office of civil rights attorney Fred Gray and gave detailed information regarding his involvement in the Tuskegee Syphilis Study; on that day Gray agreed to represent Pollard. In 1973, a $1.8 billion class action lawsuit was filed on behalf of the participants and their families. In 1974, an approximate $10 million out-of-court settlement was awarded to the participants and their families. As a result of the lawsuit, the living participants were awarded lifetime medical benefits and burial services through the Tuskegee Health Benefit Program (THBP). In 1975, the wives, widows, and offspring of the experiment participants were also afforded the opportunity to benefit from the program. The CDC stated in 1995 that the program was expanded from medical benefits to also including health benefits. According to the CDC, in 2004, the last study participant died, and the last widow to receive THBP died in 2009. There are twelve children of the participants that still receive medical and health benefits.

On May 16, 1997, former president of the United States Bill Clinton formally and publicly apologized on behalf of the nation for the Tuskegee Syphilis Study. The apology was used as an attempt to restore the trust of the African American community as a result of the Tuskegee Syphilis Study.

Reginald Barker

See also: Sexually Transmitted Infections (STIs); Syphilis.

Further Reading

Carmack, H. J., Bates, B. R., & Harter, L. M. (2008). Narrative constructions of health care issues and policies: The case of President Clinton's apology-by-proxy for the Tuskegee syphilis experiment. *Journal of Medical Humanities, 29*(2), 89–109.

Centers for Disease Control and Prevention. (2015). U.S. Public Health Service Syphilis Study at Tuskegee. Retrieved from https://www.cdc.gov/tuskegee/index.html

Centers for Disease Control and Prevention. (2019). Syphilis: Basic fact sheet. Retrieved from http://www.cdc.gov/std/syphilis/stdfact-syphilis.htm

Freimuth, V. S., Quinn, S. C., Thomas, S. B., Cole, G., Zook, E., & Duncan, T. (2001). African Americans' views on research and the Tuskegee Syphilis Study. *Social Science & Medicine, 52*(5), 797–808.

Gray, F. D. (1998). *The Tuskegee Syphilis Study: The real story and beyond.* Montgomery, AL: New South Books.

Presidential Commission for the Study of Bioethical Issues. (2012). *A study guide to "ethically impossible" STD research in Guatemala from 1946 to 1948.* Retrieved from https://bioethicsarchive.georgetown.edu/pcsbi/sites/default/files/StudyGuide_EthicallyImpossible_508_Nov26.pdf

Two-Spirit

"Two-spirit" is a term used to refer to cross-gender-identified, gender-diverse, and gender-fluid individuals who are indigenous to North America and are part of Native American or other indigenous tribes. This term was originated in 1990 at a conference of indigenous people who were upset at the use of a colonized term that settlers had been using to refer to gender-variant indigenous people. This offensive term was defined as a male prostitute, or the passive male partner in anal sex. By creating and popularizing the term "two-spirit," a term coined by indigenous people but in English, the language of the colonizers, the hope was to offer a replacement term that was less offensive. "Two-spirit" is a term that refers to gender expression and not to sexual orientation.

Originally, two-spirit was used solely to describe someone who was assigned male and embodied feminine spirit, or who was assigned female and embodied masculine spirit. However, the term is now often used as an umbrella term to refer to indigenous people who are gender diverse or gender nonconforming in a variety of ways. More than 155 North American tribes have historical accounts or retellings of the acceptance and sometimes celebration of gender-diverse individuals, including from before Europeans came to colonize the Americas. With colonization came the perpetuation of homophobia and transphobia, which infiltrated many indigenous cultures and led, in some instances, to certain tribes changing their views toward their two-spirit members. It is important to note that while many tribes acknowledge and even revere two-spirit individuals, not all tribes have the same beliefs, and different tribes may have different words naming, attitudes toward, and reactions to gender-diverse people.

In some indigenous cultures, such as the Dine (Navajo), there are four recognized genders and a term for those whose gender expression does not match the sex they were assigned at birth, *nádleeh.* The Tewa use the term *kwido* for all gender-variant people, and the Lemhi tribe use *tubasa* for both those assigned male and female at birth, while many other tribes have separate words to indicate gender-diverse people who were assigned female at birth and those who were assigned male at birth.

The roles of two-spirit individuals are different depending on the tribe. In some tribes, they are simply accepted as part of the tribe. In other tribes, two-spirit individuals are given the roles of medicine people, name givers, matchmakers, holy people, interpreters of dreams, warriors, healers, singers, or meditators. Historically, some tribes had ceremonies or other rituals for two-spirit individuals to undergo as children to assess whether their identities were truly two-spirit or whether they were only interested in masculine or feminine things. Once it was determined that they were two-spirit, they were given work traditionally assigned to their authentic gender (rather than the sex they had been assigned) and were allowed to or encouraged to wear the clothing of the gender with which they identified. In some tribes, two-spirit individuals were regarded very highly and held elevated ranks.

Shanna K. Kattari

See also: Bigender; Gender Diversity; Gender Identity; Nonbinary Gender Identities; Transgender.

Further Reading

Ansbacher, H. (Producer), Martin, R. (Producer), & Nibley, L. (Producer, Director). (2009). Two spirits [Motion picture]. Say Yes Quickly Productions. Retrieved from http://twospirits.org

Laframboise, S., & Anhorn, M. (2008). The way of the two spirited people: Native American concepts of gender and sexual orientation. Retrieved from http://www.dancingtoeaglespiritsociety.org/twospirit.php

Naswood, E., & Jim, M. (2011). Mending the rainbow: Working with LGBT/two spirit community. Presented at 12th National Indian Nations Conference, Palm Springs, CA. Retrieved from http://www.tribal-institute.org/2010/A3-EltonNaswoodPP.pdf

U

Ulrichs, Karl

Karl Heinrich Ulrichs (1825–1895) was a German poet and political activist who in the 1860s developed the first scientific theory about homosexuality and is seen today as a pioneer of the modern gay rights movement.

Ulrichs was born on August 28, 1825, in Aurich, which was part of the Kingdom of Hanover. Ulrich's childhood makes it clear where many of his ideas came from. As a young child, he wore girls' clothing and preferred playing with girls. This gravitation would later inform how he discussed queerness and how it existed in men. In 1839, at age fourteen, he had his first sexual experience when his male riding instructor sexually abused him. This experience could be a factor in his desire to separate queerness from pedophilia.

In 1846, Ulrichs graduated in law and theology from Göttingen University. From 1846 to 1848, he studied history at Berlin University, and from 1849 to 1857, he worked as an official legal adviser for the district court of Hildesheim in the Kingdom of Hanover until he was dismissed when his homosexuality became public knowledge. After his dismissal, Ulrich became more comfortable with his identity and became more vocal, opening up to his family and friends. He described himself as an "Urning," a term he created to describe men who were attracted to other men, who represented a third sex. Urnings were born that way, and their sexuality was not the result of immorality or pathology. Ulrichs believed that Urnings had a feminine quality about them to distinguish them from men who were attracted to women.

Ulrichs wrote a series of essays published under the pseudonym "Numa Numantius." Later, Ulrichs published under his real name and wrote statements of legal and moral support for men arrested for homosexual offences. In 1867, Ulrichs became the first gay man to speak publicly in defense of homosexuality and queerness when he pleaded at the Congress of German Jurists in Munich for a resolution urging the repeal of antihomosexual laws (Kennedy, 1997). Throughout the 1860s, Ulrichs's writings got him in trouble with the law. His books were banned in Saxony, Berlin, and throughout Prussia. In 1879, Ulrichs published his twelfth and final book, *Research on the Riddle of Man-Manly Love*, where he argues that homosexuality is not a disease or a sin but perfectly natural and that the strict line of differentiation between men and women has been overemphasized.

Lauren Ewaniuk

See also: Gay Rights Movement; Homosexuality; Queer.

Further Reading

Kennedy, H. (1988). *The life and works of Karl Heinrich Ulrichs: Pioneer of the modern gay movement.* Boston: Alyson.

Kennedy, H. (1997). Karl Heinrich Ulrichs, first theorist of homosexuality. In V. A. Rosario (Ed.), *Science and homosexualities* (pp. 26–45). New York: Routledge.

Yarber, W. L., Sayad, B. W., & Strong, B. (2010). *Human sexuality: Diversity in contemporary America.* New York: McGraw-Hill.

Unconsummated Marriage

"Unconsummated marriage" refers to a marriage between a man and woman in which the couple has never had sexual intercourse since marrying. In most cases, the couple has also not had intercourse previous to the marriage. Historically, nonconsummation could be grounds for marriage annulment, an official decree by the church that the marriage was not valid and that the formal relationship was over.

There is limited research about unconsummated marriages, particularly in North America, perhaps because premarital sex is more accepted. As such, most of the existing research focuses on countries where premarital sex is uncommon.

Common causes of unconsummated marriages are vaginismus (a condition where the vaginal muscles contract, causing penetration to be painful or impossible) and erectile disorder (a condition where the penis is unable to experience or sustain an erection firm enough for sexual intercourse). Other causes of unconsummated marriage include premature or early ejaculation (where the man ejaculates quickly, in this case before vaginal penetration), a thick hymen (a rare condition where a woman has an unusually thick hymen that impedes penetration), a lack of sex education, sexual aversion (where an individual experiences fear, panic, or revulsion at the thought of sex), and anxiety. In some cases, the woman may have vaginismus and after repeated unsuccessful attempts at intercourse the man develops erectile dysfunction. In other cases, one or both conditions exist from the start of the sexual relationship.

In the case of arranged marriages, the partners may face pressure to engage in sexual intercourse with someone who is almost a stranger, as they may have spent little or no time becoming acquainted before marriage. In some cultures, relatives may be nearby during the time of the expected first sexual intercourse or may require proof that consummation has occurred (such as a sheet or handkerchief stained with blood that is assumed will be produced when a virgin woman has intercourse for the first time; however, this does not always happen). This pressure-filled situation can result in anxiety leading to erectile dysfunction, causing intercourse to be impossible.

In North America, many unconsummated couples do not talk about their concerns with anyone else. The couples may have a good relationship outside of sex and may have a fulfilling sex life that simply excludes intercourse. Couples who seek treatment are often motivated by a desire to become pregnant.

Treatment of unconsummated marriage involves a detailed history of both partners to determine the factors associated with the inability to have sexual intercourse. Treatment is dependent on the factors identified as contributing to the problem and may include sex education, suggestions for self and partner exploration of the genitals, medical treatment for erectile dysfunction, pelvic floor physical therapy, surgical treatment for imperforate hymen, medication for severe premature ejaculation, and dilator use for vaginismus (the use of graduated devices to stretch the vagina and allow the woman to become accustomed to penetration). Sex therapy, a specialized type of psychotherapy or talk therapy, may be useful for all causes of unconsummated marriage. Sex therapy can provide needed sexual health information and address the psychological impact of the concern as well as any relational or psychological factors that may contribute to or maintain the problem.

Adrienne M. Bairstow

See also: Hymen; Intercourse; Marriage; Premarital Sex; Premature Ejaculation; Sexual Disorders, Female; Sexual Disorders, Male; Sexual Dysfunction, Treatment of; Vaginismus; Virginity.

Further Reading

Promodu, K. (2011). Unconsummated marriage. Retrieved from http://www.drpromodusinstitute.in/unconsummated-marriage.html

Rosenbaum, T. Y. (2015). Part 1: Couples in unconsummated marriages. Retrieved from http://www.tallirosenbaum.com/en/node/47

Urethra

The urethra is a tube that carries urine from the bladder for removal from the body. Because of anatomical differences, the urethra is very different in males and females. In males, the urethra also serves in the reproductive act by carrying semen. In females, it is used only for urination. The urethra is the site of relatively common bacterial infections, particularly in women. Other medical concerns related to the urethra include unusual development in males, cancer, and the passage of kidney stones.

The average female urethra is approximately two inches long. It runs from the bladder and exits the body between the clitoris and the vagina. The urethral sphincter muscle controls the flow of urine from the urethra. Control over the flow is made possible by the pudendal nerve. The female urethra is used only to void urine from the body.

The average male urethra is approximately eight inches long, because it runs the length of the penis. After it exits the bladder, it passes through the prostate gland. Several openings into the urethra are found here that play an important role during intercourse. The ejaculatory duct allows the entry of sperm from the vas deferens and ejaculate fluid from the seminal vesicles. Additional fluid from the prostate gland also enters at this point. The urethra then passes through the external urethral sphincter, which controls the flow of urine. The longest part of the male urethra is known as the spongy urethra and runs along the underside of the penis. When the urethra carries urine, the physiology at this point causes a spiral stream of urine. This has the effect of cleaning the inside of the urethra, reducing the likelihood of infections. The female urethra lacks a similar feature, which helps explain why urinary tract infections are more common in females.

Abnormal development of the urethra in males sometimes occurs, including the opening of the urethra being located other than at the tip of the penis. In addition, bacterial infection of the urethra, known as urethritis or a urinary tract infection, sometimes occurs. The most common symptom is a burning pain when urinating. Urethritis is usually treated with antibiotics. The passage of kidney stones down the urethra causes a great deal of pain. Cancer of the urethra may occur. It can be diagnosed by a physical examination or through testing of the urine.

Tim J. Watts

See also: Bulbourethral Glands; Penis; Prostate; Semen.

Further Reading

Mayo Clinic. (2019). Urethral structure. Retrieved from https://www.mayoclinic.org/diseases-conditions/urethral-stricture/symptoms-causes/syc-20362330

National Institutes of Health. (2019). Urethral disorders. Retrieved from https://medlineplus.gov/urethraldisorders.html

Seladi-Schulman, J. (2018). Female urethra overview. Retrieved from https://www.healthline.com/human-body-maps/female-urethra

Uterine Cancer

Uterine cancer is the abnormal, malignant (cancerous) growth of cells of the uterus, specifically the endometrium, the mucous lining of the interior walls of the uterus. Uterine cancer is also called endometrial cancer.

Uterine cancer most commonly occurs after menopause, when menstrual periods stop. The condition is most frequently diagnosed in women between the ages of fifty-five and sixty-four (making up about 34% of all cases). However, the cancer develops in some women before menopause. About 7 percent of cases are diagnosed in women between the ages of twenty and forty-four. Approximately 3 percent of women will be diagnosed as having uterine cancer at some point in their lives.

Symptoms of uterine cancer may include abnormal bleeding or other discharge from the vagina. Other symptoms are pelvic pain during urination or sexual intercourse or other unexplained pain in the pelvic region.

The causes of uterine cancer are not fully understood, but genetic factors are known to play a role in the disease. People with a family history of uterine cancer or colorectal cancer are at increased risk of uterine cancer. People are also at greater risk of uterine cancer if they have had hyperplasia, abnormally rapid cell growth in the endometrium. Even if this cell growth is benign (noncancerous), it could be an early indication of cancer development. Uterine fibroids and polyps are benign growths in uterine tissue that need to be monitored for signs of becoming malignant. Obesity further increases the risk of uterine cancer, as does estrogen-only hormone replacement therapy, use of tamoxifen to treat previous breast cancer, diabetes, high blood pressure, never having children, having menstrual periods before age twelve, and experiencing menopause after age fifty-five.

Uterine cancer is usually diagnosed with a gynecological pelvic examination (the physical inspection of the uterus, vagina, and adjacent tissues), ultrasonography examination (the use of sound waves to create images of the uterus and adjacent tissues), and biopsy (a microscopic tissue evaluation to verify the benign or malignant nature of cellular growth). Diagnosis will determine the stage of cancer development in the patient. Uterine cancer is classified in four stages—I to IV. In stage I, the cancer is confined to the endometrial and muscle layers of the uterus. In stage II, the cancer has spread to the tissue of the cervix (the neck of the uterus). Stage I and II cancers make up about 68 percent of all diagnoses. In stage III, making up 20 percent of all diagnoses, the cancer has spread beyond the uterus, to the fallopian tubes, ovaries, vagina, and regional lymph nodes. In stage IV, making up 8 percent of all diagnoses, the cancer has metastasized (spread to other parts of the body) beyond the pelvic region. The lungs are the main region to which uterine cancer spreads.

Treatment depends on the patient's specific diagnosis, including the stage of the abnormal tissue growth. Noncancerous fibroids and polyps might be treated with pain-relieving medications and surgical removal of the growths. If cancer is diagnosed in its early stages, chemotherapy (the use of medications to kill cancer cells) and/or radiation therapy could be successful treatments. Radiation to kill cancer cells can be administered externally, with a machine directing the rays at the pelvic area, or internally, with a radiation-emitting cylinder inserted inside the vagina.

Even if diagnosis indicates that the patient's condition is currently noncancerous or in the early stages of cancer, doctors may recommend a hysterectomy (surgical removal of the uterus). This surgery is the most comprehensive way to ensure removal of any dangerous or potentially dangerous tissues.

If uterine cancer is diagnosed in its later stages—when the cancer has spread to tissues beyond the uterus—treatment will most likely include surgical removal not only of the uterus but also removal of the ovaries, fallopian tubes, part of the vagina, and adjacent lymph nodes. It is important to remove the lymph nodes because once cancer cells invade the lymphatic system, they can quickly metastasize. Progesterone hormone therapy (the use of progesterone to alter the hormone balance that cancer cells use to grow) is performed for some women with advanced uterine cancer, especially women who wish to keep their uterus so that they can still become pregnant.

Chemotherapy or radiation therapy may be required after hysterectomy for patients in whom all cancerous tissue could not be surgically removed. Such follow-up treatment may also be performed to better prevent a recurrence of cancer. Additional types of follow-up treatment may be required after hysterectomy to address adverse effects, such as bleeding from the vagina, bladder, or rectum; abdominal pain or bloating; leg swelling; shortness of breath; and loss of appetite or weight. Doctors can address such postsurgery symptoms in regular checkups with the patient.

More than 80 percent of women diagnosed with uterine cancer survive at least five years after treatment. The earlier the cancer stage at diagnosis, the greater the survival rate.

A. J. Smuskiewicz

See also: Breast Cancer; Cervical Cancer; Endometrium; Hysterectomy; Ovarian Cancer; Uterus.

Further Reading

Morice, P., Leary, A., Creutzberg, C., Abu-Rustum, N., & Darai, E. (2016). Endometrial cancer. *The Lancet, 387*(10023), 1094–1108.

National Cancer Institute. (2019). Endometrial cancer treatment. Retrieved from https://www.cancer.gov/types/uterine/patient/endometrial-treatment-pdq

National Cancer Institute. (n.d.). Uterine cancer—patient version. Retrieved from https://www.cancer.gov/types/uterine

Uterus

The uterus, commonly called the womb, is a hollow female reproductive organ in which pregnancy occur and the fetus develops. It is located near the base of the abdomen and is usually about the size of a fist and the shape of an inverted pear. The lower part of the uterus is a neck-like structure called the cervix, which leads to the vagina. Sperm must make it through the cervix if fertilization is to occur. Fertilization usually occurs in a fallopian tube, one of the two tubes that leads from the ovaries, where eggs are stored and released, into the uterus. The fertilized egg implants itself in the wall of the uterus, resulting in pregnancy.

During a woman's reproductive years—which, in most women, extend from her early teens into her late forties or early fifties—the walls of the uterus prepare themselves roughly once a month to receive a fertilized egg by building up an extra lining. During this preparation, the number and extent of blood vessels, cells, and glands increase in this uterine lining. The extra lining is discharged through the vagina in menstrual bleeding (commonly called periods) if fertilization and pregnancy do not occur.

If fertilization and pregnancy do occur, the egg develops into an embryo in the uterine wall. Tissues from the embryo and the uterus grow into a placenta, a disc-shaped structure filled with blood vessels connecting the pregnant person's circulatory system to that of the fetus. The placenta provides oxygen and nutrients to the developing fetus while also carrying away wastes. A normal pregnancy lasts for nine months, during which the uterus expands to twenty-four times its usual size, as the organ's cells grow larger. During birth, the muscles of the uterus and abdomen repeatedly contract, causing the fetus to pass through the cervix and out of the vagina. Additional contractions then force out the placenta.

A number of disorders can affect the uterus, some of which can interfere with a normal pregnancy. Certain disorders cause the uterus to expel the embryo or fetus before it is able to survive on the outside. Such early ends to pregnancy are called miscarriages, or spontaneous abortions.

In endometriosis, tissue that normally lines the interior of the uterus grows in other areas, such as on the outside of the uterus, on the ovaries, or on the bladder. In adenomyosis, the tissue of the uterine lining grows within the muscular wall of the uterus. Each of these conditions may require treatment with pain medications and hormone-based therapies. Severe cases of adenomyosis may require surgery to remove the uterus, a procedure known as hysterectomy.

In a condition called hyperplasia, abnormally rapid cell growth occurs in the uterus. It may be an early indication of cancer. Uterine cancer occurs most often in those who have experienced menopause. Studies suggest that obesity and hormone replacement therapy increase the risk of uterine cancer. Treatment usually involves a hysterectomy.

Uterine fibroids, also called leiomyomas, are abnormal but noncancerous growths in the tissue of the uterus. A number of treatment options are available, ranging from "watchful waiting" (doing nothing unless symptoms become troublesome) to various pain-relieving drugs to hysterectomy. Uterine, or endometrial, polyps are abnormal growths that have the potential to spread to other parts of the body and become cancerous. Treatment may involve drugs, surgical removal of only the polyps, or hysterectomy.

A. J. Smuskiewicz

See also: Cervix; Endometriosis; Endometrium; Hysterectomy; Menstruation; Pregnancy; Uterine Cancer.

Further Reading

National Cancer Institute. (n.d.). Uterine cancer—patient version. Retrieved from https://www.cancer.gov/types/uterine

National Institutes of Health. (2019). Uterine diseases. Retrieved from https://medlineplus.gov/uterinediseases.html

Wolf, M. (2012). *Everyone has a tipped uterus: 69 things your gynecologist wishes you knew.* Indianapolis: Dog Ear Publishing.

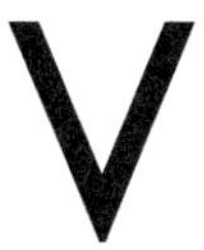

Vagina

Although medically inaccurate, the term "vagina" is popularly used to refer to the external sexual organ of females, which is actually called the vulva. It is also sometimes used, also inaccurately, in reference to the vulva and the vagina combined.

The vagina is an internal muscular and tubular organ, extending from the introitus (the opening to the vagina, situated between the urethral opening and the anus) to the cervix (the bottom portion of the uterus). The structure of the vagina expands in size and changes in shape during sexual intercourse and childbirth. The vagina is also self-lubricating, with its interior lining being formed of a mucous membrane (vaginal mucosa), and this is secreted often during sexual arousal. This helps ease sexual intercourse; however, there are some women who produce less of this than others, which can lead to discomfort or even pain when engaging in sexual activity (artificial lubrication is a simple solution to this problem). The mucosa is surrounded by layers of fibrous tissue and muscle, which assist in expansion and contraction of the vagina. The vagina also channels menstrual flow as part of the menstrual cycle.

When most females are born, the introitus is partly covered by a thin piece of tissue called the hymen. This may remain intact until first sexual intercourse; however, other nonsexual activities, such as using tampons, may also cause the hymen to rupture or tear. When this occurs, some women may experience slight bleeding and pain, but this is seldom reported to be a traumatic experience.

Unlike males, females have two external openings in their genitals. These are the urethral opening (urological tract, for urination) and the vaginal opening for the genital tract. In males, the urethral opening typically serves as the opening for both the urinary and reproductive tracts. In females, the vaginal opening is much larger than the urethral opening, with both being protected by the labia, the "lips" or folds of skin that comprise the major external parts of the vulva.

The vagina is a significant part of female sexual pleasure and sexuality. Most of the nerve endings in the vagina are situated around the introitus. In addition, located an inch or two inside the vagina on the anterior wall (toward the belly button) is the Grafenberg spot (G-spot), which may be a significant source of sexual stimulation and pleasure for some women. On either side of the introitus are the vestibular bulbs, which are made up of spongy, erectile tissue that expands in size during sexual arousal and causes the vulva to extend outward. These bulbs form the internal structure of the clitoris. During arousal and sexual stimulation, muscles in the vagina often begin to contract. However, there are fewer nerves in the top two-thirds of the vagina than in the bottom third near the introitus; as a result, penis length and width does not necessarily provide a heterosexual woman with increased pleasurable stimulation. However, since sexual stimulation and pleasurable feelings vary from person to person, different females may experience different pleasurable sensations from various forms of stimulation to their vagina (combining individual psychology and physiology).

Callum E. Cooper

See also: Grafenberg Spot (G-Spot); Hymen; Labia; Vaginal Lubrication; Vaginal Secretions; Vaginismus; Vulva.

Further Reading

Dalton, M. (2014). *Forensic gynecology*. Cambridge: Cambridge University Press.

Dutta, D. C. (2014). *Textbook of gynecology*. London: JP Medical.

Pomeroy, W. B. (1986). *Girls and sex*. Middlesex: Penguin.

Vaginal Lubrication

The vagina is the inner tube or canal leading from a female's uterus to her external genitalia. The interior of the vagina is lined with a mucosal membrane, which contributes to vaginal secretions and lubrication. Some vaginal secretions indicate a place in the menstrual cycle, while others are for cleansing purposes. Most of these secretions come from other reproductive organs such as the cervix and uterus. Some secretions have implications in sexual arousal. While some lubrication is always present, when the body is aroused the amount and process changes. During sexual arousal, the amount of lubrication in the vagina increases to facilitate penetration. This is important because if there is not sufficient lubrication, there will be too much friction in the vaginal cavity. This can cause sex to be painful and can also cause physical damage.

The vagina becomes lubricated through a process called transudation. Transudation is when fluid passes through a barrier. In sexual arousal, this process is a little different than in other instances in the body. When a person begins to feel aroused, blood rushes to their genitals. This contributes to what is described as a "full" feeling and is called vasocongestion. This is where the process of transudation becomes important. The blood in the genitals contains fluid that passes through the vaginal tissue to lubricate the cavity. This is why, after consuming alcohol, it can be difficult for a person to feel properly lubricated for penetration. Drinking alcohol dehydrates the body, and if there is little fluid in the blood, then an adequate amount cannot pass through the tissue.

Dehydration is not the only thing that can affect vaginal lubrication. Estrogen also has implications for a person's ability to produce vaginal lubrication. If a person has higher estrogen levels, which younger females tend to have, then their body will have an easier time completing this process. It is important to note that estrogen levels also fluctuate during the menstrual cycle. That means that at times in a person's cycle when their estrogen levels are lower, they might not become as wet as they might at different times in their cycle. During and after menopause, when estrogen levels are lower, people may also have difficulty with lubrication during arousal. In all cases of vaginal dryness during arousal, a person can supplement with store-bought lubricants. However, for older women, just adding lubricant may not be enough. Because hormones like estrogen also have implications in the elasticity of vaginal tissues, it might be necessary to get a prescription for a lubricant with estrogens that can keep tissues from tearing.

Rebecca Polly

See also: Arousal; Estrogen; Lubricants; Menopause; Menstruation; Vagina; Vaginal Secretions.

Further Reading

Herbenick, D. (2009). *Because it feels good: A woman's guide to sexual pleasure and satisfaction.* Emmaus, PA: Rodale Books.

Herbenick, D. (2011). *Read my lips: A complete guide to the vagina and vulva.* Lanham, MD: Rowman & Littlefield.

Vaginal Ring

In 2001, the Food and Drug Administration approved the use of the vaginal ring. It is a small, bendable ring, approximately two inches in diameter, which is placed in the vagina and releases hormones into the bloodstream to prevent pregnancy.

The vaginal ring is placed into a person's vagina, where it remains for three weeks. It releases synthetic estrogen (ethinyl estradiol) and progesterone (etonogestrel), which moves across the vaginal epithelium and enters the bloodstream. These hormones work to prevent pregnancy primarily by preventing ovulation. The hormones also thicken the cervical mucus, preventing sperm from meeting an egg. After the vaginal ring has been in the vagina for three weeks, it should be removed on the same day of the week it was inserted. The person goes without the ring for one week, and then a new one is inserted into the vagina.

In order to get a vaginal ring, a person needs to consult with a health care provider and receive a prescription. Once they have obtained the ring from a drugstore or pharmacy, a person uses their fingers to bend the sides of the ring together and pushes it inside of their vagina. It is generally placed high in the vaginal canal, back toward the cervix. At the end of three weeks, the vaginal ring is removed by hooking a finger under the rim of the ring and pulling it out of the vagina. Once removed it should be wrapped and thrown away. The person then goes without the vaginal ring for the fourth week, and this is typically when menstruation occurs. The vaginal ring can be removed during sexual intercourse for up to three hours without losing effectiveness, but it is not necessary to remove it.

The vaginal ring is known to have both positive and negative side effects. A common side effect often reported by users is lighter and shorter periods. The vaginal ring may also prevent acne and improve menstrual cramping. Some negative side effects include bleeding between periods, nausea, vomiting, and swollen or tender breasts. Typically, these side effects will cease after the first few months of use. Longer-lasting side effects might include increased vaginal discharge, vaginal irritation, or a change in sexual desire.

The vaginal ring is very effective in preventing pregnancy. It is about 99 percent effective with perfect use, meaning a ring that is kept in place for three weeks, taken out for one week, and replaced with a new one after the fourth week. This ensures the appropriate levels of hormones are circulating in a person's body. With inconsistent use, the vaginal ring is approximately 91 percent effective in preventing pregnancy. When someone chooses to stop using the vaginal ring, the ability to become pregnant returns quickly.

The vaginal ring is a relatively safe method of birth control. However, hormones affect different bodies in different ways. In some cases, and in certain bodies, using the vaginal ring may come with more severe risks. These risks are rare and can include liver tumors, gallstones, high blood pressure, or jaundice.

Sarah Gannon

See also: Cervix; Contraception; Pregnancy; Sex Hormones; Synthetic Hormones; Vagina.

Further Reading

Bedsider. (2016). The ring. Retrieved from https://www.bedsider.org/methods/the_ring#details

Jones, R. E., & Lopez, K. H. (2014). *Human reproductive biology* (4th ed.). San Diego, CA: Academic Press.

Planned Parenthood. (2019). Birth control ring. Retrieved from https://www.plannedparenthood.org/learn/birth-control/birth-control-vaginal-ring-nuvaring

Roumen, F. J. M. E., & Mishell, D. R. (2012). The contraceptive vaginal ring, NuvaRing®, a decade after its introduction. *European Journal of Contraception & Reproductive Health Care, 17*(6), 415–427.

Vaginal Secretions

Vaginal secretions are discharges of fluid from the vagina. Vaginal secretions are one way in which the body cleanses itself, maintains pH balance, and keeps skin moisturized. Vaginal discharge is a natural defense against bacteria and any potentially harmful infections.

Vaginal discharge occurs when fluid from glands inside the vagina and cervix carry away dead cells, making room for new cells to grow. Discharge comes from multiple sources, such as the vaginal wall, cervical mucous, and sweat and oil within the vulva. Vaginal discharge is a regularly occurring thing that all people with a vagina experience, and it can happen throughout the menstrual cycle. For example, discharge can appear before and after the menstrual cycle, during ovulation, and when sexually aroused. Discharge can also vary in color and texture, amount, and odor. Discharge can be clear or white and range from smooth and slippery to chunky and thick. Most healthy discharge is odorless, though smell can vary if a person is pregnant, has been exercising, or needs to take care of personal hygiene.

Clear and watery discharge can happen any time and can be especially heavy after exercising. Clear and mucous-like discharge happens during ovulation. Brown or bloody discharge is also a common occurrence, which is usually part of the menstrual cycle. Discharge before or after the menstrual cycle can be brown in color. Brown or red discharge in between periods can be the result of unprotected sexual intercourse and possibly a sign of pregnancy. Brown discharge can also be a sign of cervical cancer, but yearly pelvic exams and Pap smears can rule out cancer.

Because the vagina is self-cleaning, douches, scented menstrual products, and vaginal sprays are not necessary for maintaining a clean and healthy vagina. Some of these products can in fact lead to abnormal discharge. Overcleaning the vagina is unhealthy and can reduce naturally occurring bacteria that protect the vagina from infection. Because discharge keeps skin moisturized, constant cleaning and attempting to remove secretions can dry the vagina and lead to discomfort and itching.

Changes in odor, consistency, and color can be indications of medical conditions, especially if accompanied by vaginal itching, burning, or pain. Several factors can lead to abnormal discharge. Yeast infection is one of the most common examples of infection that can be detected through changes in secretions. Vaginal secretions during a yeast infection are most often odorless with a thick, white, cottage cheese–like consistency. Itching or burning sensations around the vagina also accompany yeast infections, and if the individual is sexually active, intercourse can be painful during a yeast infection. A number of things can cause yeast infections, including antibiotics, birth control pills, and stress. Although over-the-counter medication is available for treating yeast infections, it is best to see a doctor.

Unprotected sex can lead to sexually transmitted infections (STIs), which can cause vaginal irritation and abnormal discharge. Gonorrhea and chlamydia are two STIs that commonly include abnormal vaginal secretions. In both cases the secretions can be cloudy or yellow and sometimes gray, accompanied by a fishy odor. Both gonorrhea and chlamydia can have other symptoms as well, such as painful urination and vaginal swelling, but abnormal discharge can be one of the first signs of infection. Like yeast infections, STIs should be medically treated.

Aman Agah

See also: Bacterial Vaginosis; Cervical Mucus Method; Douching; Menstruation; Sexually Transmitted Infections (STIs); Vagina; Yeast Infection (Candidiasis).

Further Reading

Boston Women's Health Book Collective. (2011). *Our bodies, ourselves.* New York: Simon & Schuster.

Rankin, L. (2010). *What's up down there? Questions you'd only ask your gynecologist if she was your best friend.* New York: St. Martin's Press.

Vaginismus

"Vaginismus" refers to a condition wherein a woman experiences involuntary contractions of the muscles in the outer third of the vagina, causing penetration to be painful or impossible. Women with vaginismus often report that it feels like their partner is hitting a wall when they attempt penetration or that it feels like their vagina is too small.

The classification of this condition has changed over the years. In the past, vaginismus was included as a sexual pain disorder in the *Diagnostic and Statistical Manual of Mental Disorders* (*DSM*). This diagnosis required involuntary contractions of the vaginal muscles upon penetration distress or interpersonal difficulty as a result of the condition, and the condition could not be caused exclusively by a physical medical condition. Vaginismus was distinguished from another sexual pain disorder, dyspareunia (pain during intercourse without muscle spasm).

With the fifth edition of the *DSM*, the *DSM-5* (2013), the diagnoses of vaginismus and dyspareunia have been removed and replaced by genito-pelvic pain/penetration disorder. This diagnosis requires recurring difficulty with one of the following: (1) vaginal penetration during intercourse, (2) pain during vaginal intercourse or penetration attempts, (3) fear or anxiety about pain with penetration, or (4) tightening of the pelvic floor muscles during penetration attempts.

The decision to remove vaginismus from the *DSM* was prompted in part by research that demonstrated that doctors do not reliably diagnose vaginismus; if multiple doctors examine a woman with vaginismus, some will detect vaginal spasms while others will not. The change in terminology also reflects the fact that some women have a phobic response to penetration such that they are unable to attempt intercourse. Finally, there is an overlap between vaginismus and dyspareunia, in that women who have dyspareunia may then develop muscle spasms characteristic of vaginismus. Although "vaginismus" is no longer in the *DSM*, the term will likely continue to be used due to the long history of its use.

Vaginismus has also been referred to as pelvic floor dysfunction, a condition wherein the muscles supporting the reproductive organs are too loose or too tight, causing symptoms including pain during vaginal penetration. This name reflects the latest research on the biological factors involved in vaginismus, notably the tightening and spasm of the vaginal muscles.

Vaginismus interferes with sexual intercourse as well as with nonsexual activities such as gynecological exams and tampon use. Accordingly, some have argued that vaginismus and other female pelvic pain disorders such as vulvodynia (pain in the external genitals) should be considered pain disorders rather than sexual disorders.

Vaginismus may also be classified according to onset of symptoms, as either primary or secondary. "Primary vaginismus" refers to the experience of symptoms with the first attempt at intercourse or penetration. "Secondary vaginismus" refers to symptoms that arise after a period of pain-free intercourse.

The exact prevalence of vaginismus is unknown, in part due to the inconsistency of diagnosis and also to the fact that research studies use varying definitions and terminology. The American Psychiatric Association states that approximately 15 percent of North American women report recurrent pain with intercourse.

Vaginismus may have a significant impact on a woman's sex life and relationships. Women with vaginismus often experience fear and anxiety about penetration or pain with penetration. They may avoid penetrative activities such as tampon use, gynecological exams, and vaginal intercourse. Some women avoid all sexual activity out of fear that it may lead to penetrative sex. This avoidance can lead to frustration for both partners.

A commonly recommended treatment for vaginismus is the use of Kegel exercises, the contraction and release of the pelvic floor muscles. However, Kegel exercises may actually worsen vaginismus. Women with vaginismus may have underlying pelvic floor dysfunction with pelvic floor muscles that are too tight. Kegel exercises may encourage a woman to hold the muscles even tighter, thus worsening muscle tightness and spasm. It is important that a woman who is dealing with vaginismus discuss an appropriate treatment plan with her doctors, pelvic floor physiotherapist, or other health care providers.

Additional treatments include the use of dilators alone or in conjunction with pelvic floor physical therapy. Dilators are tapered devices in graduated sizes that stretch the vaginal walls and allow a woman to become used to accommodating something in the vagina. Pelvic physical therapy is a specialized type of physical therapy that involves assessment and treatment of pelvic floor dysfunction. Physical therapy may include manual stretching and trigger point release, techniques to relax the muscles, and biofeedback.

Sex therapy may also be helpful in treating vaginismus, particularly in conjunction with physical therapy. Sex therapy is a form of psychotherapy or talk therapy. Sex therapy can provide a woman with vaginismus and her partner with education about sexual response, address any negative thoughts that may contribute to the problem (such as thoughts that a woman will never be able to achieve penetration), and address any relationship dynamics that may be worsening the situation (such as conflict within the relationship).

Adrienne M. Bairstow

See also: Diagnostic and Statistical Manual of Mental Disorders (DSM); Dyspareunia; Kegel Exercises; Pelvic Floor Muscles; Psychosexual Therapy; Sexual Avoidance; Sexual Dysfunction, Treatment of; Unconsummated Marriage; Vagina; Vulvodynia.

Further Reading

American Psychiatric Association. (2000). *Diagnostic and statistical manual of mental disorders* (4th ed., Text Rev.). Washington, DC: Author.

American Psychiatric Association. (2013). *Diagnostic and statistical manual of mental disorders* (5th ed.). Washington, DC: Author.

Pelvic Health Solutions. (2019). Pelvic floor muscle tightness. Retrieved from http://www.pelvichealthsolutions.ca/for-the-patient/pelvic-floor-muscle-tightness/

Pelvic Health Solutions. (2019). What is pelvic floor physiotherapy? Retrieved from http://pelvichealthsolutions.ca/for-the-patient/what-is-pelvic-floor-physiotherapy/

Vaginitis

"Vaginitis" is the medical term for any inflammation of the vagina, whether the inflammation is from a sexually transmitted infection (STI) or a noninfectious cause such as an allergic reaction to semen or overgrowth of fungi or bacteria. The most likely causes of vaginitis include candidiasis, bacterial vaginosis (BV), and trichomonas vaginalis. Each has its own presentation, reasons why it develops, and associated treatments.

Vaginal candidiasis is an overgrowth in the vagina by the fungus *Candida*. Candidiasis is not an STI, yet many women inappropriately self-treat for yeast infections for any vaginal discharge or discomfort, leading to untreated STIs that can subsequently cause more serious complications. *Candida albicans* is responsible for 80–92 percent of vaginal candidiasis, with the remaining percentage due to other *Candida* species like *Candida glabrata* and *Candida parapsilosis*. This infection is commonly known as a yeast infection although it is truly just an overgrowth of a normal yeast within the vagina.

Vulvovaginal candidiasis occurs in approximately 20 percent of women annually. After age 17, the frequency of first vaginal candidiasis infection increases so rapidly that by the time they are 25 years, 54.7 percent of women have already experienced their first episode. There are many risk factors for vaginal candidiasis. One such risk factor is being immunocompromised. Having a decreased immune system (e.g., having HIV, being on steroids, or having uncontrolled diabetes) leaves the immune system unable to fight against this fungal infection so that the candidal fungus begins to grow more rapidly. Antibiotic use is another risk factor. Since the natural bacteria in the vagina are removed after an antibiotic is used, this destruction of the natural bacteria gives space for the *Candida* to grow, leading to a new fungal infection. *Candida* has also been found to be associated with initiation of sexual activity, oral contraceptive use, spermicide use, and previous diagnosis of vulvovaginal candidiasis in the previous year. Although it is not considered an STI since it occurs in people who do not have sex, sexual activity can still increase its spread. Other risk factors include use of vaginal sponges, intrauterine devices, and diaphragms. Overgrowth can also occur due to high estrogen levels—that is, in pregnancy, before menstruation, or if using birth control pills.

The symptoms of vaginal candidiasis include vaginal itching, swelling, and associated thick, chunky, white cottage cheese–like vaginal discharge; these symptoms can develop suddenly or progressively. Patients can also occasionally complain of burning with urination (dysuria) or seeing scaly white lesions on the labia, so a urinary tract infection and STI also need to be ruled out by a physician when these symptoms develop. During the physical examination, a pelvic exam will be performed using a speculum. This will allow the physician to view the inside of the vagina and take samples of the vaginal discharge. Physical exam can reveal redness and swelling of the vulva with associated redness of the vagina as well. The thick white discharge is usually seen on physical exam, but in some cases of non-albicans *Candida*, only mild redness of the vagina may be present.

Diagnosis of vulvovaginal candidiasis is based on history and physical and laboratory findings. The sample of vaginal discharge will be looked at under a microscope for evidence of hyphae—that is, the threadlike filaments associated with fungus formation, using a potassium hydroxide (KOH) solution, which destroys the cells and allows visualization of budding yeast. This is known as a KOH prep. The presence of these hyphae on a KOH prep underneath the microscope, along with symptoms, confirms the diagnosis and necessitates treatment. If the KOH prep is negative, as in half of cases of women with vulvovaginal candidiasis, a culture should be performed prior to treatment to avoid giving antifungals to patients who do not have the disease. Since diagnosis is based on the patient's history, plus physical exam and laboratory findings, no further imaging studies need to be performed. Self-diagnosis is not recommended given the fact that it is usually inaccurate. In a study of ninety-five women who self-treated for possible vulvovaginal infection, 33.7 percent had vulvovaginal candidiasis, 18.9 percent had BV, 21.1 percent had mixed vaginitis, 13.7 percent had normal discharge, 10.5 percent had other diagnoses, and 2.1 percent had trichomonas vaginitis. So, again, self-diagnosis is inaccurate. Going to the physician for verification of the diagnosis will ensure that the true diagnosis is revealed and treated appropriately.

Treatment of vulvovaginal candidiasis includes vaginal or oral antifungal medications that work to kill the fungus. Medications that are placed inside the vagina are available for treatment anywhere from three to fourteen days depending on the type of medication prescribed. Oral medications are available for treatment too, as a single dose or a double dosing seventy-two hours apart based on complicated or uncomplicated diagnosis. Longer therapy is required if it is a complicated infection. Complicated infections are described as those that are more frequent (more than four times per year), have higher severity of disease on physical exams or with symptoms, have uncontrolled diabetes or immunosuppression, are pregnant, or have an infection with a *Candida* species other than *Candida albicans*.

T. vaginalis is a protozoan, a single-celled organism that can move. Trichomonal infection is an STI that is spread between sexual partners, leading to the colonization of the vagina, urethra, and paraurethral glands of infected individuals. This infection is known as trichomoniasis. Trichomoniasis is prevalent in 3.1 percent of the population and has been found to account for 3–5 million cases of vaginitis per year in the United States.

Trichomonas is obtained by having sexual intercourse with an infected partner and is associated with having other STIs as well. The presence of trichomoniasis can increase the risk of acquiring HIV, worsening preterm labor, and causing a pregnant person's water to break early (preterm labor and delivery).

The classic symptoms of trichomoniasis can include large amounts of thin yellow-green frothy vaginal discharge with foul-smelling fishy odor, cramping of the uterus, painful urination, or painful sexual intercourse; bleeding after sexual intercourse can also occur. When symptoms like these begin, it is important to seek the evaluation of a physician to rule out a possible infection, especially since other infections may be present in combination with the trichomoniasis. Treatment of the *T. vaginalis* infection is with oral medications in a single-dose or multiple-dose therapy, which kill the organism; some vaginal medications are available as an alternative therapy. Treatment can range from one to seven days depending on the type of medication.

BV is an infection of the vagina by any of multiple bacteria: *Gardnerella vaginalis*, *Prevotella* species, *Porphyromonas*, *Bacteroides*, *Peptostreptococcus* species, *Mobiluncus* species, *Mycoplasma hominis*, and *Ureaplasma urealyticum*. After the normal bacteria in the vagina are altered in some way, these organisms can infect the vagina and begin to multiply. Risk factors that can lead to this alteration in normal bacteria include douching in the past six months, multiple or new sexual partners, and cigarette smoking. The most common symptom is a foul-smelling, thin, light gray vaginal discharge. After a pelvic exam is performed and a sample of fluid is placed under a microscope for analysis, the diagnosis is verified. Treatment is with either oral or vaginal medications prescribed by a doctor with 3–7 day treatment plans depending on the type of medication. BV can also resolve on its own in 13–36 percent of patients after 2–10 weeks of monitoring; however, treatment with medication is recommended if the patient is symptomatic.

Although the above three causes are responsible for most cases of vaginitis, other possible sources of inflammation exist. Allergic reaction to irritants like lotions, soaps, lubricants, and spermicides can cause inflammation, itching, and discharge. Symptoms usually occur after use of the offending product and go away after the product has been removed. Foreign bodies like retained tampons can cause the body to react by producing inflammation and vaginal discharge. STIs such as gonorrhea and chlamydia can also cause vaginitis.

Elizabeth Rodnez

See also: Bacterial Vaginosis; Sexually Transmitted Infections (STIs); Vagina; Vaginal Secretions; Yeast Infection (Candidiasis).

Further Reading

Grimes, J. A., Smith, L. A., & Fagerberg, K. (2013). *Sexually transmitted disease: An encyclopedia of diseases, prevention, treatment, and issues.* Santa Barbara, CA: Greenwood.

McAnulty, R. D., & Burnette, M. M. (Eds.). (2006). *Sex and sexuality.* Santa Barbara, CA: Praeger.

Newton, D. E. (2009). *Sexual health: A reference handbook.* Santa Barbara, CA: ABC-CLIO.

Vas Deferens

The vas deferens, from the Latin for "carrying-away vessel," is a duct or tube that carries sperm away from the epididymis to the ejaculatory ducts in the urethra. It stores sperm for up to several months in anticipation of ejaculation. The sperm are provided with nutrients in the vas deferens, and dead or damaged sperm are reabsorbed by the lining to be recycled by the body. The vas deferens is a convenient location for a contraceptive procedure known as a vasectomy.

The two vas deferens originate in the scrotum, at the lower end of the epididymis. Sperm created by the testicles moves into the epididymis and is transferred to the vas deferens. Each epididymis has a separate vas deferens. The vas deferens is about a fourth of an inch wide but nearly a foot in length. It travels up from the scrotum and into the pelvis. It then travels over the bladder and down the back side. Connective tissue holds the vas deferens in place. The lining of the vas deferens has three layers, including a thick middle layer of smooth muscle that contracts rhythmically to move the sperm along their way. The lower end of the vas deferens widens into a chamber known as the ampullae. The ampullae act as storage chambers for the sperm. The lining of the ampullae secretes several substances that join the sperm to make semen. These substances include ergothioneine, which reduces chemical compounds, and fructose, a sugar used by the sperm as a nutrient. The ampullae can hold sperm for up to several months. The ampullae join with the ducts of the seminal vesicles to form the ejaculatory ducts that allow semen to enter the urethra at the prostate.

A condition known as congenital absence of vas deferens refers to the obstruction or absence of vas deferens. This condition has been associated with cystic fibrosis. Infections can also cause obstructions of the vas deferens. The location and function of the vas deferens has also resulted in the development of medical procedures to prevent conception. The vas deferens can be cut or obstructed in a vasectomy to prevent sperm from being ejaculated. In some cases, this procedure can be reversed if the patient changes their mind.

Tim J. Watts

See also: Ejaculation; Epididymis; Semen; Sperm; Urethra; Vasectomy.

Further Reading

Barclay, T. (2017). Ductus deferens. Retrieved from http://www.innerbody.com/image_repmov/repo26-new2.html

National Institutes of Health. (2019). Congenital bilateral absence of the vas deferens. Retrieved from https://ghr.nlm.nih.gov/condition/congenital-bilateral-absence-of-the-vas-deferens

Science Direct. (2019). Vas deferens. Retrieved from https://www.sciencedirect.com/topics/agricultural-and-biological-sciences/vas-deferens

Vasectomy

Also known as male sterilization surgery, a vasectomy is a surgical procedure to prevent the release of sperm. Although there is possibility for reversal, the procedure is complicated and not guaranteed, which is why a vasectomy is viewed as a permanent form of male sterilization and birth control. It is a common procedure around the globe, and some 500,000 men undergo the procedure each year in the United States alone. Vasectomies are considered highly effective—only about 11 out of every 1,000 procedures will fail within the first two years of surgery.

Vasectomy works by cutting the vas deferens, which are the tubes that carry sperm from the testes to the urethra. Once a vasectomy has been performed, the sperm are blocked from leaving the testicle. There are two methods of performing a vasectomy, conventionally or with a "no scalpel" procedure. In a conventional procedure, a surgeon will make two small scalpel incisions in the upper part of the scrotum, which is the pouch containing the testicles. A small section of the vas deferens is removed through each of these incisions, leaving a small gap in the tube, and the remaining ends may be sealed with heat or stitches. Then, the small openings in the skin will be stitched or closed with surgical glue. In the "no scalpel" method, a surgeon will feel for the vas deferens and then hold it in place with a clamp on the outside of the skin. One small puncture will be made in the clamped skin with a sharp instrument and the vas deferens will be gently lifted out, cut and tied, and returned to the body. This method involves no interior stitches and no usage of a scalpel. Both procedures take about thirty minutes or less and are usually performed as outpatient surgery by a urologist using local anesthesia. In most cases, patients leave the surgical office within an hour or two, and full recovery takes between seven and ten days.

After a vasectomy, individuals typically experience minor bruising and discomfort, symptoms that should dissipate within two weeks of the procedure. Immediate risks following a vasectomy include the possibility of bleeding into the scrotum or infection. These issues are usually indicated with redness, swelling, or tenderness in the scrotal region. Mild abdominal pain is normal; however, more severe pain may indicate complications. Another possible complication from the surgery is the development of a small mass in the scrotum. This can occur if sperm has leaked from the cut end of the vas deferens. Although the growth is typically benign, it may be sensitive to touch. In about 10 percent of cases, a vasectomy patient will experience a chronic condition called post-vasectomy pain syndrome, in which a person experiences persistent pain in the testes for no explainable reason. In this scenario, it is generally recommended to undergo a reverse vasectomy in order to help alleviate the pain. While there has historically been some concern that having a vasectomy increases the risk of prostate cancer, most modern research shows otherwise.

A vasectomy should not affect the ability to have an erection, nor does it prevent ejaculation or sexually transmitted infections. It also does not create immediate sterilization, as the sperm count will slowly decrease with each ejaculation following a vasectomy. Studies show that after three months or twenty ejaculations, one out of five patients will still have sperm in their ejaculatory fluids. Because of this, patients are advised to continue using other forms of birth control for at least several months or until a semen analysis shows that there are no sperm in the ejaculatory fluid.

English surgeon Sir Astley Cooper is thought to have been among the first doctors to experiment with various vasectomy techniques in the late 1700s and early 1800s, performing the first vasectomy on a dog in 1823, but it was not until the twentieth century that male sterilization procedures became safely practiced and widely available. Then, in 1974, Dr. Shunqiang Li developed the "no scalpel" technique in China. The vasectomy reversal was invented and performed a year later. Nowadays, in about 10 percent of cases, those who have undergone a vasectomy will choose to reverse the procedure. While the process is similar (in reverse) to the vasectomy, the surgery is more complicated and takes more time, although many patients still return home the same day. Statistics show that if a reversal procedure is performed within three years of the original vasectomy, around 97 percent of men will have sperm in their ejaculatory fluids, and the potential pregnancy rate is about 75 percent. If the procedure is performed between three and eight years after the vasectomy, pregnancy rates drop to about 50 percent. Finally, if the procedure is performed fifteen years or more after the original surgery, the pregnancy rate falls to approximately 30 percent.

Tamar Burris

See also: Sterilization; Tubal Ligation; Vas Deferens.

Further Reading

Bullough, V. L. (2001). *Encyclopedia of birth control.* Santa Barbara, CA: ABC-CLIO.

NHS. (2018). Vasectomy (male sterilization). Retrieved from https://www.nhs.uk/conditions/contraception/vasectomy-male-sterilisation/

Urology Care Foundation. (2019). What is a vasectomy? Retrieved from https://www.urologyhealth.org/urologic-conditions/vasectomy

Zorea, A. W. (2012). *Birth control.* Westport, CT: Greenwood.

Victorian Era

During the Victorian era (named after the British monarch Queen Victoria, who ruled from 1837 to 1904), sexual behaviors were viewed though the idealized codes of conduct for being "English" or being an "Englishman." Although the common perception of these codes was described as hypocritical, narrow-minded, prudish, and stuffy, they generally only applied to the middle-class society. These idealized codes also extended to the United States.

The Victorian era was characterized by the notion that a person's gender and sexuality were the basic core of self-identity, potential, social and political standing, and personal freedom. There were different codes of conduct for the genders and different stereotypes. It was commonly thought that females were not troubled with sexual feelings, but it was acceptable for males to yield to their "baser natures" (sexual desires). For females, fidelity in marriage was the supreme virtue, and an act of adultery made them a social outcast. One factor affecting women's sexual behavior was the lack of reliable birth control, which also limited their opportunity for becoming economically independent of their husband or family if they had children. Sex was considered a woman's contractual duty to her husband. For males, sexual desire and behavior were to be diverted into disciplined aggression, such as sports, or with other alliances, such as mistresses, sex with domestic help, or prostitutes (with discretion). Not all men had sexual contact outside of their marriage, but it was a common behavior among Victorian men.

Women who did work were predominately in domestic service or factory and white-collar work; however, approximately 2–5 percent of females supported themselves with prostitution, which typically led to crime involvement, drug abuse, and sexually transmitted infections. Some women formed liaisons independently as mistresses, which generally led to social rejection, if discovered, except for those with well-placed men in society who discretely managed the alliance.

As for children and adolescents, sexual behavior, such as masturbation, was highly criticized, and a number of efforts were made to control childhood sexuality. The underlying belief was that the person who masturbated turned sexuality inward.

However, by 1895, Sigmund Freud advocated sexual expression and orgasm for both sexes among his bourgeois Victorian peers and patients but argued that female sexual satisfaction depended on the male's behavior. He claimed that if incomplete coitus or sources of sexual frustration occurred, the female might develop hysteria or nervous exhaustion. Freud argued that it became a matter of public interest for men to act with full sexual potency. Thus, sexuality became a private and a public matter. As such, sexuality also became the basis for separating the Victorian wealthy middle class from the aristocracy, peasants, and working classes in British society, and the United States' upper class, middle class, working class, and lower class.

During the middle to the end of the twentieth century, the Victorian ideals and morals gradually changed and were eventually largely discarded. However, although it may appear that American society is currently a sexually liberated culture, sexual behavior and sexual orientation are still controversial and often taboo subjects.

Joan H. Hageman

See also: Freud, Sigmund; Masturbation; Sexual Revolution; Stereotypes, Gender; Stereotypes, Sexual.

Further Reading

Acton, W. (1862). *The functions and disorders of the reproductive organs in childhood, youth, adult age, and advanced life, considered in their physiological, social, and moral relations* (3rd Ed.). London: Churchill.

Baines, B. J. (1998). Effacing rape in early modern representation. *ELH, 65*(1), 69–98.

Buckner, P. A. (2005). *Rediscovering the British world.* Calgary, Canada: Calgary University Press.

Davis, D. A. (1994). A theory for the 90s: Traumatic seduction in historical context. *Psychoanalytic Review, 81*(4), 627–640.

Freud, S. (1898). Sexuality in the etiology of the neuroses. *Smith Ely, 3*, 261–283.

Hager, K. (2010). *Dickens and the rise of divorce: The failed-marriage plot and the novel tradition.* Aldershot, England: Ashgate.

Houghton, W. (1963). *The Victorian frame of mind, 1830–1870.* New Haven, CT: Yale University Press.

Isis Creations. (n.d.). Sexuality & modernity: Victorian sexuality. Retrieved from http://www.isis.aust.com/stephan/writings/sexuality/vict.htm

Masson, J. M. (1984). *The assault on truth: Freud's suppression of the seduction theory.* New York: Farrar, Strauss, and Giroux.

Murfin, R. C., & Ray, S. M. (2003). The Bedford glossary of critical and literary terms (2nd ed.). Boston: Bedford/St. Martin's.

Virginity

Virginity is typically defined as the state of a person who has not experienced sexual intercourse. In many parts of the world, virginity has significant cultural and religious importance, particularly for women, because it is a means of controlling reproduction, property, and family caste systems. In North America today, it is still viewed as a major life event, important to identity formation as individuals transition from adolescence to adulthood.

Although there is almost unanimous agreement that penis-in-vagina intercourse defines the transition between being a virgin and a nonvirgin, other sexual behaviors are less clear. For example, 83.5 percent of participants in one study believed that a person could engage in genital touching and remain a virgin, while 70.6 percent believed a person could have oral sex and remain a virgin. Given the primacy of penile-vaginal intercourse as the transition between virgin and nonvirgin, as well as it being the behavior almost unanimously agreed on as constituting having "had sex," the term "technical virgin" has also emerged in the culture to define someone who is maintaining their virginity status by engaging in oral sex or anal sex but not engaging in penile-vaginal sex. Personal definitions of what constitutes virginity loss are often motivated by whether or not the individual thinks they would be viewed positively by the transition.

Sexual double standards still exist in North America where men's sexual agency is accepted and applauded whereas women's sexual agency is restricted and shamed. As a result, understandings of virginity and virginity loss are often different for women and men, and, consequently, sexual behaviors are influenced by these belief systems. That being said, the average age at which most North American youth have their first sexual intercourse experience is seventeen. There is no gender difference with respect to age at first intercourse. The most common relationship context in which virginity loss occurs is a romantic relationship. Condom use tends to be at its highest prevalence at first intercourse.

There are three dominant scripts with respect to how North American society understands virginity and virginity loss, including gift, stigma, and process. Some individuals see their virginity as a "gift" that they value and of which they are proud. Individuals who ascribe to a gift script want to find someone special for their first intercourse experience, someone who understands the importance of the gift and might also be able to reciprocate their virginity or an equally important relationship variable like love or commitment. Individuals who view their virginity as a "stigma," something they hide and are ashamed of, want to rid themselves of their virgin status as soon as possible. As such, the intercourse partner may not be as important as ridding oneself of the personal stigma. Individuals who are out of sync with their peers, and lose their virginity later, tend to see their virginity status as more stigmatizing and are often perceived to be less desirable as relationship partners. Finally, some individuals view their virginity as a "process" akin to a rite of passage or milestone that everyone goes through, in which people learn about themselves, their partners, and about sexuality more generally. It is viewed as a natural part of transitioning into adulthood.

When asked which of these three virginity scripts best describes their experience, 38 percent of respondents at a Canadian university viewed their virginity as a gift, 8 percent chose stigma, and 54 percent identified with the process script. However, these percentages are highly gendered. More women (40 percent) than men (23 percent) identified with the gift script, while more men (32 percent) than women (4 percent) chose the stigma script. Roughly equal numbers of men and women described themselves using the process script. This finding highlights the presence of a sexual double standard that still exists in attitudes toward virginity.

Interestingly, there are connections between how people think about their virginity and how those thoughts translate into behavior the first time someone engages in sexual intercourse. Using survey research, gift- or process-oriented individuals are more likely to report that their first partner was a *romantic* partner, while stigma-oriented individuals are equally likely to say *romantic*, *friend*, or *stranger*. In addition, gift-oriented individuals predominantly feel *love* toward their first intercourse partner, process-oriented individuals feel *love* and *like* equally, and stigma-oriented individuals feel *like* or *indifference* toward their first partner (Humphreys, 2013). Gift-oriented individuals also spend more time in a relationship with their first partners before and after their first intercourse experience than do process- and stigma-oriented individuals. Emotional outcomes connected to the experience of first intercourse also differ by virginity scripts, including gift-oriented individuals feeling more "romance" and "pleasure" than the other two groups and stigma-oriented individuals feeling more "relieved." After the first sexual intercourse, these three groups tend to engage in different sexual trajectories as well, with stigma-oriented individuals having the greatest number of lifetime sexual partners, followed by process- and then gift-oriented individuals having the fewest.

While the above discussion has focused on norms in heterosexual youth, there has been little research focused on the understanding, experience, or significance of virginity (loss) among individuals identifying as LGBTQ+. While the idea that penetration is necessary for virginity loss remains a common interpretation, qualitative research exploring LGBTQ+ definitions of virginity suggest that LGBTQ+ individuals may embrace broader definitions of virginity. Some gay men and lesbians describe the possibility of multiple virginities for different sexual behaviors. Some research has shown that more nonheterosexual individuals than heterosexuals believed that an individual could lose their virginity with a same-sex partner. Furthermore, some nonheterosexual participants indicated that, in retrospect, they considered their first same-sex sexual experience as the experience denoting their personal virginity loss, suggesting that these individuals may redefine their personal definition of virginity to make the concept more applicable to their own identity, context, and experiences. Many participants in one 2014 study spoke of the difficulty of defining virginity, particularly within the LGBTQ+ community. Due to the heterocentric nature of virginity (loss), these individuals did not feel virginity, as a concept, applied to them and their experiences.

Terry Humphreys

See also: Abstinence; Adolescent Sexuality; Anal Intercourse; Double Standards, Sexual; Intercourse; Oral Sex; Purity Pledges; Sexual Script; Sexuality across the Life Span.

Further Reading

Averett, P., Moore, A., & Price, L. (2014). Virginity meanings and definitions among the LGBT community. *Journal of Gay and Lesbian Social Services, 26*, 259–278.

Bersamin, M. M., Fisher, D. A., Walker, S., Hill, D. L., & Grube, J. W. (2007). Defining virginity and abstinence: Adolescents' interpretations of sexual behaviors. *Journal of Adolescent Health, 41*(2), 182–188.

Brückner, H., & Bearman, P. (2005). After the promise: The STD consequences of adolescent virginity pledges. *Journal of Adolescent Health, 36*(4), 271–278.

Carpenter, L. (2005). *Virginity lost: An intimate portrait of first sexual experiences*. New York: New York University Press.

Carpenter, L. M. (2001). The ambiguity of "having sex": The subjective experience of virginity loss in the United States. *The Journal of Sex Research, 38*, 127–139.

Gesselman, A. N., Webster, G. D., & Garcia, J. R. (2017). Has virginity lost its virtue? Relationship stigma associated with being a sexually inexperienced adult. *The Journal of Sex Research, 54*, 202–213.

Humphreys, T. P. (2013). Cognitive frameworks of virginity and first intercourse. *Journal of Sex Research, 50*, 664–675.

Maticka-Tyndale, E., Barrett, M., & McKay, A. (2000). Adolescent sexual and reproductive health in Canada: A review of national data sources and their limitations. *The Canadian Journal of Human Sexuality, 9*, 41–66.

Ott, M. A., & Pfeiffer, E. J. (2009). "That's nasty" to curiosity: Early adolescent cognitions about sexual abstinence. *Journal of Adolescent Health, 44*(6), 575–581.

Peterson, Z. D., & Muehlenhard, C. L. (2007). What is sex and why does it matter? A motivational approach to exploring individuals' definitions of sex. *Journal of Sex Research, 44*(3), 256–268.

Reissing, E. D., Andruff (Armstrong), H. L., & Wentland, J. J. (2012). Looking back: The experience of first sexual intercourse and current sexual adjustment in young heterosexual adults. *Journal of Sex Research, 49*(1), 27–35.

Sanders, S. A., & Reinisch, J. M. (1999). Would you say you had sex if...?. *JAMA, 281*(3), 275–277.

Schlegel, A. (1991). Status, property, and the value on virginity. *American Ethnologist, 18*(4), 719–734.

Sprecher, S. (2013). Predictors of condom use in first sexual intercourse: A consideration of individual, situational, relational, and cohort effects. *Journal of Applied Social Psychology, 43*, E71–E84.

Trotter, E. C., & Alderson, K. G. (2007). University students' definitions of having sex, sexual partner, and virginity loss: The influence of participant gender, sexual experience, and contextual factors. *Canadian Journal of Human Sexuality, 16*(1–2), 11–29.

Tsui, L., & Nicoladis, E. (2004). Losing it: Similarities and differences in first intercourse experiences of men and women. *Canadian Journal of Human Sexuality, 13*(2), 95–106.

Uecker, J. E., Angotti, N., & Regnerus, M. D. (2008). Going most of the way: "Technical virginity" among American adolescents. *Social Science Research, 37*(4), 1200–1215.

Wiederman, M. W. (2005). The gendered nature of sexual scripts. *The Family Journal, 13*(4), 496–502.

Voyeurism

Voyeurism historically has been defined narrowly as the act of achieving sexual pleasure by watching unsuspecting individuals who are naked or engaging in sexual activity. However, in modern times, this has been broadened in the public eye to mean any viewing or spying on another's life or experience. Sexual voyeurism is one of the most commonly reported paraphilic interests. However, there has been little research conducted, and there is a debate as to whether voyeuristic fantasies and desire are pathological and deviant or an aspect of normative sexual behavior. While having voyeuristic fantasies may not be problematic, if the fantasies cause distress or if they are acted on and involve people without their consent then this behavior is illegal and meets the criteria of voyeuristic disorder.

Voyeurism was first described in the academic literature at the end of the nineteenth century by Richard von Krafft-Ebing (1886) in *Psychopathia Sexualis.* In the 1910s and 1920s, several psychoanalytic theorists discussed voyeuristic behaviors, but little to no research was done.

In recent history, voyeurism has been considered a paraphilia, or sexual deviance, within the *Diagnostic and Statistical Manual of Mental Disorders* (*DSM*) and the *International Classification of Diseases* (*ICD*). Voyeuristic behavior and fantasy are considered one of the most common paraphilias and one of the less pathological, provided they are not enacted upon unknowing people who have not given their consent. Voyeurism is found predominately in males. The historical psychoanalytic theory suggested that voyeurism was the result of a rejection of castration anxiety and failure to identify with the father. Several more contemporary theories have developed but lack empirical evidence or consensus. Lovemap pathology theorizes the secondary behavior, or looking at naked others, becomes a primary erotic lovemap or sexual blueprint. Courtship disorder suggests voyeurism is a result of anomalies in the normative four-stage process of courtship: looking for and discerning potential mates, pretactile interactions with mates, tactile interactions, followed by moving to sexual intercourse.

More recently, there have been challenges to the pathologizing of sexual interests deemed not to be socially normative. With voyeurism, if the behavior is carried out illegally or involves nonconsensual viewing of others, it meets criteria for voyeuristic disorder. However, having a fantasy or desire or acting out voyeuristic behavior in a consenting manner is suggested to be within the realm of normative sexual behavior. This claim has been supported by research that has found that in general population samples, anywhere between 4 percent and 60 percent of males have admitted to being sexually aroused by secretly watching others in sexual situations. Another recent study found that in a large sample of Canadian individuals, 46 percent had voyeuristic fantasies. In particular, 60 percent of the men and 35 percent of the women surveyed endorsed voyeuristic fantasies. The authors went on to make the distinction between a paraphilic interest or fantasy and a paraphilic disorder by differentiating between intensity and the disruptive nature of the thought and frequency of actual engagement in voyeuristic behavior. When the researchers separated the sample into paraphilic interest and paraphilic disorder groups, only 9 percent of the total sample found their fantasies to be intense or disruptive, and only 3 percent endorsed engaging in voyeuristic behavior often.

Alexander Kovic

See also: Exhibitionism; Fantasy, Sexual and Erotic; Kink; Krafft-Ebing, Richard von; Paraphilias.

Further Reading

Janssen, D. F. (2018). "Voyeuristic disorder": Etymological and historical note. *Archives of Sexual Behavior, 47*(5), 1307–1311.

Joyal, C. C., & Carpentier, J. (2017). The prevalence of paraphilic interests and behaviors in the general population: A provincial survey. *The Journal of Sex Research, 54*(2), 161–171.

Joyal, C. C., Cossette, A., & Lapierre, V. (2015). What exactly is an unusual sexual fantasy? *The Journal of Sexual Medicine, 12*(2), 328–340.

Långström, N. (2010). The DSM diagnostic criteria for exhibitionism, voyeurism, and frotteurism. *Archives of Sexual Behavior, 39*(2), 317–324.

Metzl, J. (2004). From scopophilia to survivor: A brief history of voyeurism. *Textual Practice, 18*(3), 415–434.

Metzl, J. M. (2004). Voyeur nation? Changing definitions of voyeurism, 1950–2004. *Harvard Review of Psychiatry, 12*(2), 127–131.

Vulva

The vulva is the external genitalia of people who are assigned female at birth, consisting of the mons pubis (the fleshy, hair-bearing area covering the pubic bone), labia majora, labia minora, clitoris, urethral opening, and vaginal opening. The vulva is commonly mislabeled as the "vagina" by many people and the media, but they are actually two separate parts of the reproductive organs. "Vulva" is the correct term for the outer portion of the genitals, while "vagina" is the appropriate term for the vaginal entrance and the internal vaginal canal. The various structures of the vulva are homologous (developed from the same initial genital structure) to the reproductive organs of people who are assigned male at birth.

The external portion of the clitoris is a small, very sensitive area located just below the mons pubis between the labia. It can vary greatly in size, color, and appearance. This small area is full of concentrated nerve endings and has only one purpose: pleasure. The clitoris has even more nerve endings than the entire penis. The clitoris is usually partially covered by a thin "hood" of skin called the clitoral hood with the glans (head) of the clitoris protected underneath. During sexual arousal, the clitoris becomes engorged with blood and may emerge slightly from the clitoral hood. With its many sensitive nerve endings, the clitoris is the primary source of sexual stimulation and orgasm for the majority of people who have vulvas.

The labia majora (or outer lips) are the fleshy, hair-bearing pads of skin along the sides of the vulva. They are made of fatty tissue and help to protect and cover the more sensitive areas of the female genitals. There are also sweat and oil glands on this surrounding tissue, which may contribute to natural genital odors. Some people choose to remove some or all of their pubic hair on this area, and some do not.

The labia minora (or inner lips) are between the labia majora and consist of delicate, sensitive tissue that offers additional protection of the vaginal and urethral openings, helping to prevent bacteria and foreign bodies from entering. The labia minora do not grow hair. They come in many shapes, sizes, colors, and are sometimes asymmetrical, all of which are normal variations. Though sometimes less pronounced than the labia majora, the inner labia may also extend beyond the outer labia, sometimes significantly so. A rapidly growing cosmetic surgery known as labiaplasty can be performed to reduce the size of the labia minora if a person is experiencing physical discomfort due to their length. However, this surgery is most commonly performed for purely cosmetic reasons and is controversial as many people feel that women are wrongly pressured by the media and pornography to feel ashamed of their genitals or to change their appearance.

Between the labia minora and below the clitoris lies the urethral opening. The urethra is the tube responsible for the release of urine. Many people mistakenly assume that the vagina is where urine is expelled, but this is incorrect. There are separate openings for the urethra and the vagina.

Below the urethral opening is the vaginal opening. The vaginal opening is the entrance to the vagina, which is where menstrual fluid and discharge leave the body. This is also commonly where penetration takes place during sexual intercourse and where a baby is born during vaginal childbirth.

The vulva and vagina are "self-cleaning" organs, meaning that there is no need for additional cleansing beyond using a mild soap on the external parts of the genitals only. While many people are often self-conscious of their natural bodily odors, it can actually be harmful to wash between the labia minora or to douche or use other feminine hygiene products inside the vagina. This can lead to yeast or bacterial infections of the vagina.

Lyndsay Mercier

See also: Clitoris; Labia; Labiaplasty; Urethra; Vagina; Vulvodynia.

Further Reading

Boston Women's Health Book Collective. (2005). *Our bodies, ourselves.* New York: Scribner.

Herbenick, D., & Schick, V. (2011). *Read my lips: A complete guide to the vagina and vulva.* Langham, MD: Rowman & Littlefield.

Vulvodynia

Vulvodynia is a condition characterized by chronic pain in the vulva (the external female genitals including the entrance to the vagina, labia minora, labia majora, the urethra, and the clitoris). "Vulvodynia" is used as an umbrella term to describe pain, with two main subtypes: generalized vulvodynia (pain that occurs at any time, at any or all parts of the vulva, independent of whether the area is touched), and vestibulodynia (pain at the entrance or vestibule of the vagina that occurs when the area is touched, also known as provoked vestibulodynia, vestibulitis, vulvar vestibulitis, and vulvar vestibulitis syndrome). The severity and frequency of pain with vulvodynia varies among women.

The cause of vulvodynia is not known. It is not caused by a sexually transmitted or other type of infection. Although research continues in an attempt to determine the cause of vulvodynia, several possibilities have been suggested as causes or contributors to vulvodynia, including genetic predisposition to chronic pain or inflammation, injury to the nerves that transmit pain signals, increased levels of inflammation in the vulva, hypersensitivity of the vulvar cells to tissue damage or infection (including yeast infections), and pelvic floor muscle dysfunction (a condition wherein the muscles that support the reproductive organs are too tight or too weak).

Women with vulvodynia may experience interference with activities such as sitting, wearing tight clothing, tampon use, gynecological exams, and sexual activity. Although women with vulvodynia typically experience dyspareunia (pain with intercourse), they may continue sexual activity despite the pain, and they tend to engage in less frequent sexual avoidance than women with vaginismus (a condition involving spasm of the vaginal muscles and fear of pain with penetration).

Vulvodynia is a diagnosis of exclusion, meaning that it is made after other causes for the pain have been ruled out. A doctor will diagnose vulvodynia after taking a thorough medical history, completing an exam and conducting tests to rule out other possible diagnoses, and assessing the pain through what is known as a cotton-swab test. This test involves the application of gentle pressure to various points on the vulva and having the patient rate their pain for each location.

Treatment for vulvodynia involves an attempt to alleviate the pain symptoms, since the underlying cause of the condition is unknown. There are multiple treatment possibilities that have shown some effect for some women, but there is no single treatment that is effective for all women with vulvodynia. Some women may need to try multiple treatments and may only experience partial relief from pain. Treatments may include lifestyle changes (including dietary modification and elimination of possible irritants in soaps, detergents, and menstrual products), topical medication (including anesthetics to numb the pain and hormonal creams to improve the vulvar tissue), pain medications (including opioids and antidepressants that are used for their pain-blocking mechanisms in this case, rather than their effect on depression), pelvic floor physical therapy (treatment with a specially trained physical therapist to address muscles tension or weakness), surgery (for women with vestibulodynia only), and sex therapy (a form of psychotherapy that can assist women and their partners by reducing anxiety and distress that may be both a factor in the maintenance of the problem and a result of the condition). A multidisciplinary approach to treatment, including a doctor specializing in pelvic pain, a pelvic floor physical therapist, and a sex therapist, is recommended.

Adrienne M. Bairstow

See also: Dyspareunia; Pelvic Floor Muscles; Psychosexual Therapy; Sexual Avoidance; Vaginismus; Vulva.

Further Reading

American College of Obstetricians and Gynecologists. (2017). Vulvodynia. Retrieved from https://www.acog.org/Patients/FAQs/Vulvodynia

National Vulvodynia Association. (2019). What is vulvodynia? Retrieved from https://www.nva.org/what-is-vulvodynia/

Vulval Pain Society. (2019). Vulval Pain Society. Retrieved from http://www.vulvalpainsociety.org/vps/

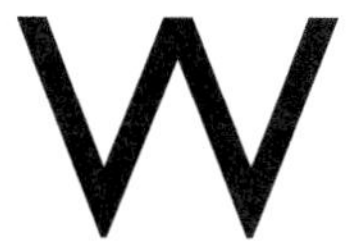

Withdrawal Method

The withdrawal method is a form of contraception used during sex, requiring the male to withdraw his penis from the female's vagina before he ejaculates. Unlike other forms of birth control, it is free and does not require the use of a device (such as condoms, birth control pills, or implants). Nonetheless, it is not a reliable form of birth control for many reasons.

Also known by the Latin term "coitus interruptus," withdrawal is one of the world's oldest documented methods of birth control, having origins in both the Old Testament and the Talmud. This practice requires that the male withdraw his penis from the female's vagina when he reaches a point in sexual excitement that he feels he is about to ejaculate. It is equally important that ejaculation occurs away from the woman's vulva, the external opening to the vagina, to keep sperm from entering the vagina and potentially causing pregnancy.

Withdrawal poses both advantages and disadvantages. Because it is free and does not require the use of a mechanism or prescription, withdrawal is viewed as a convenient form of birth control. However, some couples also feel that the withdrawal method disrupts sexual pleasure. A major disadvantage is that it does not offer protection from sexually transmitted infections, including HIV/AIDS.

Because of the risk of using withdrawal incorrectly, it is not a reliable method of birth control. In fact, research suggests that as many as twenty-eight out of one hundred women who practice the withdrawal method with their partner for one year will become pregnant, and teens represent the age group for which this method is the least effective. Many factors account for the risk of using withdrawal incorrectly. One major problem is that its success is entirely dependent on the male, requiring his motivation and willpower at the height of sexual excitement as well as a high level of knowledge and experience with his own body to predict when ejaculation will occur. Even if a male does withdraw, he might not do so quickly enough or far enough from the vulva to prevent semen from entering the vagina. Also, if sex is resumed after ejaculation, sperm may still be present in the penis, possibly resulting in pregnancy. Withdrawal will also fail in the absence of effective communication and trust between partners before and during sex or if the withdrawal method is impaired by the use of drugs or alcohol.

Linda Tancs

See also: Contraception; Ejaculation; Fertility; Fertility Awareness Methods of Contraception; Pregnancy; Teen Pregnancy.

Further Reading

American Pregnancy Association. (n.d.). Withdrawal as birth control. Retrieved from https://americanpregnancy.org/preventing-pregnancy/withdrawal-birth-control-method/

Jütte, R. (2008). *Contraception: A history.* Boston: Polity.

World Professional Association for Transgender Health (WPATH)

The World Professional Association for Transgender Health (WPATH) was created in 1979 and was originally known as the Harry Benjamin International Gender Dysphoria Association (HBIGDA). It was named after Dr. Harry Benjamin (1885–1985), one of the first physicians to work primarily with individuals who were gender dysphoric, gender diverse, or gender nonconforming, particularly in a positive, affirming way. It is now known as the World Professional Association for Transgender Health in order to better represent the mission and vision of the organization. The mission of WPATH is to "promote evidence-based care, education, research, advocacy, public policy and respect in transgender health." Their vision is to support professionals worldwide toward creating more equitable and knowledgeable practices and policies around research, education, health, equality, and respect for transsexual, transgender, and gender-variant people. As an organization, they publish the most updated versions of the standards of care; connect practicing and researching professionals doing work on, for, and with the transsexual, transgender, and gender-nonconforming communities; and work to further the treatment and understanding of gender identity disorder by various professionals.

Born in Germany, Benjamin was an endocrinologist who lived in the United States and was interested in what at the time was called transsexualism, a diagnosis in which the sex a person was assigned by a doctor at birth did not match the gender with which they identified. He was one of the first individuals to operate on the assumption that gender identity was different than sexual orientation, an assumption that was considered far ahead of his time. This recognition of gender as a different construct than sexual orientation allowed him to consider the concept of changing the body (with hormones and through surgeries) to fit the mind rather than using conversion therapy to try to make the mind fit the body. His creation of the Gender Disorientation Scale, based loosely on the Kinsey Scale (for sexual orientation) was revolutionary at the time, giving transgender and transsexual individuals the opportunity to be better understood by medical and mental health professionals.

Following his research on gender as an identity and not a subset of sexual orientation, Dr. Benjamin traveled internationally to perform what were called sex reassignment surgeries (now referred to as gender affirmation surgeries) on transgender and transsexual individuals. He was one of the first physicians to perform such surgeries and to work with psychologists and other professionals on how to support their patients throughout the process.

Based on his life work, the HBIGDA was named after Benjamin's life passion and accomplishments. One of the most well-known components of HBIGDA was to put forth the Harry Benjamin Standards of Care for Gender Identity Disorders. The first such document was published in 1979, with multiple revisions in 1980, 1981, 1990, 1998, and 2001. These standards of care were used to support health professionals around the world in better understanding how to best provide a variety of care to transgender and transsexual individuals, including therapy, hormone prescriptions, and gender affirmation surgeries. This document enumerated roles for mental health professionals, physicians, and surgeons, as well as requirements for different levels of care, including length of time living as the gender a person was transitioning to, how many letters from mental health professionals should be required for hormonal or surgical intervention, and even the treatment of adolescents who were presenting or identifying as gender diverse. For decades, until the early 2010s, this document was used as the main (and often only) guide for how to best treat patients with gender dysphoria, and many health professionals required all gender-variant patients to meet all the requirements detailed within these standards of care.

The most recent update of these standards of care, now referred to as the "Standards of Care for the Health of Transsexual, Transgender and Gender Non-Conforming People," was published by WPATH in 2012 in the *International Journal of Transgenderism*. This newest version includes a discussion on the need for flexibility in applying these guidelines, as people experience issues around gender in a variety of ways. It also centers on an informed consent and harm reduction framework, moving away from strict requirements for people to achieve in order to be allowed access to a medical- or mental health–supported transition. This newer version covers a larger variety of medical interventions and standards for providing lifelong and primary care (outside of only transition-related care), offers more suggestions from a global audience, and focuses sections on people who are intersex (also referred to as disorders of sexual development) and those who have been institutionalized, offering further access to gender-supportive care for individuals in a variety of environments.

Shanna K. Kattari

See also: Benjamin, Harry; Gender; Gender Diversity; Gender Dysphoria; Nonbinary Gender Identities; Sexual Health; Transgender; Transsexual.

Further Reading

Coleman, E., Bockting, W., Botzer, M., Cohen-Kettenis, P., DeCuypere, G., Feldman, J., … Monstrey, S. (2012). Standards of care for the health of transsexual, transgender, and gender-nonconforming people, version 7. *International Journal of Transgenderism, 13*(4), 165–232.

World Professional Association for Transgender Health. (2019). Home page. Retrieved from http://www.wpath.org/

Wyndzen, M. H. (2008). Dr. Harry Benjamin's gender disorientation scale. Retrieved from http://www.genderpsychology.org/transsexual/benjamin_gd.html

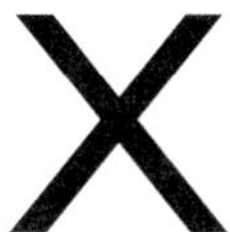

X Chromosome

The X chromosome is one of the two chromosomes that determine the biological sex of an individual, the other being the Y chromosome. The two sex chromosomes are among the forty-six chromosomes, organized into twenty-three pairs, that each person normally has inside their body cells. These microscopic thread-like structures carry the units of inheritance—genes—that determine the physical and behavioral characteristics that parents pass to their offspring. Genes are made of deoxyribonucleic acid (DNA).

Human females have a pair of X chromosomes in each of their body cells (also called somatic cells), and human males have an X chromosome paired with a Y chromosome in each of their body cells. These chromosomes are inherited from the parents when the sperm cell fertilizes the egg cell at the time of conception. Each egg cell has only one X chromosome, and each sperm cell has either an X or a Y chromosome. Thus, the sex of the child is dependent on the particular sperm cell that fertilizes the egg.

Besides determining an individual's sex, the X and Y chromosomes each carry numerous genes made of DNA codes that determine or influence other traits of the individual. These traits are either X-linked or Y-linked traits. The X chromosome has more than 800 genes, about 250 of which can cause health disorders if mutated (occurring in an abnormal form). Among the many X-linked disorders are alpha thalassemia mental retardation syndrome (a severe type of intellectual and developmental disability), androgenetic alopecia (a common form of hair loss), breast cancer, colorblindness, fragile X syndrome (a severe type of learning disability), hemophilia (a bleeding disorder resulting from an inability of the blood to clot), muscular dystrophy (progressive muscle wasting), type 1 diabetes, and certain types of deafness.

Most genes occur in pairs, called alleles, within the chromosome pair. For example, a gene will have one allele on one X chromosome and a corresponding allele on the other X chromosome within the chromosome pair of a female. One allele is inherited from the mother and the other from the father. Some alleles are dominant, while other alleles are recessive. If a gene occurs as two recessive alleles, any traits resulting from the recessive alleles will be evident in the individual. However, if a recessive allele is paired with a dominant allele, any traits coded for by the recessive allele will be blocked by the dominant allele.

Most of the genes linked to diseases and disorders on the X chromosome are in the form of recessive alleles. Thus, a female will not have the condition coded for by any of these alleles if one of her two X chromosomes has the dominant version of that allele. By contrast, because a male has only one X chromosome, there is no other dominant allele version to block the recessive allele's effects. That is why X-linked disorders are more common in males than in females.

In addition to the X-linked disorders caused by particular abnormal genes, there are other disorders caused by missing or extra X chromosomes. Turner syndrome is a developmental abnormality that occurs when only one normal X chromosome is present in cells. The other X chromosome is either missing entirely or structurally abnormal. Individuals with this syndrome are unusually short, and their ovaries do not function. Triple X syndrome, also called trisomy X, occurs when there is an extra X chromosome in the cells. Individuals with this syndrome have three X chromosomes instead of the normal two, which typically results in unusual tallness and learning disabilities.

Klinefelter syndrome occurs in individuals who have one or more extra copies of the X chromosome—for example, XXY or XXXY. The extra chromosomal material blocks the normal production of testosterone and the normal development of male sexual characteristics. As a result, these individuals typically have abnormalities in their genitals as well as female-like breast and hip development and reduced body and facial hair. Learning disabilities may also be present. The greater the number of extra X chromosomes, the greater the learning disabilities.

The presence of both an extra X chromosome and an extra Y chromosome results in a condition called 48,XXYY syndrome. As with Klinefelter syndrome, 48,XXYY syndrome is characterized by abnormal sexual development. Affected individuals have malfunctioning testes and reduced levels of testosterone.

The unusual sexual conditions caused by X-chromosome abnormalities sometimes lead to ambiguous gender appearances in affected individuals. Some individuals may be raised as one gender but as an adult identify with another gender. In certain cases, these individuals may choose to undergo gender reassignment surgery to make their physical sex conform to their psychological sex.

A. J. Smuskiewicz

See also: Chromosomal Sex; Intersexuality; Klinefelter Syndrome; Sex Chromosomes; Turner Syndrome; Y Chromosome.

Further Reading

Cover, V. I. (2012). *Living with Klinefelter Syndrome (47,XXY), Trisomy X (47,XXX), and 47,XYY: A guide for families and individuals affected by X and Y chromosome variations*. New York: Virginia Isaacs Cover.

National Institutes of Health. (2019). X chromosome. Retrieved from http://ghr.nlm.nih.gov/chromosome/X

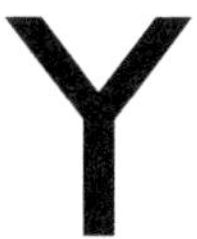

Y Chromosome

The Y chromosome is one of two chromosomes that determine the biological sex of an individual, the other being the X chromosome. The two sex chromosomes are among the forty-six chromosomes, organized into twenty-three pairs, that each person normally has inside their body cells. These microscopic threadlike structures carry the units of inheritance—genes—that determine the physical and behavioral characteristics that parents pass to their offspring. Genes are made of deoxyribonucleic acid (DNA).

Human males have an X chromosome paired with a Y chromosome in each of their body cells (also called somatic cells). Human females have a pair of X chromosomes in each of their body cells. These chromosomes are inherited from the parents when the sperm cell fertilizes the egg cell at the time of conception. Each egg cell has only one X chromosome, and each sperm cell has either an X or a Y chromosome. Thus, the sex of the child is dependent on the particular sperm cell that fertilizes the egg.

The Y chromosome has approximately sixty genes—far fewer than the 800 to 1,000 genes located on the X chromosome. The DNA of genes functions like a code, with chemical instructions for making particular proteins. These proteins, in turn, take part in biochemical reactions in the body that influence or determine particular traits of the body. The traits coded for by Y-chromosome genes are known as Y-linked traits.

Many of the genes on the Y chromosome are responsible for guiding normal male sexual development and maintaining male fertility. The main gene that prompts the development of a fetus into a male is the SRY (sex-determining region Y) gene, which codes for a protein that causes fetal precursor cells to become the cells of the testicles. Other Y-chromosome genes that have been identified include USP9Y (which plays a role in sperm cell development) and SHOX (which guides the growth and development of arm and leg bones).

Several genes on the Y chromosome can cause disorders if mutated (occurring in an abnormal form). Certain mutations in the SRY gene cause a condition called gonadal dysgenesis, also known as Swyer syndrome. Individuals with gonadal dysgenesis have XY chromosomes like a male but sex organs like a female, including a vagina, uterus, and fallopian tubes. However, instead of having ovaries or testicles, they have undeveloped masses of tissue known as streak gonads. These individuals usually live as females, but they require hormone therapy in order to develop female secondary sexual characteristics, such as breast development. Because they do not produce eggs, they cannot become pregnant naturally.

However, some individuals can become pregnant with donated eggs or donated embryos.

Another condition linked to abnormalities in the SRY gene is 46,XY sex reversal, in which the individual has XY chromosomes like a male but genitals that are sexually ambiguous. An individual may have an incompletely developed vagina as well as incompletely developed testicles. Sperm may or may not be produced, and a uterus may or may not be present. These persons may be raised as either male or female, but many eventually choose to undergo surgery so that their external genitals align with their gender identity.

Certain mutations in the SHOX gene cause conditions called Langer mesomelic dysplasia and Léri-Weill dyschondrosteosis, both of which are characterized by abnormally short leg and arm bones and other bone and muscle problems. Missing genetic material in regions of the Y chromosome called AZFA, AZFB, or AZFC lead to male infertility by causing sperm production to be absent, reduced, or abnormal.

In addition to the Y-linked disorders caused by particular abnormal genes, there are other disorders caused by missing or extra Y chromosomes. Males with XYY syndrome, also called Jacob's syndrome, have an extra Y chromosome, resulting in unusually high levels of testosterone in their bodies. As adolescents, they are typically tall and slender and have severe acne. As adults, most individuals are taller than 6 feet (1.8 meters) and live normal lives, many never even knowing that they have a unique chromosomal condition. With other polysomy Y syndromes (XYYY, XYYYY) individuals typically have skeletal abnormalities and intellectual disabilities. An extra Y chromosome together with an extra X chromosome results in a condition called 48,XXYY syndrome. Affected individuals have malfunctioning testicles and reduced levels of testosterone.

In 46,XX testicular disorder, an individual is born with the SRY gene on one of their X chromosomes. This condition occurs when the SRY gene from a Y chromosome is mistakenly transferred to an X chromosome within the sperm cell. The individual usually appears to be male but has abnormally small testicles or other testicular abnormalities. Some individuals may have genitalia that are not clearly male or female.

A. J. Smuskiewicz

See also: Chromosomal Sex; Intersexuality; Sex Chromosomes; X Chromosome.

Further Reading

Cover, V. I. (2012). *Living with Klinefelter Syndrome (47,XXY), Trisomy X (47,XXX), and 47,XYY: A guide for families and individuals affected by X and Y chromosome variations.* New York: Virginia Isaacs Cover.

National Institutes of Health. (2019). Y chromosome. Retrieved from http://ghr.nlm.nih.gov/chromosome/Y

Wade, N. (2014, April). Researchers see new importance in Y chromosome. *New York Times*, A4. Retrieved from http://www.nytimes.com/2014/04/24/science/researchers-see-new-importance-for-y-chromosome.html?_r=0

Yeast Infection (Candidiasis)

Candida are ubiquitous yeast that commonly colonize humans and are the leading fungal cause of serious infectious diseases. Several *Candida* species are part of the normal flora of the skin, mucous membranes, vagina, and gastrointestinal tract. As well as being part of the normal flora, certain species can be acquired from the environment. Candidal disease ranges from localized skin infection to life-threatening systemic disease. The growing incidence of serious infections due to *Candida* mirrors the rising numbers of immunocompromised individuals, who are at greatest risk for disease.

The earliest description of candidal infections is attributed to Hippocrates in *Epidemics* (fourth century BCE), in which he details oral candidiasis (thrush) in two patients. Thrush was again illustrated in medical reports in the late 1700s and 1800s. The fungus was first isolated in pure culture in 1844. The fungus was called by several names until 1923, when Christine M. Berkhout (1893–1932) established the genus *Candida.*

However, general interest in *Candida* remained relatively low until the second half of the twentieth century, when the incidence of invasive disease increased at a remarkable rate—by over 200 percent. This can in part be attributed to improved laboratory identification methods. However, it is largely due to advances in medicine, including chemotherapy, broad-spectrum antibiotics, intravenous catheters, and intensive care units (ICUs), resulting in increasing numbers of patients with compromised host barriers (such as the skin) and altered immunity.

The genus *Candida* currently includes more than 150 different species. However, few are usually associated with human disease. The incidence of disease caused by each species has significantly varied over the past forty years, driven by the disease spectrum of patients and the use of different antifungal drugs. *Candida albicans* remains the most common species worldwide, typically responsible for approximately 50 percent of infections. *Candida parapsilosis* and *Candida glabrata* occur at similar rates, approximately 20 percent of infections, though local variation in their rates can be quite pronounced. *Candida krusei*, *Candida tropicalis*, *Candida dubliniensis*, and *Candida lusitaniae* are less frequent, but nevertheless important, causes of invasive disease.

"Candidiasis" refers to all types of infections caused by *Candida.* The spectrum of disease is extremely broad, as infections caused by the fungus can involve virtually every tissue in the body. The most common types of candidal infections involve the skin or mucus membranes. Cutaneous infections typically occur in warm, moist regions, such as with "diaper rash" or under the breasts. These infections are characterized by a red, itchy rash, originating as either vesicles or pustules (small fluid- or pus-filled skin lesions) that then coalesce into beefy red regions with a scalloped border and frequent small satellite lesions.

Candidal infection of the tissues around nails can lead to chronic infection of the nail or nail bed (onychomycosis). Oropharyngeal (mouth and throat) candidiasis (thrush) usually occurs after antibacterial drug or steroid use and can also normally occur in newborn infants. Antibiotics and steroids primarily alter the local microbiome (group of microbes living in a region of the body) and the host response to the yeast, respectively, facilitating the growth of *Candida*. Risk factors for thrush include diabetes; leukemia or other cancers, especially patients on chemotherapy; or infection by the human immunodeficiency virus (HIV). Dentures also increase the risk of thrush. In thrush, the oral mucosa displays patchy, white lesions surrounded by red, inflamed tissue. Patients with HIV are at the greatest risk of developing a more severe form of the disease in which the esophagus is involved.

Vulvovaginal candidiasis (yeast infection) is the second most common vaginal infection in the United States. Approximately 75 percent of women of childbearing age will develop this problem, characterized by vaginal itchiness and sometimes a thick curd-like discharge.

Although less common, invasive or disseminated candidiasis is greatly feared due to the associated morbidity and mortality. Candidemia (yeast in the blood) produces illnesses that are symptomatically indistinguishable from bloodstream infections with bacteria, including fever and changes in pulse and blood pressure. Once within the bloodstream, *Candida* can localize to the heart, eyes, bone, abdominal organs, brain, or other tissues. In addition to seeding via the bloodstream, many of these tissues can also be locally infected with *Candida* after trauma, such as after intestinal perforation.

Diseases due to *Candida* most often arise from a patient's normal flora and less frequently are due to strains acquired from a health care provider or an environmental source. Important environmental sources for hospitalized patients include respirators, air-conditioning vents, foods, and countertops or floors. Candidal infections occur throughout life, and the spectrum of clinical illness primarily depends on the immune status of the host. The most important risk for severe disease is the disruption of a host's barrier, either by the placement of an intravenous catheter, damage to tissues due to surgery, trauma, or cancer, particularly in the setting of treatment with chemotherapy or radiation. Because intravenous catheters are ubiquitous in patient care, the risk of developing disseminated candidiasis is extremely high in neonatal, medical, and surgical ICUs.

Once the yeast breaches the body's natural barriers, the primary cell of the immune system that protects the infected person is the neutrophil. Therefore, conditions in which neutrophils are low (such as with leukemia, treatment of cancers, etc.) or dysfunctional (such as with steroid use, chronic granulomatous disease, Chediak-Higashi syndrome, etc.) significantly increase the risk for invasive candidiasis.

Although troublesome, cutaneous and mucocutaneous candidiasis are rarely fatal. In contrast, the mortality rate for disseminated candidiasis is about 40 percent. This is especially concerning because *Candida* species currently are the fourth most commonly isolated organism in blood cultures. In addition, it is estimated that blood cultures only detect about 70 percent of candidemias. It has been projected that the total number of hospital-acquired candidal bloodstream infections is up to 30,000 cases per year, resulting in more than 10,000 deaths annually.

Diagnosis of cutaneous and mucocutaneous candidiasis is often based on clinical presentation and generally achieved by direct observation of the fungus on a slide with staining by potassium hydroxide. Culture is performed only in refractory disease (disease resistant to treatment) or for esophageal candidiasis. The fungus grows well on a broad variety of standard mycological growth media. In blood culture, however, candidemia is missed about 30 percent of the time, and alternative testing methods have not been shown to be particularly effective.

Cutaneous candidiasis, including vaginal yeast infection, is typically treated with a short course of a topical azole (clotrimazole, miconazole), allylamine (terbinafine), or polyene (nystatin). Azoles and allylamines block ergosterol synthesis (a key component of the fungal cell membrane), polyenes disrupt the fungal cell membrane, and echinocandins inhibit cell wall synthesis in fungal cells.

Oral candidiasis is usually treated with solutions of clotrimazole or nystatin, or with the oral azole fluconazole. Esophageal candidiasis is initially treated with oral fluconazole for about two weeks, while vaginal candidiasis is treated with a single dose of oral fluconazole or with topical antifungals. Due to concerns regarding resistance, systemic infections are often initially treated intravenously with an echinocandin (caspofungin, micafungin, or anidulafungin) or the polyene amphotericin B. If the *Candida* species is susceptible, the antifungal is changed to an azole, typically fluconazole.

Handwashing is uniformly a reasonable first step in reducing infectious diseases. Keeping skin clean and dry significantly reduces the incidence of cutaneous candidiasis. Limiting the use of antibiotics also reduces the incidence of several forms of candidiasis, especially oral and vaginal disease. In certain populations, such as premature, low-birthweight newborns receiving intravenous nutrition or patients with a protracted period of neutropenia (having too few neutrophils) on chemotherapy, it is routine in many centers to administer an azole or echinocandin.

Joshua D. Nosanchuk

See also: Bacterial Vaginosis; Vagina; Vaginal Secretions; Vaginitis.

Further Reading

Calderone, R. A., & Clancy, C. J. (Eds.). (2011). *Candida and candidiasis* (2nd ed.). Washington, DC: ASM Press.

Lotz, M. M., Moses, M. A., & Pories, S. E. (2009). *Cancer.* Santa Barbara, CA: Greenwood.

Pappas, P. G., Kauffman, C. A., Andes, D., Benjamin, D. K. Jr., Calandra, T. F., Edwards, J. E., Jr., ... Reboli, A. C. (2009). Clinical practice guidelines for the management of candidiasis: 2009 update by the Infectious Diseases Society of America. *Clinical Infectious Diseases, 48*(5), 503–535.

About the Editor and Contributors

EDITOR

HEATHER L. ARMSTRONG is a lecturer (assistant professor) in sexual health at the University of Southampton. Her research focuses on improving sexual health and well-being, especially for sexual- and gender-minority folks. She has a PhD in experimental psychology from the University of Ottawa and completed postdoctoral fellowships at the U.S. Centers for Disease Control and Prevention and the University of British Columbia at the British Columbia Centre for Excellence in HIV/AIDS.

CONTRIBUTORS

JEFFREY ABRACEN is chief psychologist with Central District Parole, Correctional Service of Canada (CSC). He was employed as the clinical director of the community-based Methadone Maintenance Treatment Program operated by CSC, and until late 2011 was codirector of the Relapse Prevention Maintenance Program offered to sexual offenders in the Central District of CSC. He has provided training related to the community treatment and supervision of sexual offenders to a variety of audiences and has more than forty publications in peer-reviewed journals as well as many conference presentations. Dr. Abracen holds an adjunct faculty position at the Ontario Technology University in the Department of Psychology.

ROBERTO L. ABREU, PhD, is an assistant professor in the counseling psychology program at Tennessee State University. Dr. Abreu's research focuses on the well-being of lesbian, gay, bisexual, transgender, and queer (LGBTQ) people, people of color (POC), and LGBTQ POC. Specifically, his research has focused on Latinx LGBTQ individuals and family and community relations. Roberto's clinical experiences include working with children and adolescents diagnosed with autism spectrum disorder and other emotional behavioral disorders, LGBTQ teenagers and young adults, college students, low-income families and immigrants, incarcerated men and women with severe mental illness in state and federal prisons, and veterans with substance abuse disorders.

AMAN AGAH has published film and literary reviews in the magazines *Make/ Shift Magazine*, *Bta'arof*, and on popmatters.com. She has also cotaught Introduction to Media Literacy at George Mason University. Her areas of study and interest include film and literature with a focus on the gothic, as well as gender and queer studies. She attended George Mason University and The New School in New York.

CHRISSANDRA ANDRAE, MA, LMSW, is a queer artist and psychotherapist living in Brooklyn, New York. Chris provides kink-, poly-, trans-, and LGBQ-affirmative behavior therapy under the supervision of Dr. Dulcinea Pitagora as a member of the Manhattan Alternative Wellness Collective. Sandra was the Alec Baldwin Drama Scholar at NYU's Tisch School of the Arts as an undergraduate and a Creative Impact Scholar at the National University of Ireland: Uversity as a masters-level student. Chrissandra is a graduate of the Dialectical Behavior Therapy Training Program and Lab at the Columbia University School of Social Work.

NADAV ANTEBI-GRUSZKA is an adjunct assistant professor in the psychology department at Columbia University and the City College of New York. Nadav earned their PhD in sociomedical sciences from Columbia University, MA in human development from Cornell University, and MA in mental health counseling from City College of New York. Nadav also works at two private practices in Manhattan where they have the privilege of working with diverse clients and especially LGBTQ+ individuals. Nadav has published peer-review articles on resilience, pornography, sex work, and HIV prevention, as well as multiple encyclopedia entries and op-ed pieces about various LGBTQ+ issues. Nadav's work has been supported by numerous sources, including the American Psychological Foundation, the American Psychological Association, and the Kinsey Institute.

CASSIA ARAUJO-LANE, BA, completed her bachelor of arts in psychology at New York University in 2016. Araujo-Lane has five years' experience in harm reduction and integrated behavioral and primary care initiatives in the Bronx, Brooklyn, and Boston, Massachusetts. She completed her premedical certificate at Northeastern University in 2019 and currently works as a medical scribe at a urology clinic and a primary care clinic.

ADRIENNE M. BAIRSTOW, PhD, is a psychotherapist in Toronto, Canada, where she maintains a private practice with a focus on relationship and sex therapy. She holds a master's degree in social work from the University of Toronto, and a master's degree in education and a doctorate in human sexuality studies from Widener University.

AMANDA BAKER, LMFT, MEd, is a doctoral candidate at Widener University. She is a therapist and educator in Texas. Her therapeutic work has primarily focused on working with teenagers, military, and trauma survivors. Her research focuses on trauma and the impacts on intimate partner relationships and individuals and the impact of sexting on individuals and couples.

REGINALD BARKER is a first-year addiction studies graduate student at Governor's State University, University Park, Illinois, where he has also received a master's degree in criminal justice in May 2016. He is an investigator with the Cook County Sheriff's Department in Chicago, Illinois. He is also a varsity high school baseball assistant coach at Simeon Career Academy, also in Chicago.

KAREN S. BEALE, PhD, is an associate professor of psychology at Maryville College in Tennessee. An award-winning teacher, Karen teaches courses on human sexuality, intimate relationships, and adolescence. Her research focuses primarily on the predictors and outcomes of sex guilt, with the goal of improving sexual and relationship satisfaction.

RACHEL BECKER-WARNER is an associate professor of clinical psychology in the Program in Human Sexuality at University of Minnesota. She specializes in sexual health and gender care, focused on helping individuals across the age span establish and renew their sexual, emotional, and gender health and relational well-being. Her research and practice interests include the intersection of neuro and gender diversity, the neurobiological impact of trauma, and development of gender identity for gender-diverse people.

DIANNE BERG is an assistant professor and licensed psychologist at the Program in Human Sexuality. She has been working clinically with gender-creative children and transgender adolescents for over fifteen years and is a published scholar and invited speaker at regional and national conferences. She is the codirector of the National Center for Gender Spectrum Health, co-coordinator of the Transgender Health Services Program with a special emphasis in child and adolescent gender health, and a member of the Child and Adolescent Committee of the World Professional Association for Transgender Health, an international organization that asserts evidence-based practices through its published "Standards of Care." Dr. Berg is the coauthor of the Gender Affirmative Lifespan Approach, the theoretical framework for the clinical research program of the National Center for Gender Spectrum Health. She received her PhD in counseling psychology from the University of Illinois at Urbana-Champaign.

ILYSSA BOSESKI is a psychotherapist with experience in social work and human sexuality. She has a dual master's degree in social work and human sexuality education.

ELIZABETH R. BOSKEY, PhD, MPH, LICSW, is a research fellow and social worker with the Center for Gender Surgery at Boston Children's Hospital and has been the sexually transmitted disease expert at Verywell (formerly About.com) since 2007. She also maintains a small private practice where she focuses on working with sexual-, gender-, and relationship-minority clients. Dr. Boskey is the author of *America Debates Genetic Testing*, coauthor of *The InVision Guide to Sexual Health*, and coeditor of *The Truth about Rape*. She has contributed to the *Wiley Encyclopedia of Child Health and Human Development* and the *SAGE*

Encyclopedia of Global Health and authored numerous peer-reviewed and popular science articles on sexual and gender health.

NOVA J. BRADFORD is a graduate student in the School of Social Work at the University of Minnesota Twin Cities. Her research interests center on the relationships between sexual health, mental health, and identity development trajectories in transgender and nonbinary communities. As a mixed methodologist, she employs both quantitative and qualitative analyses to explore transgender health across the life span. As a clinical researcher, she has worked to develop and manualize gender-affirmative sex therapy techniques that are responsive to the dynamic sexual health needs of gender-diverse communities. Outside of her research, she is passionate about community organizing and policy advocacy to achieve empowerment and equity for transgender, nonbinary, and gender-nonconforming people.

RICHARD A. BRANDON-FRIEDMAN, PhD, LCSW, LCAC, is an assistant professor in the Indiana University School of Social Work. His research focuses on youth sexual identity development, sexual orientation identity, gender identity, and social and behavioral determinants of sexual health. Most of his work involves youth who identify as sexual and/or gender minorities and youth in the child welfare system. In addition to his academic work, he maintains a private clinical social work practice and serves on the board of directors for several agencies focused on serving sexual and/or gender minorities and youth in the child welfare system. Dr. Brandon-Friedman holds a bachelor of arts in psychology from the University of Notre Dame and a master's degree and PhD in social work from the Indiana University School of Social Work.

DOUGLAS BRAUN-HARVEY is a sexual health author, trainer, and psychotherapist who bridges sexual and mental health and facilitates organizational change. In 2013, Doug Braun-Harvey and Al Killen-Harvey cofounded the Harvey Institute, an international education, training, consulting, and supervision service for improving health care through integration of sexual health. Since 1993, he has been developing and implementing a sexual health–based treatment approach for men with out-of-control sexual behavior. His new book *Treating Out of Control Sexual Behavior: Rethinking Sex Addiction*, written with coauthor Michael Vigorito, was published in 2015. Previous publications include *Sexual Health in Recovery: Professional Counselor's Manual* (2011) and *Sexual Health in Drug and Alcohol Treatment: Group Facilitator's Manual* (2009). From 1987 to 2019, he provided individual and group therapy in his San Diego, California, private practice.

KELWYN BROWNE is a public health sexologist working in developing countries in the area of sexual health literacy, sexual health promotion, and sexual health education for health professionals.

TAMAR BURRIS is an independent writer and researcher. She is the owner of Tab Writers, Inc. She has worked with the Discovery Channel, PBS, ESPN, and with various educational stations, publications, and websites, as both a writer and educational curriculum expert.

LEONARDO CANDELARIO-PÉREZ, PhD, is a licensed clinical psychologist, sexual health consultant, and health care provider in urology and gynecology, as well as gender specialist for Health Partners and coeducational consultant for the National Center for Gender Spectrum Health (NCGSH). Dr. Candelario-Pérez completed their doctoral degree at Albizu University in their home country of Puerto Rico and completed a clinical postdoctoral program in 2018 at the Program in Human Sexuality at University of Minnesota. Currently, Dr. Candelario-Pérez is working on developing an integrative sexual health practice within the Health Partners' health care system. Their clinical areas of work are in sexual dysfunction, sexual pleasure, sexual and gender identity, LGBTQI+ sexual health, sexually transmitted infections and sexuality, desire discrepancy, intersections of identity, problematic sexual behaviors, and mental health and sexuality. As coeducation consultant for the NCGSH, Dr. Candelario-Pérez is involved in the development of training and educational materials for providers across the health fields. Said material is based on and promotes the use of the Gender Affirmative Life Span Approach.

KIFFER G. CARD is a Health Systems Impact Fellow with the Community-based Research Centre. He holds a BS in epidemiology and biostatistics from Brigham Young University and a PhD in health sciences from Simon Fraser University. Situated at the intersection of quantitative anthropology, social epidemiology, and behavioral science, Dr. Card's research focuses on understanding the biopsychosocial foundations of behavior and how this knowledge can be leveraged to support policies that improve the health and well-being of gay and bisexual men.

JORY M. CATALPA, MA, is a doctoral candidate and teaching and research assistant in the Family Social Science department and a research affiliate for the National Center for Gender Spectrum Health at the University of Minnesota–Twin Cities. They have published and presented in the areas of queer methods and measurement, body image, resilience, ambiguous loss, family boundary ambiguity, trans family theory, transgender community belongingness, transgender sexuality, and transgender identity development. Their queer theoretical methodology seeks to apply an antinormative framework to collecting and interpreting data and disseminating research.

STEPHANIE C. CHANDO, MEd, LSW, MSW, is a sex- and death-positive palliative care social worker and sexuality educator. She is a PhD candidate in human sexuality at Widener University, where her dissertation research focuses on the sexuality of individuals receiving hospice care. Stephanie currently serves as the social worker on the inpatient palliative care team at Pennsylvania Hospital in Philadelphia. Ms. Chando is also a part-time lecturer at the University of Pennsylvania's School of Social Policy and Practice.

CARSON CLARK is an undergraduate student at Maryville College. She is a member of the Student Judicial Board and Maryville College Democrats and is an ambassador for Maryville College. She plans to attend graduate school to study women and gender issues in the law.

ALEXANDRIA COLBURN, MS, is a doctoral student in clinical psychology at Marquette University in Milwaukee, Wisconsin, working with Ed de St. Aubin, PhD. She holds a bachelor of arts degree in psychology and women's studies from St. Catherine University and a master of science degree in clinical psychology from Marquette. She is broadly interested in conducting social justice–focused research and clinical work that supports underserved, marginalized communities. She is passionate about incorporating intersectionality theory into her work in investigating the complex underpinnings and outcomes of identity-related experiences.

CALLUM E. COOPER, PhD, is a senior lecturer of psychology at the University in Northampton, UK. He is a chartered psychologist of the British Psychological Society. He received a PhD in thanatology from the University of Northampton and a PhD in parapsychology from Manchester Metropolitan University. Dr. Cooper holds various professional positions. He is a research affiliate of Hope Studies Central (University of Alberta), a professional member of the Parapsychological Association (USA), and a Council Member of the Society for Psychical Research (UK). He has received various awards for his research in psychology and skeptical activism within science. At the University of Northampton, he lectures and conducts research on human sexual behavior, parapsychology, positive psychology, and death and bereavement. He has authored, edited, and contributed to several books, including *Paracoustics* and *Psi in Psychotherapy* (White Crow Books).

YOKO CRUME, PhD, MS, MSW, LCSW, is an international research and practice consultant specializing in aging society, long-term care, housing and environment, and mental health. Her professional experience includes an academic appointment as associate professor for the Joint Master of Social Work program (a joint venture between North Carolina A&T State University and the University of North Carolina at Greensboro) and an appointment as the lead planner and evaluator for the North Carolina Division of Aging and Adult Services. Crume was also the founding director for the Thriving Families Project, a mental health outreach program for Spanish-speaking families in Greensboro, North Carolina. Crume is licensed as a clinical social worker and publishes bilingually in English and Japanese.

MONA DALAL, MD, is a resident at the NYP/Columbia University Center of Family Medicine. She received her MD from the University of Iowa (2010) and her BS from Northwestern University (2005). She was a health educator through AmeriCorps from 2005 to 2006. Her interests include reproductive health, global health, and human rights.

SILVAIN S. DANG, MA, is a PhD candidate in clinical psychology at the University of British Columbia, in Vancouver, Canada. His dissertation research focuses on the role of cultural and interpersonal factors on the sexual experiences and functioning of Chinese and East Asian individuals in Canada. His research and clinical interests include sexual functioning; the etiology of sexual and gender diversity; and the role of culture, attachment style, and perfectionism on sexual and mental health. Silvain holds a master's degree in clinical psychology from the University of British Columbia.

CYNDI DARNELL is an Australian clinical sexologist, narrative therapist, and former psychotherapist now based in New York City. She holds multiple master's degrees in sexual health and narrative therapy from the Universities of Sydney and Melbourne, respectively, as well as graduate studies in mental health counseling and psychotherapy. She maintains a global consulting practice to individuals and couples in the areas of sex and relationships with a focus on pleasure and freedom. Her work is published in the *Journal of Sexual and Relationship Therapy* (UK) and the *Journal of Sex Education* (UK). She's presently an affiliate on the advisory board of University of Wisconsin–Stout Graduate Certificate in Sex Therapy Program and faculty on Pink Therapy's (UK) Foundation Certificate in Gender, Sexuality, and Relationship Diversity Therapy.

MELANIE DAVIS, PhD, is a certified sexuality educator, counselor, and educator supervisor through the American Association of Sexuality Educators, Counselors and Therapists. She is the Our Whole Lives program manager for the Unitarian Universalist Association and is an adjunct professor for Widener University's Center for Human Sexuality Studies. She is a founding partner in the New Jersey Center for Sexuality Education and is copresident of the Sexuality and Aging Consortium at Widener University. She is the author of *Our Whole Lives Sexuality Education for Older Adults*; *Sexuality and Our Faith: A Companion to Our Whole Lives Sexuality Education for Grades 7–9*; and *Look Within: A Woman's Journal*. She holds a master's degree and doctorate in human sexuality education from Widener University.

DAMIENE DENNER, MEd, ABD, is a doctoral candidate at Widener University in Chester, Pennsylvania, studying human sexuality education. Damiene's research focus is on sexual violence prevention, implementation fidelity, and using virtual reality as a teaching tool. Currently, Damiene works as a sexual health educator in Rochester, New York, and holds a master's in education degree from Widener University. Damiene is a student member of the American Association of Sexuality Educators, Counselors and Therapists and the Society for the Scientific Study of Sexuality.

JANNA A. DICKENSON, PhD, is a postdoctoral fellow in the program in human sexuality at the University of Minnesota. She holds a doctorate in clinical psychology from the University of Utah. Her graduate work focused on sexual fluidity and its neurobiological correlates, and she is the author of several papers on this topic. In her fellowship, she helps people who feel that their sexual behavior is out of control and researches the psychosocial factors associated with hypersexual behavior. Dr. Dickenson has also devoted her spare time to initiatives to end nonconsensual sexual interactions and has chaired a local workgroup devoted to this cause.

FRANCO DISPENZA, PhD, CRC, is an associate professor in the Department of Counseling and Psychological Services at the Georgia State University. He is a licensed psychologist and a certified rehabilitation counselor who works in the areas of multiculturalism, sexuality, and disability. Employing a variety of research and analytical methodologies (including quantitative, qualitative, and mixed methods), Dr. Dispenza has three particular lines of research that include lesbian, gay, bisexual, and transgender populations: (1) career and vocational development, (2) health and psychosocial functioning, and (3) counselor competence and counseling practice. Dr. Dispenza holds a master's degree in rehabilitation counseling and a doctorate in counseling psychology.

NICOLE C. DORIA, MA, has a BA in political science (University of Guelph), a BS in health promotion (Dalhousie University), and a MA in health promotion (Dalhousie University). Her areas of research specialization include women's health and indigenous health. Nicole holds several leadership positions with the Avalon Sexual Assault Centre board of directors in Halifax, Nova Scotia, where she works toward preventing sexual assault/abuse and changing the current sociopolitical culture that facilitates sexualized violence.

RENEE DUBIE earned a BA in philosophy from the University of California, Santa Barbara, and a MA in political science from San Diego State University.

KEVICHA ECHOLS is a full-time faculty member in health, physical education, and recreation at Kingsborough Community College in Brooklyn, New York. She is an advocate and researcher of sex workers and sex worker–related issues.

DEBBIE JOFFE ELLIS was born and raised in Melbourne, Australia. A licensed psychologist (Australia), licensed mental health counselor (New York), adjunct professor at Columbia University in New York City, presenter, and writer, for years she worked with her husband, the brilliant and renowned pioneer of modern cognitive therapies Dr. Albert Ellis, giving public presentations and professional trainings in his approach of rational emotive behavior therapy (REBT) as well as collaborating with him on writing and research projects until his death in 2007. Recognized as a world-renowned expert on REBT, she continues to present, practice, and write about his groundbreaking psychotherapeutic approach of REBT in cities throughout the United States and in countries around the globe.

LAUREN EWANIUK, PhD, is a certified secondary education teacher with nearly fifteen years of experience in the areas of social sciences and family consumer sciences. She received her BSE from Millersville University, an MEd from Gratz College, and an MEd and PhD in human sexuality from Widener University. Her areas of interest include sex and technology, child development, sexuality education for adolescents, and social movements in history. Along with her classroom experience, she has collaborated with authors on books with topics that include controversial issues in society and historical moments and figures in sexual revolutions.

ITOR FINOTELLI JR., PhD, is a psychologist and gender and sexuality specialist at Rio de Janeiro State University and has a master's degree and PhD from Sao Francisco University. Dr. Finotelli works as a clinical psychologist in the area of sexuality. Dr. Finotelli develops techniques, procedures, and measurement instruments for the assessment of human sexuality and works in projects and policies management for the promotion of sexual health and sexual rights. Dr. Finotelli is former president of the Brazilian Society for Studies of Human Sexuality and current secretary/treasurer of the World Association for Sexual Health (2017–2021).

MARISSA C. FLORO, PhD, is a postdoctoral fellow in gender and sexual identities at Stanford University and teaches about sexuality and gender issues in therapy at University of San Francisco as an adjunct faculty member in the master of marriage and family therapy graduate program. Dr. Floro's research work, clinical practice, teaching, and outreach programming focuses on the intersections of identity and how to create community, support, and belonging for those who find themselves at these intersections. Marissa holds a master's in mental health counseling from Boston College and a doctorate in counseling psychology from Loyola University Chicago.

ANNE M. FOGLE, MD, is a board-certified family physician who practices medicine in Louisville, Kentucky. She is a graduate of the University of Notre Dame and University of Louisville School of Medicine. Dr. Fogle completed her family medicine residency at the University of Nevada in Reno.

SHADEEN FRANCIS, LMFT, is a licensed marriage and family therapist, graduate professor, and author specializing in sex therapy and social justice. She has been featured as a relationship expert on national media platforms like 6abc, the *New York Times* , NBC, and *Huffington Post* , and speaks internationally on topics like sexual self-esteem, intimacy, and relationship negotiation. Shadeen got her start as a radio host and sex educator at McMaster University and eventually decided to transition her love of education to lecturer positions at Thomas Jefferson University and Lincoln University. Whether in her office, in an academic setting, or in a community space, Shadeen's work is inspired by her commitment to helping people live lives full of peace and pleasure.

ARIEL A. FRIEDMAN, MA, MEd, is a second-year PhD student at Palo Alto University, where she studies clinical psychology. She is a member of the Research on Intersectional Sexual and Gender Identity Experiences lab. Her clinical and research interests include LGBTQ+ psychology as well as complex trauma. She holds an MA and an MEd in counseling psychology from Teacher's College, Columbia University.

REBECCA FROST is a practicing clinical psychologist and the director of Benchmark Psychology in Brisbane, Australia. She is an certified emotional freedom technique couples therapist with the International Centre for Excellence in Emotionally Focused Therapy, and in her private practice she works primarily with couples and believes in supporting strong relationships of all types, including parents and their children. Rebecca completed her PhD researching the distress that can be experienced by couples as a result of sexual desire problems, and this remains a strong area of clinical interest for her. As the lead author of the Sexual and Relationship Distress Scale, Rebecca's postgraduate research has been published in leading sexual health journals, presented at international conferences, and is to be included in the newest edition of the *Handbook of Sexuality Measures*.

KARYN FULCHER is a postdoctoral fellow in the School of Public Health and Social Policy at the University of Victoria in British Columbia, Canada. Her research interests encompass a range of topics related to the sexual health and well-being of young people and sexual minorities, including pleasure-inclusive sexuality education and access to sexual health care. She takes an interdisciplinary approach to exploring these issues, drawing on anthropology, education, and public health. She holds a PhD from the Australian Research Centre in Sex, Health and Society at La Trobe University, where her research focused on the role of homophobic language use in maintaining gendered social structures among high school students.

KIMBERLY A. FULLER, PhD, is an assistant professor of social work at Cleveland State University in Cleveland, Ohio, and she maintains a private practice as a licensed independent social worker with supervisory designation and certified sex therapist. She has published several articles on the relationships of LGBTQ individuals and support. She holds two master's degrees, in social work and human sexuality education, and a doctorate in human sexuality studies from Widener University.

ALESSANDRA GALLO is a clinical psychology PhD candidate at Ryerson University in Toronto, Canada. Her research interests include forensic mental health, intellectual functioning and recidivism, and assessment and treatment of sex offenders. Alessandra is a mental health counselor at Correctional Service Canada, providing assessment and treatment services to federal offenders on conditional release. She has coauthored articles in the area of assessment and treatment of sex offenders and is a Joseph-Armand Bombardier Canada Graduate Scholar. Alessandra completed her MA in forensic psychology at John Jay College of Criminal Justice in New York City, with a focus on sexual offending.

SARAH GANNON, MEd, has been a sexuality educator, trainer, researcher, program developer, and consultant for over six years. While her recent focus has been on youth prevention programming, she has worked with people of all ages and abilities toward the goal of making healthier life choices. She has presented at several conferences, most recently at the American Association of Sexuality Educators, Counselors, and Therapists Conference, as well as the National Sex Ed Conference. She has presented on a range of topics, primarily inclusivity, removing shame and stigma, and supporting the LGBTQ+ community. She is currently the cochair for Delaware's PRIDE Council. Sarah holds a master's of education in human sexuality studies from Widener University.

ABBY GIRARD, LMFT, PsyD, is an assistant professor in the Program for Human Sexuality, Department of Family Medicine and Community Health at the University of Minnesota Medical School and is the program coordinator for the Center for Sexual Health, Relationship and Sex Therapy program. Dr. Girard specializes in couples and sex therapy and has published numerous peer-reviewed articles on sexual desire discrepancy, infidelity, consensual nonmonogamy, and compulsive sexual behavior. Girard holds a master's in marital and family therapy from the University of San Diego and a doctorate in marital and family therapy from the Alliant International University. Dr. Girard completed her postdoctoral fellowship in couple sexual health at the Program in Human Sexuality within the Department of Family Medicine and Community Health in the University of Minnesota Medical School.

CHRISTINA GIROD is author of *Indigenous Peoples of North America: Native Americans of the Southeast* (Lucent Books, 2000), *The Thirteen Colonies: Connecticut* (Lucent Books, 2001), *The Indian Americans* (Gale, 2003), and *Diseases and Disorders: Down Syndrome* (Lucent Books, 2000).

MARTHA GOLDSTEIN-SCHULTZ has a PhD in human sexuality studies and works as an educational consultant for LGBTQ+-inclusive strategies for classrooms and school environments. Sexuality Education Consulting, LLC, serves schools in Connecticut and Rhode Island. Martha has numerous years of teaching experience in secondary and higher education. She has taught life span development courses at the University of Connecticut and Quinebaug Valley Community College. Currently, Martha is designing a course in sexuality education for health and physical education teachers with Eastern Connecticut State University. She is also a social justice trainer for the National Conference for Community and Justice and a yoga instructor.

PATRICK R. GRANT, MA, MPH, is fourth-year clinical psychology doctoral candidate (PsyD) at La Salle University and a community mental health staff therapist in northeast Philadelphia, where he specializes in treating anxiety and mood disorders among special populations, which include ethnic minorities and those within the LGBT community. In 2016, he served as the creator and lead developer of the Chrome 2 Color Project—an urban-based initiative that sought to reduce rates of unintended pregnancy among LGBT-identified inner-city youth of color. He has also contributed works to numerous editions of the *Journal of Black Sexuality and Relationships* , which have centered on highlighting the nuanced experiences of black same-gender-loving men. Patrick holds a master's in public health with a completed certification in sexual health and education from Washington University of St. Louis and a master's in clinical psychology from La Salle University.

JILL A. GRIMES, MD, FAAFP, spokesperson for the American Academy of Family Physicians, is passionate about prevention of disease and patient education for all ages and body parts. She was a presidential scholar at Texas A&M University and earned her MD at Baylor College of Medicine in 1991. Dr. Grimes is an associate editor for the *5-Minute Clinical Consult,* focusing on evidence-based practical clinical information. Dr. Grimes has been on faculty for the University of Massachusetts Medical School as a clinical instructor since 2000. Her award-winning book, *Seductive Delusions: How Everyday People Catch STDs* (2008), shares stories that speak louder than statistics and is required reading in many Texas high schools. She is also the editor of ABC-CLIO's *Sexually Transmitted Disease: An Encyclopedia of Diseases, Prevention, Treatment, and Issues.* Dr. Grimes shares advice through both popular media and scholarly forums and particularly enjoys call-in radio shows.

JOAN H. HAGEMAN, PhD, is an international research scientist with multifaceted expertise in the fields of psychology, psychophysiology, neuroscience, social sciences, hypnosis, health, and biofeedback. She is the chair of research at PSYmore Research Institute, Inc., in Tampa, Florida; an adjunct professor at Saybrook University in San Francisco, California; and an associate professor with Northcentral University in Prescott Valley, Arizona. Her published works include "Phenomenological and Evidence Based Research in Ego State Therapy" (*American Journal of Clinical Hypnosis*, July 2013). Hageman holds a doctorate in psychology from Saybrook Graduate School and Research Center (now Saybrook University). Her research centers on multicultural issues in human consciousness.

VERN HARNER, MSW, is pursuing a PhD in social welfare at the University of Washington (UW). They are currently the communications coordinator for the LGBTQ Caucus of Faculty and Students in Social Work, a member of the organizing committee for UW's Inaugural Interprofessional LGBTQ Health Conference, a research associate on the *Trans Bodies, Trans Selves* research team, and a peer group facilitator with Ingersoll Gender Center. Drawing on their broad experience advocating for trans and queer issues, Vern's current work focuses on intergenerational knowledge and support within transgender communities. Vern believes that by learning how trans communities have supported one another, social workers can be better poised to create programs leveraging these strengths.

RENÉE M. HAYNES, MD, MPH, is the district health director of the North Central Health District in Georgia. As district health director, she oversees public health activities across thirteen counties in central Georgia. She completed her undergraduate work at Duke University and attended Florida International University for her master's in public health. She received her medical degree from Morehouse School of Medicine in Atlanta, Georgia. She is a family medicine physician and, prior to her current role in public health, worked for the Department of Veterans Affairs in Atlanta, Georgia.

LINDA D. HINKLE is a top undergraduate student at Maryville College. She is also a veteran, having served as a combat medical specialist in the U.S. Army for seven years. She is currently applying to graduate school and plans to work for Veterans Affairs as a counselor.

JACOB HUFF is currently an undergraduate student at Tennessee State University. His research interests include counseling of marginalized populations, major depressive disorder, community mental health, and political psychology.

TERRY HUMPHREYS, PhD, is a full professor in the Department of Psychology at Trent University, Peterborough, Ontario, Canada. He is the editor of the *Canadian Journal of Human Sexuality* and a consulting editor for the *Journal of Sex Research.* He is also the past president of the Society for the Scientific Study of Sexuality, a long-standing planning committee member of the Guelph Sexuality Conference (Canada's largest and longest-running annual sexuality conference), and a member of the advisory board of the World Association for Sexual Health. His academic and research interests lie in the broad field of sexual communication in intimate relationships. Specifically, his expertise is in the negotiation of sexual consent in multiple contexts, sexting behavior in young adults, first sexual experiences, and unwanted/coercive sexual encounters.

ALEX IANTAFFI, PhD, MS, SEP, CST, LMFT, is a certified sex therapist, family therapist, Somatic Experiencing practitioner, clinical supervisor, writer, and independent scholar. They are adjunct faculty at the University of Wisconsin–Stout and the chair elect for the trans and queer interest network of the American Association for Marriage and Family Therapy. They were the editor in chief for the *Journal of Sexual and Relationship Therapy* for eleven years and have researched, presented, and published extensively on gender, disability, sexuality, and relationships. Alex is passionate about healing justice and community-based and engaged scholarship. They are a trans masculine, nonbinary, bi queer, disabled Italian immigrant who has been living on Dakota and Anishinaabe territories, currently known as Minneapolis, Minnesota, since 2008. Alex has recently coauthored the books *How to Understand Your Gender: A Practical Guide for Exploring Who You Are* and *Life Isn't Binary* with Meg-John Barker (Jessica Kingsley Publishers). They host the podcast *Gender Stories.*

JAY A. IRWIN, PhD, is an associate professor of sociology at University of Nebraska at Omaha. Dr. Irwin's research focuses on LGBTQIA+ communities, LGBTQIA+ physical and mental health, and transgender identities. He also is involved in educational programming around LGBTQIA+ inclusion for health professionals, collegiate-level faculty and staff, and local communities broadly. Dr. Irwin is a member of the Midlands Sexual Health Research Collaborative and the Professional Transgender Resource Network, an Omaha-based collaborative effort to provide resources and education for professionals working with transgender communities. He holds a PhD in medical sociology and a graduate certificate in gerontology from the University of Alabama at Birmingham.

LAURA KABBASH, BA, is a fluently bilingual Montrealer whose passion for adolescent psychology, specifically behavioral misconduct, was kindled while directing leadership training programs at YMCA Kanawana. Following an honors psychology program at Marianopolis CEGEP in Montreal, Ms. Kabbash graduated with an honors bachelor's degree in psychology from University of British Columbia, Kelowna, while completing research on the mediating effects of personality factors on the association between child abuse experiences and adult outcomes. Ms. Kabbash is currently completing a doctorate degree in clinical psychology at the University of New Brunswick, where her research is focused on child sex trafficking and adolescent forensic populations.

RACHEL KALISH, PhD, is an assistant professor of sociology and criminology at SUNY College at Old Westbury. She received her doctorate from Stony Brook University. Her research interests include young adult sexuality, hookup culture, and gender-based violence. Prior to her graduate work, Rachel was a rape crisis counselor for ten years.

SHANNA K. KATTARI, PhD, MEd, CSE, ACS, (she/her/hers) is an assistant professor at the University of Michigan School of Social Work and Department of Women's Studies (by courtesy), core faculty at the Center for Sexuality and Health Disparities, and the director of the [Sexuality|Relationships|Gender] Research Collective. She is the author of several dozen articles on sexuality and disability, sexuality and social work, and trans experiences of health care, as well as the editor of a forthcoming book on social work and health care with trans and nonbinary individuals and communities. She is the co-chair of the Caucus of LGBTQ Social Work Faculty and PhD Students and former co-chair of the Council of Social Work Education's Council on Sexual Orientation, Gender Identity and Expressions. She holds a master's in human sexuality education from Widener University and a PhD in social work from the University of Denver.

KRISTEN KELLY, MD, is an OB/GYN resident at UMass Memorial Hospital in Worcester, Massachusetts. Dr. Kelly graduated from Jefferson Medical College (Philadelphia, Pennsylvania) and went to Middlebury College (Middlebury, Vermont) for her undergraduate degree. In between, she enjoyed teaching fifth/sixth grades for five years.

M. KILLIAN KINNEY, MSW, LSW, (they/them) is a social work doctoral candidate and associate faculty at Indiana University School of Social Work in Indianapolis, Indiana. They are an emerging empowerment and well-being scholar emphasizing the experiences of transgender and nonbinary individuals. Mx. Kinney practices at the Riley Adolescent Gender Health Clinic and provides presentations, training, and consultation on LGBTQ-affirming health care at the local, national, and international levels. They were a past president of the Indiana chapter of the National Association of Social Workers' Sexual Orientation and Gender Identity Committee and are a current member of the Council on Social Work Education's Council on Sexual Orientation and Gender Identity and Expression. Mx. Kinney is an editor and author for the upcoming book titled *Social Work and Health Care with Transgender/Nonbinary Individuals and Communities*.

ALEXANDER KOVIC, PsyD, is a postdoctoral fellow at the University of Minnesota Medical School in the program in human sexuality. He provides for individual, family, couples, and group psychotherapy for a wide range of concerns related to gender and sexual health. His training has involved work in forensic hospitals, correctional facilities, inpatient substance abuse centers, community mental health clinics, and academic centers. His areas of clinical and research interest include sexual identity and gender diversity; sexual trauma; addictive, compulsive, or risky behaviors; severe mental illness; forensic evaluation, and the management of violence. Dr. Kovic holds a doctor of psychology degree in clinical psychology and a master's in forensic psychology from the Minnesota School of Professional Psychology–Argosy University.

NATHAN LACHOWSKY employs a social justice framework to advance health equity, championing interdisciplinary community-based research. He is a social and behavioral epidemiologist with ten years of experience conducting community-based research on sexual health and HIV/AIDS with marginalized communities across Canada and New Zealand. He is an associate professor and Michael Smith Foundation for Health Research Scholar in the School of Public Health and Social Policy at the University of Victoria and research director for the Community-based Research Centre Society.

JUSTIN J. LEHMILLER, PhD, is a research fellow at the Kinsey Institute at Indiana University. He is author of the blog *Sex and Psychology* and the book *Tell Me What You Want: The Science of Sexual Desire and How It Can Help You Improve Your Sex Life*. Dr. Lehmiller has also written a textbook, *The Psychology of Human Sexuality*, that is used in college classrooms around the world to educate students about the science of sex. He maintains an active research program focused on topics including sexual fantasies, friends with benefits, and consensual nonmonogamy. Dr. Lehmiller holds a master's degree in experimental psychology from Villanova University and a doctorate in social psychology from Purdue University.

MARK A. LEVAND, PhD, MA, CSE, is an adjunct faculty member at various universities in the Philadelphia area, where he facilitates undergraduate and graduate courses in human sexuality. As a certified sexuality educator, he has taught courses at the intersection of human sexuality and counseling, education, religion, human development, and research methods. Dr. Levand often researches and writes on topics of sexuality and Catholicism, consent, and culture. He is also on the education certification committee and advocacy committee for the American Association of Sexuality Educators, Counselors and Therapists.

SYLVIE LÉVESQUE, PhD, is an associate professor at the Department of Sexology, Université du Québec in Montréal, Canada, where her time is divided between teaching, research, and community services. She is trained as a sexologist and has pursued her doctoral studies in public health (health promotion). She is a permanent researcher at the Réseau Québécois en Études Feministes and is a member of the Domestic Violence: Actors in Context and Innovative Practices Research Team. Her research interests focus on gender-based violence, intimate partner violence, reproductive coercion, promotion of reproductive and sexual health, and parenting. She holds research grants from provincial and national agencies. She has been working or doing research in these fields for the past fifteen years.

ANGELA LIBAL is a zoologist, cryptozoologist, and science writer. She has published more than four hundred articles dealing with animal husbandry, biology, and environmental science on various educational websites. She is also the author of several books, including *Forensic Anthropology* (Mason Crest, 2013), *Fingerprints, Bite Marks, Ear Prints* (Mason Crest, 2013), and *Field Guides to Finding a New Career: Science* (Ferguson, 2010). Her areas of interest include the intersection of the natural sciences, religious and ethnological history, and folklore. She holds a BA from Sarah Lawrence College.

CAMILLA LOGGINS is an undergraduate student at Maryville College in Maryville, Tennessee. Loggins is the recipient of the coveted Ledford Scholarship from the Appalachian College Association, which is funding her senior study. She is currently applying to graduate schools and plans to work in the sector of public health and human sexuality.

JAN LOOMAN completed his PhD in clinical forensic psychology at Queen's University in Kingston, Ontario, in 2000. He is currently in private practice providing assessments for sexual offenders in Kingston. Previously he worked for Correctional Services of Canada, where he supervised the delivery of the High-Intensity Sexual Offender Treatment Program at the Regional Treatment Centre (Ontario) and at Providence Care Hospital on the Forensic Psychiatric Unit. Dr. Looman's research interests include risk assessment, treatment outcomes, and psychopathy in sexual offender populations. He has published over sixty articles in peer-reviewed journals on these topics.

HOWARD W. MacLENNAN JR. is the lead physician in medical readiness standards for the North Carolina Army National Guard, where his specialties include genetics, molecular biology, and osteopathic medicine. Dr. MacLennan is a member of the American Academy of Family Physicians, American Board of Family Medicine, and American Osteopathic Association, and he has widely published in a variety of medical journals. (The views expressed by Dr. MacLennan are those of the author and do not reflect the official policy or position of the Department of the Army, Department of Defense, or U.S. government.)

CRISTINA L. MAGALHÃES, PhD, has a doctorate from Nova Southeastern University (2005) and is an associate professor of clinical psychology, associate director of the PsyD program, and coordinator of the Rockway Certificate for LGBTQ Studies at the California School of Professional Psychology at Alliant International University, Los Angeles. She is also a licensed clinical psychologist in independent practice. Dr. Magalhães's clinical, research, and teaching interests include LGBTQ health, treatment approaches for anxiety- and trauma-related disorders, and cross-cultural psychodiagnostic assessment.

JIMMIE MANNING, PhD, is a professor and chair of communication studies at the University of Nevada, Reno. His research focuses on relational discourses, especially those about sexuality, gender, love, and identity; connections between relationships and efficacy in health and organizational contexts; and digitally mediated communication. His research has been supported by funding agencies such as the National Science Foundation and Learn and Serve America, and he has accrued over thirty journal publications in outlets including *Communication Monographs*, *Journal of Social and Personal Relationships*, and *Journal of Computer-Mediated Communication*. He has authored multiple books, including *Researching Interpersonal Relationships: Qualitative Methods, Research, and Analysis* (Sage). He received his doctorate in communication studies from the University of Kansas.

AMANDA MANUEL is a counselor and psychotherapist in private practice. She holds master's degrees in arts, education in counseling psychology, and clinical human sexuality and is pursuing a PhD in clinical human sexuality.

KIM MASTERS EVANS is a freelance writer specializing in scientific topics. She has authored dozens of reference books, textbook lessons, and encyclopedia articles for students at the high school and undergraduate levels. Her published works include *Energy: Supplies, Sustainability, and Costs* (Gale, 2015); *The Environment: A Revolution in Attitudes* (Gale, 2003); and *Space Exploration: Triumphs and Tragedies* (Gale, 2007). She is also a licensed professional engineer with two decades of experience in the field of environmental engineering. Evans holds a BS in chemical engineering from Tennessee Technological University.

LAUREN G. MASUDA, PsyD, is a staff psychologist for Veterans Affairs Salt Lake City Health Care System and specializes in geropsychology and health psychology. Dr. Masuda holds a doctorate in clinical psychology from Baylor University.

ELIZABETH A. MAYNARD, PhD, is a licensed clinical psychologist whose work has explored the intersections of religion, spirituality, and sexuality. After many years in university and clinical work, she now serves as a foreign service officer for the U.S. Department of State.

MARY McCLURE, EdD, LPC, has been a counselor educator since 2009, with emphasis in teaching master's-level students seeking licensure as professional counselors. Since 2105, she has focused on counselor education in the addictions specialty area as well as on master's-level education supporting certification for alcohol and other drug addiction work. Her work includes program and course-work development and delivery in peer support recovery coaching.

MICHAEL J. McGEE, PhD, is an associate professor in health education at Borough of Manhattan Community College, City University of New York. Formerly he was the executive director of the World Association for Sexual Health.

LYNDSAY MERCIER, PhD, is a sexuality educator, author, and award-winning researcher with over fourteen years of experience working directly with adolescents and young adults surrounding healthy sexuality. She received her doctorate and master's degree in human sexuality education from Widener University.

SUSAN MILSTEIN, PhD, is an assistant professor in the Department of Public Health and Health Care Administration at California State University, Chico. She is a master certified health education specialist as well as a certified sexuality educator. Dr. Milstein is the coauthor of the fifth edition of *Human Sexuality: Making Informed Decisions* and is a former associate editor of the *American Journal of Sexuality Education*. In addition to her work at the university, Dr. Milstein is also the founder and lead consultant for Milstein Health Consulting, through which she provides sexuality education and training for professionals and the general public.

RANDI MINETOR has authored more than forty books and has served as the ghostwriter for a number of best-selling nonfiction books. She serves as a principal copywriter for the University of Rochester Medical Center patient information website. Minetor holds a master's degree in film studies from the University of Rochester and a bachelor's degree in English and psychology from the University at Buffalo.

LUCAS MIRABITO, MA, is currently a doctoral candidate in the clinical psychology program at Marquette University in Milwaukee, Wisconsin. His clinical training includes specialties in both substance abuse treatment and LGBTQ health. His research lies at the intersection of these two areas, and he is broadly interested in helping to develop and disseminate LGBTQ-adapted treatments to reduce health disparities and increase access to affirmative care in the LGBTQ community.

CAITLIN MONAHAN, BA, is a social and health psychology doctoral student at Stony Brook University. She earned her BA in psychology from New York

University in 2016. Her research interests include intergroup relations, intersectionality, and stigma of marginalized groups.

MICHELE MONTECALVO, EdD, MS, MCHES, is an assistant professor in the Department of Biology and Health Sciences at St. Francis College in Brooklyn, New York. She is the author of the forthcoming book *LGBTQ Cultural Competency for Healthcare Providers* (Peter Lang). Dr. Montecalvo uses qualitative research methods to hear the authentic voice of marginalized communities; engaging learning pedagogy, health behavior change theory, and social justice frameworks; for enhancing learning with culturally equitable programming, curricula, and policy change. Montecalvo is a master certified health education specialist, and she holds a master's in public health administration and a doctorate in health behavior studies from Teachers College, Columbia University.

TERRI NICHOLS is a freelance writer who has worked for the U.S. Forest Service, the Student Conservation Association, and the Waterkeeper Alliance. She has performed trail work, habitat restoration, and water quality monitoring in California, Montana, and Wyoming. A Michigan native, Nichols holds a bachelor's degree in journalism from Wayne State University in Detroit, Michigan. She is a coauthor of *America's Natural Places: The Midwest* (ABC-CLIO, 2009).

JOSHUA D. NOSANCHUK, MD, is senior associate dean for medical education at the Albert Einstein College of Medicine at Yeshiva University. His areas of research and expertise include medical education, fungal pathogenesis, host-pathogen biology, regenerative medicine, and innovative therapeutics.

MATTHEW NUMER is an associate professor in the School of Health and Human Performance at Dalhousie University and is cross-appointed to the Gender and Women's Studies program. He has been funded by the Canadian Institutes of Health Research and the Social Sciences and Humanities Research Council of Canada for his work in the areas of gender, sex, and sexuality. His research interests include substance use; the health of gay, bisexual, and other men who have sex with men, sexual health, online technologies, LGBTQ2S health, masculinities, indigenous boys' and men's health, and postsecondary pedagogical practices. He has received numerous awards for his interactive teaching methods and is widely known as an innovator in the classroom. He is a member of the board of directors for the Halifax Sexual Health Centre, serves on the AIDS Coalition of Nova Scotia: Gay Men's Health Advisory Committee, and is regional adviser for the Community-Based Research Centre for Gay Men's Health.

DONNA ORIOWO, PhD, MEd, MSW, is a sex and relationship therapist at her private practice, AnnodRight, in the Washington, D.C., metro area specializing in working with black women on issues related to colorism and texturism and its impacts on mental and sexual health. She is the author of *Cocoa Butter & Hair Grease: A Self Love Journey through Hair and Skin*. Dr. Donna currently serves on the Diversity, Equity, and Inclusion Committee for the American Association of Sexuality Educators, Counselors and Therapists and is a member of Women of Color Sexual Health Network. Donna holds a BS in psychology from Morgan State University, a master's in social work, a master's in education for human sexuality, and a doctorate in human sexuality from Widener University.

TORI PEÑA is a second-year cognitive science student at Stony Brook University's psychology department. She received her BS in psychology and biological anthropology from Binghamton University in May 2018. She works under Dr. Suparna Rajaram's advisement, and her current research focuses on understanding the nuances of social and nonsocial memory.

DULCINEA PITAGORA holds an MA in psychology from the New School for Social Research, an MSW from New York University, an MEd and a PhD in clinical sexology from Widener University, and is an American Association of Sexuality Educators, Counselors and Therapists–certified sex therapist. Pitagora has a practice in New York City that includes individual, couples or dyads, and multipartner therapy. Pitagora's practice is person centered and strengths based; focuses on self-determination and empowerment; and is LGBQ, trans, poly, and kink affirmative. Pitagora is an adjunct professor of sexual health at New York University and has published articles and chapters in peer-reviewed journals and books and presented at conferences on the topics of alternative sexuality and gender diversity. Pitagora conducts research, lectures, and seminars pertaining to these communities; is the founder of ManhattanAlternative.com, an alternative lifestyle–affirmative provider listing; and is a co-organizer of the AltSex NYC Conference. Pitagora is the "kink doctor" in the web series of the same name.

REBECCA POLLY is an education professional working in the greater mid-Atlantic region. Rebecca's professional interests include sexuality education in early childhood, diversity and inclusivity in trades and labor unions, and health communications and linguistics. Rebecca currently works for Job Corps, an organization within the Department of Labor, as a career transition specialist working with impoverished adolescents and emerging adults to develop long-term career success. While working with Job Corps, Rebecca designed and developed an educational series on topics such as race and identity, LGBT inclusivity, and trauma-informed youth services. She received her bachelor of science in linguistics and cognitive science from the University of Delaware in 2014. In 2017, she earned her master's of education in human sexuality at Widener University. She was recently selected to give an oral presentation at the Twenty-Fourth Congress of the World Association for Sexual Health titled "Early and Often: Sexuality Education in Early Childhood." Rebecca can be reached directly by email at reba.polly@gmail.com.

AMY REYNOLDS is a writer and editor with an MA in political science from California State University, Northridge. Her research interests include social movements and media effects.

DAVID J. REYNOLDS, PhD, is the military internship behavioral health psychologist and deputy training director at Malcolm Grow Medical Clinics and Surgery Center (MGMCSC), Joint Base Andrews, Maryland. He joined the Center for Deployment Psychology (CDP) in 2016 after retiring from the U.S. Air Force. Dr. Reynolds leads CDP's chronic pain team and is a member of the insomnia team. He facilitates training in both areas. He is also an expert in the treatment of trauma, resiliency, and relaxation. Dr. Reynolds received his bachelor's degree in psychology from State University of New York College at Brockport and his master's and doctorate degrees in clinical psychology from the University of Cincinnati. He is a 2000 graduate of the MGMCSC psychology residency program. In 2006, he completed a postdoctoral fellowship in health psychology at Wilford Hall Medical Center in San Antonio, Texas.

G. NIC RIDER, PhD, LP, is an assistant professor in the Program in Human Sexuality at the University of Minnesota Medical School and the co-associate director for research for the National Center for Gender Spectrum Health. Dr. Rider has professional interests in the areas of gender and sexual identity development, intersections of identities, discrimination and microaggressions, sexual trauma/abuse recovery, and social justice advocacy. They are on the executive board for the Asian American Psychological Association's Division on LGBTQQ Issues. Dr. Rider received a doctorate in counseling psychology from Howard University in Washington, D.C. They were also the first Randi and Fred Ettner Postdoctoral Fellow in Transgender Health at the Program in Human Sexuality, University of Minnesota Medical School.

ALEX M. RIVERA, PsyD, is a licensed psychologist who specializes in providing culturally affirming treatment for queer and trans people of color. She currently directs a group practice in the Bay Area and acts as a research consultant for the Asian Women's Health Initiative Project at Boston University. Dr. Rivera serves on the editorial board of *The Counseling Psychologist* and is the past chair of the Asian American Psychological Association Education and Training Committee. She received her doctorate from the PGSP-Stanford PsyD Consortium and has written several articles and chapters on identity and intersectionality in mental health.

ELIZABETH RODNEZ, MD, is a second-year family medicine resident at Naval Hospital Jacksonville. Having graduated from the University of Miami Miller School of Medicine, she currently works with the U.S. Navy and plans to work on medical mission trips. (The views expressed by Elizabeth Rodnez in this work are those of the author and do not necessarily reflect the official policy or position of the Department of the Navy, Department of Defense, or the U.S. government.)

SCOTT T. RONIS, PhD, is an associate professor and director of graduate studies in the Department of Psychology at the University of New Brunswick in Fredericton, New Brunswick, and he maintains a part-time private practice as a licensed psychologist, where he works with youth and adults with problem sexual behavior as well as children and families with other difficulties. His research primarily focuses on the development of problem sexual behavior, particularly among adolescents, general family relationships, and youth emotional and behavioral difficulties. Dr. Ronis holds a doctorate in clinical psychology from the University of Missouri.

DARCI SHINN graduated from Widener University in 2014 with dual master's degrees in human sexuality and social work. From 2015 to 2017, she worked as therapist for the Pennsylvania-based agency Resources for Human Development. There she worked with children in the Mastery Charter School organization who had counseling as part of their individual education plans. In 2017, Darci began working as a per diem therapist for Oaks Integrated Care. She works with clients presenting with a variety of sexual and/or mental health presenting problems. Darci recently obtained her license as a clinical social worker and is gradually working toward having her own practice. She also plans to work toward becoming certified by the American Association of Sexuality Educators, Counselors and Therapists in the near future.

LESLEY-ANN SMITH, PhD, is a senior lecturer in psychology at the University of Northampton in the United Kingdom. Dr. Smith also leads two master's programs in psychology: the MS in psychology and the MS in child and mental health at the University of Northampton. Dr. Smith is currently researching sexual grooming practices in young women and has published academic journal articles and a book chapter exploring how mental health service users experience certain spaces, (e.g., day centers, home spaces).

LORI APFFEL SMITH, MD, is an obstetrician-gynecologist in Birmingham, Alabama. She received her medical degree from Baylor College of Medicine and has been in practice for more than twenty years.

A. J. SMUSKIEWICZ is a freelance writer and editor specializing in science, health and medicine, and contemporary issues. He earned a BS in biology at Governors State University in 1988. He has worked as a biologist (including for the Environmental Protection Agency Great Lakes Monitoring Project and the Illinois Institute of Technology Research Institute), a naturalist (including for the Forest Preserve Districts of Will County and Cook County), and an artist/designer. His writing and editing experience includes staff positions with World Book Publishing and the American Osteopathic Association. In recent years, he has focused much of his writing on human sexuality and LGBT issues.

RACHEL SNEDECOR is an adolescent medicine provider and board-certified pediatrician specializing in the care of gender-diverse youth and young adults. She has worked as a health care provider in the Gender Health Program at Riley Hospital for Children and the Eskenazi Transgender Health and Wellness Program in Indianapolis. Soon, she will be joining the faculty at Cincinnati Children's Hospital. Dr. Snedecor completed her medical school training at Indiana University

School of Medicine. For her pediatric residency, she attended the University of Louisville. She finally returned to Indiana University School of Medicine for her adolescent medicine fellowship. Recently, she served as secretary of the executive board of GenderNexus, a local organization serving the transgender and nonbinary community of Indianapolis. Dr. Snedecor has also worked nationally as part of the LGBT Clinical Services Committee of the Society for Adolescent Health and Medicine. Her research areas focus on the sources of ideal body features and the actions that they inspire in gender-expansive youth and improving health care delivery to gender and sexual minority adolescents.

LEN SPERRY, MD, PhD, is a professor of mental health counseling and director of clinical training at Florida Atlantic University and clinical professor of psychiatry and behavioral medicine at the Medical College of Wisconsin. He is board certified in psychiatry, general preventive medicine, and clinical psychology. He is a fellow of the American Psychiatric Association, the American College of Preventive Medicine, and the American Psychological Association. Sperry is the editor in chief of the *American Journal of Family Therapy* and editor of *Spirituality in Clinical Practice.*

ED DE ST. AUBIN, PhD, is an associate professor of psychology at Marquette University in Milwaukee, Wisconsin. He is broadly trained in the interdisciplinary study of human development and has several intellectual interests. One topic of scholarship and teaching has been sex and gender during emerging adulthood. He and his student-colleagues have published widely in this area, and he has taught several courses in human sexuality, the queer self, and hookup campus culture, receiving several teaching grants and awards for these efforts. The threads connecting his research endeavors are the individual adult's search for meaning and the social justice dynamics that affect members of marginalized groups.

STEPHEN K. STEIN is an associate professor of history at the University of Memphis. Recent publications include *The Sea in World History: Trade, Travel, and Exploration* (2017), *Twenty-Five Years of Living in Leather: The National Leather Association, 1986–2011* (2012), and "The Greely Relief Expedition and the New Navy," *International Journal of Naval History* 5 (December 2006), which won the Rear Admiral Ernest M. Eller Prize in Naval History. He is currently working on a history of the sadism/masochism community in the United States.

JUDITH STEINHART, EdD, is a clinical sexologist who has taught human sexuality courses at the undergraduate and graduate levels in colleges and universities as well as in secondary schools. Dr. Steinhart has also provided training to health professionals and to those who work in community-based organizations. She is a popular presenter at national sexuality conferences. Dr. Steinhart has championed the cause of making the field of sexuality more inclusive by opening doors and mentoring others. She has published articles and book chapters and has been a speaker for TEDx. She co-created the first internet question-and-answer service, Go Ask Alice!, while working as a sexual health educator at Columbia University, and she coauthored the book *The "Go Ask Alice!" Book of Answers: A Guide to Your Physical, Sexual, and Emotional Health.* She is currently on the faculty of health studies, part of the Health, Physical Education, and Recreation Department, Nassau Community College, Garden City, New York.

CHUCK STEWART teaches math and statistics courses for National University and University of Phoenix and is an independent researcher and writer on LGBT topics. Formerly, he worked in aerospace. His published works include ABC-CLIO's *The Greenwood Encyclopedia of LGBT Issues Worldwide*, *Bankrupt Your Student Loans and Other Discharge Strategies*, and *Sexually Stigmatized Communities: Reducing Heterosexism and Homophobia: An Awareness Training Manual*, a manual used to create training programs for the Los Angeles Police Academy. Stewart holds a doctorate in education with a certificate in women's studies from the University of Southern California.

LARA E. STEWART, DO, MPH, is a board-certified family physician. She enjoyed focusing on the health concerns of women and young adults during her decade of clinical practice. Dr. Stewart earned her master's in public health in health care management and policy and currently works as a medical author, expert, and consultant.

VICTOR B. STOLBERG is an assistant professor and counselor at Essex County College in Newark, New Jersey, where he previously directed the Office of Disability Support Services and Office of the Substance Abuse Coordinator. He was a founding member of the CORE Institute and helped create the CORE Instrument; he is currently a board member of the Friends of the Newark Public Library and the New Jersey Community College Counselors' Association. He has delivered hundreds of workshops and other presentations across the country. He has authored, or coauthored, forty-nine scholarly articles, ninety-four encyclopedia articles, six chapters and contributed papers, and sixty-three other miscellaneous publications as well as several books, including *Painkillers: History, Science, and Issues* and *ADHD Medications: History, Science, and Issues.* This amounts to a total of over two hundred publications. He has several publications in press, including a book with ABC-CLIO titled *What You Need to Know about ADHD.* Stolberg holds nine master's degrees from Montclair State University, New Jersey Institute of Technology, Rutgers University, the State University of New York at Cortland, and the University of Buffalo.

LINDA TANCS holds a master's of law degree from Columbia University School of Law, a doctorate in law from Seton Hall University School of Law, and a bachelor of arts degree in communication from Rutgers University. Her published works include *Understanding Trademark Law: A Beginner's Guide* (Thomson Reuters, 2009), *Understanding Copyright Law: A Beginner's Guide* (Thomson Reuters, 2011), and *Understanding Patent Law: A Beginner's Guide* (Thomson Reuters, 2011).

KYNDEL L. TARZIERS, MS, is a doctoral student in counselor education and practice at Georgia State University. She currently serves as a therapist at a children's advocacy center, supporting child trauma victims. Kyndel's research interests include generational and childhood trauma, trauma-informed care and dissemination, childhood disability, and sexuality counseling. She hopes to become a counselor educator and maintain a private practice after graduation from her doctoral program. Kyndel holds a master's in clinical mental health counseling from the University of South Alabama.

DAWN S. TASILLO, MD, is an assistant professor of OB/GYN at the University of Massachusetts School of Medicine, where she has served as OB/GYN clerkship director since 2010. Her professional focus is on medical education; she has been an invited speaker in a local secondary school's bioethics class since 2009.

CHEYENNE TAYLOR, LMSW, is a licensed social worker who obtained her MSW at Fordham University in New York City. Currently, Cheyenne practices psychotherapy at the Manhattan Alternative Collective, where she specializes in issues pertaining to kink/BDSM, consensual nonmonogamy/polyamory, LGBTQ issues, issues of people of color, and sex work.

SHANE'A THOMAS, LICSW, MEd, (he/she pronouns) is a senior lecturer for the University of Southern California's Suzanne Dworak-Peck School of Social Work's Virtual Academic Center as well as a seasoned practitioner in the Washington, D.C., metro area. Clinically and educationally, Thomas commits time toward supporting LGBTQI youth and those affected by HIV/AIDS through trauma-focused care as well as training social workers, educators, and service providers around building safer therapeutic, service, and educational spaces for clients and students, especially those working and existing in communities that are underserved, people of color, and LGBTQI folks. She is an advisory board member to the National Queer and Trans Therapists of Color Network. Thomas is a proud alumnus of Virginia Tech, Howard University, and Widener University, holding a bachelor of science in psychology, a master of social work degree with a concentration in direct services (families and children), and a master of education with a concentration in human sexuality studies, as well as an advanced certificate in human sexuality studies, respectively. By 2021, Thomas will receive an EdD in organizational change and leadership through University of Southern California's Rossier's School of Education.

CASEY T. TOBIN, PhD, is an associate professor in the psychology department at the University of Wisconsin–La Crosse. Dr. Tobin's areas of interest include sexuality and sexual health, child abuse and neglect, clinical/counseling psychology, and internship and fieldwork experiences. She holds two master's degrees, one in education and one in community counseling, and a doctorate in counselor education and supervision from the University of Northern Colorado. Dr. Tobin maintains her licensure status as a licensed professional counselor, a national certified counselor, and an approved clinical supervisor.

ROSARA TORRISI, LCSWR, MEd, CST, PhD, is the director of the Long Island Institute of Sex Therapy in New York. Dr. Torrisi is a licensed clinical social worker and a certified sex therapist with the American Association of Sexuality Educators, Counselors and Therapists. She graduated from Columbia University with a master of science in social work and earned a master of education in human sexuality from Widener University, where she also earned her PhD in human sexuality. She is an adjunct professor at Widener University and guest lecturer around the country, teaching courses about sexuality, sex therapy, and disabilities. Dr. Torrisi is an Our Whole Lives comprehensive sexuality educator for youth, young adults, adults, and older adults. Dr. Torrisi is recognized as a welcoming and kink-aware therapist by the National Coalition for Sexual Freedom and is also a recommended therapist by the Long Island LGBT Network.

STEPHEN K. TRAPP, PhD, is an assistant professor with the Division of Physical Medicine and Rehabilitation at the University of Utah. He primarily conducts research on topics pertaining to rehabilitation and chronic health conditions. He also maintains a clinic devoted to the psychological needs associated with neurorehabilitation and rare health conditions. Dr. Trapp is the current chair of the Rehabilitation Technology Special Interest Group associated with the American Psychological Association's Rehabilitation Psychology Division. Trapp holds a masters in human development counseling from Vanderbilt University and a doctorate in counseling psychology from Virginia Commonwealth University.

JASON S. ULSPERGER, PhD, is a professor of sociology at Arkansas Tech University. He teaches social deviance and gerontology. He holds a master's from Arkansas State University and a doctorate from Oklahoma State University. In addition to applications of structural ritualization theory, he researches the link between sexual deviance and law formation processes. He is the coauthor of *Elder Care Catastrophe* (Routledge) and current president of the Mid-South Sociological Association. He is a recent recipient of his university's faculty awards for excellence in both scholarship and teaching.

LOUIS VARILIAS, MLIS, MS, is a recent graduate with a master's in experimental psychology from Seton University. His research interests extend beyond psychology, especially into technology, society, and other fields of science.

JENNIFER A. VENCILL, PhD, is an assistant professor, licensed psychologist, and American Association of Sexuality Educators, Counselors and Therapists–certified sex therapist at the Mayo Clinic, where she practices primarily in the Menopause and Women's Sexual Health and Transgender and Intersex Specialty Care clinics. Dr. Vencill's research interests include health disparities and minority stress in marginalized sexual and gender communities, mixed orientation relationships, and sexual health. She serves on the editorial board of the *Journal of Positive Sexuality* and is past president of the Society for the Psychology of Women's Section on Lesbian, Bisexual, and Transgender Concerns. Dr. Vencill received her PhD in counseling psychology from Texas Tech University and was the first

Michael E. Metz Postdoctoral Fellow in Couples' Sexual Health at the University of Minnesota Medical School's Program in Human Sexuality.

JAMES WADLEY, PhD, LPC (PA & NJ), NCC, CSTS, is professor and chair of the Counseling and Human Services Master of Human Services department at Lincoln University. As a scholar-practitioner, he is a licensed professional counselor and maintains a private practice in Pennsylvania and New Jersey. His recently coedited a ground-breaking book entitled *The Art of Sex Therapy Supervision* (Routledge/Taylor & Francis). He is the founding editor of the scholarly, interdisciplinary journal, *Journal of Black Sexuality and Relationships* (University of Nebraska Press). He is also the founder and principal of the Association of Black Sexologists and Clinicians, and his professional background in human sexuality education, educational leadership, and program development has enabled him to galvanize scholars and practitioners in the field of sexology across the world.

KOREY L. WATKINS, PsyD, works full time at Austin State Hospital, where he provides psychotherapy and psychological assessments to children and adolescents. He also provides forensic evaluations to children, adolescents, and adults. Dr. Watkins maintains a private practice, where he works predominantly with children, adolescents, parents, and families. He is a captain in the U.S. Army Reserves, where he serves as a clinical psychologist. Dr. Watkins holds a doctorate in clinical psychology as well as a master's degree in counseling psychology. He has several peer-reviewed publications and has presented on a variety of topics in multiple countries.

TIM J. WATTS is a content development librarian at Kansas State University, where he is responsible for content development in the social sciences, including history, political science, and psychology.

LAUREN WESLEY is a graduate of Widener University's Center for Human Sexuality Studies. Lauren also earned her MA in clinical psychology from the Chicago School of Professional Psychology and her BA from Xavier University of Louisiana. She works with African American and Latino formerly incarcerated men, helping them navigate reintegration and reunification with their families.

NICOLE WILLIAMS is a graduate student at Thomas Jefferson University, where she is pursuing a master's degree in marriage and family therapy with a concentration in sex therapy. She obtained a bachelor degree in the field of psychology at Temple University. Nicole plans on studying and specializing in the mind-body connection and incorporating yoga therapy into her treatment for her future clients.

C. MICHAEL WOODWARD, MPH, (he/him) is a LGBTQ+ inclusion consultant, writer, musician, storyteller, social justice advocate, and aging queer trans guy. Michael has published myriad books, articles, and blogs, and received the Skip

Schrader Spirit of Activism award from Equality Arizona. He contributed the title essay of the highly acclaimed anthology *Manning Up: Transsexual Men on Finding Brotherhood, Family, and Themselves* (Transgress Press, 2014). He earned an MPH in public health policy and management from the University of Arizona and a BS in communications from Butler University.

MARISSA A. WORTH, PsyD, is a clinical psychologist. She earned her master's degree in clinical psychology from Pepperdine University Graduate School of Education and Psychology and completed her doctoral studies at the California School of Professional Psychology at Alliant International University, Los Angeles. Her clinical and research interests include LGBTQ treatment and advocacy, forensic and psychodiagnostic assessment, and treatment of individuals with severe and persistent mental illnesses.

LAUREN B. YADLOSKY, MS, is a sixth-year clinical psychology doctoral student at Marquette University in Milwaukee, Wisconsin. She is currently completing her predoctoral internship at Montefiore Medical Center in the Bronx, New York, where she specializes in working with high-risk children and teens. Her research interests include applying intersectionality theory to understanding minority stress experiences and various facets of identity (e.g., race, ethnicity, gender, sexual orientation, class).

RACHAEL ZAFFIRO, LPC, NCC, is a licensed mental health counselor in the state of Ohio. She received her bachelor degree in psychology with a concentration in relationships and sexual health from Maryville College, where she completed her senior thesis on the topic of sex guilt and assisted Dr. Karen Beale with her own sex guilt research. Zaffiro received her master's in mental health counseling from the University of Cincinnati, where she was a member of the Counseling Academic and Professional Honor Society International, Chi Sigma Iota.

JUAN PABLO ZAPATA graduated with a BS (double majors in psychology and public health) from the University of South Florida in Tampa in 2016. He began the doctoral program in clinical psychology at Marquette University, working under Dr. Ed de St. Aubin. Juan's research interests include developing sustainable interventions to decrease HIV/AIDS. He is also interested in psychosocial and behavioral factors relevant to HIV/AIDS and sexual risk among Latino men who have sex with men. His research examines the role of cultural, structural, and individual characteristics on HIV risk, using various research methodological designs. He recently finished his master's thesis, which explored the psychosocial and sociocultural dimensions of PrEP use among gay and bisexual men in the Midwest. He is currently working on preparation for his dissertation, which will examine the association of PrEP and structural barriers, cultural beliefs, and HIV-related worries and concerns among Hispanic/Latino men.

Index

Note: Page numbers in **bold** indicate the location of main entries.